OCT and Imaging in Central Nervous System Diseases

Andrzej Grzybowski · Piero Barboni
Editors

OCT and Imaging in Central Nervous System Diseases

The Eye as a Window to the Brain

Third Edition

Springer

Editors
Andrzej Grzybowski
Institute for Research in Ophthalmology
Foundation for Ophthalmology
Development
Poznan, Poland

Department of Ophthalmology
University of Warmia and Mazury
Olsztyn, Poland

Piero Barboni
Studio Oculistico d'Azeglio
Bologna, Italy

ISBN 978-3-031-72158-8 ISBN 978-3-031-72156-4 (eBook)
https://doi.org/10.1007/978-3-031-72156-4

This Springer imprint is published by the registered company Springer Nature Switzerland AG
The registered company address is: Gewerbestrasse 11, 6330 Cham, Switzerland

Contents

Introduction: Retina Imaging—Past and Present

1

Andrzej Grzybowski and Piero Barboni

Abstract

The chapter presents the short description of the development of knowledge about the retina, with special recognition of early attempts of retina visualization in living animals and humans and the role of the retina in central nervous system (CNS) disorders. It also introduces to the complicated structure and physiology of the retina, and presents some of its relations to CNS, based on the use of optical coherent tomography (OCT).

Keywords

Retina • Imaging • History of ophthalmology • Fundus • Optical coherent tomography • Central nervous system • Neuro-ophthalmology • Neuro-degeneration • CNS disorders

The retina is a mysterious structure. The first use of the term comes, as to our present knowledge, from Herophilos (335–280 or 255 BC), Greek anatomist, one of founders of Greek school in Alexandria. He used two different words, arachnoeides and amfiblesteroides, for retina. For many years, both meanings were related to casting net, and retiform, a word which the modern "retina" is derived.

A. Grzybowski (✉)
University of Warmia and Mazury, Olsztyn, Poland
e-mail: ae.grzybowski@gmail.com

Institute for Research in Ophthalmology, Poznan, Poland

P. Barboni
Studio Oculistico d'Azeglio, Bologna, Italy
e-mail: p.barboni@studiodazeglio.it

Scientific Institute San Raffaele, Milan, Italy

A. Grzybowski and P. Barboni (eds.), *OCT and Imaging in Central Nervous System Diseases*, https://doi.org/10.1007/978-3-031-72156-4_1

However, as it was nicely shown recently, there might be another explanation of these original terms [1]. Amfiblesteroides meant at that time also anything that is thrown around and encircling walls. For many years it was believed, however, that the lens, not retina is the reception organ of the eye responsible for vision and there was even no agreement as to whether the eye emanated light (extramission theory) or received it (intromission theory) [2, 3]. Leonardo da Vinci (1452–1519) and Johannes Kepler (1571–1630) questioned the role of the lens in light reception. Felix Plater (1536–1614), attributed that role to the retina, what was further experimentally supported by Christopher Scheiner (1575–1650) who, by removing part of the sclera and choroids, was able to notice the reversed picture projected onto the bottom of the eye [3–6].

For the next two centuries, it was disputable weather retina or choroid was a precise structure responsible for vision reception [7]. This was finally settled by Herman von Helmholtz (1821–1894), who also constructed and popularized the first ophthalmoscope in 1851 [8]. This revolutionized the development of retinology.

The first visualization of the eye fundus of the living animal, however, was conducted by Jean Mery (1654–1718) in 1704. By plunging the head of a cat in water, Mery was able to observe the retinal vessels, the optic nerve head and the choroid (Fig. 1.1) [9]. This was later confirmed by Adolf Kussmaul in 1845 [10], Johann Nepomuk Czermak in 1851 [11] and Adolf Ernst Coccius in 1852, who introduced a water-box named "orthoscope", to neutralize the corneal curvature [12, 13]. It was, however, Johannes Purkinje (1787–1869) in 1823 who described the basics of ophthalmoscopy based on his observations living animal and human eye [14]. One of the pioneers in the use of ophthalmoscopy for the diagnosis of central nervous system disorders was Xavier Galezowski (1832–1907), who published one of early textbooks on this subject and coined a term of cerebroscopy for this examination (Fig. 1.2) [15].

The microscopical structure of the retina was described in the nineteenth century, and by the end of the twentieth century it was believed that its histological and functional characteristics was largely recognized. Then, the discovery of intrinsically photosensitive ganglion cells, a novel class of retinal photoreceptors, which express melanopsin, are sensitive to short-wavelength blue light and project throughout the brain, have presented a completely unknown area of retina-brain possible interactions [16, 17]. It is quite clear today that other cellular components of the retina, namely amacrine cells, bipolar cells and microglial cells, although somehow neglected in the past, play important functions both in physiology and pathology of the retina. For example, it was proposed that microglia are involved in the pathogenesis of several degenerative conditions of the retina, including glaucoma, age-related macular degeneration, and inherited photoreceptor degeneration [18]. Moreover, recently the evidence of retinal astrocytopathy in neuromyelitis optica spectrum disorder was provided [19].

One of the major developments in recent years in retinal imaging was the introduction of optical coherence tomography (OCT). OCT was firstly reported by Huang et al. in 1991 [20]. In vivo studies were first reported in 1993 [21, 22],

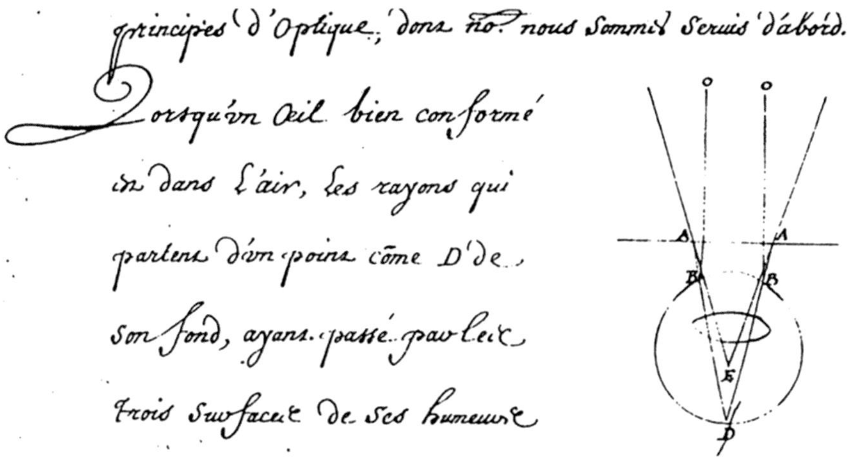

Fig. 1.1 Extract from the Proceedings of the Royal Academy of Sciences for the year 1709—Session of 20th March 1709. By this diagram, La Hire explains the visualization of the fundus of the submerged cat by the fact that the surface of the water having abolished the corneal dioptric power, the rays coming out of the eye would no longer be parallel, but would diverge and that would make the eye fundus visible to the observer. *Source* Heitz RF. Earliest Visualizations of the Living Eye's Fundus by Immersion in Water [9]

and in 1995 imaging of the normal retina [23] and macular pathology [24] was presented. OCT delivers high-resolution cross-sectional or 3-dimensional images of the retinal and choroid structures, which are generated by an optical beam scanned across the retina (and choroid). OCT testing is quick, easy and noninvasive, and pupil dilation is typically not required. Moreover, OCT yields quantitative anatomical data and is related with low variation for repeated measurements, low intra-individual and inter-individual variation and low variability across different centers using the same device.

Retinal ganglion cells axons are nonmyelinated within the retina, thus retinal nerve fiber layer (RNFL) is an optimal structure to visualize the process of neurodegeneration, neuro-protection and neuro-repair [25]. Moreover, OCT enables evaluation of retinal ganglion cells (RGC). For example, it was reported in patients with MS a dropout of RGC in 79% of eyes and inner nuclear layer atrophy (including amacrine cells and bipolar cells) in 40% of eyes [26]. It was also argued that OCT might reveal RNFL abnormalities in many patients with no clinical symptoms [27].

Retina and optic nerve originates from diencephalon, thus are a part of central nervous system (CNS). RGC present the typical morphology of CNS neurons. Optic nerve, like all fiber tracts in CNS, is covered with myelin and is unsheathed in all three meningeal layers. Insult to the optic nerve, similar to CNS, lead to retrograde and anterograde degeneration of damaged axons [28]. Because of these many similarities, it has not been very surprising that many CNS diseases can be also detected on the retina level. They include multiple sclerosis, Alzheimer

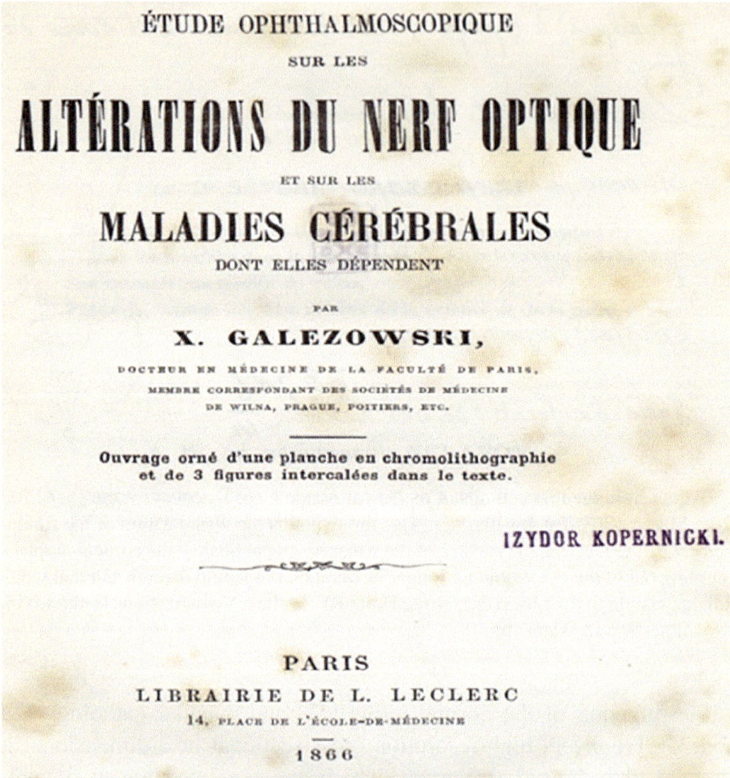

ÉTUDE OPHTHALMOSCOPIQUE

SUR LES

ALTÉRATIONS DU NERF OPTIQUE

ET SUR LES

MALADIES CÉRÉBRALES

DONT ELLES DÉPENDENT

PAR

X. GALEZOWSKI,

DOCTEUR EN MÉDECINE DE LA FACULTÉ DE PARIS,
MEMBRE CORRESPONDANT DES SOCIÉTÉS DE MÉDECINE
DE WILNA, PRAGUE, POITIERS, ETC.

Ouvrage orné d'une planche en chromolithographie
et de 3 figures intercalées dans le texte.

IZYDOR KOPERNICKI.

PARIS
LIBRAIRIE DE L. LECLERC
14, PLACE DE L'ÉCOLE-DE-MÉDECINE

1866

Fig. 1.2 Cover page of the book "Etude ophtalmoscopique sur les altérations du nerf optique et les maladies cérébrales dont elles dépenden" by Gałęzowski [15]

disease, Parkinson disease, and many others. Moreover, it was shown that there are some common degenerative mechanisms between Alzheimer disease and eye diseases, like glaucoma and age-related macular degeneration [29]. Thus, the aim of this book is to review all aspects of OCT retina studies in CNS diseases, and present some other novel and interesting techniques, including OCT angiography (OCTA), retinal amyloid imaging, retinal oximetry, and real-time imaging of single neuronal cell apoptosis. Moreover, we present and discuss how the use of machine learning (ML) algorithms trained on OCT and other fundus images of the human eye, and the animal models can be used in the studies of neurodegenerative disorders.

References

1. de Jong PT. From where does "rete" in retina originate? Graefes Arch Clin Exp Ophthalmol. 2014;252:1525–7.
2. Magnus H. Ophthalmology of the ancients, vol. 2 (Waugh RL, Translator). Oostende: Wayenborgh; 1999. p. 461–9.
3. Duke-Elder S, Wybar KC. The history of ophthalmic optics. In: Duke-Elder S, editor. System of ophthalmology, vol. 5. London: Henry Kimpton; 1970. p. 3–23.
4. Mark H. Johanees Kepler on the eye and vision. Am J Ophthalmol. 1971;72:869–78.
5. Daxecker F. Further studies by Christoph Scheiner concerning the optics of the eye. Doc Ophthalmol. 1994;86:153–61.
6. Daxecker F. Christoph Scheiner's eye studies. Doc Ophthalmol. 1992;81:27–35.
7. Grzybowski A, Aydin P. Edme Mariotte (1620–1684): pioneer of neurophysiology. Surv Ophthalmol. 2007;52:443–51.
8. Helmholtz HLFV. Beschreibung eines Augenspiegels zur Untersuchung der Netzhaut im lebenden Auge. Berlin: Forstner; 1851.
9. Heitz RF. Earliest visualizations of the living eye's fundus by immersion in water. Arch Hist Filoz Med. 2012;75:11–5.
10. Kussmaul A. Die Farben-Erscheinungen im Grunde des menschlichen Auges. Heidelberg: Groos; 1845.
11. Czermak JN. Ueber eine neue Methode zur genaueren Untersuchung des gesunden und kranken Auges. Vjschr prakt Heilk. 1851;8:154–65.
12. Coccius AE. Ueber die Ernährungsweise der Hornhaut und die Serum führenden Gefässe im menschlichen Körper. Leipzig: Muller; 1852.
13. Coccius AE. Ueber die Anwendung des Augen-Spiegels nebst Angabe eines neuen Instruments. Leipzig: Muller; 1853.
14. Reese PD. The neglect of Purkinje's technique of ophthalmoscopy prior to Helmholtz's invention of the ophthalmoscope. Ophthalmology. 1986;93:1457–60.
15. Gałęzowski X. Etude ophtalmoscopique sur les altérations du nerf optique et les maladies cérébrales dont elles dépendent. Paris: Librairie de L. Leclerc; 1866.
16. Lucas RJ, Freedman MS, Munoz M, Garcia-Fernandez JM, Foster RG. Regulation of the mammalian pineal by non-rod, non-cone, ocular photoreceptors. Science. 1999;284:505–7.
17. Schmidt TM, Chen SK, Hattar S. Intrinsically photosensitive retinal ganglion cells: many subtypes, diverse functions. Trends Neurosci. 2011;34:572–80.
18. Silverman SM, Wong WT. Microglia in the retina: roles in development, maturity, and disease. Annu Rev Vis Sci. 2018;4:45–77.
19. You Y, Zhu L, Zhang T, Shen T, Fontes A, Yiannikas C, Parratt J, Barton J, Schulz A, Gupta V, Barnett MH, Fraser CL, Gillies M, Graham SL, Klistorner A. Evidence of Müller glial dysfunction in patients with aquaporin-4 immunoglobulin G-positive neuromyelitis optica spectrum disorder. Ophthalmology. 2019. https://doi.org/10.1016/j.ophtha.2019.01.016.
20. Huang D, Swanson EZ, Lin CP, et al. Optical coherence tomography. Science. 1991;254:1178–81.
21. Swanson EA, Izatt JA, Hee MR, et al. In vivo retinal imaging by optical coherence tomography. Opt Lett. 1993;18:1864–6.
22. Fercher AF, Hitzenberger CK, Drexler W, et al. In vivo optical coherence tomography. Am J Ophthalmol. 1993;116:113–4.
23. Hee MR, Puliafito CA, Wong C, et al. Optical coherence tomography of the human retina. Arch Ophthalmol. 1995;113:325–32.
24. Puliafito CA, Hee MR, Lin CP, et al. Imaging of macular diseases with optical coherence tomography. Ophthalmology. 1995;102:217–29.
25. Galetta KM, Calabresi PA, Frohman EM, Balcer LJ. Optical coherence tomography (OCT): imaging the visual. Pathway as a model for neurodegeneration. Neurotherapeutics. 2011;8:117–32.

26. Green A, McQuaid S, Hauser SL, Allen IV, Lyness R. Ocular pathology in multiple sclerosis: retinal atrophy and inflammation irrespective of disease duration. Brain. 2010;133:1591–601.
27. Cettomai D, Hiremath G, Ratchford J, et al. Associations between retinal nerve fiber layer abnormalities and optic nerve examination. Neurology. 2010;75:1318–25.
28. London A, Benhar I, Schwartz M. The retina as a window to the brain-from eye research to CNS disorders. Nat Rev Neurol. 2013;9:44–53.
29. Sivak JM. The aging eye: common degenerative mechanisms between the Alzheimer's brain and retinal disease. Invest Ophthalmol Vis Sci. 2013;54:871–80.

OCT Technique: Past, Present and Future

2

Tigran Kostanyan, Maria de los Angeles Ramos-Cadena, Gadi Wollstein, and Joel S. Schuman

Abstract

Optical coherence tomography (OCT) has become the cornerstone technology in clinical and research imaging in the past two and half decades. OCT performs in vivo, real-time, noncontact scanning and provides cross-sectional and volumetric images with a resolution approaching that of histology. The technology has been used in various medical disciplines, but it is still most profoundly used in the field of ophthalmology where it was initially applied. OCT is continuously evolving with newly developed applications. This chapter will describe the basic principles of OCT techniques, its history, current status, major ophthalmic applications, and research that will determine the future of the technology.

Keywords

Time domain (TD-) OCT • Spectral domain (SD-) OCT • Swept source (SS-) OCT • Polarization sensitive (PS-) OCT • Adaptive optics (AO) • OCT blood flow • OCT angiography (OCTA) • Visible light (Vis-) OCT

Abbreviations

2D	Two-dimensional
3D	Three-dimensional
AO	Adaptive optics

T. Kostanyan
Department of Ophthalmology, Eye and Ear Institute, Ophthalmology and Visual Science Research Center, University of Pittsburgh School of Medicine, UPMC Eye Center, Pittsburgh, PA 15213, USA

M. de los Angeles Ramos-Cadena · G. Wollstein · J. S. Schuman (✉)
NYU Langone Eye Center, NYU Langone Health, New York, NY 10017, USA
e-mail: joel.schuman@nyu.edu

A. Grzybowski and P. Barboni (eds.), *OCT and Imaging in Central Nervous System Diseases*, https://doi.org/10.1007/978-3-031-72156-4_2

CCD	Charge-coupled device
EDI	Enhanced depth imaging
FD	Fourier domain
GCC	Ganglion cell complex
ILM	Internal limiting membrane
IPL	Inner plexiform layer
IS	Inner segment
LC	Lamina cribrosa
OCE	Optical coherence elastography
OCRT	Optical coherence refraction tomography
OCT	Optical coherence tomography
OCTA	Optical coherence tomography angiography
ONH	Optic nerve head
OS	Outer segment
PS	Polarization sensitive
RGC	Retinal ganglion cell
RNFL	Retinal nerve fiber layer
RPE	Retinal pigment epithelium
SD	Spectral domain
SS	Swept source
STOC-T	Spatio-temporal optical coherence tomography
TD	Time-domain
Vis-OCT	Visible light optical coherence tomography

2.1 Introduction

Optical coherence tomography (OCT), first developed in the 1990s, is a diagnostic imaging technology that has gained a leading position in research and clinical practice due to its ability to obtain noncontact, in vivo, high-resolution, micron-scale images of tissue structures. OCT makes in situ imaging of tissue microstructure possible with a resolution approaching that of histology [1]. The technology uses the principle of low-coherence interferometry, which was originally applied to ophthalmology for in vivo measurements of the axial length of the eye [2].

At the time of introduction, the technology was used to acquire in vivo, cross-sectional images of the anterior segment [3], and retinal pathologies. Since then, OCT has evolved significantly, with improvements in both image acquisition methods and image analysis. The evolution of OCT began with the time domain (TD) technique, followed by spectral domain (SD) and swept source (SS) [4], systems and later, newer iterations with faster acquisition speeds [5] and improved lateral resolution [6].

This chapter describes the basic principles of OCT techniques, its history, current status, major ophthalmic applications, and research that will determine the future of the technology.

2.2 Basic Principles

OCT provides cross-sectional and volumetric images of areas of interest by acquiring either the echo time delay or frequency information of back-reflected light. Differences in the optical properties of biological tissues allow the recognition of layered structures. The speed of light makes it impossible to analyze the acquired information directly, since it would be in the order of femtoseconds thus, OCT systems use the optical technique known as *interferometry*. Low-coherence interferometry enables the analysis of this information and the composition of a depth-resolved reflectivity profile (A-scan) of the scanned tissue by matching the light profiles from the scanning and reference arms.

Utilization of light provides OCT technology the ability to obtain images in a non-contact fashion and to achieve resolutions of 1–15 μm, which is 1–2 orders of magnitude finer than other conventional clinical imaging technologies such as ultrasound, computerized tomography, or magnetic resonance. Light is highly absorbed or scattered in most biological tissues, therefore the use of this technology is limited only to locations that are optically accessible or that can be imaged using devices such as endoscopes or catheters. The eye is the most optically accessible organ of the human body since the anterior and posterior segments can be visualized and imaged [7].

The key parameters that are typically used to characterize OCT technology are the center wavelength of the light source, axial and transverse resolution, scanning speed, and imaging depth.

Axial resolution determines the smallest distance along the axial direction where two adjacent points are discernable, and it is inversely related to the bandwidth of the light source. Current commercial OCT devices achieve axial resolutions up to 4 μm, and research systems can achieve up to ~ 1 μm [8]. The penetration depth (in the axial direction) is approximately 2 mm in the various OCT iterations with the exception of Visible-light OCT that does not penetrate beyond the RPE layer.

Transverse resolution is determined by the spot size projected into the eye, which is limited by the optical properties of the eye. As such, the transverse resolution of OCT ranges between 15 and 20 μm among the different generations of the technology. Improving transverse resolution requires the correction of the inherent optical aberrations of the eye using technologies such as adaptive optics.

Scanning speed is dictated by mechanical constrains and the sensitivity of the detector to the back-reflected light. As scanning speed increases, the time the detector remains in the same location is shorter, thus reducing the light that can be detected in each location. Since the power of the projected light is limited in order to remain within safety limits, faster scans require a more sensitive detector that can function with a lower level of light.

The achievable imaging depth is related to the center wavelength of the light source, with longer wavelengths providing increased imaging depth [9, 10]. However, longer wavelengths are limited by the increased optical absorption of water [11].

Currently available OCT techniques are based on several iterations of the technology: SD-OCT, also known as Fourier or frequency domain, SS-OCT, and visible-light (Vis-) OCT. The earliest iteration of the technology, time-domain (TD), is no longer manufactured for ophthalmic use and therefore will not be discussed.

SD-OCT uses a broad-bandwidth, low-coherence superluminescent diode laser light that is divided into two arms by a partially reflecting mirror (beam splitter). In the first arm light is projected toward the sampling location, while in the second arm light is projected toward a reference mirror. The backscattered light from both arms travels back to a spectrometer and recombines to form an interference pattern. Light frequency information is analyzed by Fourier transformation to encode distances within tissue microstructure [12]. SD technology allows the acquisition of information from all points along each axial scan (A-scan) simultaneously at a scanning speed of ~ 25,000–100,000 A-scans/s in clinical systems [13, 14] and up to 20 million A-scans/s in research devices [5]. A cross-sectional image, also known as a B-scan, is generated by performing fast, subsequent A-scans at adjacent transverse positions. Combining rapidly acquired subsequent cross-sectional scans allows the creation of three-dimensional (3D) datasets, enabling advanced post-processing analysis. The wide bandwidth of the SD-OCT light source facilitates an axial resolution of 3–6 μm in commercially available systems and up to 1 μm in research systems [15, 16].

SS-OCT uses a tunable laser light source that sweeps through different frequencies in rapid succession to cover the entire broad spectrum. The reflectance of the light from the scanned area is captured by a photodetector, which allows a substantially faster acquisition rate (up to 400,000 A-scans/s) than the spectrometry of SD-OCT [4, 17]. Another important advantage of SS-OCT is an improved signal-to-noise ratio and reduction in the depth dependent signal drop-off observed with SD-OCT technology [18]. Most SS-OCT devices operate with light sources centered at around 1050 nm (compared with 840 nm in the commercially available SD-OCT devices), which reduces the axial resolution to approximately 8 μm but allows for better penetration into the tissue. This combination of improved tissue penetration and reduced signal attenuation allows detailed scanning of structures such as the choroid and the lamina cribrosa (LC) within the optic nerve head (ONH).

Unlike other OCT iterations that use near infrared light sources (~800 and 1000 nm), Vis-OCT utilizes a light source with a shorter center wavelength of ~ 550 nm resulting in an improved axial resolution of < 1 μm but with reduced imaging depth [19, 20]. Using spectroscopic analysis, it is possible to quantify chromophore concentration from Vis-OCT images [20]. Retinal oximetry is one of its first applications, providing objective, functional information about retinal vasculature. Light absorbance for oxygenated and deoxygenated hemoglobin peaks in separate wavelengths, both of which are within the spectrum of Vis-OCT. Tissue oxygen consumption can be determined by extracting the venous deoxygenated level from the arterial oxygenated level. The oximetry information can be aligned

Table 2.1 Comparison of SD-OCT, SS-OCT, and Vis-OCT technologies

Technology	Light source	Primary advantages	Primary disadvantages
SD-OCT	Near infrared broadband width	High scanning speed (up to 100,000 A-scans/s in commercial ophthalmic systems); axial resolution 4–7 μm	Noticeable signal drop-off with depth
SS-OCT	Near infrared narrow bandwidth, swept through broad range	Very high scanning speeds (up to 400,000 A-scans/s in ophthalmic systems); minimal signal drop-off with depth; improved penetration into structures	Most ophthalmic systems operate at longer wavelengths (~1000 nm); with lower axial resolution than SD-OCT (7–8 μm)
Vis-OCT	Center wavelength of ~ 550 nm from incoherent light sources either spatially coherent or broadband	Highest axial resolution (<1 μm)	Limited penetration into deep tissues; slower scanning speed (up to 30,000 A-scans/s)

to the structural location observed in the same images, opening a new venue for global and local functional assessment.

The major characteristics of these 3 different OCT techniques are presented in Table 2.1.

2.3 The Past

OCT technology was first described by Huang and colleagues in 1991 [21]. The authors scanned human retinas and atherosclerotic plaques ex vivo with a prototype device using infrared light at a ~ 800 nm wavelength. The axial resolution of cross-sectional images of the retina, optic nerve, and coronary artery wall was 15 μm, which allowed the visualization of some retinal layers, ONH structures, and the composition of the coronary artery. In vivo retinal scanning was conducted using a prototype device based on a slit-lamp biomicroscope that was modified to provide a view of the fundus while scanning with OCT. The development of scan patterns that enabled the acquisition of reproducible measurements [22] led to the use of the technology in clinical practice. The first commercially available OCT, called OCT 1000, was marketed in 1996 by Zeiss (Dublin, CA). The technology went through 2 iterations, resulting in OCT 2000 in the year 2000 and then OCT 3 (Stratus), which became commercially available in 2002. Stratus OCT had an axial resolution of ~ 10 μm, a transverse resolution of 20 μm, and a scan speed of 400 A-scans/s [1, 23]. The typical cross-sectional scan was composed of 128–512 A-scans, comprising an image area of 4–6 mm.

Due to its ability to obtain quantitative and reproducible measurements of the macula [24, 25], retinal nerve fiber layer (RNFL) thickness [22, 26], and ONH [27], OCT became the gold standard clinical imaging device for posterior segment pathologies in a relatively short period of time.

Early iterations of OCT had a relatively slow acquisition rate, and therefore the conventional scan patterns were comprised of 6 radial scans through the macula (6 mm diameter) or optic nerve (4 mm) with a circular 3.4 mm diameter scan centered on the ONH. Using automated segmentation, the total macular thickness (internal limiting membrane (ILM) to the photoreceptor inner segment-outer segment (IS/OS) junction), RNFL thickness, and ONH structures were automatically quantified.

The introduction of SD-OCT facilitated a dramatic increase in scanning speed and substantially extended the clinical utility of OCT. The faster scanning speed enabled the introduction of new scanning patterns such as raster scans, where volumetric data is constructed with a rapidly acquired succession of adjacent B-scans. A 3D dataset allows a thorough sampling of the scanned region, advanced post-processing, and improved registration of consecutive scans. Another commonly used approach to improve image quality is the averaging of consecutive scans acquired at the same location.

The majority of commercial OCT systems applied SD technology for posterior eye imaging and visualization of the cross-sectional structures of the retina and optic disc [1] (Fig. 2.1). OCT has been used extensively in the diagnosis and management of a wide range of ocular pathologies including glaucoma, age-related macular degeneration, macular edema, macular holes, diabetic retinopathy, alterations in the vitreoretinal interface, papilledema, and others. In addition to acquiring tissue structural information, OCT has been incorporated into multimodal imaging systems that provide further insight into the functional characteristics of tissue [28–30].

OCT has become a key ophthalmic diagnostic imaging tool due to its ability to provide information about tissue microstructure. Over the years, it has

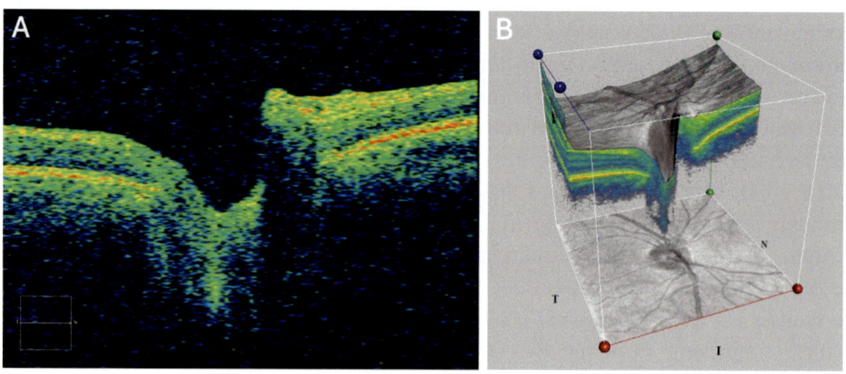

Fig. 2.1 OCT cross-sectional image of a healthy optic disc (A) and a 3D volumetric scan (B)

continuously evolved with improved visualization, new retinal imaging locations, increased reliability, and enhanced longitudinal analysis.

2.4 The Present

Since the advent of OCT, over 30 years ago, countless improvements have been implemented in an effort to acquire quantitative data with high reliability and sensitivity for precise evaluation of the structure and function of ocular structures.

2.4.1 Spectral-Domain OCT

Since the first FDA-approved SD-OCT became available in 2006, numerous improvements have enriched the capabilities of OCT. One application of advanced processing is the OCT enface image generated by integrating the information from all A-scans into an image of the surface of the retina [31]. The enface image is identical to the retinal fundus view and it can be used for subjective assessment of image quality and eye motion detection, comparison with clinical findings, and further focus on specific location within the region of interest.

Various scan patterns are available for ONH imaging from the different commercially available SD-OCT devices. This includes raster (also known as 3D or volumetric) scans, radial scans, circular scans, and a combination of radial and concentric scans. All of the devices can automatically detect the optic disc boundary as the location at which the photoreceptor layer, retinal pigment epithelium (RPE), and choriocapillaries terminate. The machine provides quantification of ONH structures such as the disc area, cup-to-disc ratio, and others along with the circumpapillary RNFL thickness measurement reported as global, quadrant, and sectoral thicknesses. Evaluation of the ONH provides important clinical information in multiple ocular and central nervous system pathologies like glaucoma and papilledema.

One of the most useful measurements provided by OCT is the circumpapillary RNFL thickness. Because the axons from retinal ganglion cells from throughout the eyeball gather to form the optic nerve, a circular scan around the ONH allows sampling of the axons from the entire retina. The limitation of this approach is that the sampling of the tissue is performed only along the circle, therefore any misplacement of the circle during consecutive scanning will result in increased measurement variability [32]. Another option is to extract the RNFL thickness from the raster scan pattern. This method can ensure that the tissue sampling location is consistent through multiple scans, as the repositioning of the circle is possible if needed during post-processing. Several devices also report the RNFL thickness as a color-coded thickness map of the peripapillary region. This map provides additive information to the circumpapillary RNFL thickness measurement, as it can highlight small, localized thinning or defects outside the circumpapillary sampling location. Furthermore, in many devices, the RNFL thickness is compared to population-derived normative data to highlight locations deviating from normal.

The Fig. 2.2A shows a Cirrus HD-OCT (Zeiss, Dublin, CA) ONH scan printout that provides the RNFL thickness map (1) and cross-Sect. 2.3. The deviation map (2) compares the RNFL measurements at each superpixel with an age-matched normative database, and locations thinner than the lowest 95% of the normal range are highlighted. In the center panel, quantitative parameters are provided for ONH structures, along with RNFL thickness presented as a thickness profile around the ONH, in quadrants and in clock hours. The background coloring reflects the comparison with the normative database, with green representing the normal range, yellow representing < 5% of the normal population, and red representing < 1% of the normal population. The right eye shows an example of eye within the normal limits while the left eye shows a glaucomatous eye with thin average RNFL, superior, inferior, and temporal thin RNFL, enlarged cup-to-disc ratio and an inferior notch. OptoVue Avanti (Visionix, North Lombard, IL) peripapillary scan (Fig. 2.2B) is created from 13 circular scans with diameters of 1.3–4.9 mm centered on the ONH. Comparison with a normative database is performed in 16 sectors and presented as the deviation map that surrounds the RNFL thickness map. Figure 2.2C shows the circumpapillary RNFL scans obtained with the Spectralis OCT (Heidelberg Engineering, Heidelberg, Germany). A retinal cross section image with delineation of RNFL boundaries is shown in (a). Note the visualization of fine details that is accomplished by averaging repetitive scans acquired in the same location while engaging eye motion tracking systems to reduce motion artifacts. Thickness measurements and color-coded comparison with normative data are presented for global average thickness, quadrants, and in six sectors (b).

The improvements introduced in SD-OCT also have a substantial impact on macular imaging. Thorough sampling of the macula, the improved visualization of the retina and choroid, and the ability to automatically segment the various layers of the retina substantially impacted clinical management. The scan patterns that are often used to image the macula include line, cross-line, raster, mesh, and radial scan patterns. Line scans are typically composed from the averaging of multiple scans at the same location. This is typically performed at a single linear location (Fig. 2.3A) or along several parallel lines (Fig. 2.3B). Line scans are clinically useful for obtaining retinal images with the highest level of detail. The principle of the volumetric cube scan is similar to the 3D ONH scan patterns described above. Volumetric macular scans are very helpful in clinical management of macular pathologies, such as macular edema, age related macular degeneration, and macular holes.

Some SD-OCT systems are capable of acquiring scans in horizontal and vertical orientations to provide a mesh scan pattern. The logic behind this scan pattern is that even at a fast scanning rate there is a relatively long temporal gap between adjacent points that are perpendicular to the scan orientation. For example, in a horizontal raster scan, the time gap between adjacent points in the horizontal direction is much shorter than the gap between adjacent points vertically. This can lead to image distortion along the slow axis of the scan. Registering the horizontal

Fig. 2.2 SD-OCT optic nerve head and retinal nerve fiber layer analysis, (A) Cirrus, (B) Avanti, and (C) Spectralis OCT

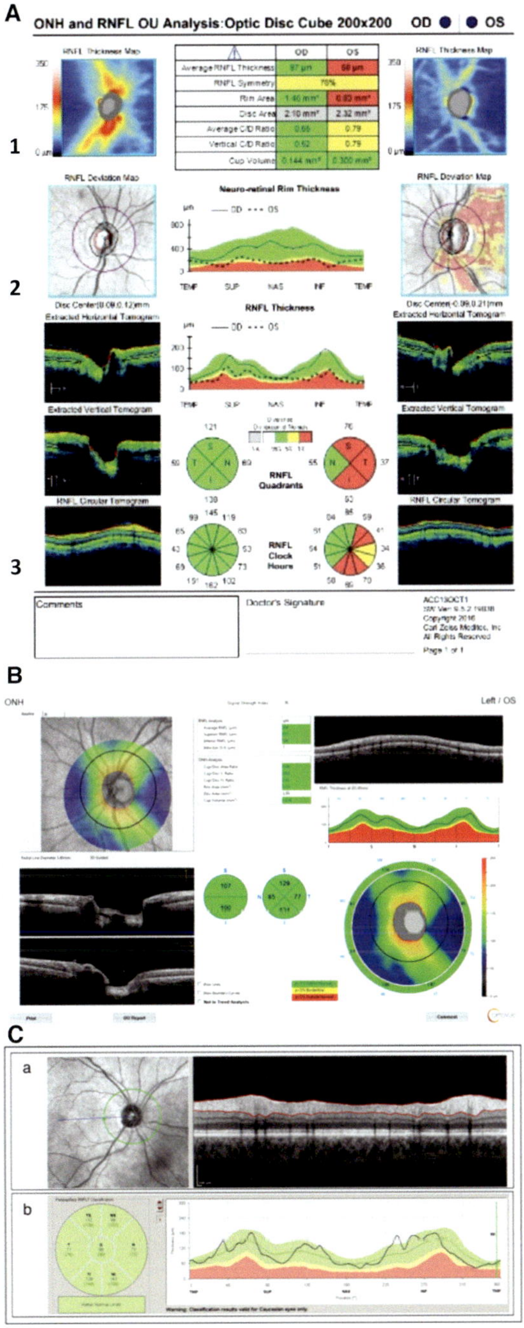

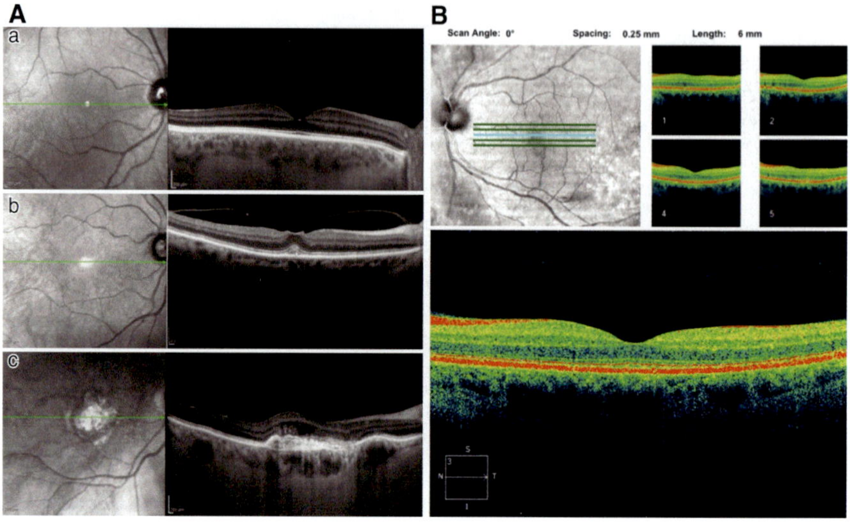

Fig. 2.3 (A) Line scans of the macular region obtained with Spectralis OCT from a healthy eye (a), an eye with vitreomacular traction (b), and wet age-related macular degeneration (c). (B) Macular five-line raster scan of a healthy eye obtained with Cirrus HD-OCT

and vertical scans together can reduce the distortion in the slow axis and improve scan quality. Figure 2.4 shows the macula thickness map acquired by a retina map scanning pattern obtained with Optovue Avanti (A) and Sperctralis OCT (B). The pattern consists of an inner, dense grid and outer grid, visible as white grid lines.

Radial scan protocols acquire multiple evenly spaced linear scans that intersect at the fovea. This pattern provides information from the entire macular region, with dense coverage near the fovea, where the lines intersect, and sparse coverage at the macula periphery.

The high resolution of SD-OCT enables automated segmentation and the analysis of individual macular layers that are of particular diagnostic interest in many ocular diseases including glaucoma and diabetic retinopathy [33–35]. Cirrus HD-OCT extracts the information from an ellipse (vertical radius of 2 mm, horizontal radius of 2.4 mm) centered on the fovea and provides a combined measurement of the retinal ganglion cell (RGC) layer and the inner plexiform layer (IPL), called the ganglion cell inner plexiform layer (GCIPL) analysis (Fig. 2.5). The macula protocol of RTVue Premier provides the ganglion cell complex (GCC), which includes the macular nerve fiber layer, RGC layer, and IPL. The data is captured from a 7 mm^2 area centered 1 mm temporal to the fovea.

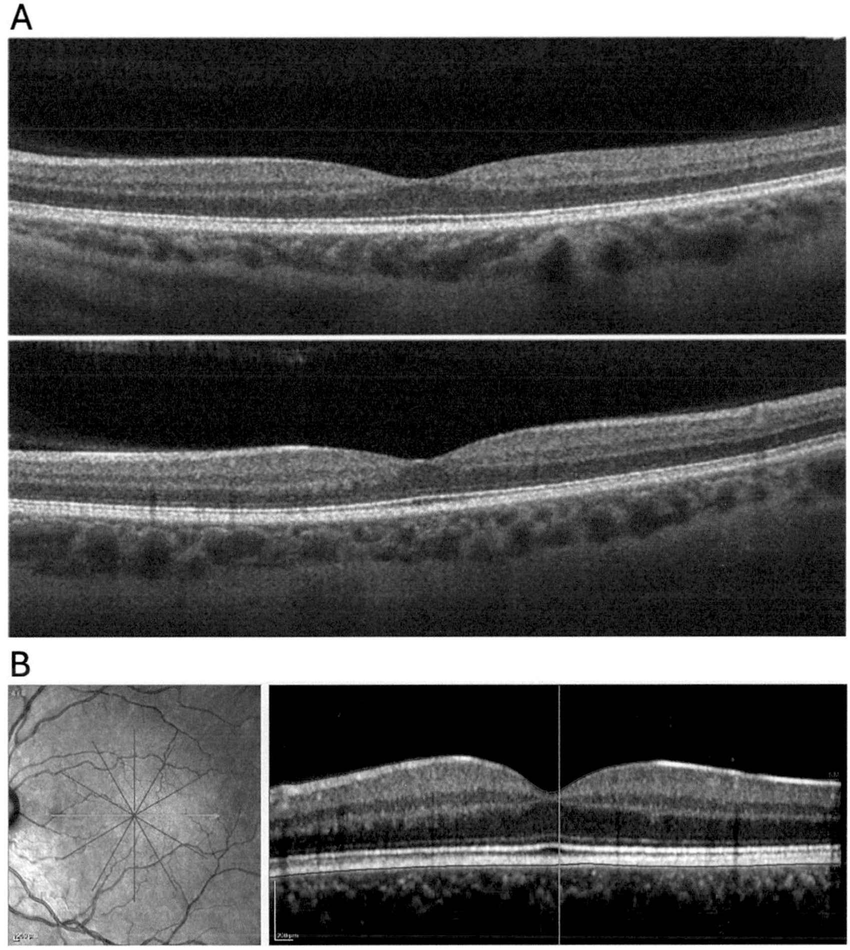

Fig. 2.4 Macular cross-hair scanning pattern obtained with Optovue Avanti with horizontal (top) and vertical (bottom) scans (A) and a Sperctralis OCT radial scan with a representative horizontal scan (B)

2.4.2 Retinal and Macular Guided Progression Analysis

The ability of OCT to provide highly reproducible, quantitative, micron-scale measurements is useful in tracking small structural changes that occur over time due to disease deterioration. Several commercial SD-OCT devices include a progression analysis tool. Automatic progression algorithms utilize trend-based analysis methods, primarily linear regression analysis, for computing the rate of change in structural parameters over time. The computed rate is compared to a no-change slope to determine if the rate is statistically significant. This rate of change is also used to predict future progression beyond the most recent visit. This prediction can

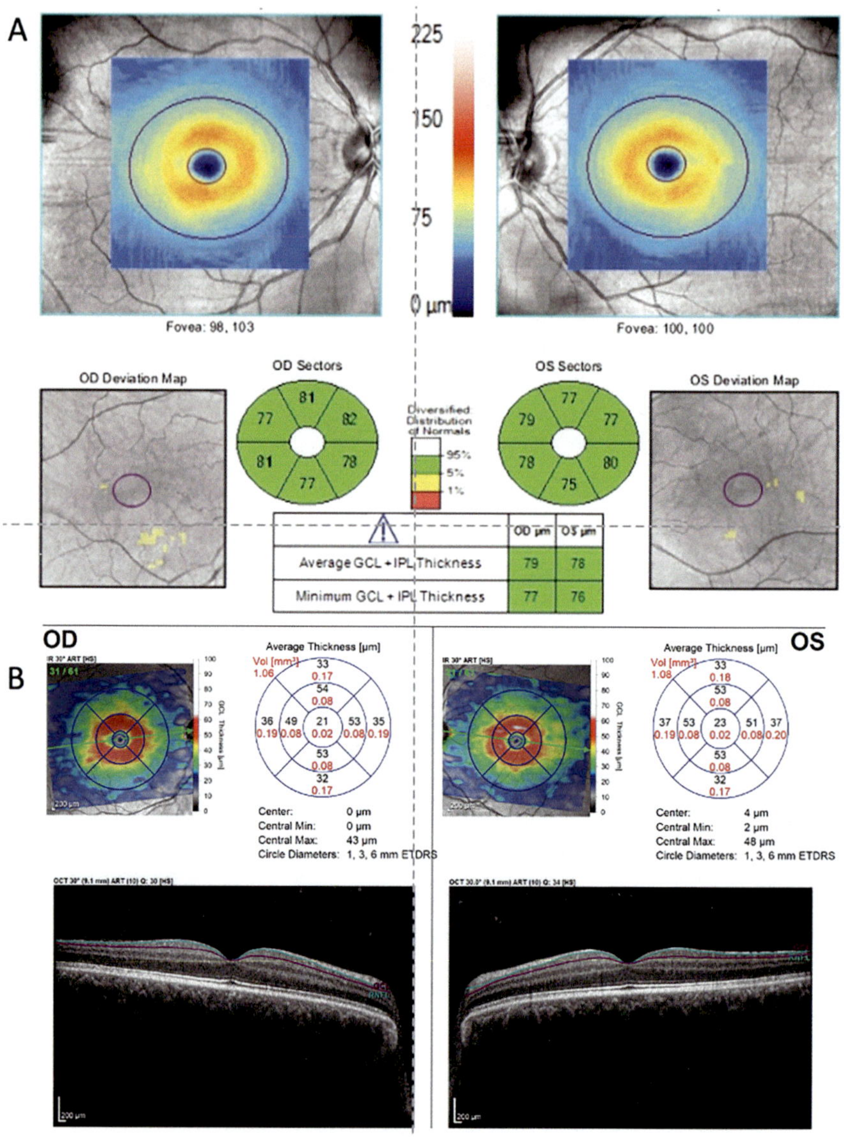

Fig. 2.5 Cirrus HD-OCT ganglion cell analysis (A) and Spectralis OCT GCC analysis (B)

be useful when discussing disease forecast with a patient or to assess the effect of treatment modification. Several commercial devices also provide event-based analysis, where a series of follow-up measurements are compared with baseline measurements and progression is defined as changes in measurements exceeding a predetermined threshold.

It has been described that the peripapillary and macular regions are both useful for detecting glaucoma progression. Glaucoma progression identification has only moderate agreement when looking at these two retinal locations, and different causal theories have been suggested, such as varying dynamic ranges of thickness measurements and minimal measurable thickness (floor effect) with different residual thickness composition (i.e., blood vessels and glial cells), or because one region is affected prior to the other [36–38].

The Fig. 2.6 shows the Cirrus HD-OCT guided progression analysis (GPA) for RNFL (A) and GCIPL (B). It provides RNFL and GCIPL event and trend analyses showing a visual display of the location of structural change. In event analysis a, baseline values are obtained by averaging the data from the first two exams. At least 20 adjacent superpixels must be flagged in the RNFL or GCIPL thickness change maps for a change to be classified as significant. If the difference from baseline is confirmed to be outside the range of test–retest variability, it is classified as "possible loss" and is color-coded in yellow; if the change is confirmed in the subsequent follow-up examination it is classified as "likely loss" and is marked in red. Trend analysis b evaluates the rate of change over time using linear regression in the GCIPL, RNFL, and ONH parameters (rim area, average cup-to-disc ratio, vertical cup-to-disc ratio, and cup volume).

Lately, it was described that macular (GCIPL average, superior, and inferior) and ONH parameters (rim area, cup volume, and cup-to-disc ratio) are sensitive biomarkers to detect glaucoma progression, even in eyes with structural glaucomatous damage, that have reached the floor effect level of RNFL OCT parameters [39].

2.4.3 Swept Source OCT

The major advantages of this OCT iteration compared to earlier ones are the faster scanning speed, deeper penetration into the tissue, and reduced signal attenuation within the scanned window. The countereffect is a reduced resolution. These properties improve visualization of choroid, sclera, and retinal sub-RPE pathologies such as central serous chorioretinopathy, AMD, choroidal tumors, and retinitis pigmentosa [40, 41]. Examination of the LC and posterior sclera will improve the understanding of the mechanical aspects of glaucoma pathogenesis. Significant differences were documented in the 3D LC microstructure between healthy and glaucomatous eyes [42, 43] as well as a more tortuous pathway of the pores in glaucomatous eyes as a potential mechanism for axonal flow obstruction and subsequent damage [44] (Figs. 2.7, 2.8, and 2.9).

2.4.4 Optical Coherence Tomography Angiography (OCTA)

OCTA is an in-vivo, non-invasive, dye-free OCT-based imaging of the blood vessels that provides volumetric vascular analysis [45]. Multiple sequential B-scans

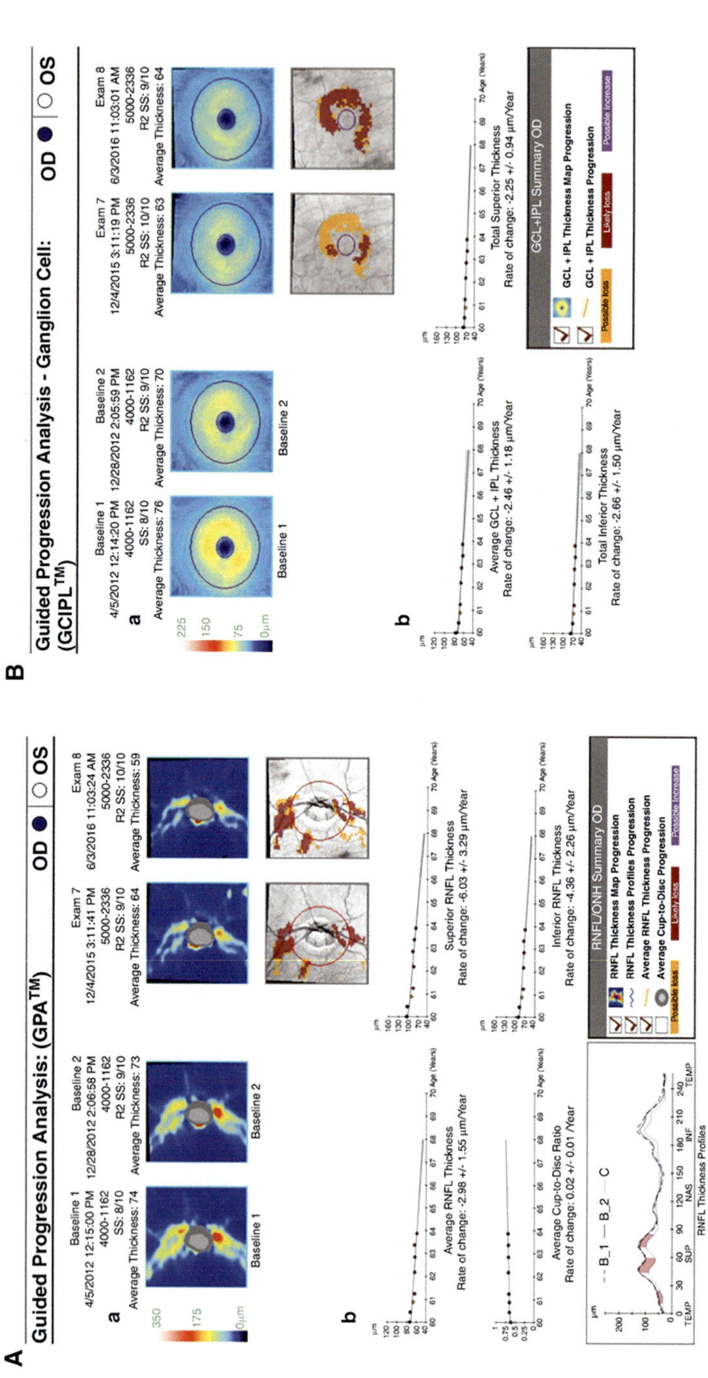

Fig. 2.6 RNFL (A) and GCIPL (B) guided progression analysis

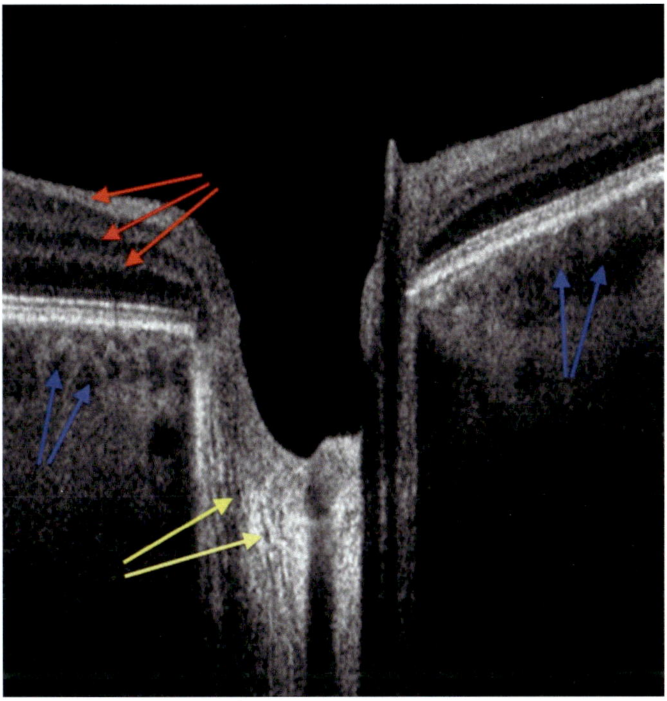

Fig. 2.7 SS-OCT cross section where retinal layers (red arrows), lamina cribrosa (yellow arrows), and choroidal vessels (blue arrows) are all captured in the same scan because this technology is less prone to signal drop-off in comparison with other OCT iterations

are acquired in rapid succession and then compared [41]. The dynamic motion of red blood cells from one image to the other causes a decorrelation signal which is detected by the machine to generate three-dimensional angiograms of the retinal, ONH and choroidal vasculature [41, 45]. It should be noted that this method only provides the anatomical location of blood vessels with flow within a predefined range. Vessels with fast or slow flow outside of this range will not be detected. Furthermore, the device does not report the actual flow within the vessels. The device provides the visualization of blood vessel networks and quantitative analysis of the blood vessel density in the scanned region. OCTA can be performed using both SD-OCT and SS-OCT technologies.

The Fig. 2.10 shows the SD-OCTA Angioplex (Zeiss) report of both ONH and macula angiography scans. The report includes the enface angiography images at different depths on the left, the superficial vascular network and cross-sectional scan overlaid with the location of detected vessels in the middle, and the vessel density analysis by region in the inferior right corner.

The Fig. 2.11 shows the ONH SS-OCT Triton (Topcon, Oakland, NJ) angiography report. The top row of the report shows the angiography analysis in different depths starting with the innermost section closest to the ILM (labeled as the "nerve

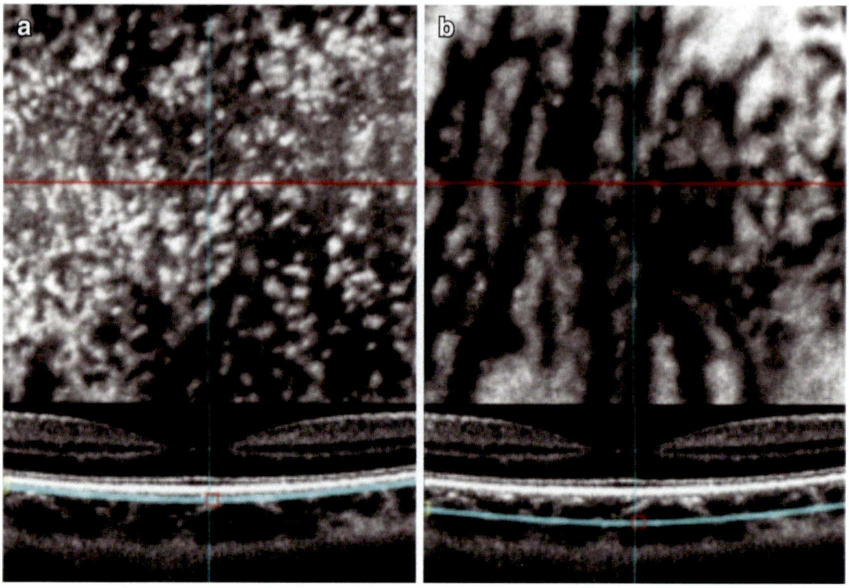

Fig. 2.8 Upper panel demonstrates enface images of SS-OCT of choriocapillaries (**a**) and the large vessels of the choroid (**b**). Bottom panel shows the corresponding cross-sectional scans with the turquoise lines marking the plane where the enface image was acquired

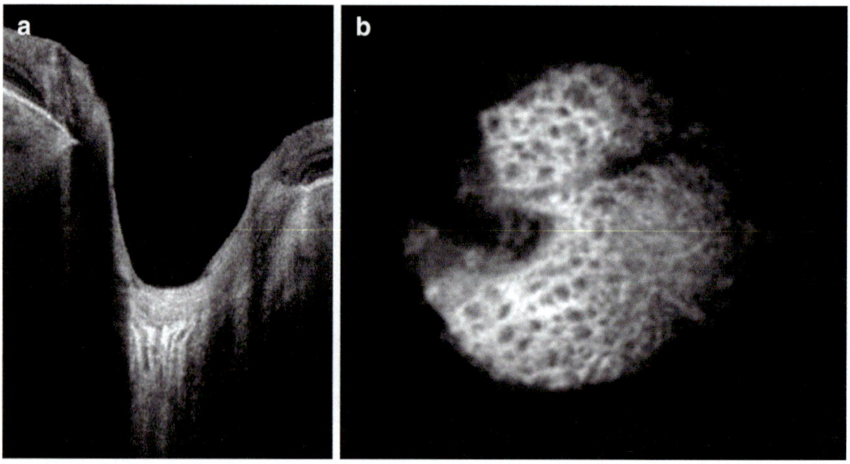

Fig. 2.9 Swept-source OCT cross-section image of the optic nerve head region (**a**). Enface image at the lamina cribrosa level demonstrating the intricate structure of the hyper-reflective beams (white) and hypo-reflective pores (black) (**b**)

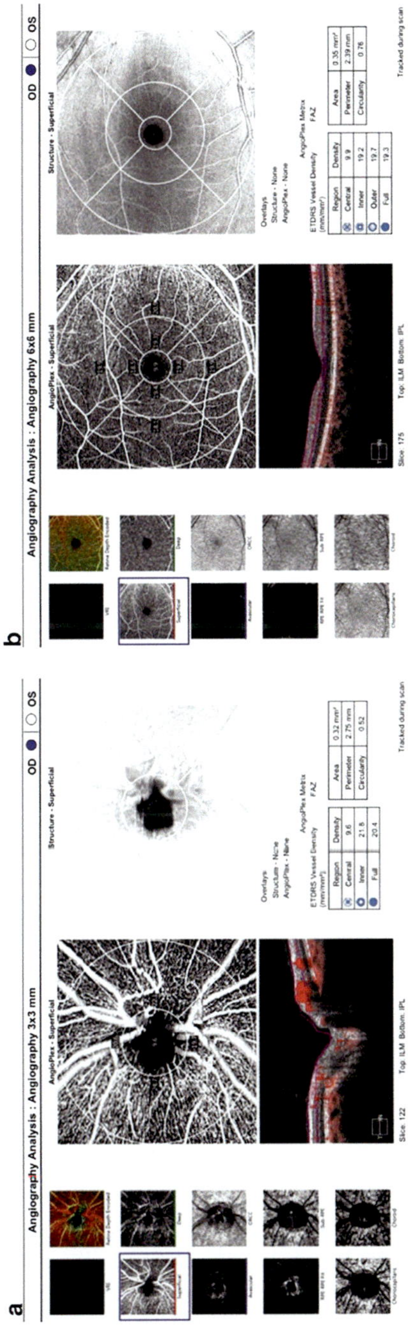

Fig. 2.10 Angioplex angiography with the 3 × 3 ONH (**a**) and 6 × 6 macula (**b**) report

head"), followed by an intermediary depth (vitreous), then the analysis at the level of retinal photoreceptor cells (RPC), and ending closest to the choroid (choroid disc). The inferior row shows on the left a cross-sectional image of the optic nerve and in the middle a color-coded vessel density map.

2.4.5 Doppler Optical Coherence Tomography

This technique allows for determining arterial and venous blood flow through spectral-domain and swept-source based Doppler OCT [46]. Using the Doppler shift detected in the OCT signal, this method can determine depth-resolved retinal vessels flow without the use if dye [47]. However, a notable drawback of this method is that it cannot detect flow if the vessels are perpendicular to the incident OCT beam or in smaller size vessels [48]. While Doppler OCT retinal blood flow measurements showed good repeatability and excellent correlation with clinical presentations of retinal diseases, the role of this technique in disease detection and monitoring is yet to be determined [48].

2.5 The Future

As technology keeps evolving, several innovative OCT iterations are being tested. The following sections will provide a brief description of some of the most promising developments.

2.5.1 Adaptive Optics

Adaptive optics (AO) is an optical method designed to dynamically adjust monochromatic aberrations in optical systems. AO was initially used in astronomy for correcting distortions of light passing through the atmosphere. The first in vivo examination of the retina with an AO fundus camera using a wave front sensor and a deformable mirror was introduced in 1997 [49]. A few years later, AO was combined with scanning laser ophthalmoscope [50] and OCT systems [51]. As discussed above, the transverse resolution of all conventional OCT systems is limited to the range of 15–20 μm due to the optical aberrations of light beams when passing through various media in the eye. AO measures and corrects the optical aberrations, reduces the projected spot size, and improves the transverse resolution from 20 μm to the range of 5–10 μm [51]. This resolution allows the acquisition of highly detailed images, enabling the visualization of fine details such as the retinal microvasculature, photoreceptor mosaic [52, 53], LC, and microstructures within the RNFL [6, 54] and ganglion cell layer. The ability to acquire highly detailed in vivo images of these structures allow further insight into ocular anatomy in health and disease, providing the opportunity to expand the understanding of pathologic processes in the eye.

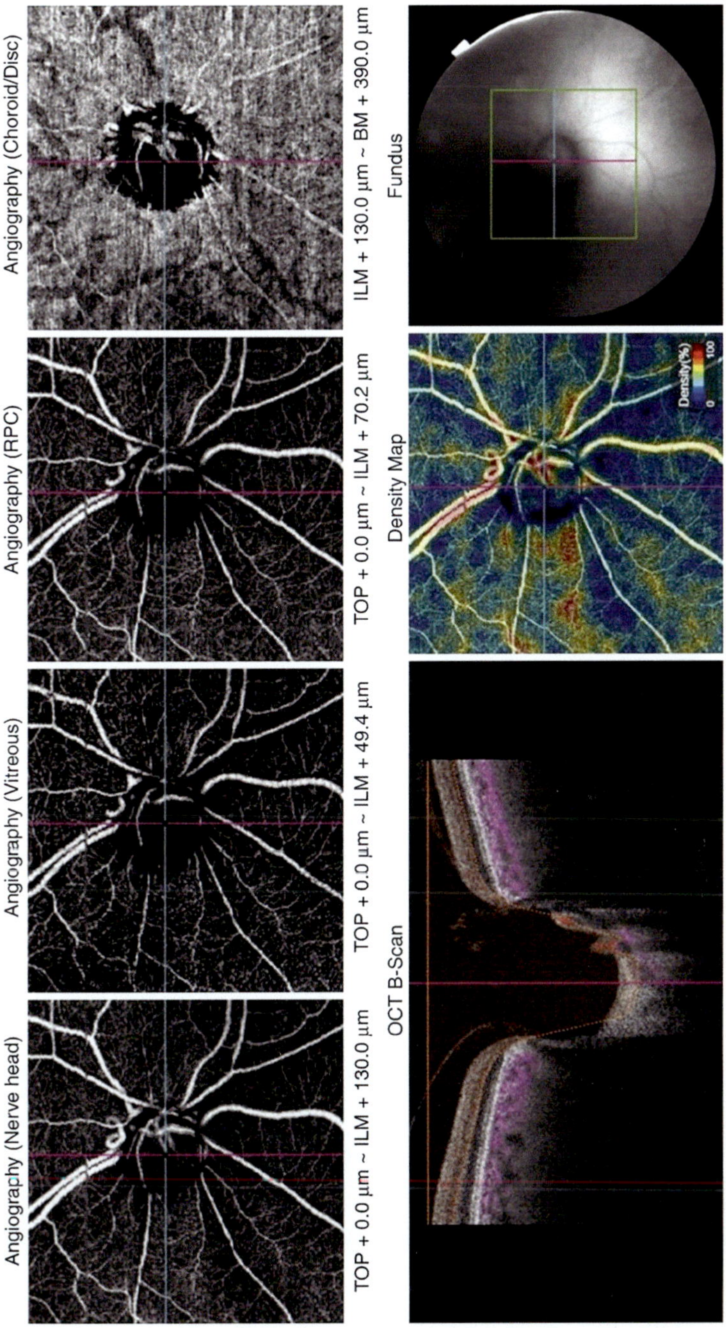

Fig. 2.11 Triton ONH angiography report

Alternatives to hardware-based AO OCT systems have been developed, including Computational AO and Sensorless AO. Computational AO, which modifies the phase of OCT data in the spectral domain to reduce aberrations. While image quality may be compromised, the advantage of this approach is to minimize the need for expensive hardware by correcting distortions in post-processing [55, 56]. Sensorless AO relies on analyzing properties of the acquired images rather than utilizing a wavefront sensor to measure and correct aberrations [57]. Various optimization methods and algorithms have been developed for Sensorless AO, including Zernike Mode Hill Climbing [58], stochastic parallel gradient descent [59, 60], deep reinforcement learning [61], and others.

The major limitation of the AO technique is the small field of view, which is restricted to approximately 1–3°. The use of an eye-tracking system to acquire a series of neighboring scans to cover a larger volume can resolve this limitation, though the longer scanning time might prohibit large scale clinical use [62]. Similarly, the focusing depth of the AO technique is also limited, and therefore acquiring high quality images of thick structures such as the choroid and retina in the same image is difficult to obtain. It may be possible to address this limitation by varying the focal plane while scanning in depth [63]. The volume of data needed for image processing and advanced analysis requirements are also limiting factors for commercialization of the technology. Datasets are 100 times larger than the conventional OCT counterparts, and therefore storage and accessibility of the information are challenging [64].

2.5.2 Visible-Light OCT

Switching to light sources in the visible light wavelength (~550 nm), instead of near infrared wavelengths, allows further improvement in axial resolution to the level of < 1 μm and the extraction of spectroscopic information that is registered to the structural information. The higher scattering coefficients of biological tissue with visible light improves imaging contrast, but at the expense of reduced imaging depth (Fig. 2.12) [20]. Speckle noise reduction techniques can be applied to reduce background noise level and further improve image quality.

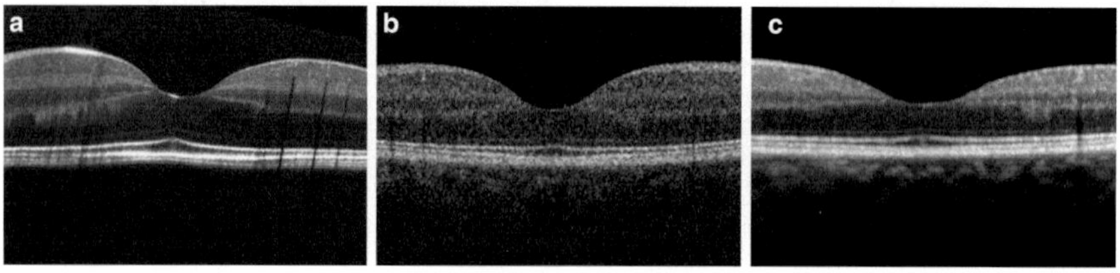

Fig. 2.12 Macula scan of the same subject with Vis-OCT with speckle reduction (**a**) Cirrus OCT (**b**), and Spectralis OCT (**c**). Note the improved visualization with the Vis-OCT and the distinct interface between retinal layers without the need of averaging of multiple images

The evaluation of oxygen saturation through spectroscopy analysis is one of the most promising applications of the Vis-OCT system [20]. By taking advantage of the distinct light absorption of oxygenated and de-oxygenated hemoglobin within the visible spectral range it is possible to determine the oxygen consumption of tissue in a given region [19]. The role of oxygen saturation and consumption by the ocular tissue for diagnosing and monitoring various ophthalmic disease is currently being examined. Other chromatophores indicating metabolic and biochemical tissue activity are also being initially evaluated.

Adaptive spectroscopic Vis-OCT, a recent modification to the technique, is capable of further improving the potential clinical utility of Vis-OCT by making it possible to remove spectral contaminants from human images and accurately measure sO_2 by conforming measurements to the specific conditions of each vessel [65].

2.5.3 Polarization Sensitive OCT

Polarization sensitive OCT (PS-OCT) uses the polarization state of polarized light for the assessment of tissue function. Different ocular structures and tissues alter the polarization state of light in different ways, such as through birefringence (sclera, RNFL), polarization-preservation (photoreceptors), and depolarization (RPE) (Fig. 2.13). PS-OCT estimates these light state alterations by simultaneously measuring intensity, retardation, and optic axis information. The technology was initially incorporated into TD-OCT system, with subsequent introduction into all known OCT iterations such as SD-OCT [66], SS-OCT [30], and AO-OCT [67]. A few studies demonstrated that alteration in the polarization of ocular tissues might precede the occurrence of structural alteration, thus evaluation of the functional properties of the RNFL [68], sclera, and RPE [69] using PS-OCT technology could be an attractive candidate for improving the detection of ocular pathologies such as glaucoma and age-related macular degeneration.

2.5.4 Phase Sensitive OCT

The Phase Sensitive OCT technique is able to provide in vivo information on micron scale movements or vibrations within the tissue [70]. The technology analyzes the phase information of the back-reflected light beam, which is typically ignored in conventional OCT systems. OCT phase imaging has been demonstrated with SD-OCT [71] and SS-OCT [72] technologies. Phase sensitive OCT offers the advantage of simultaneously assessing both the structural and functional information of the scanned tissue. The device has been shown to capture the retinal pigment epithelium layer, Henle's loop of the macula and retinal nerve fiber layer [73–76]. PS-OCT might be clinically useful in the context of glaucoma, AMD and potentially multiple sclerosis [73, 75, 77], but the clinical application is challenging because it is very sensitive to eye motion.

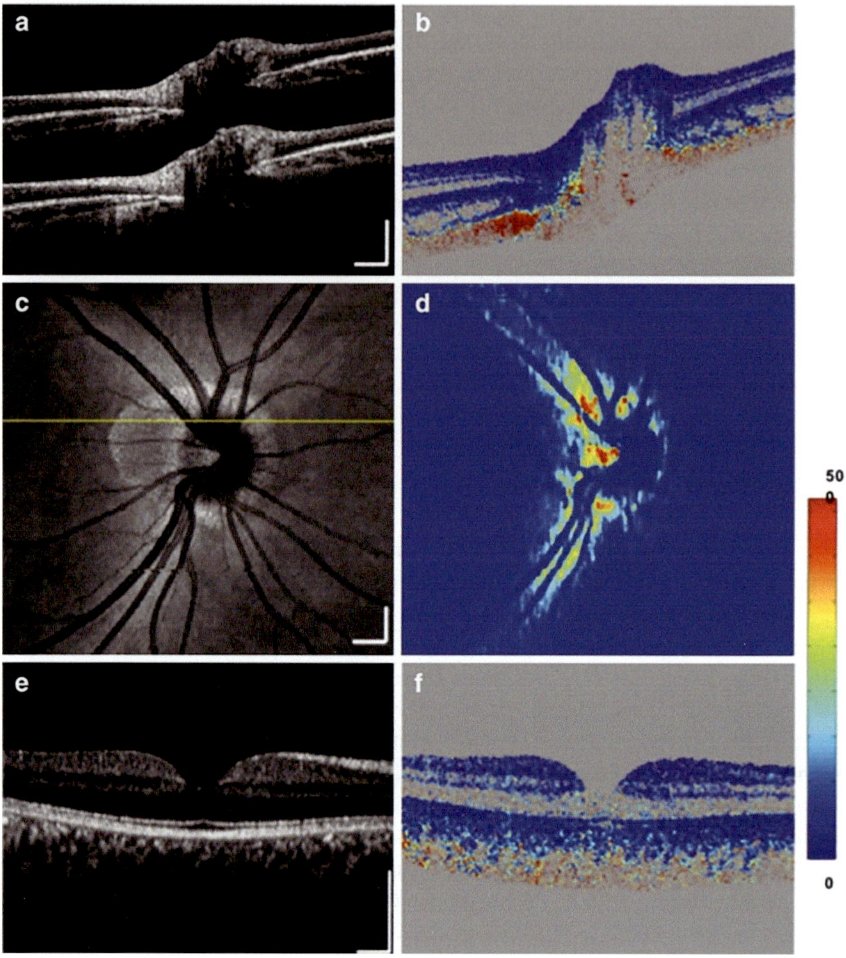

Fig. 2.13 PS-OCT optic nerve head and retinal imaging in healthy subjects. (**a**) A cross-sectional intensity image with two depth-encoded copies of the optic nerve head region. (**b**) Corresponding PS-OCT image shows high retardance in the RNFL and sclera. (**c**) OCT fundus image. (**d**) Corresponding PS-OCT map shows high retardance around the optic nerve head region. (**e**) A cross-sectional intensity image at the fovea region. (**f**) Corresponding PS-OCT image shows low retardance in the retinal layers

2.5.5 3D Optical Coherence Refraction Tomography (3D OCRT)

3D optical coherence refraction tomography (3D OCRT) offering improved imaging capabilities for biomedical samples [78]. 3D OCRT has been demonstrated to be capable of capturing 5D plenoptic datasets (multiple 3D volumes acquired in two rotation axes) and computationally synthesizing 3D contrast without any movement of the sample being imaged [79]. By incorporating a parabolic mirror into the optical design, 3D OCRT overcomes limitations of acquiring high-resolution OCT images over a wide field of view in all directions simultaneously. The method combines multiple views into a single high-quality 3D image, correcting for distortions, noise, and imperfections to generate detailed images and reveal features that are challenging to observe with traditional OCT. Similar to the parabolic mirror approach, other conic-section mirror-based imaging systems may be used for high-speed multiview imaging [80]. 3D OCRT has broad applicability, offering the possibility of in vivo diagnostic imaging. The technology is currently available at a microscope setting but can be miniaturized into endoscopes for accessing different parts of the body, creating additional opportunities for medical diagnostics.

With improvements including faster sources, the introduction of anticonjugate galvanometers instead of 2D translation, and the capability to generate image contrast from multi-angle data, 3D OCRT has the potential to be used in the field of in vivo biomedical imaging [79].

2.5.6 Optical Coherence Elastography (OCE)

Optical coherence elastography [OCE), is an emerging technique for characterizing the mechanical properties of ocular tissues [81]. Compared to traditional elastography techniques, OCE capitalizes on the superior resolution of OCT imaging while also facing limitations in the depth of tissue penetration. OCE operates at a "meso-scale" resolution range, probing groups of cells while bridging the gap between individual cells and whole tissues [82]. The manipulation of parameters, including length scale, time scale, and source type, offer a range of choices for OCE methodology [83, 84]. Common methods involve either quasi-static compression or shear/surface wave generation. Compressive OCE utilizes a compressor to capture images before and after compression, enabling the determination of local axial strain [85]. Shear and surface waves can be produced through contact or non-contact means. Ongoing research in OCE focuses on addressing measurement accuracy and challenges in modeling. Recent advancements in imaging techniques, including multi-excitation "M-B mode" imaging, hold promise for enhancing the capabilities of OCE [84].

Various ocular diseases, including keratoconus, presbyopia, glaucoma, and arteriosclerosis, are closely linked to alterations in tissue elasticity. OCE provides a reliable and non-contact approach to measure tissue elasticity in vivo, potentially enabling earlier disease detection even before structural changes are observable with conventional OCT imaging. Different methods, such as static force, sinusoidal vibration, and fast transient excitation have been tested. Non-contact techniques, such as air-puff application [86, 87] or focused ultrasound excitation [88, 89], demonstrate promise for clinical use.

2.5.7 Spatio-Temporal Optical Coherence Tomography (STOC-T)

Using light with controlled spatial and temporal coherence in conjunction with signal processing, spatio-temporal optical coherence tomography (STOC-T) is a novel technique designed for optoretinography the chorioretinal complex [90, 91]. Advancements in STOC-T have enabled high-resolution imaging of the retina and choroid at varying depths. The advantages of STOC-T include uniform 5 μm resolution imaging of the chorioretinal complex, > 1 mm axial imaging range with full-field detection and digital defocus correction, high contrast coronal projections of the choroid at depth of choice, and deriving quantitative morphometry metrics from generated choriocapillaris images [90]. STOC-T overcomes some of the limitations of conventional OCT by offering a broader depth-of-field and enhanced lateral resolution. In addition, STOC-T manipulation has the capability of enhancing SS-OCT imaging by suppressing cross-talk-generated noise without compromising transversal resolution [92]. Notably, this technology has successfully demonstrated the ability to differentiate and non-invasively visualize morphological layers of the chorioretinal complex, including the Sattler, Haller, and choriocapillaris layers [90].

2.5.8 At-Home OCT

In response to the necessity of frequent monitoring and imaging in the management of some retinal diseases such as neovascular AMD, At-Home OCT devices has been developed. At-Home OCT provides the option of daily self-imaging for subjects with or at risk for the progression of retinal disease without the need for additional clinical visits. At-Home SD-OCT system, has demonstrated the production of high-quality images and good agreement with in-clinic OCT scans, as well as between independent graders [93–95]. Longitudinal testing over a three month follow-up observed excellent usage with a self-imaging rate of 5.7 scans per week [95]. The integration of artificial intelligence has further improved the capabilities of At-Home imaging, allowing for an accurate automation of retinal fluid identification [93, 96]. Although additional validation is warranted, At-Home OCT may become a reliable alternative to conventional testing in-clinic.

In conclusion, OCT has an important clinical role in the diagnosis of ocular diseases and in tracking changes overtime, leading to improved clinical management and better insight into pathophysiology of diseases. The constant enhancement of this technology ensures that clinicians will have an indispensable diagnostic tool in their armament.

References

1. Fujimoto JG, Brezinski ME, Tearney GJ, Boppart SA, Bouma B, Hee MR, et al. Optical biopsy and imaging using optical coherence tomography. Nat Med. 1995;1(9):970–2.
2. Fercher AF, Mengedoht K, Werner W. Eye-length measurement by interferometry with partially coherent light. Opt Lett. 1988;13(3):186–8.
3. Izatt JA, Hee MR, Swanson EA, Lin CP, Huang D, Schuman JS, et al. Micrometer-scale resolution imaging of the anterior eye in vivo with optical coherence tomography. Arch Ophthalmol. 1994;112(12):1584–9.
4. Potsaid B, Baumann B, Huang D, Barry S, Cable AE, Schuman JS, et al. Ultrahigh speed 1050nm swept source/Fourier domain OCT retinal and anterior segment imaging at 100,000 to 400,000 axial scans per second. Opt Express. 2010;18(19):20029–48.
5. Wieser W, Biedermann BR, Klein T, Eigenwillig CM, Huber R. Multi-megahertz OCT: High quality 3D imaging at 20 million A-scans and 4.5 GVoxels per second. Opt Express. 2010;18(14):14685-704.
6. Kocaoglu OP, Cense B, Jonnal RS, Wang Q, Lee S, Gao W, et al. Imaging retinal nerve fiber bundles using optical coherence tomography with adaptive optics. Vision Res. 2011;51(16):1835–44.
7. Lavinsky F, Lavinsky D. Novel perspectives on swept-source optical coherence tomography. Int J Retina Vitreous. 2016;2:25.
8. Kuroda H, Baba M, Suzuki M, Yoneya S. A high speed three-dimensional spectral domain optical coherence tomography with < 2 μm axial resolution using wide bandwidth femtosecond mode-locked laser. Appl Phys Lett. 2013;102(25).
9. Unterhuber A, Povazay B, Hermann B, Sattmann H, Chavez-Pirson A, Drexler W. In vivo retinal optical coherence tomography at 1040 nm—enhanced penetration into the choroid. Opt Express. 2005;13(9):3252–8.
10. Yasuno Y, Hong Y, Makita S, Yamanari M, Akiba M, Miura M, et al. In vivo high-contrast imaging of deep posterior eye by 1-microm swept source optical coherence tomography and scattering optical coherence angiography. Opt Express. 2007;15(10):6121–39.
11. Hale GM, Querry MR. Optical constants of Water in the 200-nm to 200-microm wavelength region. Appl Opt. 1973;12(3):555–63.
12. Fercher AF, Hitzenberger CK, Drexler W, Kamp G, Sattmann H. In vivo optical coherence tomography. Am J Ophthalmol. 1993;116(1):113–4.
13. Ahlers C, Schmidt-Erfurth U. Three-dimensional high resolution OCT imaging of macular pathology. Opt Express. 2009;17(5):4037–45.
14. Kim JS, Ishikawa H, Sung KR, Xu J, Wollstein G, Bilonick RA, et al. Retinal nerve fibre layer thickness measurement reproducibility improved with spectral domain optical coherence tomography. Br J Ophthalmol. 2009;93(8):1057–63.
15. Drexler W, Morgner U, Kärtner FX, Pitris C, Boppart SA, Li XD, et al. In vivo ultrahigh-resolution optical coherence tomography. Opt Lett. 1999;24(17):1221–3.
16. Lim H, Jiang Y, Wang Y, Huang YC, Chen Z, Wise FW. Ultrahigh-resolution optical coherence tomography with a fiber laser source at 1 microm. Opt Lett. 2005;30(10):1171–3.
17. Huber R, Adler DC, Fujimoto JG. Buffered Fourier domain mode locking: unidirectional swept laser sources for optical coherence tomography imaging at 370,000 lines/s. Opt Lett. 2006;31(20):2975–7.
18. Yaqoob Z, Wu J, Yang C. Spectral domain optical coherence tomography: a better OCT imaging strategy. Biotechniques. 2005;39(6 Suppl):S6-13.
19. Yi J, Wei Q, Liu W, Backman V, Zhang HF. Visible-light optical coherence tomography for retinal oximetry. Opt Lett. 2013;38(11):1796–8.
20. Shu X, Beckmann L, Zhang H. Visible-light optical coherence tomography: a review. J Biomed Opt. 2017;22(12):1–14.
21. Huang D, Swanson EA, Lin CP, Schuman JS, Stinson WG, Chang W, et al. Optical coherence tomography. Science. 1991;254(5035):1178–81.

22. Schuman JS, Pedut-Kloizman T, Hertzmark E, Hee MR, Wilkins JR, Coker JG, et al. Reproducibility of nerve fiber layer thickness measurements using optical coherence tomography. Ophthalmology. 1996;103(11):1889–98.
23. Hee MR, Izatt JA, Swanson EA, Huang D, Schuman JS, Lin CP, et al. Optical coherence tomography of the human retina. Arch Ophthalmol. 1995;113(3):325–32.
24. Otani T, Kishi S, Maruyama Y. Patterns of diabetic macular edema with optical coherence tomography. Am J Ophthalmol. 1999;127(6):688–93.
25. Sánchez-Tocino H, Alvarez-Vidal A, Maldonado MJ, Moreno-Montañés J, García-Layana A. Retinal thickness study with optical coherence tomography in patients with diabetes. Invest Ophthalmol Vis Sci. 2002;43(5):1588–94.
26. Medeiros FA, Zangwill LM, Bowd C, Weinreb RN. Comparison of the GDx VCC scanning laser polarimeter, HRT II confocal scanning laser ophthalmoscope, and stratus OCT optical coherence tomograph for the detection of glaucoma. Arch Ophthalmol. 2004;122(6):827–37.
27. Paunescu LA, Schuman JS, Price LL, Stark PC, Beaton S, Ishikawa H, et al. Reproducibility of nerve fiber thickness, macular thickness, and optic nerve head measurements using StratusOCT. Invest Ophthalmol Vis Sci. 2004;45(6):1716–24.
28. Srinivasan VJ, Wojtkowski M, Fujimoto JG, Duker JS. In vivo measurement of retinal physiology with high-speed ultrahigh-resolution optical coherence tomography. Opt Lett. 2006;31(15):2308–10.
29. Kagemann L, Wollstein G, Wojtkowski M, Ishikawa H, Townsend KA, Gabriele ML, et al. Spectral oximetry assessed with high-speed ultra-high-resolution optical coherence tomography. J Biomed Opt. 2007;12(4): 041212.
30. Yamanari M, Makita S, Lim Y, Yasuno Y. Full-range polarization-sensitive swept-source optical coherence tomography by simultaneous transversal and spectral modulation. Opt Express. 2010;18(13):13964–80.
31. Wojtkowski M, Srinivasan V, Fujimoto JG, Ko T, Schuman JS, Kowalczyk A, et al. Three-dimensional retinal imaging with high-speed ultrahigh-resolution optical coherence tomography. Ophthalmology. 2005;112(10):1734–46.
32. Leung CK, Cheung CY, Weinreb RN, Qiu Q, Liu S, Li H, et al. Retinal nerve fiber layer imaging with spectral-domain optical coherence tomography: a variability and diagnostic performance study. Ophthalmology. 2009;116(7):1257–63, e1–2.
33. Tan O, Li G, Lu AT, Varma R, Huang D. Mapping of macular substructures with optical coherence tomography for glaucoma diagnosis. Ophthalmology. 2008;115(6):949–56.
34. Tan O, Chopra V, Lu AT, Schuman JS, Ishikawa H, Wollstein G, et al. Detection of macular ganglion cell loss in glaucoma by Fourier-domain optical coherence tomography. Ophthalmology. 2009;116(12):2305–14.e1–2.
35. Asrani S, Rosdahl JA, Allingham RR. Novel software strategy for glaucoma diagnosis: asymmetry analysis of retinal thickness. Arch Ophthalmol. 2011;129(9):1205–11.
36. Kim KE, Park KH, Jeoung JW, Kim SH, Kim DM. Severity-dependent association between ganglion cell inner plexiform layer thickness and macular mean sensitivity in open-angle glaucoma. Acta Ophthalmol. 2014;92(8):e650–6.
37. Belghith A, Medeiros FA, Bowd C, Liebmann JM, Girkin CA, Weinreb RN, et al. Structural Change Can Be Detected in Advanced-Glaucoma Eyes. Invest Ophthalmol Vis Sci. 2016;57(9):Oct511–8.
38. Bowd C, Zangwill LM, Weinreb RN, Medeiros FA, Belghith A. Estimating optical coherence tomography structural measurement floors to improve detection of progression in advanced glaucoma. Am J Ophthalmol. 2017;175:37–44.
39. Lavinsky F, Wu M, Schuman JS, Lucy KA, Liu M, Song Y, et al. Can macula and optic nerve head parameters detect glaucoma progression in eyes with advanced circumpapillary retinal nerve fiber layer damage? Ophthalmology. 2018;125(12):1907–12.
40. Keane PA, Ruiz-Garcia H, Sadda SR. Clinical applications of long-wavelength (1,000-nm) optical coherence tomography. Ophthalmic Surg Lasers Imaging. 2011;42(Suppl):S67-74.
41. Yasin Alibhai A, Or C, Witkin AJ. Swept source optical coherence tomography: a review. Curr Ophthalmol Rep. 2018;6(1):7–16.

42. Wang B, Nevins JE, Nadler Z, Wollstein G, Ishikawa H, Bilonick RA, et al. In vivo lamina cribrosa micro-architecture in healthy and glaucomatous eyes as assessed by optical coherence tomography. Invest Ophthalmol Vis Sci. 2013;54(13):8270–4.
43. Omodaka K, Maekawa S, An G, Tsuda S, Shiga Y, Takada N, et al. Pilot study for three-dimensional assessment of laminar pore structure in patients with glaucoma, as measured with swept source optical coherence tomography. PLoS ONE. 2018;13(11): e0207600.
44. Wang B, Lucy KA, Schuman JS, Sigal IA, Bilonick RA, Lu C, et al. Tortuous pore path through the glaucomatous lamina cribrosa. Sci Rep. 2018;8(1):7281.
45. Hou H, Moghimi S, Zangwill LM, Shoji T, Ghahari E, Penteado RC, et al. Macula vessel density and thickness in early primary open-angle glaucoma. Am J Ophthalmol. 2019;199:120–32.
46. Leitgeb RA, Werkmeister RM, Blatter C, Schmetterer L. Doppler optical coherence tomography. Prog Retin Eye Res. 2014;41(100):26–43.
47. Werkmeister RM, Dragostinoff N, Pircher M, Götzinger E, Hitzenberger CK, Leitgeb RA, et al. Bidirectional doppler fourier-domain optical coherence tomography for measurement of absolute flow velocities in human retinal vessels. Opt Lett. 2008;33(24):2967–9.
48. Wang Y, Fawzi AA, Varma R, Sadun AA, Zhang X, Tan O, et al. Pilot study of optical coherence tomography measurement of retinal blood flow in retinal and optic nerve diseases. Invest Ophthalmol Vis Sci. 2011;52(2):840–5.
49. Liang J, Williams DR, Miller DT. Supernormal vision and high-resolution retinal imaging through adaptive optics. J Opt Soc Am A Opt Image Sci Vis. 1997;14(11):2884–92.
50. Roorda A, Romero-Borja F, Donnelly Iii W, Queener H, Hebert T, Campbell M. Adaptive optics scanning laser ophthalmoscopy. Opt Express. 2002;10(9):405–12.
51. Hermann B, Fernández EJ, Unterhuber A, Sattmann H, Fercher AF, Drexler W, et al. Adaptive-optics ultrahigh-resolution optical coherence tomography. Opt Lett. 2004;29(18):2142–4.
52. Kocaoglu OP, Lee S, Jonnal RS, Wang Q, Herde AE, Derby JC, et al. Imaging cone photoreceptors in three dimensions and in time using ultrahigh resolution optical coherence tomography with adaptive optics. Biomed Opt Express. 2011;2(4):748–63.
53. Shirazi MF, Brunner E, Laslandes M, Pollreisz A, Hitzenberger CK, Pircher M. Visualizing human photoreceptor and retinal pigment epithelium cell mosaics in a single volume scan over an extended field of view with adaptive optics optical coherence tomography. Biomed Opt Express. 2020;11(8):4520–35.
54. Takayama K, Ooto S, Hangai M, Ueda-Arakawa N, Yoshida S, Akagi T, et al. High-resolution imaging of retinal nerve fiber bundles in glaucoma using adaptive optics scanning laser ophthalmoscopy. Am J Ophthalmol. 2013;155(5):870–81.
55. Akyol E, Hagag AM, Sivaprasad S, Lotery AJ. Adaptive optics: principles and applications in ophthalmology. Eye. 2021;35(1):244–64.
56. Adie SG, Graf BW, Ahmad A, Carney PS, Boppart SA. Computational adaptive optics for broadband optical interferometric tomography of biological tissue. Proc Natl Acad Sci. 2012;109(19):7175–80.
57. Liu L, Wu Z, Qi M, Li Y, Zhang M, Liao D, et al. Application of adaptive optics in ophthalmology. Photonics. 2022;9(5):288.
58. Camino A, Ng R, Huang J, Guo Y, Ni S, Jia Y, et al. Depth-resolved optimization of a real-time sensorless adaptive optics optical coherence tomography. Opt Lett. 2020;45(9):2612–5.
59. Hofer H, Sredar N, Queener H, Li C, Porter J. Wavefront sensorless adaptive optics ophthalmoscopy in the human eye. Opt Express. 2011;19(15):14160–71.
60. Zhu D, Wang R, Žurauskas M, Pande P, Bi J, Yuan Q, et al. Automated fast computational adaptive optics for optical coherence tomography based on a stochastic parallel gradient descent algorithm. Opt Express. 2020;28(16):23306–19.
61. Durech E, Newberry W, Franke J, Sarunic MV. Wavefront sensor-less adaptive optics using deep reinforcement learning. Biomed Opt Express. 2021;12(9):5423–38.
62. Burns SA, Tumbar R, Elsner AE, Ferguson D, Hammer DX. Large-field-of-view, modular, stabilized, adaptive-optics-based scanning laser ophthalmoscope. J Opt Soc Am A Opt Image Sci Vis. 2007;24(5):1313–26.

63. Zawadzki RJ, Choi SS, Fuller AR, Evans JW, Hamann B, Werner JS. Cellular resolution volumetric in vivo retinal imaging with adaptive optics-optical coherence tomography. Opt Express. 2009;17(5):4084–94.
64. Jonnal RS, Kocaoglu OP, Zawadzki RJ, Liu Z, Miller DT, Werner JS. A Review of Adaptive Optics Optical Coherence Tomography: Technical Advances, Scientific Applications, and the Future. Invest Ophthalmol Vis Sci. 2016;57(9):Oct51–68.
65. Rubinoff I, Kuranov RV, Fang R, Ghassabi Z, Wang Y, Beckmann L, et al. Adaptive spectroscopic visible-light optical coherence tomography for clinical retinal oximetry. Commun Med. 2023;3(1):57.
66. Götzinger E, Pircher M, Baumann B, Ahlers C, Geitzenauer W, Schmidt-Erfurth U, et al. Three-dimensional polarization sensitive OCT imaging and interactive display of the human retina. Opt Express. 2009;17(5):4151–65.
67. Cense B, Gao W, Brown JM, Jones SM, Jonnal RS, Mujat M, et al. Retinal imaging with polarization-sensitive optical coherence tomography and adaptive optics. Opt Express. 2009;17(24):21634–51.
68. Liu S, Wang B, Yin B, Milner TE, Markey MK, McKinnon SJ, et al. Retinal nerve fiber layer reflectance for early glaucoma diagnosis. J Glaucoma. 2014;23(1):e45-52.
69. Michels S, Pircher M, Geitzenauer W, Simader C, Götzinger E, Findl O, et al. Value of polarisation-sensitive optical coherence tomography in diseases affecting the retinal pigment epithelium. Br J Ophthalmol. 2008;92(2):204–9.
70. Choma MA, Ellerbee AK, Yang C, Creazzo TL, Izatt JA. Spectral-domain phase microscopy. Opt Lett. 2005;30(10):1162–4.
71. Joo C, Akkin T, Cense B, Park BH, de Boer JF. Spectral-domain optical coherence phase microscopy for quantitative phase-contrast imaging. Opt Lett. 2005;30(16):2131–3.
72. Sarunic MV, Weinberg S, Izatt JA. Full-field swept-source phase microscopy. Opt Lett. 2006;31(10):1462–4.
73. Ju MJ, Hong YJ, Makita S, Lim Y, Kurokawa K, Duan L, et al. Advanced multi-contrast Jones matrix optical coherence tomography for doppler and polarization sensitive imaging. Opt Express. 2013;21(16):19412–36.
74. Cense B, Wang Q, Lee S, Zhao L, Elsner AE, Hitzenberger CK, et al. Henle fiber layer phase retardation measured with polarization-sensitive optical coherence tomography. Biomed Opt Express. 2013;4(11):2296–306.
75. Braaf B, Vermeer KA, de Groot M, Vienola KV, de Boer JF. Fiber-based polarization-sensitive OCT of the human retina with correction of system polarization distortions. Biomed Opt Express. 2014;5(8):2736–58.
76. Wang Z, Lee HC, Ahsen OO, Lee B, Choi W, Potsaid B, et al. Depth-encoded all-fiber swept source polarization sensitive OCT. Biomed Opt Express. 2014;5(9):2931–49.
77. Jiang H, Chen W, Delgado S, Liu Y, Lin Y, Wang J. Altered birefringence of peripapillary retinal nerve fiber layer in multiple sclerosis measured by polarization sensitive optical coherence tomography. Eye Vis (Lond). 2018;5:14.
78. Zhou KC, Qian R, Degan S, Farsiu S, Izatt JA. Optical coherence refraction tomography. Nat Photonics. 2019;13(11):794–802.
79. Zhou KC, McNabb RP, Qian R, Degan S, Dhalla A-H, Farsiu S, et al. Computational 3D microscopy with optical coherence refraction tomography. Optica. 2022;9(6):593–601.
80. Zhou KC, Dhalla A-H, McNabb RP, Qian R, Farsiu S, Izatt JA. High-speed multiview imaging approaching 4pi steradians using conicsection mirrors: theoretical and practical considerations. J Opt Soc Am A. 2021;38(12):1810–22.
81. Larin KV, Sampson DD. Optical coherence elastography—OCT at work in tissue biomechanics [Invited]. Biomed Opt Express. 2017;8(2):1172–202.
82. Kennedy BF, Wijesinghe P, Sampson DD. The emergence of optical elastography in biomedicine. Nat Photonics. 2017;11(4):215–21.
83. Liu CH, Nevozhay D, Schill A, Singh M, Das S, Nair A, et al. Nanobomb optical coherence elastography. Opt Lett. 2018;43(9):2006–9.

84. Zvietcovich F, Pongchalee P, Meemon P, Rolland JP, Parker KJ. Reverberant 3D optical coherence elastography maps the elasticity of individual corneal layers. Nat Commun. 2019;10(1):4895.
85. Kennedy KM, Chin L, McLaughlin RA, Latham B, Saunders CM, Sampson DD, et al. Quantitative micro-elastography: imaging of tissue elasticity using compression optical coherence elastography. Sci Rep. 2015;5:15538.
86. Sinha Roy A, Kurian M, Matalia H, Shetty R. Air-puff associated quantification of nonlinear biomechanical properties of the human cornea in vivo. J Mech Behav Biomed Mater. 2015;48:173–82.
87. Wang S, Larin KV, Li J, Vantipalli S, Manapuram RK, Aglyamov S, et al. A focused air-pulse system for optical-coherence-tomography-based measurements of tissue elasticity. Laser Phys Lett. 2013;10(7).
88. Kirby MA, Pelivanov I, Song S, Ambrozinski Ł, Yoon SJ, Gao L, et al. Optical coherence elastography in ophthalmology. J Biomed Opt. 2017;22(12):1–28.
89. Ambroziński Ł, Song S, Yoon SJ, Pelivanov I, Li D, Gao L, et al. Acoustic micro-tapping for non-contact 4D imaging of tissue elasticity. Sci Rep. 2016;6:38967.
90. Auksorius E, Borycki D, Wegrzyn P, Sikorski BL, Lizewski K, Zickiene I, et al. Spatiotemporal optical coherence tomography provides full thickness imaging of the chorioretinal complex. iScience. 2022;25(12):105513.
91. Tomczewski S, Wegrzyn P, Auksorius E, Ciacka P, Borycki D, Lizewski K, et al., editors. Optoretinography with use of spatio-temporal optical coherence tomography STOC-T. European Conferences on Biomedical Optics 2021 (ECBO); 2021 2021/06/20; Munich: Optica Publishing Group.
92. Borycki D, Hamkało M, Nowakowski M, Szkulmowski M, Wojtkowski M. Spatiotemporal optical coherence (STOC) manipulation suppresses coherent cross-talk in full-field swept-source optical coherence tomography. Biomed Opt Express. 2019;10(4):2032–54.
93. Nahen K, Benyamini G, Loewenstein A. Evaluation of a self-imaging SD-OCT system for remote monitoring of patients with neovascular age related macular degeneration. Klin Monbl Augenheilkd. 2020;237(12):1410–8.
94. Kim JE, Tomkins-Netzer O, Elman MJ, Lally DR, Goldstein M, Goldenberg D, et al. Evaluation of a self-imaging SD-OCT system designed for remote home monitoring. BMC Ophthalmol. 2022;22(1):261.
95. Liu Y, Holekamp NM, Heier JS. Prospective, longitudinal study: daily self-imaging with home OCT for neovascular age-related macular degeneration. Ophthalmol Retina. 2022;6(7):575–85.
96. Chakravarthy U, Goldenberg D, Young G, Havilio M, Rafaeli O, Benyamini G, et al. Automated identification of lesion activity in neovascular age-related macular degeneration. Ophthalmology. 2016;123(8):1731–6.

3 The APOSTEL Recommendations

Aykut Aytulun, Andrés Cruz-Herranz, Lisanne Balk,
Alexander U. Brandt, and Philipp Albrecht

Abstract

With continuous development of optical coherence tomography (OCT) devices and analysis software as well as an increasing number of quantitative OCT studies, there is an obvious need for standardized reporting recommendations. The Advised Protocol for OCT Study Terminology and Elements (APOSTEL) recommendations were developed by a panel of experienced OCT researchers

A. Aytulun
Department of Neurology, Medical Faculty, Heinrich Heine University Düsseldorf, Moorenstr. 5, 40225 Düsseldorf, Germany
e-mail: ahmetaykut.aytulun@med.uni-duesseldorf.de

A. Cruz-Herranz
Department of Neurology, University of California, San Francisco, CA 94143, USA
e-mail: Andres.CruzHerranz@ucsf.edu

L. Balk
Departments of Neurology and Ophthalmology, VU University Medical Centre, Amsterdam, The Netherlands
e-mail: l.balk@vumc.nl

A. U. Brandt
NeuroCure Clinical Research Center, Charité-Universitätsmedizin Berlin, Freie Universität Berlin, Humboldt-Universität zu Berlin and Berlin Institute of Health, Berlin, Germany
e-mail: alexander.brandt@charite.de

Department of Neurology, University of California, Irvine, CA, USA

P. Albrecht (✉)
Department of Neurology, University Clinic and Medical Faculty, Heinrich Heine University Düsseldorf, Moorenstr. 5, 40225 Düsseldorf, Germany
e-mail: philipp.albrecht@mariahilf.de; philipp.albrecht@med.uni-duesseldorf.de

Department of Neurology, Maria Hilf Clinic Moenchengladbach, Viersener Str. 450, 41063 Mönchengladbach, Germany

A. Grzybowski and P. Barboni (eds.), *OCT and Imaging in Central Nervous System Diseases*, https://doi.org/10.1007/978-3-031-72156-4_3

in order to harmonize and improve the quality of reporting in quantitative OCT studies. They include a 9-point checklist of relevant aspects for reporting of quantitative OCT studies covering the areas of study protocol, acquisition device, acquisition settings, scanning protocol, fundoscopic imaging, post-acquisition data selection and analysis, recommended nomenclature, and statistical analysis. The recommendations help to improve the completeness of reporting of quantitative OCT studies, increasing the generalizability and interpretability in line with existing standards for reporting research in other biomedical areas.

Keywords

Reporting recommendations • Quantitative OCT studies • Neurodegeneration • Standardization • Quality assurance

As the number of quantitative OCT studies rapidly increases, there is an obvious need for standardization on how these studies should be performed and reported. Important steps for standardization were the development of quality control criteria and of a consensus on the nomenclature of retinal structures accessible to OCT imaging. The OSCAR-IB Consensus Criteria for Retinal OCT Quality Assessment [1] were developed to validate the accuracy and quality of peripapillary ring scans assessing the retinal nerve fiber layer (RNFL) in multiple sclerosis (MS). The majority of these criteria not only apply to imaging of the peripapillary RNFL in MS but can also be used to rate e.g. macular scans or be applied in other conditions associated with quantitative changes of retinal layers (e.g. neurodegenerative disorders). The International Nomenclature for Optical Coherence Tomography (INOCT) Panel has proposed a consensus nomenclature for the classification of retinal and choroidal layers and bands visible on spectral-domain optical coherence tomography (SD-OCT) images of a normal eye [2].

However, despite these recommendations, imprecise reporting of quantitative OCT studies has sometimes led to uncertainty about methodological aspects, such as scan protocols, analysis software, the use of quality control criteria and inclusion or exclusion of patients and/or eyes. This impacts the interpretability and generalizability of these reports. Therefore, a panel of experts from the International MS Visual (IMSVISUAL) consortium convened at two international meetings in 2015 to develop the Advised Protocol for OCT Study Terminology and Elements recommendations ("APOSTEL recommendations"). These recommendations include a checklist of nine items of particular relevance when reporting quantitative OCT studies (Table 3.1).

Table 3.1 9-point APOSTEL checklist (adapted from [3])

Item		Recommendation	
1	Study protocol	(a) Describe how many OCT operating sites and graders were included	☐
		(b) Report the timing of OCT compared to other measurements (same day, delayed)	☐
		(c) Describe the inclusion and exclusion criteria	☐
2	Acquisition device	For all OCT devices used, report data on	
		(a) Manufacturer	☐
		(b) Model	☐
		(c) Version	☐
		(d) Software version	☐
3	Acquisition settings	Clearly describe the settings in which OCT scans were obtained	
		(a) Room light conditions	☐
		(b) Pupils dilated before exam (y/n)	☐
		(c) Number of operators and devices	☐
4	Scanning protocol	Clearly describe the scanning protocol, including	
		(a) Type of scan (circular, volume, star, line, other)	☐
		(b) Location (area of interest, macula, optic nerve head, papillo-macular bundle, other?)	☐
		(c) Scan parameters (with or without eye tracking)	☐
		• *Volume scan: size of scan area (degrees or mm), number of B-scans, alignment of B-scans, number of A-scans per B-scan*	
		• *Radial scan: size of scan area (degrees or mm), number of B-scans, alignment of B-scans, number of A-scans per B-scan*	
		• *Ring scan: diameter, A-scans/B-scan, manual or automatic placement of ring or method of centering, depth resolution*	
		• *Line scan: angle, location, number of A-scans, depth resolution*	
5	Fundoscopic imaging	(a) Report other imaging modalities used in addition to OCT (fundoscopy, CSLO, retinal angiography, autofluorescence imaging, etc.)	☐
		(b) Describe acquisition protocol, including	☐

(continued)

Table 3.1 (continued)

Item		Recommendation	
		1. Excitation wavelength	
		2. Filter sets	
		3. Number of frames averaged (if applicable)	
6	Post-acquisition data selection	Describe image selection process including	
		(a) Quality control criteria (i.e. OSCAR-IB [1] or other criteria)	☐
		(b) Post-acquisition discard (number and criteria)	☐
		(c) Eye selection strategy (if applicable)	☐
7	Post-acquisition analysis	Describe all post-acquisition steps	
		(a) Software used for processing scans and segmentation (may be different from acquisition software)	☐
		(b) Which individual retinal layers were segmented/included	☐
		(c) Method of segmentation (automated, semi-automated or manually)	☐
		(d) How potential bias was addressed in the case of manual segmentation (masking)	☐
		(e) Grid used for data-extraction (size, shape, selected sections)	☐
8	Nomenclature and abbreviations	Define	
		(a) Anatomical structures analyzed	☐
		(b) Units of provided measurements (e.g. volume or thickness)	☐
9	Statistical approach	Describe	
		(a) Statistical models used for the analyses of OCT data	☐
		(b) Whether data was analyzed by eye or by patient	☐

In the following, a short overview of the nine items is provided:

1. Describe the study protocol

The study design should be reported in line with the applicable guidelines STROBE, CONSORT or CARE [3]. Additionally, for OCT studies, authors should define if inclusion and exclusion criteria were applied at the eye or patient level and if/how confounding ocular pathologies, e.g. as listed in the OSCAR-IB criteria [1], were ruled out. Reporting the history of and time span from events of particular relevance for the OCT outcomes at study, i.e. optic neuritis (ON) in neuroinflammatory diseases or first symptoms in Leber's hereditary optic neuropathy, is of major importance.

2. State the acquisition device type, name and version

As OCT technology is continuously evolving, it is important to provide not only the specifications of the devices used (manufacturer, model, interferometric technique) but also the exact version of the software used for the acquisition.

3. Define the acquisition setting

The exact conditions, under which and how OCT measurements were performed, should be reported, including the use of methods to facilitate imaging such as the use of device-specific control for movement artifacts or pupil dilation.

4. Define the OCT scanning protocol

It is essential to report the target structures imaged and the exact acquisition parameters of the full measurement protocol, including a detailed description of all scan types employed in a study.

5. Define fundoscopic imaging

In case additional fundus imaging modalities such as confocal scanning laser ophthalmoscopy (cSLO), retinal angiography and auto-fluorescence imaging are reported, these should be described. Likewise, the acquisition protocol, including the excitation wavelength, filter sets and the number of frames averaged (if applicable), should be indicated.

6. Describe post-acquisition data selection

A crucial point of all studies is the quality of the scans, which can have a major impact on the results and their interpretation. If strategies to select or exclude scans from analyses were applied, these should be described in detail. In order to ensure a high quality of scans and interpretability of the results, the use of quality control criteria is recommended. For example, an extensive set of quality control criteria has been published in the form of the OSCAR-IB criteria [1, 4].

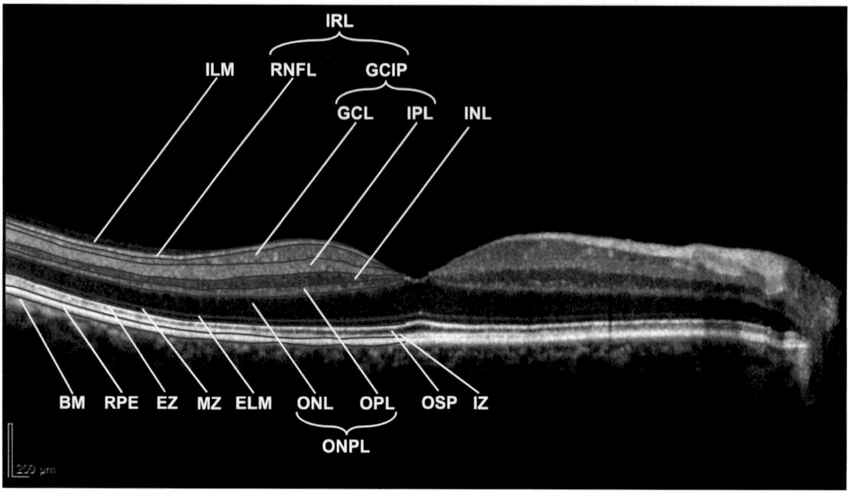

Fig. 3.1 The consensus nomenclature for retinal structures

7. Describe post-acquisition data analysis

Authors should precisely report how the post-processing analysis (e.g. intraretinal layer segmentation) was performed (e.g. fully automated, semi-automated with manual correction of obvious errors or fully manual) [5].

To obtain thickness or volume data from volume scans, differently sized and/or shaped grids can be employed, such as the ring-shaped grid defined for the Early Treatment of Diabetic Retinopathy Study (ETDRS) [6]. Area shape and size of these analysis grids should be reported in addition to the size and location of the source scan (see scanning protocol) [7].

8. Use common nomenclature and abbreviations

All structures analyzed should be precisely defined and described ideally using the recommended nomenclature proposed by the IN-OCT consortium (Fig. 3.1) [2]. If additional (composite) structures are reported, these should clearly be defined.

9. Define the statistical approach with exact model description

Reporting of statistical analyses should adhere to the applicable reporting guidelines [3]. As data for both eyes of each subject are usually available in OCT studies, it is important to describe how the inter-eye within-patient dependencies are accounted for. Strategies to deal with this include either randomly selecting one eye, calculating the mean of both eyes or applying statistical methods accounting for these dependencies, such as general mixed effects models or generalized estimating equation models (GEE). Specific questions may require different strategies [8] and advanced statistical models should be reported in sufficient detail.

3.1 Outlook/Future Development

Shortly after their publication, a letter to the editor by James Cameron has commented on the retinal layer nomenclature proposed by the APOSTEL recommendations. He pointed out that additional structures can be described below the external limiting membrane (ELM), which have been detailed in the International Nomenclature for Optical Coherence Tomography (IN-OCT) consensus paper. Between the inner segment/outer segment junction (ISOS) and the ELM, a myoid zone can be defined; between the ISOS and the outer photoreceptor tips (OPT), an ellipsoid zone; and between the OPT and the retinal pigment epithelium (RPE), an interdigitation zone. These structures are already included in the figure. The APOSTEL recommendations are currently being revised using the formalized consensus finding approach of a Delphi process involving a large public of neurologists and ophthalmologists. The nomenclature proposed by the revised recommendations will be harmonized with the IN-OCT consensus.

The different layers (and their borders) are illustrated in a central vertical scan through the middle of the foveola. Abbreviations of retinal structures and layers: ILM (Inner limiting membrane), RNFL (Retinal nerve fiber layer), GCL (Ganglion cell layer), IPL (Inner plexiform layer), INL (Inner nuclear layer), OPL (Outer plexiform layer), ONL (Outer nuclear layer), ELM (External limiting membrane), MZ (Myoid Zone), EZ (Ellipsoid Zone) (Inner and Outer segment Junction), OSP (Outer segment of photoreceptors), IZ (Interdigitation zone), RPE (Retinal pigment epithelium), BM (Bruch's Membrane). Compound layers are Ganglion cell and inner plexiform layer (GCIP) composite of macular GCL and IPL, Inner retinal layers (IRL) composite of macular RNFL, GCL and IPL, and Outer nuclear and plexiform layer (ONPL) composite of ONL and OPL. (Image courtesy of Philipp Albrecht and Aykut Aytulun).

References

1. Tewarie P, Balk L, Costello F, Green A, Martin R, Schippling S, Petzold A. The OSCAR-IB consensus criteria for retinal OCT quality assessment. PLoS One. 2012;7:e34823. Available at http://www.pubmedcentral.nih.gov/articlerender.fcgi?artid=3334941&tool=pmcentrez&rendertype=abstract. Accessed May 20, 2014.
2. Staurenghi G, Sadda S, Chakravarthy U, Spaide RF. Proposed lexicon for anatomic landmarks in normal posterior segment spectral-domain optical coherence tomography: the IN• OCT consensus. Ophthalmology. 2014;121:1572–8. Available at https://doi.org/10.1016/j.ophtha.2014.02.023.
3. Pandis N, Fedorowicz Z. The international EQUATOR network: enhancing the quality and transparency of health care research. J Appl Oral Sci. 2011;19. Available at http://www.ncbi.nlm.nih.gov/pubmed/21986662. Accessed November 24, 2018.

4. Schippling S, Balk L, Costello F, Albrecht P, Balcer L, Calabresi P, Frederiksen J, Frohman E, Green A, Klistorner A, Outteryck O, Paul F, Plant G, Traber G, Vermersch P, Villoslada P, Wolf S, Petzold A. Quality control for retinal OCT in multiple sclerosis: validation of the OSCAR-IB criteria. Mult Scler. 2014.
5. Oberwahrenbrock T, Traber GL, Lukas S, Gabilondo I, Nolan R, Songster C, Balk L, Petzold A, Paul F, Villoslada P, Brandt AU, Green AJ, Schippling S. Multicenter reliability of semiautomatic retinal layer segmentation using OCT. Neurol Neuroimmunol Neuroinflamm. 2018;5:e449. Available at https://doi.org/10.1212/NXI.0000000000000449.
6. Anon. Photocoagulation for diabetic macular edema. Early treatment diabetic retinopathy study report number 1. Early treatment diabetic retinopathy study research group. Arch Ophthalmol. 1985;103:1796–806.
7. Oberwahrenbrock T, Weinhold M, Mikolajczak J, Zimmermann H, Paul F, Beckers I, Brandt AU. Reliability of intra-retinal layer thickness estimates. PLoS ONE. 2015;10:e0137316.
8. Fan Q, Teo Y-Y, Saw S-M. Application of advanced statistics in ophthalmology. Invest Ophthalmol Vis Sci. 2011;52:6059–65. Available at http://www.ncbi.nlm.nih.gov/pubmed/21807933. Accessed November 5, 2014.
9. Cruz-Herranz A, Balk LJ, Oberwahrenbrock T, Saidha S, Martinez-Lapiscina EH, Lagreze WA, Schuman JS, Villoslada P, Calabresi P, Balcer L, Petzold A, Green AJ, Paul F, Brandt AU, Albrecht P. The APOSTEL recommendations for reporting quantitative optical coherence tomography studies. Neurology. 2016;86.
10. Anon. (n.d.). The EQUATOR network. Enhancing the quality and transparency of health research.

4 OCT Angiography: Guidelines for Analysis and Interpretation

Andrea Servillo, Riccardo Sacconi, Marco Battista, and Giuseppe Querques

Abstract

The recent introduction of optical coherence tomography angiography (OCTA) has remarkably expanded our knowledge of the ocular vascularization. Furthermore, this imaging modality has been widely spread adopted to investigate different ocular and systemic diseases. In this chapter, a review of the salient anatomical features of the ocular vascularization is followed by a discussion of the fundamental principles of OCTA and the application of this imaging modality to study the retinal and choroidal vessels. A proper comprehension of this imaging modality is essential for the interpretation of OCTA imaging applications in neurological and optic nerve disorders.

Keywords

Optical coherence tomography angiography • Retinal vessels • Choroid • Choriocapillaris • Image analysis

4.1 Introduction

Optical coherence tomography angiography (OCTA) is an emerging noninvasive imaging technique that allows for rapidly producing three-dimensional angiographic images of the eye [1, 2]. The basic concept of OCTA is to detect the movement of erythrocytes within vasculature as an intrinsic contrast agent. To obtain this, several repeated OCT B-scans are performed in the same location and

A. Servillo · R. Sacconi · M. Battista · G. Querques (✉)
Department of Ophthalmology, San Raffaele University Hospital, Milan, Italy
e-mail: querques.giuseppe@unisr.it

A. Grzybowski and P. Barboni (eds.), *OCT and Imaging in Central Nervous System Diseases*, https://doi.org/10.1007/978-3-031-72156-4_4

are compared in order to detect differences, or decorrelation, in the blood flow signal. Since repeated B-scans are executed at successively locations, this generates volumetric OCTA data.

OCTA has several potential advantages, including the absence of a dye administration, a fast acquisition time, and the ability to perform depth-resolved analysis of the vasculature. Despite its many advantages, OCTA is not without limitation. Therefore, some issues should be considered during the analysis and interpretation of OCTA images, including lack of information on flow or filling speed, and different artifacts which may affect the images [1].

In this chapter, we will describe the basic principles of OCTA technology, its advantages and limitations in comparison with dye angiographic techniques, and the approaches to analyze the OCTA images, quantifying OCTA variables. This chapter is thus intended to help better guide clinicians on how to interpret OCTA findings.

4.2 Ocular Vascularization

The ophthalmic artery provides the vascular supply to the eye. This artery arises, from the internal carotid artery and divides to constitute the central retinal artery, the short and long posterior ciliary arteries (SPCAs and LPCAs, respectively), and the anterior ciliary arteries [3].

The central retinal artery is contained in the optic nerve and from the optic nerve head to the retinal periphery progressively branches into smaller retinal arterioles. These retinal arterioles supply the inner retina, while the outer retina is supplied by the choroid. The central retinal vein drains the retinal tissue and leaves the eye through the optic nerve. Importantly, histological studies of the human retina have demonstrated that retinal vessels constitute three distinct capillary layers: the superficial (SCP), middle (MCP), and deep capillary (DCP) plexuses [4, 5]. In addition, a fourth vascular layer, the radial peripapillary capillary plexus (RPCP), is mainly located within the superficial nerve fiber layer (NFL) surrounding the optic disc [4, 5]. In the latter vascular plexus, long capillary segments are oriented parallel to the direction of retinal ganglion cell axons. Noteworthy, the retinal capillaries are featured by walls without fenestrations and by tight junctions constituting the inner blood-retinal barrier which is impermeable to even small molecules.

The choroid is supplied by the short and long posterior ciliary arteries. Some branches of the SPCAs also supply the optic disc via an anastomotic ring named the circle of Zinn-Haller. Histological studies have demonstrated that the choroid is constituted of five sublayers: Bruch's membrane, the choriocapillaris (CC), Haller's and Sattler's layers, and the suprachoroidal space [6]. The Haller's and Sattler's layers contain larger diameter vessels which are directly supplied by the SPCAs and LPCAs. Conversely, the choriocapillaris is a highly anastomosed network of capillaries arising from the arterioles in Sattler's layer and is located between Bruch's membrane and the medium-sized choroidal vessels. This vascular layer is organized into a series of hexagonal-shaped lobules, which were demonstrated to be progressively larger toward the periphery [6]. In contrast with the retinal vessels, the CC is unique in that it is fenestrated and this facilitates the movement of even large macromolecules into the extra-capillary compartment [7].

The LPCAs run anteriorly between the sclera and choroid and connect to the anterior ciliary arteries shaping the major arterial circle of the iris [3]. The anterior ciliary arteries reach the sclera near the limbus after travelling with the extraocular muscles [3].

4.3 Optical Coherence Tomography Angiography

4.3.1 Overview on Technical Aspects

Structural OCT can acquire volumetric images of the retina by executing successive single B-scans at different retinal locations. Conversely, OCTA devices perform several repeated B-scans at the same retinal location and the obtained structural information are compared to detect signal changes secondary to flowing erythrocytes (motion contrast). Furthermore, each B-scan is composed of several A scans that are acquired at sequential positions to cover the whole B-scan size. The A-scan rate is dependent on the OCT instrument and is typically comprised between 70,000 A-scans per second (spectral domain devices) and 100,000 A-scans per second (swept source instruments). Of note, faster acquisition speeds may characterize research instruments.

The interscan time, which represents the delay between two B-scan repeated at the same retinal location, has a crucial role. Therefore, while a longer interscan time may increase sensitivity to motion, this also increase the occurrence of parasitic eye motion which can defeat the motion signal [8].

In order to detect the motion contrast, three different methodologies may be used by OCTA devices, as follows: (i) phase based; (ii) amplitude-based; and (iii) complex amplitude-based, in which OCTA algorithm uses both phase and amplitude information. The OCTA signal is typically normalized between 0 and 1. The interscan time and the background noise determine the slowest detectable flow. Erythrocytes must move a sufficient distance within repeated B-scans to be detected. In addition, differences in signal must be higher than the background noise to be detected as flow. This causes an intrinsic limitation to current OCTA technology which may not be able to distinguish the absence of flow from slow flow below a detectable threshold range [8].

Optical coherence tomography angiography may be captured with spectral domain OCT (SD OCT), which in commercial devices employs a wavelength at around 840nm, or with swept-source OCT (SS OCT), which uses a longer wavelength (~ 1050 nm).

4.3.2 Visualization of the OCTA Images

While OCT is considered a cross-sectional imaging modality, OCTA images are mainly displayed with *en face* visualization. The *en face* approach combines the 3-dimensional volumetric information obtained from previously established OCT techniques for the automated segmentation of anatomic reference planes, which allow the definition of "slabs" and the segmentation of the volumetric OCTA scans at specific depths. Using this strategy, the flow data within any slab are summed or projected into a two-dimensional *en face* image that can be viewed and studied.

The creation of the 2-dimensional OCTA *en face* images can be obtained with different methods. The "maximal intensity projection" process projects the maximal intensity pixel from each column onto a flat two-dimensional summary. While the advantage of this strategy is that it detects the smaller vessels, an increased sensitivity to noise may occur. Other processes to obtain the 2-dimensional OCTA images include the "average intensity projection" process, which is less sensitive to noise and small vessels.

Importantly, 2-dimensional images are more susceptible to segmentation artifacts.

Indeed, the creation of 2-dimensional en face images may result in an undervaluation of flow as overlapping vessels segmented in the same space may erroneously be merged [9, 10]. An additional limitation of 2-dimensional images is that retinal vessels crossing different slabs may also be erroneously visualized twice on two different OCTA images [11]. For this reason, cross-sectional OCTA scans may be helpful for studying these eyes. These OCTA B-scans typically show flow in red over the grayscale OCT image.

These limitations have been overcome with 3-dimensional OCTA images, that are independent of data segmentation. The 3-dimensional analysis provided a way to investigate the spatial orientation of vascular alteration with respect to the retinal layers [11]. It could be useful in vascular optic nerve head diseases where 2-dimensional image may not always distinguish the origin of alteration, given the anastomosis between SPCAs and retinal vasculature [12, 13].

4.3.3 Comparison with Previous Dye-Based Imaging Techniques

Fluorescein angiography (FA) and indocyanine green angiography (ICGA) have traditionally been considered the gold standard for clinical assessment of the retinal and choroidal vasculature in vivo. Even though dye administration is generally safe in patients, serious allergic reactions may occur, and these techniques are considered invasive and require considerable patient cooperation. On contrary, OCTA provides non-invasive assessment of the retinal and choroidal vasculatures [15]. Moreover, OCTA has the additional advantage of depth-resolution with improved visualization of the deeper vascular plexuses. Despite these limitations, dye-based imaging provides other advantages including dynamic estimation of dye transit and dye leakage in diseases affecting the blood-retinal barrier (e.g. diabetic retinopathy).

In addition, FA has some limitations in the assessment of the retinal vessels, given that visibility of the capillaries is lower with increasing distance from the fovea and for smaller vessels [16]. Furthermore, FA has significant deficiencies in the visualization of the choroid, given that fluorescein is a small molecule which rapidly leaks from the choroidal vessels. In contrast to FA, ICGA grants an improved visualization of the choroid. ICGA employs an alternative dye that is significantly (99%) bound to plasma lipoproteins thus limiting CC leakage [17]. Furthermore, ICGA uses a longer excitation wavelength and emits fluorescence in the 800–860 nm range, allowing a more efficient penetration through RPE and other ocular pigments [18].

4.3.4 Limitations and Artifacts

Imaging the vascular plexuses with OCTA may also be challenging because of different artifacts which may alter their visualization.

Low signal strength may significantly affect the quality of the OCTA images. The ratio between the signal (signal to noise ratio), which is the information component dependent on the imaged tissue, and the non-signal component (or noise), is a mathematical relationship which may influence the image quality. As an example, media opacities may reduce the signal to noise ratio by decreasing the OCT signal. A decreased signal to noise ratio leads to an adjustment of the grayscale range with a consequent increase in image noise and false OCTA signal. Averaging of multiple *en face* OCTA images may reduce noise, as well as significantly improve qualitative and quantitative measurements [19, 20].

False OCTA signals may be also generated by movement of the eye, head, or body [21]. Recent advancements in eye tracking systems have however significantly decreased the impact of these artifacts in OCTA imaging. Using eye tracking, the retina position is rapidly tracked and corrective movements are applied.

Segmentation error represents a significant and recurring OCTA artifact [14, 21]. As discussed above, *en face* OCTA images are displayed by locating two boundaries throughout the retinal and/or choroidal structure and vessels are therefore visualized using different available processes. These boundaries may be set by selecting pre-defined layers which can be differentiated on the basis of reflectivity, texture, or other attributes. The main problem with this strategy is that these parameters used to differentiate retinal and choroidal layers may be significantly modified in pathological conditions [14]. As an example, the automatic segmentation of vascular layers may be challenging in eyes with myopia, even in the absence of chorioretinal complications. Of note, many OCTA devices employ software enabling manual correction of segmentation errors and propagation of corrections throughout multiple B-scans, but this process may result extremely time-consuming.

Projection artifacts, also known as decorrelation tails, may affect the visualization of the deeper vascular layers (ICP, DCP, and CC). In order to image the deeper structures, the OCT beam passes through the retinal layers, and vessels included in these layers may be falsely detected in the deeper layers, even in the absence of real flow in these slabs. Since the transmitted light diffuses through flowing blood, the deeper layers are thus reached by fluctuating light which can create a decorrelation between two successive B-scans at the same location. The projection artifact may also occur at high reflective layers, such as the RPE. In addition, projection artifacts from the retina are attenuated by the RPE, thereby limiting this confounding problem in the choroid. Several strategies have been evolved to limit projection artifacts [22, 23]. One of the easiest strategists is to subtract the SCP OCTA *en face* image from the deeper layers. Using this strategy, the bright projections from the superficial retinal vessels are replaced with dark versions of the vessels. However, unintentional removal of real blood flow from the resultant images can represent a relevant limit of this strategy.

Shadowing artifact represents another important artifact in the visualization of the deeper vascular layers. This artifact occurs when OCT beam is attenuated or blocked thereby impeding its passage to the deeper layers of the retina/choroid. This may occur due to the presence of different structures, including vitreous opacities, hemorrhage, drusen. SS-OCTA systems have partially overcome this limitation, since a longer wavelength limits attenuation from media opacities and improves penetration into the deeper retinal and choroidal layers. However, this light is known to be more scattered by water absorption in the vitreous [24–26].

OCTA is still limited in the visualization of the larger vessels of the choroid. This limitation is secondary to the signal attenuation due to scattering by the RPE and by the CC vessels [2]. In consequence of this, choroidal vessels may be typically displayed as silhouettes with complete loss of signal at greater depths [27, 28].

4.3.5 OCTA Quantitative Metrics

Various commercial devices use different algorithms to obtain OCTA images and quantifiable metrics applied to these images were demonstrated to be not comparable between devices [29]. However, different studies have used quantitative variables to quantify the retinal and choroidal vasculature with OCTA.

OCTA *en face* images are composed of pixels which may be in a grayscale range of possible values from 0 to 255, where typically 0 is taken to be black, and 255 is taken to be white. In order to obtain quantitative analysis, a threshold may be applied to these images. Thresholding is used to create binary images (in which pixels over the applied threshold are displayed as white and pixels falling under the threshold are shown as black) from grayscale images. Moreover, thresholding may be obtained using different methodologies that were demonstrated to significantly influence the final quantification [30]. The binarized OCTA images may be also skeletonized, in order to obtain an image in which vessels are visualized as tracings of 1 pixel in width [31].

Remarkably, Rabiolo et al. demonstrated that the quantification of retinal perfusion is strictly dependent on the OCTA *en face* image's size [32].

Binarized and skeletonized OCTA images may be used to provide different quantitative parameters:

- *Perfusion density* can be calculated as a unitless proportion of the number of pixels over the threshold divided by the total number of pixels in the analyzed area on the binarized image.
- *Vessel length density (VD)* is defined as the total length of the perfused vasculature divided by the total number of pixels in the analyzed area on the skeletonized image.
- *Vessel diameter index*, which represents the average vessel caliber, may be calculated by dividing the total vessel area in the binarized image by the total vessel length in the skeletonized image [33].
- *Fractal dimension*, which is a mathematical parameter that describes the complexity of the biological structure [34].
- Vessel tortuosity (VT), a measure of the degree of vessel distortion [35].
- *Foveal avascular zone (FAZ) size,* the central area containing no blood vessels, surrounded by a continuous network of capillaries [34].

These metrics have been widely employed in recent years to assess retinal vasculature in diabetic retinopathy [34].

Furthermore, quantitative OCTA parameters could also provide very useful information regarding structural and vascular impairment of optic nerve head [12]. In a recent study Pierro et al. analyze OCTA quantitative parameters differences in representative cases of arteritic anterior ischemic optic neuropathy (AAION) and non arteritic ischemic optic neuropathy (NAION) [36]. Particularly VD and VT values for RPCP and SCP were significantly reduced in AAION and NAION in comparison with healthy subjects. On the other hands, VT values were considerably lower in AAION than NAION for SCP, DCP, and RPCP, demonstrating more vascular abnormality in AAION than NAION, which may be justified by more swelling of the optic disc characterizing AAION. Noteworthy, these OCTA metrics show an excellent matching with RNFL and visual field damages, confirmed by correlation analyses [12].

4.3.6 Wide Field Optical Coherence Tomography Angiography

Many OCTA devices have been implemented with the capability to capture WF images of the retinal and choroidal vasculature [11]. The latest ultra-wide field OCTA devices allow to obtain an image of a 24 mm × 20 mm area with a total field of view (FOV) of 120° in a single scan [39]. This employment makes the OCTA a powerful tool to characterize vascular alterations in retinal vasculopathies (e.g. diabetic retinopathy). Furthermore, several studies proved the utility of WF OCTA in uveitis, considering that the onset and progression of these disease often involve the midperiphery and periphery [40, 41].

Implementation of the widest possible FOV in OCTA is also of great importance for optic nerve diseases, such as glaucoma [42]. Wide-field montage OCTA can visualize the expansion of the RPCP network. Recent studies showed that the RPCP density on OCTA correlated well with the RNFL thickness in glaucoma patients [42–44].

A recent study by Kim et al. present study evaluated the diagnostic accuracy of WF OCTA for the detection of glaucomatous defects in high myopic patients, demonstrating the clinical utility of WF OCTA for the diagnosis of open-angle glaucoma in high myopic patients [42].

In addition, Jia and colleagues illustrated an association between perfusion in RPCP vascular network and nerve fiber layer thickness using WF OCTA [45].

The WF OCTA evaluation is still limited by artifacts and by the inability in assessing dynamic information (leakage, staining), as compared with WF FA [1, 46].

4.4 Evaluation of the Vascular Layers with OCTA

4.4.1 The Retinal Vessels

OCTA has significantly improved our knowledge on the organization of the retinal vessels. The retinal vascularization may be separated into the following plexuses: the superficial capillary plexus, the middle capillary plexus, the deep capillary plexus, and the radial peripapillary capillary plexus (Figs. 4.1 and 4.2) [47–50]. The RPCP is unique in that it is mainly located within the superficial nerve fiber layer surrounding the optic disc and is therefore discussed separately.

Since the introduction of OCTA, a number of models have been proposed regarding connections among the retinal vascular plexuses.

The SCP is a dense meshwork of vessels accommodated in the retinal ganglion cell layer (GCL). The small capillaries arise from SCP arterioles and drain into SCP venules. Using OCTA, SCP arterioles were demonstrated to be located more superficially than SCP venules [50]. The SCP capillaries were shown to be arranged in a centripetal pattern in the macula and to converge on the parafoveal capillary ring [49]. In the periphery, the superior and inferior circulations converge in an interleaved comb pattern [49].

The SCP capillaries are connected with the other two layers of vessels at the inner plexiform layer/inner nuclear layer (IPL/INL) border (MCP) and inner nuclear layer/outer plexiform layer (INL/OPL) border (DCP). While the MCP colocalizes with the bipolar cell processes and amacrine cells, the DCP colocalizes with horizontal cells. These two plexuses are thus close to the high oxygen

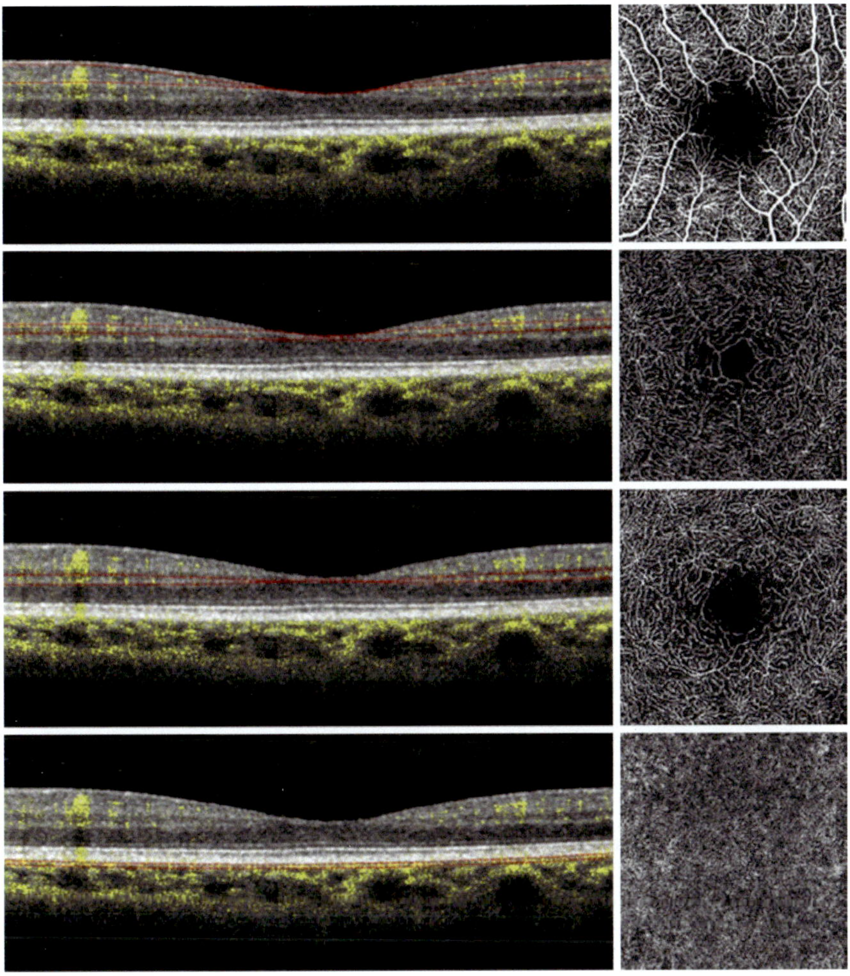

Fig. 4.1 **Optical coherence tomographic angiographic image of the macula of a healthy subject**. The retinal vascularization at the macula includes four different plexuses: the superficial (SCP—top line), middle (MCP—second from top), deep (DCP—third from top) retinal capillary plexuses, and choriocapillaris (CC—bottom). OCTA images are mainly displayed with *en face* visualization (images on the right) which is obtained by segmenting the volumetric OCTA scans at specific depths. Using this strategy, the flow data within any slab, whose boundaries are red in the left images, are summed or projected into a two-dimensional *en face* image that can be viewed and studied. (PLEX Elite 9000; Carl Zeiss Meditec Inc., Dublin, CA, USA)

demand synapses of the IPL and OPL, respectively. The capillaries of the MCP and DCP have a lobular configuration without directional preference within their laminar planes [49]. Because the middle and deep capillary plexuses consist of capillaries of uniform size and are separated by only a small distance, they are often grouped together as the deep vascular complex (DVC).

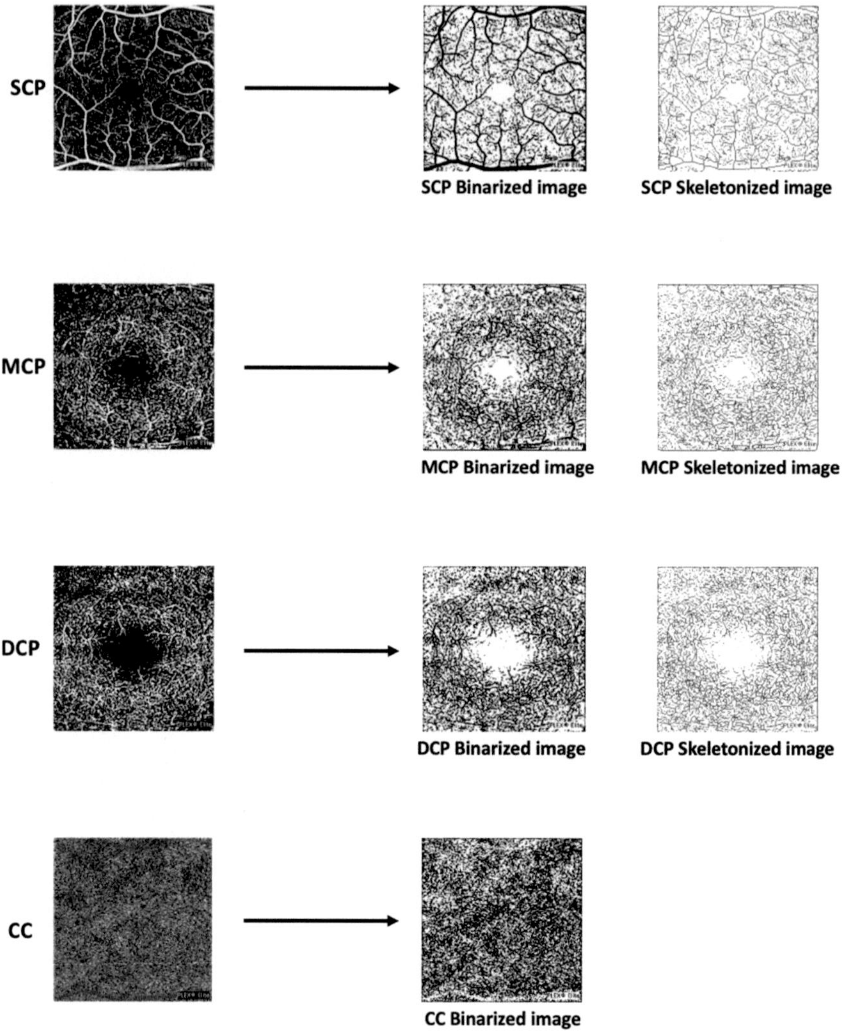

Fig. 4.2 **Main OCTA metrics to quantify the retinal and choroidal vasculature**. The OCTA images can be thresholded to obtain binarized and skeletonized images which are utilized to provide a quantitative analysis. (PLEX Elite 9000; Carl Zeiss Meditec Inc., Dublin, CA, USA)

Around the FAZ, these three retinal capillary plexuses converge to form a single parafoveal capillary loop and collectively define the borders of the FAZ [49].

Recently, using higher axial resolution OCTA technology, Nesper and Fawzi [50] identified distinct vascular connections from large-caliber arterioles and venules in the SCP to each of the three retinal capillary plexuses in healthy subjects. This organization accounts for the high oxygen demand of the plexiform layers that need highly oxygenated (arteriolar) blood in the MCP and DCP. Furthermore, they provided further evidence for the presence of vortices in the DCP, these draining into conduits which are straightly connected to venules in the SCP. Interestingly, collateral vessels crossing the horizontal raphe were identified at the DCP level. These crossing vessels were speculated to represent an alternative pathway of least resistance in the event of occlusive diseases.

In conclusion, these imaging evidences support the theory that each of the three plexuses has its own arteriolar supply and venular drainage, which would theoretically allow each neurovascular unit to have independent control of its vascular supply under physiologic conditions.

Recently, using a full-spectrum probabilistic OCTA with a novel algorithm for 3-D projection artifact removal (PAR), Hirano and colleagues [51] investigated the retinal microcirculation. Since full-spectrum OCTA algorithms improve axial resolution, the authors provided important insights into the 3-D architecture of the retinal vasculature. Remarkably, unlike the MCP and DCP, the location of the SVP significantly varied among retinal regions. In all parafoveal regions tested, the SVP was featured by a small peak at the NFL-GCL junction and a larger, broader peak within the GCL. Conversely, the perifovea had only a single SVP peak. Furthermore, this peak was closer to the ILM in the perifoveal nasal, superior, and inferior quadrants. The authors presumed that this displacement was secondary to the thicker NFL associated with the arcuate and papillo-macular bundles in these regions.

4.4.2 The Radial Peripapillary Capillary Plexus

The nerve fibers in the retina are unmyelinated and they thus require large amounts of energy to maintain ion concentration gradients [52]. The retinal nerve fiber layer contains the radial peripapillary capillary network to supply oxygen and metabolites to the optic nerve axons. The RPCP is composed of long, straight vessels with infrequent anastomoses. These capillaries arise from peripapillary retinal arterioles, extend radially from the optic disc in parallel with the nerve fiber axons, farthest along the temporal arcades [53].

Since OCTA grants a reliable visualization of the capillaries in the optic nerve head and peripapillary regions, OCTA has been extensively used to characterize the RPCP in healthy eyes and to assess microvascular changes occurring in various optic nerve and neurological disorders.

As stated above, Jia and colleagues [45] examined the RPCP flow characteristics in 10 eyes of 10 healthy patients and illustrated an association between perfusion in this vascular network and nerve fiber layer thickness. The perfusion of these regions may thus serve as a surrogate measure for the metabolic activity of the ganglion cell axons.

The analysis of RPCP is of paramount relevance also in patients with optic nerve head edema. The key features of these patients are (1) tortuosity and dilatation of RPCP, that appear similar to "tangled ball or bushy"; (2) potential dropout in very severe edema or chronic stages due to compression or becoming undetectable by the slow flow [12].

RPCP measurements have the potential of providing key functional information in disease processes such as glaucoma and other optic neuropathies.

4.4.3 The Choriocapillaris

Given that previous imaging techniques have significant limitations for the evaluation of the CC, OCTA has been becoming a key technology for investigation of the CC [2, 37, 38].

En face OCTA images of the CC are generated by segmenting a thin slab with a thickness of 10–30-μm starting at Bruch's membrane. In these OCTA CC *en face* images, small dark regions (called flow voids or signal voids) [54, 55] alternate with granular bright areas, the latter thought to represent CC flow, and the former more likely to be secondary to CC vascular dropout or flow reduction [55]. Signal voids seem to represent the inter-capillary spaces which have been characterized in histological studies on the CC [56]. However, this typical single en face CC image with a granular appearance makes it difficult to distinguish the capillary detail. In addition, histological images of the CC are slightly similar to the OCTA versions. Different strategies have been adopted in order to enhance the representation of the choriocapillaris such as the averaging of the multiple *en face* image [57]. The registration and averaging of sequential *en face* OCTA images was shown to transform the poorly defined granular appearance of the CC displayed with OCTA to a morphologic pattern that more closely represented the meshwork pattern observed on histology. Notably, not only did averaging improve CC visualization, but more precise quantitative measures of the CC were obtained.

Another important issue in the analysis of the CC is the correct segmentation due to the variability of the thickness of CC and the possible presence of pathology along the RPE. Thus, Therefore, it is important to cheque all segmentation lines in the cross-sectional image and adjust as required.

4.4.4 The Choroid

Although the OCTA is still limited in the analysis of the choroid, the ultrahigh-speed SS OCTA instrument seems to be partially overcome these limitation [27]. A novel research device with a Fourier-domain mode-locked laser system operating with a 1.7-MHz sweep rate (1.7 million A-scans/s), at a 1065-nm center wavelength, has been used to image the choroid [28]. This instrument was demonstrated to be able to obtain an improved visualization of the medium and larger-sized choroidal vessels. Noteworthy, this device was demonstrated to be even better than ICGA in the visualization of the medium-sized choroidal vessels.

4.5 Conclusions

OCTA is an evolving technology that has significantly enhanced the visualization of the retinal and choroidal vessels. However, major limitations still affect its widespread application. The employment of OCTA to study ocular and systemic diseases, along with advancements of this technology, will certainly expand our knowledge of optic nerve and neurological disorders.

Acknowledgements None.

Funding This paper was not funded.

Declaration of Interest Riccardo Sacconi is consultant for Allergan Inc, Bayer Shering-Pharma, Medivis, Novartis, and Zeiss. Giuseppe Querques is consultant for Alimera Sciences, Allergan Inc, Amgen, Bayer Shering-Pharma, Heidelberg, KBH, LEH Pharma, Lumithera, Novartis, Sandoz, Sifi, Sooft-Fidea, and Zeiss. The authors have no other relevant affiliations or financial involvement with any organization or entity with a financial interest in or financial conflict with the subject matter or materials discussed in the manuscript apart from those disclosed.

References

1. Spaide RF, Fujimoto JG, Waheed NK, Sadda SR, Staurenghi G. Optical coherence tomography angiography. Prog Retin Eye Res. 2018;64:1–55. https://doi.org/10.1016/j.preteyeres.2017.11.003.
2. Borrelli E, Sarraf D, Freund KB, Sadda SR. OCT angiography and evaluation of the choroid and choroidal vascular disorders. Prog Retin Eye Res. 2018. https://doi.org/10.1016/j.preteyeres.2018.07.002.
3. Kiel JW. The ocular circulation. In: Colloquium series on integrated systems physiology: from molecule to function; 2011. https://doi.org/10.4199/C00024ED1V01Y201012ISP012.
4. Tan PEZ, Yu PK, Balaratnasingam C, et al. Quantitative confocal imaging of the retinal microvasculature in the human retina. Invest Ophthalmol Vis Sci. 2012. https://doi.org/10.1167/iovs.12-10017.
5. Chan G, Balaratnasingam C, Yu PK, et al. Quantitative morphometry of perifoveal capillary networks in the human retina. Invest Ophthalmol Vis Sci. 2012. https://doi.org/10.1167/iovs.12-10265.
6. Olver JM. Functional anatomy of the choroidal circulation: Methyl methacrylate casting of human choroid. Eye. 1990;4(2):262–72. https://doi.org/10.1038/eye.1990.38.
7. De Stefano ME, Mugnaini E. Fine structure of the choroidal coat of the avian eye. Vascularization, supporting tissue and innervation. Anat Embryol. 1997;195(5):393–418. https://doi.org/10.1007/s004290050060.
8. Spaide R, Fujimoto JG, Waheed NK, Sadda SR, Staurenghi G. Optical coherence tomography angiography. Prog Retin Eye Res. 2017. https://doi.org/10.1016/j.preteyeres.2017.11.003.
9. Spaide RF, Suzuki M, Yannuzzi LA, Matet A, Behar-Cohen F. Volume-rendered angiographic and structural optical coherence tomography angiography of macular telangiectasia type 2. Retina. 2017;37(3):424–35. https://doi.org/10.1097/IAE.0000000000001344.
10. Borrelli E, Sacconi R, Brambati M, Bandello F, Querques G. In vivo rotational three-dimensional OCTA analysis of microaneurysms in the human diabetic retina. Sci Rep. 2019;9(1). https://doi.org/10.1038/S41598-019-53357-1.

11. Querques G, Borrelli E, Battista M, Sacconi R, Bandello F. Optical coherence tomography angiography in diabetes: focus on microaneurysms. Eye. 2021;35(1):142–8. https://doi.org/10.1038/s41433-020-01173-7.
12. Karrabi N, Hooshmandi S, Amirabadi A, Roshandel D, Hassanpour K, Pakravan M. The role of optical coherence tomography angiography in optic nerve head edema: a narrative review. J Ophthalmol. 2022;2022. https://doi.org/10.1155/2022/5823345.
13. Abri Aghdam K, Ashraf Khorasani M, Soltan Sanjari M, et al. Optical coherence tomography angiography features of optic nerve head drusen and nonarteritic anterior ischemic optic neuropathy. Can J Ophthalmol. 2019;54(4):495–500. https://doi.org/10.1016/J.JCJO.2018.08.002.
14. Ghasemi Falavarjani K, Al-Sheikh M, Akil H, Sadda SR. Image artefacts in swept-source optical coherence tomography angiography. Br J Ophthalmol. 2016. https://doi.org/10.1136/bjophthalmol-2016-309104.
15. Jia Y, Tan O, Tokayer J, et al. Split-spectrum amplitude-decorrelation angiography with optical coherence tomography. Opt Express. 2012;20(4):4710–25.
16. Weinhaus RS, Burke JM, Delori FC, Snodderly DM. Comparison of fluorescein angiography with microvascular anatomy of macaque retinas. Exp Eye Res. 1995. https://doi.org/10.1016/S0014-4835(95)80053-0.
17. Mames RN, Shady-McCoy L, Guy J. Central retinal and posterior ciliary artery occlusion after particle embolization of the external carotid artery system. Ophthalmology. 1991;98(4):527–31. https://doi.org/10.1016/S0161-6420(91)32261-9.
18. Ozawa G. Fundus fluorescein and indocyanine green angiography: a textbook and atlas, vol. 86; 2009. https://doi.org/10.1097/OPX.0b013e3181b31a29.
19. Uji A, Balasubramanian S, Lei J, Baghdasaryan E, Al-Sheikh M, Sadda SR. Impact of multiple en face image averaging on quantitative assessment from optical coherence tomography angiography images. Ophthalmology. 2017. https://doi.org/10.1016/j.ophtha.2017.02.006.
20. Uji A, Balasubramanian S, Lei J, et al. Multiple enface image averaging for enhanced optical coherence tomography angiography imaging. Acta Ophthalmol. 2018. https://doi.org/10.1111/aos.13740.
21. Spaide RF, Fujimoto JG, Waheed NK. Image artifacts in optical coherence tomography angiography. Retina. 2015;35(11):2163–80. https://doi.org/10.1097/IAE.0000000000000765.
22. Long AW, Zhang J, Granick S, Ferguson AL. Machine learning assembly landscapes from particle tracking data. Soft Matter. 2015;11(41):8141–53. https://doi.org/10.1039/C5SM01981H.
23. Zhang M, Hwang TS, Campbell JP, et al. Projection-resolved optical coherence tomographic angiography. Biomed Opt Express. 2016;7(3):816. https://doi.org/10.1364/BOE.7.000816.
24. Povazay B, Bizheva K, Hermann B, et al. Enhanced visualization of choroidal vessels using ultrahigh resolution ophthalmic OCT at 1050 nm. Opt Express. 2003;11(17):1980–6. https://doi.org/10.1364/OE.11.001980.
25. Považay B, Hermann B, Unterhuber A, et al. Three-dimensional optical coherence tomography at 1050 nm versus 800 nm in retinal pathologies: enhanced performance and choroidal penetration in cataract patients. J Biomed Opt. 2007;12(4):041211. https://doi.org/10.1117/1.2773728.
26. Unterhuber A, Povazay B, Hermann B, Sattmann H, Chavez-Pirson A, Drexler W. In vivo retinal optical coherence tomography at 1040 nm—enhanced penetration into the choroid. Opt Express. 2005;13(9):3252. https://doi.org/10.1364/OPEX.13.003252.
27. Choi W, Mohler KJ, Potsaid B, et al. Choriocapillaris and choroidal microvasculature imaging with ultrahigh speed OCT angiography. PLoS ONE. 2013;8(12):e81499. https://doi.org/10.1371/journal.pone.0081499.
28. Poddar R, Migacz J V., Schwartz DM, Werner JS, Gorczynska I. Challenges and advantages in widefield optical coherence tomography angiography imaging of the human retinal and choroidal vasculature at 1.7-MHz A-scan rate. J Biomed Opt. 2017;20(10):1–14. https://doi.org/10.1117/1.JBO.22.10.106018.
29. Corvi F, Pellegrini M, Erba S, Cozzi M, Staurenghi G, Giani A. Reproducibility of vessel density, fractal dimension, and foveal avascular zone using 7 different optical coherence

tomography angiography devices. Am J Ophthalmol. 2018. https://doi.org/10.1016/j.ajo.2017.11.011.
30. Rabiolo A, Gelormini F, Sacconi R, et al. Comparison of methods to quantify macular and peripapillary vessel density in optical coherence tomography angiography. PLoS One. 2018;13(10):e0205773. https://doi.org/10.1371/journal.pone.0205773.
31. Durbin MK, An L, Shemonski ND, et al. Quantification of retinal microvascular density in optical coherence tomographic angiography images in diabetic retinopathy. JAMA Ophthalmol. 2017;135(4):370. https://doi.org/10.1001/jamaophthalmol.2017.0080.
32. Rabiolo A, Gelormini F, Marchese A, et al. Macular perfusion parameters in different angiocube sizes: does the size matter in quantitative optical coherence tomography angiography? Invest Ophthalmol Vis Sci. 2018. https://doi.org/10.1167/iovs.17-22359.
33. Borrelli E, Balasubramanian S, Triolo G, Barboni P, Sadda SR, Sadun AA. Topographic macular microvascular changes and correlation with visual loss in chronic leber hereditary optic neuropathy. Am J Ophthalmol. 2018;192:217–28. https://doi.org/10.1016/j.ajo.2018.05.029.
34. Battista M, Borrelli E, Sacconi R, Bandello F, Querques G. Optical coherence tomography angiography in diabetes: a review. Eur J Ophthalmol. 2020;30(3):411–6. https://doi.org/10.1177/1120672119899901.
35. Yao X, Alam MN, Le D, Toslak D. Minireview quantitative optical coherence tomography angiography: a review. Exp Biol Med. 2020;245:301–12. https://doi.org/10.1177/1535370219899893.
36. Pierro L, Arrigo A, Aragona E, Cavalleri M, Bandello F. Vessel density and vessel tortuosity quantitative analysis of arteritic and non-arteritic anterior ischemic optic neuropathies: an optical coherence tomography angiography study. J Clin Med. 2020;9(4). https://doi.org/10.3390/JCM9041094.
37. Sacconi R, Borrelli E, Corbelli E, et al. Quantitative changes in the ageing choriocapillaris as measured by swept source optical coherence tomography angiography. Br J Ophthalmol. 2018. https://doi.org/10.1136/bjophthalmol-2018-313004.
38. Nassisi M, Baghdasaryan E, Tepelus T, Asanad S, Borrelli E, Sadda SR. Topographic distribution of choriocapillaris flow deficits in healthy eyes. PLoS One. 2018;13(11):e0207638. https://doi.org/10.1371/journal.pone.0207638.
39. Liu X, Chen S, Leng H, et al. New findings on choroidal features in healthy people by ultra-widefield swept-source optical coherence tomography angiography. Sci Rep. 2023;13(1):9215. https://doi.org/10.1038/S41598-023-36374-Z.
40. Pichi F, Salas EC, D De Smet M, Gupta V, Zierhut M, Munk MR. Standardisation of optical coherence tomography angiography nomenclature in uveitis: first survey results. Br J Ophthalmol. 2021;105(7):941–7. https://doi.org/10.1136/BJOPHTHALMOL-2020-316881.
41. Kalra G, Pichi F, Kumar Menia N, et al. Recent advances in wide field and ultrawide field optical coherence tomography angiography in retinochoroidal pathologies. Expert Rev Med Devices. 2021;18(4):375–86. https://doi.org/10.1080/17434440.2021.1902301.
42. Kim YJ, Na KI, Lim HW, Seong M, Lee WJ. Combined wide-field optical coherence tomography angiography density map for high myopic glaucoma detection. Sci Rep. 2021;11(1). https://doi.org/10.1038/S41598-021-01661-0.
43. Mase T, Ishibazawa A, Nagaoka T, Yokota H, Yoshida A. Radial peripapillary capillary network visualized using wide-field montage optical coherence tomography angiography. Invest Ophthalmol Vis Sci. 2016;57(9):504–10. https://doi.org/10.1167/IOVS.15-18877.
44. Jeong Kim Y, Ik Na K, Woong Lim H, Seong M, June Lee W. Combined wide-field optical coherence tomography angiography density map for high myopic glaucoma detection. Scientific Reports. 2021;11:22034. https://doi.org/10.1038/s41598-021-01661-0.
45. Jia Y, Simonett JM, Wang J, et al. Wide-field OCT angiography investigation of the relationship between radial peripapillary capillary plexus density and nerve fiber layer thickness. Invest Ophthalmol Vis Sci. 2017. https://doi.org/10.1167/iovs.17-22593.
46. Servillo A, Sacconi R, Querques G. Fluorescein angiography in the era of octa this tried-and-true imaging modality remains an asset in the retina clinic for several conditions. 34 Retina Today. 2022.

47. Savastano MC, Lumbroso B, Rispoli M. In vivo characterization of retinal vascularization morphology using optical coherence tomography angiography. Retina. 2015. https://doi.org/10.1097/IAE.0000000000000635.
48. Garrity ST, Paques M, Gaudric A, Freund KB, Sarraf D. Considerations in the understanding of venous outflow in the retinal capillary plexus. Retina. 2017. https://doi.org/10.1097/IAE.0000000000001784.
49. Campbell JP, Zhang M, Hwang TS, et al. Detailed vascular anatomy of the human retina by projection-resolved optical coherence tomography angiography. Sci Rep. 2017. https://doi.org/10.1038/srep42201.
50. Nesper PL, Fawzi AA. Human parafoveal capillary vascular anatomy and connectivity revealed by optical coherence tomography angiography. Invest Ophthalmol Vis Sci. 2018. https://doi.org/10.1167/iovs.18-24710.
51. Hirano T, Chanwimol K, Weichsel J, Tepelus T, Sadda S. Distinct retinal capillary plexuses in normal eyes as observed in optical coherence tomography angiography axial profile analysis. Sci Rep. 2018. https://doi.org/10.1038/s41598-018-27536-5.
52. Carelli V, La Morgia C, Sadun AA. Mitochondrial dysfunction in optic neuropathies: animal models and therapeutic options. Curr Opin Neurol. 2013. https://doi.org/10.1097/WCO.0b013e32835c5f0b.
53. Henkind P. Radial peripapillary capillaries of the retina. I. Anatomy: human and comparative. Br J Ophthalmol. 1967. https://doi.org/10.1136/bjo.51.2.115.
54. Choi W, Moult EM, Waheed NK, et al. Ultrahigh-speed, swept-source optical coherence tomography angiography in nonexudative age-related macular degeneration with geographic atrophy. Ophthalmology. 2015;122(12):2532–44. https://doi.org/10.1016/j.ophtha.2015.08.029.
55. Spaide RF. Choriocapillaris signal voids in maternally inherited diabetes and deafness and in pseudoxanthoma elasticum. Retina. 2017:1. https://doi.org/10.1097/IAE.0000000000001497.
56. Seddon JM, McLeod DS, Bhutto IA, et al. Histopathological insights into choroidal vascular loss in clinically documented cases of age-related macular degeneration. JAMA Ophthalmol. 2016. https://doi.org/10.1001/jamaophthalmol.2016.3519.
57. Uji A, Balasubramanian S, Lei J, Baghdasaryan E, Al-Sheikh M, Sadda SR. Choriocapillaris imaging using multiple en face optical coherence tomography angiography image averaging. JAMA Ophthalmol. 2017. https://doi.org/10.1001/jamaophthalmol.2017.3904.

5 Seeing the Brain Through the Eye: What is Next for Neuroimaging and Neurology Applications

Delia Cabrera DeBuc, Gábor Márk Somfai, Irene Newman Jimenez, Gabriella Szatmáry, Carolina CruzVal O'Reilly, Ignacio Anzola De Goiricelaya, Jorge A. Jimenez, Edmund Arthur, Carlos Mendoza-Santiesteban, and Andrzej Grzybowski

Abstract

The changes of the retinal structure and microvasculature are seemingly correlated with neurodegenerative and cerebrovascular lesions, which in turn

D. C. DeBuc (✉) · I. N. Jimenez · C. C. O'Reilly · I. A. De Goiricelaya · J. A. Jimenez · E. Arthur · C. Mendoza-Santiesteban
Bascom Palmer Eye Institute, University of Miami Miller School of Medicine, Miami, FL, USA
e-mail: dcabrera2@med.miami.edu

I. A. De Goiricelaya
e-mail: iaa56@miami.edu

J. A. Jimenez
e-mail: jjimenez@umc.edu

E. Arthur
e-mail: exa647@med.miami.edu

C. Mendoza-Santiesteban
e-mail: cxm1244@med.miami.edu

G. M. Somfai
Department of Ophthalmology City Hospital Waid and Triemli, Zurich, Switzerland

Department of Ophthalmology, Semmelweis University, Budapest, Hungary

G. Szatmáry
Hattiesburg Clinic, Hattiesburg, MS, USA

I. N. Jimenez
University of Mississippi School of Medicine, Jackson, MS, USA

A. Grzybowski
Department of Ophthalmology, University of Warmia and Mazury, Olsztyn, Poland

Institute for Research in Ophthalmology, Foundation for Ophthalmology Development, Poznań, Poland

A. Grzybowski and P. Barboni (eds.), *OCT and Imaging in Central Nervous System Diseases*, https://doi.org/10.1007/978-3-031-72156-4_5

supports the view that the retina may serve as a window to the brain. It can be postulated that retinal microvascular structure could be mirroring that of the brain while the substructure of the retina may be like the structure of the brain. Both features of the central nervous system are difficult and costly to assess, whereas retinal imaging could provide a meaningful and low-cost means to provide surrogate markers for disease detection and disease management that could be valuable assets for the neurologists and general doctors at primary clinical care settings. In the long run, retinal imaging could replace or complement neuroimaging techniques and could contribute to a better understanding of disease etiology of cerebrovascular and neurodegenerative disorders. In this chapter, we will give an overview of Optical Coherence Tomography as an emerging technology in neurology applications and express our view about how retinal imaging could serve the above goals and open a window, which could serve as a direct view to the brain.

Keywords

Eye • Brain • Connectome • Neuroimaging • Optical coherence tomography • Neurology

5.1 Introduction

"*We can only see what we expect to see*", or "*the eyes see what the mind knows*" by Johann Wolfgang von Goethe. These sayings highlight the fundamental challenge that we face in exploring the function of the mind while also confined by the limitations of the mind, through its major sensory input, vision. Increasing evidence suggests that the conditions of retinal morphology and microvascular network are indicators to a variety of cerebrovascular, neurodegenerative, psychiatric, and developmental diseases [1]. Visual function is indeed often affected in subjects with cerebrovascular and neurodegenerative diseases, including ocular motility abnormalities, visual loss, contrast sensitivity changes, and defects in color vision [1].

The changes of the retinal structure and microvasculature are seemingly correlated with neurodegenerative and cerebrovascular lesions, which in turn supports the view that the retina may serve as a window to the brain. It can be postulated that retinal microvascular structure could be mirroring that of the brain while the sub-structure of the retina may be like the structure of the brain. Both features of the central nervous system (CNS) are difficult and costly to assess, whereas retinal imaging could provide a meaningful and low-cost means to provide surrogate markers for disease detection and disease management that could be valuable assets for the neurologists and general doctors at primary clinical care settings. In the long run, retinal imaging could replace or complement neuroimaging techniques and could contribute to a better understanding of disease etiology of cerebrovascular and neurodegenerative disorders.

The area of optical imaging of the retina is progressing rapidly, enabling the noninvasive quantitative and qualitative assessment and follow-up of the retina and its changes. Optical coherence tomography (OCT) is a noninvasive imaging technique routinely used in ophthalmology to visualize and quantify eye structures (e.g., retinal and corneal tissue). Considering the pathophysiological complexity of cere-brovascular and neurodegenerative diseases, the targets for surrogate markers should come from combined diagnostic modalities that could even facilitate the early screening efforts or the prediction of prognosis. Once these ophthalmic bio-markers are combined with the standard clinical toolkit used for the clinical workup of neurological changes in various CNS pathologies, a powerful clinical tool could be developed to reduce the otherwise heavy burden of these diseases.

In this chapter, we will give an overview of OCT as an emerging technology in neurology applications and express our view about how retinal imaging could serve the above goals and open a window, which could serve as a direct view to the brain.

5.2 Eye-Brain Connectome

Investigating the eye-brain connections may unravel the relationship between the connecting pathways of neurons in the brain and eye. This undertaking may help us to determine how vision impairment affects the brain, and facilitate a better explanation about how changes in the brain might influence the outcome of potential therapeutic approaches targeting vision restoration. Connectomics is the science to map out connections, extensively used in brain research to obtain its wiring diagram to better understand patterns in brain connectivity (Fig. 5.1) [2]. Interestingly, determining the circuit diagram of the retina, considering that a little piece of neural tissue such as the photoreceptor segments sense light and sends visual information to the brain, will be valuable to help to decode novel medical treatments yet undiscovered. Therefore, the idea that patients may respond to treatment differently based on how their eye-brain connections are wired and not only on the specific conditions of the eye disease is provocative and deserves attention.

Our understanding of the path the retinal neurons take to the primary visual cortex (V1) and the extrastriate areas has come a long way from early human cadaver and staining studies to a much sophisticated and audacious approach of tracing the path of each specific retinal location in the brain termed the human connectome project [3–6]. The audacious goal of these projects is to find the precise mapping of the retinal neural fibers in the brain that may help us to identify the corresponding brain locations of specific retinal locations with pathology in the eye. This mapping could be useful to investigate whether treatment of a specific retinal disease influences their unique brain locations [3–6]. For example, the connection between the eye and the brain is evident in parts of V1 not developed in amblyopia during the critical period of the infant eye development as certain parts of the retina are not 67 stimulated by light (e.g., in deprivational amblyopia) and hence the corresponding points in the brain are not developed. The question of whether

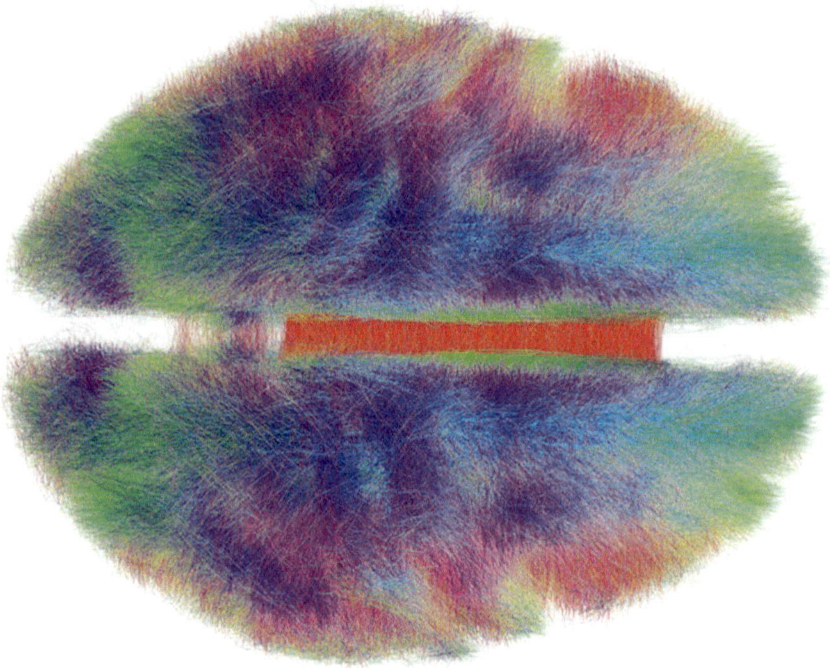

Fig. 5.1 Typical wiring diagram used in connectomics to better understand patterns in the brain connectivity (*image source labeled for reuse*: https://hu.wikipedia.org/wiki/Konnektom)

the visual areas in the brain are rewired and developed during vision therapy or when the cause of amblyopia such as refractive error, strabismus, and cataract is removed has been the focus of many researchers for decades [7]. The more peculiar question in this perspective is whether there is rewiring of the neurons in V1 and the extrastriate areas of the brain beyond the critical period of the infant eye development. The above questions are bolstered by the fact there is evidence in the literature that wearing customized therapeutic eyeglasses in a participant with refractive error reduces the deviations in the electroencephalogram (EEG) and the quantitative EEG recordings towards normative values [8]. Perhaps, this evidence may point researchers in the right direction of how the decline in vision affects the brain and how the changes in the brain may eventually affect the outcome of treatments aimed at restoring vision.

The human connectome project which also revolves around the eye-brain connectome has been the major focus of many researchers [4–6]. The audacious goal is to link every diseased point in the retina to a corresponding point in the brain, and this may be possible using advanced brain imaging modalities such as the Siemens 3T Prism Scanner, which is the most preferred MRI scanner for the human connec-tome project [4]. The idea is that these fine eye-brain connections will help optimize vision restoration treatments such as the Argus II implants for patients with Retinitis Pigmentosa (RP) and to investigate the effect of stem cell treatment for age-related macular degeneration (AMD) [4]. Both RP and AMD have been extensively investigated using OCT technology which may enrich the eye-brain connectome research quest by providing additional information on the retinal neural layers involved in such pathological eye conditions [9–12].

Also, it is well established in the literature that the mapping of the brain neurons (brain connectome) is disrupted in Alzheimer's disease (AD) [13]. Alzheimer's disease is the most common form of dementia and a public health burden as the life expectancy of the aged is increased. Although there are no current drugs to completely treat AD, there are anti-amyloid drugs that can slow the progression of the disease and hence the early detection of the disease is imperative. Classically AD is diagnosed when amyloid plaques and Tau proteins are seen in the brain and the cerebrospinal fluid respectively using expensive and invasive methods such as Positron Emission Tomography (PET) and spinal tap, respectively. The retina of the human eye thus offers a potential window to study AD as it can be imaged with noninvasive imaging modalities and hence aid in the early detection of the disease. Peripheral drusen are observed in the eyes of AD patients and may serve as a potential retinal biomarker for AD (Fig. 5.2) [14–21]. AD is classified by 3 stages including the preclinical, mild cognitive impairment (MCI, prodromal), and the cognitive impairment stages. Much research aimed towards detecting the disease in the MCI and preclinical stages is based on the idea that there is ongoing neurodegeneration occurring in the brain; however, there are no active corresponding symptoms. Perhaps, the human connectome project aimed at mapping the retina and brain will elucidate much better the potential of retinal biomarkers for early detection of AD.

As the human connectome project progresses with the advent of sophisticated brain mapping and imaging techniques, the specific location of each retinal pathology may be traced to a corresponding location in the brain. This project may improve our understanding of the effect of the use of therapeutic glasses on neural activities in the brain and help elucidate whether vision therapy treatment aid in the rewiring of brain neurons not developed during the critical period of the infant eye development. It may also help optimize current and future vision restoration treatments and improve our understanding of whether treatment modalities for eye diseases such asstem cell treatment has any effect on rewiring of the brain neurons in the visualcortex. It may also help improve our understanding of potential retinal biomarkers for the detection of AD and other neurodegenerative diseases such as PD and multiple sclerosis (MS). Perhaps; the next decade holds much excitement for our understanding of the above eye-brain connections as the human connectome project progresses.

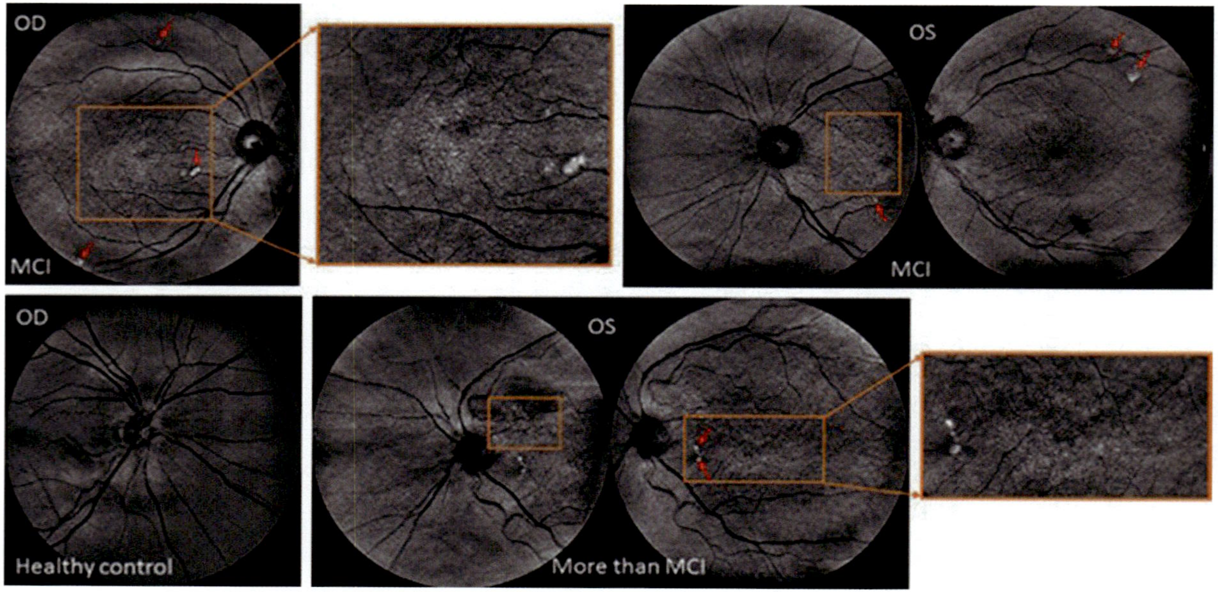

Fig. 5.2 Retinal topographical features observed in individuals with mild cognitive impairment. *Top row*: Central and nasal infrared light-images obtained from a female subject (79 years old) with MCI showing extramacular features such as drusen-like regions depicted by irregularly shaped bright spots in the periphery of the superior quadrant as well as with pigment dispersion in both eyes. *Bottom image*: *Right*—Central and nasal infrared light-images obtained from a female subject (81 years old) with MCI showing tortuous vessels, extramacular features such as drusen- like regions along with pigment dispersion in the left eye. *Left*—Nasal infrared-light image obtained from a healthy control (71 years old). All images were acquired with the EasyScan Unit (i-Optics Corporation, The Netherlands). The EasyScan camera is a dual color confocal SLO: Infrared (785 nm) and pure green (532 nm). The different colors are related to different penetration depth. The red arrows indicate the location of the drusen and white spots observed at extramacular locations. The ROIs enclosed by the orange rectangles indicate the locations where pigment dispersion was observed. The green light-image is reflected at the retinal nerve fiber layer (RNFL) showing the vascular structure up to the 4th bifurcation. The infrared light-image is reaching the choroidal vessel layer (*Image Courtesy of Delia Cabrera DeBuc, Ph.D.*)

5.3 Homology Between the Eye and Brain

The retina and optic nerve extend from the diencephalon during their embryonic development. Thus, both are part of the central nervous system (CNS). The retina contains various neural elements, which are interconnected with each other and play a crucial role in visual processing, beginning already at the retinal level [22]. The final processing stage occurs at the level of the retinal ganglion cells (RGCs), and the axons of many RGCs are collected in a bundle to form the optic nerve. The optic nerve, similarly to all fiber tracts in the CNS, is covered with oligodendrocyte- produced myelin and is being sheathed by all three meningeal layers.

However, it is not only the neural structure that shares similarities with the CNS [23, 24]. Like the CNS, the eye, and the retina has a unique relationship with the immune system that involves specialized barriers, such as the inner blood-retinal barrier, the retinal analog of the blood–brain barrier (BBB) [25]. This analogy is in great part due to the same radial pattern of vascularization during development that is driven in part by the expression of vascular endothelial growth factors (VEGFs) and other growth factors [25–28]. Accordingly, the retinal vasculature shares certain features with the vasculature of the brain because both networks must provide sufficient levels of oxygen and substrates to the large demand of the tissues supplied. It is known that cerebral capillary density mirrors the metabolic demand and activity of the given brain regions [29, 30]. Accordingly, retinal capillary density is greatest in the central, macular area, whereas the peripheral retina is practically avascular (Fig. 5.3). It is important to note that the retinal capillary networks consist of two distinct beds: the superficial capillary layer in the ganglion cell layer (GCL), and the deeper capillary layer at the level of the outer plexiform layer (OPL) (Fig. 5.3) [31]. Interestingly, these capillaries are smaller than cerebral capillaries, with a diameter of approximately 5 μm [32, 33].

It is noteworthy that retinal blood vessels are so-called end arteries and arte rioles having no anastomotic connections, and thus occlusion of these vessels leads to infarction and atrophy of the inner retina [34]. In contrast, cerebral microvasculartture, similarly to most human organs (except the heart), has enough collateral vessels [32]. Also, unlike cerebral arterioles, retinal arterioles often show sharp, 90° branching patterns allowing substantial plasma skimming, i.e. separation of plasma and cellular elements of blood, providing flow-perfusion through the smaller size of capillaries in the retina [32].

As mentioned above, the blood-retina barrier (BRB) is very similar to its cerebral counterpart, protecting the neural tissue of the retina from various large molecules and hematogenous cells. The BRB consists of both mechanical (tight junctional complexes) and metabolic components (metabolic transport acting as a metabolic barrier), similarly to the BBB [35, 36]. Early ultrastructural studies in both brain and retinal vessels showed the presence of caveolae (also called plasmalemma vesicles) and specific membrane enzymes at the abluminal plasma membrane of endothelial cells. These vesicles are static structures, facilitating the transport of small ions and solutes across the BRB and BBB. The number of

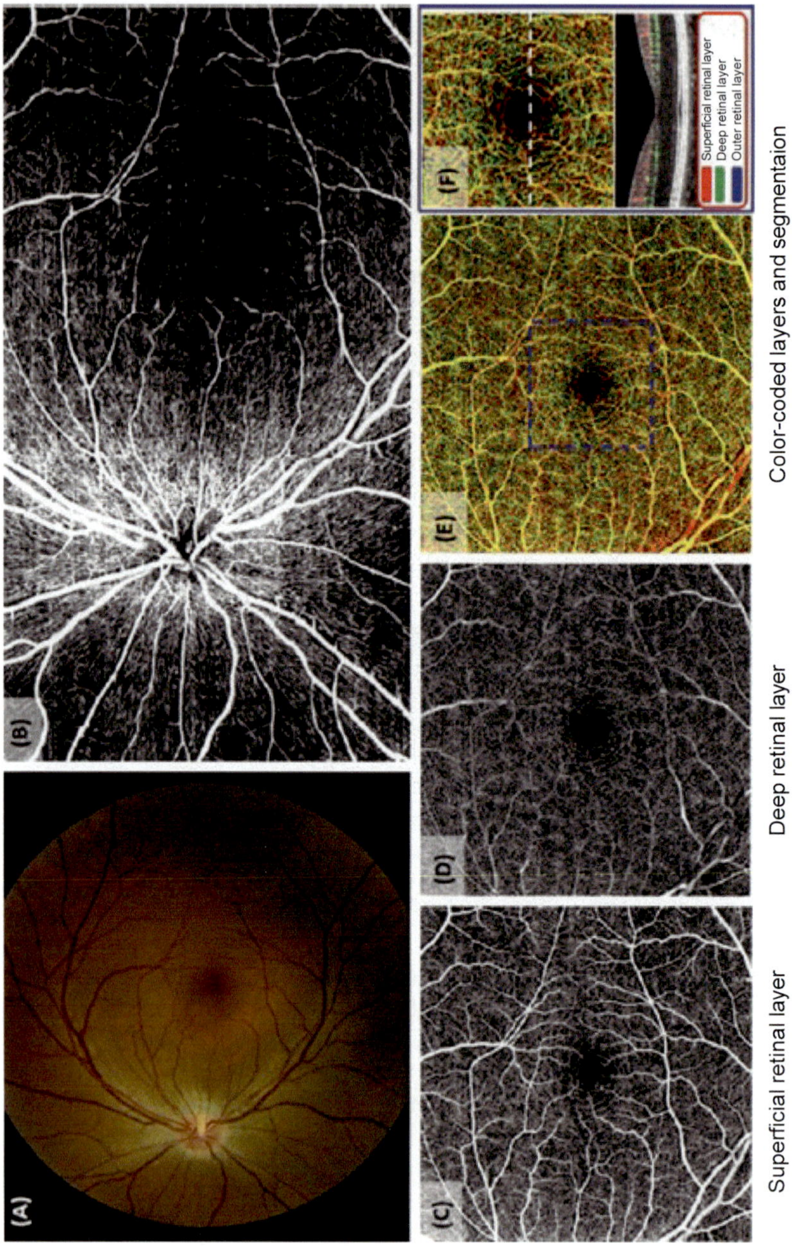
(A)
(B)
(C)
(D)
(E)
(F)
Superficial retinal layer
Deep retinal layer
Outer retinal layer
Superficial retinal layer
Deep retinal layer
Color-coded layers and segmentaion

◀**Fig. 5.3** Details of the retinal microvasculature. (**a**) Fundus photograph of a healthy eye allowing visualization of the entire posterior pole of the ocular fundus, including the optic nerve, the macula, and the major retinal vessels. (**b**) Montage of images of the nerve fiber layer obtained by wide- field optical coherence tomography based microangiography (OMAG) for the same eye. Note the radial pericapillary network within the RNFL. (**c**) The superficial retinal layer slab contains the vascular network within the ganglion cell layer (GCL) and the outer plexiform layer (OPL). Both the arcade vessels and the fine capillaries are shown. (**d**) The deep retinal layer demonstrates deeper capillary network. (**e**) The whole retinal layer slab composed of the superficial retinal layer, the deep retinal layer, and the outer retinal layer allows visualization of the shallow, intermediate, and deep retinal capillary plexuses. Different colors identify various levels of the retina. (**f**) The magnified image of the central macula (identified as in the blue box from (**e**)). The cross-sectional flow image of the area marked with a white dashed line on the magnified OMAG image. Blood flow detected in the superficial retinal layer, the deep retinal layer, and the outer retinal layer (ORL) in red, green, blue; respectively. Note that flow can be detected in the ORL (*Images adapted with permission from Scientific Reports 6, Article number: 22017 (2016)*) vesicles and their polarity are similar in retinal and cerebral microvessels and likely contribute to their barriers, further supporting the idea that the two systems resemble each other [37].

The micro-vessels of the retina contain non-fenestrated endothelial cells and pericytes, both playing an important role in the maintenance of the BRB [31]. Also, the retinal microvasculature includes many perivascular end-feet (also called astrocytic processes) that are actively involved in the regulation of barrier properties and the release of various pericyte-derived factors, which also influence angiogenesis, stabilize micro-vessels and contribute to vasomotor control and neurovascular coupling [31, 38–40].

Finally, because both organs are enclosed in hard capsules, both cerebral and the retinal microcirculation have mechanisms to control vascular resistance in the face of changing systemic blood pressure (and flow) to maintain a relatively constant blood flow called autoregulation [41]. Like the brain, in the eye, the autoregulation is supported by the retinal pericytes and the vascular smooth muscles, in part by the myogenic and perhaps flow sensitive mechanisms [42, 43]. Nevertheless, locally there is still sufficient room for metabolic factors to couple regulation of blood flow to regional neuronal activity—neurovascular coupling [44, 45]. Indeed, the temporal retina that contains the macula has a greater blood flow compared to the nasal retina, reflecting the differences in metabolic activity [46]. It is worth noting that both the retina and the brain are non-homogeneous organs frequently exhibiting similar microvascular pathology suggesting that both bodies undergo similar disease developments.

Although there is no clear evidence regarding a neurogenic control of blood flow in the retina, there are data on the neurogenic control of cerebral blood flow (CBF). Under normal physiological conditions gas, chemical and metabolic vasomotor controls are dominant in the brain; whereas in severely challenging circumstances, such as delayed cerebral ischemia following subarachnoidal hemorrhage, these local mechanisms are suppressed, increasing the relative importance of neurogenic, sympathetic control of CBF [47].

5.4 OCT Challenges in Neuroimaging

The importance and challenges of exploring the function of the brain is highlighted by the concerted efforts of scientists around the world and huge financial investments like the Human Connectome Project and Allen Brain Atlas [48, 49]. It is of utmost importance to be mindful of the major technical and clinical limitations of OCT and to use OCT-based imaging judiciously, correlating it continuously with the clinical findings. Therefore, it is helpful to consider its challenges by comparing it to the most frequently used neuro-imaging modality, MRI. As future technological advances translate from bench to bedside, it is critical to bear in mind the limitations of these tools.

5.4.1 Challenges of OCT as a Neuro-Imaging Tool Using the MRI Simile

Challenges of optical coherence tomography-based imaging can be divided into technical and clinical (Table 5.1). The technical aspect is defined by the laws of physics and this has been reviewed by several excellent publications [50–53].

Therefore, this will only be reviewed briefly here and the emphasis will be placed on the clinical scenarios where expectations from OCT-based imaging are reasonable but still pending.

The first challenge is to become more familiar with the wide spectrum of pre-disease neuro-retinal findings that potentially affect OCT measurements after disease onset, so as not to label a "normal variant" as abnormal. Secondly, to understand the relevance of eye structural and functional findings in both health and disease of the brain. Because understanding the normal spectrum is a prerequisite to disentangle disease states, we must first better define the former to tackle the latter.

Presently, there are several unknown physiological variables that limit understanding cause and effect relationships between retinal measurements and brain states. For example, inability to determine the translaminar gradient across the lamina cribrosa due to the invasiveness of intracranial pressure (ICP) measurements results in uncertainty of its direct and indirect effect on OCT measurements [54]. Recently, promising MRI-based techniques in patients with idiopathic intracranial hypertension (IIH) have been described for indirect measurement of ICP [55, 56]. Additionally, another mechanical factor that likely affects RNFL, and perhaps gan-glion cell complex (GCC: GCL-IPL) thickness, is repetitive traction at the optic nerve head during eye movements, which has been implicated to cause peripapillary temporal choroidal atrophy and possibly normal tension glaucoma [57].

Furthermore, there is lack of information on *anatomical* variables due to great inter-individual variability in the number of retinal ganglion cells, which is estimated to vary between 0.7 to 1.5 million in the human retina [58]. Moreover, there could be structure and function discrepancy in the spectrum of normality, exemplified by the so-called normal neuroanatomical variants or incidentalomas on MRI brain scan, such as pineal cysts or enlarged cisterna magna that are often clinically insignificant [59]. Therefore, in the era of personalized, so-called precision medicine, ophthalmo-anatomical variants must be defined. Although, some findings that were previously considered to be incidental on brain MRI, such as so-called Virchow-Robin or enlarged perivascular spaces, have later been implicated as pathological and possibly indicative of mild cognitive impairment [60]. Therefore, the most important challenge is to determine if a finding is clinically significant (contributory or relevant to the present clinical complaint and examination findings) or incidental. This is exemplified in considering patients who have an empty sella on brain MRI. An empty sella can represent a secondary finding, an epiphenomenon, as in the case of IIH or it can be a normal variant, as in the case of patients with normal ICP [61]. Ultimately, this neuro-imaging finding must

Table 5.1 Challenges of OCT: technical and clinical with risk of misinterpretation

Technical challenges	Comments
Reduced signal strength due to media opacity and operator dependence	Example: dry eyes, cataracts
Truncation due to decentering scan in the z-axis	RNFL thickness can only drop to about 30–40 μm
Effects of refractive error	Need to adjust for ocular magnification
Effects of eye's axial length	• Longer associated with thinner RNFL • Manufacturers normal population database excludes subjects with high refractive error
Effects of cyclotorsion	Shift in the RNFL-TSNIT profile on OCT
Segmentation algorithm failure of RNFL in disease states	• In peripapillary atrophy (e.g., glaucoma)
	• In optic disc edema (e.g., papilledema)
Segmentation algorithm failure of GCC (GCL + IPL)	GCC more prone to segmentation failure than RNFL
Artificial increase in RNFL thickness	In gliosis, myelinated nerve fibers, optic disc edema
Structural abnormalities of the outer retina affect segmentation of the inner retinal layers	Outer retina not routinely segmented
Different algorithms used by different vendors	Data is not comparable between OCT brands, even between same brand but different software
Effects of the scanning distance	Boundary detection errors predominant in the peripheral regions of the macula
Suboptimal repeatability	To improve implement gaze tracker, faster scanning
Clinical challenges	*Comments*
Non-specific findings	• Differential diagnosis of incidental optic neuropathy • Similar findings in neurodegenerative disorders: • AD, MS, NMO, MOG, PD
Non-localizing	ON reflects pathology of the entire retina, thus RNFL is less localizing than GCC
Unable to differentiate antegrade from retrograde degeneration	RNFL and GCC affected by antegrade and retrograde degeneration, even trans-synaptic retrograde degeneration from retro-chiasmal lesion can develop even in few months

(continued)

Table 5.1 (continued)

Technical challenges	Comments
Unable to differentiate congenital versus acquired abnormality	Unable to assess acquired on the top of congenital variant, an example: myelinated nerve fiber layer and papilledema

be interpreted within the clinical context, such as cases of normal opening pressure on lumbar puncture in patients with typical phenotypes and clinical history for the disease and who also have optic nerve head (ONH) swelling on fundus examination. Thus, in this example, the neuro-imaging information adds to the diagnosis of probable IIH (see Chap. 7: OCT and Optic disc edema). Another frequently encountered example of this non-specificity of neuro-imaging on brain MRI is the so-called non-specific white matter disease (WMD) [62]. Often, this finding does not correlate with the patient's symptoms but rather represents a wide differential diagnosis that ranges in severity from the more "severe" demyelinating or microvascular etiologies to the more "benign" etiologies such as migraine. Therefore, having the knowledge of patient specific symptoms and physical examination findings in combination with multi-modal imaging offers the best available option to address the underlying patho-physiology. Analogy between OCT and MRI, particularly in the use of CNS disorders is helpful to address the need for OCT as a neuroimaging tool. For example, perhaps the microvascular rarefaction seen on OCTA in several neurodegenerative disorders is the retinal correlate of brain WMD [63–65].

In determining clinical significance, OCT findings are confounded by intra-individual (inter-eye) structural variability in the number of ganglion cells and their axons that make up the optic nerve and their correlation to the approximately 10, times more brain neurons [66]. In addition, the optic nerve is not only made of gan-glion cell axons but are outnumbered by glial cells, similar to the brain where it is estimated that the ratio of glial cells to neurons is 10 to 1 [48].

5.4.2 Multimodal Imaging Advantage

One way to partially overcome some of these shortcomings of OCT-based imaging is to follow a multimodal approach, with the aim of subtracting complementary information about the clinical problem [67, 68]. However, the imaging-based information will need to be integrated with neuro-ophthalmic history and physical examination findings to decide whether it is relevant to the presenting complaint. While deciphering the eye and brain connections (structure) and visual perception (function), we rely on a growing number of sophisticated imaging technologies such as adaptive optics, computer tomography, fundus imaging (including autofluorescence, infrared reflectance, hyperspectral cameras), MRI, OCT, optogenetics, calcium imaging with the utilization of 3D photon imaging of neuronal and dendritic spine assemblies of the visual cortex, scanning laser ophthalmoscopy, ultrasonography, and/or a combination of these tools [67–78]. These methods rely on the function of our own visual system; therefore, they are subject to its limitations. However, when we combine ophthalmic and neuro-imaging structural with functional tools, such as electrophysiology (electroretinography, pupillometry, visual evoked potentials) [79], functional MRI (fMRI), OCTA, and visual field testing, there is a higher likelihood that the limitations of each of these methods are overcome, or at least decreased. Texture analysis of CT, PET, and MRI images in combination with OCT results can additionally serve to decrease possible limitations that may arise from using one imaging method alone [80]. In OCT, noise-robust texture analysis approaches are most appropriate due to the speckle noise that may occur in these scans [80]. Bernardes et al. demonstrated that texture metrics of OCT imaging showing differences between wild-type control mice and AD groups were found for all neuroretinal layers, with the RNFL layer presenting the most significant metrics [81]. The most significant differences were observed between the groups at two months old, with fewer measures displaying differences at eight months old and onward [81]. This study helps to illustrate the ability of texture metrics in discriminating the retinas of AD mice from the control group based on OCT imaging [81].

Therefore, both the neurology and the ophthalmology community has been using some combination of complementary technologies. A frequent but difficult neuro-ophthalmic complaint is monocular transient visual loss [82], when evaluation of orbital vascular supply is of interest but is a particularly difficult area to assess. The use of OCT and OCTA is limited in this area secondary to its poor penetrance. Ultrasonography has better penetrance but limited field of view. Traditional magnetic resonance angiography (MRA), like 2D-and 3D time-of-flight sequences are limited by suboptimal resolution and the fact that orbital adipose tissue, in which the vasculature is buried, has short T1 and long T2 relaxation times and therefore appears bright (hyperintense) on both T1- and T2 weighted sequences. Moreover, the usually applied fat suppression methods have significant artifacts that make them suboptimal for the assessment of small vessels such as the central retinal and medial and lateral posterior ciliary arteries that supply the retina and optic nerve, as well as having great inter-individual variability (see Sect. 5.3 above).Therefore, to achieve maximal MRA contrast between arteries and fat in retrobulbar space, the ideal way is to completely suppress fat signal while leaving blood signal high. Moreover, high resolution imaging is needed to reduce partial volume effects on small branches of the vessels [83]. MRA, even with the above limitations, complements OCTA in the visualization of the vascular network of the eye, especially with the use of contrast agents that improve vessel signals.

In daily clinical practice, there is also lack of sensitivity of these methods compared to the ideal research environment due to subject-based technical limitations, such as degraded quality due to inability to cooperate resulting in poor fixation and motion-induced artifacts, which is a major issue in patients with neurodegenerative disorders and visual fixation instability due to underlying disease such as optic neuropathy [84].

Also, a major drawback of OCT-based neuroimaging is lack of specificity for not only a particular disorder but even for underlying pathophysiology such as compressive–infiltrative, hereditary, degenerative, inflammatory-infectious, traumatic, and vascular etiologies [85, 86].

Moreover, another defy is associated to normal changes in the anatomy of the retina and optic nerve due to aging, and that the retina might not entirely reveal the extent of neurological damage because of the characteristic diffuse manner in which typically neurodegenerative diseases occur in the CNS.

Other major clinical disadvantages of OCT are that it is likely to miss early changes [87], thereby limiting its role in determining the time course of disease, and that it provides nonlocalizing information (e.g., symptoms and signs suggestive of orbital disease: localizing versus nonlocalizing) [88–90]. Therefore, correlation with other structural and functional studies, such as visual field testing, is needed to localize and determine etiology [91, 92]. When evaluating complex neurodegenerative disorders, it is important to segment the entire retina and not only the neuro- retina, as outer retinal changes have already been described [93]. Also, subtracting additional information from the available datasets, such as shape, texture, and other voxel-based morphometry is necessary due to the limited information thickness provides [94].

5.4.3 OCT Challenges in the Brain

Regarding the cerebral cortex, OCT-based imaging has the capability to visualize cortical neurons and microvasculature, especially of the deeper layers that are presently inaccessible by existing methods such as MRA and fMRI. Cortical neurons are assembled into functional units consisting of horizontal layers and vertical columns, an example of such architecture is the interdigitated column system of the V1 (see Sect. 5.3 above). The superficial cortical layers are supplied by the so-called microvascular lobules [95]. Horton et al. raised the question as to how the so-called cytochrome oxidase (CO) patches that define the metabolic activity of neurons are able to maintain a 49% higher mean firing rate without having a richer microcirculation. The answer is not yet known but it is hypothesized that it is secondary to faster blood flow and/or a higher oxygen extraction ratio compared to other areas. Because of this discrepancy, fMRI findings may not necessarily correlate with increased neuronal activity. Perhaps this question is best addressed in humans through multimodal manners, such as by combining in vivo non-invasive fMRI, 3D-photon microscopy, and even OCT and OCT-angiography (OCTA) [96–98].

A major advantage of OCT and OCTA over MRI is lower cost and therefore easier accessibility, and as such would be an ideal screening tool in neurodegenerative disorders. However, presently, high cost is still a limiting factor to academic research centers in some of the newer methods, such as OCTA (Fig. 5.4).

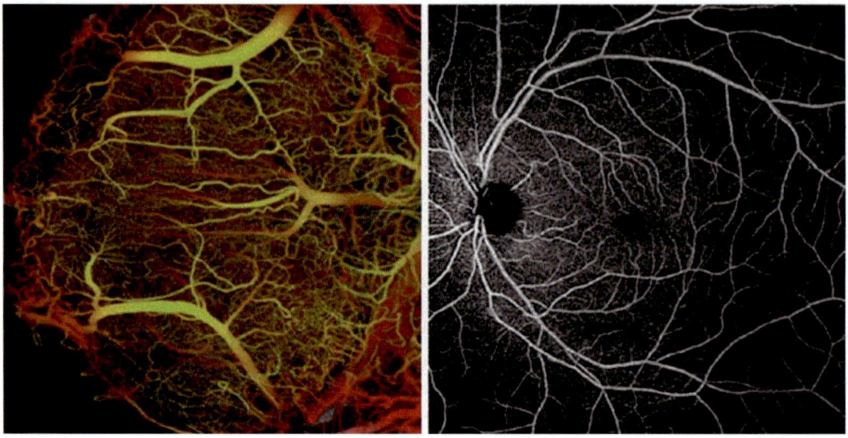

Fig. 5.4 OCT-angiography images. (**Left**) Three-dimensional cerebral vascular map (mouse, *image courtesy of Nishan Mohan, Ph.D., Wasatch Photonics, Inc.*). The depth location of the vessels is color-coded from superficial green to deepest red colors. (**Right**) OCTA image form a glaucomatous' patients (*image courtesy of Luis Vazques, MD*)

5.5 Emerging Applications of OCT in Neurology

Imaging of the eye is increasingly investigated as a potential tool for discovering ocular biomarkers of primarily non-ophthalmic disorders, ranging from neurovascular and neurodegenerative diseases to cardiovascular disease [17]. As reported by the World Health Organization, millions of individuals around the world have various types of neurological disorders, including 326 million who suffer from migraines and 24 million that suffer from AD [99]. These neurological diseases affect vision and originate eye complaints characterized by ocular symptoms that can range from double vision to dry eye to legal blindness. The eye complaints related to neurologic disorders include primary glaucomatous optic nerve disease, ischemic optic neuropathy, and optic neuritis, whereas those related to systemic neurologic diseases such as Alzheimer's and Parkinson's diseases have ocular signs associated to decline of the brain' function. Also, visual problems are often reported in patients after stroke due to the associated neurologic damage. Numerous studies have revealed that many brain diseases like AD could be reflected in retinal alterations, and therefore could also be correlated with structural changes in the retinal neural layers and [17]. For example, it has been hypothesized that if an association can be made between the amyloid in the brain and the amyloid in the eye, then it would be feasible to diagnose AD by looking into the eye. This evidence has progressively accumulated, supporting the hypothesis that the retina may be a window to the brain [1, 17, 18].

Various publications using OCT suggest that several neurologic ailments have pathologic changes in the RNFL of the eye, proposing that the RNFL thickness could be a potential surrogate marker for neurodegeneration [17]. For example,

Fig. 5.5 shows the exponential loss of the RNFL in the affected eye of a subject with acute ON. Also, several studies have reported the atrophy of the RNFL around the optic disc in patients with MS with and even without optic neuritis (ON) in medical history [100–105]. The mean overall circumpapillary RNFL (cpRNFL) thickness and the cpRNFL thickness in each quadrant has been found significantly lower in the eyes of MS patients with a history of ON compared to the non ON-affected eyes and in comparison, with healthy eyes except for the nasal quadrant [106]. However, the cpRNFL thickness is decreased only in the temporal quadrant of the nonaffected eyes of MS patients compared to healthy eyes [106]. A strong correlation with disease severity measured by the EDSS score was also obtained in the case of the GCC thickness which implies that this parameter might also be useful in the estimation of disease progression as a surrogate marker. Similarly, the most pronounced reduction in the thickness of cpRNFL (27% and 17% in the ON-affected and non-affected eyes, respectively) was also observed in the temporal quadrant [106]. These findings agree with previous OCT studies confirming that the fibers of the papillomacular bundle are the most susceptible to damage in ON [103, 107]. One important aspect of this fact, as it has been widely reported in glaucomatous damage, is that the evaluation of the sectoral thickness values could provide the possibility to discriminate the RNFL atrophy caused by glaucomatous damage and other disorders affecting the optic nerve, such as MS [100].

OCT examination additionally provides differentiation between MS and Susac's Syndrome (SS) by comparing RNFL thickness damage [108]. SS is a rare autoimmune vascular occlusive disease where the vascular endothelium is injured by surrounding antibodies, resulting in arterial microinfarcts affecting the central nervous system, inner ear, and retina [109]. Diagnosis for SS includes brain involvement, vestibucochlear involvement, and retinal involvement, i.e., branch retinal artery occlusion (BRAO) or arteriolar wall hyper-fluorescence [109]. Macular OCT scans can be used to assess two important aspects of SS (see Fig. 5.5). First, they can evaluate regions where the RNFL to the outer plexiform layer shows hyper-reflexive thickening indicative of tissue swelling due to acute BRAO [138]. Secondly, this imaging can also identify areas where these layers have thinned, indicating previous ischemic damage [109].

Differentiation between MS and SS is imperative as a treatment for MS may exacerbate SS [110]. This worsening may be due to changes in the immune system under the effect of treatment applied in MS [111]. Diagnostic criteria for MS and SS include visual disturbance, with the specifics of each differing slightly. Patients with SS have visual disturbances as a result of BRAO [111]. However, patients with MS demonstrate ocular manifestations, including pars planitis, peripheral vasculitis, and ocular motility dysfunction manifesting as nystagmus or diplopia [111].

OCT imaging can allow for differentiation between the two, as MS patients present with patchy reductions of peripapillary RNFL and the total macular volume compared with healthy controls [112]. Additionally, MS patients exhibit dispersed RNFL thickness thinning, specifically in the temporal quadrant after optic neuritis [108]. This trend is compatible with the segmental involvement of retinal arterioles

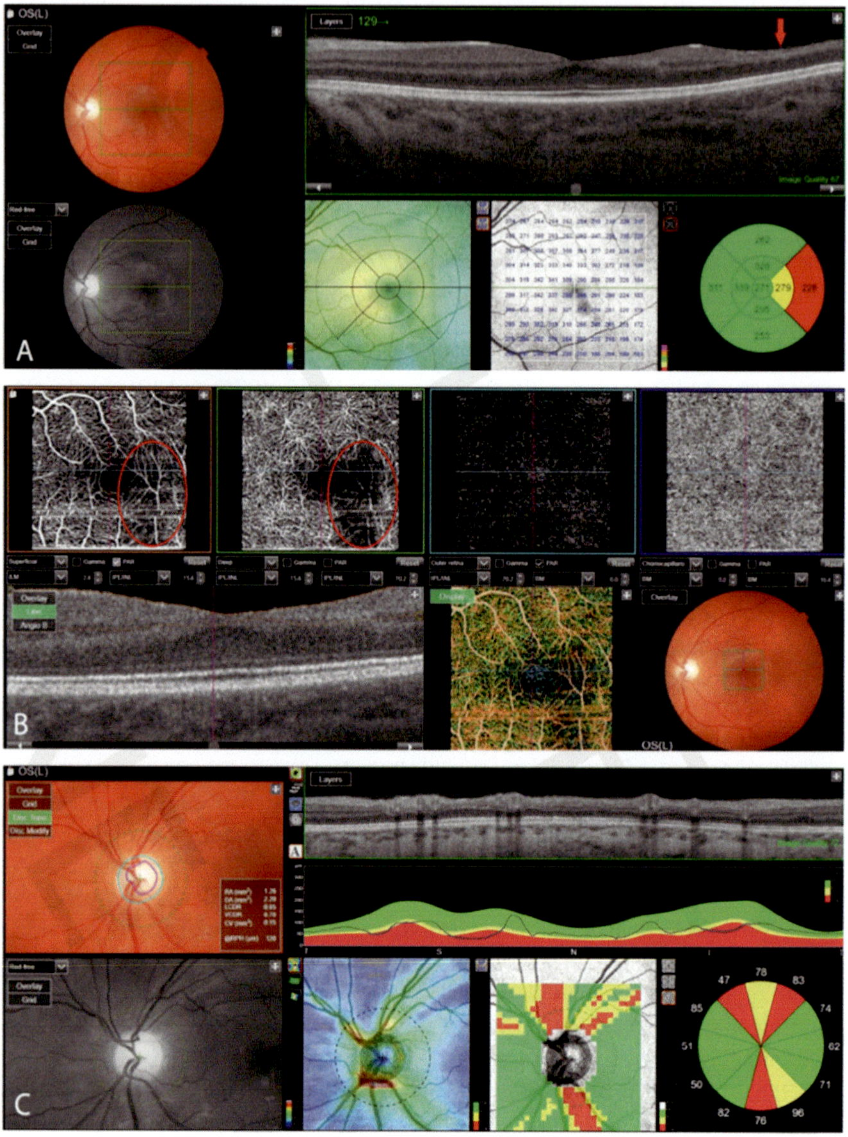

Fig. 5.5 Findings for an SS patient months after initial presentation. (**A**) OCT image of atrophic inner retina thinning (as indicated by the arrow). (**B**) OCTA of severely affected deep retinal plexus (ischemic areas marked by a circle). (**C**) OCT image of sectoral RNFL thickness decrease. [108]

in SS [108]. However, much of the OCT imaging that revealed this differentiation was done months after diagnosis, and therefore the described changes do not apply to the initial stages of these diseases [108]. Still, there retinal layer changes in the prognosis of SS demonstrate the usefulness of OCT imaging for evaluating this disease.

Also, OCT has been very useful in identifying maculopathy that mimics optic neuropathy in the neuro-ophthalmic practice (Fig. 5.6). As a matter of fact, OCT offers evidence of normality in the retinal structure when there may be functional or fictitious loss of vision and may be relied upon when there has been long-standing functional loss of vision [113–118]. Moreover, OCT has been useful in dealing with a range of conditions related with optic disc swelling, including papilledema, pseudo papilledema, and anterior ischemic optic neuropathy (AION). OCT can also be useful in toxic, hereditary and nutritional neuropathy as well as in many cases of optic atrophy, including optic neuritis and optic nerve compression [113–122]. It has been also noted that OCT may not always reflect the overall degree of demyelination occurring in individuals with ON, although OCT can serve as a biomarker for the progression of demyelinating disease [123–126]. This can include neuromyelitis optica spectrum disorder (NMOSD) [127]. NMOSD is a group of autoimmune conditions primarily affecting the optic nerves and spinal cord [127]. In ~ 80% of patients diagnosed with NMOSD, initial clinical manifestation included optic neuritis and a seropositive result for an antibody against the water channel aquaporin-4 (AQP4) [127]. OCT imaging has revealed a thinner RNFL in AQP4 antibody-positive NMOSD patients (AQP4-NMOSD) compared to MS patients [128]. Additionally, when comparing relapse-remitting MS with AQP4-NMOSD, ganglion cell inner-plexiform layer (GCIPL) thickness was lower in AQP4-NMOSD [129]. This differentiation of retinal layer thickening illustrates the usefulness of OCT as a diagnostic tool for NMOSD.

OCT could also aid in diagnosing amyotrophic lateral sclerosis (ALS), though there are generally conflicting findings on the relationship between retinal layer thinning and ALS [130]. ALS is a neurodegenerative disease that provokes motor neuronal death in the primary motor cortex, brainstem, and spinal cord [130]. Though some patients with ALS present with visual disturbance, there is contradictory evidence as to whether pRNFL thickness decreases in ALS and whether this correlates to functional measures [131]. Some studies have found significant pRNFL thinning in patients with ALS compared to controls [131], but others failed to find a significant difference [132]. Other macular OCT parameters, including whole retinal thickness, GCIPL, and mGCL, have been reported as statistically equivalent between patients with ALS and control [133]. While OCT displays the potential to contribute to the evaluation of ALS, further research that yields consistent findings on assessment parameters is essential to ensure the utility of OCT in ALS.

Recent studies of the retina using OCT have also being helpful in revealing atrophy of the peripapillary RNFL and to a lesser extent the macular GCL in patients with multiple system atrophy (MSA) which rarely have visual complaints (Fig. 5.7)

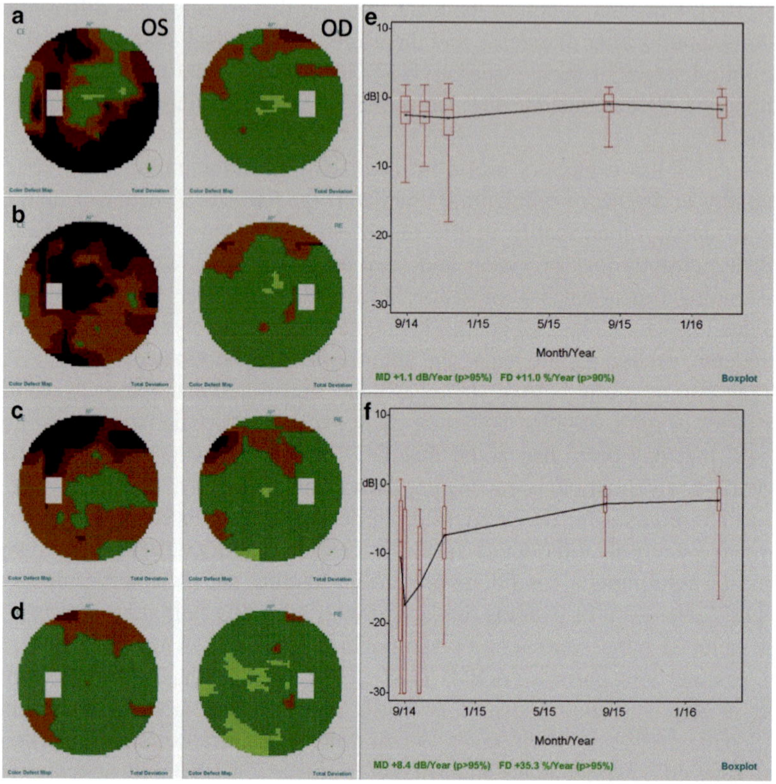

Fig. 5.6 Follow-up of a 38-year-old female patient with acute optic neuritis (ON) in the left eye. The patient presented with mild visual symptoms in the left eye with a VA of 0.6 and a visual field seen on (**a**). The ON that progressed within 2 weeks to a total loss of the visual field with VA 0.1 left (**b**). Three months after presentation her visual acuity and visual field began to improve (**c**, VA 0.8), whereas 1 year after the onset of symptoms her visual field was almost preserved with full visual function (**d**, VA 1.0). Figures (**e**) and (**f**) are showing the changes in the MD (mean defect) value in the right and left eye, respectively. Figures (**g**) and (**h**) are showing the circumpapillary RNFL measurements obtained during follow-up. In the right eye (**g**) the values are unchanged, in the affected left eye (**h**) there is an exponential decrease in the amount of nerve fibers. Please note that the baseline values are similar in both eyes. Figures (**i–k**) are showing images from the 1-year follow-up of the patient. (Please note that for the easier reading of the figure we are showing the two eyes similarly to the visual field data, with the left eye being on the left, unlike the way OCT readings are presented.) In the right eye there is a marked, diffuse reduction of RNFL thickness (**i**), with all sectors being markedly reduced as compared to the right eye but still within normal limits, except for the global thickness values. Figure (**k**) is showing the global and fine structural changes of the inner retina in both eyes. In the right eye there is a marked, diffuse thinning of the macula, reflected in the macular volume; also, the RNFL, the GCL and the IPL layers are similarly diffusely thinner in the affected left eye (see also the layer volume data in red) indicating the neurodegenerative changes in the inner retina. It is of note that despite the observed changes the visual field is showing only minimal changes and the visual function is also full. (The reason for the latter is that visual acuity is routinely assessed by full acuity and not contrast sensitivity tests that would be more sensitive for such changes.) The patient had relapsing–remitting MS for which the findings of relatively mild changes after one ON episode are quite typical (*Image courtesy of Gabor Mark Somfai, M.D., Ph.D.*)

Fig. 5.6 (continued)

g h i j

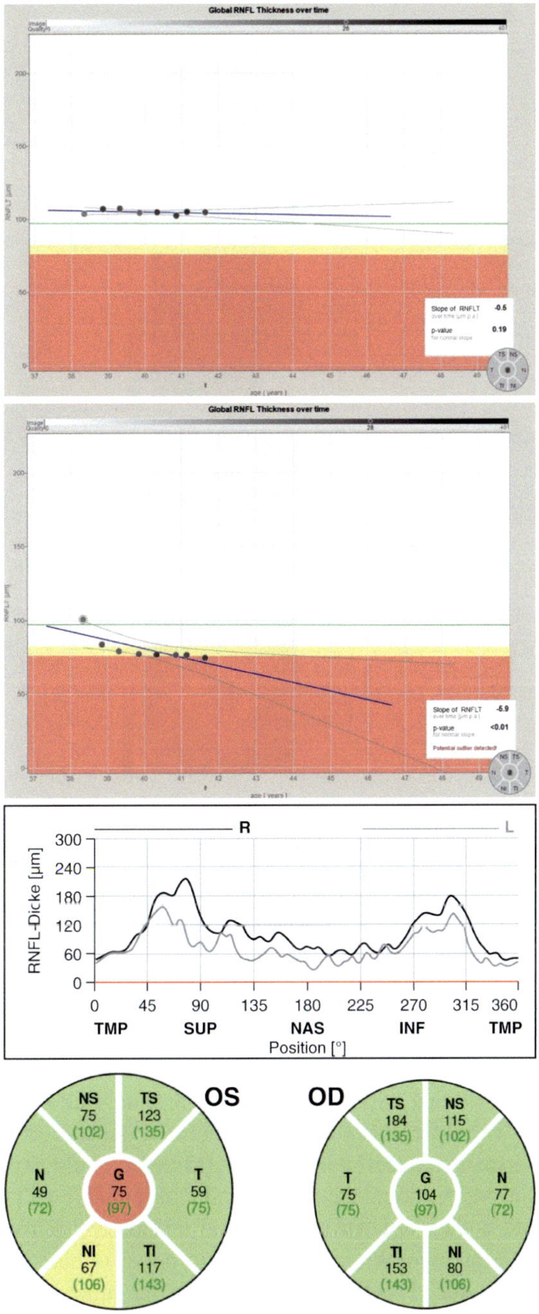

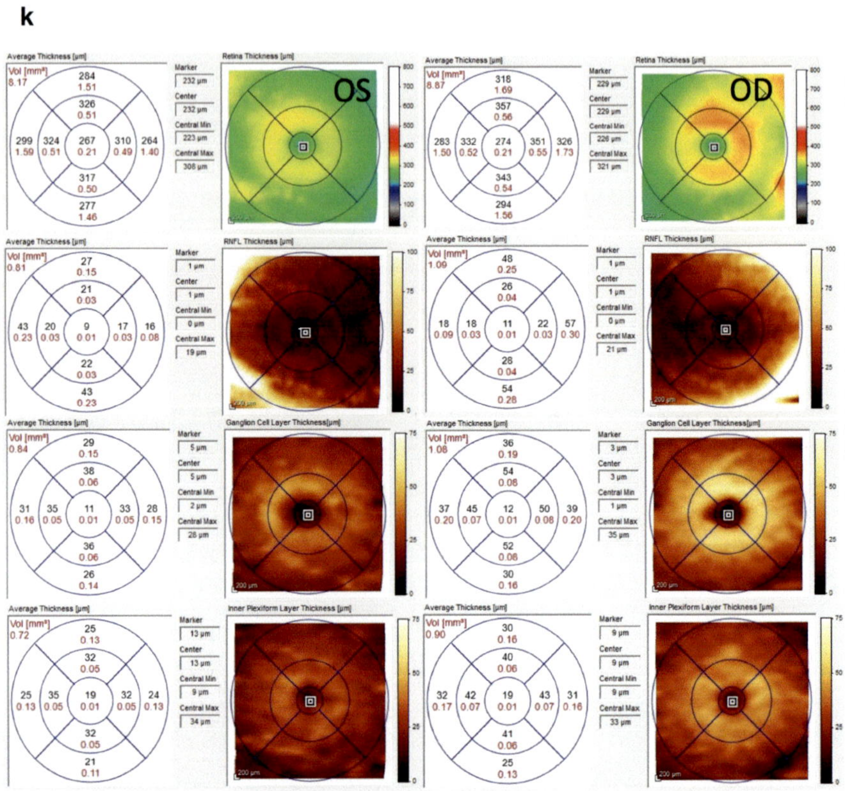

Fig. 5.6 (continued)

[134]. OCT imaging in this rare, adult-onset, rapidly progressive fatal synucleinopathy that primarily affects oligodendroglial cells in the brain, has shown that the retinal damage in patients with MSA appears to follow a different pattern to that observed in those with Parkinson's disease (PD) (Fig. 5.8). Whereas in individuals with PD the atrophy of temporal RNFL sectors and internal retinal layers (i.e., GCC) at the parafoveal region are prominent, in subjects with MSA the inferior, superior and nasal RNFL sectors are more affected than in PD.

The differences in the preferential damage of parvocellular pathway (P-cells) versus magnocellular pathway (M-cells) could explain dissimilarities between PD and MSA patients at the clinical and retinal level [135]. Axons from M-cells (with cell bodies situated in peripheral macula and retina) are in the superior, nasal, and inferior regions around the optic nerve (where the RNFL is measured). On the other side, P-cells predominate in the central macular region (where the macular GCC is measured), their axons project to the temporal portion of the RNFL and they are highly related to color discrimination, visual acuity, central visual field sensitivity, and contrast sensitivity for high spatial frequencies. These M-cells

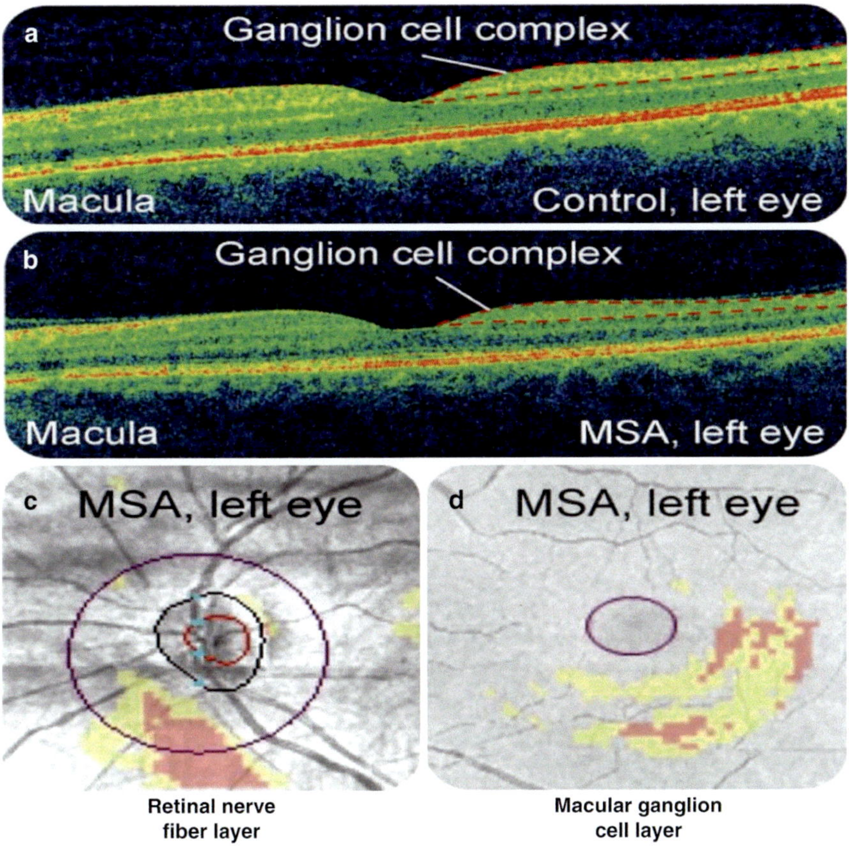

Fig. 5.7 OCT imaging in a control eye and a patient with MSA showing OCT macular sections where the different layers of the retina can be appreciated. The ganglion cell layer (GCL) complex (delimited with a dashed red line) is thinner in a patient with MSA (**b**) compared to an age-matched normal control (**a**). In the same patient with MSA, the thickness of the inferior quadrant of the retinal nerve fiber layer (**c**) and the macular ganglion cell complex layer (**d**), measured by OCT, are substantially reduced (reduced thickness identified in yellow and red) (*Image courtesy of Carlos Mendoza-Santiesteban, M.D.*)

relay information about achromatic vision, motion detection, peripheral visual field sensitivity and contrast sensitivity for low spatial frequencies.

The fact that MSA patients typically have normal visual acuity and color vision in combination with inferior RNFL atrophy may indicate that, in MSA, M-cells are more affected than P-cells. This contrasts with PD patients, who have preferential atrophy of temporal RNFL sectors and higher central macular GCC atrophy (compared to MSA), and is in keeping with their relatively frequent complains of visual problems, such as decreased visual acuity, impaired color discrimination, defective motion perception, and visual hallucinations. The hypothesis of a preferential injury of P-cells in PD and M-cells in MSA is still unproven, but it may

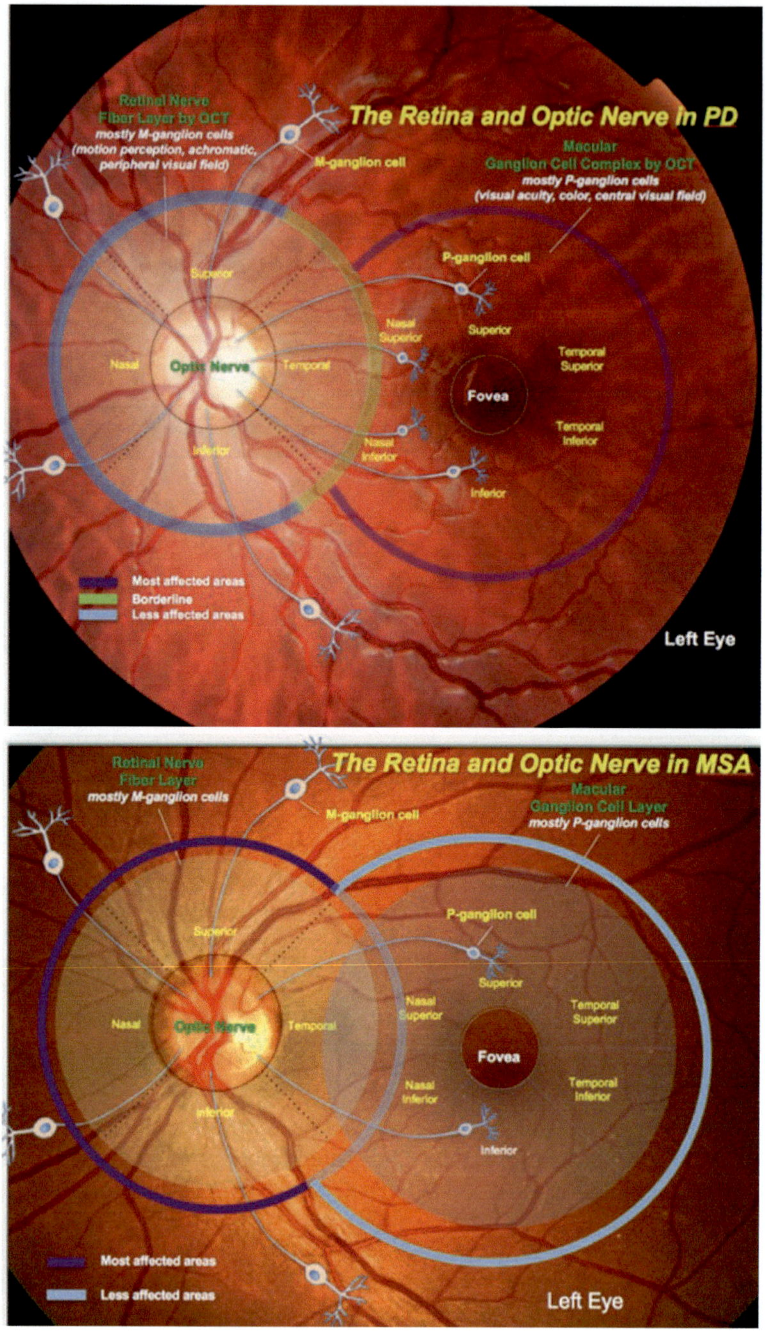

Fig. 5.8 Differences in the preferential damage of parvocellular pathway (P-cells) versus magnocellular pathway (M-cells) in PD and MSA (*Image courtesy of Carlos Mendoza-Santiesteban, M.D.*)

be related to a predominant damage of optic nerve axons in MSA that being especially coarse and myelinated (like those from M-cells) require high support from oligodendrocytes.

In addition, by using OCT to analyze peripapillary RNFL (pRNFL) thickness in the context of mGCC thickness, objective measurements of optic nerve damage can aid in diagnosing idiopathic intracranial hypertension (IIH) [127]. In cases of papilledema caused by IIH, OCT can aid in evaluating these patients, as OCT metrics can identify early optic neuropathy due to IIH [127]. Thinning in the GCL-IPL layer is suggestive of optic neuropathy, which may manifest in chronic, refractory, or fulminant IIH cases [87]. Therefore, the observed GCL-IPL thickness on OCT macular scans can predict outcomes of patients with optic neuropathy alone or a combination of optic neuropathy caused by IIH [87].

OCT can be a valuable tool in determining the timing of a previous stroke, as pRNFL and mGCIPL thinning has been observed approximately one month after pre-geniculate lesions and five months following post-geniculate lesions [127]. In the case of homonymous hemiatrophy, pRNFL and GCIPL analysis combined have a greater sensitivity than either examination alone [136]. Abegg et al. showed that thinning of the GCIPL in 20% of the patients with a pRNFL in the normal range suggests a slightly better sensitivity of GCIPL hemianopia than with pRNFL analysis [136]. Employing OCT examinations for focal retinal layer thinning can assist in identifying previous retinal arterial occlusion and facilitate the assessment of further embolic examinations [127].

OCT additionally enables the detection of longitudinal pattern changes associated with the mitochondrial disorder Leber's hereditary optic neuropathy (LHON). LHON is the most common mitochondrial genetic disease, and this mitochondrial dysfunction results in selective neurodegeneration of RGCs in the papillomacular bundle [127]. Papillary OCT shows pRNFL thickening and subsequent thinning beginning in the temporal quadrant, progressing to inferior and superior sectors, and eventually spreading to the nasal quadrant [137]. Though patients may have different mitochondrial DNA mutations, different degrees of RNFL swelling in terms of quality and duration, and different duration and types of treatment, many consistently follow this pattern [138]. The mGCIPL seems to be affected later, with mGCIPL thickness reduction beginning in the inner ring of nasal sectors, where the RGC bodies that contribute to the papillomacular bundle fibers are contained [139]. These mGCIPL changes, however, do not occur in the phases preceding clinical onset and seem to become significant after the onset of visual loss when a significant reduction of thickness is evident [138]. The pattern of mGCIPL thinning follows a centrifugal and spiral pattern resembling the anatomic distribution of the papillomacular bundle fibers [139]. This mGCIPL thinning after this pRNFL thickening can initially affect the nasal quadrant, which can propagate to other quadrants [127]. Thus, OCT can be a beneficial tool for identifying and monitoring these retinal layer alterations associated with LHON (Fig. 5.9).

The link between retina pathology and a variety of neurodegenerative and cerebrovascular diseases has been established in various OCT studies which are also well detailed in different chapters of this book [17, 140, 141]. Particularly, this

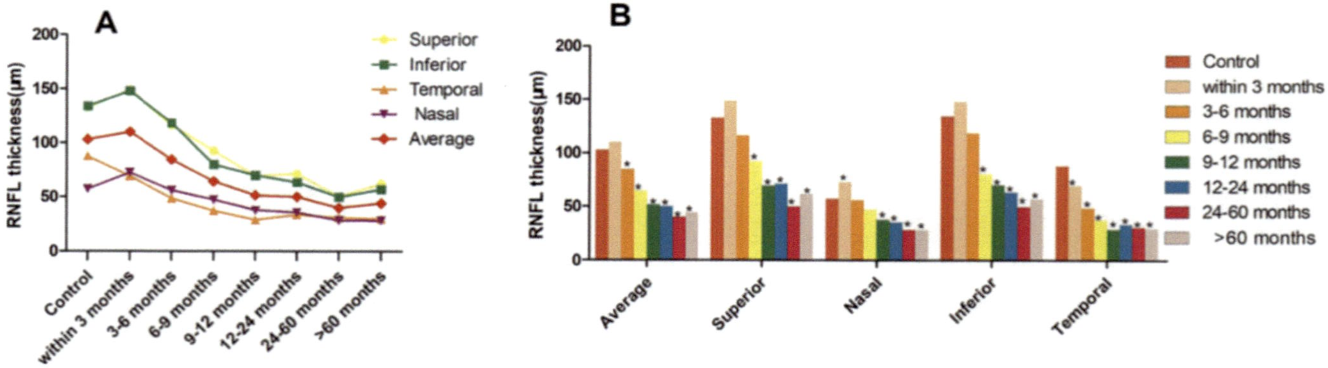

Fig. 5.9 Disease progression in Leber's hereditary optic neuropathy (LHON) patients. A. The figure shows that temporal pRNFL thickness decreased within three months of onset and gradually progressed, while pRNFL in other quadrants thickened and thinned. B. figure demonstrates that compared with the healthy control group, temporal pRNFL thickness decreased within three months of onset with a statistically significant difference. The superior, inferior, nasal, and average pRNFL thickness showed an initial increase, with nasal pRNFL thickness showing a statistically significant difference. With disease progression at 3–6 months, pRNFL thickness of all quadrants decreased; average pRNFL thickness decreased and showed a statistical difference. At 6–9 months, superior and inferior pRNFL thickness decreased and showed a significant difference at 9–12 months. Nasal pRNFL thickness at 9–12 months had decreased and showed significant differences. *$P < 0.05$ when compared with healthy controls [137]

link reinforces the use of retinal microvasculature and neural layers as biomarkers to assess the condition of the cerebral vessels supplying the neurons in the brain. Therefore, examining pathologic alterations of the retinal tissue using OCT technology may be valuable for understanding the etiology of brain disorders.

5.6 Controversies and Challenges in Neurology

A great challenge exists to understanding how changes in the retinal neurovascular unit reflect neurovascular pathology in the brain, which seems to play a critical role to understand cerebral neurovascular pathogenesis. Another challenge is the variations in retinal structural and vascular features between individuals due to aging along with the existing confounding variables that may also result in retinal changes. Also, in the case of AD, it has been reported that amyloid deposition can be identified among cognitively normal elderly persons during life and the prevalence of asymptomatic amyloid deposition may be like that of symptomatic amyloid deposition. An early study has shown that in a group of participants without clinically significant impairment, amyloid deposition was not associated with worse cognitive function, suggesting that an elderly person with a significant amyloid burden can remain cognitively normal [142]. Therefore, OCT algorithms and potential OCT- base biomarkers should carefully consider potential pitfalls related to both con- founding factors and asymptomatic amyloid deposition features.

The use of different OCT instruments or technologies to collect imaging data for neurologic applications is another major limitation affecting the integration and correlation of ocular and brain data [143, 144]. Therefore, improved software analysis considering different OCT imaging technologies and magnification correction factors would allow for better data structure and standardization once an efficient strategy is in place for better comparability between different imaging instruments. The quality assurance of the data and algorithms precision to extract image-based features are additional important factors to consider when using OCT imaging in neurologic applications.

Another imperative consideration is to carefully collect OCT imaging data from healthy subjects without subtle brain abnormalities. In general, it is unknown whether healthy subjects included in normative databases of OCT imaging devices may have focal discrete lesions (i.e. mild signs) in the brain without visible or detectable ocular manifestations. Thus, caution should be exercised when considering normative data from OCT imaging, particularly if considering them for OCT applications of neurologic conditions with complications in the eye. Also, it is important to consider the variance of normal healthy OCT findings because there is anatomical variability between normal healthy eyes of different people as well as differences between the normal healthy findings between the right and left eyes of everyone. This consideration may be useful to better demarcate pathological asymmetry. A valid example of this respect being the OCT recent findings revealing that thinning of the foveal region was more prominent in the eye opposite the side of the body extremely affected by tremor in patients with PD as well as subjects with essential tremor [141].

Additional aspects to be considered in the detection and evaluation of features for OCT imaging in neurology are the differences in phenotyping, the velocity of disease development in patients, the disease duration and impact of age, the subclinical retinal damage, and the practicality of features to be confirmed in independent populations. Also, we note that the OCT biomarkers at the population level may not apply to all individuals and that large-scale studies are frequently needed. Although OCT imaging has expanded our understanding of the pathology of numerous diseases of the retina and optic nerve, differential diagnosis and cellular distinction-based pathology are still needed to determine the role that OCT may play in the diagnosis and monitoring of neurological diseases in the future.

5.7 Advantages in Seeing the Brain Through the Eye

The use of OCT technology as a non-invasive technique to extract important information from the brain in certain neurological conditions has gained much attention recently. Current procedures, such as neuroimaging methods (e.g., MRI and PET) are very high-priced, extremely invasive, lacking in specificity and not readily accessible to most clinicians and affected individuals. The average cost of an MRI exam is about $2175 and a PET scan can cost up to $4000 depending of the scan type needed. Particularly, for a new, state-of-the-art 3 T MRI machine the price can reach $3 million. The room that houses the machine can cost hundreds of thousands more because safety features must be built in to protect the outside personnel from the magnetic field. Add in patient support areas and installation costs, and a suite with just one machine can cost anywhere from $3 million to $5 million. In contrast, OCT imaging is a low-cost and user-friendly approach that can advance research in many brain disorders and eye diseases as well as enhance healthcare even at points of care representing a significant cost reduction when compared to the current standard care in brain diseases. This simplified yet effective technique has the potential to change the way we diagnose certain neurological conditions. But more importantly perhaps, this could possibly be done at the level of geriatric clinics and primary health care facilities, such as day hospitals and community clinics. In this perspective, OCT imaging can possibly provide an affordable and faster option, potentially replacing or complementing the current expensive neuroimaging methods.

5.8 Final Remarks and Future Directions

In summary, OCT has already proven to offer invaluable information in several retinal and optic nerve head disorders that is not available by any other method to date and has improved patient management and outcomes [142]. Also, OCT might facilitate earlier detection of axonal loss than visual field testing or funduscopic examination and could be used to monitor patients with optic neuropathies as well as neurologic disorders affecting the anterior visual pathways. However, OCT-based imaging in the realm of complex brain anatomy, physiology, and pathophysiology, presently offers nonspecific, non-localizing, and sometimes contradictory information emphasizing its limitations by only offering one piece of the puzzle. In the era of precision medicine, future well-designed, prospective, controlled, and longitudinal studies with homogeneous populations are needed in both health and disease to be able to answer patient specific questions while filling out the current gaps of knowledge by utilizing high quality standardized scanning protocols and reporting [142, 143]. The future is bright as pieces of the brain-eye connection puzzle are falling into place through technologies such as OCT-based neuro-imaging and minimally invasive theranostics [143–146]. Keeping in mind though that the usefulness of these tools in clinical practice requires familiarity with detailed anatomy and physiology and pathophysiology of the entire visual system. Moreover, the acquired high quality OCT data to be clinically useful (establish cause and effect relationship, provide prognostic value, follow treatment effect) needs to be scrutinized and correlated with clinical findings [147–148]. Accordingly, it is important to note the following future directions needed to improve the use of the OCT technology as a neuroimaging tool:

- The manufacturer's normative database needs to be routinely corrected for refractive errors, AL, and ophthalmo-anatomical variants
- Individual eye and brain layers should not be looked at in isolation
- To assess the past, present and predict the future of eye and brain states by OCT, longitudinal studies and correlation with histopathology and in vivo multimodal imaging is needed
- Disease process specific and localizing neuro-imaging markers are needed

Ultimately, the continuous improvement and development of novel applications of the OCT technology could allow us to further characterize eye-brain signatures that may facilitate a more comprehensive assessment of the effect of both age- decline and impairment ailments on ocular and cerebral function at the early stage.

References

1. London A, Benhar I, Schwartz M. The retina as a window to the brain-from eye research to CNS disorders. Nat Rev Neurol. 2013;9:44–53. https://doi.org/10.1038/nrneurol.2012.227.
2. Seung S. Tracing the wires of the brain. In: Connectomics. 2018. http://dana.org/Cerebrum/2008/ConnectomicsTracing_the_Wires_of_the_Brain/. Accessed 6 Dec 2018.
3. Schmolesky M. The primary visual cortex. In: The organization of the retina and visual system. 2018. https://webvision.med.utah.edu/book/part-ix-psychophysics-of-vision/the-primary-visual-cortex/. Accessed 6 Dec 2018.
4. USC Eye Institute. USC Eye Institute researchers use Human Connectome Project brain mapping techniques to unlock mysteries that can lead to vision-restoring therapies. 2018.

https://www.prnewswire.com/news-releases/usc-eye-institute-researchers-use-human-connectome-project-brain-mapping-techniques-to-unlock-mysteries-that-can-lead-to-vision-restoring-therapies-300226553.html. Accessed 6 Dec 2018.
5. Chen C, Bickford ME, Hirsch JA. Untangling the web between eye and brain. Cell. 2016;165:20–1. https://doi.org/10.1016/j.cell.2016.03.010.
6. Seung S. Connectome: how the brain's wiring makes us who we are. Boston: HMH; 2012.
7. Joly O, Frankó E. Neuroimaging of amblyopia and binocular vision: a review. Front Integr Neurosci. 2014;8:62. https://doi.org/10.3389/fnint.2014.00062.
8. Zelinsky D, Feinberg C. Quantitative electroencephalograms and neuro-optometry: a case study that explores changes in electrophysiology while wearing therapeutic eyeglasses. Neurophotonics. 2017;4: 011013. https://doi.org/10.1117/1.NPh.4.1.011013.
9. Vámos R, Tátrai E, Németh J, Holder GE, DeBuc DC, Somfai GM. The structure and function of the macula in patients with advanced retinitis pigmentosa. Invest Ophthalmol Vis Sci. 2011;52:8425–32. https://doi.org/10.1167/iovs.11-7780.
10. Liu G, Liu X, Li H, Du Q, Wang F. Optical coherence tomographic analysis of retina in retinitis pigmentosa patients. Ophthalmic Res. 2016;56:111–22. https://doi.org/10.1159/000445063.
11. Bhende M, Shetty S, Parthasarathy MK, Ramya S. Optical coherence tomography: a guide to interpretation of common macular diseases. Indian J Ophthalmol. 2018;66:20–35. https://doi.org/10.4103/ijo.IJO_902_17.
12. Garcia-Layana A, Ciuffo G, Zarranz-Ventura J, Alvarez-Vidal A. Optical coherence tomography in age-related macular degeneration. 2018. http://amdbook.org/content/optical-coherence-tomography-age-related-macular-degeneration. Accessed 10 Dec 2018.
13. Wang J, Zuo X, Dai Z, Xia M, Zhao Z, Zhao X, et al. Disrupted functional brain connectome in individuals at risk for Alzheimer's disease. Biol Psychiatry. 2013;73:472–81. https://doi.org/10.1016/j.biopsych.2012.03.026.
14. Duke Science Review. 2018. http://dukesciencereview.com/content/2-issues/4-issue-4/issue4.pdf. Accessed 6 Dec 2018.
15. Cabrera DeBuc D, Somfai GM, Arthur E, Kostic M, Oropesa S, Mendoza-Santiesteban C. Investigating multimodal diagnostic eye biomarkers of cognitive impairment by measuring vascular and neurogenic changes in the retina. Front Physiol. 2018;9:1721. https://doi.org/10.3389/fphys.2018.01721.
16. Berisha F, Feke GT, Trempe CL, Mcmeel JW, Schepens CL. Retinal abnormalities in early Alzheimer's disease. Invest Ophthalmol Vis Sci. 2007;48:2285–9. https://doi.org/10.1167/iovs.06-1029.
17. Cabrera DeBuc D, Somfai GM, Koller A. Retinal microvascular network alterations: potential biomarkers of cerebrovascular and neural diseases. Am J Physiol Heart Circ Physiol. 2017;312:H201–12. https://doi.org/10.1152/ajpheart.00201.2016.
18. Cheung CY, Ong YT, Ikram MK, Ong SY, Li X, Hilal S, et al. Microvascular network alterations in the retina of patients with Alzheimer's disease. Alzheimers Dement. 2014;10:135–42. https://doi.org/10.1016/j.jalz.2013.06.009.
19. Koronyo Y, Biggs D, Barron E, Boyer DS, Pearlman JA, Au WJ, et al. Retinal amyloid pathology and proof-of-concept imaging trial in Alzheimer's disease. JCI Insight. 2017;2:pii: 93621. https://doi.org/10.1172/jci.insight.93621
20. Koronyo Y, Salumbides BC, Black KL, Koronyo-Hamaoui M. Alzheimer's disease in the retina: imaging retinal abeta plaques for early diagnosis and therapy assessment. Neurodegener Dis. 2012;10:285–93. https://doi.org/10.1159/000335154.
21. Koronyo-Hamaoui M, Koronyo Y, Ljubimov AV, Miller CA, Ko MK, Black KL, et al. Identification of amyloid plaques in retinas from Alzheimer's patients and noninvasive in vivo optical imaging of retinal plaques in a mouse model. NeuroImage. 2011;54:S204–17. https://doi.org/10.1016/j.neuroimage.2010.06.020

22. Patton N, Aslam T, Macgillivray T, Pattie A, Deary IJ, Dhillon B. Retinal vascular image analysis as a potential screening tool for cerebrovascular disease: a rationale based on homology between cerebral and retinal microvasculatures. J Anat. 2005;206:319–48. https://doi.org/10.1111/j.1469-7580.2005.00395.x.
23. Murray CD. The physiological principle of minimum work: I. The vascular system and the cost of blood volume. Proc Natl Acad Sci USA. 1926;12:207–14.
24. Zamboni P, Galeotti R, Menegatti E, Malagoni AM, Tacconi G, Dall'Ara S, et al. Chronic cerebrospinal venous insufficiency in patients with multiple sclerosis. J Neurol Neurosurg Psychiatry. 2009;80:392–9. https://doi.org/10.1136/jnnp.2008.157164
25. Gariano RF, Gardner TW. Retinal angiogenesis in development and disease. Nature. 2005;438:960–6. https://doi.org/10.1038/nature04482.
26. Haigh JJ, Morelli PI, Gerhardt H, Haigh K, Tsien J, Damert A, et al. Cortical and retinal defects caused by dosage-dependent reductions in VEGF-A paracrine signaling. Dev Biol. 2003;262:225–41.
27. Hughes S, Yang H, Chan-Ling T. Vascularization of the human fetal retina: roles of vasculogenesis and angiogenesis. Invest Ophthalmol Vis Sci. 1997;41:1217–28.
28. Risau W. Mechanisms of angiogenesis. Nature. 1997;386:671–4.
29. Gjedde A, Diemer NH. Double-tracer study of the fine regional blood-brain glucose transfer in the rat by computer-assisted autoradiography. J Cereb Blood Flow Metab. 1985;5:282–9. https://doi.org/10.1038/2Fjcbfm.1985.36.
30. Klein B, Kuschinsky W, Schrock H, Vetterlein F. Interdependency of local capillary den- sity, blood flow, and metabolism in rat brains. Am J Phys. 1986;251:H1333–40. https://doi.org/10.1152/ajpheart.1986.251.6.H1333
31. Toussaint D, Kuwabara T, Cogan DG. Retinal vascular patterns. II. Human retinal vessels studied in three dimensions. Arch Ophthalmol. 1961;65:575–81.
32. Cogan DG, Kuwabara T. Comparison of retinal and cerebral vasculature in trypsin digest preparations. Br J Ophthalmol. 1984;68:10–2.
33. Zirkulations TL. Ernahrungsverhaltnisse des Auges. In: Graefe AST, editor. Handbuch der Gesamten Augenheilkunde. Leipzig: Springer-Verlag; 1903.
34. Wong TY, Klein R, Sharrett AR, Couper DJ, Klein BE, Liao DP, et al. Cerebral white matter lesions, retinopathy, and incident clinical stroke. JAMA. 2002;288:67–74.
35. Neuwelt EA. Implications of the blood-brain barrier and its manipulation. New York: Plenum; 1989.
36. Tornquist P, Alm A. Carrier-mediated transport of amino acids through the blood-retinal and the blood-brain barriers. Graefes Arch Clin Exp Ophthalmol. 1986;224:21–5.
37. Sagaties MJ, Raviola G, Schaeffer S, Miller C. The structural basis of the inner blood-retina barrier in the eye of Macaca mulatta. Invest Ophthalmol Vis Sci. 1987;28:2000–14.
38. Zhang Y, Stone J. Role of astrocytes in the control of developing retinal vessels. Invest Ophthalmol Vis Sci. 1997;38:1653–66.
39. Janzer RC. The blood-brain barrier: cellular basis. J Inherit Metab Dis. 1993;16:639–47.
40. Abbott NJ, Revest PA, Romero IA. Astrocyte-endothelial interaction: physiology and pathology. Neuropathol Appl Neurobiol. 1992;18:424–33.
41. Koller A, Toth P. Contribution of flow-dependent vasomotor mechanisms to the autoregulation of cerebral blood flow. J Vasc Res. 2012;49:375–89. https://doi.org/10.1159/000338747.
42. Wallis SJ, Firth J, Dunn WR. Pressure-induced myogenic responses in human isolated cerebral resistance arteries. Stroke. 1996;27:2287–90. Discussion 2291.
43. Yu DY, Su EN, Cringle SJ, Yu PK. Isolated preparations of ocular vasculature and their applications in ophthalmic research. Prog Retin Eye Res. 2003;22:135–69.

44. Leenders KL, Perani D, Lammertsma AA, Heather JD, Buckingham P, Healy MJ, et al. Cerebral blood flow, blood volume and oxygen utilization. Normal values and effect of age. Brain. 1990;113:27–47.
45. Hoge RD, Atkinson J, Gill B, Crelier GR, Marrett S, Pike GB. Linear coupling between cerebral blood flow and oxygen consumption in activated human cortex. Proc Natl Acad Sci USA. 1999;96:9403–8.
46. Rassam SM, Patel V, Chen HC, Kohner EM. Regional retinal blood flow and vascular autoregulation. Eye. 1996;10:331–7.
47. ter Laan M, van Dijk JM, Elting JW, Staal MJ, Absalom AR. Sympathetic regulation of cerebral blood flow in humans: a review. Br J Anaesth. 2013;111:361–7. https://doi.org/10.1093/bja/aet122.
48. Fields RD. Map the other brain. Nature. 2013;501:25–7.
49. Gilbert TL. The Allen brain atlas as a resource for teaching undergraduate neuroscience. J Undergrad Neurosci Educ. 2018;16:A261–7.
50. Chen JJ, Kardon RH. Avoiding clinical misinterpretation and artifacts of optical coherence tomography analysis of the optic nerve, retinal nerve fiber layer, and ganglion cell layer. J Neuroophthalmol. 2016;364:417–38. https://doi.org/10.1097/WNO.0000000000000422.
51. Coric D, Petzold A, Uitdehaag BMJ, Balk LJ. Software updates of OCT segmentation algorithms influence longitudinal assessment of retinal atrophy. J Neurol Sci. 2018;387:16–20. https://doi.org/10.1016/j.jns.2018.01.020.
52. Lang A, Carass A, Al-Louzi O, Bhargava P, Solomon SD, Calabresi PA, et al. Combined registration and motion correction of longitudinal retinal OCT data. Proc SPIE Int Soc Opt Eng. 2016;9784:97840X. https://doi.org/10.1117/12.2217157.
53. Watson GM, Keltner JL, Chin EK. Comparison of retinal nerve fiber layer and central macular thickness measurements among five different optical coherence tomography instruments in patients with multiple sclerosis and optic neuritis. J Neuroophthalmol. 2011;31:110–6. https://doi.org/10.1097/WNO.0b013e3181facbbd.
54. Lee SH, Kim TW, Lee EJ, Girard MJ, Mari JM, Ritch R. Ocular and clinical characteristics associated with the extent of posterior lamina cribrosa curve in normal tension glaucoma. Sci Rep. 2018;8:961. https://doi.org/10.1038/s41598-018-19321-1.
55. Hu R, Holbrook J, Newman NJ, Biousse V, Bruce BB, Qiu D, et al. Cerebrospinal fluid pressure reduction results in dynamic changes in optic nerve angle on magnetic resonance imaging. J Neuroophthalmol. 2018. https://doi.org/10.1097/WNO.0000000000000643.
56. Saindane AM, Qiu D, Oshinski JN, Newman NJ, Biousse V, Bruce BB, et al. Noninvasive assessment of intracranial pressure status in idiopathic intracranial hypertension using displacement encoding with stimulated echoes (DENSE) MRI: a prospective patient study with contemporaneous CSF pressure correlation. Am J Neuroradiol. 2018;392:311–6. https://doi.org/10.3174/ajnr.A5486
57. Suh SY, Le A, Shin A, Park J, Demer JL. Progressive deformation of the optic nerve head and peripapillary structures by graded horizontal duction. Invest Ophthalmol Vis Sci. 2017;58:5015–21. https://doi.org/10.1167/iovs.17-22596.
58. Kolb H, Fernandez E, Nelson R. The Organization of the Retina and Visual System. Salt Lake City: University of Utah Health Sciences Center; 2018. https://webvision.med.utah.edu. Accessed 11 Dec 2018.
59. Ramji S, Touska P, Rich P, MacKinnon AD. Normal neuroanatomical variants that may be misinterpreted as disease entities. Clin Radiol. 2017;72:810–25. https://doi.org/10.1016/j.crad.2017.06.118.
60. Niazi M, Karaman M, Das S, Zhou XJ, Yushkevich P, Cai K. Quantitative MRI of perivascular spaces at 3T for early diagnosis of mild cognitive impairment. Am J Neuroradiol. 2018;39:1622–8. https://doi.org/10.3174/ajnr.A5734.
61. Saindane AM, Bruce BB, Riggeal BD, Newman NJ, Biousse V. Association of MRI findings and visual outcome in idiopathic intracranial hypertension. Am J Roentgenol. 2013;201:412–8. https://doi.org/10.2214/AJR.12.9638.

62. Habes M, Erus G, Toledo JB, Zhang T, Bryan N, Launer LJ, et al. White matter hyperintensities and imaging patterns of brain ageing in the general population. Brain. 2016;139:1164–79. https://doi.org/10.1093/brain/aww008.
63. Wang L, Murphy O, Caldito NG, Calabresi PA, Saidha S. Emerging applications of optical coherence tomography angiography (OCTA) in neurological research. Eye Vis (Lond). 2018;5:11. https://doi.org/10.1186/s40662-018-0104-3.
64. Lanzillo R, Cennamo G, Criscuolo C, Carotenuto A, Velotti N, Sparnelli F, et al. Optical coherence tomography angiography retinal vascular network assessment in multiple sclerosis. Mult Scler. 2018;24:1706–14. https://doi.org/10.1177/1352458517729463.
65. Spain RI, Liu L, Zhang X, Jia Y, Tan O, Bourdette D, et al. Optical coherence tomography angiography enhances the detection of optic nerve damage in multiple sclerosis. Br J Ophthalmol. 2018;102:520–4. https://doi.org/10.1136/bjophthalmol-2017-310477.
66. Herculano-Houzel S. The human brain in numbers: a linearly scaled-up primate brain. Front Hum Neurosci. 2009;3:31. https://doi.org/10.3389/neuro.09.031.2009.
67. Saidha S, Al-Louzi O, Ratchford JN, Bhargava P, Oh J, Newsome SD, et al. Optical coherence tomography reflects brain atrophy in multiple sclerosis: a four-year study. Ann Neurol. 2015;78:801–13. https://doi.org/10.1002/ana.24487.
68. Kuo AN, Verkicharla PK, McNabb RP, Cheung CY, Hilal S, Farsiu S, et al. Posterior eye shape measurement with retinal OCT compared to MRI. Invest Ophthalmol Vis Sci. 2016;57:OCT196–203. https://doi.org/10.1167/iovs.15-18886
69. Meixner E, Michelson G. Measurement of retinal wall-to-lumen ratio by adaptive optics retinal camera: a clinical research. Graefes Arch Clin Exp Ophthalmol. 2015;253:1985–95. https://doi.org/10.1007/s00417-015-3115-y.
70. Zwillinger S, Paques M, Safran B. In vivo characterization of lamina cribrosa pore mor- phology in primary open-angle glaucoma. J Fr Ophtalmol. 2016;39:265–71. https://doi.org/10.1016/j.jfo.2015.11.006.
71. Szatmáry G. Imaging of the orbit. Neurol Clin. 2009;27:251–84. https://doi.org/10.1016/j.ncl.2008.09.008.
72. More SS, Beach JM, Vince R. Early detection of amyloidopathy in Alzheimer's mice by hyperspectral endoscopy. Invest Ophthalmol Vis Sci. 2016;57:3231–8. https://doi.org/10.1167/iovs.15-17406.
73. Szatmáry G. Imaging in patients with visual symptoms. Continuum (Minneap Minn). 2016;22:1499–528. https://doi.org/10.1212/CON.0000000000000375.
74. Mokbul MI. Optical coherence tomography: basic concepts and applications in neuroscience research. J Med Eng. 2017;2017:3409327. https://doi.org/10.1155/2017/3409327.
75. Oberwahrenbrock T, Traber GL, Lukas S, Gabilondo I, Nolan R, Songster C, et al. Multicenter reliability of semiautomatic retinal layer segmentation using OCT. Neurol Neuroimmunol Neuroinflamms. 2018;5: e449. https://doi.org/10.1212/NXI.0000000000000449.
76. Roska B, Sahel JA. Restoring vision. Nature. 2018;557:359–67. https://doi.org/10.1038/s41586-018-0076-4.
77. Hillier D, Fiscella M, Drinnenberg A, Trenholm S, Rompani SB, Raics Z, et al. Causal evidence for retina-dependent and -independent visual motion computations in mouse cortex. Nat Neurosci. 2017;20:960–8. https://doi.org/10.1038/nn.4566.
78. Mallery RM, Poolman P, Thurtell MJ, Full JM, Ledolter J, Kimbrough D, et al. Visual fixation instability in multiple sclerosis measured using SLO-OCT. Invest Ophthalmol Vis Sci. 2018;59:196–201. https://doi.org/10.1167/iovs.17-22391.
79. Meltzer E, Sguigna PV, Subei A, Beh S, Kildebeck E, Conger D, et al. Retinal architecture and melanopsin-mediated pupillary response characteristics: a putative pathophysiologic signature for the retino-hypothalamic tract in multiple sclerosis. JAMA Neurol. 2017;74:574–82. https://doi.org/10.1001/jamaneurol.2016.5131.
80. Bernardes R, Ghalati M, Ferreira H, Martins J, Guimarães P, Moreira P, Ambrósio A, Castelo-Branco M, Serranho P. Longitudinal OCT texture analysis to assess the retinal changes in the triple-transgenic mouse model of Alzheimer's disease. Acta Ophthalmologica. 2022;100(S275). https://doi.org/10.1111/j.1755-3768.2022.0173

81. Bernardes R, Ghalati MK, Nunes A, Ferreira H, Serranho P. Texture analysis and its applications in biomedical imaging: a survey. IEEE Rev Biomed Eng. 2021;15:222–46. https://doi.org/10.1109/RBME.2021.3115703.
82. Biousse V, Nahab F, Newman NJ. Management of acute retinal ischemia: follow the guidelines! Ophthalmology. 2018;125:1597–607. https://doi.org/10.1016/j.ophtha.2018.03.054.
83. Graessl A, Muhle M, Schwerter M, Rieger J, Oezerdem C, Santoro D, et al. Ophthalmic magnetic resonance imaging at 7 T using a 6-channel transceiver radiofrequency coil array in healthy subjects and patients with intraocular masses. Investig Radiol. 2014;49:260–70. https://doi.org/10.1097/RLI.0000000000000049.
84. Mallery RM, Poolman P, Thurtell MJ, Wang JK, Garvin MK, Ledolter J, et al. The pattern of visual fixation eccentricity and instability in optic neuropathy and its spatial relationship to retinal ganglion cell layer thickness. Invest Ophthalmol Vis Sci. 2016;57:OCT429–37. https://doi.org/10.1167/iovs.15-18916
85. Szatmáry G. Neuroimaging in the diagnostic evaluation of eye pain. Curr Pain Headache Rep. 2016;20:52. https://doi.org/10.1007/s11916-016-0582-8.
86. Chen JJ, AbouChehade JE, Iezzi R Jr, Leavitt JA, Kardon RH, et al. Optical coherence angiographic demonstration of retinal changes from chronic optic neuropathies. Neuroophthalmology. 2017;4:76–83. https://doi.org/10.1080/01658107.2016.1275703.
87. Kupersmith MJ, Garvin MK, Wang JK, Durbin M, Kardon R. Retinal ganglion cell layer thinning within one month of presentation for optic neuritis. Mult Scler. 2016;22:641–8. https://doi.org/10.1177/1352458515598020.
88. Al-Louzi O, Button J, Newsome SD, Calabresi PA, Saidha S. Retrograde trans-synaptic visual pathway degeneration in multiple sclerosis: a case series. Mult Scler. 2017;23:1035–9. https://doi.org/10.1177/1352458516679035.
89. Vislisel JM, Chen JJ, Kardon RH. Localizing the lesion in Foster Kennedy syndrome from hemiretinal atrophy at the macula. J Neuroophthalmol. 2014;34:422–5. https://doi.org/10.1097/WNO.0000000000000168
90. Zehnder S, Wildberger H, Hanson JV, Lukas S, Pelz S, Landau K, et al. Retinal ganglion cell topography in patients with visual pathway pathology. J Neuroophthalmol. 2018;38:172–8. https://doi.org/10.1097/WNO.0000000000000589.
91. Blanch RJ, Micieli JA, Oyesiku NM, Newman NJ, Biousse V. Optical coherence tomography retinal ganglion cell complex analysis for the detection of early chiasmal compression. Pituitary. 2018;21:515–23. https://doi.org/10.1007/s11102-018-0906-2.
92. Micieli JA, Newman NJ, Biousse V. Retinal imaging of an optic tract lesion: OCT angiography of structural and functional defects. Ophthalmology. 2018;125:756. https://doi.org/10.1016/j.ophtha.2018.01.027
93. Al-Louzi OA, Bhargava P, Newsome SD, Balcer LJ, Frohman EM, Crainiceanu C, et al. Outer retinal changes following acute optic neuritis. Mult Scler. 2016;22:362–72. https://doi.org/10.1177/1352458515590646
94. Wang JK, Kardon RH, Ledolter J, Sibony PA, Kupersmith MJ, Garvin MK. Peripapillary retinal pigment epithelium layer shape changes from acetazolamide treatment in the idiopathic intracranial hypertension treatment trial. Invest Ophthalmol Vis Sci. 2017;58:2554–65. https://doi.org/10.1167/iovs.16-21089.
95. Adams DL, Piserchia V, Economides JR, Horton JC. Vascular supply of the cerebral cortex is specialized for cell layers but not columns. Cereb Cortex. 2015;25:3673–81. https://doi.org/10.1093/cercor/bhu221.
96. Chen W, You J, Gu X, Du C, Pan Y. High-speed swept source optical coherence Doppler 6tomography for deep brain microvascular imaging. Sci Rep. 2016;6:38786. https://doi.org/10.1038/srep38786.
97. Merkle CW, Srinivasan VJ. Laminar microvascular transit time distribution in the mouse 7somatosensory cortex revealed by dynamic contrast optical coherence tomography. Neuroimage. 2016;125:350–62. https://doi.org/10.1016/j.neuroimage.2015.10.017.
98. Drexler W, Liu M, Kumar A, Kamali T, Unterhuber A, Leitgeb RA. Optical coherence tomography today: speed, contrast, and multimodality. J Biomed Opt. 2014;19: 071412.

99. World Health Organization. Neurological disorders: public health challenges. 2018. https://www.who.int/mental_health/neurology/neurological_disorders_report_web.pdf. Accessed 12 Dec 2018.
100. Bock M, Brandt AU, Dorr J, Kraft H, Weinges-Evers N, Gaede G, et al. Patterns of retinal nerve fiber layer loss in multiple sclerosis patients with or without optic neuritis and glaucoma patients. Clin Neurol Neurosurg. 2010;112:647–52. https://doi.org/10.1016/j.clineuro.2010.04.014.
101. Fjeldstad C, Bemben M, Pardo G. Reduced retinal nerve fiber layer and macular thickness in patients with multiple sclerosis with no history of optic neuritis identified by the use of spectral domain high-definition optical coherence tomography. J Clin Neurosci. 2011;18:1469–72. https://doi.org/10.1016/j.jocn.2011.04.008
102. Parisi V, Manni G, Spadaro M, Colacino G, Restuccia R, Marchi S, et al. Correlation between morphological and functional retinal impairment in multiple sclerosis patients. Invest Ophthalmol Vis Sci. 1999;40:2520–7.
103. Pueyo V, Martin J, Fernandez J, Almarcegui C, Ara J, Egea C, et al. Axonal loss in the retinal nerve fiber layer in patients with multiple sclerosis. Mult Scler. 2018;14:609–14. https://doi.org/10.1177/1352458507087326.
104. Sepulcre J, Murie-Fernandez M, Salinas-Alaman A, García-Layana A, Bejarano B, Villoslada P. Diagnostic accuracy of retinal abnormalities in predicting disease activity in MS. Neurology. 2007;68:1488–94. https://doi.org/10.1212/01.wnl.0000260612.51849.ed.
105. Tegetmeyer H, Kuhn E. Quantitative analysis of changes in macular layers following optic neuritis. Neuro-Ophthalmol. 2011;35:101–7.
106. Tatrai E, Simo M, Iljicsov A, Nemeth J, Debuc DC, Somfai GM. In vivo evaluation of retinal neurodegeneration in patients with multiple sclerosis. PLoS One. 2012;7:e30922. https://doi.org/10.1371/journal.pone.0030922.
107. Klistorner A, Arvind H, Nguyen T, Garrick R, Paine M, Graham S, et al. Multifocal VEP and OCT in optic neuritis: a topographical study of the structure-function relationship. Doc Ophthalmol. 2009;118:129–37. https://doi.org/10.1007/s10633-008-9147-4.
108. Odrobina D, Roskal-Wałek J, Mackiewicz J, Wypchło Ł, Biskup M. Susac's syndrome—the crucial role of imaging tests for proper diagnosis. Annals of Agricul Environ Med. 2022;29(2):190–200. https://doi.org/10.26444/aaem/149954
109. Habot-Wilner Z, Zur D, Goldstein M, Barequet D, Oron Y, Elkayam O, Karni A, Wilf-Yarkoni A, Regev K. Susac's syndrome—a new ocular finding and disease outcome. Eye. 2022;36(4):Article 4. https://doi.org/10.1038/s41433-021-01464-7
110. Odrobina D, Roskal-Wałek J, Biskup M, Dolecka-Ślusarczyk M, Rosołowska A, Jaroszyński A. Manifestation of Susac syndrome during interferon beta-1a and glatiramer acetate treatment for misdiagnosed multiple sclerosis: a case report. BMC Ophthalmol. 2021;21(1):352. https://doi.org/10.1186/s12886-021-02101-3.
111. Hardy TA, Buzzard KA, Reddel SW, Yiannikas C, Sean Riminton D, Barnett MH. Distinguishing Susac's syndrome from multiple sclerosis. J Neurol. 2015;262(7):1613–21. https://doi.org/10.1007/s00415-014-7628-9.
112. Brandt AU, Zimmermann H, Kaufhold F, Promesberger J, Schippling S, Finis D, Aktas O, Geis C, Ringelstein M, Ringelstein EB, Hartung H-P, Paul F, Kleffner I, Dörr J. Patterns of retinal damage facilitate differential diagnosis between susac syndrome and MS. 2012;7(6):e38741. https://doi.org/10.1371/journal.pone.0038741.
113. Johnson LN, Diehl ML, Hamm CW, Sommerville DN, Petroski GF. Differentiating optic disc edema from optic nerve head drusen on optical coherence tomography. Arch Ophthalmol. 2009;127:45–9. https://doi.org/10.1001/archophthalmol.2008.524.
114. Hoye VJ, Berrocal AM, Hedges TR, Amaro-Quireza ML. Optical coherence tomography demonstrates subretinal macular edema from papilledema. Arch Ophthalmol. 2001;119:1287–90.

115. Hedges TR, Vuong LN, Gonzalez-Garcia AO, Mendoza-Santiesteban CE, Amaro-Quiereza AL. Subretinal fluid from anterior ischemic optic neuropathy demonstrated by opti- cal coherence tomography. Arch Ophthalmol. 2008;126:812–5. https://doi.org/10.1001/archopht.126.6.812.
116. Hedges TR, Flattem NL, Bagga A. Vitreopapillary traction confirmed by optical coherence tomography. Arch Ophthalmol. 2006;124:279–81. https://doi.org/10.1001/archopht.124.2.279.
117. Kanamori A, Nakamura M, Matsui N, Nagai A, Nakanishi Y, Kusuhara S, et al. Optical coherence tomography detects characteristic retinal nerve fiber layer thickness correspond- ing to band atrophy of the optic discs. Ophthalmology. 2004;111:2278–83. https://doi.org/10.1016/j.ophtha.2004.05.035.
118. Monteiro MLR, Leal BC, Rosa AAM, Bronstein MD. Optical coherence tomography analysis of axonal loss in band atrophy of the optic nerve. Br J Ophthalmol. 2004;88:896–9. https://doi.org/10.1136/bjo.2003.038489.
119. Barboni P, Savini G, Valentino ML, Montagna P, Cortelli P, De Negri AM, et al. Retinal nerve fiber layer evaluation by optical coherence tomography in Leber's hereditary optic neuropathy. Ophthalmology. 2005;112:120–6. https://doi.org/10.1016/j.ophtha.2004.06.034.
120. Barboni P, Carbonelli M, Savini G, Ramos CVF, Carta A, Berezovsky A, et al. Natural history of Leber's hereditary optic neuropathy: longitudinal analysis of the retinal nerve fiber layer by optical coherence tomography. Ophthalmology. 2010;113:623–7. https://doi.org/10.1016/j.ophtha.2009.07.026.
121. Savini G, Barboni P, Valentino ML, Montagna P, Cortelli P, De Negri AM, et al. Retinal nerve fiber layer evaluation by optical coherence tomography in unaffected carriers with Leber hereditary optic neuropathy mutations. Ophthalmology. 2005;112:127–31. https://doi.org/10.1016/j.ophtha.2004.09.033.
122. Chicani CM, Carelli V, Berezovsky A. Leber's hereditary optic neuropathy: Project Brazil/LHON—8-year summary. Vision Panamerican. 2009:170–7.
123. Zaveri MS, Conger A, Salter A, Frohman TC, Galetta SL, Markowitz CE, et al. Retinal imaging by laser polarimetry and optical coherence tomography evidence of axonal degeneration in multiple sclerosis. Arch Neurol. 2008;65:924–8. https://doi.org/10.1001/archneur.65.7.924.
124. Frohman EM, Dwyer MG, Frohman T, Cox JL, Salter A, Greenberg BM, et al. Relationship of optic nerve and brain conventional and non-conventional MRI measures and retinal nerve fiber layer thickness, as assessed by OCT and GDx: a pilot study. J Neurol Sci. 2009;282:96.
125. Costello F, Hodge W, Pan YI, Eggenberger E, Coupland S, Kardon RH. Tracking retinal nerve fiber layer loss after optic neuritis: a prospective study using optical coherence tomography. Mult Scler. 2008;14:893–905. https://doi.org/10.1177/1352458508091367.
126. Xie JS, Donaldson L, Margolin E. The use of optical coherence tomography in neurology: a review. Brain. 2022;145(12):4160–77. https://doi.org/10.1093/brain/awac317.
127. Zéphir H, Outteryck O, Majed B, Defoort-Dhellemmes S, Vermersch P. A comparative optical coherence tomography study in neuromyelitis optica spectrum disorder and multiple sclerosis. Multiple Sclerosis J. 2015;21(14):1781–93. https://doi.org/10.1177/1352458515578888.
128. Ciccarelli O, Cortese R, Carrasco FP, Tur C, Bianchi A, Brownlee W, Angelis FD, Paz IDL, Grussu F, Haider L, Jacob A, Kanber B, Magnollay L, Nicholas RS, Trip A, Yiannakas M, Toosy AT, Hacohen Y, Barkhof F. Differentiating multiple sclerosis from AQP4-neuromyelitis optica spectrum disorder and MOG-antibody disease with imaging. Neurology. 2023;100(3):e308–23. https://doi.org/10.1212/WNL.0000000000201465.
129. Vlad Marin A. Observing the brain through the eye' A longitudinal study on amyotrophic lateral sclerosis patients using optical coherence tomography and magnetic resonance imaging [Doctoral Dissertation, Department of Neurology—Ulm University] 2020. https://www.semanticscholar.org/paper/Observing-the-brain-through-the-eye%3A-a-longitudinal-Marin/5f214918a68db05c822079dadb0517b10fb593c1

130. Pinkhardt EH, Hübers A, Müller HP, Dreyhaupt J, Böhm K, Lauda F, Tumani H, Kassubek J, Ludolph AC. Retinal involvement in amyotrophic lateral sclerosis: a study with optical coherence tomography and diffusion tensor imaging. J Neural Transmission. 2016;123(3):281–7. https://doi.org/10.1007/s00702-015-1483-4.
131. Pinkhardt EH, Abdelhak A, Hübers A, Böhm K, Ludolph AC, Kassubek J. In vivo assessment of retinal vessel pathology in amyotrophic lateral sclerosis. J Neurol. 2018;265(4):949–53. https://doi.org/10.1007/s00415-018-8787-x.
132. Ramírez JM, Rojas P, de Hoz R, Ramírez AI, Ferreras A, Salobrar-Garcia E, Muñoz-Blanco JL, Urcelay-Segura JL, Salazar JJ. Changes in retinal OCT and their correlations with neurological disability in early ALS patients, a follow-up study. Brain Sci. 2019;9(12), Article 12. https://doi.org/10.3390/brainsci9120337
133. Mendoza-Santiesteban CE, Gabilondo I, Palma JA, Norcliffe-Kaufmann L, Kaufmann H. The retina in multiple system atrophy: systematic review and meta-analysis. Front Neurol. 2017;8:206. https://doi.org/10.3389/fneur.2017.00206.
134. Mendoza-Santiesteban CE, Palma JA, Martinez J, Norcliffe-Kaufmann L, Hedges TR III, Kaufmann H. Progressive retinal structure abnormalities in multiple system atrophy. Mov Disord. 2015;30:1944–53. https://doi.org/10.1002/mds.26360.GreenbergBM.
135. Abegg M, Mühlemann F, Grabe H, Fok A, Wagner F, Brügger D, Sheldon CA. Homonymous hemiatrophy of ganglion cell layer from retrochiasmal lesions in the visual pathway. Neurology. 2020;94(3):e323–9. https://doi.org/10.1212/WNL.0000000000008738.
136. Wang D, Liu H-L, Du Y-Y, Yuan J, Li X, Tian Z, Zhou H, Wang S, Song L, Sun J, Xiao X, Wang Z-T, Li B. Characterisation of thickness changes in the peripapillary retinal nerve fibre layer in patients with Leber's hereditary optic neuropathy. British J Ophthalmol. 2021;105(8):1166–71. https://doi.org/10.1136/bjophthalmol-2020-316573.
137. Barboni P, Balducci N, Carbonelli M, Morgia CL, Romagnoli M, Amore G, D'Agati P, Valentino ML, Caporali L, Cascavilla ML, Battista M, Borrelli E, Renzo AD, Parisi V, Carelli V. Capturing the pattern of transition from carrier to affected in leber hereditary optic neuropathy. Amer J Ophthalmol. 2022;241:71–9. https://doi.org/10.1016/j.ajo.2022.04.016.
138. Balducci N, Savini G, Cascavilla ML, Morgia CL, Triolo G, Giglio R, Carbonelli M, Parisi V, Sadun AA, Bandello F, Carelli V, Barboni P. Macular nerve fibre and ganglion cell layer changes in acute Leber's hereditary optic neuropathy. British J Ophthalmol. 2016;100(9):1232–7. https://doi.org/10.1136/bjophthalmol-2015-307326.
139. Greenberg BM, Frohman E. Optical coherence tomography as a potential readout in clinical trials. Ther Adv Neurol Disord. 2010;3:153–60. https://doi.org/10.1177/1756285610368890.
140. Bodis-Wollner I, Miri S, Glazman S. Venturing into the no-man's land of the retina in Parkinson's disease. Mov Disord. 2014;29:15–22. https://doi.org/10.1002/mds.25741.
141. Malmqvist L, Sibony PA, Fraser CL, Wegener M, Heegaard S, Skougaard M, et al. Peripapillary ovoid hyperreflectivity in optic disc edema and pseudopapilledema. Ophthalmology. 2018;125:1662–4. https://doi.org/10.1016/j.ophtha.2018.04.036.
142. Cruz-Herranz A, Balk LJ, Oberwahrenbrock T, Saidha S, Martinez-Lapiscina EH, Lagreze WA, et al. The APOSTEL recommendations for reporting quantitative optical coherence tomography studies. Neurology. 2016;86:2303–9. https://doi.org/10.1212/WNL.000000000 0002774.
143. Baran U, Wang RK. Review of optical coherence tomography based angiography in neuroscience. Neurophotonics. 2016;3: 010902. https://doi.org/10.1117/1.NPh.3.1.010902.
144. Kut C, Chaichana KL, Xi J, Raza SM, Ye X, McVeigh ER, et al. Detection of human brain cancer infiltration ex vivo and in vivo using quantitative optical coherence tomography. Sci Transl Med. 2015;7:292ra100. https://doi.org/10.1126/scitranslmed.3010611

145. Fan Y, Zhang B, Chang W, Zhang X, Liao H. A novel integration of spectral-domain optical coherence tomography and laser-ablation system for precision treatment. Int J Comput Assist Radiol Surg. 2018;13(3):411–23. https://doi.org/10.1007/s11548-017-1664-8.
146. Chen JJ, Thurtell MJ, Longmuir RA, Garvin MK, Wang JK, Wall M, et al. Causes and prognosis of visual acuity loss at the time of initial presentation in idiopathic intracranial hypertension. Invest Ophthalmol Vis Sci. 2015;56:3850–9. https://doi.org/10.1167/iovs.15-16450.
147. Button J, Al-Louzi O, Lang A, Bhargava P, Newsome SD, Frohman T, et al. Disease modifying therapies modulate retinal atrophy in multiple sclerosis: a retrospective study. Neurology. 2017;88:525–32. https://doi.org/10.1212/WNL.0000000000003582.
148. Feucht N, Maier M, Lepennetier G, Pettenkofer M, Wetzlmair C, Daltrozzo T, et al. Optical coherence tomography angiography indicates associations of the retinal vascular network and disease activity in multiple sclerosis. Mult Scler. 2018. https://doi.org/10.1177/1352458517750009.

Imaging Alzheimer's Retinopathy

6

Bhakta Prasad Gaire, Yosef Koronyo, Haoshen Shi, Altan Rentsendorj, Oana M. Dumitrascu, Jean-Philippe Vit, Jonah Doustar, Keith L. Black, Dieu-Trang Fuchs, and Maya Koronyo-Hamaoui

Abstract

Growing evidence suggests that Alzheimer's disease (AD) pathology is not confined to the brain but also appears in the neurosensory retina. The retina, viewed as an extension of the brain, is a neural tissue easily accessible for direct and noninvasive imaging at the vascular, cellular, and molecular resolution. Postmortem examinations of AD patients' retinas, including those in early stages, have identified Aβ accumulations, vascular $A\beta_{40}$ and $A\beta_{42}$ deposits, hyperphosphorylated tau inclusions, microgliosis, astrogliosis, Müller glia changes, abnormal electroretinography patterns, and neuronal degeneration. Several studies further provided data suggesting that the brain and retina follows a similar trajectory during AD progression, possibly due to their common embryonic origin and anatomical proximity. In vivo fundus imaging, optical coherence tomography (OCT), and OCT-angiopathy have detected various retinal vascular abnormalities in preclinical AD, mild cognitively impaired (MCI), and AD dementia patients, including reduced blood flow, blood vessel tortuosity, and increased foveal avascular zone and arteriole-to-venule ratio. Moreover, histological analyses of postmortem retinas of MCI and AD patients revealed early and progressive vascular platelet-derived growth factor receptor-β (PDGFRβ) and pericyte losses along with endothelial tight-junction deficiencies. Retinal

B. P. Gaire · Y. Koronyo · H. Shi · A. Rentsendorj · O. M. Dumitrascu · J.-P. Vit · J. Doustar · K. L. Black · D.-T. Fuchs · M. Koronyo-Hamaoui (✉)
Department of Neurosurgery, Maxine Dunitz Neurosurgical Research Institute, Cedars-Sinai Medical Center, 127 S. San Vicente Blvd., Los Angeles, CA 90048, USA
e-mail: maya.koronyo@csmc.edu

M. Koronyo-Hamaoui
Department of Biomedical Sciences, Division of Applied Cell Biology and Physiology, Cedars-Sinai Medical Center, 127 S. San Vicente Blvd., Los Angeles, CA 90048, USA

Department of Neurology, Cedars-Sinai Medical Center, 127 S. San Vicente Blvd., Los Angeles, CA 90048, USA

A. Grzybowski and P. Barboni (eds.), *OCT and Imaging in Central Nervous System Diseases*, https://doi.org/10.1007/978-3-031-72156-4_6

vascular damage was closely associated with increased retinal vascular amyloidosis, cerebral amyloid angiopathy, and cognitive deficits. Proteomics profiling has revealed common molecular signatures in the AD retina and brain, with enriched pathways related to inflammatory, vascular, mitochondrial, and photoreceptor vulnerability. Notably, novel imaging techniques, such as curcumin fluorescence of retinal Aβ deposits detected by scanning laser ophthalmoscope and hyperspectral imaging indicated increased retinal amyloid burden in AD, which was correlated with hippocampal atrophy and brain amyloid-PET load, and together with vascular changes, was predictive of cognitive decline. This book chapter provides an overview of the evidence of AD pathology in the retina, AD-related visual dysfunctions, and ophthalmic imaging modalities, while also highlighting the current gaps in knowledge that should be addressed in future studies. With recent advances in anti-Aβ immunotherapies for early AD cases, noninvasive retinal imaging strategies may fundamentally transform the feasibility for early screening and monitoring of AD.

Keywords

Alzheimer's disease • Retina • Amyloidosis • Tauopathy • Vasculopathy • Inflammation • Ocular pathology • Optical imaging • Fluorescence imaging

6.1 Introduction

Alzheimer's disease (AD) is an age-dependent neurodegenerative disorder that is characterized by progressive and relentless cognitive decline. An estimated 6.7 million elderly Americans are afflicted by AD dementia, and it is considered the seventh leading cause of death in the United States [1]. Globally, over 55 million people live with AD and related dementia, resulting in annual associated costs of more than 1 trillion dollars [2–4]. As the elderly population continues to grow, this number is projected to reach approximately 139 million by 2050, making AD a serios health and economic challenge. Despite advances in understanding AD pathogenesis, there are still limited therapies [5] and significant challenges in the feasibility of early and accurate AD detection and monitoring in the clinical settings [6]. Indeed, with the sharp rise in current AD cases, there is an urgent, unmet need for a dependable, noninvasive, and affordable diagnostic technique suitable for widespread clinical use.

The characteristic signs of AD neuropathology include the early accumulation of misfolded amyloid beta-protein (Aβ) in plaques and subsequent neurofibrillary tangles (NFTs) comprised of hyperphosphorylated tau (pTau) protein, which are prerequisites for a definitive AD diagnosis [7, 8]. Along with these core AD hallmarks, low-grade chronic inflammation and vascular abnormalities are recognized as additional pathogenic features that ultimately lead to severe synaptic and neuronal loss [9–20]. Longitudinal biomarker studies have demonstrated that the accumulation of Aβ pathology occurs as early as 20 years before the onset of clinical dementia, in insidious phases denoted as preclinical and prodromal AD [21–24]. Aβ pathology is thought to drive tauopathy and its spread throughout the brain, inducing reactive astrogliosis and microgliosis [13, 25–27], which contributes to neurodegeneration and eventually dementia [16, 28]. Indeed, the accumulation of misfolded Aβ and tau species during AD progression is associated with aberrant activation of glial cells, vascular damage, and peripheral immune cell infiltration, which may either facilitate resolution or further aggravate neuroinflammation and neurodegeneration [13, 29, 30].

Emerging experimental and translational studies indicate that the neurosensory retina is deleteriously affected during AD pathogenesis. Multiple pieces of evidence from histological, biochemical, and *in vivo* imaging studies demonstrate that the pathological hallmarks of AD, Aβ deposits and pTau inclusions, extend beyond the brain and also manifest in the retinas of AD patients at the preclinical, prodromal, and clinical stages [31–62]. Concomitant with these pathological hallmarks, other key signs of AD, such as gliosis, vasculopathy, optic nerve degeneration, retinal neuronal degeneration, and thinning, have been detected in the retina of patients with mild cognitive impairment (MCI) and AD [39, 45, 47, 56, 58, 62–76] (see a summary illustration in Fig. 6.1). Experimental studies in the retina of AD animal models have further described a plethora of AD-specific signs and associated inflammation, metabolic changes, vascular, and neurodegeneration [31, 33, 41, 46, 54, 61, 77–102].

The retina is a sensory extension of the brain and the only central nervous system (CNS) tissue not shielded by bone, making it feasible for direct, noninvasive, and repeated imaging with ultra-high spatial resolution [103–106]. As a tissue derived from the embryonic diencephalon, the retina contains high-density neuronal cells and fibers [104, 106, 107]. Furthermore, the axons of retinal ganglion cells (RGCs) form the optic nerve that directly connects the retina and brain. The optic nerves from both eyes converge at the optic chiasm, and from this point, most optic tract fibers establish synapses connecting to the visual cortex via the optic nerve and the lateral geniculate nucleus (LGN) of the thalamus. From the LGN, these projections extend into the optic radiation and further project to various executive regions of the brain. A distinct subset of cells known as melanopsin-containing or intrinsically photosensitive RGCs project their axons in a monoaxonal manner directly to the suprachiasmatic nucleus (or SCN) located within the hypothalamus. In the context of AD, the optic nerve may facilitate vesicular transportation of Aβ precursor protein (AβPP), which is synthesized by RGCs [108]. Retinal neurons and glia also secrete proteins that are related to the amyloid cascade (e.g., BACE1, γ-secretase, ApoE, and clusterin) [109–113]. Importantly, retinal Aβ accumulation seems to follow a similar trajectory to that of brain Aβ burden during disease progression [44, 45, 58]. A recent report suggested that retinal $A\beta_{42}$, S100 calcium-binding protein B^+ macrogliosis, and atrophy correlated with the severity of brain Aβ pathology, tauopathy (NFTs and Braak stage), and atrophy [45]. Additionally, retinal Aβ burden, including oligomeric Aβ, retinal gliosis, and retinal atrophy, was correlated with cognition [45]. Furthermore, retinal pTau (Ser202/Thr205 and Thr217) were correlated with brain pTau (cortical

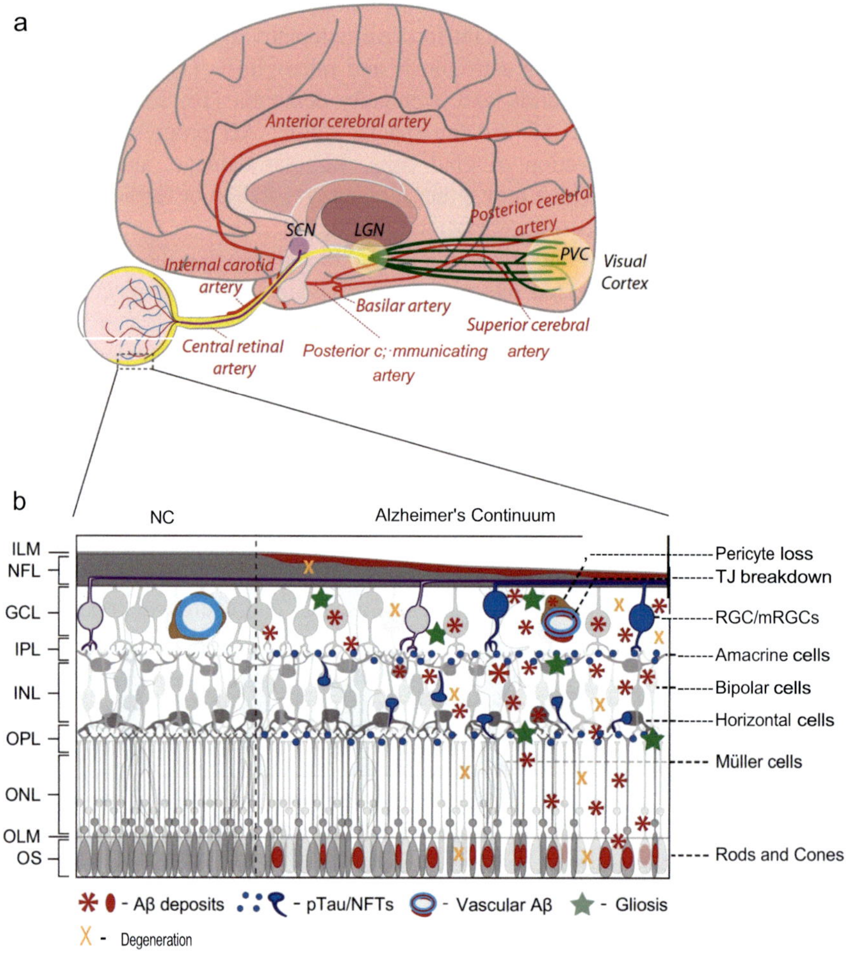

Fig. 6.1 Retinal projections into the brain and AD pathological progression in retinal tissue. (**a**) An illustration of the primary visual pathway with axonal projections to the lateral geniculate nucleus (LGN; yellow), proceeding to the primary visual cortex (PVC; green). Photosensitive retinal ganglion cells (RGCs), such as melanopsin (m)RGCs, form the retinohypothalamic tract (purple) and synapse with three other locations in the brain for specific visual regulations: the pretectal nucleus, midbrain nuclei, and suprachiasmatic nucleus (SCN). (**b**) Schematic illustration of retinal pathology in the retina of AD patients. A comparison between cognitively normal control (NC) and AD retinas along a continuum. AD-attributed retinal pathology includes the accumulation of Aβ and phosphorylated-tau proteins, degeneration, and subsequent thinning, and an inflammatory response. AD retinal vessels display substantial thinning and pericyte loss alongside Aβ protein deposition. Aβ, Amyloid-β protein; GCL, ganglion cell layer; ILM, inner limiting membrane; INL, inner nuclear layer; IPL, inner plexiform layer; mRGCs, melanopsin-containing retinal ganglion cells; NFL, nerve fiber layer; NFTs, neurofibrillary tangles; OPL, outer plexiform layer; ONL, outer nuclear layer; OLM, outer limiting membrane; OS, outer segment; RGCs, retinal ganglion cells; pTau, hyperphosphorylated Tau; TJ, tight junction. The illustration in panel **b** is reproduced from Mirzaei et al., Front Neurosci 2020 [50]

and hippocampal Ser202/Thr205) and Braak stage for NFTs [42]. However, future studies with larger cohorts are required to establish the relationship between retinal and brain pathologies in AD.

The feasibility of detecting retinal amyloid deposits through noninvasive retinal optical imaging was shown in human trials. The amyloid load was found to be greater in MCI and AD patients compared to individuals with normal cognition [37, 38, 41, 49, 51, 52, 60, 114]. Importantly, a growing number of experimental and clinical studies have reported that AD-specific signs occur in the retina at the onset of functional impairment (MCI) and before symptom manifestation. These signs can be detected prior to their appearance in the brain, suggesting that the pathological processes of AD can be detected earlier in the retina [37–39, 45, 46, 51, 52, 56, 58, 60, 65, 69, 86, 90, 98, 99, 115–123]. Overall, these findings support the use of the retina as an appealing and unparalleled CNS site for early AD screening of at-risk populations and for monitoring its progression [43, 50, 57].

The mounting evidence of parallel AD pathologies in both the brain and retina, observed in patients and animal models [44, 45, 55, 86, 101, 124], coupled with the availability of retinal imaging modalities in the clinical setting providing ultra-high resolution spatial information on the vascular, cellular, and molecular levels [125–131], emphasized the urgency of expanding research on distinct neuropathological signs of AD in the retina. This chapter highlights findings related to AD pathology in the retina, with a focus on characteristic Aβ and tau accumulations, as well as emerging new retinal amyloid imaging modalities that offer new hope for advancing highly specific and sensitive methods for early AD detection and monitoring.

6.2 Histopathological Evidence of AD Hallmarks in the Retina

6.2.1 Retinal Aβ Pathology in AD Patients

In the early 1900s, plaques and tangles were discovered in the postmortem brain of Auguste Deter, the first known AD patient, and subsequently, these plaques were shown to contain Aβ aggregates [132–135]. A century later, in 2010, Koronyo-Hamaoui et al., identified the presence of AD hallmark pathology, Aβ deposits, in retinal tissues extracted from patients with definite AD diagnosis at early and late disease stages [46]. These human samples were characterized by both pre-mortem cognitive evaluations and extensive post-mortem neuropathological analyses. Comparisons against a cohort of age- and sex-matched cognitively normal controls revealed a substantial difference in the observed Aβ pathology between the two diagnostic groups [46]. Since then, a growing number of studies have demonstrated the accumulation of $A\beta_{40}$ and $A\beta_{42}$ peptides and Aβ plaque aggregates in retinal flat mounts and cross-sections of the post-mortem retina of AD patients [31, 33, 35, 38, 39, 41, 44, 45, 47–49, 51–53, 55, 56, 58–62]. Aβ immunoreactivity and deposits were detected in various retinal layers, particularly in the inner layers, with intracellular deposits localized within ganglion, amacrine, horizontal, and Müller cells [35, 45, 48, 62]. Extracellular and vascular Aβ deposits were also found preferentially in the superior temporal retina [35, 44, 45, 48, 56, 58]. These studies involved various fluorescence and non-fluorescence histological and biochemical techniques that demonstrated Aβ accumulation in the human retina, using numerous monoclonal antibodies recognizing diverse epitopes within the Aβ sequence and Aβ-labeling compounds, such as curcumin, thioflavin-S, Gallyas silver, and Congo red [31, 33, 35, 36, 39, 44–48, 53, 55, 56, 58, 62]. Such findings have led to a stronger understanding of the spatial distribution and subtypes of Aβ aggregates in the human retina. Figure 6.2 displays the geographical distribution and morphology of Aβ plaques in AD retinal flatmounts, and Fig. 6.3 displays histological examination in AD retinal cross-sections, revealing the layer and cellular distribution of Aβ deposits. Aβ manifests in the human retina as diffuse, immature, or mature-classic morphology, and appears unevenly distributed across geometric regions and cell layers [36, 39, 44, 45, 47, 48, 62]. Although Aβ plaques in the retina are generally smaller in size compared to brain plaques, they are structurally and biochemically similar (Fig. 6.4). A few studies, however, were not able to confirm the presence of Aβ plaques in the retina [136, 137], possibly due to reliance on traditional tissue processing, suboptimal protocols, and/or incomplete tissue screening of anatomical regions more impacted in AD. However, to date, the vast majority of peer-reviewed publications using rigorous biochemical, histological, and/or in vivo retinal amyloid imaging techniques in humans have reproduced the findings of Aβ pathology in the AD retina [31, 33, 35–39, 41, 44–46, 48, 49, 51–53, 55, 56, 58, 60, 62, 138]. Furthermore, studies employing comparable tissue processing methodologies, including vitreous body removal and optimal staining protocols employing antigen retrievals, have shown great similarities between retinal Aβ plaques in flatmounts (en face visualization) and brain Aβ plaques (Figs. 6.4a–c and 6.5a, b), while Aβ deposits in retinal cross-sections (vertical visualization) appear morphologically different (see TEM image in Fig. 6.3g).

Among the different Aβ alloforms, the amyloidogenic 42-residue-long ($A\beta_{42}$) peptide is regarded as the most pathognomonic in AD and has been shown to disrupt brain synaptic integrity and long-term potentiation [18, 139–143]. In AD postmortem tissues, the retinal flatmounts showed a significant increase in $A\beta_{42}$ plaques' immunoreactive area in AD patients compared to the individuals with normal cognition (NC) and strongly correlated with the severity of brain Aβ plaque pathology [44]. Moreover, a recent study [45] revealed a significant increase of $A\beta_{42}$ alloform in the superior and inferior temporal retinal cross-sections from MCI and AD patients compared to NC subjects, with a strong correlation to brain Aβ plaque, Braak stage, retinal micro- and macrogliosis, and a strong inverse correlation to retinal thickness and cognition. Furthermore, synaptotoxic intraneuronal Aβ oligomers [17, 144] were identified in the retina with significant increases in MCI and AD patients compared to NC subjects (Fig. 6.5) and were closely associated with exacerbated retinal macrogliosis, tissue atrophy, and cognition [45].

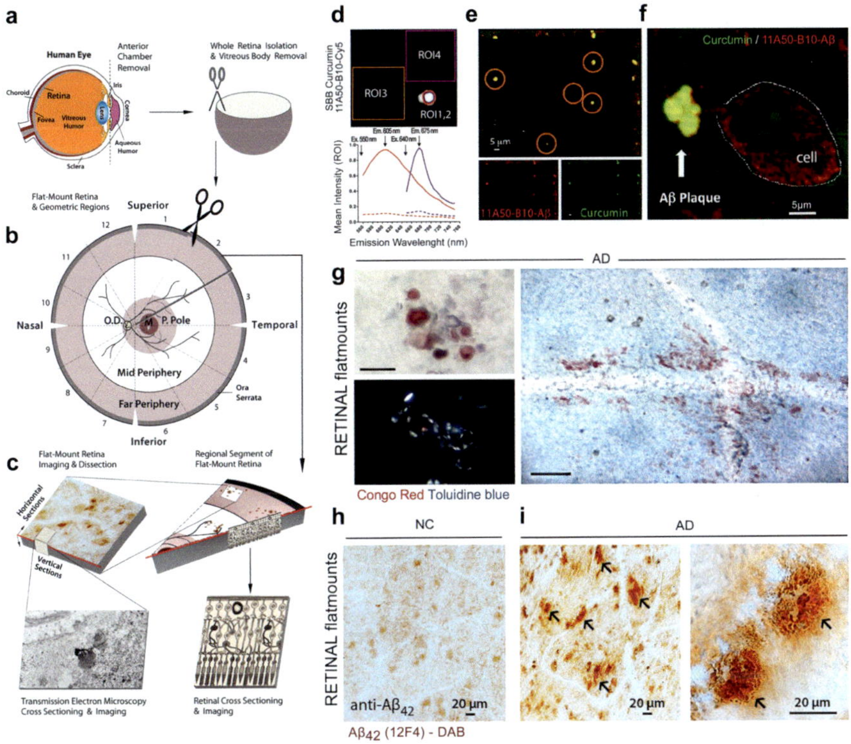

Fig. 6.2 Identification and characterization of Aβ pathology in retinal flatmounts from NC and AD patients. (**a**–**c**) Schematic illustrations of donor eye dissection, retinal isolation, and tissue processing for histological analysis. Whole retinas were isolated, and flatmount and cross-sections were processed in pre-defined geometric regions. Immunohistochemical and transmission electron microscopy (TEM) analyses were conducted. P. Pole, posterior pole; O.D., optic disc; M, macula; F, fovea. (**d**) Representative image and spectral curves of retinal Aβ plaque double-labeled with Sudan Black B (SBB) and curcumin (ROI1; orange line) and with Cy5-antibody 11A50-B10 conjugate (ROI2; purple line), and corresponding background areas (ROI3 and ROI4; dashed lines), at excitation wavelengths of 550 nm (for curcumin spectra) and 640 nm (for 11A50-B10-Cy5 conjugate). Peak wavelengths for curcumin and Cy5-antibody captured in the same individual Aβ plaque are distinct and separable; they remain the same as after single staining. (**e**) Representative images of whole-mount retinas of AD patients following curcumin and anti-human Aβ$_{40}$ mAb (11A50-B10) staining. Clear Aβ plaques were found in AD retinas. Scale bar: 5 μm. (**f**) Aβ plaque at higher magnification. Extracellular Aβ plaque with a compacted large cluster is indicated by an arrow (intracellular Aβ$_{40}$ demarcated by a dotted line). Scale bar: 5 μm. (**g**) Congo red amyloid deposits staining with toluidine blue counterstain in flatmount retinas of AD patients (top left). Birefringence (apple-green) of Congo red-stained retinas under polarized light indicates the presence of amyloid fibrils (bottom left). Scale bar: 25 μm. Congo red-positive amyloid plaques in AD patient retinas (right). Scale bar: 100 μm. Two intersecting blood vessels surrounded (along blood vessels and perivascular) by extensive Congo red-positive staining. (**h**) Representative microscopic images from a definite AD patient and an age- and sex-matched NC individual stained for Aβ$_{42}$ with 12F4 mAb and visualized with peroxidase-based 3,3′ diaminobenzidine (DAB) labeling. Blood vessel structures are seen as lighter lanes. Classical mature Aβ plaques are observed along a retinal blood vessel (right). Scale bar: 20 μm. Illustrations and images in panels **a**-**c**, and **g** are adapted from Koronyo et al., JCI Insight 2017 [44], panels **d**-**f** are reproduced from Koronyo-Hamaoui et al., Neuroimage 2011 [46], and panel **h** is adapted from La Morgia et al., Ann Neurol 2016 [47]

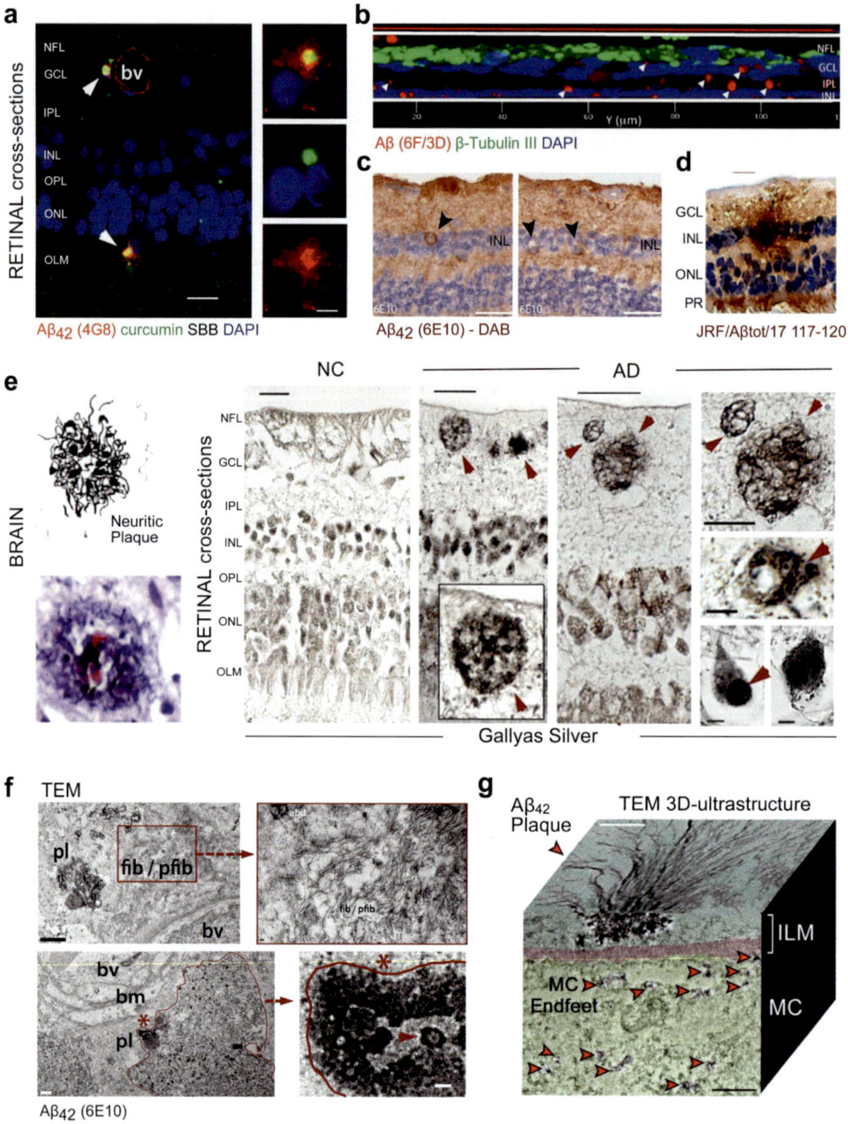
a
RETINAL cross-sections
NFL
GCL
bv
IPL
INL
OPL
ONL
OLM
Aβ42 (4G8) curcumin SBB DAPI
b
NFL
GCL
IPL
INL
Y (μm)
Aβ (6F/3D) β-Tubulin III DAPI
c
INL
Aβ42 (6E10) - DAB
d
GCL
INL
ONL
PR
JRF/Aβtot/17 117-120
e
BRAIN
Neuritic Plaque
NC
AD
Gallyas Silver
f
TEM
pl
fib / pfib
bv
bm
Aβ42 (6E10)
g
Aβ42 Plaque
TEM 3D-ultrastructure
ILM
MC Endfeet
MC

◀**Fig. 6.3** Identification and characterization of Aβ pathology in retinal cross-sections from MCI and AD patients. (**a**) Representative fluorescent images of retinal cross-sections showing Aβ deposits detected in the ONL, and in the GCL near and inside blood vessel walls (bv). Left scale bar: 20 μm. Colocalization of curcumin and 4G8 in a retinal Aβ plaque near DAPI nuclear staining demonstrates each unique staining pattern; right scale bar: 5 μm. (**b**) An orthogonal view of a set of images from an AD eye wholemount Z-stack demonstrates Cy3 (red) Aβ immunofluorescence (arrows) in the NFL, GCL, IPL, and INL. The green fluorescence is β-tubulin III immunoreactivity demonstrating neuronal processes associated with RGC axons in the NFL. (**c**) Representative images of retinal cross-sections showing Aβ plaques around amacrine cells (left) and horizontal cells (right) in the INL region. Scale bar: 50 μm. (**d**) Micrographs of retinal cross-section from an MCI patient that was stained with JRF/Aβtot/17 117–120 mAb (specific to the N¢-terminus of Aβ) with peroxidase-based DAB. Retinal Aβ plaques are seen in the INL. Scale bar: 20 μm. (**e**) Illustration of cerebral senile/neuritic plaque (top left) and Gallyas silver stain (bottom left) with subsequent immunochemistry of neuritic plaque in the hippocampus of an AD patient. Paraffin-embedded retinal cross-sections from AD and NC subjects (right). Scale bar: 20 μm. NC exhibited intact retinal tissue. AD-associated neuropathologies in the AD retina (red arrowheads) were notably observed in the GCL (left). A classic Aβ plaque and compact deposits are shown with a higher-magnification image in the inset. Neuritic components of senile plaques in GCL at higher magnification; top right scale bar: 10 μm. Soma-positive silver stain aggregates and nuclear-dominant silver stain (red arrowheads) are observed in GCL and INL. Lower right scale bar: 5 μm. (**f**) TEM analyses of vertical and en face (horizontal) retinal sections from AD patients. Retinas were pre-stained with 12F4 immunoperoxidase-based system and DAB substrate chromogen. Top left: TEM image showing the ultrastructure of Aβ plaque (pl), fibrils (fib), and protofibrils (pfib) near a blood vessel (bv) in vertical sections. Scale bar: 1 μm. Higher-magnification image (top right), indicating the presence of 10- to 150-nm-wide Aβ fibrils as well as protofibrils and Aβ deposits (abd). Scale bar: 50 nm. Bottom left: Aβ plaque-like structure, marked by an asterisk and bordering red line, near the basement membrane (bm) of a blood vessel (scale bar: 0.5 μm). Higher-magnification image (bottom right) showing the Aβ plaque-like area, with structures resembling paranuclei containing annular oligomers (arrowhead; scale bar: 40 nm). (**g**) 3D-reconstruction of vertical/en face TEM images shows retinal $A\beta_{42}$ plaque ultrastructure with fibril arms emanating from its dense core and Aβ-containing deposits (red arrowheads). ILM: Inner limiting membrane, MC: Müller cell. Scale bar: 1 μm. Images in panels **a**, **e**, and **f** are reproduced from Koronyo et al., JCI Insight 2017 [44], panel **b** is adapted from Lee et al., Front Neurosci, 2020 [48], panel **c** is adapted from den Hann et al., Acta Neuropathol Commun 2018 [35], panels **d** and **g** are reproduced from Koronyo et al., Acta Neuropathol 2023 [45]

Retinal $A\beta_{1\text{-}42}$ and $A\beta_{1\text{-}40}$ detected by ELISA showed a significant (6- and 1.8-fold respectively) increase in AD retina compared to NC retina [45, 58]. Moreover, another study detected higher levels of retinal high-molecular-weight (HMW) $A\beta_{42}$ and $A\beta_{40}$ in AD patients with high cerebral Aβ plaque scores, and those who were apolipoprotein E ε4 allele (APOEε4) carriers [55]. Importantly, the levels of retinal $A\beta_{42}$- and $A\beta_{40}$-HMW were significantly correlated with respective levels in the hippocampus as well as with cerebral NFT scores [55]. $A\beta_{40}$ and $A\beta_{42}$ alloforms were also identified in retinal blood vessel walls and perivascular regions [44, 56, 58]. The deposits of these Aβ alloform were identified in the tunica intima, media, and adventitia of the blood vessel walls [58]. Evaluation of postmortem retinas revealed an early and progressive decrease in vascular PDGFRβ in MCI and AD compared to NC. Retinal PDGFRβ loss significantly associated with increased retinal vascular $A\beta_{40}$ and $A\beta_{42}$ burden. Vascular $A\beta_{40}$ levels in pre-defined retinal

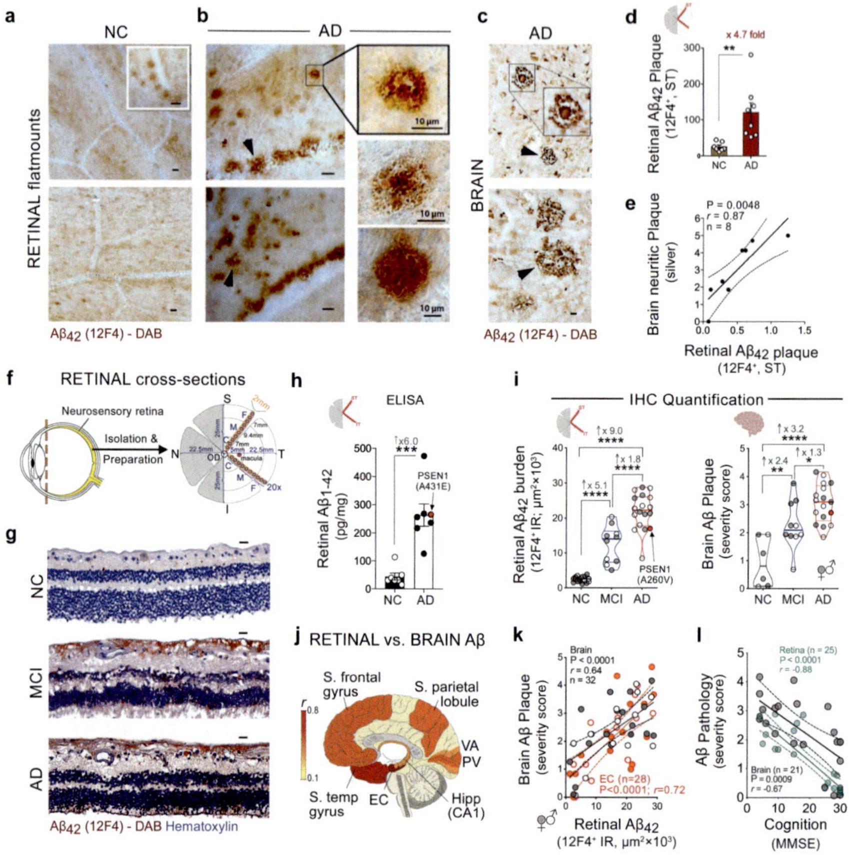
a
NC
RETINAL flatmounts
Aβ42 (12F4) - DAB
b
AD
10 μm
c
AD
BRAIN
Aβ42 (12F4) - DAB
d
x 4.7 fold
Retinal Aβ42 Plaque (12F4⁺, ST)
NC
AD
e
P = 0.0048
r = 0.87
n = 8
Brain neuritic Plaque (silver)
Retinal Aβ42 plaque (12F4⁺, ST)
f
RETINAL cross-sections
Neurosensory retina
Isolation & Preparation
g
NC
MCI
AD
Aβ42 (12F4) - DAB Hematoxylin
h
ELISA
Retinal Aβ1-42 (pg/mg)
PSEN1 (A431E)
NC
AD
i
IHC Quantification
Retinal Aβ42 burden (12F4⁺ IR; μm²×10³)
PSEN1 (A260V)
Brain Aβ Plaque (severity score)
NC
MCI
AD
j
RETINAL vs. BRAIN Aβ
S. frontal gyrus
S. parietal lobule
VA
PV
S. temp gyrus
EC
Hipp (CA1)
k
Brain
P < 0.0001
r = 0.64
n = 32
EC (n=28)
P<0.0001; r=0.72
Brain Aβ Plaque (severity score)
Retinal Aβ42 (12F4⁺ IR, μm²×10³)
l
Retina (n = 25)
P < 0.0001
r = -0.88
Brain (n = 21)
P = 0.0009
r = -0.67
Aβ Pathology (severity score)
Cognition (MMSE)

◀**Fig. 6.4** Parallels between retinal and brain Aβ pathology in MCI and AD patients. Representative micrographs from flatmount retinas (**a–b**) and brains (**c**) of AD patients and age- and sex-matched NC stained with 12F4 using peroxidase-DAB labeling. Scale bar: 20 μm. High-magnification images display diverse Aβ aggregate morphology, including diffuse, compact, and "classical" mature plaques. Scale bar: 10 μm. (**d**) Quantitative 12F4-immunoreactive area of $A\beta_{42}$-containing plaques (geometric region: superotemporal ST1xx-3) in a subset of confirmed AD patients and age- and sex-matched NC. (**e**) Pearson's r correlation analysis between retinal $12F4^{+}$-plaque burden and cerebral plaques. (**f**) Schematic representation of analyzed retinal cross-sections in predefined geometrical regions, including superior- and inferior temporal (ST/IT) strips (orange), extending from the optic disc (OD) to the ora serrata and separated into subregions: central (C), mid-periphery (M), and far periphery (F). (**g**) Representative micrographs of retinal cross-sections from MCI and AD patients compared to NC controls immunolabeled with $12F4^{+}$-$A\beta_{42}$ using peroxidase-based DAB and hematoxylin counterstaining. Scale bar: 20 μm. (**h**) Retinal $A\beta_{1\text{-}42}$ levels determined by ELISA are shown in a cohort of NC and autosomal-dominant AD patients (patient with *PSEN1*-A431E mutation, red circle). (**i**) Violin plots display quantitative-IHC analysis of retinal $A\beta_{42}$-immunoreactive area in age- and sex-matched patients with premortem clinical diagnoses of NC, MCI, or AD, and paired-brain Aβ-plaque severity scores in NC, MCI, and AD patients. The red circle represents an autosomal-dominant AD patient with an A260V mutation in *PSEN1*. (**j**) Mid-sagittal brain illustration shows color-grading magnitude of Pearson's correlation coefficient (r) values between retinal $A\beta_{42}$ burden and brain pathology in the hippocampus (Hipp), superior (S.) frontal gyrus and temporal (temp) gyrus, S. parietal lobule, entorhinal cortex (EC), primary visual (PV), and visual association (VA) cortices. (**k**) Scatterplot presents correlations between retinal $A\beta_{42}$ area and Aβ plaques in the brain (gray) or EC (orange). (**l**) Pearson's correlations between retinal $A\beta_{42}$ area (green) or brain Aβ burden (gray) and the Mini-Mental State Examination (MMSE)-cognitive scores. $^{*}P < 0.05$, $^{**}P < 0.01$, $^{***}P < 0.001$, $^{****}P < 0.0001$, by one-way ANOVA and Tukey's post hoc multiple comparison test, or by two-tailed paired Student's t test. Images and data in panels **a–e** are reproduced from Koronyo et al., JCI Insight 2017 [44], illustrations, images, and data in panels **f–l** are reproduced from Koronyo et al., Acta Neuropathol 2023 [45]

subregions indicated that certain geometrical and cellular layers are more susceptible to AD pathology. $A\beta_{42}$ deposits were identified in pericytes. Furthermore, correlations were identified between retinal vascular abnormalities and cerebral Aβ burden, cerebral amyloid angiopathy (CAA), and clinical status [58]. Retinal arterioles $A\beta_{40}$ deposits were correlated with a severe decrease in retinal vascular tight junction, zonula occludens-1 (ZO-1), and claudin-5, and the deficiency in retinal claudin-5 was strongly associated with CAA, while ZO-1 defects correlated with brain pathology and cognitive status [56].

The development of noninvasive *in vivo* retinal amyloid imaging using oral curcumin administration shows the feasibility of detecting retinal amyloid deposits. In vivo curcumin imaging revealed increased amyloid deposits in asymptomatic AD with high cerebral amyloid, MCI, and AD patients compared to NC subjects [37, 38, 44, 52, 60]. Additionally, several studies reported label-free hyperspectral imaging methods to identify and quantify amyloid deposits in the retina by capturing the spectral signatures of retinal amyloid aggregates [36, 41, 49, 51, 90, 145]. These independent studies reported the potential of hyperspectral imaging as an amyloid retinal imaging modality to screen AD, as retinal amyloid scores were correlated with brain Aβ loads and spectral deviations from NC subjects, obtained at the MCI stage with MMSE scores ≥ 22 [41, 51]. Moreover, the ex-vivo study by

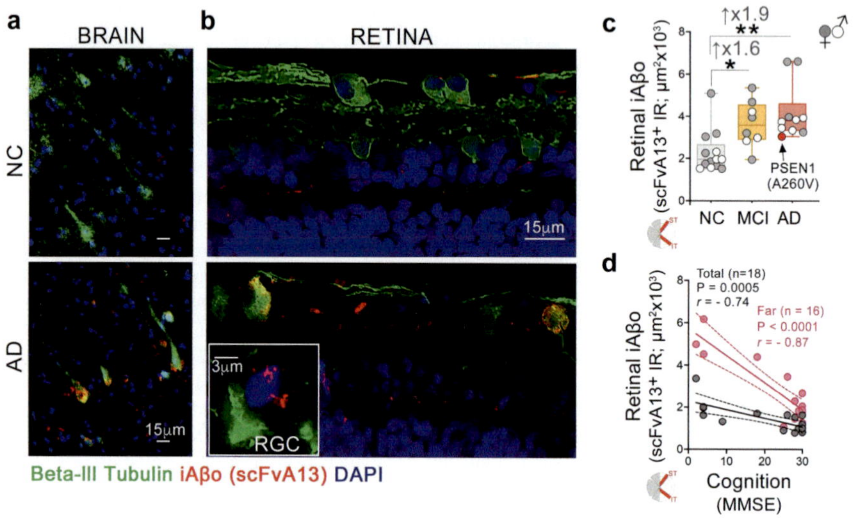

Fig. 6.5 Discovery of retinal Aβ oligomers in AD patients. (**a**) Representative microscopic images of postmortem brain cross-sections show the existence of intracellular Aβ oligomers (iAβO) detected by scFvA13 (red), selectively recognizing AD-relevant Aβ oligomers inside cortical pyramidal neurons in AD patients with minimal signal in NC controls. Scale bar: 15 μm. (**b**) Microscopic images of retinal cross-sections showing iAβO inside β-III-tubulin$^+$-ganglion cells and nerve fibers (green) in AD patients, while less so in NC controls. Scale bar: 15 μm. Insert image: iAβO$^+$-RGC. Scale bar: 3 μm. (**c**) A quantitative analysis of scFvA13$^+$-iAβO-immunoreactive area in ST/IT retina in MCI and AD patients versus NC controls (red circle, an autosomal-dominant AD patient with *PSEN1*-A260V mutation). (**d**) Pearson's correlations of ST/IT retinal iAβO versus MMSE cognitive scores. $^*P < 0.05$, $^{**}P < 0.01$, by one-way ANOVA with Tukey's post hoc multiple comparison test. All panels are reproduced from Koronyo et al., Acta Neuropathol 2023 [45]

Du et al., revealed the feasibility of detecting the signature of retinal pTau, besides Aβ signatures, and demonstrated an accurate prediction of Aβ and pTau distribution powered by deep learning prediction [36]. Overall, these mounting studies from AD patients confirm the presence of AD-specific Aβ species in the retina and highlight the significant similarities between retinal and brain vulnerability to AD pathology.

6.2.2 Retinal Aβ Pathology in Animal Models of AD

In line with findings in MCI and AD human subjects, numerous studies examining the retina of sporadic and transgenic AD (ADtg) animal models have reported the deposition of soluble and insoluble Aβ, often associated with local inflammation, RGC degeneration, and visual deficits. These AD animal models include a large group of ADtg rodent models, such as Tg2576, $APP_{SWE}/PS1_{\Delta E9}$, APP/PS1, 3xTg,

5xFAD mice, the TgF344-AD rat, and *Octodon (O.) degus* [31, 41, 46, 61, 80–82, 88, 90–92, 101, 146–149]. A few of these studies reported an increase in the production of the most pathognomonic forms of Aβ, $A\beta_{40}$ and particularly $A\beta_{42}$, in the retina of rodent AD models [31, 61, 80, 81, 88, 101, 146, 147, 149] and even in ADtg drosophila [150, 151]. Insoluble Aβ formations and plaque deposits have been observed in the retinas of transgenic 2576, $APP_{SWE}/PS1_{\Delta E9}$, $APP_{SWE}/PS1_{M146L/L286V}$, 3xTg, and 5xFAD mice, as well as *O. degus* [31, 46, 80, 82, 88, 90–92, 100, 101, 119, 149, 152]. Cross-sectional analysis of tg2576 mouse retinas identified plaque pathology in ~85% of transgenic mice, as opposed to a consistent absence in wild-type (WT) controls. These plaques were primarily reported in the various nuclear retinal layers (NFL, GCL, INL, and ONL) [88, 149]. However, one study reported minimal to no detection of retinal Aβ pathology in a tg2576 mouse positive for cerebral amyloid burden under enzyme-linked immunosorbent assay (ELISA) and Western blot [81]. Studies on 5xFAD mice, ADtg mice expressing both amyloid and tau-associated pathologies, showed detectable levels of $A\beta_{42}$ and $A\beta_{40}$ in a number of ocular tissues, including the retina, and revealed notable increases in $A\beta_{40}$ in the non-neural RPE [41, 146, 147]. The sporadic, naturally occurring *O. degus* model of AD appears to display a progressive abundance of Aβ deposition, initially arising in the NFL, GCL, and photoreceptors, then spreading to the remaining retinal layers. Histological examination of whole retinas showed Aβ oligomer expression and Aβ peptides in the inner and outer segments of the photoreceptors, the NFL, and GCL, while the greatest plaque burden was detected in the central regions, determined via a number of Aβ-specific staining methods, except Congo red [80].

The transmembrane amyloid precursor protein (APP), the source of the toxic Aβ protein, has been identified in the retinas of numerous transgenic animal models for AD, including drosophila, and various mouse and rat models (Tg2576, $hTgAPP^{tg/tg}$, $APP_{SWE}/PS1_{\Delta E9}$, and $APP_{SWE}/PS1_{M146L/L286V}$, TgF344-AD), as well as the non transgenic, sporadic rodent strain *O. degus* [61, 80, 81, 88, 91, 153]. Analysis of cytoplasmic APP levels in retinal layers revealed a marked increase in ADtg models [81, 91], while the sporadic *O. degus* shows a reduction with age [81]. A study by Ning et al., in 2008 identified APP immunoreactivity within cells of the GCL and INL but not the ONL. Additionally, the neuropil of the inner and outer plexiform layers (IPL and OPL) as well as the outer segment (OS) and retinal pigmented epithelium (RPE) displayed elevated APP levels. These regions exhibited elevated APP immunoreactivity with age [91]. Interestingly, retinal Aβ plaque and Aβ oligomer formations were also detected prior to the corresponding brain burden [46, 86]. Studies on the positive effects of therapy on cerebral Aβ and tauopathy burden of ADtg animal models have also described similar responses observed in the respective retina [46, 88, 101, 119, 147, 152, 154, 155]. These findings have not only been invaluable in understanding the disease characteristics and progression but have also provided the foundation for the potential role of the retina as a measure of therapeutic efficacy.

One of the most studied ADtg model is the double transgenic $APP_{SWE}/PS1_{\Delta E9}$ mouse strain. A study by Koronyo-Hamaoui et al., utilized curcumin-specific staining of Aβ to visualize retinal plaque distribution [46]. Interestingly, this highly specific protocol for both human and mouse tissue revealed Aβ accumulation in whole-mount retinas prior to its deposition in the corresponding cerebral tissue. When 2.5-month-old mice were intravenously injected with curcumin, curcumin-positive Aβ deposits were detected in isolated retinal flatmounts, further confirmed as Aβ-specific deposits by *ex vivo* 4G8 monoclonal antibody staining, and were observed prior to their appearance in the respective brains. Retinal cross-section analysis demonstrated the presence of Aβ deposits in the innermost retinal layers of adult ADtg mice, as well as in the choroid and surrounding scleral tissue, with minimal to no fluorescence in non-ADtg controls [46]. Another study also revealed that retinal Aβ immunoreactivity was present in the inner retinal layers and consisted of small speck-like extracellular deposits and intracellular labeling in the cytoplasm of a subset of RGCs. *In vivo* retinal fluorescence with curcumin injection was significantly greater in older mice (11–19 months) than in younger mice (5–9 months) in both ADtg and WT groups and was significantly greater in ADtg than in WT in older mice (ages 11–19 months). Importantly, this study also revealed a stronger correlation between *in vivo* retinal fluorescence with curcumin injection and Aβ immunoreactivity in the cortex of ADtg compared to WT groups [96]. Similar findings were reported in a number of other studies using the same mouse model and 344F-ADtg rats, which share the same double transgenes [61, 88, 91, 92]. In agreement with the above-mentioned studies, a study by Grimaldi et al., reported the presence of retinal Aβ plaques and tau tangles in the RGC layer of young, pre-symptomatic 3xTg mice [102].

Noninvasive *in vivo* retinal imaging has provided the opportunity to monitor alterations in amyloid burden following therapeutic intervention. Studies aimed at determining co-reactions between retinal and cerebral amyloid burden in response to therapies provide valuable insight into the applicability of retinal imaging as a tool for measuring therapeutic efficacy. In 2009, Liu et al., reported the retinal response to subcutaneous amyloid-peptide vaccination in tg2576 mice. Specifically, islet amyloid polypeptide and Aβ oligomer immunizations resulted in significant reductions in histological examinations of retinal amyloid burden. Interestingly, retinal amyloid angiopathy was markedly increased with these treatments, along with microglial and astroglial reactivity. Retinal thickness was greater with treatment compared to sham-controls, but still displayed thinning compared to non-treated WT [88].

One of these therapies involves the FDA-approved drug, glatiramer acetate (GA; brand name Copaxone), currently deployed for treating remitting-relapsing multiple sclerosis and repurposed for studies on the effects of immunomodulation in AD. Over the past few years, the Koronyo-Hamaoui group has published their findings on the beneficial effects of GA and a similar myelin-derived therapy, modified myelin oligodendrocyte glycoprotein-derived peptide (MOG45D), which was loaded onto dendritic cells (DC-45D) [46, 119]. Their initial investigation of MOG45D treatment on APP/PS1 mice in 2010 reported a remarkable

69% reduction of curcumin- and 4G8-positive retinal Aβ area assessed ex vivo. Importantly, this retinal response was comparable to the attenuation of the corresponding cerebral burden [46]. Subsequent studies utilizing GA produced the first *in vivo* assessment of retinal Aβ deposition, revealing decreased deposition following 1- and 2-month regimens [119]. In addition, Doustar et al., reported that GA immunomodulation significantly reduced the expression of APP/Aβ both in the brain and retina in a cohort of old, late-stage ADtg mice [101]. An additional study by Yang et al., on bone marrow transplantation in APP/PS1 mice showed significant reductions of retinal and cerebral amyloid plaque burden when compared to non-treated controls [152]. Importantly, Kile et al., reported that intravenous immunoglobulin treatment in MCI subjects over 2 months led to the reduction in amyloid deposits both in the brain and retina [156], suggesting its potential therapeutic value in AD patients. These similar therapeutic responses in AD brain and retina could be because of the similarity in the degree and progression of AD pathogenesis in the brain and retina. Indeed, parallel changes in proteome signatures have been recently reported [45] from the temporal cortex and the retina of AD patient as compared to cognitively normal individuals.

Collectively, the abundance of studies published in the past decade strongly supports the retina as an extension of the brain in the context of AD. It may faithfully function as a reliable tool for measuring disease progression and therapeutic response.

6.2.3 Retinal Tauopathy in AD Patients

Aberrant hyperphosphorylation of tau and its NFT inclusions are key characteristic signs of AD that strongly reflect neuronal injury and cognitive decline [157–160]. In 2012, the disease-associated pTau, tau phosphorylated at Ser202/Thr205 (AT8), was first described in post-mortem retinas from confirmed AD cases, while other phosphorylation sites yielded negative results [54]. Recently, different groups have reported site-specific pTau in the AD retina, such as pThr181 (AT270), pThr212/pSer214 (AT100), pThr217 (T217), pSer396 (pS396), and pSer202/pThr205 (AT8) [35, 36, 39, 42]. However, these studies were unable to report tau fibrils or NFTs in the AD retina. These pTau species were principally found in the diverse retinal layers, particularly in the synaptic dense regions as IPL and OPL of AD patients [35, 36, 39, 42, 54]. Importantly, pTau (AT8) staining was more apparent in the superior retina than in the medial retina, with a positive gradient towards the periphery [35].

A recent finding revealed that retinal pTau (Ser202/Thr205 and Thr217) was found in amacrine and horizontal cells of the INL, and both markers showed significant discrimination between AD and other tauopathies, as well as non-tauopathy cases, including controls. However, there were no differences in the immunopositivity of other pTau epitopes (Thr212/Ser214, Thr181, and Ser396) between the groups. Importantly, the presence of retinal pTau Ser202/Thr205 and Thr217 correlated with the Braak stage for NFTs and with the presence of pTau Ser202/Thr205 in hippocampus and cortical brain regions [42]. A few studies were not able to confirm the findings of pTau in the human retina [136, 137], possibly due to the methodological issues.

To date, there have been no studies related to noninvasive *in vivo* imaging of human retinal tauopathy. However, a recent study identified the specific optical signature of retinal pTau (pTauS396) that can be detected label-free in histologically stained human retinal tissue using hyperspectral imaging, and further confirmed by deep-learning prediction of unstained tissue [36]. This pTauS396 optical signature, along with other disease-associated pTau signatures that may be developed in the future, can serve as a marker for retinal noninvasive hyperspectral imaging in AD. The known tauopathy-related changes in the human AD retina are depicted in Fig. 6.6.

Different pTau species have been identified in the post-mortem retina of AD patients; however, only one study detected NFT-like structures in AD retinas using Gallyas silver staining [44]. Nevertheless, the colocalization of pTau and sites of neuronal loss in the human AD retina [39, 44] indicates a similar pathophysiological vulnerability to pTau accumulation in the retina and brain. Despite this, there is still a limited understanding of the impact of retinal tauopathy in humans, its association with other retinal AD findings, and how this correlates with the complexities of AD pathology in the brain, ultimately resulting in cognitive impairment.

6.2.4 Retinal Tauopathy in Animal Models of AD

Increased retinal tauopathy has also been observed in AD animal models. Zhao et al., [100] reported elevated levels of different epitopes of phosphorylated tau (i.e., at Thr231, Thr205, or Ser396) in the retinas of double transgenic APP/PS1 mice, as shown by Western blot analysis, along with NFTs through immunohistochemical analysis. Interestingly, this increased hyperphosphorylated tau in the retina of APP/PS1 ADtg mice is related with the upregulation of p35/p25 and activation of cyclin-dependent kinase 5, which is mediated by calpain [100]. Another study in 3xTg-AD mice detected pTau: pSer202/pThr205 (AT8) pS199 (PS199), and pS396/S404 (PHF1), which correlated with AD severity, and visualization of Western blots probed with AT8 or PHF1 revealed an increase in pTau at these epitopes in 3-month-old 3xTg retinas. The study revealed tau accumulation in the soma and dendrites of RGCs, which surprisingly preceded cerebral accumulation [115]. Notably, retinal tau is distributed in the soma, dendrites, and intraretinal axons of RGCs but is markedly decreased in the optic nerve axons in 3xTg-AD mice, suggesting that in early-stage AD, tau accumulation is lower in RGC axons within the optic nerve [115]. Anterograde transport from RGCs to the superior colliculus in the brain is significantly higher in 3-month-old 3xTg-AD mice treated with tau-targeting siRNA, suggesting that the reduction of retinal tau partially restores RGC axonal transport [115]. Similarly, in a rat model of hyperhomocysteinemia, Guo et al. reported increased levels of Ser262 hyperphosphorylated tau

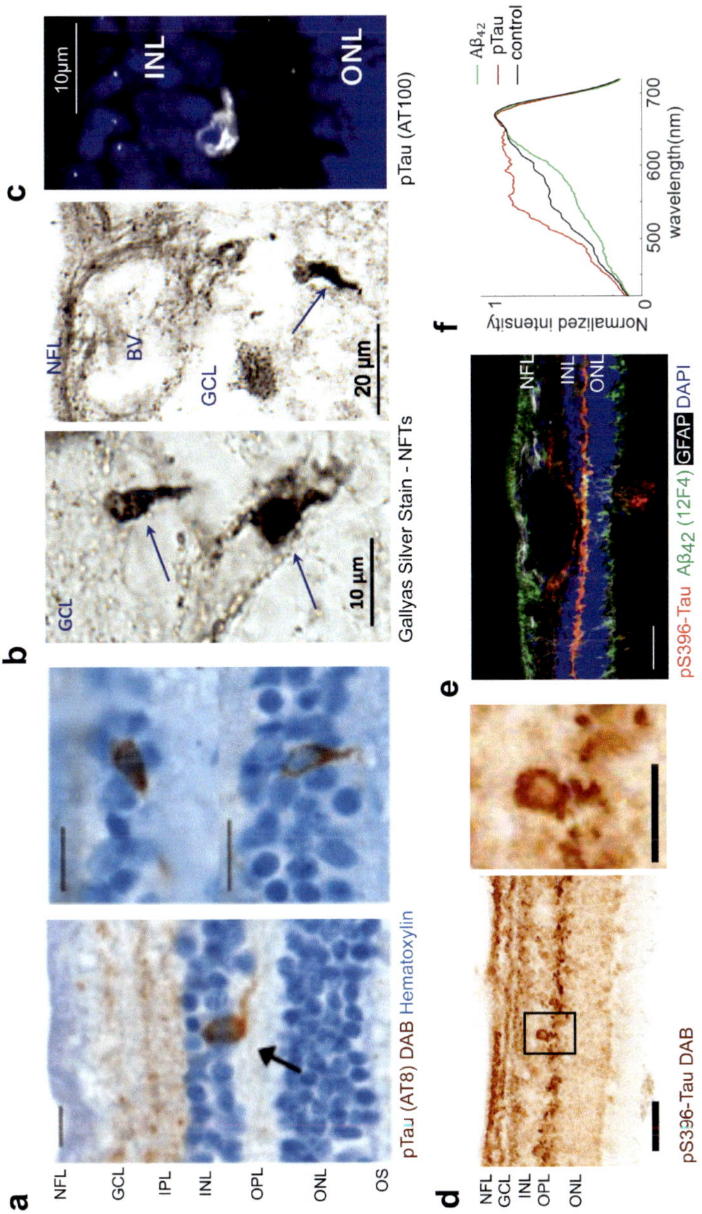
a
NFL
GCL
IPL
INL
OPL
ONL
OS
pTau (AT8) DAB Hematoxylin
b
GCL
10 µm
Gallyas Silver Stain - NFTs
NFL
BV
GCL
20 µm
c
10µm
INL
ONL
pTau (AT100)
d
NFL
GCL
INL
OPL
ONL
pS396-Tau DAB
e
NFL
INL
ONL
pS396-Tau Aβ42 (12F4) GFAP DAPI
f
Normalized intensity
0
1
500
600
700
wavelength(nm)
Aβ42
pTau
control

◀**Fig. 6.6** Retinal tauopathy in MCI and AD patients. (**a**) Representative images from retinal cross-sections of AD patients showing (p)tau (AT8) cells in the INL (arrow) and staining of the plexiform layers and GCL (left), and higher magnification images of individual $AT8^+$ cells in the INL (right). Scale bars: 10 μm. (**b**) Neurofibrillary tangles (NFTs) in retinal cross-sections of definite AD patients. Gallyas Silver staining shows intraneuronal positive staining resembling NFTs, especially in the retinal GCL (marked with blue arrows). (**c**) A (p)tau $(AT100)^+$ cell in retinal INL from an AD patient. (**d**) Immunostaining for pS396-Tau and peroxidase labeling (brown) in retinal cross-section from an AD patient, demonstrating intracellular and intra-processes pS396-tau aggregates in the OPL and NFL to IPL. High-magnification image showing a retinal NFT-like structure. (**e**) Immunofluorescence staining showing positive signals for 12F4-$A\beta_{42}$ (green), pS396-tau (red), $GFAP^+$ astrocytes (white), and DAPI nuclei (blue) in a retinal cross-section of an AD patient. (**f**) Hyperspectral imaging identifies the spectral signatures of $A\beta_{42}$ (green line) and pS396-tau (red line) in the human AD retina. BV, Blood vessel. Panel **a** is adapted from Schön et al., PLoS One 2012 [54], panel **b** is reproduced from Koronyo et al., JCI Insight 2017 [44], panel **c** is from Koronyo-Hamaoui Lab (Unpublished Data), and panels **d**-**f** are reproduced from Du et al., PNAS Nexus 2022 [36] in the retina earlier than in the hippocampus [161]. Importantly, a few other reports suggested the presence of tangles of hyperphosphorylated tau in the retina of ADtg mice [100, 102]. More recently, Rodrigues-Neves et al., [162] corroborated previous results by reporting an increase in phosphorylated tau at Ser396 in the retina of 3xTg-AD mice at both 4 and 8 months of age. Du et al., detected increased tau phosphorylation of pSer202/pThr205 (AT8) and pS235 in the retina of aging *O. degus*, a sporadic AD rodent model [80]. The NH2htau, a truncated tau fragment, immunoreactivity appeared to be significantly increased in postnatal (p28) reelin-deficient mice retina compared to WT controls [163]. Similarly, a study revealed that an N-terminal-domain truncated tau is associated with the degeneration of the retina in transgenic 2576 mice (carrying a mutant form of APP linked to early-onset familial AD), highlighting the role of other post-transcriptional modifications of tau during AD progression [164]. Increased tau phosphorylation was observed in retinal photoreceptor cells stimulated by $A\beta_{1-42}$ fragment in culture [165].

Several studies have revealed that tau accumulation in the retina is associated with retinal neurodegeneration, as evidenced by RGC death, neurotrophic dysfunction, and impairment of glutamatergic photoreceptor synapse during tauopathy in AD animal models [100, 115, 166, 167]. Similarly, tau hyperphosphorylation was associated with retinal neurotoxicity in Drosophila [168] and triggered the post-synaptic toxicity of APP/$A\beta_{1-42}$, the causative agents of AD, in the neuromuscular junction [169]. Ngolab et al., found that mutant 3R tau can mediate toxicity in RGCs by promoting caspase-2 expression, which results in RGC degeneration in animal models of Pick's disease [170].

Tau oligomers have been associated with increased inflammatory responses in the retina of mice with tauopathy and in neurodegenerative diseases. In P301L transgenic mice compared to WT controls, the tau oligomers co-localize with astrocytes, microglia, and HMGB1, a pro-inflammatory cytokine [167]. Grimaldi et al., reported the significant elevation of hyperphosphorylated tau in the retina of 3xTg-AD mice. Importantly, during the pre symptomatic (5–20 weeks) and late disease (50–80 weeks) stages, tau distribution was significantly higher in the inner retina. However, during the early disease stage (30–40 weeks), a similar tau distribution was observed in both the inner and outer retinal layers, suggesting the profound tau distribution in the retina during different disease stages [102]. In the transgenic CRND8 mouse model of AD, Buccarello et al., reported increased tau hyperphosphorylation in the retina, which correlated with increased C-JUN and JNK phosphorylation and reduced NFL/GCL thickness. Their results suggest that degenerative changes in the retina of the AD mouse model mirror the events observed in the brain parenchyma [171]. Additionally, retinal vascular abnormalities, such as decreased vessel density and increased acellular capillary formation indicating vascular degeneration, were reported in the mouse model of tauopathy [172]. Despite hyperphosphorylated tau being pathogenic in AD, tau protein is essential for normal tissue homeostasis. Loss of tau has been associated with progressive neurodegeneration and defects in retinal photoreceptor development [173]. Collectively, profound tauopathy has been reported in the retina of AD animal models.

6.2.5 Retinal Degeneration in AD Patients

The pathological hallmarks of AD in the brain are hypothesized to induce and amplify neuroinflammation and vascular abnormalities, eventually leading to neurodegeneration and cognitive decline. In alignment with the observed distribution of retinal Aβ deposits and pTau in AD patients, mounting histological reports indicate structural damage in the AD retina, leading to retinal atrophy. This includes optic nerve atrophy, macular degeneration, NFL thinning, and RGC degeneration, particularly in the superior quadrant of the retina [44, 45, 47, 63, 66–68, 71, 76]. Clinical and histopathological findings both suggest primary impairment of larger the caliber magnocellular pathway that specializes in contrast sensitivity and motion detection [174]. Koronyo et al., provided evidence for substantial neuronal degeneration (22–29%) across several retinal layers, including the GCL, INL, and ONL in AD patients compared to age-matched controls. Importantly, such neurodegeneration was observed at sites of Aβ deposition [44]. The same group recently reported the comparable extent of tissue atrophy in the brain and retina, revealing the parallel neurodegeneration [45]. Retinal thickness was strongly correlated with retinal $A\beta_{42}$/oligomeric-Aβ and brain Aβ plaques and cognition [45]. In addition, a morphometric analysis of post-mortem retinas indicated increased retinal atrophy across retinal layers in AD patients relative to cognitively normal controls [63]. Retinal NFL thinning was most pronounced superotemporally and in the peripapillary region. Importantly, this pattern of retinal layer atrophy was very similar to the distribution of retinal amyloid deposits observed in the mid- and far-periphery of the superior retinal quadrant of AD patients [37, 44, 45, 47]. Furthermore, RGC dysfunction was identified by electroretinography in early-stage preclinical AD patients, preceding cognitive decline [175]. These studies reveal profound neurodegeneration in the AD retina, which can function as potential markers of cerebral neurodegeneration.

Histopathological examination of the AD retina revealed significant degeneration of melanopsin-containing RGCs (mRGCs), closely linked to Aβ accumulation within and around these cells [47]. This subpopulation of RGCs influences photoentrainment and project their axons to the SCN, a brain region that controls circadian rhythms. Thus, mRGCs are thought to be vital to regulating sleep–wake cycles. The selective loss of mRGCs may indicate that Aβ is particularly detrimental to certain retinal cell subtypes, providing the first potential retina-based mechanistic explanation for the circadian rhythm disturbances observed in AD patients [176]. Figures 6.7 and 6.8 summarize the findings on retinal degeneration in AD patients. Overall, the accumulation of retinal Aβ and pTau, together with inflammatory cascades and vascular dysfunction, ultimately leads to irreversible neurodegeneration in the retina of AD patients, possibly contributing to visual dysfunction and circadian disturbances. Indeed, a recent study revealed that retinal atrophy correlated with brain AD pathology and atrophy [45].

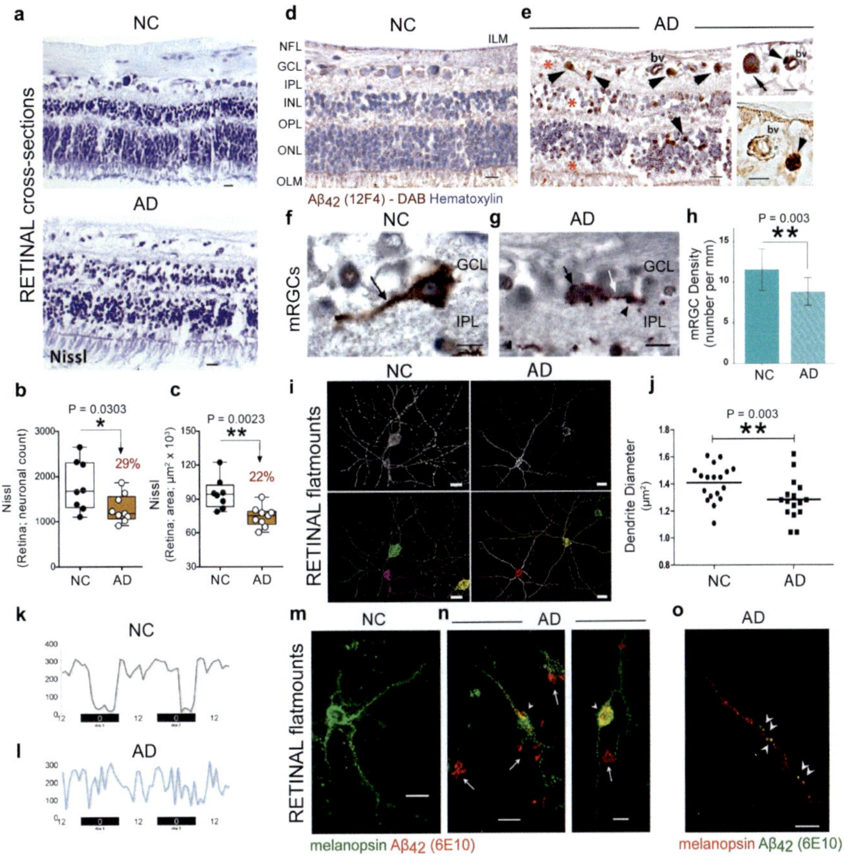

a
NC
AD
RETINAL cross-sections
Nissl
d
NC
NFL
GCL
IPL
INL
OPL
ONL
OLM
ILM
e
AD
bv
Aβ42 (12F4) - DAB Hematoxylin
f
NC
mRGCs
GCL
IPL
g
AD
GCL
IPL
h
P = 0.003
**
mRGC Density (number per mm)
NC
AD
b
P = 0.0303
*
29%
Nissl (Retina; neuronal count)
NC
AD
c
P = 0.0023
**
22%
Nissl (Retina; area; μm² x 10³)
NC
AD
i
NC
AD
RETINAL flatmounts
j
P = 0.003
**
Dendrite Diameter (μm²)
NC
AD
k
NC
l
AD
m
NC
RETINAL flatmounts
melanopsin Aβ42 (6E10)
n
AD
o
AD
melanopsin Aβ42 (6E10)

◂**Fig. 6.7** Retinal neurodegeneration in AD patients. (**a**) Representative images of Nissl staining of retinal cross-sections from a definite AD patients and age- and sex-matched NC subjects. Altered Nissl neuronal staining is observed in AD patients; changes in cytoplasmic staining patterns (chromatolysis) that could be associated with neuronal loss are observed in the retinal GCL, INL, and ONL. Scale bar: 20 μm. (**b–c**) Quantitative Nissl neuronal count and total area in a subset of AD patients and age- and sex-matched NC. Percentage change compared with NC is in red. (**d–e**) Paraffin-embedded retinal cross-sections from superior quadrants of AD patients and matched NCs stained with 12F4 and peroxidase-based labeling (brown) followed by hematoxylin counter stain for nuclei (violet). Retinas of AD patients contained a multitude of Aβ deposits (arrowheads), especially in the GCL. Marked loss of retinal cells is apparent in the GCL, INL, and ONL; areas of nuclei loss are indicated by asterisks. Scale bar: 20 μm. Higher-magnification images are shown. Intracellular cytoplasmic Aβ (top; arrow). Aβ deposits near and inside blood vessel walls (bottom; bv; arrowheads); these vascular and perivascular deposits are frequent in GCL. Scale bar: 10 μm. (**f–g**) Single mRGC in the GCL of a NC and AD retina. Note the homogeneous staining of the cell body and dendrite (arrow) in the NC and the patchy staining of melanopsin in the cell body (black arrow) of the AD. A single dendrite can be seen with a focal attenuation (white arrow) and varicosity (arrowhead). (**h**) Quantification of mRGC density in NC and AD patients. (**i**) Morphological analysis of NC (top left) and AD (top right) mRGCs. Stacks of images of mRGCs were generated, and a 3-dimensional reconstruction was performed followed by analysis of the processes using the filament trace module in Imaris (Bitplane). Three cells (green, purple, and yellow) and their dendritic processes are visualized (bottom images). Scale bars: 25 μm. (**j**) Quantitative analysis of dendrite diameter demonstrating a significant reduction of dendrite diameter in AD patients. (**k–l**) Representative actigraphic profiles are shown for a NC, and an AD patient with a severe disruption of the rest–activity circadian rhythm. (**m**) Representative micrograph from a NC individual demonstrates an intact mRGC having long dendrites without the presence of Aβ. (**n**) Representative micrographs from AD patients demonstrating intracellular Aβ deposition in mRGCs (arrowheads) as well as extracellular Aβ (arrows). (**o**) An example of an mRGC neurite from an AD retina showing colocalization with Aβ (arrowheads). Scale bars: 20 μm. $*P < 0.05$, $**P < 0.01$, by Student's t-test. Images and data in panels **a–e** are reproduced from Koronyo et al., JCI Insight 2017 [44], panels **f–o** are reproduced from La Morgia et al., Ann Neurol 2016 [47]

6.2.6 Retinal Degeneration in Animal Models of AD

Degeneration of retinal cells is extensively reported in rodent models of AD [85, 91, 177]. For instance, apoptotic cells were detected in the RGC layer of $APP_{SWE}/PS1_{M146L}$ and $APP_{SWE}/PS1_{\Delta E9}$ double transgenic mice [91]. Additionally, a significant reduction in retinal thickness was detected from the RGC layer to the ONL in ADtg mice compared with their WT counterparts [91]. A decrease in retinal thickness indicates the loss of either the photoreceptor cells (rods and cones) in the ONL or neuronal cells in the inner retinal layers (RGCs, bipolar cells, horizontal cells, or amacrine cells). A recent study employing 5xFAD mice with different age groups revealed a close association between retinal neurodegeneration and amyloid pathology, following a progressive pattern in the retina similar to that of the brain [87]. Amyloid deposition in the retina also leads to axonal neurodegeneration in the GCL. As the disease progresses, more widespread retinal dysfunction is observed, manifested by the degeneration of photoreceptors, interneurons, and other inner retinal structures [87]. These multiple studies in AD murine models clearly demonstrate a profound and complex pattern of degeneration that extends across retinal layers and negatively impacts a diverse array of retinal functions.

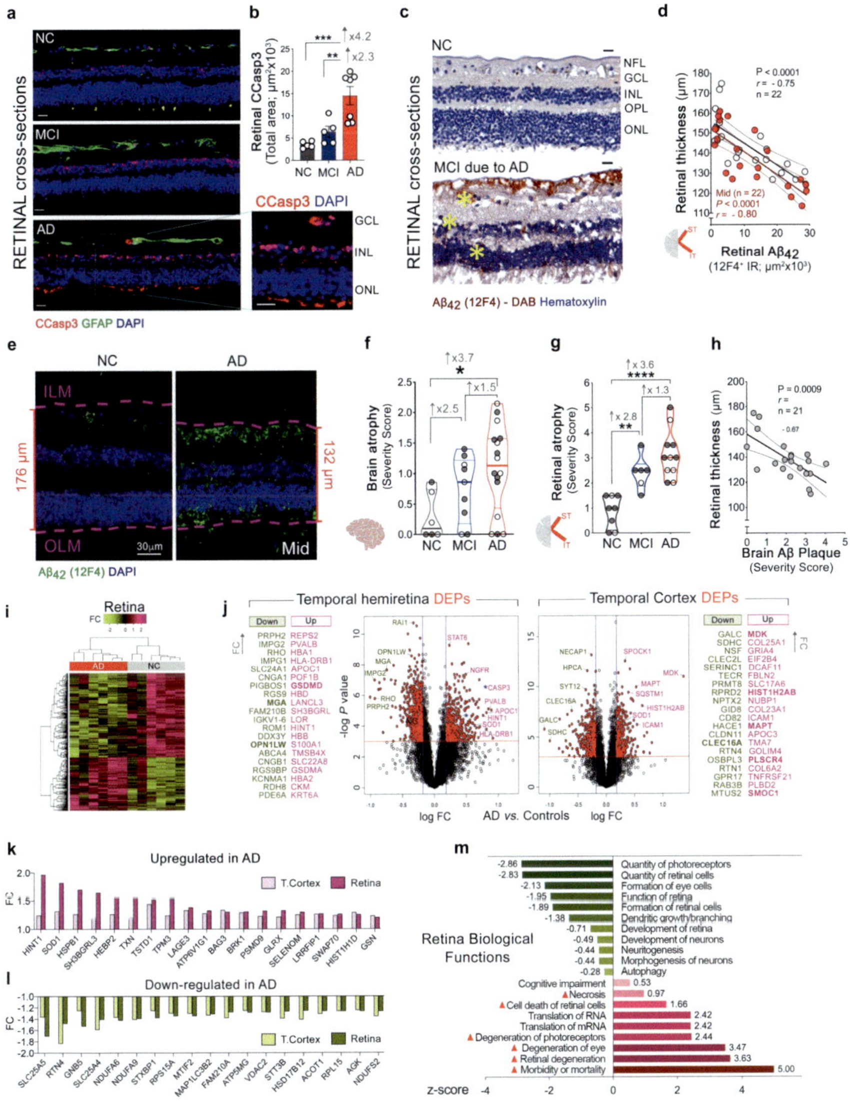

a
RETINAL cross-sections
NC
MCI
AD
CCasp3 GFAP DAPI
b
Retinal CCasp3 (Total area; μm²x10³)
x4.2
x2.3
NC MCI AD
CCasp3 DAPI
GCL
INL
ONL
c
RETINAL cross-sections
NC
NFL
GCL
INL
OPL
ONL
MCI due to AD
Aβ42 (12F4) - DAB Hematoxylin
d
Retinal thickness (μm)
P < 0.0001
r = -0.75
n = 22
Mid (n = 22)
P < 0.0001
r = -0.80
Retinal Aβ42
(12F4⁺ IR; μm²x10³)
e
NC
AD
ILM
OLM
176 μm
132 μm
30μm
Mid
Aβ42 (12F4) DAPI
f
Brain atrophy (Severity Score)
x3.7
x2.5
x1.5
NC MCI AD
g
Retinal atrophy (Severity Score)
x 3.6
x 2.8
x 1.3
NC MCI AD
h
Retinal thickness (μm)
P = 0.0009
r = -0.67
n = 21
Brain Aβ Plaque
(Severity Score)
i
Retina
FC
AD
NC
j
Temporal hemiretina DEPs
Temporal Cortex DEPs
Down
Up
-log P value
log FC
AD vs. Controls
k
Upregulated in AD
T.Cortex
Retina
l
Down-regulated in AD
T.Cortex
Retina
m
Retina Biological Functions
Quantity of photoreceptors
Quantity of retinal cells
Formation of eye cells
Function of retina
Formation of retinal cells
Dendritic growth/branching
Development of retina
Development of neurons
Neuritogenesis
Morphogenesis of neurons
Autophagy
Cognitive impairment
Necrosis
Cell death of retinal cells
Translation of RNA
Translation of mRNA
Degeneration of photoreceptors
Degeneration of eye
Retinal degeneration
Morbidity or mortality
z-score

◀**Fig. 6.8** Retinal atrophy correlates with retinal and cerebral Aβ burden and is identified by proteomics in AD patients. (**a**) Representative retinal cross-sections labeled for cleaved caspase-3 (CCasp3; red), early apoptotic marker, GFAP (green), and DAPI nuclei (blue) in NC, MCI, or AD patients. Zoomed-in inserts illustrate the presence of $CCasp3^+$ cells within the INL and GCL. Scale bar: 20 μm. (**b**) Quantitative CCasp3-immunoreactive area in the ST/IT retina. (**c**) Representative images of retinal cross-sections from NC and MCI due to AD patient containing a multitude of Aβ deposits (asterisk), especially in GCL. Marked loss of retinal cells is apparent in the GCL, INL, and ONL; areas of nuclei loss are indicated by asterisks. Scale bar: 20 μm. (**d**) Scatterplots display Pearson's correlations between retinal thickness and retinal $A\beta_{42}$ burden. (**e**) A reduction in tissue thickness is shown in representative retinal cross-sections from an AD patient (132 μm) versus NC control (176 μm). Thickness was measured from ILM to OLM (purple dashed lines) in the mid-periphery (mid) retinal region. Scale bar: 30 μm. (**f–g**) Quantitative analysis of (**f**) brain atrophy severity scores in a subset of human donors with AD, MCI, or NC, and (**g**) ST/IT retinal atrophy scores for an overlapping subset of patients with AD, MCI, or NC. (**h**) Pearson's correlation between retinal thickness and brain Aβ plaques. (**i**) Heatmap displays the proteomics profiling of retinal tissues with detectable protein hierarchies from the ST/IT temporal hemiretina. (**j**) Volcano plots of the top 20 up- or downregulated differentially expressed proteins (DEPs) organized by fold change (lowest *P* values highlighted in bold) in retinas and temporal cortices of AD versus NC (DEPs marked by red circles). Common (**k**) up- or (**l**) downregulated proteins between the retina and temporal cortex in AD patients versus NCs. (**m**) Ingenuity pathway analysis of the top up- and downregulated biological functions in AD versus NC retinas. $^*P < 0.05$, $^{**}P < 0.01$, $^{***}P < 0.001$, $^{****}P < 0.0001$ by one-way ANOVA and Tukey's post-hoc multiple comparison test. All panels are reproduced from Koronyo et al., Acta Neuropathol 2023 [45]

6.2.7 Retinal Vasculopathy in AD Patients

Accumulating evidence from previous studies indicates that AD pathogenesis is associated with severe effects on cerebral vasculature [15, 178–180]. The vascular complications associated with AD pathogenesis in humans include CAA [181–183], vascular nonperfusion [184–186], uncoupling and degeneration of the neurovascular unit [187–189], aberrant angiogenesis [190, 191], distortions of small blood vessels [192–195], breakdown of the blood–brain barrier (BBB) [196–201], dysregulated glucose metabolism [202, 203], vascular neuroinflammation [204, 205], hypertension [206], atherosclerosis [207], hypercholesterolemia [208], and notably, an accumulation of vascular tau [209, 210].

Similar to the AD brain, numerous studies have described diverse parameters of vascular dysfunction in the AD retina, including decreased blood flow [65, 211], macular degeneration, and Foveal Avascular Zone (FAZ) enlargement [212], compromised microvascular networks [65, 69, 116, 211–217], vein narrowing [65, 69, 211, 213, 215], distorted vascular branching complexity and capillary neovascularization [69, 215], and increased vascular tortuosity [215]. Several studies have reported a significant correlation between retinal vascular damage and AD susceptibility. Nevertheless, these discoveries have provided abundant potential of retinal vascular targets for AD monitoring and diagnosis. Unfortunately, there is a substantial lack of understanding regarding the precise cellular and molecular mechanisms involved in retinal vascular AD pathology because most prior studies extensively focused on live imaging of retinal blood flow dynamics in AD patients.

A few studies addressed this gap in the literature by highlighting the existence of vascular $A\beta_{40}$ and $A\beta_{42}$ deposits in the post-mortem retinas of MCI and AD patients, localized at both perivascular regions and within vessel walls. These deposits involve the tunica intima, media, and adventitia outside the basement membrane [44, 56, 58]. These findings were consistent with known cerebrovascular Aβ pathology [218–222]. Transmission electron microscopy (TEM) analysis confirmed the ultrastructure of retinal $A\beta_{42}$ fibrils near a blood vessel basal membrane (10–15 nm wide) with typical antiparallel β-sheets and in retinal pericytes [44, 58]. Notably, in the brains of APP-overexpressing mice, vascular amyloidosis was found to increase the rigidity of blood vessels and decrease blood flow [223]. These studies suggest profound vascular amyloidosis in AD. The triggered vascular amyloidosis in the AD retina is shown in Fig. 6.9.

The BBB is composed of endothelial cells firmly joined by tight junction (TJ) proteins forming vessel walls, astroglial end-feet, and supporting pericytes in the basement membrane. Similarly, in the retina, the blood-retinal barrier (BRB) is comprised of an inner barrier with vascular endothelial cells and an outer barrier with epithelial cells. Both include TJ proteins and supporting pericytes [224–226]. It is well established that compromised BBB vascular networks in AD are likely an important cause of cerebral amyloid deposition due to impaired Aβ removal to the circulating blood [227–232]. An early and progressive deficiency of vascular PDGFRβ (vPDGFRβ) and apoptotic loss of pericytes in post-mortem retinas of MCI and AD patients were reported, which were mapped across four retinal quadrants [58]. Retinal vPDGFRβ loss was closely associated with the accumulation of retinal $A\beta_{40}$ and $A\beta_{42}$ deposits, as well as reactive astrocytes. Intriguingly, retinal vPDGFRβ expression levels were correlated with cerebral Aβ-plaque burden, CAA scores, and cognitive deficit assessed by the Mini-Mental State Examination (MMSE) [58]. Shi et al., recently reported the significant loss of retinal vascular zonula occludens-1 (ZO-1) and claudin-5, correlating with abundant arteriolar $A\beta_{40}$ deposition identified in MCI and AD patients. Retinal claudin-5 deficiency was strongly associated with CAA, whereas ZO-1 defects correlated with cerebral pathology and cognitive deficits [56]. AD-related retinovascular degeneration and TJ protein loss are depicted in Fig. 6.10. Overall, profound vascular impairment has been reported during AD pathogenesis, indicating that monitoring retinal vascular abnormalities is a possible strategy for AD diagnosis.

6.2.8 Retinal Vasculopathy in Animal Models of AD

As in humans, a few studies in AD animal models have also revealed the vascular abnormalities in the retina during AD pathogenesis. One recent study employing a mouse model of AD revealed retinal capillary and PDGFRβ losses and vascular Aβ deposits in young and adult AD mice, which were associated with inner BRB TJ changes and BRB leakage [94]. In transgenic $APP_{SWE}/PS1_{\Delta E9}$ mice models of AD, increased retinal capillary degeneration was associated with vPDGFRβ loss, vascular Aβ deposits, and BRB damage due to TJ [i.e., claudin-1 and zonula

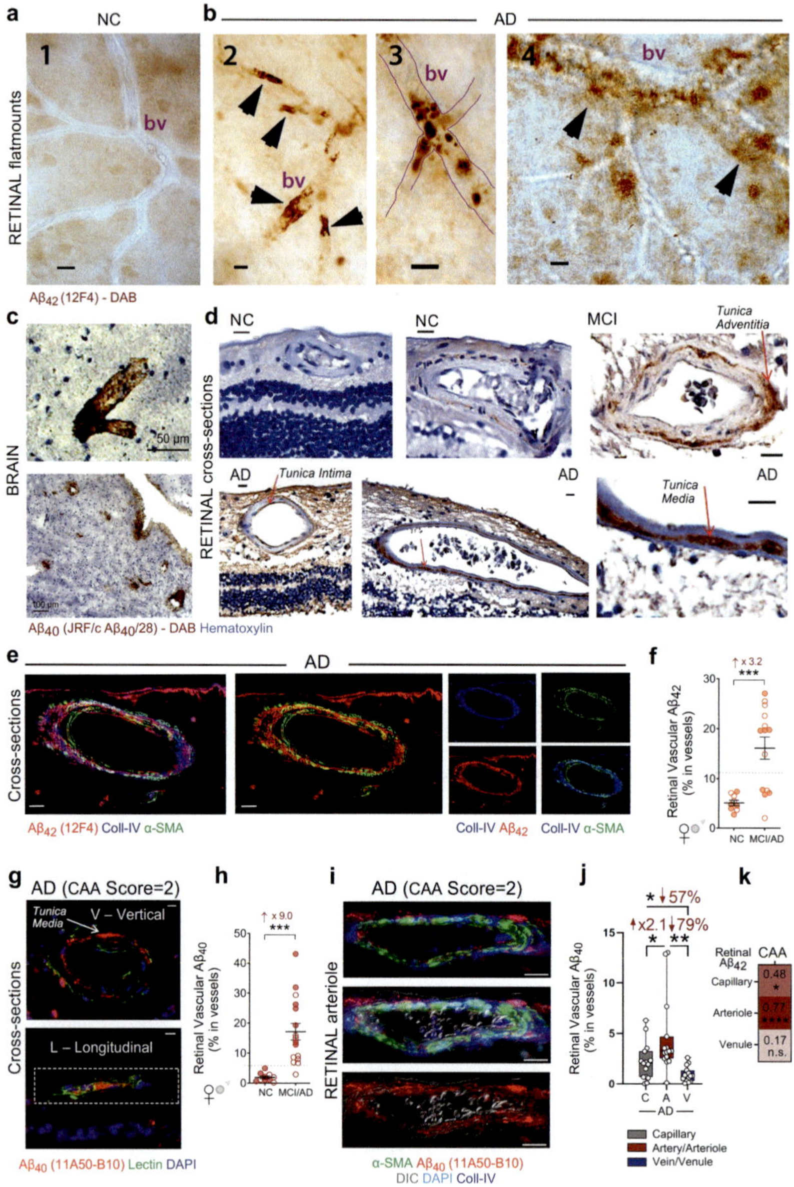
a
NC
b
AD
RETINAL flatmounts
bv
Aβ42 (12F4) - DAB
c
BRAIN
50 µm
100 µm
Aβ40 (JRF/c Aβ40/28) - DAB Hematoxylin
d
NC
MCI
Tunica Adventitia
RETINAL cross-sections
AD
Tunica Intima
Tunica Media
e
Cross-sections
Aβ42 (12F4) Coll-IV α-SMA
Coll-IV Aβ42
Coll-IV α-SMA
f
↑ x 3.2
***
Retinal Vascular Aβ42 (% in vessels)
NC
MCI/AD
g
AD (CAA Score=2)
V – Vertical
L – Longitudinal
Aβ40 (11A50-B10) Lectin DAPI
h
↑ x 9.0
Retinal Vascular Aβ40 (% in vessels)
i
RETINAL arteriole
α-SMA Aβ40 (11A50-B10)
DIC DAPI Coll-IV
j
* ↓57%
↑x2.1 ↓79%
Retinal Vascular Aβ40 (% in vessels)
C A V
AD
Capillary
Artery/Arteriole
Vein/Venule
k
Retinal Aβ42
CAA
Capillary
0.48 *
Arteriole
0.77 ****
Venule
0.17 n.s.

◀**Fig. 6.9** Retinal amyloid vasculopathy and increased arterial Aβ_{40} deposits predict CAA in MCI and AD patients. (**a–b**) Representative images of NC and AD retinal flatmounts stained with 12F4 and peroxidase-based labeling. The NC retina is clear of Aβ deposits in blood vessels (bv) compared to AD (arrowheads). Retinal Aβ deposits are apparent inside bv, perivascular, and along the vessel walls. Scale bar: 20 μm. (**c–d**) Representative images of brain and retinal sections immunostained against Aβ_{40} (JRF/cAβ_{40}/28) with DAB labeling and hematoxylin counterstain in cohorts of NC, MCI, and AD human subjects. Arrows indicate vascular Aβ_{40} staining in tunica media, adventitia, or intima; right bottom image is an enlargement of the area indicated by the arrow from the middle image. Scale bar: 20 μm. (**e**) Representative images of immunofluorescent staining for 12F4 (Aβ_{42}, red) in a retinal blood vessel (arteriole), α-SMA (green), Coll-IV (blue), and DAPI (cyan) on postmortem retinal cross-sections from AD patients. Scale bar: 20 μm. (**f**) Quantitative analysis of total retinal vascular Aβ_{42}. (**g**) Representative immunofluorescence images of paraffin-embedded retinal cross-sections isolated from human donors with AD and stained for Aβ_{40} (11A50–B10, red), blood vessels (lectin, green), and nuclei (DAPI, blue) in vertical (V; up) and longitudinal (L; bottom) retinal blood vessels. Dashed geometric white shapes indicate pre-defined areas of analysis. Scale bars: 10 μm. (**h**) Quantitative analysis of retinal vascular total Aβ_{40}. (**i**) Representative images of immunofluorescent staining for 11A50-B10 (Aβ_{40}, red) in a retinal blood vessel (arteriole), α-SMA (green), Coll-IV (blue), and DAPI (cyan) with a differential interference contrast (DIC) channel on postmortem retinal cross-sections from AD patients. Scale bars: 20 μm. (**j**) Quantitative analysis of retinal vascular Aβ_{40} immunoreactivity stratified by blood vessel types in AD group. (**k**) Pearson's correlations between retinal Aβ_{40} by 11A50-B10 in capillaries, arterioles, and venules versus brain CAA score. $^*P < 0.05$, $^{**}P < 0.01$, $^{***}P < 0.001$, determined by two-tailed student's t-test or two-way analysis of variance with Tukey's post hoc multiple comparison. Images in panels **a** and **b** are reproduced from Koronyo et al., JCI Insight 2017 [44], panels **c-g** are reproduced from Shi et al., Acta Neuropathol 2020 [58], and panels **h–k** are reproduced from Shi et al., Alzheimers Dement 2023 [56]

occuludens-1 (ZO-1)] alterations, enhanced inflammation (NF-κB p65 phosphorylation), and BRB leakage [94]. In addition, increased retinal MGnD microglia that were identified in the murine $APP_{SWE}/PS1_{L166P}$ models of AD were associated with an increased retinal pro-inflammatory profile, vascular amyloidosis, and BRB impairment [95] (Fig. 6.11). BRB permeability changes, measured using intravenously injected fluorescein (322 Da), Texas-Red-dextran (3 kDa), and FITC-dextran molecules (2000 kDa) in $APP_{SWE}/PS1_{\Delta E9}$ (ADtg) mice, occurred even earlier than the respective cerebral leakage [233]. One recent study in an animal model of prion disease [234] also revealed that the progression of perivascular amyloid can be directly monitored in the eye by live imaging, illustrating the utility of this technology for diagnosing and monitoring the progression of CAA. Overall, these findings suggest that several BRB compartments are affected during AD progression. It is unclear whether BRB pathology, including TJ changes, occurs in human AD and is potentially associated with inflammation, vascular amyloidosis, and tauopathy.

6.2.9 Retinal Inflammation in AD Patients

A low-grade chronic inflammation in the brain typically involves molecular mediators and cellular processes such as astrogliosis, microgliosis, and infiltration

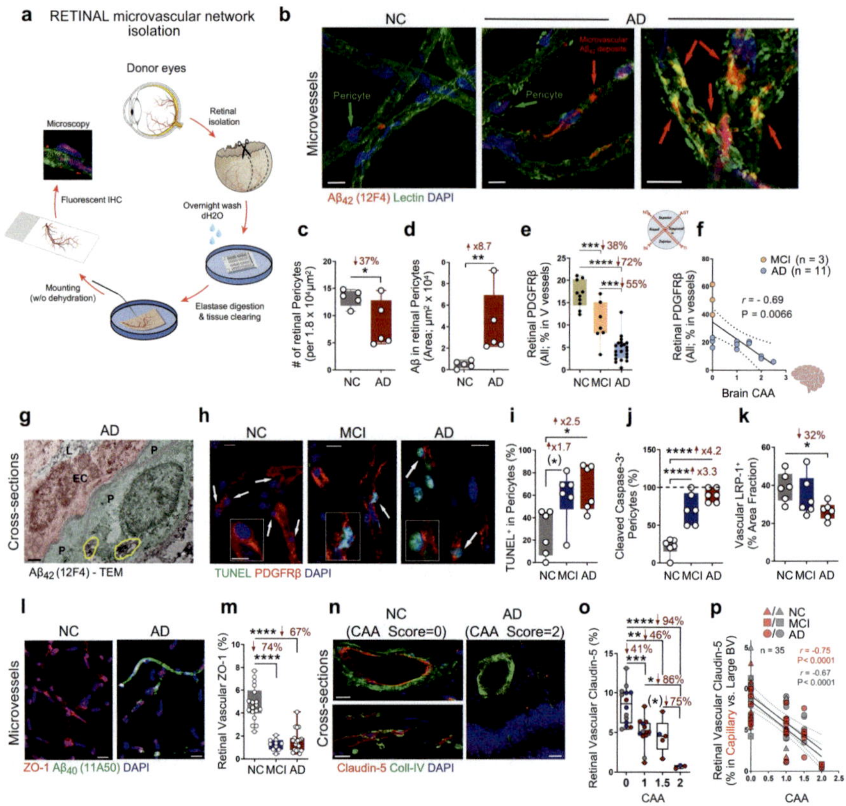
a
RETINAL microvascular network isolation
Donor eyes
Retinal isolation
Overnight wash dH2O
Elastase digestion & tissue clearing
Mounting (w/o dehydration)
Fluorescent IHC
Microscopy
b
NC
AD
Microvessels
Pericyte
Pericyte
Aβ42 (12F4) Lectin DAPI
c
# of retinal Pericytes (per 1.8 x 10⁴μm²)
↓37%
*
NC AD
d
Aβ in retinal Pericytes (Area; μm² x 10⁴)
↑x8.7
**
NC AD
e
Retinal PDGFRβ (All; % in V vessels)
***↓38%
****↓72%
***↓55%
NC MCI AD
f
MCI (n = 3)
AD (n = 11)
r = - 0.69
P = 0.0066
Retinal PDGFRβ (All; % in vessels)
Brain CAA
g
AD
Cross-sections
L
EC
P
P
P
Aβ42 (12F4) - TEM
h
NC
MCI
AD
TUNEL PDGFRβ DAPI
i
TUNEL⁺ in Pericytes (%)
↑x2.5
↑x1.7
(*)
NC MCI AD
j
Cleaved Caspase-3⁺ Pericytes (%)
****↑x4.2
****↑x3.3
NC MCI AD
k
Vascular LRP-1⁺ (% Area Fraction)
↓32%
*
NC MCI AD
l
NC
AD
Microvessels
ZO-1 Aβ40 (11A50) DAPI
m
Retinal Vascular ZO-1 (%)
****↓67%
↓74%
****
NC MCI AD
n
NC (CAA Score=0)
AD (CAA Score=2)
Cross-sections
Claudin-5 Coll-IV DAPI
o
Retinal Vascular Claudin-5 (%)
****↓94%
**↓46%
↓41%
***
*↓86%
(*)↓75%
0 1 1.5 2
CAA
p
NC
MCI
AD
n = 35
r = -0.75
P< 0.0001
r = -0.67
P< 0.0001
Retinal Vascular Claudin-5 (% in Capillary vs. Large BV)
CAA

◀**Fig. 6.10** Retinal pericytes and tight junctions deficiency in capillaries predicts CAA in MCI and AD patients. (**a**) Schema of modified retinal vascular network isolation and immunofluorescent staining. (**b**) Representative immunofluorescence images of isolated retinal microvasculature stained for $A\beta_{42}$ (12F4, red), blood vessels (lectin, green), and nuclei (DAPI, blue) in age- and sex-matched human donors with AD and NC. Red arrows indicate microvascular $A\beta_{42}$ deposits in capillaries of AD retina. A zoomed-in image (right) shows co-localization of $A\beta_{42}$ with the retinal vascular wall (yellow spot) or pericytes (green arrow). Scale bar: 10 μm. Quantitative analyses of: (**c**) mean number of retinal pericytes in each microscopic visual field (1.8×10^4 μm^2 area), (**d**) Aβ immunoreactive area within pericytes, and (**e**) percent PDGFRβ immunoreactive area in vertical (V) blood vessels, in NC, MCI, and AD human donors. (**f**) Pearson's coefficient (r) correlation between the percent retinal PDGFRβ immunoreactive area in the sum of vertical and longitudinal blood vessels against CAA scores in AD and MCI human donors. (**g**) TEM image showing retinal $A\beta_{42}$ deposits within pericytes, detected in the cytoplasm and adjacent to mitochondria, as well as on the vessel's outer surface external to the pericytes. Scale bar: 0.5 μm. (**h**) Representative fluorescent images of paraffin-embedded retinal cross-sections isolated from NC, MCI, or AD subjects, stained for PDGFRβ (red), TUNEL (green), and nuclei (DAPI, blue). Insets show zoomed-in retinal $TUNEL^+$ pericytes from the original images of subjects. All scale bars: 10 μm. Quantitative analysis of percent (**i**) retinal $TUNEL^+$ pericytes, and (**j**) cleaved caspase-3^+ pericytes in 10–15 pericytes counted. The dashed line represents the 100% reference point. (**k**) Quantitative analysis of percent LRP-1 immunoreactive area in retinal blood vessels in NC, MCI, and AD subjects. (**l**) Representative images of immunofluorescent staining for ZO-1 (red), $A\beta_{40}$-11A50 (green), and DAPI (blue) on isolated postmortem retinal blood vessels from an AD patient versus an age and sex-matched NC control. Scale bars: 20 μm. (**m**) Quantitative analysis of retinal vascular ZO-1 immunoreactivity separately in capillaries and large blood vessels in NC, MCI, and AD subjects. (**n**) Representative images of immunofluorescent staining for claudin-5 (red), collagen IV (Coll-IV, green), and DAPI (blue) on cross-sections of retina from NC subjects and AD with different degrees of CAA severity scores. Scale bars: 20 μm. (**o**) Quantitative analysis of retinal vascular claudin-5 immunoreactivity in capillaries in NC, MCI, and AD subjects stratified by CAA severity scores. (**p**) Pearson's coefficient (r) correlation between CAA severity scores and claudin-5 in retinal capillaries (red) and large blood vessels (gray). $*P < 0.05$, $**P < 0.01$, $***P < 0.001$, $****P < 0.0001$ by two-tailed student's t-test or one-way ANOVA and Tukey's post-hoc multiple comparison test. Images and data in panels **a-k** are reproduced from Shi et al., Acta Neuropathol 2020 [58] and panels **l-p** are reproduced from Shi et al., Alzheimers Dement 2023 [56]

of immune cells [29]. Recent genome-wide studies, histological, proteomic, and single-cell RNA sequencing (RNAseq) analyses indicate that innate immune processes are central to AD pathogenesis [13, 235, 236]. Neuroinflammation in AD is associated with increased astrocyte and microglia activation, seeding, aggregation, and propagation of Aβ and tau; as well as microglia-mediated excessive synaptic pruning [29, 237–243]. These mechanisms conspire to result in neurotoxicity. An RNAseq analysis further identified a distinct neurodegenerative microglial phenotype that was closely associated with cerebral Aβ plaques and is regulated via the activation of the triggering receptor expressed on the myeloid cells 2-APOE [114, 244].

A few previous histological studies have reported inflammation in the retina of AD patients [39, 45, 62, 67]. Koronyo et al., recently reported augmented gliosis in MCI and AD retinas compared to retinas from individuals with normal cognition [45] (Fig. 6.12). Increased microgliosis was observed at the synaptic-rich plexiform layers (IPL and OPL) in the AD retina, suggesting their potential involvement in synaptic pruning and functional impairment. Importantly, microglia in MCI and

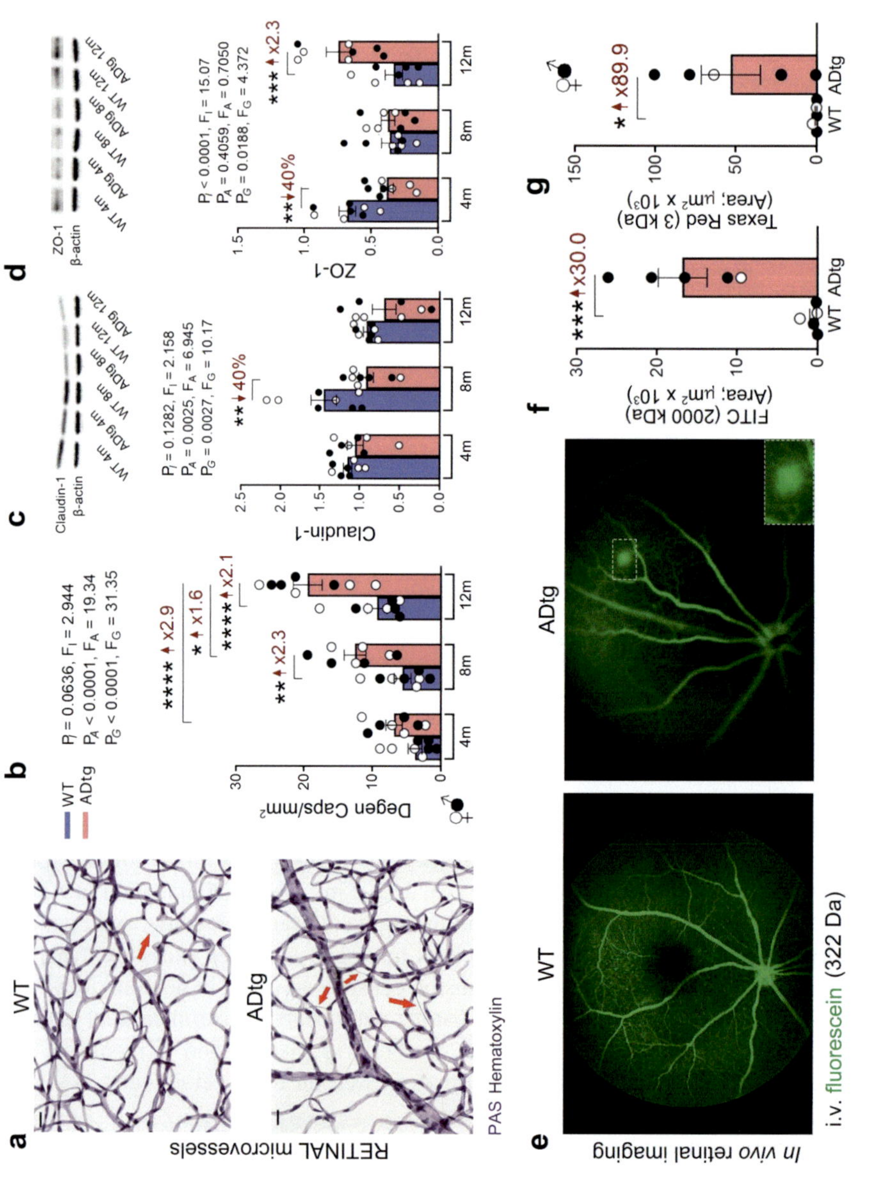
a
RETINAL microvessels
WT
ADtg
PAS Hematoxylin
b
WT
ADtg
Degen Caps/mm²
P_I = 0.0636, F_I = 2.944
P_A < 0.0001, F_A = 19.34
P_G < 0.0001, F_G = 31.35
4m
8m
12m
c
Claudin-1
β-actin
WT 4m
ADtg 4m
WT 8m
ADtg 8m
WT 12m
ADtg 12m
P_I = 0.1282, F_I = 2.158
P_A = 0.0025, F_A = 6.945
P_G = 0.0027, F_G = 10.17
d
ZO-1
β-actin
P_I < 0.0001, F_I = 15.07
P_A = 0.4059, F_A = 0.7050
P_G = 0.0188, F_G = 4.372
e
In vivo retinal imaging
i.v. fluorescein (322 Da)
WT
ADtg
f
FITC (2000 kDa)
(Area; µm² x 10³)
g
Texas Red (3 kDa)
(Area; µm² x 10³)

◀**Fig. 6.11** Retinal capillary and tight junction protein loss along with blood-retinal barrier breakdown in ADtg mice. Retinal capillary degeneration was identified in $APP_{SWE}/PS1_{\Delta E9}$ (ADtg) mice and intensified during disease progression. ADtg mice and their age- and sex-matched wild-type (WT) littermates, both males and females in equal numbers, were used in this study at the ages of 4, 8, and 12 months. (**a**) Representative images of isolated retinal microvasculature from ADtg and matched WT, stained with periodic acid-Schiff (PAS) and hematoxylin. Acellular degenerated retinal capillaries are indicated by red arrows. (**b**) Numbers of degenerated retinal capillaries (Degen Caps) stratified by mouse genotypes, WT or ADtg, and age groups of 4, 8, and 12 months. (**c, d**) Representative Tris–glycine gel images showing Western blot protein bands and their densitometric analyses for (**c**) claudin-1 and (**d**) zonula occludin-1 (ZO-1) from retinal lysates of ADtg mice and age- and sex-matched WT. (**e**) Representative images of noninvasive retinal microvascular imaging after intravenous fluorescein injection in 12-month-old WT and ADtg mice. Images show intact retinal microvasculature in WT and leakage in ADtg mice. (**f, g**) Quantitative analysis of FITC or Texas Red-stained areas of retinal flatmounts from 7-month-old WT or ADtg mice that received intravenous tail injections of FITC-dextran and Texas Red-dextran. Black-filled circles represent males, and clear circles represent females. $^{*}P < 0.05$, $^{**}P < 0.01$, $^{***}P < 0.001$, $^{****}P < 0.001$, determined by unpaired 2-tailed Student *t*-test or two-way ANOVA with Tukey's post hoc multiple comparison test. *P* and F values of two-way ANOVA refer to comparisons of age groups (P_A, F_A), ADtg versus WT genotype groups (P_G, F_G), interactions (P_I, F_I). Fold changes are shown in red. All images and data panels are reproduced from Shi et al., Acta Neuropathol Commun 2020 [94]

AD retinas often surround Aβ deposits and are directly involved in Aβ uptake, as that reported in the AD brain. Interestingly, this study revealed substantially fewer retinal microglial cells internalizing $A\beta_{42}$ in MCI and AD patients compared to retinas from cognitively normal individuals, suggesting that despite the increased presence of microglia in the retinas of patients with MCI or AD, there are 80% decreases in the relative number of microglia engaging in Aβ phagocytosis. This could be because microglia become dysfunctional and unable to effectively clear Aβ, resulting in its accumulation in these patients [45]. Intriguingly, significantly higher retinal microgliosis was observed in female AD patients than in males, which correlated with cognitive deficits. They also reported profound $GFAP^{+}$-gliosis in the inner retina and $S100\beta^{+}$-gliosis across the retinal layers, implicating the activation of several glial cell populations during AD pathogenesis [45]. Blanks et al., also discovered increased GFAP expression in retinal astrocytes and Müller cells in the GCL of the AD retina [67]. More recently, reactive astrocytes and microglial activation were observed along with Aβ plaques and pTau in post-mortem retinal tissues of a small cohort of AD patients [39]. Notably, molecular mediators of innate immunity, including interleukin-1β (IL-1β), complement component 3, osteopontin, and TREM2, were found to be upregulated in the retinal tissues of AD patients [39]. Recent studies by Xu et al., also reported findings of glial activation in the AD retina [62]. In agreement with previous reports, they found that microglial immunoreactivity was significantly increased in the INL and OPL of the mid-peripheral retinal zone [62]. The findings from this study suggest extensive microgliosis and Müller cell degeneration in the retina of AD patients [62].

6.2.10 Retinal Inflammation in Animal Model of AD

Despite limited studies in human subjects, various studies employing AD animal models have provided evidence and insights into retinal inflammation in AD [82, 88, 91, 92, 95, 102, 148, 152, 154, 245]. A recent study employing 3xTg AD mice further described morphological changes in retinal microglia consistent with inflammatory phenotypes [93]. Compared to age-matched animals, the retina of 3xTg-AD mice presents a higher number of microglial cells and a thicker microglial cell body area. Moreover, the microglia migrate, reorient, and retract their processes, changing their localization from a parallel to a perpendicular position relative to the retinal surface [93]. Increased astrogliosis, as well as activation of Müller cells, were also reported in these mouse models [82]. Another recent study discovered the existence of a neurodegenerative or disease-associated microglial state (MGnD/DAM) that was increased in the retina of $APP_{SWE}/PS1_{L166P}$ ADtg mice [95]. Further, transcriptional regulation of retinal MGnD microglial phenotype through depletion of micro-RNA (miR)-155 not only limited retinal inflammation but also reduced vascular amyloidosis and protected

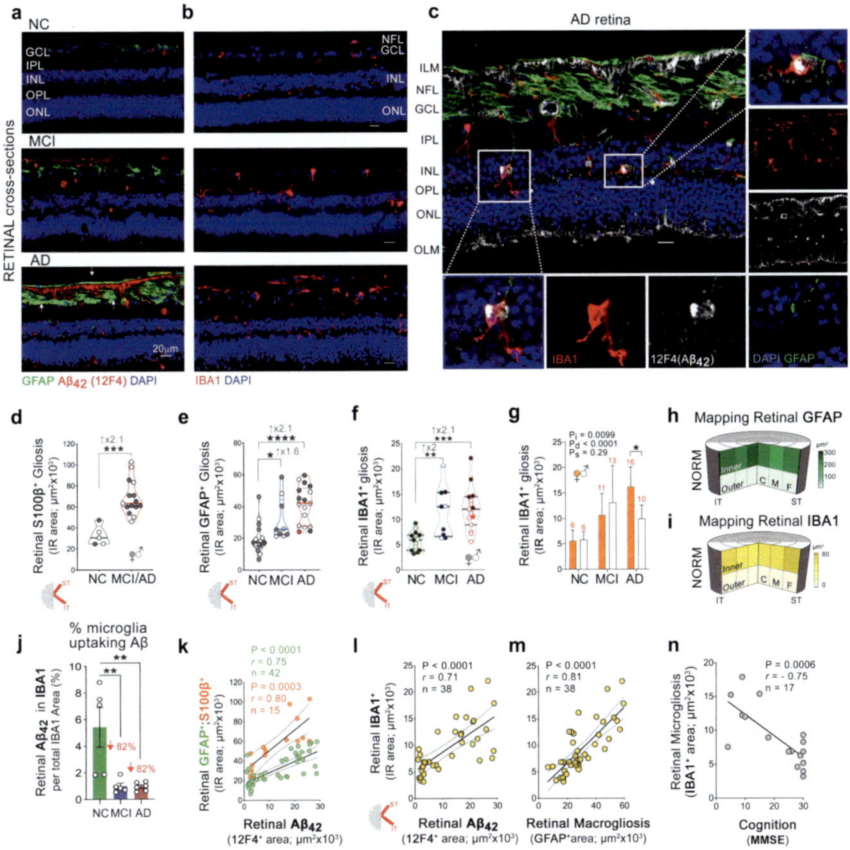
a
b
c
NC
MCI
AD
AD retina
RETINAL cross-sections
GCL
IPL
INL
OPL
ONL
NFL
ILM
OLM
20μm
GFAP Aβ42 (12F4) DAPI
IBA1 DAPI
IBA1
12F4(Aβ42)
DAPI GFAP
d
e
f
g
h
i
Retinal S100β⁺ Gliosis
(IR area; μm²x10³)
Retinal GFAP⁺ Gliosis
Retinal IBA1⁺ gliosis
↑x2.1
↑x1.6
↑x2
NC MCI/AD
NC MCI AD
Pi = 0.0099
Pd < 0.0001
Ps = 0.29
Mapping Retinal GFAP
Mapping Retinal IBA1
NORM
Inner
Outer
C M F
IT
ST
j
k
l
m
n
% microglia uptaking Aβ
Retinal Aβ42 in IBA1
per total IBA1 Area (%)
82%
82%
Retinal GFAP⁺;S100β⁺
P < 0.0001
r = 0.75
n = 42
P = 0.0003
r = 0.80
n = 15
Retinal Aβ42
(12F4⁺ area; μm²x10³)
Retinal IBA1⁺
P < 0.0001
r = 0.71
n = 38
r = 0.81
Retinal Macrogliosis
(GFAP⁺area; μm²x10³)
Retinal Microgliosis
(IBA1⁺ area; μm²x10³)
P = 0.0006
r = - 0.75
n = 17
Cognition
(MMSE)

◀**Fig. 6.12** Macrogliosis and microgliosis in the retina of MCI and AD patients. (**a**) Representative fluorescence micrographs of retinal cross-sections immunolabeled for $GFAP^+$ (green), markers of reactive astrocytes and Müller glia. Retinal $GFAP^+$ macrogliosis is detected surrounding sites of $12F4^+$-$A\beta_{42}$ deposits (red), especially in the GCL in patients with MCI or AD versus NC. White arrows indicate Aβ colocalized within retinal $GFAP^+$ macroglia. Scale bar: 20 μm. (**b**) Representative fluorescence micrographs showing retinal $IBA1^+$ microgliosis (red) in cross-sections from NC, MCI, and AD patients. Scale bar: 20 μm. (**c**) Fluorescence micrograph shows retinal $IBA1^+$ microgliosis (red) colocalized at sites of $12F4^+$-$A\beta_{42}$ deposits (white) with $GFAP^+$ macrogliosis (green) and DAPI nuclei (blue). Scale bar: 20 μm. Retinal $IBA1^+$ microglia often internalize $A\beta_{42}$ (enlarged images). (**d-f**) Violin plots display quantitative IHC analyses of (**d**) retinal S100β, (**e**) retinal GFAP, and (**f**) retinal IBA1-immunoreactive areas in NC, MCI, and AD (red circle, an ADAD patient with *PSEN1*-A260V mutation). (**g**) Bar graph displays retinal $IBA1^+$ microgliosis by sex in NC, MCI, and AD groups. (**h, i**) Pie charts show (**h**) retinal $GFAP^+$ macrogliosis and (**i**) retinal $IBA1^+$ microgliosis distributions (normalized to tissue thickness) in the inner and outer retina, and in C, M, and F subregions; higher burden shown by darker color. (**j**) Quantitative analysis of percent retinal $12F4^+$-$A\beta_{42}$ puncta count co-localized with $IBA1^+$ microglia of total retinal $IBA1^+$ microglia. (**k**) Pearson's correlations of retinal $S100\beta^+$ or $GFAP^+$ macrogliosis against retinal $A\beta_{42}$-immunoreactive area. (**l, m**) Pearson's correlations between retinal $IBA1^+$ immunoreactive area against (**l**) retinal $A\beta_{42}$ and (**m**) retinal $GFAP^+$ immunoreactive area. (**n**) Scatterplot displays of Pearson's correlation between retinal $IBA1^+$ microgliosis and MMSE cognitive scores. Data points are presented with group means ± SEMs. Filled and empty circles represent women and men, respectively. Median and lower and upper quartiles are indicated on each violin plot. *P*d, diagnostic groups; *P*s, sex groups; *P*i, interactions. $^*P < 0.05$, $^{**}P < 0.01$, $^{***}P < 0.001$, $^{****}P < 0.0001$ by one-way or two-way ANOVA and Tukey's post hoc multiple comparison test. All images and data panels are reproduced from Koronyo et al., Acta Neuropathol 2023 [45]

inner BRB integrity in these AD-model mice [95] (Fig. 6.13). Undoubtedly, evidence for inflammation and glial responses in the retina is a key area of further research in AD.

6.3 Retinal Imaging in AD

Retinal optical imaging techniques have developed rapidly over the last few decades; consequently, the retinal microvasculature and neuronal structure can now be visualized easily and non-invasively [32, 36–38, 41, 44, 49, 51, 59, 74, 125, 129, 131, 246–256]. Pilot studies have found that the retinal amyloid load is significantly greater in patients with preclinical AD, MCI, or AD dementia than in individuals with normal cognition [37, 38, 41, 44, 49, 51, 52, 60]. Additionally, the degree of retinal amyloid burden has been found to correlate with cerebral amyloid load, as measured by positron emission tomography (PET), as well as hippocampal and whole gray matter atrophy and verbal memory deficits [37, 38, 52, 60]. PET imaging offered significant differences in reflectance spectra between individuals with Aβ-positive MCI and age-matched Aβ-negative controls [41]. Functional carbon quantum dots (CDs) may be used to assess retinal Aβ deposits as they can colocalize with Aβ aggregates [257]. Optical coherence tomography (OCT), OCT angiography, fundus photography, and dynamic vessel analyzer (DVA) are useful imaging methods providing quantitative assessment of retinal structural and

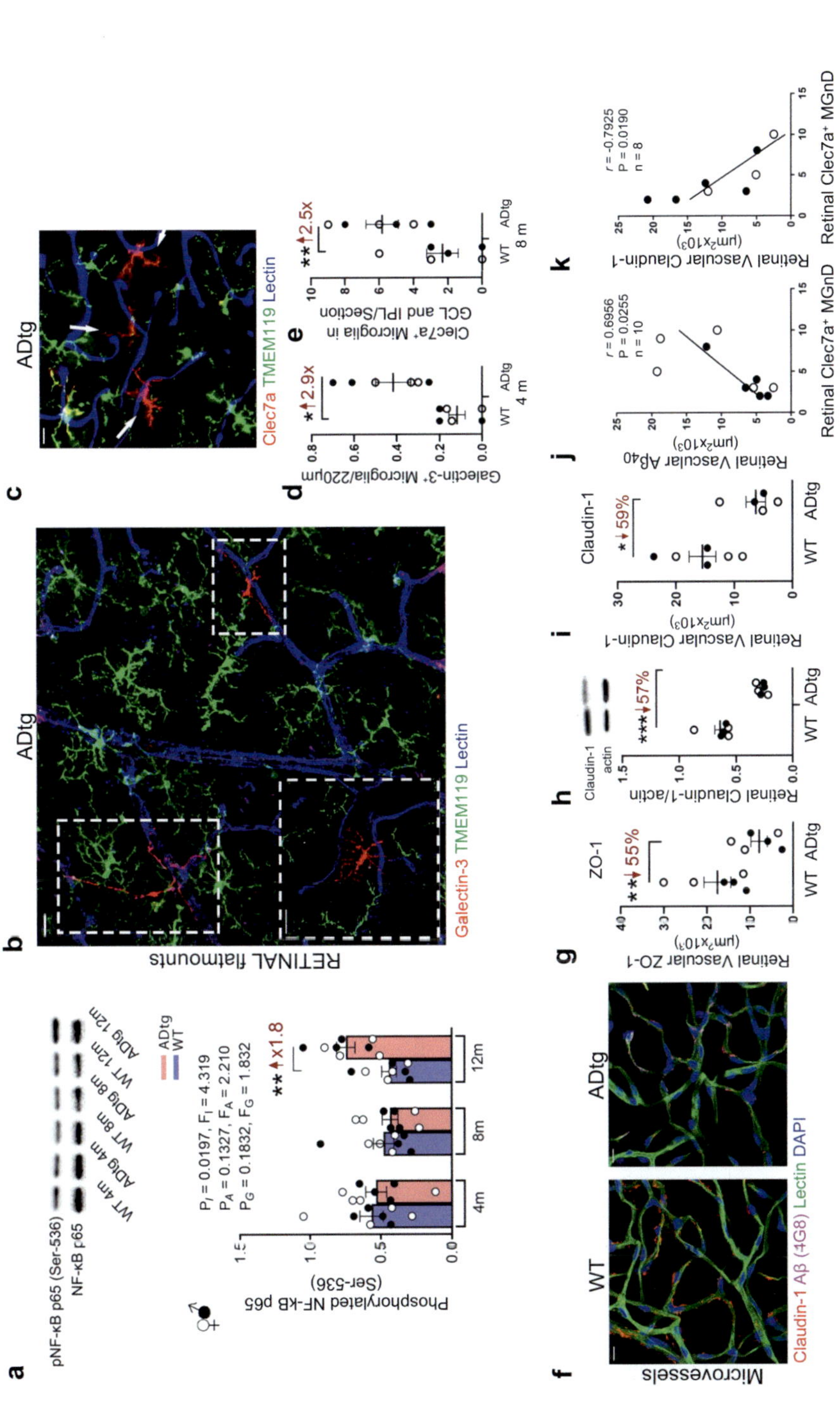
a
pNF-κB p65 (Ser-536)
NF-κB p65
WT 4m
ADtg 4m
WT 8m
ADtg 8m
WT 12m
ADtg 12m
ADtg
WT
$P_I = 0.0197, F_I = 4.319$
$P_A = 0.1327, F_A = 2.210$
$P_G = 0.1832, F_G = 1.832$
** ↑x1.8
Phosphorylated NF-κB p65 (Ser-536)
4m
8m
12m
b
RETINAL flatmounts
ADtg
Galectin-3 TMEM119 Lectin
c
ADtg
Clec7a TMEM119 Lectin
d
Galectin-3⁺ Microglia/220μm
* ↑2.9x
WT ADtg 4 m
e
Clec7a⁺ Microglia in GCL and IPL/Section
** ↑2.5x
WT ADtg 8 m
f
Microvessels
WT
ADtg
Claudin-1 Aβ (4G8) Lectin DAPI
g
ZO-1
** ↓55%
Retinal Vascular ZO-1 (μm²x10³)
WT ADtg
h
Claudin-1
actin
*** ↓57%
Retinal Claudin-1/actin
WT ADtg
i
Claudin-1
* ↓59%
Retinal Vascular Claudin-1 (μm²x10³)
WT ADtg
j
r = 0.6956
P = 0.0255
n = 10
Retinal Vascular Aβ40 (μm²x10³)
Retinal Clec7a⁺ MGnD
k
r = -0.7925
P = 0.0190
n = 8
Retinal Vascular Claudin-1 (μm²x10³)
Retinal Clec7a⁺ MGnD

◀**Fig. 6.13** Retinal neurodegenerative microglia is linked to tight junction loss in ADtg mice. (**a**) Representative Tris–glycine gel images showing Western blot protein bands and their densitometric analyses for pNF-κB p65 normalized by total NF-κB p65 from retinal lysates of ADtg mice and age- and sex-matched WT. (**b, c**) Representative images of immunofluorescent staining for (**b**) Galectin-3^+ microglia (red) and (**c**) Clec7a^+ microglia (red) with Tmem119^+ microglia (green) and lectin for blood vessels (blue) on retinal flatmounts from ADtg mice. Dashed-line rectangles highlight Galectin-3^+ microglia. Arrows indicate Clec7a^+ microglia. Scale bars: 10 μm. (**d, e**) Manual counting of (**d**) Galectin-3^+ microglia and (**e**) Clec7a^+ microglia in each retinal cross-section from 4- and 8-month-old ADtg and WT mice, respectively. (**f**) Representative images of immunofluorescent staining for 4G8^+-$A\beta_{42}$ (magenta), claudin-1 (red), lectin for blood vessels (green), and DAPI (blue) on isolated retinal blood vessels from ADtg and WT mice. (**g**) Quantitative analysis of ZO-1 immunoreactivity in isolated retinal blood vessels from 8-month-old WT and ADtg mice. (**h**) Densitometric analysis of Western blotting protein bands of claudin-1 normalized by β-actin control for retinal lysates from 8-month-old WT and ADtg mice. (**i**) Quantitative analysis of claudin-1-immunoreactivity in isolated retinal blood vessels from 8-month-old WT and ADtg mice. (**j, k**) Pearson's coefficient (r) correlation between retinal Clec7a^+ microglia and (**j**) retinal vascular $A\beta_{40}$ and (**k**) retinal vascular claudin-1 immunoreactivity. $^*P < 0.05$, $^{**}P < 0.01$, $^{***}P < 0.001$, by one-way or two-way ANOVA and Tukey's post hoc multiple comparison test. *P* and F values of two-way ANOVA refer to comparisons of age groups (PA, FA), ADtg versus WT genotype groups (PG, FG), interactions (PI, FI). Fold changes are shown in red. Data in panel **a** are reproduced from Shi et al., Acta Neuropathol Commun 2020 [94] Images and data of panels **b–k** are reproduced from Shi et al., Acta Neuropathol Commun 2022 [95] vascular indicators, such as thickness of the inner retinal layers, retinal vessel density, foveal avascular zone area, tortuosity, and fractal dimension of retinal vessels, and microvascular dysfunction, for cognitive impairment and dementia [258]. Advances in retinal imaging techniques have improved the screening, diagnosis, and management of retinal diseases such as diabetic retinopathy, age-related macular degeneration, and AD [40, 125, 128, 249, 258–262]. These retinal imaging techniques have been utilized to assess the hallmarks of AD pathogenesis in the retina [256]. Imaging of retinal degeneration, amyloid deposition, and retinal vasculature are the most common techniques employed in retinal imaging in AD patients.

6.3.1 Imaging Retinal Degeneration in AD

A growing body of recent studies employing cross-sectional imaging by OCT or OCTA has revealed consistent structural abnormalities and neurodegeneration in the AD retina [250, 261, 263–270]. In addition, analysis of blue-light high-resolution fundus photography in AD patients indicates thinner retinal NFL, a higher cup-to-disc ratio, and either diffuse optic atrophy or temporal pallor [138, 271]. However, these are non-specific changes due to the normal age-associated loss of axons in the human optic nerve [121, 272, 273]. A meta-analysis of OCT studies that included reports from AD and MCI patients showed a marked decline in the peripapillary retinal NFL as well as loss of macular thickness and volume in AD subjects compared to controls [248]. These changes were progressive from MCI to severe AD. Similarly, employing OCT imaging, Asanad et al., revealed that retinal NFL thickness predicts CSF amyloid/tau levels before cognitive decline [274]. Marquié et al., investigated the association of retinal thickness quantified by OCT with Aβ accumulation and conversion to MCI over 24 months in individuals with subjective cognitive decline (SCD). They found that subtle retinal thickness changes in the macular region are already present in SCD and correlate with Aβ uptake [275]. OCT imaging also revealed the significant attenuation of retinal choroidal thickness in the AD group compared to the control group [276].

A longitudinal study conducted by Santos et al., found a decrease in macular NFL, ONL, and IPL volumes over a 27-month follow-up period in preclinical AD relative to controls. Moreover, the reduction in macular NFL was related to increased neocortical amyloid-β accumulation observed by PET imaging. They concluded that the attenuation of macular retinal NFL might be the earliest anatomic marker of retinal neuronal loss in the preclinical stage of AD [277]. Retinal thickness changes in AD patients were almost universal despite the use of different commercially available OCT devices. Intriguingly, another study utilizing OCT revealed a significant correlation between inclusion bodies in the retina and amyloid burden in the cortex in pre-clinical patients via florbetapir PET imaging and multiple retinal spectral domain OCT aggregation markers of possible disease burden [255]. Significant thinning of GCL and the NFL was reported in pTau-positive individuals in OCT measurements [278]. Reduction of these retinal layers was significantly correlated with the hippocampal volume, suggesting pTau-associated neurodegeneration in the retina [278]. Dumitrascu et al., detected the significant inverse correlation between retinal amyloid count (RAC) and hippocampal volume loss in the patients with cognitive decline in laser ophthalmoscopy following specific amyloid-binding fluorophore curcumin administration [37, 38]. In addition, the proximal mid-periphery (PMP) RAC and retinal amyloid areas were significantly greater in patients with Montreal Cognitive Assessment (MOCA) scores < 26. PMP showed significantly more RAC and area in subjects with amnestic MCI and AD compared to the cognitively normal [37]. Jorge et al., measured the retinal and primary visual cortex (V1) thicknesses, along with V1 Aβ retention using combined OCT, magnetic resonance, and PET imaging. They found that V1 showed increased amyloid-binding potential and a positive association between the synapse-rich IPL and V1 in AD patients [279]. These diverse imaging techniques offer an avenue for non-invasive, more cost-effective, and precise imaging of retinal neurodegeneration, potentially allowing for the early diagnosis of AD even before overt clinical changes manifest.

Imaging of retinal degeneration has also been observed in animal models of AD. OCT imaging revealed significant retinal thinning in 3xTg-AD mice compared to WT. Significant retinal thinning was observed as early as 1 month of age in transgenic mice and lasted up to 12 months [280]. Yap et al., used the DARC (Detection of Apoptosing Retinal Cells) live imaging technique to detect apoptotic cells in the retina of mice with glaucoma [281]. As apoptosis is the critical neurodegenerative feature in AD [282, 283], this technology could also be employed to monitor AD progression. Georgevsky et al., revealed the significant retinal thinning in both the inner retina and outer retina of APP/PS1 mice at different ages using OCT, suggesting profound neurodegeneration in AD [83]. Taken together, studies in AD patients and animal models reveal the utility of imaging techniques to identify retinal degeneration during AD progression.

6.3.2 Retinal Amyloid Imaging in AD

The eye's optical accessibility has inspired the use of non-invasive imaging to detect amyloid burden in the retina, offering a clinically feasible approach with potentially improved precision, sensitivity, and cost compared to PET imaging. The first *in vivo* imaging of amyloid pathology was demonstrated by Koronyo et al., in living AD patients utilizing a modified confocal scanning laser ophthalmoscope following oral administration of highly bioavailable Longvida curcumin [44] (Figs. 6.14 and 6.15). Importantly, this study revealed a significantly higher retinal amyloid index in AD patients when compared to age-matched healthy controls [44]. Subsequent studies have also reported the feasibility of noninvasive detection and quantification of augmented retinal amyloid burden in MCI and AD patients [37, 38, 52, 60]. Additionally, increased retinal amyloid deposits, especially those in the proximal mid-periphery of the superior-temporal retina, have been correlated with hippocampal volume loss and whole gray matter atrophy [37,

60]. These observations, along with venular tortuosity, were predictive of verbal memory deficit [38]. Various methods have been applied to detect Increased retinal amyloidosis in AD patients, such as fundus autofluorescence imaging with OCT and retinal hyperspectral imaging [36, 41, 49, 51, 284]. Using cerebral PET imaging validation, the retinal imaging scores were greatly correlated with brain Aβ burden [41]. Moreover, several studies have demonstrated techniques for fluorescent detection of specific Aβ deposits, which allows for longitudinal monitoring of these deposits and their rate of clearance over the course of disease progression [33, 44, 119, 285]. A robust methodology for assessing amyloid deposition in the retina could offer clinicians an early window into cerebral amyloid burden and could help stratify at-risk patients who may benefit from further cerebral amyloid PET imaging. This ultimately could lead to early identification of patients who could be treated with amyloid-clearing therapeutics. Additionally, tracking amyloid burden over time could allow dynamic assessment of the response to these therapeutics.

Retinal amyloid imaging has also been successfully employed in living AD animal models [33, 46, 96, 119, 286, 287]. The first *in vivo* imaging of AD amyloid pathology was initially developed and tested in transgenic murine models of AD by Koronyo-Hamaoui et al., [46, 119] (Figs. 6.16 and 6.17). The researchers paired curcumin – a natural and safe fluorochrome that labels Aβ fibrils and oligomers with high affinity and specificity – with a modified rodent retinal optical imaging microscope. In addition, Chibhabha et al., [286] found that the staining of the curcumin micelles is colocalized with $A\beta_{42}$ in the hippocampal sections and retina of $APP_{SWE}/PS1_{\Delta E9}$ transgenic mice. This study provides a basis for optical imaging of retinal amyloid plaques through the eye *in vivo*. Hoh Kam et al., also observed the progressive accumulation of Aβ deposits on outer segments using scanning electron microscopy, revealing age-related changes in Aβ accumulation. Fundus autofluorescence images taken using the confocal scanning laser ophthalmoscope at 3, 6, 12 and 24 months revealed an age-dependent increase in the number of hyperautofluorescence spots in sub-retinal regions. These spots were identified as macrophage/microglia cells, with over 95% of these cells containing Aβ. The amount of Aβ in these cells appeared to increase with age [287]. Cao et al., detected amyloid aggregates in the retina during antemortem imaging following the intraperitoneal administration of the amyloid-targeting fluorescent dye, ARCAM-1 [33]. These studies suggest an efficient and non-invasive means of amyloid imaging in the AD retina.

6.3.3 Retinal Tau Imaging in AD

To date, there have been no reports revealing live tau imaging in the retina of AD patients or AD animal models. However, Schön et al., successfully detected fibrillar tau aggregates in the retinas of living transgenic mice expressing human mutant P301S tau using a modified scanning laser ophthalmoscopy [54]. Further

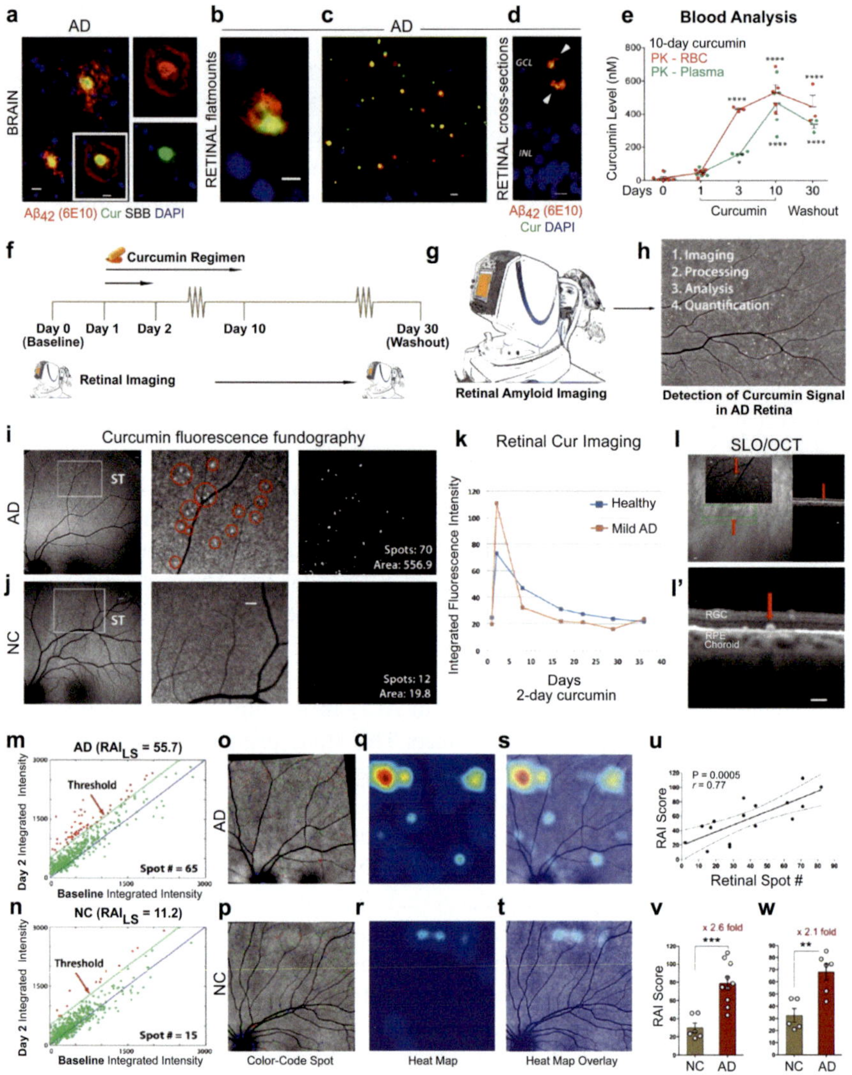
Blood Analysis
Curcumin fluorescence fundography
Retinal Cur Imaging
SLO/OCT
Curcumin Regimen
Retinal Imaging
Retinal Amyloid Imaging
Detection of Curcumin Signal in AD Retina
Color-Code Spot
Heat Map
Heat Map Overlay

◂**Fig. 6.14** Development of the first retinal amyloid imaging method, using curcumin labeling and a non-invasive, high-resolution ophthalmic imaging device: proof-of-concept trial for detecting and quantifying sub-cellular size retinal amyloid deposits in living patients. (**a, b**) Brain and retinal tissue taken from the same subset of AD patients stained with fluorescent 6E10 antibody for Aβ (red) and Longvida curcumin (Cur-green) after treatment with Sudan Black B (SBB) to minimize autofluorescence. Scale bar: 10 μm (brain); 5 μm (retina). (**c, d**) Distribution of Aβ deposition in (**c**) large retinal whole-mount regions and (**d**) cross-section retinal layers. (**e**) Pharmacokinetic analyses of Longvida curcumin plasma and red blood cell (RBC) levels in living healthy controls during 10-day trial administration. Peak plasma and RBC levels reached at 10 days prior to washout. (**f, g**) Administration timeline of oral Longvida curcumin intake (two or ten days) and retinal imaging via modified retinal ophthalmoscope. (**h**) Representative retinal image and curcumin Aβ fluorescence in an AD patient. (**i, j**) Representative detection of retinal curcumin$^+$ spots in (**i**) an AD patient and (**j**) a healthy NC patient given curcumin under the same regimen. Scale bar: 400 μm. Curcumin fluorescence fundography of the superior temporal region (ST) reveals preferential Aβ deposition in the periphery. High magnification images displaying regions of interest determined by white square and further post-processing of curcumin fluorescence with respective spot count and area (μm^2). Scale bar: 400 μm. (**k**) Quantitative longitudinal assessment of retinal curcumin fluorescent intensity in a healthy NC and mild AD patient following a 2-day curcumin regimen. Exponential decay of integrated fluorescent intensity (IFI) after day 2. Decay rate = 10.4% per day, half-life = 6.3 days, offset IFI = 21.5. (**l, l′**) Tracing certain retinal amyloid plaques, indicated by a red arrow, under curcumin fluorescence fundography and optical coherence tomography (OCT) segmentation. Retinal cross-section imaging by OCT reveals Aβ plaque in the outer retinal layers above the retinal pigment epithelium (RPE). Scale bar: 200 μm. (**m, n**) Threshold defining increased curcumin fluorescent signal in the left eye superior hemisphere (LS) of a representative mild AD patient and an age-matched NC. Blue lines indicate a 1:1 reference, and green lines represent the threshold level, with red spots denoting above threshold. (**o, p**) Color-coded spot overlay images determined by the threshold established in (**m, n**). Red spots are above the threshold and considered curcumin-positive amyloid deposits. (**q–t**) Heatmap images with high fluorescence red spot centroids (left side). Overlay images of heatmap and regional fundus imaging displaying overlap with regions high in above-threshold spots (right side) in a mild AD patient (top) and healthy NC (bottom). The same automated image processing and analysis were applied to all human subjects. (**u**) Pearson's r correlation between Retinal amyloid index (RAI) scores and retinal spot number in the entire data set. (**v, w**) Comparison between RAI scores of AD patients and non-age-matched NC (left) and between a subgroup of AD patients age-matched against NC (right). $^*P < 0.05$, $^{**}P < 0.01$, $^{***}P < 0.001$, $^{****}P < 0.0001$, determined by unpaired 2-tailed Student's t- test. SLO: Scanning laser ophthalmoscope. All panels are adapted from Koronyo et al., JCI Insight 2017 [44]

investigation is needed for retinal tau to explore the disease stage-specific tau distribution in the retina of AD patients. Lastly, the development of new fluorescent labeling against pTau holds promise for future applications.

6.3.4 Retinal Vascular Imaging in AD

Numerous clinical imaging studies employing color fundus photography, Doppler or confocal scanning laser ophthalmoscopy, OCTA, and dynamic vessel analysis have demonstrated multiple vascular changes in AD subjects compared to controls. These include vascular (venular) caliber and density, retinal and choroidal blood flow, and retinal vascular branching complexity [59, 69, 252, 288–291]. While

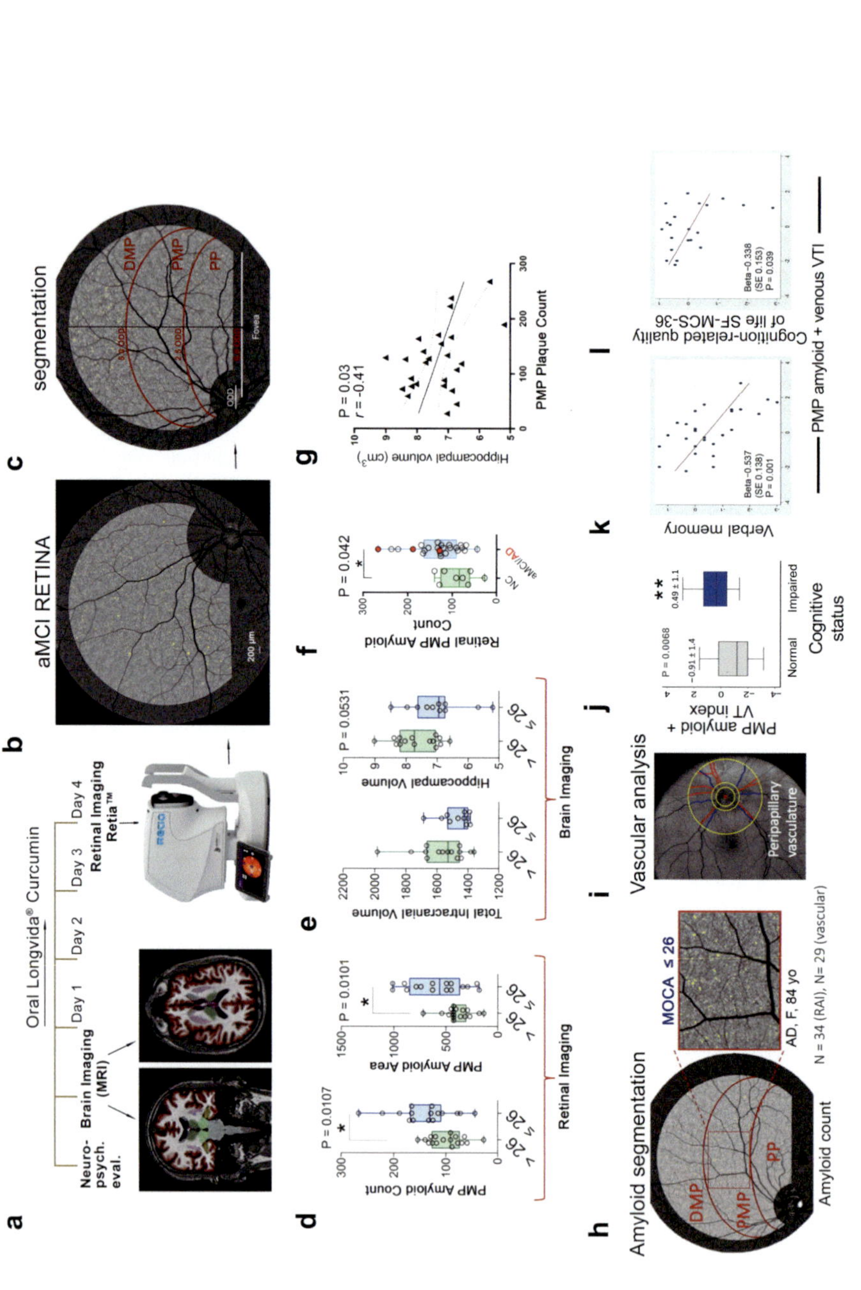
a
Oral Longvida® Curcumin
Neuro-psych. eval.
Brain Imaging (MRI)
Day 1
Day 2
Day 3
Day 4
Retinal Imaging Retia™
b
aMCI RETINA
200 µm
c
segmentation
DMP
PMP
PP
Fovea
d
PMP Amyloid Count
P = 0.0107
PMP Amyloid Area
P = 0.0101
Retinal Imaging
e
Total Intracranial Volume
Hippocampal Volume
P = 0.0531
Brain Imaging
f
Retinal PMP Amyloid Count
P = 0.042
NC
aMCI/AD
g
Hippocampal volume (cm³)
P = 0.03
r = -0.41
PMP Plaque Count
h
Amyloid segmentation
MOCA ≤ 26
AD, F, 84 yo
Amyloid count
N = 34 (RAI), N= 29 (vascular)
i
Vascular analysis
Peripapillary vasculature
j
PMP amyloid + VT index
P = 0.0068
-0.91 ± 1.4
0.49 ± 1.1
Normal
Impaired
Cognitive status
k
Verbal memory
Beta -0.537
(SE 0.138)
P = 0.001
l
Cognition-related quality of life SF-MCS-36
Beta -0.338
(SE 0.153)
P = 0.039
PMP amyloid + venous VTI

◄**Fig. 6.15** Sectoral retinal amyloid burden, jointly with venular tortuosity, correlates with hippocampal volume and cognition. (**a**) Study timeline schema and representative images of brain magnetic resonance imaging (MRI). (**b**) Post-processed image of the retinal superotemporal quadrant from a subject with amnestic mild cognitive impairment (aMCI). (**c**) Region of interest from the retinal superotemporal quadrant and its predefined divisions used for the quantification of the retinal amyloid plaque burden; topographical segmentation methodology for retinal amyloid analysis in an image from an MCI patient; DMP, distal mid-periphery; ODD, optic disc diameter; PMP, proximal mid-periphery; PP, posterior pole. (**d–e**) Quantitative analysis of the differences in (**d**) retinal PMP amyloid count and area and (**e**) total intracranial volume and hippocampal volume in the patients stratified by MOCA score threshold of 26. (**f**) The graph shows the differences in retinal amyloid count in the PMP. (**g**) Pearson's r correlation analysis between hippocampal volume and retinal PMP amyloid count. (**h**) A representative fluorescent fundus image of retinal amyloid plaques (yellow dots) per topographical region for an AD patient with a MOCA score lower than 26. (**i**) Illustration of the region of interest used for the retinal vascular analysis. The red circle indicates the center of the optic nerve-head, and the smallest yellow circle shows the optic nerve-head area. The two larger circles indicate the region of interest for the vascular analysis, which were 1.5 and 4 times the diameter of the optic disc. The branching angle and tortuosity of vessels within the region of interest were calculated. Arteries and veins are outlined by red and blue lines, respectively. (**j**) Quantitative analysis of the combined retinal PMP amyloid and venous vessel tortuosity (VT) index when patients are stratified by cognitive status (normal vs. impaired). (**k, l**) Pearson's correlations of the combined PMP amyloid and venous VT index (VTI) with (**k**) verbal memory or (**l**) cognitive-related quality-of-life Z-scores. $*P < 0.05$, $**P < 0.01$, determined by two-tailed unpaired Student t-test. Panels **a–h** are reproduced from Dumitrascu et al., Alzheimers Dement 2020 [37]. Panels **i–l** are reproduced from Dumitrascu et al., Cells 2021 [38]

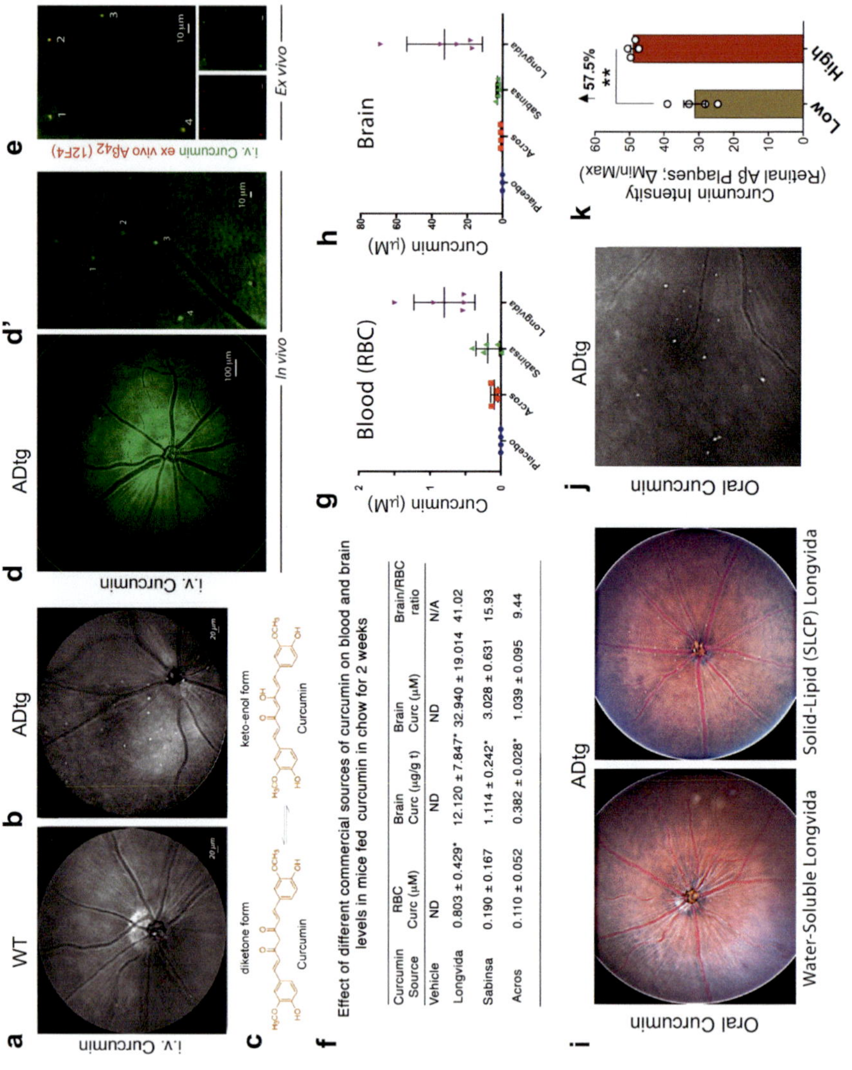

Effect of different commercial sources of curcumin on blood and brain levels in mice fed curcumin in chow for 2 weeks

Curcumin Source	RBC Curc (μM)	Brain Curc (μg/g t)	Brain Curc (μM)	Brain/RBC ratio
Vehicle	ND	ND	ND	N/A
Longvida	0.803 ± 0.429*	12.120 ± 7.847*	32.940 ± 19.014	41.02
Sabinsa	0.190 ± 0.167	1.114 ± 0.242*	3.028 ± 0.631	15.93
Acros	0.110 ± 0.052	0.382 ± 0.028*	1.039 ± 0.095	9.44

◂**Fig. 6.16** Live imaging detection of curcumin-bound Aβ in retina of ADtg mice. (**a, b**) Representative fundus retinal images from ADtg and WT mice capturing specific curcumin fluorescence bound to Aβ deposits following an intravenous (i.v.) injection of curcumin (Sigma-Aldrich; 7.5 mg/Kg once a day for 2 days). (**c**) Curcumin tautomeric forms. (**d, d′**) Representative images demonstrating in vivo detection of curcumin-labeled plaques in the retinas of 8-month-old ADTg mice, following a single i.v. injection of curcumin (7.5 mg/kg) two hours prior to imaging. (d′) Enlarged image of the selected area from (**d**). Note that blood vessels appear unstained (dark), possibly due to blood flow in the live mouse. (**e**) Whole-mount retina prepared from the same in vivo imaged mouse eye as in (d), following perfusion. An additional ex vivo staining with anti-human $A\beta_{42}$ mAb (12F4) further confirmed the specificity of curcumin signals (captured by Micron II) to Aβ plaques (indicated by the numbers 1–4). Bottom panels show separate channels for each staining. (**f**) Three different commercial formulations of curcumin were fed to WT mice *ad libitum* for 14 days. The table shows group means and standard deviations of RBC and brain levels [grams wet tissue (g t) or mM]. ND, not detectable; N/A, not applicable. Asterisks signify differences between the source curcumin (within tissue compartments). Note that concentrations in the brain are at least 9 times higher than in the blood. (**g, h**) The scattergram plots show individual values, means, and standard deviation in (**g**) RBC and (**h**) brain tissue. (**i**) Fundus bright-field images of live ADtg mouse retinas after oral administration of water-soluble or non-water-soluble proprietary SLCP (Solid lipid curcumin particle) Longvida (optimized curcumin). (**j**) Fluorescent signal of retinal Aβ deposits following high-dose SLCP Longvida. (**k**) Quantitative analysis showing increased mean curcumin-labeled plaque intensity fluorescent signals following high- versus low-dose curcumin oral administration. Five plaques per image were analyzed for each mouse using ImageJ delta Min/Max ROI values. $^{**}P < 0.01$ by two-tailed unpaired t-test. Panels **a–c** and **f–k** are reproduced from Koronyo et al., JCI Insight 2017 [44]. Panels **d** and **e** are reproduced from Koronyo et al., Neuroimage 2011 [46]

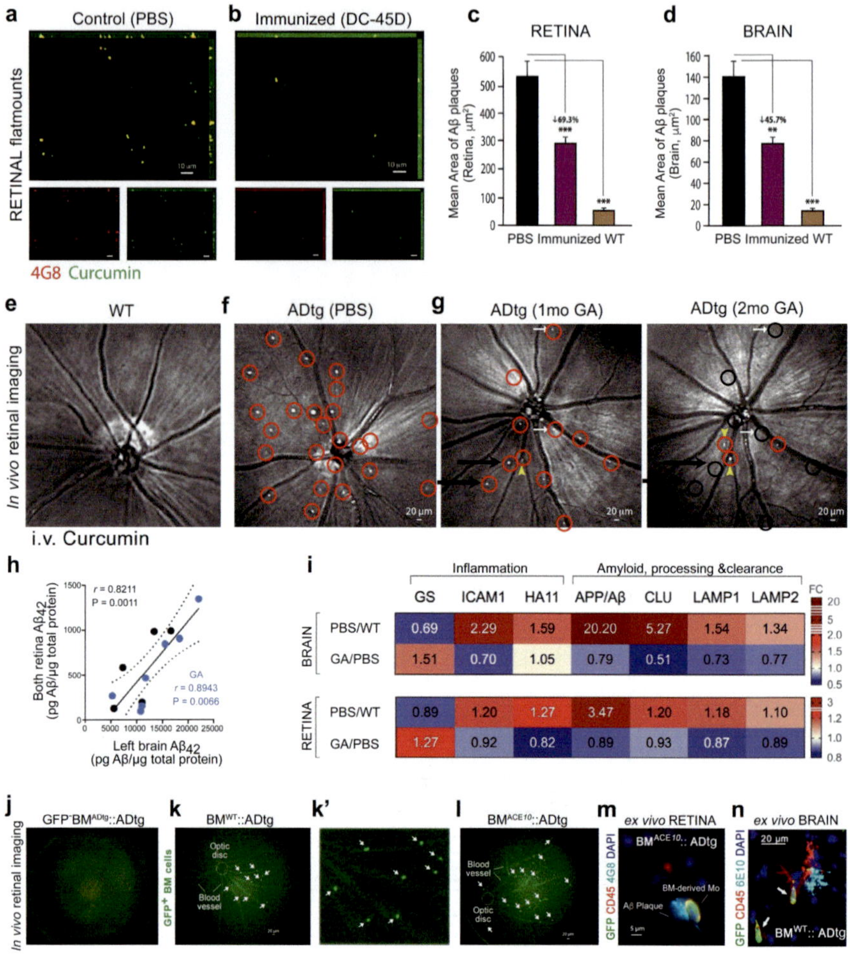
a Control (PBS)
b Immunized (DC-45D)
RETINAL flatmounts
4G8 Curcumin
c RETINA
Mean Area of Aβ plaques (Retina, μm²)
↓69.3% ***
***
PBS Immunized WT
d BRAIN
Mean Area of Aβ plaques (Brain, μm²)
↓45.7% **
***
PBS Immunized WT
e WT
f ADtg (PBS)
g ADtg (1mo GA)
ADtg (2mo GA)
In vivo retinal imaging
i.v. Curcumin
20 μm
h
r = 0.8211
P = 0.0011
GA
r = 0.8943
P = 0.0066
Both retina Aβ42 (pg Aβ/μg total protein)
Left brain Aβ42 (pg Aβ/μg total protein)
i
Inflammation
Amyloid, processing &clearance
GS ICAM1 HA11 APP/Aβ CLU LAMP1 LAMP2
BRAIN PBS/WT 0.69 2.29 1.59 20.20 5.27 1.54 1.34
BRAIN GA/PBS 1.51 0.70 1.05 0.79 0.51 0.73 0.77
RETINA PBS/WT 0.89 1.20 1.27 3.47 1.20 1.18 1.10
RETINA GA/PBS 1.27 0.92 0.82 0.89 0.93 0.87 0.89
FC
j GFP⁻BM^ADtg::ADtg
k BM^WT::ADtg
k'
l BM^ACE10::ADtg
Optic disc
Blood vessel
GFP⁺ BM cells
m ex vivo RETINA
BM^ACE10:: ADtg
BM-derived Mo
Aβ Plaque
GFP CD45 4G8 DAPI
n ex vivo BRAIN
BM^WT:: ADtg
GFP CD45 6E10 DAPI
20 μm

◂**Fig. 6.17** Parallels in retina and brain response to immunomodulation in ADtg mice. (**a, b**) Representative z-axis projection images of whole-mount retinas from (**a**) PBS-treated control (WT) and (**b**) MOG45D-vaccinated ADtg mice, stained ex vivo with curcumin (green) and anti-human Aβ mAb (4G8; red). (**c, d**) Quantitative analysis of the mean area of Aβ plaque in the retina and brain of WT and ADtg mice following immunization. A significant reduction in mean curcumin-positive plaque number and area was observed in (**c**) retinas and (**d**) brain hippocampus and cortex from MOG45D-vaccinated ADtg mice compared to PBS-treated WT controls. Curcumin staining revealed the same decrease in plaque burden following vaccination in the retina and in the brain, while Aβ mAbs confirmed its specificity to Aβ, suggesting that curcumin is a suitable dye for monitoring Aβ plaque changes. (**e–g**) Real-time monitoring of retinal Aβ plaque dynamics in (**e**) PBS-treated WT control mice, (**f**) PBS-treated ADtg mice, and (**g**) GA-immunized ADtg mice after 1 month and 2 months of treatment. Representative appearance and clearance of retinal Aβ plaques: arrows indicate the existence and removal of the same Aβ plaques, while arrowheads indicate newly formed Aβ plaques. (**h**) Pearson's *r* correlations between levels of $A\beta_{42}$ in the left brain and the average of both retinas in 20-month-old WT and ADtg mice. Strong correlations in $A\beta_{1-42}$ burden between brain and retinal tissues are especially apparent following GA immunization (blue). (**i**) Heatmap displaying relative fold change of significantly changed proteins in mass spectrometry analysis in the same cohort. Highlighted are AD-related amyloid-associated markers (amyloid-β A4 protein—APP/Aβ, clusterin—CLU, lysosomal-associated membrane protein 1 and 2—LAMP1/2) and inflammatory markers (glutamine synthetase—GS, intercellular adhesion molecule 1—ICAM1, h-2 class I histocompatibility antigen—HA11) that were significantly up- or down-regulated in brain and retinal tissues of PBS-control ADtg mice versus naïve WT mice and/or GA-immunized versus PBS-control ADtg mice. (**j–n**) To explore the unique immunomodulatory functions of myelomonocytes overexpressing angiotensin-converting enzyme (ACE10 mouse model) that possess unique enhanced neuroprotective properties in the context of AD, 2-month-old double transgenic ADtg recipient mice underwent irradiation. Their bone marrow (BM) was then reconstituted by an intravenous injection of BM from ADtg, WT, and ACE10 donor mice. The generated chimeric mice underwent retinal imaging at the age of 7 months. Representative non-invasive retinal fluorescence imaging of infiltrating GFP^+ BM cells in living ADtg chimeric mice are shown from (**j**) a control ADtg mouse that underwent BM transplantation of GFP^-BM^{ADtg} (GFP^-BM^{ADtg}::ADtg), (**k**) a GFP^+BM^{WT}::ADtg mouse (**k′**, enlarged image), (**l**) a GFP^+BM^{ACE10}::ADtg mouse (arrows indicate GFP^+BM cells). Scale bar: 20 μm (**m**) Representative microscopic image of a retina extracted from a BM^{ACE10}::ADtg mouse, *ex vivo* staining with antibodies against GFP (green), CD45 (red), 4G8 (cyan), and DAPI (blue), validating the homing of GFP^+ACE^{10} monocytes to retinal Aβ plaques. Scale bar: 5 μm. (**n**) Representative fluorescence micrograph of the BM^{WT}::AD^+ chimeric mouse brain showing infiltrating monocytes ($GFP^+/CD45^{hi}$; arrows) near a $6E10^+$ Aβ plaque site. Scale bar: 20 μm. $^{**}P < 0.005$, $^{***}P < 0.0001$, analyzed by one-way ANOVA followed by Bonferroni multiple comparison post-test. Panels **a–d** are reproduced from Koronyo et al., Neuroimage 2011 [46]. Panels **e–g** are reproduced from Koronyo et al., Neurodegener Dis 2012 [119]. Panels **h–i** are reproduced from Doustar et al., Aging cell 2020 [101]. Panels **j–n** are reproduced from Koronyo et al., Brain 2020 [385]

there is significant data demonstrating correlation of retinal artery and venous caliber assessed by color fundus images of the retina in subjects with dementia [252, 292], a recent meta-analysis suggests inconsistency in the results, perhaps due to variability in the underlying definition of AD [253]. A significant association between vascular caliber, branching complexity, and amyloid plaque burden in the brain has been demonstrated [69, 253], and a significant increase in vessel density has been reported among asymptomatic monozygotic twins with amyloid-positive status compared to those with non-amyloid positive status [293]. Importantly, in a well-characterized cohort of cerebral amyloid-positive AD patients, perifoveal capillary density on OCTA was significantly lower in the AD cohort and correlated with the Fazekas scale [294], and was associated with the cerebrovascular lesions in AD. Another study using multimodal imaging also supports the association between retinal geometric vascular and functional parameters and physiological changes in the retina of cognitively impaired individuals [213]. Laser Doppler and other retinal imaging modalities demonstrate a decrease in blood column diameter, blood velocity, capillary vessel density, and blood flow, as well as altered vessel pulsatility and reactivity, which is more severe in subjects with a clinical diagnosis of AD [65, 211, 289, 295]. The reported changes in retinal vascular caliber and geometry suggest that there may be concomitant changes in blood flow in patients with presumed AD.

According to a report investigating OCTA parameters in AD subjects – presented by Bulut et al., – the superficial retinal capillary vessel density is significantly decreased, and the FAZ area is significantly larger in patients with AD compared to normal controls [263]. This FAZ enlargement in AD patients possibly occurs due to decreased angiogenesis owing to the binding of VEGF to Aβ and the accumulation of Aβ deposits in the internal vessel walls, resulting in occlusion of the vascular structures and reduced blood flow. Lahme et al., also showed reduced vessel density in the superficial retinal vascular layer (SVP) and in the radial peripapillary capillary layer. They found an association between decreased retinal flow density and vascular cerebral lesions in AD [294]. Additionally, O'Bryhim et al., observed capillary dropout areas specifically within the fovea, leading to an increased FAZ area in the biomarker-positive ($A\beta^+$) group compared to controls ($A\beta^-$). They concluded that cognitively healthy individuals with $A\beta^+$, preclinical AD might have retinal vascular and architectural alterations even before the onset of clinically detectable cognitive symptoms [212]. Similarly, another study successfully distinguished cerebral $A\beta^+$ subjects from $A\beta^-$ subjects with 85% accuracy based on retinal vascular measures, including vessel tortuosity and diameter [296]. Jiang et al., described reduced retinal vessel density not only at the level of the superficial but also in the deep retinal vascular plexus (DVP) in MCI and AD patients. In contrast to SVP, retinal vessel density of DVP was correlated with GCL-IPL thickness in AD [297]. AD patients are characterized by a significant impairment of the retinal neurovascular structures, as evidenced by decreased arterial dilation. The reaction amplitude was decreased both in AD and MCI subjects compared with controls [295]. Nevertheless, during dynamic vessel analysis, the arterial dilation was decreased in the AD group, and the reaction amplitude was reduced both in AD and MCI compared to controls [295]. Another study by Csincsik et al., identified peripheral biomarkers, including an increased number of drusen deposits, increased venular widening, and decreased arterial fractal dimension in AD patients [298].

OCTA technology has enabled visualization of various vascular abnormalities in the retina, such as microaneurysms, retinal vascular non-perfusion, neovascularization, reduced vascular density, and modified FAZ [247, 299, 300]. The significant potential of this novel technology has recently led to a surge of investigations exploring its utility in detecting retinal biomarkers in AD. To date, OCTA case-controlled studies seem to be consistent in demonstrating retinal vascular loss and increased FAZ area in AD patients, but they differ in identifying the exact vascular areas affected, such as the superficial versus deep or parafoveal versus perifoveal vessels [123, 258, 291, 294, 301–304]. OCT-adaptive optics is a promising new advancement of this technology that provides ultra-high-resolution images, including images of blood vessel walls, which warrants further testing in the AD retina [59]. Collectively, these studies suggest the applicability of OCTA retinal imaging for the diagnosis of AD.

Studies in AD patients have consistently supported the notion that these vascular abnormalities in the retina can predict cognitive decline [213, 305, 306]. Recent progress in retinal amyloid imaging [37, 38, 44, 52, 60, 254], including clinically available fundus fluorescein angiography and OCTA microvascular imaging [307–309] are promising tools to aid in detection of pathological vascular features of AD in an outpatient clinical setting. In future practice, the recently developed OCT-Leakage method to assess vascular circulation, BRB permeability, and edema [310, 311], along with the potential of pericyte imaging by adaptive optics [262], should allow for a comprehensive assessment of retinal Aβ pathology and BRB damage. These methodologies, enabling dynamic and *in vivo* assessment of evolving AD pathology, combined with validated cognitive testing and advanced cerebral imaging techniques, have the potential to revolutionize AD diagnostics and provide a novel way to track disease progression.

AD-related vascular impairment is also evident in murine models of AD. Shi et al., recently reported a dramatic alteration in BRB permeability in the retina of $APP_{SWE}/PS1_{\Delta E9}$ mice compared to WT counterparts, as evidenced by leakage in the retinal microvessels [94]. Using the noninvasive Micron-III retinal imaging microscope, Shi et al., observed fluorescein leakage in 12-month-old ADtg mice [94]. Overall, findings from AD patients and animal models suggest that imaging the retinal vasculature could provide valuable insights into monitoring AD progression.

6.4 Visual and ERG Pattern Deficits in AD

A variety of visual and ERG pattern abnormalities have been reported in both MCI and AD patients. These include loss of contrast sensitivity and color discrimination, narrowed field of view, difficulties with depth and motion perception, as well as irregularities in circadian rhythm and sleep patterns [43, 175, 268, 312–331]. These disturbances can be attributed to the retinal damage found in these patients. Importantly, retinal changes in AD patients, such as RGC degeneration, reduced NFL thickness, and decreased blood circulation, have been linked to specific visual and ocular disturbances [47, 65, 67, 68, 71, 267, 319, 329, 332].

Alzheimer's hallmark pathologies, Aβ deposits and tauopathy, provide a link between AD-related retinal neuropathology and the visual deficits reported in living patients. For instance, histological examination of retinal tissue reveals the accumulation of pTau and Aβ in regions associated with RGC loss [35, 39, 44, 45, 47, 63]. In particular, the degeneration of RGCs would undoubtedly compromise their essential role in receiving sensory input from photoreceptors via bipolar cells, and in the initial stages of visual information processing and transmission to the brain [333]. Supporting this notion, a recent study utilizing OCT and pattern ERG in AD patients showed a linear relationship between NFL thickness and the bioelectrical integrity of RGCs and their nerve fibers, which are vital for afferent signal transduction [334].

There is growing evidence indicating functional retinal impairments in pattern ERG, which suggests significant amplitude reductions in patients with MCI and AD as compared to the age-matched control subjects. These reductions in ERG amplitude were associated with dysfunction of RGCs. Notably, these abnormalities were also observed in preclinical AD cases [175, 320, 322, 331]. ERG analysis in preclinical AD patients demonstrated marked RGC dysfunction relative to healthy controls [175]. Intriguingly, preclinical AD eyes with normal retinal morphology by OCT exhibited significant retinal dysfunction when analyzed with ERG relative to control eyes [175]. Krasodomska et al., found increased implicit time of the P50-wave in early-stage AD patients compared to the controls in PERG examination, whereas amplitudes of P50- and N95-waves were significantly reduced in AD patients. This could be attributed to RGC and optic nerve dysfunction in early-stage AD patients [335]. Ngoo et al., further confirmed these PERG findings of reduced P50- and N95-waves amplitudes in AD patients [334]. Similarly, Parisi et al., found a significant delay in N35, P50, and N95 implicit times, as well as a reduction in N35-P50 and P50-N95 amplitudes in PERG analysis of AD patients compared to the age-matched control subjects [267]. Another study further reported that the mean amplitude in the re-test PERG was significantly lower in the AD group than in the control, while the intrinsic variability of the second harmonic phase was significantly higher in the AD group than in the control group [322]. These findings indicate early-stage alteration of pattern ERG in AD. Additionally, a few independent studies also revealed significant reduction of multifocal ERG wave amplitudes with delayed implicit times in AD patients, which were significantly correlated with the inner retinal layer thinning and poorer disease severity scores [246, 331, 336, 337].

In addition to ERG, visual evoked potential (VEP) is another crucial electrophysiological process affected in AD patients [320, 329, 334–336, 338–340]. VEP is the expression of the electrical activity of the visual pathways, from the optic nerve to the calcarine cortex, measuring the electrical signal generated at the visual cortex in response to visual stimulation [341, 342]. Mounting evidence suggests a range of functional retinal impairments in pattern VEP latency and amplitude waves in MCI and AD patients. One study found a significant increase in the latency for yellow-black N-wave, whereas its amplitude was reduced in AD patients compared to the controls [340]. Interestingly, there were no differences in the latencies and amplitudes for red-green and blue-yellow N-waves in AD and control groups. The abnormalities in yellow-black N-waves VEP in AD patients suggest a specific impairment of the magnocellular stream in AD patients

[340]. Similarly, Stothart et al., found a significant reduction of P1 and N1 VEP amplitudes in AD patients, whereas amnestic MCI patients showed a reduction in N1 amplitude compared to healthy older adults. The reduction in P1 amplitude in AD patients was associated with the degree of cognitive impairment (MMSE) [338]. Despite no difference in amplitude, Krasodomska et al., found a significant increase in the latency of the P100 wave in early-stage AD patients compared to controls [335]. Taken together, the altered latencies and amplitudes of diverse waves in pattern VEP might contribute to the visual disturbances experienced by AD patients.

Color impairment and contrast sensitivities are frequent visual deficits reported in AD patients. AD patients experience altered color vision with a selective and severity-independent deficiency in blue hue discrimination [343–345]. Additionally, AD patients suffer from impaired color selections. Pache et al., found that AD patients made significantly more unspecific errors in the Ishihara PV-16 choice test than the controls, suggesting an unspecific color vision deficiency in AD [325]. Moreover, impaired contrast sensitivity in AD patients is associated with poor visual acuity [316, 346]. Diminished contrast sensitivity, altered motion and depth perception, as well as sleep and oculomotor disturbances in AD patients, are partially attributed to a preferential loss of the functionally-relevant magnocellular RGCs (M-cells) and their nerve fibers [47, 76, 347, 348]. Furthermore, impaired contrast sensitivity in MCI and AD patients is sensitive to early AD-associated changes [327]. Given the higher concentration of rods in the peripheral retina and their importance in motion and depth perception, low-contrast sensitivity, and peripheral vision, it is not surprising that these visual functions may be adversely influenced by increased levels of Aβ deposits and pTau in the periphery [42, 45, 62, 174, 326].

AD patients are also reported to have visual deficits related to lower thresholds for motion detection [174] and difficulty maintaining fixation on objects [117], along with impaired semantic memory [349, 350], slower reaction times [351], and reduced stereopsis [352, 353]. More complex visual functions, such as reading and object/face recognition, can also be affected in AD. This is likely a combination of poor transmission of raw visual information via defunct retinal ganglion cells to higher cortical centers, along with dysfunction of higher cortical processing centers [354]. In addition, AD patients often suffer from reading impairment, which may result from neuropathological changes in the occipital lobes and the left temporal region, which are specialized in the high-level visual processing of the written word [355]. An attenuation in reading speed has also been reported in AD patients, particularly at lower contrast [356]. Notably, reading latency is increased among AD patients, particularly when irregular words are present in the text [357]. These studies further suggest that vision-related functional deficits occur in AD patients.

The spatial distribution of retinal AD pathology may indicate specific functional deficits. Regionally, both Aβ and pTau pathologies appear to predominately affect the peripheral superior and inferior retinal quadrants in AD patients [35, 42, 44–47]. In a recent study by Risacher et al., a significant association was identified between the temporal distribution of Aβ and pTau with contrast sensitivity in MCI and AD patients [327] (Fig. 6.18a–f). Increased retinal Aβ and tauopathy, along with consistent neuronal loss, degeneration of mRGCs and RGCs, and NFL thinning in these specific peripheral regions, could underlie visual abnormalities such as contrast sensitivity, motion perception, and circadian rhythms described in AD [44, 45, 47, 67, 68, 72, 74, 121, 250, 326, 331, 337, 358, 359]. Beyond AD-related manifestations predominantly in the inner layers and peripheral retinal regions, deposits of Aβ were found in close proximity to blood vessels and within vessel walls [44, 46, 47, 56, 58]. These findings, together with altered retinal neurovascular coupling and structural vascular changes in clinically diagnosed MCI and AD patients [65, 69, 295], implicate retinal vascular-associated Aβ in causing or amplifying retinal metabolic dysfunctions and impaired clearance pathways. These factors may lead to functional-visual abnormalities.

Abnormalities in efferent ocular pathways, in conjunction with retinal abnormalities, have been associated with altered pupillary light response (PLR) in patients. These alterations include increased latency of pupillary constriction to light, decreased constriction amplitude, faster re-dilation after light offset, decreased maximum constriction velocity, and acceleration [360]. Additionally, pupil dilation response during cognitive tasks was found to be altered in some studies [361, 362]. Therefore, there is a growing interest in exploring various aspects of pupillary responses using specialized pupillometry tools in both pre-clinical and clinically diagnosed AD patients. PLR is governed not only by both the sympathetic and parasympathetic systems but is also regulated by retinal rods, cones, and mRGCs [363]. In line with this, altered PLR in AD patients was found to be associated with retinal mRGC loss [364], highlighting the consequences of retinal AD pathology for various ocular and visual dysfunctions. Moreover, these intrinsically photosensitive RGCs are also reported to regulate light photoentrainment of circadian rhythms by tightly communicating with photoreceptors and projecting to the central circadian clock in the hypothalamic suprachiasmatic nucleus [365–368]. Therefore, retinal mRGC loss is suggested to play a key role in the sleep–wake cycle dysfunctions observed in AD patients [47, 347]. Sleep abnormalities reported in MCI and AD patients include prolonged sleep latency, reduced total sleep duration and rapid eye movement sleep, sleep fragmentation, frequent awakenings, lower melatonin levels at night, and daytime somnolence [47, 347, 369–373]. Intriguingly, there are reports of sleep disturbances exacerbating or even preceding the cognitive impairments [374–376]. The essential discovery that Aβ accumulates within or in close proximity to mRGCs, leading to their degeneration and dendrite diameter loss, at least in part, can explain impaired sleep patterns and altered pupil dilation in AD patients [47]. These findings also suggest that certain retinal cells are more susceptible to Aβ-induced neurotoxicity and propose the first retinal damage-based mechanism for functional disturbances commonly seen in AD patients.

AD-associated visual abnormalities have been extensively studied in animal models as well. A recent study in monkeys has provided evidence for the involvement of mRGCs in blue color sensitivity [377]. In animal AD models, including drosophila, AD pathophysiology has been linked to visual impairments and ERG

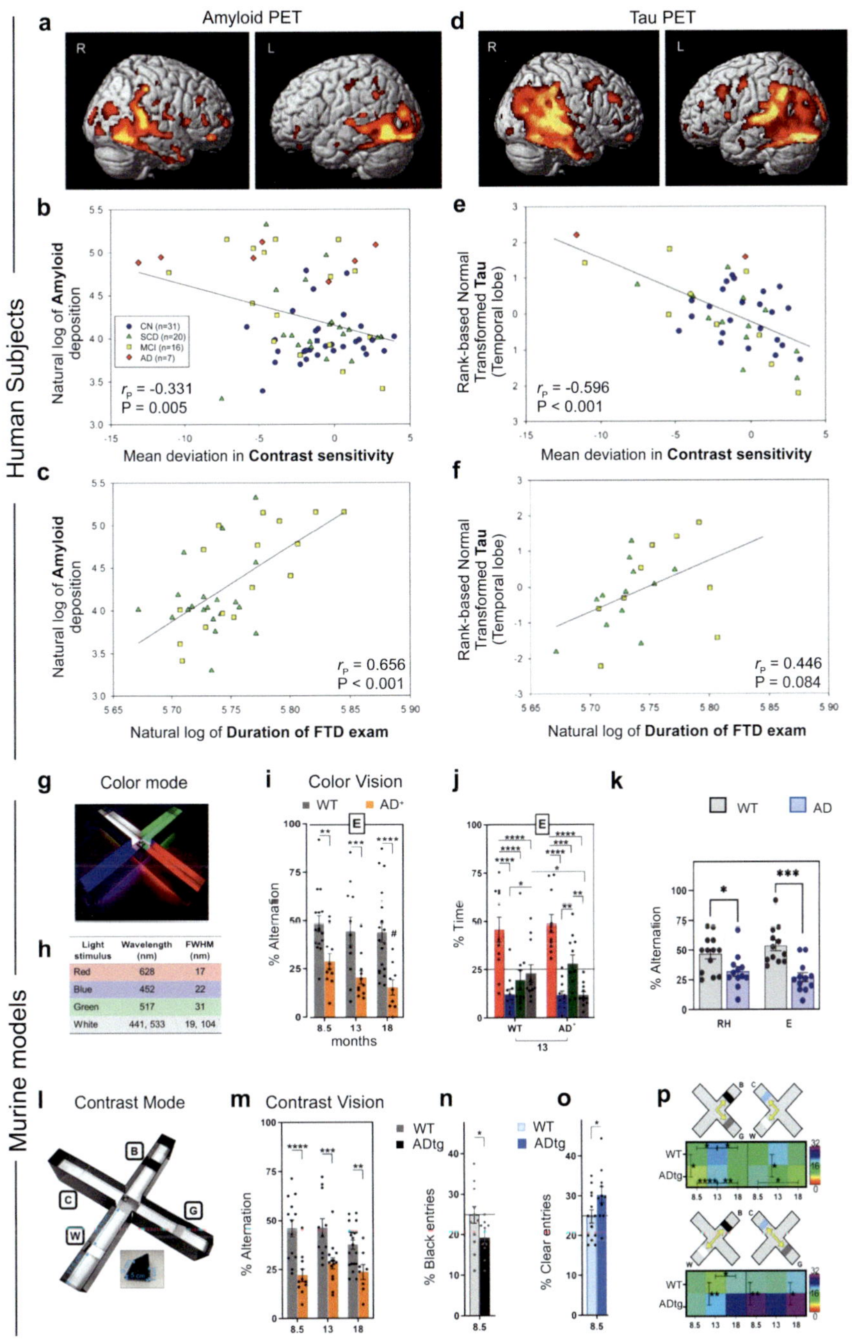
Human Subjects
a
Amyloid PET
R
L
d
Tau PET
R
L
b
Natural log of Amyloid deposition
CN (n=31)
SCD (n=20)
MCI (n=16)
AD (n=7)
rP = -0.331
P = 0.005
Mean deviation in Contrast sensitivity
e
Rank-based Normal Transformed Tau (Temporal lobe)
rP = -0.596
P < 0.001
Mean deviation in Contrast sensitivity
c
Natural log of Amyloid deposition
rP = 0.656
P < 0.001
Natural log of Duration of FTD exam
f
Rank-based Normal Transformed Tau (Temporal lobe)
rP = 0.446
P = 0.084
Natural log of Duration of FTD exam
Murine models
g
Color mode
h
Light stimulus | Wavelength (nm) | FWHM (nm)
Red | 628 | 17
Blue | 452 | 22
Green | 517 | 31
White | 441, 533 | 19, 104
i
Color Vision
WT
AD+
% Alternation
months
j
% Time
WT
AD+
k
WT
AD
% Alternation
RH
E
l
Contrast Mode
B
C
G
W
m
Contrast Vision
% Alternation
n
WT
ADtg
% Black entries
o
WT
ADtg
% Clear entries
p
WT
ADtg

◂**Fig. 6.18** Contrast and color loss is associated with cerebral Aβ and tau. (**a–f**) Visual contrast sensitivity was assessed in human subjects with different degrees of AD pathologies, such as subjective cognitive decline (SCD), MCI, AD, compared to NC subjects using MRI scans and amyloid PET imaging. (**a**) Visual contrast sensitivity is associated with voxel-wise cerebral amyloid deposition. On the voxel-wise analysis, significant associations between visual contrast sensitivity (examination duration) and amyloid deposition in the medial and lateral temporal lobes were observed. Examination duration (indicated as the natural log of seconds needed to complete the examination) is a measure of contrast sensitivity performance as the test is iterative and those with poorer contrast sensitivity take longer on the examination, and lower mean deviation scores represent poorer contrast sensitivity performance. (**b**) Scatter plot shows the significant association between visual contrast sensitivity and regional cerebral amyloid deposition. (**c**) In SCD and MCI individuals only, significant associations were observed between cortical amyloid and examination duration. (**d**) Visual contrast sensitivity is associated with voxel-wise cerebral tau deposition. Significant associations between mean deviation in visual contrast sensitivity and tau deposition in the lateral and medial temporal lobes were observed. (**e**) Scatter plot shows the significant association between visual contrast sensitivity and regional cerebral tau deposition. (**f**) In SCD and MCI participants only, the mean deviation in visual contrast sensitivity is significantly associated with normal transformed tau in the temporal lobe. (**g-p**) In murine models, the Visual X maze, or Visual-Stimuli 4-arm Maze (ViS4M) is used to quantitatively study color and contrast vision along with cognitive function. (**g**) Photograph of the ViS4M in color mode showing the illuminated arms. (**h**) Table showing the characteristics of the light stimuli (peak wavelength, FWHM). (**i**) Percent alternation in the Equal (E) condition of the color mode in 8.5-, 13-, and 18-month-old WT and ADtg mice. (**j**) Percentage of time spent in each colored arm under the E condition in 13-month-old mice. (**k**) Percent alternation in the red high (RH) and the E light intensity conditions in old WT and ADtg mice. (**l**) Visual X maze in the contrast mode: the arms include either black, grey, white, or clear objects against the white floor and black walls. (**m**) Percentage of alternation under the contrast mode setting in 8.5-, 13-, and 18-month-old WT versus ADtg mice. (**n, o**) Percentage of entries in the arm containing (**n**) the black object and (**o**) the clear object in 8.5-month-old mice. (**p**) Rainbow heatmap illustrating the percentage of bidirectional transitions between arms with grey and black objects, white and clear objects, white and black objects, and grey and clear objects. The color gradient bar shows the range of percent transitions (from lowest in red to highest in purple). $^{*}P < 0.05$, $^{**}P < 0.01$, $^{***}P < 0.001$, $^{****}P < 0.0001$, analyzed by two-way ANOVA followed by post-hoc Fisher's LSD test. FDT, frequency doubling technology; FWHM, full width at half-maximum; LTL, lateral temporal lobe. Panels **a–f** are adapted from Risacher et al., Brain Commun 2020 [327]. Panels **g–o** are reproduced from Vit et al., Bio Protoc 2021 [380] and Sci Rep 2021 [379]

disturbances in animal AD models, including drosophila [83, 87, 378–384]. Our group has specifically demonstrated color and contrast vision deficits in young and old transgenic murine models of AD [379, 380] (Fig. 6.18g–p). Therefore, visual abnormalities in elderly individuals may serve as an indicator of AD pathogenesis.

Despite numerous recent reports, the field of AD retinopathy is still in its infancy, and more studies focusing on dysfunction and pathomechanisms are necessary to determine the connection between specific retinal pathologies, neuronal subtype impairments, and visual-functional deficits.

6.5 Conclusion

Emerging evidence indicates the presence of AD hallmark pathology and associated degeneration, inflammation, and vasculopathy in the retina, mirroring that seen in the brain, as described here. This field is currently under intense investigation. As the number of individuals suffering from AD is quickly rising – expected to more than double by 2050 – there is an urgent unmet need for a noninvasive, affordable, and accurate method of diagnosis and disease monitoring.

The previously demonstrated capacity to detect and quantify Aβ deposits, and possibly vascular Aβ pathology in the future, using noninvasive retinal amyloid imaging, may offer an exceptional modality for early and specific diagnosis of AD, as well as monitoring the response to therapies. Currently, there is no clinical method for non-invasive imaging of CNS tissue with such high resolution and specificity. The studies discussed in this chapter, along with related future research, may pave the way towards translation. To conclude, the retina could become an important site for screening and monitoring AD pathogenesis beyond the brain.

Acknowledgements This work was funded by National Institute of Health NIA R01AG056478 (MKH), NIA R01AG055865 (MKH), NIA R41AG044897 (MKH), NIA R01AG075998 (MKH), Alzheimer's Association Research Fellowship to Promote Diversity, AARFD-21-851509 (HS), the Haim Saban, the Susan and David Wilstein, the Tom Gordon, and the Maurice Marciano Foundations (MKH). We thank Elijiah Maxfield for help in editing this chapter.

Dedication This article is dedicated to the memories of Dr. Salomon Moni Hamaoui and Lillian Jones Black, both of whom died from Alzheimer's disease.

References

1. Alzheimer's A. Alzheimer's disease facts and figures. Alzheimers Dement. 2023;19(4):1598–695.
2. Gauthier S, Webster C, Servaes S, Morais JA, Rosa-Neto P. World Alzheimer report 2022: life after diagnosis: navigating treatment, care and support. London, England: Alzheimer's Disease International; 2022.
3. Wiese LAK, Gibson A, Guest MA, Nelson AR, Weaver R, Gupta A, et al. Global rural health disparities in Alzheimer's disease and related dementias: state of the science. Alzheimers Dement. 2023.
4. Collaborators GBD. Global mortality from dementia: application of a new method and results from the global burden of disease study 2019. Alzheimers Dement. 2021;7(1):e12200.
5. Liu KY, Villain N, Ayton S, Ackley SF, Planche V, Howard R, et al. Key questions for the evaluation of anti-amyloid immunotherapies for Alzheimer's disease. Brain Commun. 2023;5(3):fcad175.
6. Porsteinsson AP, Isaacson RS, Knox S, Sabbagh MN, Rubino I. Diagnosis of early Alzheimer's disease: clinical practice in 2021. J Prev Alzheimers Dis. 2021;8(3):371–86.
7. Jack CR Jr, Bennett DA, Blennow K, Carrillo MC, Dunn B, Haeberlein SB, et al. NIA-AA research framework: toward a biological definition of Alzheimer's disease. Alzheimers Dement. 2018;14(4):535–62.

8. Jack CR Jr, Bennett DA, Blennow K, Carrillo MC, Feldman HH, Frisoni GB, et al. A/T/N: An unbiased descriptive classification scheme for Alzheimer disease biomarkers. Neurology. 2016;87(5):539–47.
9. Akiyama H, Barger S, Barnum S, Bradt B, Bauer J, Cole GM, et al. Inflammation and Alzheimer's disease. Neurobiol Aging. 2000;21(3):383–421.
10. Baker-Nigh A, Vahedi S, Davis EG, Weintraub S, Bigio EH, Klein WL, et al. Neuronal amyloid-beta accumulation within cholinergic basal forebrain in ageing and Alzheimer's disease. Brain. 2015;138(Pt 6):1722–37.
11. Bettcher BM, Tansey MG, Dorothee G, Heneka MT. Peripheral and central immune system crosstalk in Alzheimer disease—a research prospectus. Nat Rev Neurol. 2021;17(11):689–701.
12. Guo T, Zhang D, Zeng Y, Huang TY, Xu H, Zhao Y. Molecular and cellular mechanisms underlying the pathogenesis of Alzheimer's disease. Mol Neurodegener. 2020;15(1):40.
13. Heneka MT, Carson MJ, El Khoury J, Landreth GE, Brosseron F, Feinstein DL, et al. Neuroinflammation in Alzheimer's disease. Lancet Neurol. 2015;14(4):388–405.
14. Jackson J, Jambrina E, Li J, Marston H, Menzies F, Phillips K, et al. Targeting the synapse in Alzheimer's disease. Front Neurosci. 2019;13:735.
15. Nelson AR, Sweeney MD, Sagare AP, Zlokovic BV. Neurovascular dysfunction and neurodegeneration in dementia and Alzheimer's disease. Biochim Biophys Acta. 2016;1862(5):887–900.
16. Ratan Y, Rajput A, Maleysm S, Pareek A, Jain V, Pareek A, et al. An insight into cellular and molecular mechanisms underlying the pathogenesis of neurodegeneration in Alzheimer's disease. Biomedicines. 2023;11(5).
17. Selkoe DJ. Soluble oligomers of the amyloid beta-protein impair synaptic plasticity and behavior. Behav Brain Res. 2008;192(1):106–13.
18. Shankar GM, Li S, Mehta TH, Garcia-Munoz A, Shepardson NE, Smith I, et al. Amyloid-beta protein dimers isolated directly from Alzheimer's brains impair synaptic plasticity and memory. Nat Med. 2008;14(8):837–42.
19. Tzioras M, McGeachan RI, Durrant CS, Spires-Jones TL. Synaptic degeneration in Alzheimer disease. Nat Rev Neurol. 2023;19(1):19–38.
20. Wu M, Zhang M, Yin X, Chen K, Hu Z, Zhou Q, et al. The role of pathological tau in synaptic dysfunction in Alzheimer's diseases. Transl Neurodegener. 2021;10(1):45.
21. Beason-Held LL, Goh JO, An Y, Kraut MA, O'Brien RJ, Ferrucci L, et al. Changes in brain function occur years before the onset of cognitive impairment. J Neurosci. 2013;33(46):18008–14.
22. Bilgel M, An Y, Zhou Y, Wong DF, Prince JL, Ferrucci L, et al. Individual estimates of age at detectable amyloid onset for risk factor assessment. Alzheimers Dement. 2016;12(4):373–9.
23. Perrin RJ, Fagan AM, Holtzman DM. Multimodal techniques for diagnosis and prognosis of Alzheimer's disease. Nature. 2009;461(7266):916–22.
24. Vermunt L, Sikkes SAM, van den Hout A, Handels R, Bos I, van der Flier WM, et al. Duration of preclinical, prodromal, and dementia stages of Alzheimer's disease in relation to age, sex, and APOE genotype. Alzheimers Dement. 2019;15(7):888–98.
25. Bellaver B, Povala G, Ferreira PCL, Ferrari-Souza JP, Leffa DT, Lussier FZ, et al. Astrocyte reactivity influences amyloid-beta effects on tau pathology in preclinical Alzheimer's disease. Nat Med. 2023.
26. Dani M, Wood M, Mizoguchi R, Fan Z, Walker Z, Morgan R, et al. Microglial activation correlates in vivo with both tau and amyloid in Alzheimer's disease. Brain. 2018;141(9):2740–54.
27. Ismail R, Parbo P, Madsen LS, Hansen AK, Hansen KV, Schaldemose JL, et al. The relationships between neuroinflammation, beta-amyloid and tau deposition in Alzheimer's disease: a longitudinal PET study. J Neuroinflamm. 2020;17(1):151.
28. Crews L, Masliah E. Molecular mechanisms of neurodegeneration in Alzheimer's disease. Hum Mol Genet. 2010;19(R1):R12-20.

29. Wyss-Coray T. Inflammation in Alzheimer disease: driving force, bystander or beneficial response? Nat Med. 2006;12(9):1005–15.
30. Zuroff L, Daley D, Black KL, Koronyo-Hamaoui M. Clearance of cerebral Abeta in Alzheimer's disease: reassessing the role of microglia and monocytes. Cell Mol Life Sci. 2017;74(12):2167–201.
31. Alexandrov PN, Pogue A, Bhattacharjee S, Lukiw WJ. Retinal amyloid peptides and complement factor H in transgenic models of Alzheimer's disease. NeuroReport. 2011;22(12):623–7.
32. Ashraf G, McGuinness M, Khan MA, Obtinalla C, Hadoux X, van Wijngaarden P. Retinal imaging biomarkers of Alzheimer's disease: A systematic review and meta-analysis of studies using brain amyloid beta status for case definition. Alzheimers Dement. 2023;15(2): e12421.
33. Cao KJ, Kim JH, Kroeger H, Gaffney PM, Lin JH, Sigurdson CJ, et al. ARCAM-1 facilitates fluorescence detection of amyloid-containing deposits in the retina. Transl Vis Sci Technol. 2021;10(7):5.
34. den Haan J, Hart de Ruyter FJ, Lochocki B, Kroon M, Kemper EM, Teunissen CE, et al. No difference in retinal fluorescence after oral curcumin intake in amyloid-proven AD cases compared to controls. Alzheimers Dement. 2022;14(1):e12347.
35. den Haan J, Morrema THJ, Verbraak FD, de Boer JF, Scheltens P, Rozemuller AJ, et al. Amyloid-beta and phosphorylated tau in post-mortem Alzheimer's disease retinas. Acta Neuropathol Commun. 2018;6(1):147.
36. Du X, Koronyo Y, Mirzaei N, Yang C, Fuchs DT, Black KL, et al. Label-free hyperspectral imaging and deep-learning prediction of retinal amyloid beta-protein and phosphorylated tau. PNAS Nexus. 2022;1(4):pgac164.
37. Dumitrascu OM, Lyden PD, Torbati T, Sheyn J, Sherzai A, Sherzai D, et al. Sectoral segmentation of retinal amyloid imaging in subjects with cognitive decline. Alzheimers Dement. 2020;12(1):e12109.
38. Dumitrascu OM, Rosenberry R, Sherman DS, Khansari MM, Sheyn J, Torbati T, et al. Retinal venular tortuosity jointly with retinal amyloid burden correlates with verbal memory loss: a pilot study. Cells. 2021;10(11).
39. Grimaldi A, Pediconi N, Oieni F, Pizzarelli R, Rosito M, Giubettini M, et al. Neuroinflammatory processes, A1 astrocyte activation and protein aggregation in the retina of Alzheimer's disease patients, possible biomarkers for early diagnosis. Front Neurosci. 2019;13:925.
40. Gupta VB, Chitranshi N, den Haan J, Mirzaei M, You Y, Lim JK, et al. Retinal changes in Alzheimer's disease-integrated prospects of imaging, functional and molecular advances. Prog Retin Eye Res. 2021;82:100899.
41. Hadoux X, Hui F, Lim JKH, Masters CL, Pebay A, Chevalier S, et al. Non-invasive in vivo hyperspectral imaging of the retina for potential biomarker use in Alzheimer's disease. Nat Commun. 2019;10(1):4227.
42. Hart de Ruyter FJ, Morrema THJ, den Haan J, Netherlands Brain B, Twisk JWR, de Boer JF, et al. Phosphorylated tau in the retina correlates with tau pathology in the brain in Alzheimer's disease and primary tauopathies. Acta Neuropathol. 2023;145(2):197–218.
43. Hart NJ, Koronyo Y, Black KL, Koronyo-Hamaoui M. Ocular indicators of Alzheimer's: exploring disease in the retina. Acta Neuropathol. 2016;132(6):767–87.
44. Koronyo Y, Biggs D, Barron E, Boyer DS, Pearlman JA, Au WJ, et al. Retinal amyloid pathology and proof-of-concept imaging trial in Alzheimer's disease. JCI Insight. 2017;2(16).
45. Koronyo Y, Rentsendorj A, Mirzaei N, Regis GC, Sheyn J, Shi H, et al. Retinal pathological features and proteome signatures of Alzheimer's disease. Acta Neuropathol. 2023;145(4):409–38.
46. Koronyo-Hamaoui M, Koronyo Y, Ljubimov AV, Miller CA, Ko MK, Black KL, et al. Identification of amyloid plaques in retinas from Alzheimer's patients and noninvasive in vivo optical imaging of retinal plaques in a mouse model. Neuroimage. 2011;54(Suppl 1):S204–17.
47. La Morgia C, Ross-Cisneros FN, Koronyo Y, Hannibal J, Gallassi R, Cantalupo G, et al. Melanopsin retinal ganglion cell loss in Alzheimer disease. Ann Neurol. 2016;79(1):90–109.

48. Lee S, Jiang K, McIlmoyle B, To E, Xu QA, Hirsch-Reinshagen V, et al. Amyloid beta immunoreactivity in the retinal ganglion cell layer of the Alzheimer's eye. Front Neurosci. 2020;14:758.
49. Lemmens S, Van Craenendonck T, Van Eijgen J, De Groef L, Bruffaerts R, de Jesus DA, et al. Combination of snapshot hyperspectral retinal imaging and optical coherence tomography to identify Alzheimer's disease patients. Alzheimers Res Ther. 2020;12(1):144.
50. Mirzaei N, Shi H, Oviatt M, Doustar J, Rentsendorj A, Fuchs DT, et al. Alzheimer's retinopathy: seeing disease in the eyes. Front Neurosci. 2020;14:921.
51. More SS, Beach JM, McClelland C, Mokhtarzadeh A, Vince R. In vivo assessment of retinal biomarkers by hyperspectral imaging: early detection of Alzheimer's disease. ACS Chem Neurosci. 2019;10(11):4492–501.
52. Ngolab J, Donohue M, Belsha A, Salazar J, Cohen P, Jaiswal S, et al. Feasibility study for detection of retinal amyloid in clinical trials: the anti-amyloid treatment in asymptomatic alzheimer's disease (A4) trial. Alzheimers Dement. 2021;13(1):e12199.
53. Qiu Y, Jin T, Mason E, Campbell MCW. Predicting thioflavin fluorescence of retinal amyloid deposits associated With Alzheimer's disease from their polarimetric properties. Transl Vis Sci Technol. 2020;9(2):47.
54. Schon C, Hoffmann NA, Ochs SM, Burgold S, Filser S, Steinbach S, et al. Long-term in vivo imaging of fibrillar tau in the retina of P301S transgenic mice. PLoS ONE. 2012;7(12):e53547.
55. Schultz N, Byman E, Netherlands Brain B, Wennstrom M. Levels of retinal amyloid-beta correlate with levels of retinal IAPP and hippocampal amyloid-beta in neuropathologically evaluated individuals. J Alzheimers Dis. 2020;73(3):1201–9.
56. Shi H, Koronyo Y, Fuchs DT, Sheyn J, Jallow O, Mandalia K, et al. Retinal arterial Abeta(40) deposition is linked with tight junction loss and cerebral amyloid angiopathy in MCI and AD patients. Alzheimers Dement. 2023.
57. Shi H, Koronyo Y, Rentsendorj A, Fuchs DT, Sheyn J, Black KL, et al. Retinal vasculopathy in Alzheimer's disease. Front Neurosci. 2021;15:731614.
58. Shi H, Koronyo Y, Rentsendorj A, Regis GC, Sheyn J, Fuchs DT, et al. Identification of early pericyte loss and vascular amyloidosis in Alzheimer's disease retina. Acta Neuropathol. 2020;139(5):813–36.
59. Snyder PJ, Alber J, Alt C, Bain LJ, Bouma BE, Bouwman FH, et al. Retinal imaging in Alzheimer's and neurodegenerative diseases. Alzheimers Dement. 2021;17(1):103–11.
60. Tadokoro K, Yamashita T, Kimura S, Nomura E, Ohta Y, Omote Y, et al. Retinal amyloid imaging for screening Alzheimer's disease. J Alzheimers Dis. 2021;83(2):927–34.
61. Tsai Y, Lu B, Ljubimov AV, Girman S, Ross-Cisneros FN, Sadun AA, et al. Ocular changes in TgF344-AD rat model of Alzheimer's disease. Invest Ophthalmol Vis Sci. 2014;55(1):523–34.
62. Xu QA, Boerkoel P, Hirsch-Reinshagen V, Mackenzie IR, Hsiung GR, Charm G, et al. Muller cell degeneration and microglial dysfunction in the Alzheimer's retina. Acta Neuropathol Commun. 2022;10(1):145.
63. Asanad S, Ross-Cisneros FN, Nassisi M, Barron E, Karanjia R, Sadun AA. The retina in Alzheimer's disease: histomorphometric analysis of an ophthalmologic biomarker. Invest Ophthalmol Vis Sci. 2019;60(5):1491–500.
64. Ascaso FJ, Cruz N, Modrego PJ, Lopez-Anton R, Santabarbara J, Pascual LF, et al. Retinal alterations in mild cognitive impairment and Alzheimer's disease: an optical coherence tomography study. J Neurol. 2014;261(8):1522–30.
65. Berisha F, Feke GT, Trempe CL, McMeel JW, Schepens CL. Retinal abnormalities in early Alzheimer's disease. Invest Ophthalmol Vis Sci. 2007;48(5):2285–9.
66. Blanks JC, Hinton DR, Sadun AA, Miller CA. Retinal ganglion cell degeneration in Alzheimer's disease. Brain Res. 1989;501(2):364–72.
67. Blanks JC, Schmidt SY, Torigoe Y, Porrello KV, Hinton DR, Blanks RH. Retinal pathology in Alzheimer's disease. II. Regional neuron loss and glial changes in GCL. Neurobiol Aging. 1996;17(3):385–95.

68. Blanks JC, Torigoe Y, Hinton DR, Blanks RH. Retinal pathology in Alzheimer's disease. I. Ganglion cell loss in foveal/parafoveal retina. Neurobiol Aging. 1996;17(3):377–84.
69. Frost S, Kanagasingam Y, Sohrabi H, Vignarajan J, Bourgeat P, Salvado O, et al. Retinal vascular biomarkers for early detection and monitoring of Alzheimer's disease. Transl Psychiatry. 2013;3:e233.
70. Gao L, Liu Y, Li X, Bai Q, Liu P. Abnormal retinal nerve fiber layer thickness and macula lutea in patients with mild cognitive impairment and Alzheimer's disease. Arch Gerontol Geriatr. 2015;60(1):162–7.
71. Hinton DR, Sadun AA, Blanks JC, Miller CA. Optic-nerve degeneration in Alzheimer's disease. N Engl J Med. 1986;315(8):485–7.
72. Kesler A, Vakhapova V, Korczyn AD, Naftaliev E, Neudorfer M. Retinal thickness in patients with mild cognitive impairment and Alzheimer's disease. Clin Neurol Neurosurg. 2011;113(7):523–6.
73. Kim HM, Han JW, Park YJ, Bae JB, Woo SJ, Kim KW. Association between retinal layer thickness and cognitive decline in older adults. JAMA Ophthalmol. 2022;140(7):683–90.
74. Kirbas S, Turkyilmaz K, Anlar O, Tufekci A, Durmus M. Retinal nerve fiber layer thickness in patients with Alzheimer disease. J Neuroophthalmol. 2013;33(1):58–61.
75. Marziani E, Pomati S, Ramolfo P, Cigada M, Giani A, Mariani C, et al. Evaluation of retinal nerve fiber layer and ganglion cell layer thickness in Alzheimer's disease using spectral-domain optical coherence tomography. Invest Ophthalmol Vis Sci. 2013;54(9):5953–8.
76. Sadun AA, Bassi CJ. Optic nerve damage in Alzheimer's disease. Ophthalmology. 1990;97(1):9–17.
77. Araya-Arriagada J, Bello F, Shivashankar G, Neira D, Duran-Aniotz C, Acosta ML, et al. Retinal ganglion cells functional changes in a mouse model of Alzheimer's disease are linked with neurotransmitter alterations. J Alzheimers Dis. 2021;82(s1):S5–18.
78. Chang LY, Ardiles AO, Tapia-Rojas C, Araya J, Inestrosa NC, Palacios AG, et al. Evidence of synaptic and neurochemical remodeling in the retina of aging degus. Front Neurosci. 2020;14:161.
79. Cutler T, Sarkar A, Moran M, Steffensmeier A, Puli OR, Mancini G, et al. Drosophila eye model to study neuroprotective role of CREB binding protein (CBP) in Alzheimer's disease. PLoS ONE. 2015;10(9):e0137691.
80. Du LY, Chang LY, Ardiles AO, Tapia-Rojas C, Araya J, Inestrosa NC, et al. Alzheimer's disease-related protein expression in the retina of octodon degus. PLoS ONE. 2015;10(8):e0135499.
81. Dutescu RM, Li QX, Crowston J, Masters CL, Baird PN, Culvenor JG. Amyloid precursor protein processing and retinal pathology in mouse models of Alzheimer's disease. Graefes Arch Clin Exp Ophthalmol. 2009;247(9):1213–21.
82. Edwards MM, Rodriguez JJ, Gutierrez-Lanza R, Yates J, Verkhratsky A, Lutty GA. Retinal macroglia changes in a triple transgenic mouse model of Alzheimer's disease. Exp Eye Res. 2014;127:252–60.
83. Georgevsky D, Retsas S, Raoufi N, Shimoni O, Golzan SM. A longitudinal assessment of retinal function and structure in the APP/PS1 transgenic mouse model of Alzheimer's disease. Transl Neurodegener. 2019;8:30.
84. Guo L, Ravindran N, Shamsher E, Hill D, Cordeiro MF. Retinal changes in transgenic mouse models of Alzheimer's disease. Curr Alzheimer Res. 2021;18(2):89–102.
85. Gupta VK, Chitranshi N, Gupta VB, Golzan M, Dheer Y, Wall RV, et al. Amyloid beta accumulation and inner retinal degenerative changes in Alzheimer's disease transgenic mouse. Neurosci Lett. 2016;623:52–6.
86. Habiba U, Merlin S, Lim JKH, Wong VHY, Nguyen CTO, Morley JW, et al. Age-specific retinal and cerebral immunodetection of amyloid-beta plaques and oligomers in a rodent model of Alzheimer's disease. J Alzheimers Dis. 2020;76(3):1135–50.
87. Lim JKH, Li QX, He Z, Vingrys AJ, Chinnery HR, Mullen J, et al. Retinal functional and structural changes in the 5xFAD mouse model of Alzheimer's disease. Front Neurosci. 2020;14:862.

88. Liu B, Rasool S, Yang Z, Glabe CG, Schreiber SS, Ge J, et al. Amyloid-peptide vaccinations reduce {beta}-amyloid plaques but exacerbate vascular deposition and inflammation in the retina of Alzheimer's transgenic mice. Am J Pathol. 2009;175(5):2099–110.
89. Matei N, Leahy S, Blair NP, Burford J, Rahimi M, Shahidi M. Retinal vascular physiology biomarkers in a 5XFAD mouse model of Alzheimer's disease. Cells. 2022;11(15).
90. More SS, Vince R. Hyperspectral imaging signatures detect amyloidopathy in Alzheimer's mouse retina well before onset of cognitive decline. ACS Chem Neurosci. 2015;6(2):306–15.
91. Ning A, Cui J, To E, Ashe KH, Matsubara J. Amyloid-beta deposits lead to retinal degeneration in a mouse model of Alzheimer disease. Invest Ophthalmol Vis Sci. 2008;49(11):5136–43.
92. Perez SE, Lumayag S, Kovacs B, Mufson EJ, Xu S. Beta-amyloid deposition and functional impairment in the retina of the APPswe/PS1DeltaE9 transgenic mouse model of Alzheimer's disease. Invest Ophthalmol Vis Sci. 2009;50(2):793–800.
93. Salobrar-Garcia E, Rodrigues-Neves AC, Ramirez AI, de Hoz R, Fernandez-Albarral JA, Lopez-Cuenca I, et al. Microglial activation in the retina of a triple-transgenic Alzheimer's disease mouse model (3xTg-AD). Int J Mol Sci. 2020;21(3).
94. Shi H, Koronyo Y, Fuchs DT, Sheyn J, Wawrowsky K, Lahiri S, et al. Retinal capillary degeneration and blood-retinal barrier disruption in murine models of Alzheimer's disease. Acta Neuropathol Commun. 2020;8(1):202.
95. Shi H, Yin Z, Koronyo Y, Fuchs DT, Sheyn J, Davis MR, et al. Regulating microglial miR-155 transcriptional phenotype alleviates Alzheimer's-induced retinal vasculopathy by limiting Clec7a/Galectin-3(+) neurodegenerative microglia. Acta Neuropathol Commun. 2022;10(1):136.
96. Sidiqi A, Wahl D, Lee S, Ma D, To E, Cui J, et al. In vivo retinal fluorescence imaging with curcumin in an Alzheimer mouse model. Front Neurosci. 2020;14:713.
97. Tams ALM, Sanz-Morello B, Westi EW, Mouhammad ZA, Andersen JV, Freude KK, et al. Decreased glucose metabolism and glutamine synthesis in the retina of a transgenic mouse model of Alzheimer's disease. Cell Mol Neurobiol. 2022;42(1):291–303.
98. Zhang J, Gao F, Ma Y, Xue T, Shen Y. Identification of early-onset photoreceptor degeneration in transgenic mouse models of Alzheimer's disease. iScience. 2021;24(11):103327.
99. Zhang M, Zhong L, Han X, Xiong G, Xu D, Zhang S, et al. Brain and retinal abnormalities in the 5xFAD mouse model of Alzheimer's disease at early stages. Front Neurosci. 2021;15:681831.
100. Zhao H, Chang R, Che H, Wang J, Yang L, Fang W, et al. Hyperphosphorylation of tau protein by calpain regulation in retina of Alzheimer's disease transgenic mouse. Neurosci Lett. 2013;551:12–6.
101. Doustar J, Rentsendorj A, Torbati T, Regis GC, Fuchs DT, Sheyn J, et al. Parallels between retinal and brain pathology and response to immunotherapy in old, late-stage Alzheimer's disease mouse models. Aging Cell. 2020:e13246.
102. Grimaldi A, Brighi C, Peruzzi G, Ragozzino D, Bonanni V, Limatola C, et al. Inflammation, neurodegeneration and protein aggregation in the retina as ocular biomarkers for Alzheimer''s disease in the 3xTg-AD mouse model. Cell Death Dis. 2018;9(6):685.
103. Purves D, Fitzpatrick D. In: Dale Purves GJA, David Fitzpatrick, Lawrence C Katz, Anthony-Samuel LaMantia, James O McNamara, and S Mark Williams, editors. The Retina. 2nd ed Sunderland (MA): Sinauer Associates; 2001.
104. Byerly MS, Blackshaw S. Vertebrate retina and hypothalamus development. Wiley Interdisc Rev Syst Biol Med. 2009;1(3):380–9.
105. Trost A, Lange S, Schroedl F, Bruckner D, Motloch KA, Bogner B, et al. Brain and retinal pericytes: origin, function and role. Front Cell Neurosci. 2016;10:20.
106. Sadda SV, Schachat A, Wilkinson C, Hinton D, Wiedemann P, Freund KB, et al. Ryan's retina 7th ed. Elsevier (eBook ISBN: 9780323722148; Hardcover ISBN: 9780323722131); 2022. p. 3.
107. Maude RJ, Dondorp AM, Abu Sayeed A, Day NP, White NJ, Beare NA. The eye in cerebral malaria: what can it teach us? Trans R Soc Trop Med Hyg. 2009;103(7):661–4.

108. Morin PJ, Abraham CR, Amaratunga A, Johnson RJ, Huber G, Sandell JH, et al. Amyloid precursor protein is synthesized by retinal ganglion cells, rapidly transported to the optic nerve plasma membrane and nerve terminals, and metabolized. J Neurochem. 1993;61(2):464–73.
109. Li L, Luo J, Chen D, Tong JB, Zeng LP, Cao YQ, et al. BACE1 in the retina: a sensitive biomarker for monitoring early pathological changes in Alzheimer's disease. Neural Regen Res. 2016;11(3):447–53.
110. Cai J, Qi X, Kociok N, Skosyrski S, Emilio A, Ruan Q, et al. Beta-secretase (BACE1) inhibition causes retinal pathology by vascular dysregulation and accumulation of age pigment. EMBO Mol Med. 2012;4(9):980–91.
111. Vecino E, Rodriguez FD, Ruzafa N, Pereiro X, Sharma SC. Glia-neuron interactions in the mammalian retina. Prog Retin Eye Res. 2016;51:1–40.
112. Johnson LV, Leitner WP, Rivest AJ, Staples MK, Radeke MJ, Anderson DH. The Alzheimer's A beta-peptide is deposited at sites of complement activation in pathologic deposits associated with aging and age-related macular degeneration. Proc Natl Acad Sci USA. 2002;99(18):11830–5
113. Frost GR, Li YM. The role of astrocytes in amyloid production and Alzheimer's disease. Open Biol. 2017;7(12).
114. Krasemann S, Madore C, Cialic R, Baufeld C, Calcagno N, El Fatimy R, et al. The TREM2-APOE pathway drives the transcriptional phenotype of dysfunctional microglia in neurodegenerative diseases. Immunity. 2017;47(3):566–81 e9.
115. Chiasseu M, Alarcon-Martinez L, Belforte N, Quintero H, Dotigny F, Destroismaisons L, et al. Tau accumulation in the retina promotes early neuronal dysfunction and precedes brain pathology in a mouse model of Alzheimer's disease. Mol Neurodegener. 2017;12(1):58.
116. Frost S, Martins RN, Kanagasingam Y. Ocular biomarkers for early detection of Alzheimer's disease. J Alzheimers Dis. 2010;22(1):1–16.
117. Gaynor LS, Curiel Cid RE, Penate A, Rosselli M, Burke SN, Wicklund M, et al. Visual object discrimination impairment as an early predictor of mild cognitive impairment and Alzheimer's disease. J Int Neuropsychol Soc. 2019;25(7):688–98.
118. Habiba U, Descallar J, Kreilaus F, Adhikari UK, Kumar S, Morley JW, et al. Detection of retinal and blood Abeta oligomers with nanobodies. Alzheimers Dement. 2021;13(1):e12193.
119. Koronyo Y, Salumbides BC, Black KL, Koronyo-Hamaoui M. Alzheimer's disease in the retina: imaging retinal abeta plaques for early diagnosis and therapy assessment. Neurodegener Dis. 2012;10(1–4):285–93.
120. Laatu S, Revonsuo A, Jaykka H, Portin R, Rinne JO. Visual object recognition in early Alzheimer's disease: deficits in semantic processing. Acta Neurol Scand. 2003;108(2):82–9.
121. Lu Y, Li Z, Zhang X, Ming B, Jia J, Wang R, et al. Retinal nerve fiber layer structure abnormalities in early Alzheimer's disease: evidence in optical coherence tomography. Neurosci Lett. 2010;480(1):69–72.
122. Tadokoro K, Yamashita T, Fukui Y, Nomura E, Ohta Y, Ueno S, et al. Early detection of cognitive decline in mild cognitive impairment and Alzheimer's disease with a novel eye tracking test. J Neurol Sci. 2021;427:117529.
123. Zhang YS, Zhou N, Knoll BM, Samra S, Ward MR, Weintraub S, et al. Parafoveal vessel loss and correlation between peripapillary vessel density and cognitive performance in amnestic mild cognitive impairment and early Alzheimer's Disease on optical coherence tomography angiography. PLoS ONE. 2019;14(4):e0214685.
124. Mei X, Yang M, Zhu L, Zhou Q, Li X, Chen Z, et al. Retinal levels of amyloid beta correlate with cerebral levels of amyloid beta in young APPswe/PS1dE9 transgenic mice before onset of Alzheimer's disease. Behav Neurol. 2020;2020:1574816.
125. Burns SA, Elsner AE, Sapoznik KA, Warner RL, Gast TJ. Adaptive optics imaging of the human retina. Prog Retin Eye Res. 2019;68:1–30.
126. Corvi F, Corradetti G, Parrulli S, Pace L, Staurenghi G, Sadda SR. Comparison and repeatability of high resolution and high speed scans from spectralis optical coherence tomography angiography. Transl Vis Sci Technol. 2020;9(10):29.

127. Gao M, Guo Y, Hormel TT, Sun J, Hwang TS, Jia Y. Reconstruction of high-resolution 6x6-mm OCT angiograms using deep learning. Biomed Opt Exp. 2020;11(7):3585–600.
128. Hampson KM, Turcotte R, Miller DT, Kurokawa K, Males JR, Ji N, et al. Adaptive optics for high-resolution imaging. Nat Rev Methods Primers. 2021;1.
129. Lai-Tim YM, Krafft L, Chen A, Petit C, Mecê P, Grieve K, Paques M, Meimon S. Super-resolution in vivo retinal imaging using structured illumination ophthalmoscopy (2020). arXiv preprint arXiv:200716028
130. Xie F, Luo W, Zhang Z, Sun D. In vivo molecular imaging in retinal disease. J Ophthalmol. 2012;2012:429387.
131. Xiao PMV, Grieve K, Sahel J-A, Fink M, Boccara AC. In vivo high-resolution human retinal imaging with wavefront-correctionless full-field OCT. Optica. 2018;5(4):409–12.
132. Alzheimer A, Stelzmann RA, Schnitzlein HN, Murtagh FR. An English translation of Alzheimer's 1907 paper, "Uber eine eigenartige Erkankung der Hirnrinde." Clin Anat. 1995;8(6):429–31.
133. Hippius H, Neundorfer G. The discovery of Alzheimer's disease. Dialogues Clin Neurosci. 2003;5(1):101–8.
134. Masters CL, Simms G, Weinman NA, Multhaup G, McDonald BL, Beyreuther K. Amyloid plaque core protein in Alzheimer disease and Down syndrome. Proc Natl Acad Sci U S A. 1985;82(12):4245–9.
135. Alzheimer A. Über einen eigenartigen schweren Erkrankungsprozeβ der Hirnrincle. Neurol Central. 1906;25:1134.
136. Ho CY, Troncoso JC, Knox D, Stark W, Eberhart CG. Beta-amyloid, phospho-tau and alpha-synuclein deposits similar to those in the brain are not identified in the eyes of Alzheimer's and Parkinson's disease patients. Brain Pathol. 2014;24(1):25–32.
137. Williams EA, McGuone D, Frosch MP, Hyman BT, Laver N, Stemmer-Rachamimov A. Absence of Alzheimer disease neuropathologic changes in eyes of subjects With Alzheimer disease. J Neuropathol Exp Neurol. 2017;76(5):376–83.
138. Tsai CS, Ritch R, Schwartz B, Lee SS, Miller NR, Chi T, et al. Optic nerve head and nerve fiber layer in Alzheimer's disease. Arch Ophthalmol. 1991;109(2):199–204.
139. Barucker C, Bittner HJ, Chang PK, Cameron S, Hancock MA, Liebsch F, et al. Abeta42-oligomer Interacting Peptide (AIP) neutralizes toxic amyloid-beta42 species and protects synaptic structure and function. Sci Rep. 2015;5:15410.
140. Cohen SI, Linse S, Luheshi LM, Hellstrand E, White DA, Rajah L, et al. Proliferation of amyloid-beta42 aggregates occurs through a secondary nucleation mechanism. Proc Natl Acad Sci USA. 2013;110(24):9758–63.
141. Lee A, Kondapalli C, Virga DM, Lewis TL Jr, Koo SY, Ashok A, et al. Abeta42 oligomers trigger synaptic loss through CAMKK2-AMPK-dependent effectors coordinating mitochondrial fission and mitophagy. Nat Commun. 2022;13(1):4444.
142. Pauwels K, Williams TL, Morris KL, Jonckheere W, Vandersteen A, Kelly G, et al. Structural basis for increased toxicity of pathological abeta42:abeta40 ratios in Alzheimer disease. J Biol Chem. 2012;287(8):5650–60.
143. Varga E, Juhasz G, Bozso Z, Penke B, Fulop L, Szegedi V. Amyloid-beta1-42 disrupts synaptic plasticity by altering glutamate recycling at the synapse. J Alzheimers Dis. 2015;45(2):449–56.
144. Li S, Hayden EY, Garcia VJ, Fuchs DT, Sheyn J, Daley DA, et al. Activated bone marrow-derived macrophages eradicate Alzheimer's-related abeta(42) oligomers and protect synapses. Front Immunol. 2020;11:49.
145. More SS, Beach JM, Vince R. Early detection of amyloidopathy in Alzheimer's mice by hyperspectral endoscopy. Invest Ophthalmol Vis Sci. 2016;57(7):3231–8.
146. Park SW, Kim JH, Mook-Jung I, Kim KW, Park WJ, Park KH. Intracellular amyloid beta alters the tight junction of retinal pigment epithelium in 5XFAD mice. Neurobiol Aging. 2014;35(9):2013–20.

147. Parthasarathy R, Chow KM, Derafshi Z, Fautsch MP, Hetling JR, Rodgers DW, et al. Reduction of amyloid-beta levels in mouse eye tissues by intra-vitreally delivered neprilysin. Exp Eye Res. 2015;138:134–44.
148. Pogue AI, Dua P, Hill JM, Lukiw WJ. Progressive inflammatory pathology in the retina of aluminum-fed 5xFAD transgenic mice. J Inorg Biochem. 2015.
149. Williams PA, Thirgood RA, Oliphant H, Frizzati A, Littlewood E, Votruba M, et al. Retinal ganglion cell dendritic degeneration in a mouse model of Alzheimer's disease. Neurobiol Aging. 2013;34(7):1799–806.
150. Carmine-Simmen K, Proctor T, Tschape J, Poeck B, Triphan T, Strauss R, et al. Neurotoxic effects induced by the Drosophila amyloid-beta peptide suggest a conserved toxic function. Neurobiol Dis. 2009;33(2):274–81.
151. Greeve I, Kretzschmar D, Tschape JA, Beyn A, Brellinger C, Schweizer M, et al. Age-dependent neurodegeneration and Alzheimer-amyloid plaque formation in transgenic Drosophila. J Neurosci. 2004;24(16):3899–906.
152. Yang Y, Shiao C, Hemingway JF, Jorstad NL, Shalloway BR, Chang R, et al. Suppressed retinal degeneration in aged wild type and APPswe/PS1DeltaE9 mice by bone marrow transplantation. PLoS ONE. 2013;8(6):e64246.
153. Deacon RM, Altimiras FJ, Bazan-Leon EA, Pyarasani RD, Nachtigall FM, Santos LS, et al. Natural AD-Like neuropathology in octodon degus: impaired burrowing and neuroinflammation. Curr Alzheimer Res. 2015;12(4):314–22.
154. Gao L, Chen X, Tang Y, Zhao J, Li Q, Fan X, et al. Neuroprotective effect of memantine on the retinal ganglion cells of APPswe/PS1DeltaE9 mice and its immunomodulatory mechanisms. Exp Eye Res. 2015;135:47–58.
155. He Y, Zhao H, Su G. Ginsenoside Rg1 decreases neurofibrillary tangles accumulation in retina by regulating activities of neprilysin and PKA in retinal cells of AD mice model. J Mol Neurosci. 2014;52(1):101–6.
156. Kile S, Au W, Parise C, Sohi J, Yarbrough T, Czeszynski A, et al. Reduction of amyloid in the brain and retina after treatment with IVIG for mild cognitive impairment. Am J Alzheimers Dis Other Demen. 2020;35:1533317519899800.
157. Ballatore C, Lee VM, Trojanowski JQ. Tau-mediated neurodegeneration in Alzheimer's disease and related disorders. Nat Rev Neurosci. 2007;8(9):663–72.
158. Hanseeuw BJ, Betensky RA, Jacobs HIL, Schultz AP, Sepulcre J, Becker JA, et al. Association of amyloid and Tau with cognition in preclinical Alzheimer disease: a longitudinal study. JAMA Neurol. 2019;76(8):915–24.
159. Jadhav S, Cubinkova V, Zimova I, Brezovakova V, Madari A, Cigankova V, et al. Tau-mediated synaptic damage in Alzheimer's disease. Transl Neurosci. 2015;6(1):214–26.
160. Zhang H, Cao Y, Ma L, Wei Y, Li H. Possible mechanisms of tau spread and toxicity in Alzheimer's disease. Front Cell Dev Biol. 2021;9:707268.
161. Guo J, Xu C, Ni S, Zhang S, Li Q, Zeng P, et al. Elevation of pS262-Tau and demethylated PP2A in retina occurs earlier than in hippocampus during hyperhomocysteinemia. J Alzheimers Dis. 2019;68(1):367–81.
162. Rodrigues-Neves AC, Carecho R, Correia SC, Carvalho C, Campos EJ, Baptista FI, et al. Retina and brain display early and differential molecular and cellular changes in the 3xTg-AD mouse model of Alzheimer's disease. Mol Neurobiol. 2021;58(7):3043–60.
163. Balzamino BO, Esposito G, Marino R, Calissano P, Latina V, Amadoro G, et al. Morphological and biomolecular targets in retina and vitreous from Reelin-deficient mice (Reeler): potential implications for age-related macular degeneration in Alzheimer's dementia. Front Aging Neurosci. 2022;14:1015359.
164. Latina V, Giacovazzo G, Cordella F, Balzamino BO, Micera A, Varano M, et al. Systemic delivery of a specific antibody targeting the pathological N-terminal truncated tau peptide reduces retinal degeneration in a mouse model of Alzheimer's Disease. Acta Neuropathol Commun. 2021;9(1):38.

165. Deng L, Pushpitha K, Joseph C, Gupta V, Rajput R, Chitranshi N, et al. Amyloid beta induces early changes in the ribosomal machinery, cytoskeletal organization and oxidative phosphorylation in retinal photoreceptor cells. Front Mol Neurosci. 2019;12:24.
166. Arouche-Delaperche L, Cadoni S, Joffrois C, Labernede G, Valet M, Cesar Q, et al. Dysfunction of the glutamatergic photoreceptor synapse in the P301S mouse model of tauopathy. Acta Neuropathol Commun. 2023;11(1):5.
167. Nilson AN, English KC, Gerson JE, Barton Whittle T, Nicolas Crain C, Xue J, et al. Tau oligomers associate with inflammation in the brain and retina of tauopathy mice and in neurodegenerative diseases. J Alzheimers Dis. 2017;55(3):1083–99.
168. Reinecke JB, DeVos SL, McGrath JP, Shepard AM, Goncharoff DK, Tait DN, et al. Implicating calpain in tau-mediated toxicity in vivo. PLoS ONE. 2011;6(8):e23865.
169. Lee S, Wang JW, Yu W, Lu B. Phospho-dependent ubiquitination and degradation of PAR-1 regulates synaptic morphology and tau-mediated Abeta toxicity in Drosophila. Nat Commun. 2012;3:1312.
170. Ngolab J, Canchi S, Rasool S, Elmaarouf A, Thomas K, Sarsoza F, et al. Mutant three-repeat tau expression initiates retinal ganglion cell death through caspase-2. Neurobiol Dis. 2021;152:105277.
171. Buccarello L, Sclip A, Sacchi M, Castaldo AM, Bertani I, ReCecconi A, et al. The c-jun N-terminal kinase plays a key role in ocular degenerative changes in a mouse model of Alzheimer disease suggesting a correlation between ocular and brain pathologies. Oncotarget. 2017;8(47):83038–51.
172. Buscho S, Palacios E, Xia F, Shi S, Li S, Luisi J, et al. Longitudinal characterization of retinal vasculature alterations with optical coherence tomography angiography in a mouse model of tauopathy. Exp Eye Res. 2022;224:109240.
173. Bolkan BJ, Kretzschmar D. Loss of Tau results in defects in photoreceptor development and progressive neuronal degeneration in Drosophila. Dev Neurobiol. 2014;74(12):1210–25.
174. Gilmore GC, Wenk HE, Naylor LA, Koss E. Motion perception and Alzheimer's disease. J Gerontol. 1994;49(2):P52–7.
175. Asanad S, Felix CM, Fantini M, Harrington MG, Sadun AA, Karanjia R. Retinal ganglion cell dysfunction in preclinical Alzheimer's disease: an electrophysiologic biomarker signature. Sci Rep. 2021;11(1):6344.
176. Oh AJ, Amore G, Sultan W, Asanad S, Park JC, Romagnoli M, et al. Pupillometry evaluation of melanopsin retinal ganglion cell function and sleep-wake activity in pre-symptomatic Alzheimer's disease. PLoS ONE. 2019;14(12):e0226197.
177. Chiu K, Chan TF, Wu A, Leung IY, So KF, Chang RC. Neurodegeneration of the retina in mouse models of Alzheimer's disease: what can we learn from the retina? Age. 2012;34(3):633–49.
178. Chakraborty A, de Wit NM, van der Flier WM, de Vries HE. The blood brain barrier in Alzheimer's disease. Vascul Pharmacol. 2017;89:12–8.
179. Di Marco LY, Venneri A, Farkas E, Evans PC, Marzo A, Frangi AF. Vascular dysfunction in the pathogenesis of Alzheimer's disease—a review of endothelium-mediated mechanisms and ensuing vicious circles. Neurobiol Dis. 2015;82:593–606.
180. Govindpani K, McNamara LG, Smith NR, Vinnakota C, Waldvogel HJ, Faull RL, et al. Vascular dysfunction in Alzheimer's disease: a prelude to the pathological process or a consequence of it? J Clin Med. 2019;8(5).
181. Arvanitakis Z, Leurgans SE, Wang Z, Wilson RS, Bennett DA, Schneider JA. Cerebral amyloid angiopathy pathology and cognitive domains in older persons. Ann Neurol. 2011;69(2):320–7.
182. Ellis RJ, Olichney JM, Thal LJ, Mirra SS, Morris JC, Beekly D, et al. Cerebral amyloid angiopathy in the brains of patients with Alzheimer's disease: the CERAD experience. Part XV Neurology. 1996;46(6):1592–6.
183. Viswanathan A, Greenberg SM. Cerebral amyloid angiopathy in the elderly. Ann Neurol. 2011;70(6):871–80.

184. Binnewijzend MA, Benedictus MR, Kuijer JP, van der Flier WM, Teunissen CE, Prins ND, et al. Cerebral perfusion in the predementia stages of Alzheimer's disease. Eur Radiol. 2016;26(2):506–14.
185. Bonte FJ, Ross ED, Chehabi HH, Devous MD Sr. SPECT study of regional cerebral blood flow in Alzheimer disease. J Comput Assist Tomogr. 1986;10(4):579–83.
186. Hirsch C, Bartenstein P, Minoshima S, Mosch D, Willoch F, Buch K, et al. Reduction of regional cerebral blood flow and cognitive impairment in patients with Alzheimer's disease: evaluation of an observer-independent analytic approach. Dement Geriatr Cogn Disord. 1997;8(2):98–104.
187. Claudio L. Ultrastructural features of the blood-brain barrier in biopsy tissue from Alzheimer's disease patients. Acta Neuropathol. 1996;91(1):6–14.
188. Higuchi Y, Miyakawa T, Shimoji A, Katsuragi S. Ultrastructural changes of blood vessels in the cerebral cortex in Alzheimer's disease. Jpn J Psychiatry Neurol. 1987;41(2):283–90.
189. Vinters HV, Secor DL, Read SL, Frazee JG, Tomiyasu U, Stanley TM, et al. Microvasculature in brain biopsy specimens from patients with Alzheimer's disease: an immunohistochemical and ultrastructural study. Ultrastruct Pathol. 1994;18(3):333–48.
190. Biron KE, Dickstein DL, Gopaul R, Jefferies WA. Amyloid triggers extensive cerebral angiogenesis causing blood brain barrier permeability and hypervascularity in Alzheimer's disease. PLoS ONE. 2011;6(8):e23789.
191. Desai BS, Schneider JA, Li JL, Carvey PM, Hendey B. Evidence of angiogenic vessels in Alzheimer's disease. J Neural Transm. 2009;116(5):587–97.
192. Beskow J, Hassler O, Ottosson JO. Cerebral arterial deformities in relation to senile deterioration. Acta Psychiatr Scand Suppl. 1971;221:111–9.
193. Fischer VW, Siddiqi A, Yusufaly Y. Altered angioarchitecture in selected areas of brains with Alzheimer's disease. Acta Neuropathol. 1990;79(6):672–9.
194. Hassler O. Vascular changes in senile brains. A micro-angiographic study. Acta Neuropathol. 1965;5(1):40–53.
195. Kalaria RN, Kroon SN. Expression of leukocyte antigen CD34 by brain capillaries in Alzheimer's disease and neurologically normal subjects. Acta Neuropathol. 1992;84(6):606–12.
196. Bell RD, Zlokovic BV. Neurovascular mechanisms and blood-brain barrier disorder in Alzheimer's disease. Acta Neuropathol. 2009;118(1):103–13.
197. Ryu JK, McLarnon JG. A leaky blood-brain barrier, fibrinogen infiltration and microglial reactivity in inflamed Alzheimer's disease brain. J Cell Mol Med. 2009;13(9A):2911–25.
198. Sengillo JD, Winkler EA, Walker CT, Sullivan JS, Johnson M, Zlokovic BV. Deficiency in mural vascular cells coincides with blood-brain barrier disruption in Alzheimer's disease. Brain Pathol. 2013;23(3):303–10.
199. van de Haar HJ, Burgmans S, Jansen JF, van Osch MJ, van Buchem MA, Muller M, et al. Blood-brain barrier leakage in patients with early Alzheimer disease. Radiology. 2016;281(2):527–35.
200. van de Haar HJ, Jansen JFA, van Osch MJP, van Buchem MA, Muller M, Wong SM, et al. Neurovascular unit impairment in early Alzheimer's disease measured with magnetic resonance imaging. Neurobiol Aging. 2016;45:190–6.
201. Zipser BD, Johanson CE, Gonzalez L, Berzin TM, Tavares R, Hulette CM, et al. Microvascular injury and blood-brain barrier leakage in Alzheimer's disease. Neurobiol Aging. 2007;28(7):977–86.
202. Harik SI. Changes in the glucose transporter of brain capillaries. Can J Physiol Pharmacol. 1992;70(Suppl):S113–7.
203. Kalaria RN, Harik SI. Reduced glucose transporter at the blood-brain barrier and in cerebral cortex in Alzheimer disease. J Neurochem. 1989;53(4):1083–8.
204. Grammas P, Ovase R. Inflammatory factors are elevated in brain microvessels in Alzheimer's disease. Neurobiol Aging. 2001;22(6):837–42.

205. Tripathy D, Thirumangalakudi L, Grammas P. Expression of macrophage inflammatory protein 1-alpha is elevated in Alzheimer's vessels and is regulated by oxidative stress. J Alzheimers Dis. 2007;11(4):447–55.
206. Gabin JM, Tambs K, Saltvedt I, Sund E, Holmen J. Association between blood pressure and Alzheimer disease measured up to 27 years prior to diagnosis: the HUNT Study. Alzheimers Res Ther. 2017;9(1):37.
207. Yarchoan M, Xie SX, Kling MA, Toledo JB, Wolk DA, Lee EB, et al. Cerebrovascular atherosclerosis correlates with Alzheimer pathology in neurodegenerative dementias. Brain. 2012;135(Pt 12):3749–56.
208. Matsuzaki T, Sasaki K, Hata J, Hirakawa Y, Fujimi K, Ninomiya T, et al. Association of Alzheimer disease pathology with abnormal lipid metabolism: the Hisayama Study. Neurology. 2011;77(11):1068–75.
209. Castillo-Carranza DL, Nilson AN, Van Skike CE, Jahrling JB, Patel K, Garach P, et al. Cerebral microvascular accumulation of tau oligomers in alzheimer's disease and related tauopathies. Aging Dis. 2017;8(3):257–66.
210. Williams S, Chalmers K, Wilcock GK, Love S. Relationship of neurofibrillary pathology to cerebral amyloid angiopathy in Alzheimer's disease. Neuropathol Appl Neurobiol. 2005;31(4):414–21.
211. Feke GT, Hyman BT, Stern RA, Pasquale LR. Retinal blood flow in mild cognitive impairment and Alzheimer's disease. Alzheimers Dement. 2015;1(2):144–51.
212. O'Bryhim BE, Apte RS, Kung N, Coble D, Van Stavern GP. Association of preclinical alzheimer disease with optical coherence tomographic angiography findings. JAMA Ophthalmol. 2018;136(11):1242–8.
213. Cabrera DeBuc D, Somfai GM, Arthur E, Kostic M, Oropesa S, Mendoza SC. Investigating multimodal diagnostic eye biomarkers of cognitive impairment by measuring vascular and neurogenic changes in the retina. Front Physiol. 2018;9:1721.
214. Abbasi J. A retinal scan for Alzheimer disease. JAMA. 2017;318(14):1314.
215. Cheung CY, Ong YT, Ikram MK, Ong SY, Li X, Hilal S, et al. Microvascular network alterations in the retina of patients with Alzheimer's disease. Alzheimers Dement. 2014;10(2):135–42.
216. Einarsdottir AB, Hardarson SH, Kristjansdottir JV, Bragason DT, Snaedal J, Stefansson E. Retinal oximetry imaging in Alzheimer's disease. J Alzheimers Dis. 2016;49(1):79–83.
217. Williams MA, McGowan AJ, Cardwell CR, Cheung CY, Craig D, Passmore P, et al. Retinal microvascular network attenuation in Alzheimer's disease. Alzheimers Dement. 2015;1(2):229–35.
218. Bakker EN, Bacskai BJ, Arbel-Ornath M, Aldea R, Bedussi B, Morris AW, et al. Lymphatic clearance of the brain: perivascular, paravascular and significance for neurodegenerative diseases. Cell Mol Neurobiol. 2016;36(2):181–94.
219. Engelhardt B, Carare RO, Bechmann I, Flugel A, Laman JD, Weller RO. Vascular, glial, and lymphatic immune gateways of the central nervous system. Acta Neuropathol. 2016;132(3):317–38.
220. Vinters HV, Gilbert JJ. Cerebral amyloid angiopathy: incidence and complications in the aging brain. II. The distribution of amyloid vascular changes. Stroke. 1983;14(6):924–8.
221. Vinters HV. Cerebral amyloid angiopathy. A critical review. Stroke. 1987;18(2):311–24.
222. Bennett D. Public health importance of vascular dementia and Alzheimer's disease with cerebrovascular disease. Int J Clin Pract Suppl. 2001;120:41–8.
223. Kimbrough IF, Robel S, Roberson ED, Sontheimer H. Vascular amyloidosis impairs the gliovascular unit in a mouse model of Alzheimer's disease. Brain. 2015;138(Pt 12):3716–33.
224. Campbell M, Humphries P. The blood-retina barrier: tight junctions and barrier modulation. Adv Exp Med Biol. 2012;763:70–84.
225. Zenaro E, Piacentino G, Constantin G. The blood-brain barrier in Alzheimer's disease. Neurobiol Dis. 2017;107:41–56.
226. Cai Z, Qiao PF, Wan CQ, Cai M, Zhou NK, Li Q. Role of blood-brain barrier in Alzheimer's disease. J Alzheimers Dis. 2018;63(4):1223–34.

227. Zlokovic BV, Ghiso J, Mackic JB, McComb JG, Weiss MH, Frangione B. Blood-brain barrier transport of circulating Alzheimer's amyloid beta. Biochem Biophys Res Commun. 1993;197(3):1034–40.
228. Do TM, Dodacki A, Alata W, Calon F, Nicolic S, Scherrmann JM, et al. Age-dependent regulation of the blood-brain barrier influx/efflux equilibrium of amyloid-beta peptide in a mouse model of Alzheimer's disease (3xTg-AD). J Alzheimers Dis. 2015;49(2):287–300.
229. Banks WA, Robinson SM, Verma S, Morley JE. Efflux of human and mouse amyloid beta proteins 1–40 and 1–42 from brain: impairment in a mouse model of Alzheimer's disease. Neuroscience. 2003;121(2):487–92.
230. DeMattos RB, Bales KR, Cummins DJ, Paul SM, Holtzman DM. Brain to plasma amyloid-beta efflux: a measure of brain amyloid burden in a mouse model of Alzheimer's disease. Science. 2002;295(5563):2264–7.
231. Sweeney MD, Sagare AP, Zlokovic BV. Blood-brain barrier breakdown in Alzheimer disease and other neurodegenerative disorders. Nat Rev Neurol. 2018;14(3):133–50.
232. Zhao Z, Sagare AP, Ma Q, Halliday MR, Kong P, Kisler K, et al. Central role for PICALM in amyloid-beta blood-brain barrier transcytosis and clearance. Nat Neurosci. 2015;18(7):978–87.
233. Lahiri S, Regis GC, Koronyo Y, Fuchs DT, Sheyn J, Kim EH, et al. Acute neuropathological consequences of short-term mechanical ventilation in wild-type and Alzheimer's disease mice. Crit Care. 2019;23(1):63.
234. Aguilar-Calvo P, Sevillano AM, Rasool S, Cao KJ, Randolph LM, Rissman RA, et al. Non-invasive antemortem detection of retinal prions by a fluorescent tracer. J Alzheimers Dis. 2022;88(3):1137–45.
235. Calsolaro V, Edison P. Neuroinflammation in Alzheimer's disease: current evidence and future directions. Alzheimers Dement. 2016;12(6):719–32.
236. Karch CM, Goate AM. Alzheimer's disease risk genes and mechanisms of disease pathogenesis. Biol Psychiatry. 2015;77(1):43–51.
237. Friker LL, Scheiblich H, Hochheiser IV, Brinkschulte R, Riedel D, Latz E, et al. β-Amyloid clustering around ASC fibrils boosts its toxicity in microglia. Cell Rep. 2020;30(11):3743-54.e6.
238. Fuhrmann M, Bittner T, Jung CK, Burgold S, Page RM, Mitteregger G, et al. Microglial Cx3cr1 knockout prevents neuron loss in a mouse model of Alzheimer's disease. Nat Neurosci. 2010;13(4):411–3.
239. Ising C, Venegas C, Zhang S, Scheiblich H, Schmidt SV, Vieira-Saecker A, et al. NLRP3 inflammasome activation drives tau pathology. Nature. 2019;575(7784):669–73.
240. Lee S, Varvel NH, Konerth ME, Xu G, Cardona AE, Ransohoff RM, et al. CX3CR1 deficiency alters microglial activation and reduces beta-amyloid deposition in two Alzheimer's disease mouse models. Am J Pathol. 2010;177(5):2549–62.
241. Rajendran L, Paolicelli RC. Microglia-mediated synapse loss in Alzheimer's disease. J Neurosci. 2018;38(12):2911–9.
242. Salter MW, Stevens B. Microglia emerge as central players in brain disease. Nat Med. 2017;23(9):1018–27.
243. Wyss-Coray T, Rogers J. Inflammation in Alzheimer disease—a brief review of the basic science and clinical literature. Cold Spring Harb Perspect Med. 2012;2(1):a006346-a.
244. Keren-Shaul H, Spinrad A, Weiner A, Matcovitch-Natan O, Dvir-Szternfeld R, Ulland TK, et al. A unique microglia type associated with restricting development of Alzheimer's disease. Cell. 2017;169(7).1276–90 e17.
245. Antes R, Salomon-Zimri S, Beck SC, Garcia Garrido M, Livnat T, Maharshak I, et al. VEGF mediates ApoE4-induced neovascularization and synaptic pathology in the choroid and retina. Curr Alzheimer Res. 2015;12(4):323–34.
246. Byun MS, Park SW, Lee JH, Yi D, Jeon SY, Choi HJ, et al. Association of retinal changes with Alzheimer disease neuroimaging biomarkers in cognitively normal individuals. JAMA Ophthalmol. 2021;139(5):548–56.

247. Cheung CY, Mok V, Foster PJ, Trucco E, Chen C, Wong TY. Retinal imaging in Alzheimer's disease. J Neurol Neurosurg Psychiatry. 2021;92(9):983–94.
248. Coppola G, Di Renzo A, Ziccardi L, Martelli F, Fadda A, Manni G, et al. Optical coherence tomography in Alzheimer's disease: a meta-analysis. PLoS ONE. 2015;10(8):e0134750.
249. Doustar J, Torbati T, Black KL, Koronyo Y, Koronyo-Hamaoui M. Optical coherence tomography in Alzheimer's disease and other neurodegenerative diseases. Front Neurol. 2017;8:701.
250. Kromer R, Serbecic N, Hausner L, Froelich L, Aboul-Enein F, Beutelspacher SC. Detection of retinal nerve fiber layer defects in Alzheimer's disease using SD-OCT. Front Psychiatry. 2014;5:22.
251. Zhang Y, Wang Y, Shi C, Shen M, Lu F. Advances in retina imaging as potential biomarkers for early diagnosis of Alzheimer's disease. Transl Neurodegener. 2021;10(1):6.
252. Cheung CY, Ikram MK, Chen C, Wong TY. Imaging retina to study dementia and stroke. Prog Retin Eye Res. 2017;57:89–107.
253. McGrory S, Cameron JR, Pellegrini E, Warren C, Doubal FN, Deary IJ, et al. The application of retinal fundus camera imaging in dementia: a systematic review. Alzheimers Dement. 2017;6:91–107.
254. Ong SS, Proia AD, Whitson HE, Farsiu S, Doraiswamy PM, Lad EM. Ocular amyloid imaging at the crossroad of Alzheimer's disease and age-related macular degeneration: implications for diagnosis and therapy. J Neurol. 2019;266(7):1566–77.
255. Snyder PJ, Johnson LN, Lim YY, Santos CY, Alber J, Maruff P, et al. Nonvascular retinal imaging markers of preclinical Alzheimer's disease. Alzheimers Dement. 2016;4:169–78.
256. Vij R, Arora S. A systematic survey of advances in retinal imaging modalities for Alzheimer's disease diagnosis. Metab Brain Dis. 2022.
257. Kumar VB, Sher I, Rencus-Lazar S, Rotenstreich Y, Gazit E. Functional carbon quantum dots for ocular imaging and therapeutic applications. Small. 2023;19(7):e2205754.
258. Czako C, Kovacs T, Ungvari Z, Csiszar A, Yabluchanskiy A, Conley S, et al. Retinal biomarkers for Alzheimer's disease and vascular cognitive impairment and dementia (VCID): implication for early diagnosis and prognosis. Geroscience. 2020;42(6):1499–525.
259. Fenner BJ, Wong RLM, Lam WC, Tan GSW, Cheung GCM. Advances in retinal imaging and applications in diabetic retinopathy screening: a review. Ophthalmol Ther. 2018;7(2):333–46.
260. Riazi Esfahani P, Reddy AJ, Thomas J, Sommer DA, Nguyen A, Farasat V, et al. An analysis of the usage of retinal imaging technology in the detection of age-related macular degeneration. Cureus. 2023;15(6):e40527.
261. Polans J, Keller B, Carrasco-Zevallos OM, LaRocca F, Cole E, Whitson HE, et al. Wide-field retinal optical coherence tomography with wavefront sensorless adaptive optics for enhanced imaging of targeted regions. Biomed Opt Express. 2017;8(1):16–37.
262. Schallek J, Geng Y, Nguyen H, Williams DR. Morphology and topography of retinal pericytes in the living mouse retina using in vivo adaptive optics imaging and ex vivo characterization. Invest Ophthalmol Vis Sci. 2013;54(13):8237–50.
263. Bulut M, Kurtulus F, Gozkaya O, Erol MK, Cengiz A, Akidan M, et al. Evaluation of optical coherence tomography angiographic findings in Alzheimer's type dementia. Br J Ophthalmol. 2018;102(2):233–7.
264. Cunha LP, Almeida AL, Costa-Cunha LV, Costa CF, Monteiro ML. The role of optical coherence tomography in Alzheimer's disease. Int J Retina Vitreous. 2016;2:24.
265. Ferrari L, Huang SC, Magnani G, Ambrosi A, Comi G, Leocani L. Optical coherence tomography reveals retinal neuroaxonal thinning in frontotemporal dementia as in Alzheimer's disease. J Alzheimers Dis. 2017;56(3):1101–7.
266. Janez-Escalada L, Janez-Garcia L, Salobrar-Garcia E, Santos-Mayo A, de Hoz R, Yubero R, et al. Spatial analysis of thickness changes in ten retinal layers of Alzheimer's disease patients based on optical coherence tomography. Sci Rep. 2019;9(1):13000.
267. Parisi V, Restuccia R, Fattapposta F, Mina C, Bucci MG, Pierelli F. Morphological and functional retinal impairment in Alzheimer's disease patients. Clin Neurophysiol. 2001;112(10):1860–7.

268. Polo V, Rodrigo MJ, Garcia-Martin E, Otin S, Larrosa JM, Fuertes MI, et al. Visual dysfunction and its correlation with retinal changes in patients with Alzheimer's disease. Eye. 2017;31(7):1034–41.
269. Rotenstreich Y, Sharvit-Ginon I, Sher I, Zloto O, Fabian ID, Abd-Elkader A, et al. Thicker macula in asymptomatic APOE E4 middle-aged adults at high AD risk. Alzheimers Dement. 2022;14(1):e12275.
270. Salobrar-Garcia E, de Hoz R, Ramirez AI, Lopez-Cuenca I, Rojas P, Vazirani R, et al. Changes in visual function and retinal structure in the progression of Alzheimer's disease. PLoS ONE. 2019;14(8):e0220535.
271. Hedges TR 3rd, Perez Galves R, Speigelman D, Barbas NR, Peli E, Yardley CJ. Retinal nerve fiber layer abnormalities in Alzheimer's disease. Acta Ophthalmol Scand. 1996;74(3):271–5.
272. Coleman-Belin J, Harris A, Chen B, Zhou J, Ciulla T, Verticchio A, et al. Aging effects on optic nerve neurodegeneration. Int J Mol Sci. 2023;24(3).
273. Repka MX, Quigley HA. The effect of age on normal human optic nerve fiber number and diameter. Ophthalmology. 1989;96(1):26–32.
274. Asanad S, Fantini M, Sultan W, Nassisi M, Felix CM, Wu J, et al. Retinal nerve fiber layer thickness predicts CSF amyloid/tau before cognitive decline. PLoS ONE. 2020;15(5):e0232785.
275. Marquie M, Valero S, Castilla-Marti M, Martinez J, Rodriguez-Gomez O, Sanabria A, et al. Association between retinal thickness and beta-amyloid brain accumulation in individuals with subjective cognitive decline: Fundacio ACE Healthy Brain Initiative. Alzheimers Res Ther. 2020;12(1):37.
276. Asanad S, Ross-Cisneros FN, Barron E, Nassisi M, Sultan W, Karanjia R, et al. The retinal choroid as an oculovascular biomarker for Alzheimer's dementia: a histopathological study in severe disease. Alzheimers Dement. 2019;11:775–83.
277. Santos CY, Johnson LN, Sinoff SE, Festa EK, Heindel WC, Snyder PJ. Change in retinal structural anatomy during the preclinical stage of Alzheimer's disease. Alzheimers Dement. 2018;10:196–209.
278. Lopez-de-Eguileta A, Lopez-Garcia S, Lage C, Pozueta A, Garcia-Martinez M, Kazimierczak M, et al. The retinal ganglion cell layer reflects neurodegenerative changes in cognitively unimpaired individuals. Alzheimers Res Ther. 2022;14(1):57.
279. Jorge L, Canario N, Martins R, Santiago B, Santana I, Quental H, et al. The retinal inner plexiform synaptic layer mirrors grey matter thickness of primary visual cortex with increased amyloid beta load in early Alzheimer's disease. Neural Plast. 2020;2020:8826087.
280. Batista A, Guimarães P, Serranho P, Nunes A, Martins J, Moreira PI, Ambrósio AF, Morgado M, Castelo-Branco M, Bernardes R. Retinal imaging in animal models: Searching for biomarkers of neurodegeneration. Front Ophthalmol. 2023;3.
281. Yap TE, Davis BM, Guo L, Normando EM, Cordeiro MF. Annexins in Glaucoma. Int J Mol Sci. 2018;19(4).
282. Obulesu M, Lakshmi MJ. Apoptosis in Alzheimer's disease: an understanding of the physiology, pathology and therapeutic avenues. Neurochem Res. 2014;39(12):2301–12.
283. Overmyer M, Kraszpulski M, Helisalmi S, Soininen H, Alafuzoff I. DNA fragmentation, gliosis and histological hallmarks of Alzheimer's disease. Acta Neuropathol. 2000;100(6):681–7.
284. Kayabasi U, Sergott R, Rispoli M. Retinal examination for the diagnosis of Alzheimer's disease. Int J Ophthal Pathol. 2014;3(4).
285. Barton SM, To E, Rogers BP, Whitmore C, Uppal M, Matsubara JA, et al. Inhalable thioflavin S for the detection of amyloid beta deposits in the retina. Molecules. 2021;26(4).
286. Chibhabha F, Yang Y, Ying K, Jia F, Zhang Q, Ullah S, et al. Non-invasive optical imaging of retinal Abeta plaques using curcumin loaded polymeric micelles in APPswe/PS1DeltaE9 transgenic mice for the diagnosis of Alzheimer's disease. J Mater Chem B. 2020;8(33):7438–52.
287. Hoh Kam J, Lenassi E, Jeffery G. Viewing ageing eyes: diverse sites of amyloid beta accumulation in the ageing mouse retina and the up-regulation of macrophages. PLoS ONE. 2010;5(10).

288. Chua J, Hu Q, Ke M, Tan B, Hong J, Yao X, et al. Retinal microvasculature dysfunction is associated with Alzheimer's disease and mild cognitive impairment. Alzheimers Res Ther. 2020;12(1):161.
289. Golzan SM, Goozee K, Georgevsky D, Avolio A, Chatterjee P, Shen K, et al. Retinal vascular and structural changes are associated with amyloid burden in the elderly: ophthalmic biomarkers of preclinical Alzheimer's disease. Alzheimers Res Ther. 2017;9(1):13.
290. Liew G, Wang JJ, Mitchell P, Wong TY. Retinal vascular imaging: a new tool in microvascular disease research. Circ Cardiovasc Imaging. 2008;1(2):156–61.
291. Yoon SP, Grewal DS, Thompson AC, Polascik BW, Dunn C, Burke JR, et al. Retinal microvascular and neurodegenerative changes in Alzheimer's disease and mild cognitive impairment compared with control participants. Ophthalmol Retina. 2019;3(6):489–99.
292. Lesage SR, Mosley TH, Wong TY, Szklo M, Knopman D, Catellier DJ, et al. Retinal microvascular abnormalities and cognitive decline: the ARIC 14-year follow-up study. Neurology. 2009;73(11):862–8.
293. van de Kreeke JA, Nguyen HT, Konijnenberg E, Tomassen J, den Braber A, Ten Kate M, et al. Optical coherence tomography angiography in preclinical Alzheimer's disease. Br J Ophthalmol. 2020;104(2):157–61.
294. Lahme L, Esser EL, Mihailovic N, Schubert F, Lauermann J, Johnen A, et al. Evaluation of ocular perfusion in Alzheimer's disease using optical coherence tomography angiography. J Alzheimers Dis. 2018;66(4):1745–52.
295. Querques G, Borrelli E, Sacconi R, De Vitis L, Leocani L, Santangelo R, et al. Functional and morphological changes of the retinal vessels in Alzheimer's disease and mild cognitive impairment. Sci Rep. 2019;9(1):63.
296. Sharafi SM, Sylvestre JP, Chevrefils C, Soucy JP, Beaulieu S, Pascoal TA, et al. Vascular retinal biomarkers improves the detection of the likely cerebral amyloid status from hyperspectral retinal images. Alzheimers Dement. 2019;5:610–7.
297. Jiang H, Wei Y, Shi Y, Wright CB, Sun X, Gregori G, et al. Altered macular microvasculature in mild cognitive impairment and Alzheimer disease. J Neuroophthalmol. 2018;38(3):292–8.
298. Csincsik L, MacGillivray TJ, Flynn E, Pellegrini E, Papanastasiou G, Barzegar-Befroei N, et al. Peripheral retinal imaging biomarkers for Alzheimer's disease: a pilot study. Ophthalmic Res. 2018;59(4):182–92.
299. Kashani AH, Chen CL, Gahm JK, Zheng F, Richter GM, Rosenfeld PJ, et al. Optical coherence tomography angiography: a comprehensive review of current methods and clinical applications. Prog Retin Eye Res. 2017;60:66–100.
300. Wang X, Zhao Q, Tao R, Lu H, Xiao Z, Zheng L, et al. Decreased retinal vascular density in Alzheimer's disease (AD) and Mild Cognitive Impairment (MCI): an optical coherence tomography angiography (OCTA) study. Front Aging Neurosci. 2020;12:572484.
301. Lee JY, Kim JP, Jang H, Kim J, Kang SH, Kim JS, et al. Optical coherence tomography angiography as a potential screening tool for cerebral small vessel diseases. Alzheimers Res Ther. 2020;12(1):73.
302. Rifai OM, McGrory S, Robbins CB, Grewal DS, Liu A, Fekrat S, et al. The application of optical coherence tomography angiography in Alzheimer's disease: a systematic review. Alzheimers Dement. 2021;13(1):e12149.
303. Wu J, Zhang X, Azhati G, Li T, Xu G, Liu F. Retinal microvascular attenuation in mental cognitive impairment and Alzheimer's disease by optical coherence tomography angiography. Acta Ophthalmol. 2020;98(6):e781–7.
304. Zabel P, Kaluzny JJ, Wilkosc-Debczynska M, Gebska-Toloczko M, Suwala K, Zabel K, et al. Comparison of retinal microvasculature in patients With Alzheimer's disease and primary open-angle glaucoma by optical coherence tomography angiography. Invest Ophthalmol Vis Sci. 2019;60(10):3447–55.
305. Deal JA, Sharrett AR, Rawlings AM, Gottesman RF, Bandeen-Roche K, Albert M, et al. Retinal signs and 20-year cognitive decline in the atherosclerosis risk in communities study. Neurology. 2018;90(13):e1158–66.

306. Baker ML, Marino Larsen EK, Kuller LH, Klein R, Klein BE, Siscovick DS, et al. Retinal microvascular signs, cognitive function, and dementia in older persons: the cardiovascular health study. Stroke. 2007;38(7):2041–7.
307. La Mantia A, Kurt RA, Mejor S, Egan CA, Tufail A, Keane PA, et al. Comparing fundus fluorescein angiography and swept-source optical coherence tomography angiography in the evaluation of diabetic macular perfusion. Retina. 2019;39(5):926–37.
308. Memon AS, Memon NA, Mahar PS. Role of optical coherence tomography angiography to differentiate intraretinal microvascular abnormalities and retinal neovascularization in diabetic retinopathy. Pak J Med Sci. 2022;38(1):57–61.
309. Mochi T, Anegondi N, Girish M, Jayadev C, Sinha RA. Quantitative comparison between optical coherence tomography angiography and fundus fluorescein angiography images: effect of vessel enhancement. Ophthalmic Surg Lasers Imaging Retina. 2018;49(11):e175–81.
310. Marmor MF, Ravin JG. Fluorescein angiography: insight and serendipity a half century ago. Arch Ophthalmol. 2011;129(7):943–8.
311. Cunha-Vaz J, Santos T, Alves D, Marques I, Neves C, Soares M, et al. Agreement between OCT leakage and fluorescein angiography to identify sites of alteration of the blood-retinal barrier in diabetes. Ophthalmol Retina. 2017;1(5):395–403.
312. Armstrong R, Kergoat H. Oculo-visual changes and clinical considerations affecting older patients with dementia. Ophthal Physiol Opt J Brit College Ophthal Opt. 2015;35(4):352–76.
313. Cerquera-Jaramillo MA, Nava-Mesa MO, González-Reyes RE, Tellez-Conti C, de-la-Torre A. Visual features in Alzheimer's disease: from basic mechanisms to clinical overview. Neural Plast. 2018;2018:2941783.
314. Chang LY, Lowe J, Ardiles A, Lim J, Grey AC, Robertson K, et al. Alzheimer's disease in the human eye. Clinical tests that identify ocular and visual information processing deficit as biomarkers. Alzheimers Dement. 2014;10(2):251–61.
315. Colligris P, Perez de Lara MJ, Colligris B, Pintor J. Ocular manifestations of Alzheimer's and other neurodegenerative diseases: the prospect of the eye as a tool for the early diagnosis of Alzheimer's disease. J Ophthalmol. 2018;2018:8538573.
316. Cormack FK, Tovee M, Ballard C. Contrast sensitivity and visual acuity in patients with Alzheimer's disease. Int J Geriatr Psychiatry. 2000;15(7):614–20.
317. Cronin-Golomb A. Vision in Alzheimer's disease. Gerontologist. 1995;35(3):370–6.
318. Cronin-Golomb A, Rizzo JF, Corkin S, Growdon JH. Visual function in Alzheimer's disease and normal aging. Ann NY Acad Sci. 1991;640:28–35.
319. Javaid FZ, Brenton J, Guo L, Cordeiro MF. Visual and ocular manifestations of Alzheimer's disease and their use as biomarkers for diagnosis and progression. Front Neurol. 2016;7:55.
320. Katz B, Rimmer S, Iragui V, Katzman R. Abnormal pattern electroretinogram in Alzheimer's disease: evidence for retinal ganglion cell degeneration? Ann Neurol. 1989;26(2):221–5.
321. Lakshminarayanan V, Lagrave J, Kean ML, Dick M, Shankle R. Vision in dementia: contrast effects. Neurol Res. 1996;18(1):9–15.
322. Mavilio A, Sisto D, Prete F, Guadalupi V, Dammacco R, Alessio G. RE-PERG in early-onset Alzheimer's disease: a double-blind, electrophysiological pilot study. PLoS ONE. 2020;15(8):e0236568.
323. Ng S, Villemagne VL, Berlangieri S, Lee ST, Cherk M, Gong SJ, et al. Visual assessment versus quantitative assessment of 11C-PIB PET and 18F-FDG PET for detection of Alzheimer's disease. J Nucl Med Off Publ Soc Nucl Med. 2007;48(4):547–52.
324. Nolan JM, Loskutova E, Howard AN, Moran R, Mulcahy R, Stack J, et al. Macular pigment, visual function, and macular disease among subjects with Alzheimer's disease: an exploratory study. J Alzheimers Dis. 2014;42(4):1191–202.
325. Pache M, Smeets CH, Gasio PF, Savaskan E, Flammer J, Wirz-Justice A, et al. Colour vision deficiencies in Alzheimer's disease. Age Ageing. 2003;32(4):422–6.
326. Risacher SL, Wudunn D, Pepin SM, MaGee TR, McDonald BC, Flashman LA, et al. Visual contrast sensitivity in Alzheimer's disease, mild cognitive impairment, and older adults with cognitive complaints. Neurobiol Aging. 2013;34(4):1133–44.

327. Risacher SL, WuDunn D, Tallman EF, West JD, Gao S, Farlow MR, et al. Visual contrast sensitivity is associated with the presence of cerebral amyloid and tau deposition. Brain Commun. 2020;2(1):fcaa019.
328. Rizzo M, Anderson SW, Dawson J, Nawrot M. Vision and cognition in Alzheimer's disease. Neuropsychologia. 2000;38(8):1157–69.
329. Sadun AA, Borchert M, DeVita E, Hinton DR, Bassi CJ. Assessment of visual impairment in patients with Alzheimer's disease. Am J Ophthalmol. 1987;104(2):113–20.
330. Salamone G, Di Lorenzo C, Mosti S, Lupo F, Cravello L, Palmer K, et al. Color discrimination performance in patients with Alzheimer's disease. Dement Geriatr Cogn Disord. 2009;27(6):501–7.
331. Trick GL, Barris MC, Bickler-Bluth M. Abnormal pattern electroretinograms in patients with senile dementia of the Alzheimer type. Ann Neurol. 1989;26(2):226–31.
332. Iseri PK, Altinas O, Tokay T, Yuksel N. Relationship between cognitive impairment and retinal morphological and visual functional abnormalities in Alzheimer disease. J Neuroophthalmol. 2006;26(1):18–24.
333. Demb JB, Singer JH. Functional circuitry of the retina. Annu Rev Vis Sci. 2015;1:263–89.
334. Ngoo QZ, Wan Hitam WH, Ab RA. Evaluation of retinal nerve fiber layer thickness, electroretinogram and visual evoked potential in patients with Alzheimer's disease. J Ophthalmol. 2019;2019:6248185.
335. Krasodomska K, Lubinski W, Potemkowski A, Honczarenko K. Pattern electroretinogram (PERG) and pattern visual evoked potential (PVEP) in the early stages of Alzheimer's disease. Doc Ophthalmol. 2010;121(2):111–21.
336. Sen S, Saxena R, Vibha D, Tripathi M, Sharma P, Phuljhele S, et al. Detection of structural and electrical disturbances in macula and optic nerve in Alzheimer's patients and their correlation with disease severity. Semin Ophthalmol. 2020;35(2):116–25.
337. Moschos MM, Markopoulos I, Chatziralli I, Rouvas A, Papageorgiou SG, Ladas I, et al. Structural and functional impairment of the retina and optic nerve in Alzheimer's disease. Curr Alzheimer Res. 2012;9(7):782–8.
338. Stothart G, Kazanina N, Naatanen R, Haworth J, Tales A. Early visual evoked potentials and mismatch negativity in Alzheimer's disease and mild cognitive impairment. J Alzheimers Dis. 2015;44(2):397–408.
339. Crow RW, Levin LB, LaBree L, Rubin R, Feldon SE. Sweep visual evoked potential evaluation of contrast sensitivity in Alzheimer's dementia. Invest Ophthalmol Vis Sci. 2003;44(2):875–8.
340. Sartucci F, Borghetti D, Bocci T, Murri L, Orsini P, Porciatti V, et al. Dysfunction of the magnocellular stream in Alzheimer's disease evaluated by pattern electroretinograms and visual evoked potentials. Brain Res Bull. 2010;82(3–4):169–76.
341. Baiano C, Zeppieri M. Visual evoked potential. StatPearls. Treasure Island (FL) ineligible companies. Disclosure: Marco Zeppieri declares no relevant financial relationships with ineligible companies; 2023.
342. Celesia GG. Anatomy and physiology of visual evoked potentials and electroretinograms. Neurol Clin. 1988;6(4):657–79.
343. Boedeker S, Halstenberg E, Schulz P, Beblo T, Kreisel S, Driessen M, et al. Impaired color discrimination in Alzheimer disease dementia. Alzheimer Dis Assoc Disord. 2022;36(1):22–8.
344. Cronin-Golomb A, Sugiura R, Corkin S, Growdon JH. Incomplete achromatopsia in Alzheimer's disease. Neurobiol Aging. 1993;14(5):471–7.
345. Wijk H, Berg S, Sivik L, Steen B. Colour discrimination, colour naming and colour preferences among individuals with Alzheimer's disease. Int J Geriatr Psychiatry. 1999;14(12):1000–5.
346. Hutton JT, Morris JL, Elias JW, Poston JN. Contrast sensitivity dysfunction in Alzheimer's disease. Neurology. 1993;43(11):2328–30.
347. La Morgia C, Ross-Cisneros FN, Sadun AA, Carelli V. Retinal ganglion cells and circadian rhythms in Alzheimer's disease, Parkinson's disease, and beyond. Front Neurol. 2017;8:162.

348. Fiorentini A, Porciatti V, Morrone MC, Burr DC. Visual ageing: unspecific decline of the responses to luminance and colour. Vision Res. 1996;36(21):3557–66.
349. Rogers SL, Friedman RB. The underlying mechanisms of semantic memory loss in Alzheimer's disease and semantic dementia. Neuropsychologia. 2008;46(1):12–21.
350. Chertkow H, Bub D. Semantic memory loss in dementia of Alzheimer's type. What do various measures measure? Brain. 1990;113(Pt 2):397–417.
351. Crawford TJ, Devereaux A, Higham S, Kelly C. The disengagement of visual attention in Alzheimer's disease: a longitudinal eye-tracking study. Front Aging Neurosci. 2015;7:118.
352. Kim NG, Lee HW. Stereoscopic depth perception and visuospatial dysfunction in Alzheimer's disease. Healthcare. 2021;9(2).
353. Lee CN, Ko D, Suh YW, Park KW. Cognitive functions and stereopsis in patients with Parkinson's disease and Alzheimer's disease using 3-dimensional television: a case controlled trial. PLoS ONE. 2015;10(3):e0123229.
354. Armstrong RA. Alzheimer's disease and the eye. J Optom. 2009;2(3):103–11.
355. Glosser G, Baker KM, de Vries JJ, Alavi A, Grossman M, Clark CM. Disturbed visual processing contributes to impaired reading in Alzheimer's disease. Neuropsychologia. 2002;40(7):902–9.
356. Gilmore GC, Groth KE, Thomas CW. Stimulus contrast and word reading speed in Alzheimer's disease. Exp Aging Res. 2005;31(1):15–33.
357. Passafiume D, Di Giacomo D, Giubilei F. Reading latency of words and nonwords in Alzheimer's patients. Cortex. 2000;36(2):293–8.
358. Ju YE, Lucey BP, Holtzman DM. Sleep and Alzheimer disease pathology—a bidirectional relationship. Nat Rev Neurol. 2014;10(2):115–9.
359. Trick GL, Trick LR, Morris P, Wolf M. Visual field loss in senile dementia of the Alzheimer's type. Neurology. 1995;45(1):68–74.
360. Chougule PS, Najjar RP, Finkelstein MT, Kandiah N, Milea D. Light-Induced pupillary responses in Alzheimer's disease. Front Neurol. 2019;10:360.
361. Granholm EL, Panizzon MS, Elman JA, Jak AJ, Hauger RL, Bondi MW, et al. Pupillary responses as a biomarker of early risk for Alzheimer's disease. J Alzheimers Dis. 2017;56(4):1419–28.
362. Kremen WS, Panizzon MS, Elman JA, Granholm EL, Andreassen OA, Dale AM, et al. Pupillary dilation responses as a midlife indicator of risk for Alzheimer's disease: association with Alzheimer's disease polygenic risk. Neurobiol Aging. 2019;83:114–21.
363. Hattar S, Lucas RJ, Mrosovsky N, Thompson S, Douglas RH, Hankins MW, et al. Melanopsin and rod-cone photoreceptive systems account for all major accessory visual functions in mice. Nature. 2003;424(6944):76–81.
364. Romagnoli M, Stanzani Maserati M, De Matteis M, Capellari S, Carbonelli M, Amore G, et al. Chromatic pupillometry findings in Alzheimer's disease. Front Neurosci. 2020;14:780.
365. Gooley JJ, Lu J, Fischer D, Saper CB. A broad role for melanopsin in nonvisual photoreception. J Neurosci. 2003;23(18):7093–106.
366. Berson DM, Dunn FA, Takao M. Phototransduction by retinal ganglion cells that set the circadian clock. Science. 2002;295(5557):1070–3.
367. Markwell EL, Feigl B, Zele AJ. Intrinsically photosensitive melanopsin retinal ganglion cell contributions to the pupillary light reflex and circadian rhythm. Clin Exp Optom. 2010;93(3):137–49.
368. Chen SK, Badea TC, Hattar S. Photoentrainment and pupillary light reflex are mediated by distinct populations of ipRGCs. Nature. 2011;476(7358):92–5.
369. Feng R, Li L, Yu H, Liu M, Zhao W. Melanopsin retinal ganglion cell loss and circadian dysfunction in Alzheimer's disease (review). Mol Med Rep. 2016;13(4):3397–400.
370. Ju YE, McLeland JS, Toedebusch CD, Xiong C, Fagan AM, Duntley SP, et al. Sleep quality and preclinical Alzheimer disease. JAMA Neurol. 2013;70(5):587–93.
371. Peter-Derex L, Yammine P, Bastuji H, Croisile B. Sleep and Alzheimer's disease. Sleep Med Rev. 2015;19:29–38.

372. Petit D, Gagnon JF, Fantini ML, Ferini-Strambi L, Montplaisir J. Sleep and quantitative EEG in neurodegenerative disorders. J Psychosom Res. 2004;56(5):487–96.
373. Weissová K, Bartoš A, Sládek M, Nováková M, Sumová A. Moderate changes in the circadian system of Alzheimer's disease patients detected in their home environment. PLoS ONE. 2016;11(1):e0146200.
374. Lim AS, Kowgier M, Yu L, Buchman AS, Bennett DA. Sleep fragmentation and the risk of incident Alzheimer's disease and cognitive decline in older persons. Sleep. 2013;36(7):1027–32.
375. Kang JE, Lim MM, Bateman RJ, Lee JJ, Smyth LP, Cirrito JR, et al. Amyloid-beta dynamics are regulated by orexin and the sleep-wake cycle. Science. 2009;326(5955):1005–7.
376. Benito-Leon J, Bermejo-Pareja F, Vega S, Louis ED. Total daily sleep duration and the risk of dementia: a prospective population-based study. Eur J Neurol. 2009;16(9):990–7.
377. Dacey DM, Liao HW, Peterson BB, Robinson FR, Smith VC, Pokorny J, et al. Melanopsin-expressing ganglion cells in primate retina signal colour and irradiance and project to the LGN. Nature. 2005;433(7027):749–54.
378. Raudino F. Ocular and visual manifestation of the Alzheimer's Disease: a literature review, part I: animal models and human pathology. Arch Neurosci. 2018;5(4):e74225.
379. Vit JP, Fuchs DT, Angel A, Levy A, Lamensdorf I, Black KL, et al. Color and contrast vision in mouse models of aging and Alzheimer's disease using a novel visual-stimuli four-arm maze. Sci Rep. 2021;11(1):1255.
380. Vit JP, Fuchs DT, Angel A, Levy A, Lamensdorf I, Black KL, et al. Visual-stimuli four-arm maze test to assess cognition and vision in mice. Bio Prot. 2021;11(22):e4234.
381. Parnell M, Guo L, Abdi M, Cordeiro MF. Ocular manifestations of Alzheimer's disease in animal models. Int J Alzheimers Dis. 2012;2012:786494.
382. O'Leary TP, Brown RE. Visuo-spatial learning and memory impairments in the 5xFAD mouse model of Alzheimer's disease: Effects of age, sex, albinism, and motor impairments. Genes Brain Behav. 2022;21(4):e12794.
383. O'Leary TP, Brown RE. Visuo-spatial learning and memory deficits on the Barnes maze in the 16-month-old APPswe/PS1dE9 mouse model of Alzheimer's disease. Behav Brain Res. 2009;201(1):120–7.
384. Chouhan AK, Guo C, Hsieh YC, Ye H, Senturk M, Zuo Z, et al. Uncoupling neuronal death and dysfunction in Drosophila models of neurodegenerative disease. Acta Neuropathol Commun. 2016;4(1):62.
385. Koronyo-Hamaoui M, Sheyn J, Hayden EY, Li S, Fuchs DT, Regis GC, et al. Peripherally derived angiotensin converting enzyme-enhanced macrophages alleviate Alzheimer-related disease. Brain. 2020;143(1):336–58.

Real-Time Imaging of Single Neuronal Cell Apoptosis (DARC)

7

Timothy E. Yap, Monica Kelada, Azeem Sher, Maja Szymanska, Radhika Pooja Patel, and M. Francesca Cordeiro

Abstract

Retinal imaging techniques of the macula and optic nerve head are becoming a mainstay in the management of ophthalmic and neurodegenerative diseases. The ability to monitor the change in individual cellular populations over time can provide information on disease activity and the need for intervention. As we approach implementing cellular-resolution imaging into clinical practice, the ability to image retinal cellular activity remains an unmet clinical need. Detection of Apoptosing Retinal Cells (DARC) technology offers the potential to detect live apoptosis in-vivo at a cellular level, given the clear optical media of the eye. This uses a fluorescent annexin-A5 marker of early apoptosis that has been studied in both animals and humans, with promising results. The hope is that with further study, this technique can be used to provide real-time information on neurodegenerative disease activity both in glaucoma and CNS conditions such as Alzheimer's disease, where apoptosis is thought to play a key role. The ability of DARC to reflect disease progression would provide a useful surrogate marker in clinical trials, expediting the availability of novel treatments to protect against sight loss and cognitive decline.

T. E. Yap · R. P. Patel · M. F. Cordeiro (✉)
The Western Eye Hospital, Imperial College Healthcare NHS Trust (ICHNT), 153-173 Marylebone Rd, Marylebone, London NW1 5QH, UK
e-mail: m.cordeiro@imperial.ac.uk

T. E. Yap · M. Kelada · A. Sher · M. Szymanska · R. P. Patel · M. F. Cordeiro
The Imperial College Ophthalmic Research Group (ICORG), Imperial College, London NW1 5QH, UK

M. F. Cordeiro
Glaucoma and Retinal Neurodegenration Group, Department of Visual Neuroscience, UCL Institute of Ophthalmology, London EC1V 9EL, UK

A. Grzybowski and P. Barboni (eds.), *OCT and Imaging in Central Nervous System Diseases*, https://doi.org/10.1007/978-3-031-72156-4_7

Keywords

Retinal ganglion cell imaging • Detection of Apoptosing Retinal Cells (DARC) technology • Glaucoma

7.1 Mechanisms of Cell Death and Apoptosis

Amongst the distinct pathways through which cells are believed to die, increased rates of apoptosis are thought to play a key role in glaucoma and other neurodegenerative conditions such as Alzheimer's disease, Parkinson's disease and motor neurone disease [1]. 'Apoptosis' from the Greek for 'falling off' represents the pathway of programmed cell death by which cells can die in order to make way for new cells, without triggering inflammation that may threaten the health and function of neighbouring cells. The rate of this stereotyped behaviour is important when considering the requirement of some neuronal cells to last an organism's lifetime in order to maintain learnt neurological functions, memories or motor units [1]. It follows that minimising the triggers of this process may prolong visual, neurological or neuromuscular function in certain neurodegenerative conditions. It is believed apoptosis is triggered by a combination of genetic susceptibility and environmental factors, progressing downstream to a highly conserved intracellular apoptotic pathway. Well-studied examples of chemical activation signals include lack of neurotrophic factor support, glutamate excitotoxicity, and oxidative, metabolic, and environmental stresses [1]. It is becoming increasingly apparent that mitochondrial events may also be important in apoptosis initiation [2]. Early cellular signals associated with an activated apoptosis pathway include the pro- and anti-apoptotic members of the B-cell lymphoma-2 (Bcl-2) regulator protein family, upstream and downstream apoptosis-activating caspases, and telomerase activity [3]. The ensuing morphological changes involve cellular shrinkage, membrane blebbing, chromatin condensation and the development of pyknotic neuclei [4]. This apoptotic pathway is distinct from primary necrosis in which immediate, unregulated cell death occurs in response to extreme stress, causing mass release of intracellular molecules, damage-associated molecular patterns (DAMPs) [5] and recruitment of cells mediating an acute inflammatory response. Less acute events sufficient to cause necrosis with delayed rupture of the cell membrane allow modification of intracellular components prior to release, presumably to prune the inflammatory response [6].

Phosphatidylserine (PS) is a marker of early apoptosis of particular interest in diagnostics. This anionic phospholipid is usually maintained in an asymmetric distribution across the cell membrane by ATP-dependent flippases located on the inner leaflet of the cell membrane, in physiologic conditions [7]. In apoptotic conditions, flippases are downregulated which causes the increased externalisation of PS on the outer leaflet of the cell membrane. Scramblase proteins are another type of cell membrane protein thought to induce this change, enlisting their ability to facilitate bi-directional, non-specific movement of phospholipids across bilayers in a calcium-dependent manner [8].

In glaucoma in particular, apoptosis is believed to be the predominant mechanism of ganglion cell layer (GCL) loss in glaucoma. Ganglion cells reside in the inner retina, with their dendrites forming the inner plexiform layer and axons projecting over the inner surface of the retina, forming the retinal nerve fibre layer. Studies have also confirmed neurodegeneration extending further into the central nervous system, specifically the lateral geniculate nucleus and visual cortex [9, 10]. Typically difficult to image due to their low-contrast edges, retinal ganglion cells (RGCs) vary in density across the retina, peaking at around 32,000-38,000 cells/mm^2 in the perifoveal region [11], whilst also varying in number throughout development and lifespans, and between healthy individuals. Unsatisfactorily, the evidence for RGC apoptosis is provided by the absence of features of necrosis, such as ATP depletion, cell lysis and acute inflammation. However, in addition to this observation, primate studies have attempted to show DNA fragmentation typical of apoptosis in ocular hypertension models. However these are hampered by the low number of cells thought to be undergoing apoptosis at any one time [12]. Detection of the typical 180-200 base pair fragments created in apoptosis has proven a slightly more successful way forward with TUNEL (Terminal transferase dUTP Nick End Labelling), showing significantly increased levels in experimental glaucoma eyes in comparison to their healthy, contralateral counterparts [13]. Such results have also since been replicated in humans [14–16]. The trigger for apoptosis in the setting of glaucoma has been widely debated and may indeed be multi-factorial, with several prominent theories. Deprivation of neurotrophic factor support (e.g brain derived neurotrophic factor, BDNF) due to intraocular pressure (IOP) related congestion and restricted axoplasmic transport at the lamina cribrosa where the optic nerve exits the globe, has been proposed. Similarly, the vascular hypothesis implicating optic nerve head vaso-dysregulation [17] has been proposed to cause deficiencies in neurotrophic factor support. Glutamate excitotoxicity via NMDA receptor over-activation is another theory behind the basis for novel neuroprotective therapies. Conflicting findings exist with regards to whether glutamate is present in raised levels in the vitreous of glaucoma patients [18–22], and indeed the significance of this measure in the context of the overall theory [23]. Oxidative stress [24] and immunological factors [25, 26] amy also be important in triggering apoptotic cascades.

7.2 DARC Technology

The molecular basis of DARC uses the affinity annexin A5 has for PS, therefore lending itself well to the application of labelling cells in the early phases of apoptosis. Annexin A5 is a 36 kDa protein that is ubiquitously expressed in humans. Its unique function is unclear, with possible roles in membrane repair and permeability [27, 28], autophagy [29], and anti-endotoxin activities [30], as well as working in combination with C1q complement protein as a ligand in the induction of apoptosis [31]. Annexin A5 electrostatically binds PS in a strong but reversible, calcium-dependent fashion, taking advantage of the local high calcium (Ca^{2+}) concentrations found near the negatively charged cell surface [32, 33]. In-vitro use of fluorescently-labelled or biotinylated annexin A5 has therefore been used to detect apoptosing cells with both imaging and flow cytometry [34]. When used in combination with propidium iodide (PI), cells undergoing necrosis (annexin A5+/PI+) or apoptosis (annexin A5+/PI−) can be successfully identified. The high affinity with PS also brings about high levels of sensitivity for early apoptosis which favours annexin A5 as a detector of apoptosis, such that it has been translated into human studies as a radiolabelled marker investigating diseases where rates of apoptosis are altered such as malignancy [35–38], stroke, myocardial infarction [39, 40], organ transplantation [41] and inflammatory bowel disease [42]. However, in many of these applications, resolution and localisation is limited by tissue opacity. In contrast, the transparent media of the eye including the cornea, aqueous humour, lens and vitreous body allow direct visualisation of fluorescent markers in the retina, permitting cellular-resolution imaging using DARC, amongst other techniques [43, 44].

DARC technology uses Annexin A5 conjugated with either a 488 nm (ANX488) or 776 nm (ANX776) fluorophore to visualise apoptosing retinal cells. These probes have have been administered intravitreally in animals [45] and intravenously in humans [46] as a novel type of contrast agent for detecting retinal cell apoptosis. ANX488 has excitation/emission wavelengths of 495/519 nm, and ANX776, excitation/emission wavelengths in the near-infrared spectrum of 771/793 nm. ANX776 was developed using a human variant annexin molecule (RhAnnexin V128) permitting a single covalent bond between the maleimide form of Dy776 fluorescent marker (Dy-776-mal) and RhAnnexin V128. This provided a similar excitation/emission profile to indocyanine green (ICG), for which imaging is widely available in clinical practice.

Confocal scanning laser ophthalmoscopy is an imaging technique that is able to provide high resolution imaging with depth selectivity in order to form optical cross-sections. The axial volume required is selected by passing the reflected light through an adjustable pinhole aperture, therefore improving axial resolution by minimising optical cross-talk [47]. For acquiring DARC images using ANX488, illumination with argon laser of 488 nm in conjunction with a wide band-pass filter with short wavelength cut-off at 521 nm to select out the fluorescent signal has been used. Using ANX776 however, ICG settings with diode laser illumination of 786 nm and a 800 nm barrier filter was possible. The resultant images show 'DARC spots' 12–16 μm in diameter that can be counted using an automated system based on a template-matching approach [48], after transformations to take into account large non-enhancing structures such as blood vessels and non-linear optical distortions. To maximise signal-to-noise ratio, the manufacturer's eye tracking technology was used in combination with 100-frame averaging.

7.3 DARC Investigating Disease Pathogenesis

DARC imaging has been used in animal models of several neurodegenerative diseases including glaucoma, Alzheimer's disease, Parkinson's disease and diabetes mellitus (Table 7.1). The first study published in 2004 used rodent and primate glaucoma models to demonstrate proof of concept. The rat models included the Morrison's chronic ocular hypertension model involving episcleral vein injections of hypertonic saline resulting in chronic ocular hypertension (OHT), another model using intravitreal injections of staurosporine, a non-selective protein kinase inhibitor causing neuronal cell death [49], and a further optic nerve transection (ONT) model of secondary neurodegeneration [50, 51]. DARC imaging was combined with histological analysis to determine the identity of DARC spots. Rats received intravitreal injections of ANX488 and retrograde labelling of RGCs was carried out using an injection of DiAsp (4-(4-(didecylamino)styryl)-*N*-methylpyridinium iodide) to the superior colliculi of rats. After sacrifice, subsequent histological staining using Cy5-labeled anti-caspase-3 antibodies confirmed apoptosing cells. Anatomical reconstructions of in-vivo imaging and histological studies showed good correlation between staining patterns and DARC spots, supporting the identity of DARC spots as apoptosing RGCs [50]. DARC count was highest at 7 days in ONT and peaked between 3 and 4 weeks in the OHT model. A correlation between the number of apoptosing cells and the magnitude of ocular hypertensive or staurosporine dose-related insult was also seen. Furthermore, using spectrally distinct fluorescent markers of early and late apoptosis, DARC was shown to longitudinally image the same cells through time [52]. Thus, the ability of DARC to both identify and quantify retinal cell apoptosis suggested its capability as an outcome measure in future studies.

The relationship with intraocular pressure (IOP) was confirmed in a further study investigating the effect of raised IOP on apoptosis of RGCs and expression of specific extracellular matrix (ECM) components in a rat ocular hypertension model. Results showed a strong correlation between DARC count and the magnitude of IOP elevation. This study also demonstrated IOP-related alterations in extra-cellular matrix components including a positive correlation with matrix metalloproteinase-9 activity (MMP-9), tissue inhibitor of matrix metalloproteinase (TIMP-1) and collagen I, and negative correlations with laminin and TGF-beta2 deposition in the RGC layer [53] supporting the theory of glaucomatous RGC apoptosis relating to ECM remodelling, and the retina being the primary site of glaucomatous injury.

Another study of glaucoma pathogenesis examined the role of amyloid beta (Aβ) peptide in glaucoma, the production and deposition of which drives the pathogenesis of Alzheimer's disease (AD) [54, 55]. AD is characterised histologically by the deposition of beta amyloid plaques in the brain and neurofibrillary tangles formed by the aggregation of tau [56]. These substances are thought to contribute to disease pathophysiology by causing altered mitochondrial dysregulation and altered neurotransmission [57], and have been detected in the retinas of animal models [58] and some AD patients [59–61] potentially prior to changes seen in

Table 7.1 Summary of DARC studies showing proof-of-concept and investigating pathogenesis

Factor of interest	Findings	Citations
Proof of concept	DARC demonstrating in-vivo apoptosing retinal cells using ANX488	[50]
Intraocular pressure	Correlation of DARC with intraocular pressure and changes in the extracellular matrix	[53]
DMSO	DMSO toxicity demonstrated with in-vivo DARC imaging and in-vitro studies	[112]
Staurosporine model	Staurosporine (SSP) induced RGC apoptosis confirmed with histological analysis	[73]
Partial optic nerve transection	Retinal apoptosis detected following pONT	[86]
Alzheimer's model	Triple transgenic model of Alzheimer's disease	[52]
Amyloid-β	Amyloid-β induction of RGC apoptosis and co-localization with DARC	[54]
Diabetic retinopathy	Raised DARC count in transgenic diabetic mice	[63]
Laser damage	Inner nuclear layer damage from lasers demonstrated with DARC	[64]
Blue light exposure	Photoreceptor death in response to blue light exposure investigated with DARC	[65]
Parkinson's model	DARC imaging used in a rotenone-induced model of Parkinson's disease.	[82]
Proof-of-concept	Longitudinal DARC using spectrally distinct fluorophores to image multiple phases of cell death in rats	[52]
Phase I clinical trial	Demonstration of DARC spot visualisation in humans, including demonstration of the safety and efficacy of intravenous ANX776	[46]
Phase II clinical trial	Demonstration of an automatic CNN-aided algorithmic method of DARC spot detection to enable prediction of glaucoma progression	[96]

the brain [62]. This study found that in a rat ocular hypertension model, amyloid beta not only co-localized with RGCs undergoing apoptosis, but also significantly contributed to their apoptosis in a time and dose-dependent manner. These findings suggested that the amyloid beta pathway could be a therapeutic target in glaucoma, together with in-vivo DARC imaging to assess the efficacy of treatment [54].

In addition to glaucoma, DARC has been used to study the pathogenesis of other diseases in which neurodegeneration is implicated. DARC was able to provide the first in-vivo visualisation of apoptosing RGCs in a transgenic mouse model of diabetic retinopathy. This study suggested that the rate of apoptosis was highest early in the lifecycle of this model (8 weeks), suggesting DARC may have a future role as a detector of early diabetic retinopathy [63].

Retinal damage using Nd:YAG laser has also been examined with DARC. This study found that the damage to the inner nuclear layer of rats was correlated with the power and duration of the laser insult, with DARC spot density showing a dose-dependent correlation with laser exposure [64]. Blue light damage has also been studied, with DARC demonstrating damage to the outer retinal layers, as confirmed by histological studies finding photoreceptor death [65].

7.4 DARC Investigating Novel Therapeutics

DARC has been used in pre-clinical studies to assess the neuroprotective efficacy of several novel therapeutic agents and new formulations of drugs already in clinical use (Table 7.2). In relation to glaucoma, the alpha agonist brimonidine has been suggested to have neuroprotective actions in addition to its anti-ocular hypertensive actions [66]. However, the human studies supporting this theory are plagued with difficulties surrounding high attrition rates due to drop intolerance [67]. Using DARC, systemic brimonidine and clonidine were shown to reduce apoptosis in a rodent model by 92.8% and 92.3% respectively, via the non-amyloidogenic Aβ and secreted amyloid precursor protein α (sAPPα) pathways suggesting these drugs may have a role to play in other pathologies involving Aβ toxicity such as Alzheimer's disease [68]. In contrast to clonidine, no significant IOP lowering effect was seen with brimonidine supporting the hypothesis of an IOP-independent neuroprotective mechanism.

Glutamate-induced excitotoxicity implicated in Alzheimer's disease [69] is also likely to play a role in glaucoma, causing RGC death. Furthermore, blocking N-Methyl-D-aspartate (NMDA) receptors has been reported to reduce RGC apoptosis

Table 7.2 Summary of DARC studies as an outcome measure

Factor of interest	Findings	Citations
NMDA receptor antagonists	DARC used to investigate NMDA receptor antagonism to target glutamate excitotoxicity as a neuroprotective strategy in rat models of glaucoma	[73]
Amyloid-β	Investigation of MRZ-99030, an amyloid-β aggregator	[78]
Schwann cell delivery	DARC used to help evaluate the efficacy of a novel direct Schwann cell delivery method in a partial optic nerve transection model	[86]
Adenosine A3 agonism	Selective adenosine A3 agonism by 2-Cl-IB-MECA investigated with DARC as a neuroprotective treatment strategy	[75]
Rosiglitazone	The neuroprotective potential of liposome-encapsulated rosiglitazone investigated with DARC	[82]
Alpha-agonists	DARC used to demonstrate IOP-independent neuroprotection	[68]
Coenzyme Q10	Topical coenzyme Q10 investigated in an ocular hypertension model	[85]
Curcumin	The efficacy of neuroprotective agent, Curcumin, against Alzheimer's disease	[79]

[70–72]. Targeting the role glutamate excitotoxicity may play in glaucoma, non-selective (MK801) and selective (ifenprodil) NMDA receptor antagonists and a metabotropic glutamate receptor agonist (mGluR Group II, LY354740) were used in a study on rat models of glaucoma. All the glutamate modulation strategies employed were shown to have efficacy in neuroprotection in the staurosporine model seen with both in-vivo imaging and histological analysis, in a dose-dependent manner. MK801 was shown to have greater efficacy than ifenprodil, however due to MK801's neurotoxic side effects, best results were achieved with low-dose MK801 combined with LY354740 [73]. Treatments were administered to an OHT model using DARC as an outcome measure, demonstrating maximal neuroprotective efficacy at the start of IOP elevation.

There is some evidence suggesting that targeting adenosine A1 receptors (A1Rs) may be a useful neuroprotective strategy [74], in at least part due to its inhibitory effect on glutaminergic activity. 2-Cl-IB-MECA, a selective (A3R) agonist was trialled with DARC in models of partial optic nerve transection (pONT). DARC showed significantly increased apoptosis after pONT, an effect reduced by intravitreal 2-Cl-IB- MECA [75].

The commonality in the excitotoxic pathogenesis of both glaucoma and Alzheimer's disease has led to the same drugs being trialled in both diseases [76]. Similarly, amyloid-beta (Aβ) central to the amyloid hypothesis of Alzheimer's disease [77], has been proposed as a potential therapeutic target in glaucoma. In a rat model of ocular hypertension, DARC imaging was used as an outcome measure in combination with histological studies to demonstrate the Aβ aggregation modulator MRZ-99030 could achieve dose-dependent neuroprotection, with MRZ-99030 achieving a 33% reduction of apoptosis without exhibiting any effect on the IOP [78].

Intranasal delivery of annexin has been investigated as an alternative, technically less demanding route [79, 80]. Shamsher *et al.* evaluated the efficacy of curcumin nanoparticles (CNs), a natural polyphenol which has been advocated as a potential neuroprotectant [79]. Transgenic mice were treated intranasally for 3 months (5 days per week) with either 3 μL of CN ($n = 7$) or vehicle only ($n = 6$). DARC imaging was performed after the treatment course. Mice receiving CN were found to have a significant reduction in DARC count compared to vehicle control ($p < 0.05$). In vitro, R28 cells showed the CN formulation was well tolerated and it protected against glutamate excitotoxicity and hypoxia mimetic, cobalt chloride. Their results suggest that CN has potential therapeutic effect against AD, which can be assessed through the eye using DARC. Hill et al. [80] used 10 female triple transgenic mice (3xTg-AD) as a model of retinal cell death and 10 healthy controls. Retinas were imaged in-vivo at baseline and 2 h after intranasal DARC administration, and ex-vivo. A significantly higher spot count in diseased animals was found compared to healthy animals both in- and ex-vivo. Although images were of similar quality to those acquired from intravitreal DARC, a higher intranasal DARC dose was required (approximately 10-fold increase).

DARC has also been used to study drugs more commonly used in another neurodegenerative condition, Parkinson's disease (PD). Using a rotenone-induced rat model, animals were treated with liposome-encapsulated rosiglitazone, a peroxisome proliferator-activated receptor gamma (PPAR-gamma) agonist [81]. The results of the treatment versus vehicle-only controls demonstrated a neuroprotective effect of intraperitoneal rosiglitazone in this formulation. More importantly for DARC, in-vivo apoptosis imaging detected a peak in counts at 20 days after rotenone administration in comparison to pathological studies at day 60. The earlier appearance of a significant rise in DARC count compared to the pathological finding of dopaminergic loss from the substantia nigra further supports the role of DARC as a useful tool for early diagnosis [82].

The role of impaired mitochondrial function and oxidative stress in triggering RGC apoptosis has been examined with DARC. Coenzyme Q10 (CoQ10) is a mitochondrial antioxidant, key to the normal function of the electron transport chain. CoQ10 has been shown to play a neuroprotective role in neurological conditions such as AD, PD, Huntington's disease [83] and experimental glaucoma [84]. In a rat OHT model, the effect of topically applied CoQ10 was examined, in a micellular α-tocopherol polyethylene glycol succinate (TPGS) formulation. DARC imaging revealed a significantly lower number of apoptosing retinal cells in those animals treated with CoQ10 compared to the TPGS-only controls at 3 weeks [85], suggesting translational therapeutic promise for this formulation of CoQ10.

A novel cell-based therapy using Schwann cells has also been investigated with DARC technology, comparing direct optic nerve sheath application (DONS) versus intravitreal injections, in a pONT model. Although both methods showed a significantly increased proportion of RGCs remaining at certain time points, the DONS method demonstrated delayed but longer-lasting effects at 56 days. These histological results using Brn-3a-labelling were mirrored by using DARC, demonstrating significantly reduced rates of apoptosis in the DONS group compared to those untreated at days 7 and 21. Using DARC to provide in-vivo observation of retinal cell apoptosis in this manner facilitated the comparison of effect on secondary degeneration through multiple time intervals in the same subject, instead of requiring sacrifice in order to complete histological analysis at each timepoint [86].

RGC apoptosis is thought to account for RNFL thinning seen in patients with optic neuritis (ON) [87]. Immunisation of animals with myelin proteins induces experimental autoimmune encephalomyelitis (EAE) [88]. Guan et al. utilised this rat model with the aim of investigating the relationship of inflammation with RGC loss during ON [89]. Retinas were examined for the number of fluorescent-labelled RGCs in each field, and the optic nerve was examined for the presence of inflammatory cell infiltration. The study demonstrated that neuronal loss was not detected at day 10, while histopathological ON had begun suggesting neuronal loss likely occurs secondary to inflammation. These findings have been corroborated by similar studies using immunisation induced EAE in mice [90].

Dutt et al. investigated the timing of steroid treatment in EAE mice with two corticosteroids before and after optic nerve inflammation [91]. Their study found that early treatment with corticosteroids prevented the development of optic neuritis and prevented RGC loss. As DARC technology can be used to track retinal apoptosis and RNFL changes over time, it can be feasibly applied with the same principles to optic neuritis to determine MS activity. By identifying patients who are at high risk of permanent vision loss, it may be possible to stratify patients and determine who can be targeted with immunotherapies to prevent this.

7.5 DARC in Humans

DARC has now been translated into investigating human disease, with a Phase I trial published in 2017 [46]. This study set out to examine the safety and tolerability of DARC using intravenous ANX776. The study population included eight glaucoma subjects proven to demonstrate disease progression, and eight healthy volunteers. Inclusion of glaucoma patients was based on having at least one progressing index from visual field testing or OCT/HRT (optical coherence imaging/Heidelberg retinal tomography) imaging. A storer design was used to allocate 4 groups of subjects to each dose of ANX776. Each group consisted of 2 glaucoma and 2 healthy subjects. The doses given were 0.1 mg, 0.2 mg, 0.4 mg and 0.5 mg. The results showed that no serious adverse event occurred, with the six reported adverse events deemed not related to the ANX776 itself. Pharmacokinetic experiments showed a dose-dependent relationship with ANX776 administration. Clearance of the drug was also found to be high, with no drug accumulation. With regards to efficacy, DARC spots were successfully seen appearing in humans as in animals previously (Figure 7.1). At the 0.4 mg dose, significantly more spots were seen in the glaucomatous group compared to healthy controls ($n = 4$, $p < 0.005$). DARC count was also seen to be significantly correlated with reduced central corneal thickness ($R = -0.68$, $p = 0.006$) and increased cup-to-disc ratio ($R = 0.47$, $p = 0.038$). Further post-hoc analysis was carried out using clinical follow-up data for these subjects, demonstrating that the DARC count was significantly higher in those subjects who underwent increased rates of disease progression following ANX776 administration, compared to healthy controls.

Phase II of the DARC project included a wider spectrum of neurodegenerative conditions and healthy controls. Five subject groups were included in this study; healthy volunteers, progressive glaucoma patients, optic neuritis (ON) patients, age-related macular degeneration patients (AMD), and subjects with Down syndrome (a condition found to demonstrate similar CNS pathology to Alzheimer's disease) [92]. This was a single-centre, open-label study in which all subjects received a single intravenous injection of 0.4mg of ANX776. The outcomes from 40 healthy eyes and 20 eyes with glaucoma were published in 2020, demonstrating the use of artificial intelligence (AI) to count DARC spots [93]. Inclusion of glaucoma subjects was based on having at least one eye demonstrating disease progression on visual field testing or imaging. Rates of glaucoma progression were defined by serial OCT scans 18 months after DARC.

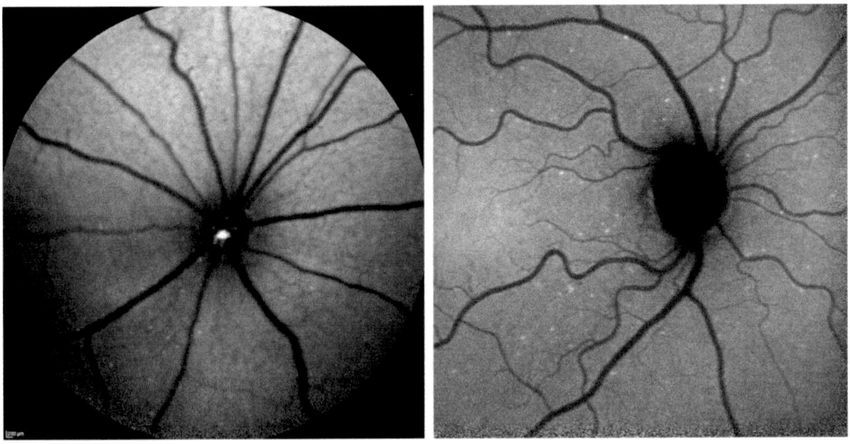

Fig. 7.1 DARC images from a rat model (left) and human (right) demonstrating DARC spots (Unpublished data reproduced with permission from Prof. M. F. Cordeiro)

To generate the AI-assisted DARC count, anonymised images were randomised and reviewed by five masked operators who manually identified spots. An automated convolutional neural network (CNN) was trained and validated using the manual counts from the healthy subjects. When compared to manual grading, the algorithm had 97.0% accuracy, 91.1% sensitivity and 97.1% specificity to detect positive spots in healthy eyes. The CNN was then applied to the images from the glaucoma cohort to determine if the DARC count was predictive for glaucoma progression at 18 months. A DARC count of greater than 24 was associated with a maximal sensitivity (85.7%) and specificity (91.7%) with an AUROC (area under the ROC curve) of 0.88 (likelihood ratio 8.57) for the CNN algorithm. Alternatively, the maximal sensitivity for the manual count was 71.4% and specificity of 87.5% with an AUC of 0.79 (likelihood ratio of 4.76) for DARC count greater than 11, showing superior performance of the CNN counts compared to the manual observer counts.

The Phase II results in subjects with AMD have also been published [94]. Two forms of AMD exist; 'wet' and 'dry' characterised by the presence or absence of choroidal neovascularisation (CNV) and the formation of subretinal or intraretinal fluid (SRF or IRF) [95]. Nineteen subjects (29 eyes) with either form of AMD were recruited and underwent DARC imaging, after which they were followed up with OCT imaging for 36 months. The same CNN algorithm described above was used to detect DARC spots [93]. At 36 months, 7 eyes had developed new SRF for the first time. A CNN DARC count >5 was associated with SRF development ($p = 0.02$). All 7 eyes that developed new SRF had CNN DARC counts >5. At 6 months, DARC count >5 had a specificity of 90%, and a sensitivity of 83% [positive predictive value (PPV) = 70%, negative predictive value (NPV) = 95%]. A peak PPV of 86% was achieved at 30 months. DARC counts overlying SRF were also seen to correlate with SRF size.

Analysis with regards to geographic atrophy (GA) has also been performed [96]. GA is end stage AMD that leads to blindness, characterised by demarcated atrophy of the RPE, photoreceptors, and choriocapillaris [97, 98]. A significant association between the Euclidean distance from DARC spots and new areas of expanded atrophy was found, compared to non-DARC areas. Any eye with a mean DARC distance of <12 pixels developed a large final area of GA ($p = 0.014$). DARC activity at baseline was shown to be predictive of GA activity at a mean of 29.3 months [96].

Detecting human DARC spots has also shown promise in the optic neuritis cohort of 12 optic neuritis subjects all given ANX776 [99]. The study results demonstrated a significant difference in the number of DARC spots compared to healthy eyes. Although larger studies are needed to replicate this finding, these results suggests a wider use of DARC technology.

7.6 Potential Implications for Clinical Practice in Glaucoma and Beyond

Neurodegenerative diseases have inherent challenges in their diagnosis, monitoring and treatment that may be overcome if DARC technology is able to be successfully translated to clinic and human research. In the case of glaucoma, subtle early visual field defects not affecting central vision are rarely noticed by patients, with incidental findings of raised IOP, family history or fundus examination detecting more advanced disease all more common methods of presentation. The biomarker most commonly considered is intraocular pressure (IOP). IOP is carefully monitored, and the sole target of current glaucoma therapies. However its reliability is under constant scrutiny as measurements can vary by technique, corneal thickness and time of day, amongst other variables [100]. Also, deciding how low an individual's IOP should be is often a clinical decision that can influence whether a patient undergoes procedures that may involve laser or intraocular surgery. Further complexity lies in the fact that intraocular pressure is not a universal surrogate marker for disease progression. From the Ocular Hypertension Treatment Study [101], we have learnt that lowering IOP reduces the rate of conversion to glaucoma in patients with ocular hypertension to glaucoma (number needed to treat, NNT = 20). However, the fact remains that the majority of those with high IOP will not develop glaucomatous damage, and a small proportion of those with sufficiently treated IOP will still progress. As a further complexity, the Collaborative Normal-Tension Glaucoma Study (CNTGS) has also shown that reducing IOP still reduces disease progression in 'normal-tension' glaucoma (NTG), where IOP is thought to be within 'normal' range.

Visual field tests are currently the gold standard investigation in glaucoma, demonstrating the extent and location of functional loss a patient is experiencing. As is the case with IOP, many variables affect the test reliability, with patient technique, good concentration and steady fixation required for up to 4–5 minutes at a time. This can be challenging for patients, especially those with musculoskeletal or cognition-related health problems that are common in the glaucoma population. Such is the difficulty many patients experience carrying out these tests, a significant 'learning effect' takes place whereby the first few visual fields may paradoxically improve with increasing reliability parameters [102]. There is also believed to be a significant lag between the onset of glaucoma and the appearance of visual field defects, with an estimated 20–30% RGC loss prior to the development of 'perimetric' glaucoma. This is also dependent on the test sensitivity, with studies suggesting that the standard 24-2 visual field testing algorithm may not detect early visual field defects [103]. A further limiting factor in visual field testing is the slow rate at which many patients progress [104], thus making the use of visual fields as a primary outcome in clinical trials expensive. Concomitant ophthalmic pathology may also affect visual field testing that may mask glaucomatous change in a subset of patients. These factors have led to most glaucoma treatments proven on the efficacy of IOP-lowering alone. The first large placebo-controlled study demonstrating visual field-sparing efficacy of a topical glaucoma therapy was published in 2015 [105].

OCT imaging in glaucoma has shown great promise in detecting 'pre-perimetric glaucoma' in patients who are yet to develop detectable visual field defects. This period is reported to last between 2 and 8 years in the cohorts studied [106, 107]. Due to individual variation in optic disc and posterior pole morphologies, rate of progression indicated by longitudinal change is thought to be a good predictor of future visual field progression [107] but requires multiple timepoints for reliable trends to be detected, during which RGC loss may be continuing. OCT imaging in other neurodegenerative conditions where apoptosis has been implicated is also starting to be recognised, especially in the field of dementia. Alzheimer's disease similarly has a lag-time between disease onset and diagnosis due to a non-specific early prodrome of symptoms. Both retinal nerve fibre layer (RNFL) and ganglion cell layers have been demonstrated to display thinning, especially in the superior and inferior peripapillary quadrants and may be used as part of a diagnostic or monitoring tool to provide easily accessible information on disease severity and progression [108]. However, in a similar manner to glaucoma, rate of progression is likely to be slow and require multiple visits to assess.

The placing of DARC in human research or clinical practice is still yet to be fully clarified. What is very promising for the future is the first demonstration of in-vivo visualisation of apoptosing retinal cells in humans using a method that is easily achievable in most clinical environments. Additionally, the ANX776 has been shown to be safe for use in humans with no adverse events thought to be related to the agent itself. The concepts of primary and secondary neurodegeneration suggest that early treatment in a range of diseases is crucial to have a hope of reducing increasingly convergent secondary pathways [68, 109–111]. Given our current lack of ability to confidently diagnose early neurodegeneration, DARC is attempting to meet a unmet clinical need both in terms of patient management and surrogate markers. The future for DARC will involve further demonstrating what DARC spots mean in humans, and whether this helps to reduce morbidity from visual or cognitive decline with early treatment, or facilitate the study of novel therapeutics in order to abate neurodegenerative processes.

References

1. Mattson MP. Apoptosis in neurodegenerative disorders. Nat Rev Mol Cell Biol. 2000;1:120–9. https://doi.org/10.1038/35040009.
2. Kroemer G, Dallaporta B, Resche-Rigon M. The mitochondrial death/life regulator in apoptosis and necrosis. Annu Rev Physiol. 1998;60:619–42. https://doi.org/10.1146/annurev.physiol.60.1.619.
3. Liu JP. Studies of the molecular mechanisms in the regulation of telomerase activity. FASEB J. 1999;13:2091–104.
4. Zhang Y, Chen X, Gueydan C, et al. Plasma membrane changes during programmed cell deaths. Cell Res. 2018;28:9–21. https://doi.org/10.1038/cr.2017.133.
5. Schaefer L. Complexity of danger: the diverse nature of damage-associated molecular patterns. J Biol Chem. 2014;289:35237–45. https://doi.org/10.1074/jbc.R114.619304.
6. Sachet M, Liang YY, Oehler R. The immune response to secondary necrotic cells. Apoptosis. 2017;22:1189–204. https://doi.org/10.1007/s10495-017-1413-z.
7. Daleke DL. Phospholipid flippases. J Biol Chem. 2007;282:821–5. https://doi.org/10.1074/jbc.R600035200.
8. Hankins HM, Baldridge RD, Xu P, et al. Role of flippases, scramblases and transfer proteins in phosphatidylserine subcellular distribution. Traffic. 2015;16:35–47. https://doi.org/10.1111/tra.12233.
9. Danesh-Meyer HV, Levin LA. Glaucoma as a neurodegenerative disease. J Neuroophthalmol. 2015;35(Suppl1):S22-28. https://doi.org/10.1097/WNO.0000000000000293.
10. Gupta N, Ang LC, Noel de Tilly L, et al. Human glaucoma and neural degeneration in intracranial optic nerve, lateral geniculate nucleus, and visual cortex. Br J Ophthalmol. 2006;90:674–8. https://doi.org/10.1136/bjo.2005.086769.
11. Curcio CA, Allen KA. Topography of ganglion cells in human retina. J Comp Neurol. 1990;300:5–25. https://doi.org/10.1002/cne.903000103.
12. Nickells RW. Retinal ganglion cell death in glaucoma: the how, the why, and the maybe. J Glaucoma. 1996;5:345–56.
13. Quigley HA, Nickells RW, Kerrigan LA, et al. Retinal ganglion cell death in experimental glaucoma and after axotomy occurs by apoptosis. Invest Ophthalmol Vis Sci. 1995;36:774–86.
14. Kyrylkova K, Kyryachenko S, Leid M, et al. Detection of apoptosis by TUNEL assay. Methods Mol Biol. 2012;887:41–7. https://doi.org/10.1007/978-1-61779-860-3_5.
15. Okisaka S, Murakami A, Mizukawa A, et al. Apoptosis in retinal ganglion cell decrease in human glaucomatous eyes. Jpn J Ophthalmol. 1997;41:84–8.
16. Kerrigan LA, Zack DJ, Quigley HA, et al. TUNEL-positive ganglion cells in human primary open-angle glaucoma. Arch Ophthalmol. 1997;115:1031–5.
17. Flammer J, Konieczka K, Flammer AJ. The primary vascular dysregulation syndrome: implications for eye diseases. EPMA J. 2013;4:14. https://doi.org/10.1186/1878-5085-4-14.
18. Dreyer EB, Zurakowski D, Schumer RA, et al. Elevated glutamate levels in the vitreous body of humans and monkeys with glaucoma. Arch Ophthalmol. 1996;114:299–305.
19. Brooks DE, Garcia GA, Dreyer EB, et al. Vitreous body glutamate concentration in dogs with glaucoma. Am J Vet Res. 1997;58:864–7.
20. Honkanen RA, Baruah S, Zimmerman MB, et al. Vitreous amino acid concentrations in patients with glaucoma undergoing vitrectomy. Arch Ophthalmol. 2003;121:183–8.
21. Levkovitch-Verbin H, Martin KR, Quigley HA, et al. Measurement of amino acid levels in the vitreous humor of rats after chronic intraocular pressure elevation or optic nerve transection. J Glaucoma. 2002;11:396–405.

22. Wamsley S, Gabelt BT, Dahl DB, et al. Vitreous glutamate concentration and axon loss in monkeys with experimental glaucoma. Arch Ophthalmol. 2005;123:64–70. https://doi.org/10.1001/archopht.123.1.64.
23. Salt TE, Cordeiro MF. Glutamate excitotoxicity in glaucoma: throwing the baby out with the bathwater? Eye (Lond). 2006; 20:730–731; author reply 731–732. https://doi.org/10.1038/sj.eye.6701967
24. Izzotti A, Bagnis A, Sacca SC. The role of oxidative stress in glaucoma. Mutat Res. 2006;612:105–14. https://doi.org/10.1016/j.mrrev.2005.11.001.
25. Rieck J. The pathogenesis of glaucoma in the interplay with the immune system. Invest Ophthalmol Vis Sci. 2013;54:2393–409. https://doi.org/10.1167/iovs.12-9781.
26. Tezel G. The immune response in glaucoma: a perspective on the roles of oxidative stress. Exp Eye Res. 2011;93:178–86. https://doi.org/10.1016/j.exer.2010.07.009.
27. Bouter A, Gounou C, Berat R, et al. Annexin-A5 assembled into two-dimensional arrays promotes cell membrane repair. Nat Commun. 2011;2:270. https://doi.org/10.1038/ncomms1270.
28. Creutz CE, Hira JK, Gee VE, et al. Protection of the membrane permeability barrier by annexins. Biochemistry. 2012;51:9966–83. https://doi.org/10.1021/bi3013559.
29. Ghislat G, Aguado C, Knecht E. Annexin A5 stimulates autophagy and inhibits endocytosis. J Cell Sci. 2012;125:92–107. https://doi.org/10.1242/jcs.086728.
30. Park JH, Jang JH, Choi EJ, et al. Annexin A5 increases survival in murine sepsis model by inhibiting HMGB1-mediated pro-inflammation and coagulation. Mol Med. 2016;22:424–36. https://doi.org/10.2119/molmed.2016.00026.
31. Martin M, Leffler J, Blom AM. Annexin A2 and A5 serve as new ligands for C1q on apoptotic cells. J Biol Chem. 2012;287:33733–44. https://doi.org/10.1074/jbc.M112.341339.
32. Meers P, Mealy T. Calcium-dependent annexin V binding to phospholipids: stoichiometry, specificity, and the role of negative charge. Biochemistry. 1993;32:11711–21.
33. Andree HA, Reutelingsperger CP, Hauptmann R, et al. Binding of vascular anticoagulant alpha (VAC alpha) to planar phospholipid bilayers. J Biol Chem. 1990;265:4923–8.
34. Schutte B, Nuydens R, Geerts H, et al. Annexin V binding assay as a tool to measure apoptosis in differentiated neuronal cells. J Neurosci Methods. 1998;86:63–9.
35. Hofstra L, Dumont EA, Thimister PW, et al. In vivo detection of apoptosis in an intracardiac tumor. JAMA. 2001;285:1841–2.
36. Belhocine T, Steinmetz N, Hustinx R, et al. Increased uptake of the apoptosis-imaging agent (99m)Tc recombinant human Annexin V in human tumors after one course of chemotherapy as a predictor of tumor response and patient prognosis. Clin Cancer Res. 2002;8:2766–74.
37. Kartachova M, Haas RL, Olmos RA, et al. In vivo imaging of apoptosis by 99mTc-Annexin V scintigraphy: visual analysis in relation to treatment response. Radiother Oncol. 2004;72:333–9. https://doi.org/10.1016/j.radonc.2004.07.008.
38. Vermeersch H, Ham H, Rottey S, et al. Intraobserver, interobserver, and day-to-day reproducibility of quantitative 99mTc-HYNIC annexin-V imaging in head and neck carcinoma. Cancer Biother Radiopharm. 2004;19:205–10. https://doi.org/10.1089/108497804323071986.
39. Thimister PW, Hofstra L, Liem IH, et al. In vivo detection of cell death in the area at risk in acute myocardial infarction. J Nucl Med. 2003;44:391–6.
40. Hofstra L, Liem IH, Dumont EA, et al. Visualisation of cell death in vivo in patients with acute myocardial infarction. Lancet. 2000;356:209–12.
41. Narula J, Acio ER, Narula N, et al. Annexin V imaging for noninvasive detection of cardiac allograft rejection. Nat Med. 2001;7:1347–52. https://doi.org/10.1038/nm1201-1347.
42. Van den Brande JM, Koehler TC, Zelinkova Z, et al. Prediction of antitumour necrosis factor clinical efficacy by real-time visualisation of apoptosis in patients with Crohn's disease. Gut. 2007;56:509–17. https://doi.org/10.1136/gut.2006.105379.
43. Yap TE, Donna P, Almonte MT, et al. Real-time imaging of retinal ganglion cell apoptosis. Cells. 2018. https://doi.org/10.3390/cells7060060.

44. Dong ZM, Wollstein G, Wang B, et al. Adaptive optics optical coherence tomography in glaucoma. Prog Retin Eye Res. 2017;57:76–88. https://doi.org/10.1016/j.preteyeres.2016.11.001.
45. Yap TE, Davis BM, Guo L, et al. Annexins in glaucoma. Int J Mol Sci. 2018. https://doi.org/10.3390/ijms19041218.
46. Cordeiro MF, Normando EM, Cardoso MJ, et al. Real-time imaging of single neuronal cell apoptosis in patients with glaucoma. Brain. 2017;140:1757–67. https://doi.org/10.1093/brain/awx088.
47. Webb RH, Hughes GW, Delori FC. Confocal scanning laser ophthalmoscope. Appl Opt. 1987;26:1492–9. https://doi.org/10.1364/AO.26.001492.
48. Brunelli R. Template matching techniques in computer vision: theory and practice. New York, NY: Wiley; 2009.
49. Koh JY, Wie MB, Gwag BJ, et al. Staurosporine-induced neuronal apoptosis. Exp Neurol. 1995;135:153–9. https://doi.org/10.1006/exnr.1995.1074.
50. Cordeiro MF, Guo L, Luong V, et al. Real-time imaging of single nerve cell apoptosis in retinal neurodegeneration. Proc Natl Acad Sci USA. 2004;101:13352–6. https://doi.org/10.1073/pnas.0405479101.
51. Levkovitch-Verbin H, Quigley HA, Martin KR, et al. A model to study differences between primary and secondary degeneration of retinal ganglion cells in rats by partial optic nerve transection. Invest Ophthalmol Vis Sci. 2003;44:3388–93.
52. Cordeiro MF, Guo L, Coxon KM, et al. Imaging multiple phases of neurodegeneration: a novel approach to assessing cell death in vivo. Cell Death Dis. 2010;1: e3. https://doi.org/10.1038/cddis.2009.3.
53. Guo L, Moss SE, Alexander RA, et al. Retinal ganglion cell apoptosis in glaucoma is related to intraocular pressure and IOP-induced effects on extracellular matrix. Invest Ophthalmol Vis Sci. 2005;46:175–82. https://doi.org/10.1167/iovs.04-0832.
54. Guo L, Salt TE, Luong V, et al. Targeting amyloid-beta in glaucoma treatment. Proc Natl Acad Sci USA. 2007;104:13444–9. https://doi.org/10.1073/pnas.0703707104.
55. Murphy MP, LeVine H 3rd. Alzheimer's disease and the amyloid-beta peptide. J Alzheimers Dis. 2010;19:311–23. https://doi.org/10.3233/JAD-2010-1221.
56. Weller J, Budson A. Current understanding of Alzheimer's disease diagnosis and treatment. F1000Research 2018; 7:1161. https://doi.org/10.12688/f1000research.14506.1
57. Wong KY, Roy J, Fung ML, et al. Relationships between mitochondrial dysfunction and neurotransmission failure in Alzheimer's disease. Aging Dis. 2020;11(1291–1316):20201001. https://doi.org/10.14336/AD.2019.1125.
58. Koronyo-Hamaoui M, Koronyo Y, Ljubimov AV, et al. Identification of amyloid plaques in retinas from Alzheimer's patients and noninvasive in vivo optical imaging of retinal plaques in a mouse model. *Neuroimage* (2011); 54 Suppl 1: S204–S217. https://doi.org/10.1016/j.neuroimage.2010.06.020
59. Ho CY, Troncoso JC, Knox D, et al. Beta-amyloid, phospho-tau and alpha-synuclein deposits similar to those in the brain are not identified in the eyes of Alzheimer's and Parkinson's disease patients. Brain Pathol. 2014;24(25–32):20130628. https://doi.org/10.1111/bpa.12070.
60. Koronyo Y, Salumbides BC, Black KL, et al. Alzheimer's disease in the retina: imaging retinal abeta plaques for early diagnosis and therapy assessment. Neurodegener Dis. 2012;10(285–293):20120210. https://doi.org/10.1159/000335154.
61. Koronyo Y, Biggs D, Barron E, et al. Retinal amyloid pathology and proof-of-concept imaging trial in Alzheimer's disease. JCI Insight. 2017. https://doi.org/10.1172/jci.insight.93621.
62. More SS, Vince R. Hyperspectral imaging signatures detect amyloidopathy in Alzheimer's mouse retina well before onset of cognitive decline. ACS Chem Neurosci. 2015;6(306–315):20141126. https://doi.org/10.1021/cn500242z.
63. Borrie SC, Cheung W, Guo L, et al. Diabetic retinal neurodegeneration: in vivo imaging of retinal ganglion cell apoptosis in the Ins2Akita/J mouse. Invest Ophthalmol Visual Sci. 2008;49:4924–4924.

64. Schmitz-Valckenberg S, Guo L, Maass A, et al. Real-time in vivo imaging of retinal cell apoptosis after laser exposure. Invest Ophthalmol Vis Sci. 2008;49:2773–80. https://doi.org/10.1167/iovs.07-1335.
65. Schmitz-Valckenberg S, Guo L, Cheung W, et al. In vivo imaging of retinal cell apoptosis following acute light exposure. Ophthalmologe. 2010;107:22–9. https://doi.org/10.1007/s00347-009-1952-y.
66. Saylor M, McLoon LK, Harrison AR, et al. Experimental and clinical evidence for brimonidine as an optic nerve and retinal neuroprotective agent: an evidence-based review. Arch Ophthalmol. 2009;127:402–6. https://doi.org/10.1001/archophthalmol.2009.9.
67. Krupin T, Liebmann JM, Greenfield DS, et al. A randomized trial of brimonidine versus timolol in preserving visual function: results from the Low-Pressure Glaucoma Treatment Study. Am J Ophthalmol. 2011;151:671–81. https://doi.org/10.1016/j.ajo.2010.09.026.
68. Nizari S, Guo L, Davis BM, et al. Non-amyloidogenic effects of alpha2 adrenergic agonists: implications for brimonidine-mediated neuroprotection. Cell Death Dis. 2016;7: e2514. https://doi.org/10.1038/cddis.2016.397.
69. Hynd MR, Scott HL, Dodd PR. Glutamate-mediated excitotoxicity and neurodegeneration in Alzheimer's disease. Neurochem Int. 2004;45:583–95. https://doi.org/10.1016/j.neuint.2004.03.007.
70. WoldeMussie E, Yoles E, Schwartz M, et al. Neuroprotective effect of memantine in different retinal injury models in rats. J Glaucoma. 2002;11:474–80.
71. Hare WA, WoldeMussie E, Lai RK, et al. Efficacy and safety of memantine treatment for reduction of changes associated with experimental glaucoma in monkey, I: Functional measures. Invest Ophthalmol Vis Sci. 2004;45:2625–39. https://doi.org/10.1167/iovs.03-0566.
72. Hare WA, WoldeMussie E, Weinreb RN, et al. Efficacy and safety of memantine treatment for reduction of changes associated with experimental glaucoma in monkey, II: Structural measures. Invest Ophthalmol Vis Sci. 2004;45:2640–51. https://doi.org/10.1167/iovs.03-0567.
73. Guo L, Salt TE, Maass A, et al. Assessment of neuroprotective effects of glutamate modulation on glaucoma-related retinal ganglion cell apoptosis in vivo. Invest Ophthalmol Vis Sci. 2006;47:626–33. https://doi.org/10.1167/iovs.05-0754.
74. Cunha RA. Neuroprotection by adenosine in the brain: from A(1) receptor activation to A(2A) receptor blockade. Purinergic Signal. 2005;1:111–34. https://doi.org/10.1007/s11302-005-0649-1.
75. Galvao J, Elvas F, Martins T, et al. Adenosine A3 receptor activation is neuroprotective against retinal neurodegeneration. Exp Eye Res. 2015;140:65–74. https://doi.org/10.1016/j.exer.2015.08.009.
76. Weinreb RN, Liebmann JM, Cioffi GA, et al. Oral memantine for the treatment of glaucoma: design and results of 2 randomized, placebo-controlled, phase 3 studies. Ophthalmology. 2018;125:1874–85. https://doi.org/10.1016/j.ophtha.2018.06.017.
77. Selkoe DJ. Toward a comprehensive theory for Alzheimer's disease. Hypothesis: Alzheimer's disease is caused by the cerebral accumulation and cytotoxicity of amyloid beta-protein. Ann N Y Acad Sci. 2000;924:17–25.
78. Salt TE, Nizari S, Cordeiro MF, et al. Effect of the Abeta aggregation modulator MRZ-99030 on retinal damage in an animal model of glaucoma. Neurotox Res. 2014;26:440–6. https://doi.org/10.1007/s12640-014-9488-6.
79. Shamsher E, Guo L, Davis BM, et al. Curcumin nanoparticles are neuroprotective in a mouse model of Alzheimer's disease. Invest Ophthalmol Vis Sci. 2019; 60.
80. Hill D, Luong V, Guo L, Cordeiro MF. Establishing intranasal administration as an alternative to intravitreal delivery of fluorescent annexin. Acta Ophthalmol. 2022;100:S267. https://doi.org/10.1111/j.1755-3768.2022.140.
81. Bove J, Perier C. Neurotoxin-based models of Parkinson's disease. Neuroscience. 2012;211:51–76. https://doi.org/10.1016/j.neuroscience.2011.10.057.
82. Normando EM, Davis BM, De Groef L, et al. The retina as an early biomarker of neurodegeneration in a rotenone-induced model of Parkinson's disease: evidence for a neuroprotective

effect of rosiglitazone in the eye and brain. Acta Neuropathol Commun. 2016;4:86. https://doi.org/10.1186/s40478-016-0346-z.
83. McMonnies C. Reactive oxygen species, oxidative stress, glaucoma and hyperbaric oxygen therapy. J Optom. 2018;11:3–9. https://doi.org/10.1016/j.optom.2017.06.002.
84. Nucci C, Tartaglione R, Cerulli A, et al. Retinal damage caused by high intraocular pressure-induced transient ischemia is prevented by coenzyme Q10 in rat. Int Rev Neurobiol. 2007;82:397–406. https://doi.org/10.1016/S0074-7742(07)82022-8.
85. Davis BM, Tian K, Pahlitzsch M, et al. Topical coenzyme Q10 demonstrates mitochondrial-mediated neuroprotection in a rodent model of ocular hypertension. Mitochondrion. 2017;36:114–23. https://doi.org/10.1016/j.mito.2017.05.010.
86. Guo L, Davis B, Nizari S, et al. Direct optic nerve sheath (DONS) application of Schwann cells prolongs retinal ganglion cell survival in vivo. Cell Death Dis. 2014;5: e1460. https://doi.org/10.1038/cddis.2014.399.
87. Garcia-Martin E, Rodriguez-Mena D, Satue M, et al. Electrophysiology and optical coherence tomography to evaluate Parkinson disease severity. Invest Ophthalmol Vis Sci. 2014;55(696–705):20140204. https://doi.org/10.1167/iovs.13-13062.
88. Kornek B, Storch MK, Weissert R, et al. Multiple sclerosis and chronic autoimmune encephalomyelitis: a comparative quantitative study of axonal injury in active, inactive, and remyelinated lesions. Am J Pathol. 2000;157:267–76. https://doi.org/10.1016/S0002-9440(10)64537-3.
89. Guan Y, Shindler KS, Tabuena P, et al. Retinal ganglion cell damage induced by spontaneous autoimmune optic neuritis in MOG-specific TCR transgenic mice. J Neuroimmunol. 2006;178(40–48):20060707. https://doi.org/10.1016/j.jneuroim.2006.05.019.
90. Shindler KS, Ventura E, Dutt M, et al. Inflammatory demyelination induces axonal injury and retinal ganglion cell apoptosis in experimental optic neuritis. Exp Eye Res. 2008;87(208–213):20080603. https://doi.org/10.1016/j.exer.2008.05.017.
91. Dutt M, Tabuena P, Ventura E, et al. Timing of corticosteroid therapy is critical to prevent retinal ganglion cell loss in experimental optic neuritis. Invest Ophthalmol Vis Sci. 2010;51(1439–1445):20091105. https://doi.org/10.1167/iovs.09-4009.
92. Cork LC. Neuropathology of Down syndrome and Alzheimer disease. Am J Med Genet Suppl. 1990;7:282–6.
93. Normando EM, Yap TE, Maddison J, et al. A CNN-aided method to predict glaucoma progression using DARC (Detection of Apoptosing Retinal Cells). Expert Rev Mol Diagn. 2020;20(737–748):20200503. https://doi.org/10.1080/14737159.2020.1758067.
94. Corazza P, Maddison J, Bonetti P, et al. Predicting wet age-related macular degeneration (AMD) using DARC (detecting apoptosing retinal cells) AI (artificial intelligence) technology. Expert Rev Mol Diagn. 2021;21(109–118):20201228. https://doi.org/10.1080/14737159.2020.1865806.
95. Grossniklaus HE, Green WR. Choroidal neovascularization. Am J Ophthalmol. 2004;137:496–503. https://doi.org/10.1016/j.ajo.2003.09.042.
96. Cordeiro MF, Hill D, Patel R, et al. Detecting retinal cell stress and apoptosis with DARC: progression from lab to clinic. Prog Retin Eye Res. 2022;86(100976):20210605. https://doi.org/10.1016/j.preteyeres.2021.100976.
97. Sacconi R, Corbelli E, Querques L, et al. A review of current and future management of geographic atrophy. Ophthalmol Ther. 2017;6(69–77):20170408. https://doi.org/10.1007/s40123-017-0086-6.
98. Boyer DS, Schmidt-Erfurth U, van Lookeren Campagne M, et al. The pathophysiology of geographic atrophy secondary to age-related macular degeneration and the complement pathway as a therapeutic target. Retina. 2017;37:819–35. https://doi.org/10.1097/IAE.0000000000001392.
99. Choi S MJ, Nicholas R, et al. Characterising DARC (Detecting Apoptosing Retinal Cells) spots in optic neuritis. J Neurol Neurosurg Psychiatry. 2022; 93

100. Yap TE, Normando EM, Cordeiro MF. Redefining clinical outcomes and endpoints in glaucoma. Exp Rev Ophthalmol. 2018;13:113–27. https://doi.org/10.1080/17469899.2018.1465820.
101. Kass MA, Heuer DK, Higginbotham EJ et al. The Ocular Hypertension Treatment Study: a randomized trial determines that topical ocular hypotensive medication delays or prevents the onset of primary open-angle glaucoma. Arch Ophthalmol 2002;120:701–13; discussion 829–730
102. Castro DP, Kawase J, Melo LA Jr. Learning effect of standard automated perimetry in healthy individuals. Arq Bras Oftalmol. 2008;71:523–8.
103. De Moraes CG, Hood DC, Thenappan A, et al. 24–2 visual fields miss central defects shown on 10–2 tests in glaucoma suspects, ocular hypertensives, and early glaucoma. Ophthalmology. 2017;124(1449–1456):20170524. https://doi.org/10.1016/j.ophtha.2017.04.021.
104. Heijl A, Buchholz P, Norrgren G, et al. Rates of visual field progression in clinical glaucoma care. Acta Ophthalmol. 2013;91:406–12. https://doi.org/10.1111/j.1755-3768.2012.02492.x.
105. Garway-Heath DF, Crabb DP, Bunce C, et al. Latanoprost for open-angle glaucoma (UKGTS): a randomised, multicentre, placebo-controlled trial. Lancet. 2015;385:1295–304. https://doi.org/10.1016/S0140-6736(14)62111-5.
106. Kuang TM, Zhang C, Zangwill LM, et al. Estimating lead time gained by optical coherence tomography in detecting glaucoma before development of visual field defects. Ophthalmology. 2015;122:2002–9. https://doi.org/10.1016/j.ophtha.2015.06.015.
107. Yu M, Lin C, Weinreb RN, et al. Risk of visual field progression in glaucoma patients with progressive retinal nerve fiber layer thinning: a 5-year prospective study. Ophthalmology. 2016;123:1201–10. https://doi.org/10.1016/j.ophtha.2016.02.017.
108. Chan VTT, Sun Z, Tang S, et al. Spectral-domain OCT measurements in Alzheimer's disease: a systematic review and meta-analysis. Ophthalmology. 2018. https://doi.org/10.1016/j.ophtha.2018.08.009.
109. Glass CK, Saijo K, Winner B, et al. Mechanisms underlying inflammation in neurodegeneration. Cell. 2010;140:918–34. https://doi.org/10.1016/j.cell.2010.02.016.
110. Gauthier SG. Alzheimer's disease: the benefits of early treatment. Eur J Neurol. 2005;12(Suppl3):11–6. https://doi.org/10.1111/j.1468-1331.2005.01322.x.
111. Heijl A, Leske MC, Bengtsson B, et al. Reduction of intraocular pressure and glaucoma progression: results from the Early Manifest Glaucoma Trial. Arch Ophthalmol. 2002;120:1268–79.
112. Galvao J, Davis B, Tilley M, et al. Unexpected low-dose toxicity of the universal solvent DMSO. FASEB J. 2014;28:1317–30. https://doi.org/10.1096/fj.13-235440.

Retinal Oximetry in Central Nervous System Diseases

8

Anna Bryndis Einarsdottir, Olof Birna Olafsdottir, and Sveinn Hakon Hardarson

Abstract

Metabolic imaging with retinal oximetry involves noninvasive spectrophotometric imaging of retinal blood vessels. Retinal oximetry imaging demonstrates metabolic abnormalities in central nervous system diseases, such as Alzheimer's disease, mild cognitive impairment and multiple sclerosis. Retinal oximetry correlates with cerebral oxygen saturation. Retinal oximetry offers insights into the pathophysiology of central nervous system diseases and is a potential biomarker for diagnosis of CNS diseases and evaluation of progression.

Keywords

Retinal oximetry • Biomarker • Retina • Oxygen • Metabolic imaging • Central nervous system • Alzheimer's disease • Mild cognitive impairment • Multiple sclerosis • Optic neuritis

A. B. Einarsdottir (✉)
Department of Neurology, Landspitali University Hospital, Reykjavik, Iceland
e mail: annabei@landspitali.is

O. B. Olafsdottir
Department of Ophthalmology, Landspitali University Hospital, Reykjavik, Iceland

S. H. Hardarson
Department of Physiology, University of Iceland, Reykjavik, Iceland

A. Grzybowski and P. Barboni (eds.), *OCT and Imaging in Central Nervous System Diseases*, https://doi.org/10.1007/978-3-031-72156-4_8

8.1 Introduction

Retinal imaging is gaining interest for diagnostics of central nervous system (CNS) diseases and to evaluate progression of CNS diseases. The retina is part of the central nervous system and is the only part of the CNS that can be visualized non-invasively with visible light. It is easy to image structural and metabolic changes in the retina, which reflect abnormalities in the CNS.

The notion of using the eye to learn about the brain dates back to ancient Rome and the proverb "the eyes are the mirror of the soul" exists in many languages. It is however only recently that modern imaging technologies have realized this potential. Optical coherence tomography images the structure of the retina and retinal oximetry documents the oxygen metabolism and both reflect changes in the wider central nervous system.

Optical coherence tomography of the retina has demonstrated changes in the retinal structure in central nervous system diseases. Thinning of the retinal nerve fiber layer and other structural anomalies in the retina has been found in Alzheimer's disease [1, 2], mild cognitive impairment [3, 4], multiple sclerosis (MS) [5, 6] and Parkinson's disease [7] and suggest that OCT imaging may help to diagnose and evaluate progression of central nervous system disease.

The fundus of the eye provides direct view of retinal blood vessels, which are part of central nervous system vasculature. Imaging them provides information on oxygen saturation in central nervous system vessels. Metabolic imaging with retinal oximetry involves noninvasive spectrophotometric imaging of retinal blood vessels. This fairly new clinical technology has led to discovery of new biomarkers in several eye diseases, such as diabetic retinopathy [8, 9], glaucoma [10–12], central retinal vein occlusion [13], age-related macular degeneration [14], retinitis pigmentosa [15, 16], and central nervous system diseases, such as Alzheimer's disease [17], mild cognitive impairment [18] and MS [19, 20].

8.2 Retinal Oximetry—The Technology

Retinal oximetry is an imaging technique that allows the visualization and measurement of oxygen saturation of hemoglobin in retinal arterioles and venules. The most common form of retinal oximetry uses conventional fundus cameras to image retinal vessels. The only inconvenience for the patient is pupil dilation and the light flash, which can be less intense than in conventional fundus photography [21, 22].

The technology has been described in detail [23]. Retinal oximetry typically involves specialized optics and camera(s) that are coupled to a fundus camera to capture images at two different wavelengths simultaneously. Analysis at two wavelengths measures the ratio of oxy- and deoxyhemoglobin light absorption in retinal vessels (optical density ratio, ODR). If one of the wavelengths is relatively insensitive to oxygen and the other is sensitive, there is a nearly linear relationship between hemoglobin oxygen saturation and the optical density ratio.

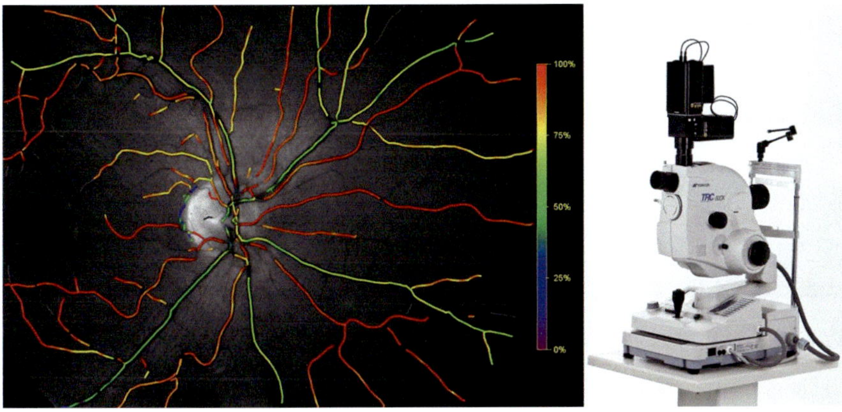

Fig. 8.1 Left: retinal oximetry image of a normal fundus. Color indicates oxygen saturation in retinal vessels (pseudocolor scale to the right of the image; red is fully saturated, blue and purple is low oxygen saturation). Right: dual wavelength non-invasive retinal oximeter Oxymap T1 (Oxymap ehf., Reykjavik, Iceland) coupled to a fundus camera (Topcon TRC-50DX) [25]

Analysis software displays the results as a pseudocolor fundus image as shown in Fig. 8.1. This approach to oximetry has been commercialized by two companies, Oxymap in Reykjavik, Iceland, and Imedos in Jena, Germany. Retinal oximetry is as easy and safe to perform as regular fundus photography and provides robust and reproducible data on retinal oxygen metabolism [24].

8.3 Retinal Oximetry is Affected in Alzheimer's Disease

Einarsdottir et al. were first to report oximetry abnormalities in retinas of individuals with moderate stage Alzheimer's disease compared with a healthy cohort [17]. Alzheimer's patients showed increased oxygen saturation in retinal arterioles and venules compared to healthy individuals (Fig. 8.2) [17]. While the oximetry findings in Alzheimer's disease are similar to diabetic retinopathy [8, 9] and neovascular age-related macular degeneration [14], the biological basis behind these findings has not been fully elucidated and need not be the same for all diseases.

Cerebrovascular dysfunction is evident early in Alzheimer's disease. One of the major pathologies of Alzheimer's disease is accumulation of amyloid beta on the vascular wall, or cerebral amyloid angiopathy [26]. This leads to thickening of vessel walls and to decreased diffusion of glucose and oxygen from the vessels, which could increase venular oxygen saturation. This could also explain the measured increase in arteriolar oxygen saturation, as arterioles lose oxygen by diffusion and this loss would decrease with thicker walls. Similar results have been demonstrated in diabetic retinopathy (increased arteriolar and venular oxygen saturation), and it has been suggested that thickening of the vessel wall could partly explain those results [27]. Another possible explanation for increased arteriolar

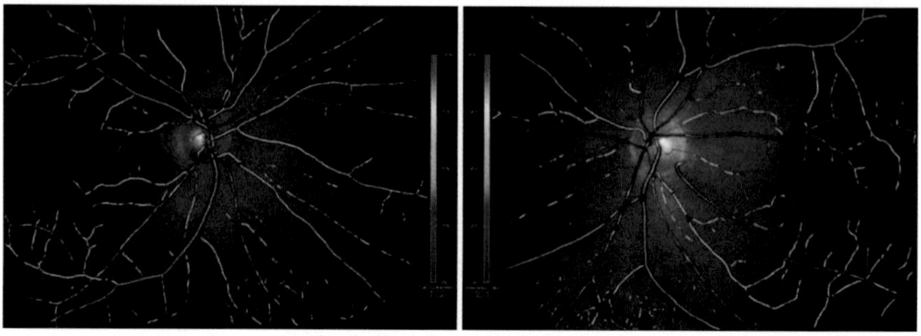

Fig. 8.2 Oximetry fundus images from healthy subject (left image) and patient with Alzheimer's disease (right image). Color indicates oxygen saturation in retinal vessels (pseudocolor scale to the right of the image; red is fully saturated, blue and purple is low oxygen saturation) [17]

oxygen saturation could be an effect from atrophy and a thinner retinal nerve fiber layer and a resultant decreased oxygen consumption and uptake by tissue adjacent to an arteriole. Decreased difference of oxygen concentration between the arterioles (arteries) and adjacent venules (veins) could also decrease counter current diffusion of oxygen between these arterioles and venules. This would result in increased arterial levels.

Retinal oximetry studies on Alzheimer's patients indicate that retinal oxygen metabolism is affected in patients with Alzheimer's disease and could therefore be a useful objective biomarker for Alzheimer's disease. Further and larger studies are needed to confirm these findings.

8.4 Retinal Oxygen Metabolism Changes in Mild Cognitive Impairment

The findings from retinal oximetry in Alzheimer's disease have been confirmed and extended to individuals with mild cognitive impairment. Olafsdottir et al. showed increased retinal arteriolar and venular oxygen saturation and decreased arteriovenous difference in individuals with mild cognitive impairment compared to healthy subjects (Fig. 8.3) [18]. These changes could reflect decreased oxygen extraction by retinal tissue in individuals with mild cognitive impairment, compared with healthy subjects. Fluorodeoxyglucose positron emission tomography studies have showed that metabolism could be decreased in the brain of individuals with mild cognitive impairment [28, 29]. The findings by Olafsdottir et al. could indicate less metabolic activity in the retinal tissue due to atrophy and thinner retinal nerve fiber layer and less metabolically active retina in mild cognitive impairment [18].

Retinal oxygen metabolism is affected in patients with Alzheimer's disease and mild cognitive impairment. The value of these biomarkers in clinical practice remains to be elucidated as well as what insights this provides into the pathophysiology of these disorders.

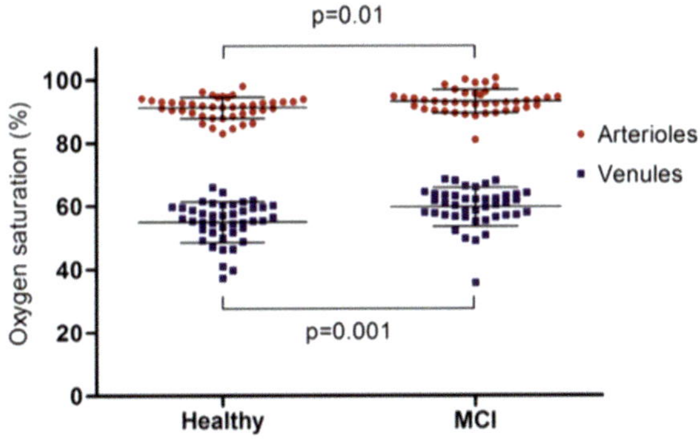

Fig. 8.3 Oxygen saturation in retinal arterioles and venules in patients with mild cognitive impairment (MCI) and healthy controls [18]

8.5 Retinal Oxygen Metabolism is Affected in Multiple Sclerosis and Optic Neuritis

Studies have shown that retinal oxygen metabolism is abnormal in individuals with MS [19, 20]. Lucero et al. reported oximetry abnormalities in retinas of individuals with MS compared to healthy subjects [20]. Einarsdottir et al. showed increased venular oxygen saturation and decreased arteriovenous difference in patients with MS compared to healthy individuals [19]. These results may indicate reduced oxygen uptake, which may be due to less oxygen demand following retinal atrophy.

Optic neuritis is a common presenting symptom of MS [30]. In 1989 Sebag et al. studied retinal oxygen saturation in individuals with optic neuritis with an early prototype retinal oximeter [31]. They compared eyes with optic neuritis with the healthy fellow eye and found optic neuritis eyes to have increased arteriovenous difference and reduced blood flow. The net result of these changes was decreased oxygen delivery. A recent study by Svrčinová et al. assessed acute optic neuritis in individuals with MS [32]. They found increased arteriovenous difference in eyes affected by optic neuritis in MS compared to patients' unaffected eye. This is in accordance with report by Sebag et al. [31]. A follow-up study six months after acute optic neuritis in patients with MS showed decreased arteriovenous difference and thinning of retinal nerve fiber layer in optic neuritis affected eye compared to healthy fellow eye [33]. Decreased arteriovenous difference may indicate reduced oxygen uptake or decreased oxygen consumption, which may be due to retinal atrophy in patients with MS. This could suggest that in acute optic neuritis there is increased oxygen consumption during acute inflammation, followed by tissue atrophy and reduced oxygen consumption [33].

It remains to be seen whether the retinal oximetry findings in Alzheimer's disease, mild cognitive impairment and multiple sclerosis are a consequence of tissue atrophy and reduced oxygen consumption and thereby a simple consequence of the disease processes; or whether they reflect metabolic changes earlier in the pathophysiological process.

8.6 Good Correlation Between Retinal and Transcranial Oximetry

Cerebral ischemia and hypoxia may exist in the absence of systemic hypoxia and there is a need for selective assessment of central nervous system oxygenation [34, 35]. Non-invasive techniques to measure cerebral vessel saturation exist, but they have some drawbacks. Transcranial near-infrared spectroscopy (NIRS) can be used to measure cerebral vessel saturation, but the oxygen saturation is affected by superficial peripheral circulation. Also, oxygen saturation measured by NIRS is a combination of arterial, capillary and venous blood.

The retina offers an opportunity to evaluate central nervous system vasculature and oxygen metabolism. Embryologically, the retina is an extension of the diencephalon and the retina and cerebral circulation share a common anatomical and physiological background. Retinal oximetry can measure arterial and venous oxygen saturation separately without being affected by superficial peripheral circulation. Van Keer et al. reported a positive correlation between transcranial oxygen blood vessel saturation and retinal arteriolar and venular saturation [36]. Retinal oximetry may be useful to estimate cerebral oxygen saturation in clinical settings such as intensive care and with major surgery and injuries.

8.7 Conclusion

Retinal oximetry and metabolic imaging of the retina show abnormalities in central nervous system diseases, such as Alzheimer's disease, mild cognitive impairment and multiple sclerosis.

The pathophysiological mechanism behind these changes is not fully elucidated. Comparable abnormalities are found in vascular physiology and oxygen metabolism in the brain and retina in Alzheimer's disease and to some degree in mild cognitive impairment and MS. The retinal oximetry findings may be a simple consequence of tissue atrophy and reduced oxygen consumption. Alternatively, they may be more directly linked with the pathophysiological process and reflect features such as vessel wall thickening and changes in energy metabolism.

There is a correlation between oxygen metabolism in the brain and retina. This may be useful to monitor brain oxygenation in intensive care, surgery and major injuries.

Retinal oximetry may offer insights into the pathophysiology of central nervous system diseases. It has the potential to provide biomarkers to help diagnose central nervous system diseases and evaluate their progression. More extensive studies are indicated to realize this potential.

References

1. Bambo MP, Garcia-Martin E, Pinilla J, Herrero R, Statue M, Otin S, et al. Detection of retinal nerve fiber layer degeneration in patients with Alzheimer's disease using optical coherence tomography: searching new biomarkers. Acta Ophthalmol. 2014;92(7):e581–2.
2. Marziani E, Pomati S, Ramolfo P, Cigada M, Giani A, Mariani C, et al. Evaluation of retinal nerve fiber layer and ganglion cell layer thickness in Alzheimer's disease using spectral-domain optical coherence tomography. Invest Ophthalmol Vis Sci. 2013;54(9):5953–8.
3. Lad EM, Mukherjee D, Stinnett SS, Cousins SW, Potter GG, Burke JR, et al. Evaluation of inner retinal layers as biomarkers in mild cognitive impairment to moderate Alzheimer's disease. PLoS ONE. 2018;13(2):e0192646.
4. Paquet C, Boissonnot M, Roger F, Dighiero P, Gil R, Hugon J. Abnormal retinal thickness in patients with mild cognitive impairment and Alzheimer's disease. Neurosci Lett. 2007;420(2):97–9.
5. Garcia-Martin E, Pablo LE, Herrero R, Ara JR, Martin J, Larrosa JM, et al. Neural networks to identify multiple sclerosis with optical coherence tomography. Acta Ophthalmol. 2013;91(8):e628–34.
6. Park KA, Kim J, Oh SY. Analysis of spectral domain optical coherence tomography measurements in optic neuritis: differences in neuromyelitis optica, multiple sclerosis, isolated optic neuritis and normal healthy controls. Acta Ophthalmol. 2014;92(1):e57-65.
7. Lee JY, Ahn J, Kim TW, Jeon BS. Optical coherence tomography in Parkinson's disease: is the retina a biomarker? J Parkinsons Dis. 2014;4(2):197–204.
8. Hammer M, Vilser W, Riemer T, Mandecka A, Schweitzer D, Kühn U, et al. Diabetic patients with retinopathy show increased retinal venous oxygen saturation. Graefes Arch Clin Exp Ophthalmol. 2009;247(8):1025–30.
9. Hardarson SH, Stefánsson E. Retinal oxygen saturation is altered in diabetic retinopathy. Br J Ophthalmol. 2012;96(4):560–3.
10. Olafsdottir OB, Hardarson SH, Gottfredsdottir MS, Harris A, Stefánsson E. Retinal oximetry in primary open-angle glaucoma. Invest Ophthalmol Vis Sci. 2011;52(9):6409–13.
11. Olafsdottir OB, Vandewalle E, Abegão Pinto L, Geirsdottir A, De Clerck E, Stalmans P, et al. Retinal oxygen metabolism in healthy subjects and glaucoma patients. Br J Ophthalmol. 2014;98(3):329–33.
12. Vandewalle E, Abegão Pinto L, Olafsdottir OB, De Clerck E, Stalmans P, Van Calster J, et al. Oximetry in glaucoma: correlation of metabolic change with structural and functional damage. Acta Ophthalmol. 2014;92(2):105–10.
13. Hardarson SH, Stefánsson E. Oxygen saturation in central retinal vein occlusion. Am J Ophthalmol. 2010;150(6):871–5.
14. Geirsdottir A, Hardarson SH, Olafsdottir OB, Stefánsson E. Retinal oxygen metabolism in exudative age-related macular degeneration. Acta Ophthalmol. 2014;92(1):27–33.
15. Eysteinsson T, Hardarson SH, Bragason D, Stefánsson E. Retinal vessel oxygen saturation and vessel diameter in retinitis pigmentosa. Acta Ophthalmol. 2014;92(5):449–53.
16. Türksever C, Valmaggia C, Orgül S, Schorderet DF, Flammer J, Todorova MG. Retinal vessel oxygen saturation and its correlation with structural changes in retinitis pigmentosa. Acta Ophthalmol. 2014;92(5):454–60.
17. Einarsdottir AB, Hardarson SH, Kristjansdottir JV, Bragason DT, Snaedal J, Stefánsson E. Retinal oximetry imaging in Alzheimer's disease. J Alzheimers Dis. 2016;49(1):79–83.
18. Olafsdottir OB, Saevarsdottir HS, Hardarson SH, Hannesdottir KH, Traustadottir VD Karlsson RA, et al. oxygen metabolism in patients with mild cognitive impairment. Alzheimers Dement (Amst). 2018;10:340–45.
19. Einarsdottir AB, Olafsdottir OB, Hjaltason H, Hardarson SH. Retinal oximetry is affected in multiple sclerosis. Acta Ophthalmol. 2018;96(5):528–30.

20. Lucero M, Conger A, Conger D, Sobhanian M, Stokes V, Frohman T, et al. Retinal oximetry-derived biomarkers of metabolic dysfunction in MS. Neurology. 2015;84(14 Supplement):P5.307.
21. Geirsdottir A, Palsson O, Hardarson SH, Olafsdottir OB, Kristjansdottir JV, Stefánsson E. Retinal vessel oxygen saturation in healthy individuals. Invest Ophthalmol Vis Sci. 2012;53(9):5433–42.
22. Hardarson SH, Harris A, Karlsson RA, Halldorsson GH, Kagemann L, Rechtman E, et al. Automatic retinal oximetry. Invest Ophthalmol Vis Sci. 2006;47(11):5011–6.
23. Beach J. Pathway to retinal oximetry. Transl Vis Sci Technol. 2014;3(5):2.
24. Palsson O, Geirsdottir A, Hardarson SH, Olafsdottir OB, Kristjansdottir JV, Stefánsson E. Retinal oximetry images must be standardized: a methodological analysis. Invest Ophthalmol Vis Sci. 2012;53(4):1729–33.
25. Stefánsson E, Olafsdottir OB, Einarsdottir AB, Eliasdottir TS, Eysteinsson T, Vehmeijer W, et al. Retinal oximetry discovers novel biomarkers in retinal and brain diseases. Invest Ophthalmol Vis Sci. 2017;58(6):BIO227–33.
26. Thal DR, Griffin WS, de Vos RA, Ghebremedhin E. Cerebral amyloid angiopathy and its relationship to Alzheimer's disease. Acta Neuropathol. 2008;115(6):599–609.
27. Hardarson SH, Olafsdottir OB, Karlsson RA, Beach JM, Eysteinsson T, Benediktsson JA, et al. Retinal vessel oxygen saturation in patients with diabetic retinopathy. Invest Ophthalmol Vis Sci. 2009;50:1328.
28. Mosconi L, Tsui WH, Herholz K, Pupi A, Drzezga A, Lucignani G, et al. Multicenter standardized 18F-FDG PET diagnosis of mild cognitive impairment, Alzheimer's disease, and other dementias. J Nucl Med. 2008;49(3):390–8.
29. Perani D, Della Rosa PA, Cerami C, Gallivanone F, Fallanca F, Vanoli EG, et al. Validation of an optimized SPM procedure for FDG-PET in dementia diagnosis in a clinical setting. Neuroimage Clin. 2014;6:445–54.
30. Sørensen TL, Frederiksen JL, Brønnum-Hansen H, Petersen HC. Optic neuritis as onset manifestation of multiple sclerosis: a nationwide, long-term survey. Neurology. 1999;53(3):473–8.
31. Sebag J, Delori FC, Feke GT, Weiter JJ. Effects of optic atrophy on retinal blood flow and oxygen saturation in humans. Arch Ophthalmol. 1989;107(2):222–6.
32. Svrčinová T, Mareš J, Chrapek O, Šínová I, Rybariková M, Otruba P, et al. Changes in oxygen saturation and the retinal nerve fibre layer in patients with optic neuritis—a pilot study. Acta Ophthalmol. 2018;96(3):e309–14.
33. Svrčinová T, Hok P, Šínová I, Dornák T, Král M, Hubnerová P, et al. Changes in oxygen saturation and the retinal nerve fiber layer in patients with optic neurits associated with multiple sclerosis in a 6-month follow-up. Acta Ophthalmol. 2020;98(8):841–7.
34. Hadolt I, Litscher G. Noninvasive assessment of cerebral oxygenation during high altititude trekking in the Nepal Himalayas. Neurol Res. 2003;25:183–8.
35. Yeh T Jr, Gouldman J, Auden SM, Seremet V, Edmonds HL Jr, Cerrito PB, et al. Mixed venous oxygen saturation does not adequately predict cerebral perfusion during pediatric cardiopulmonary bypass. J Thorac Cardiovasc Surg. 2001;122(1):192–3.
36. Van Keer K, Van Keer J, Barbosa Bred J, Nassiri V, De Deyne C, Genbrugge C, et al. Noninvasive assessment of cerebral oxygenation: a comparison of retinal and transcranial oximetry. PLoS ONE. 2018;13(1):e0190612.

Optical Coherence Tomography in Optic Disc Edema

9

Steffen Hamann and Fiona Costello

Abstract

Optical coherence tomography (OCT) continues to advance our understanding of the various diseases characterized by optic disc edema. In acute papilledema or nonarteritic anterior ischemic optic neuropathy, OCT has demonstrated subretinal fluid extending from the optic disc towards the subfoveal region, assisting in our understanding of the pathophysiology of vision loss in these cases. In evolving cases of optic disc edema, OCT of the peripapillary retinal nerve fiber layer (pRNFL) can thus be an objective measurement of nerve swelling. By analyzing the macular ganglion cell-inner plexiform layer complex (mGCIPL), OCT can now help detect early axonal damage in optic nerve disease, even when the RNFL is edematous, which may be helpful in predicting visual outcomes. Finally, OCT of the optic nerve head has proven to be a reliable tool in assisting clinicians in differentiating between cases of frank papilledema and pseudopapilledema, including that which occurs in optic disc drusen, vitreopapillary traction, Bergmeister papilla and myelinated nerve fiber layer.

S. Hamann (✉)
Department of Ophthalmology, Rigshospitalet, University of Copenhagen, Copenhagen, Denmark
e-mail: steffen.ellitsgaard.hamann@regionh.dk

F. Costello
Departments of Clinical Neurosciences and Surgery Cumming School of Medicine, University of Calgary, Calgary, Canada

A. Grzybowski and P. Barboni (eds.), *OCT and Imaging in Central Nervous System Diseases*, https://doi.org/10.1007/978-3-031-72156-4_9

Keywords

Papilledema • Pseudopapilledema • Increased intracranial pressure • Optic nerve sheath meningioma • Optic disc edema • Vitreopapillary traction • Bergmeister papilla • Myelinated nerve fiber layer • Nonarteritic anterior ischemic optic neuropathy (NAION) • Optic disc drusen • Peripapillary retinal nerve fiber layer (pRNFL) • Macular ganglion cell layer-inner plexiform layer (mGCIPL) • Leber hereditary optic neuropathy (LHON)

9.1 Introduction

Optic disc edema can be defined as axoplasmic flow stasis in the optic nerve fibers in the surface retinal nerve fiber layer and in the prelaminar region of the optic nerve head [1]. The appearance of optic disc edema occurs with a number of clinical conditions including raised intracranial pressure (papilledema), ischemia (anterior ischemic optic neuropathy), and inflammation (optic neuritis or papillitis). Optic disc edema has classically been identified with ophthalmoscopy or fundus photography; both techniques detect optic disc elevation, blurring of the optic disc margins, venous tortuosity, and, when present, peripapillary hemorrhages. Due to the common denominator of axoplasmic flow stasis, it is not possible to determine the etiology of optic disc edema from ophthalmoscopy alone. Furthermore, mere fundoscopic observation of an optic disc does not provide you with any quantitative information regarding the extent of optic nerve injury.

In recent years, optical coherence tomography (OCT) of the optic nerve head and peripapillary region has evolved as an increasingly important tool for detecting and elucidating different types of optic disc edema. Specifically, OCT may be used to establish the diagnosis of optic disc edema, to differentiate between true optic disc edema and pseudo-disc edema, to assist in identifying etiology, to quantify axonal damage exerted by the edema, and to monitor disease progression across a spectrum of optic neuropathies.

This chapter begins with an in-depth description of the various OCT measures of interest that are currently used to diagnose and manage optic disc edema. This overview will provide a conceptual framework for later sections that discuss the role of OCT in evaluating optic disc edema (versus pseudopapilledema) from raised intracranial pressure (ICP), ischemia, and inflammation. Our goal is to provide a basic and practical knowledge platform, which can be used in the daily application and interpretation of OCT in the context of suspected optic disc edema.

9.2 Measures of Interest and Their Specific Use

When faced with a suspected optic disc edema, it is first important to perform a thorough history and a careful neuroophthalmic examination to guide the diagnostic evaluation. Optical coherence tomography can provide structural measures of inner retinal integrity and vascular supply that correlate with visual outcomes. In this manner, OCT can quantify the impact of neuroaxonal injury on visual recovery. The use of the various OCT modalities in the workup of suspected optic disc edema is summarized in Table 9.1.

9.2.1 OCT of the Peripapillary Region

A classic ring scan can be performed on most commercial OCT machines to provide a measure of peripapillary retinal nerve fiber layer (pRNFL) thickness. Spectral domain OCT quantifies the global pRNFL thickness with a resolution of 3–5 μm in the range from 50–600 μm. As a marker of axonal structure, pRNFL thickness increases in optic disc edema and subsequently regresses with its resolution [2]. Depending on the extent and etiology of the initial insult, the pRNFL thickness might not only normalize, but thin with evolving optic atrophy. Decreasing pRNFL values can be a good sign (resolving optic disc edema) or a bad sign (evolving optic nerve atrophy), therefore additional information is needed.

It is important to note, with respect to optic disc edema, that the automatic segmentation algorithm may fail when the edema is moderate to severe (pRNFL thickness > 200 μm). In such cases it is important to check for accuracy on the line that defines the RNFL on the circular tomogram, and if needed, perform manual segmentation [3].

A more detailed assessment of the peripapillary region in form of a radial circle optic nerve head scan can be provided, with some OCT machines, Fig. 9.1. In this scan type the OCT beam is directed radially, which provides images that are displayed in a 'radar-like' circular plot. The radial circle optic nerve head scan takes a series of 6–24 radial scans centered on the optic nerve head. Three scan circles (3.5, 4.1, and 4.7 mm in diameter) can be used to measure the pRNFL thickness. In addition to this, this scan type provides you with a possibility of assessing the Bruch's membrane and the Bruch's membrane opening (BMO). Notably, the diameter of the latter provides a surrogate measure of the size of the scleral canal. Also, by aligning the color fundus image and the OCT volumes obtained with the radial scan, the optic disc margin can be accurately defined. The radial circle scan can be used for assessing Bruch's membrane morphology and angulation, but more information regarding these parameters and with relevance for suspected optic disc edema can be obtained from the transverse axial scan of the optic nerve head (see below). A radial circle optic nerve head scan can also be used to detect and to measure the volume of a peripapillary hyperreflective ovoid mass-like structures (PHOMS), if present, as an anatomical biomarker of axoplasmic flow stasis. The PHOMS are described in detail below.

Table 9.1 Multimodal optical coherence tomography of optic disc edema from various etiologies

Suspected etiology	Peripapillary OCT	Macular OCT	Optic nerve head OCT	OCT angiography
Raised ICP	RNFL thickness increased in true papilledema (100-300 μm: beware of pseudopapilledema, >300 μm: certain papilledema) RNFL thickness decreased in postpapilledema optic atrophy	mGCIPL thinning in chronic papilledema represents retinal ganglion cell and optic nerve injury Macular pathologies including subretinal fluid	Detection of ODD co-existing with papilledema or causing pseudo-edema PHOMS usually present Lamina cribrosa anteriorly displaced Peripapillary wrinkles and folds on en face OCT AI may differentiate between papillededema and pseudopapilledema	Clinical marker for early optic nerve damage
Ischemia	RNFL thickness increased in AION and decreased post-insult	mGCIPL thinning in post-insult represents retinal ganglion cell and optic nerve injury Macular pathologies including subretinal fluid, sometimes seen in NA-AION, and PAMM, seen in A-AION but not in NA-AION	Detection of ODD in young patients with NA-AION or older NA-AION patients without vascular risk factors	Can probably be used to differentiate NA-AION from optic neuritis with or without AI
Inflammation	RNFL often slightly increased in the acute stage of an apparent retrobulbar optic neuritis RNFL thickness more severely increased in MOGAD and NMOSD	mGCIPL thinning represents retinal ganglion cell and optic nerve injury and often precedes RNFL thickness increase Subretinal fluid in neuroretinitis Macular pathologies	Of limited value except for the detection of ODD in middle-aged individuals where ODD-AION may be a differential diagnosis	May be helpful in the differentiation between neuroinflammatory disorders

OCT = optical coherence tomography; ICP = intracranial pressure; RNFL = retinal nerve fiber layer, mGCIPL = macular ganglion cell-inner plexiform layer; ODD = optic disc drusen; PHOMS = peripapillary hyperreflective ovoid mass-like structure; AION = anterior ischemic optic neuropathy, NA-AION = nonarteritic AION; PAMM = paracentral acute middle maculopathy; A-AION = arteritic AION; AI = artificial intelligence; MOGAD = myelin oligodendrocyte glycoprotein antibody disease; NMOSD = neuromyelitis optica spectrum disorder; ODD-AION = AION caused by ODD

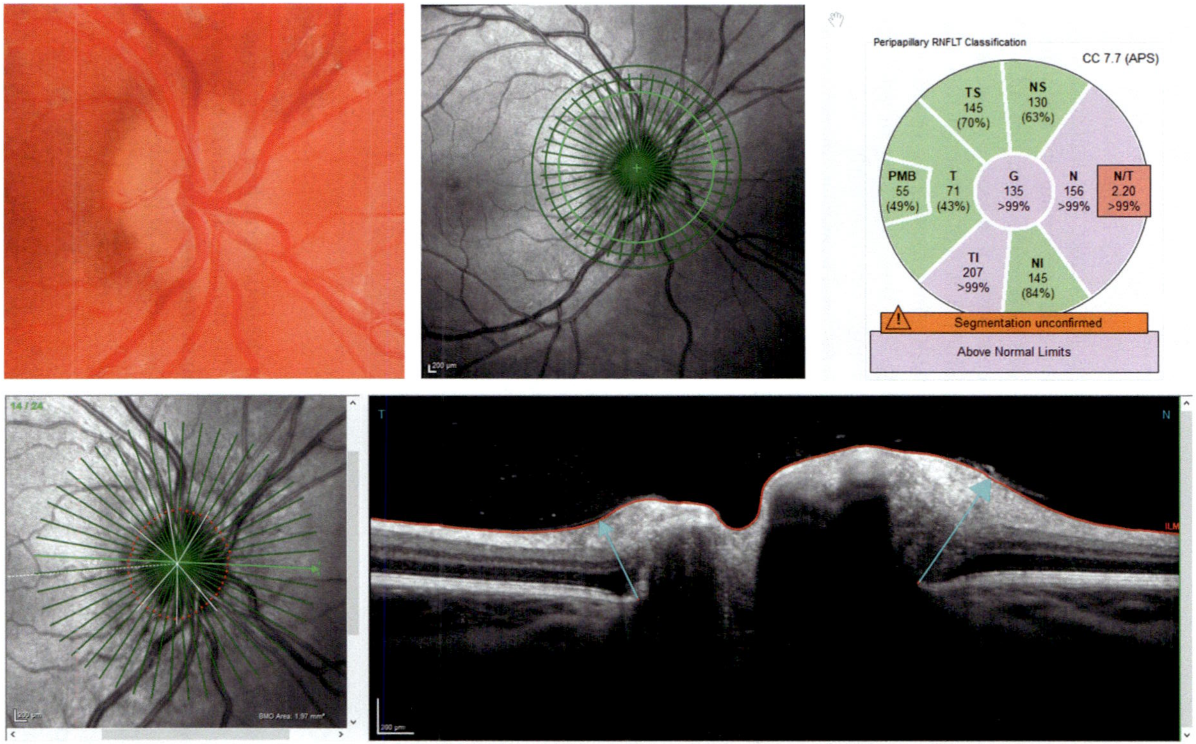

Fig. 9.1 Fundus photo and corresponding radial circle optic nerve head optical coherence tomography scan of the right eye from a 19-year-old woman with idiopathic intracranial hypertension and Frisén grade 1 papilledema. In addition to the peripapillary retinal nerve fiber layer thickness (upper panel, right), this scan type provides the Bruch's membrane opening diameter, which can be measured as a line connecting the two small red dots marking the end of Bruch's membrane on each side of the optic disc (lower panel, right). The blue arrows are measuring the total retinal height perpendicular to the inner limiting membrane automatically

9.2.2 OCT of the Macula

Performing a macular OCT volume scan with a scan area of approximately 30 × 25 degree centered over the macula, is standard and should be systematically obtained in the OCT evaluation of any patient with a suspected optic neuropathy. It provides the thickness of the macular ganglion cell–inner plexiform layer (mGCIPL) which is a surrogate measure of the retinal ganglion cell integrity in the visual afferent pathway. Therefore, mGCIPL values may be used to detect neuronal loss in the atrophic stages of any optic neuropathy, including a demyelinating optic neuritis or compressive optic nerve lesion [4]. It is important to note however, that mGCIPL loss in optic disc edema only refers to a subacute onset of at least 3–4 weeks or previous, ipsilateral episodes of optic neuropathy [5]. Used in conjunction with pRNFL, mGCIPL values are important for longitudinal monitoring of treatment response in cases of papilledema. Specifically, new onset thinning of mGCIPL values, in the setting of elevated pRNFL measures, provides early evidence of neuroaxonal injury. This observation may herald the need to escalate therapy, either by augmenting medical management or performing a CSF diversion procedure. One challenge, however, is that like pRNFL thickness, mGCIPL measures are impacted by floor effects. Hence, it can be difficult to detect new mGCIPL or pRNFL thinning in cases of significant pre-existing optic nerve injury.

From a practical perspective it is important to exclude co-existing macular pathology such as epiretinal membranes, edema, pigment epithelial detachments, and choroidal neovascular membrane(s). The observation of macular fluid is relevant to the evaluation of optic disc edema, because it may help explain central vision loss and provide clues to the underlying basis of optic disc swelling. OCT of the macula can also be used to detect microcystic macular edema, also known as retrograde maculopathy, the pathogenesis of which, however, is debated [6]. This finding seems to be a marker of severe optic nerve atrophy irrespective of underlying cause [7].

9.2.3 OCT of the Optic Nerve Head

A dense, cross-sectional transverse axial scan of the optic nerve head may be used to diagnose optic disc drusen (ODD), and in this manner, differentiate cases of true optic disc edema from mimics. The main indication for performing the test is to determine whether the optic disc elevation could be due to pseudo-disc edema versus true disc edema, Fig. 9.2.

9.2.3.1 Optic Disc Drusen

Spectral domain OCT of the optic nerve head, with enhanced depth imaging (EDI), is the gold standard for detection of ODD, and provides more accurate information than B-scan ultrasonography, fundus photography, and fundus autofluorescence [8]. The reason for enabling EDI is the added possibility of visualizing structures 500–800 μm deeper than with conventional OCT [9]. On a dense, transverse axial

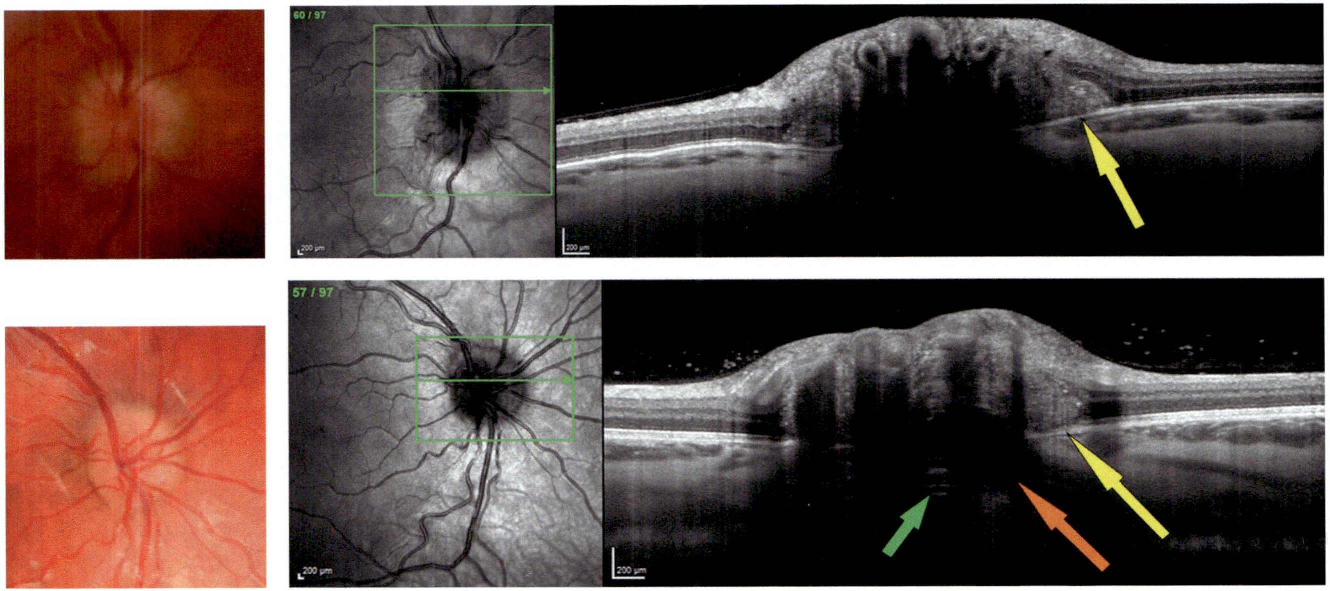

Fig. 9.2 Upper panel: Fundus photo and corresponding enhanced depth imaging optical coherence tomography scan of the optic nerve head from the right eye of a 44-year-old woman with idiopathic intracranial hypertension and Frisén grade 2 papilledema. The yellow arrow points at a peripapillary hyperreflective ovoid mass-like structure (PHOMS). Lower panel: Fundus photo and corresponding enhanced depth imaging optical coherence tomography scan of the optic nerve head from the right eye of a 12-year-old girl with buried optic disc drusen (orange arrow) and a peripapillary hyperreflective ovoid mass-like structure (yellow arrow) causing the appearance of pseudopapilledema on the fundus photo. The green arrows point at prelaminar hyperreflective lines

EDI-OCT scan of the optic nerve head, ODD appear as hyporeflective, rounded structures, oftentimes with hyperreflective margins, most pronounced anteriorly [10], Fig. 9.2. Both size and location of ODD can be assessed with OCT. For example, ODD can be readily classified as large (> 200 μm) or small (< 200 μm) on a single OCT image. Sometimes ODD are too small to separate and cluster in conglomerates [10]. Using manual segmentation tools, it is possible to estimate the three-dimensional ODD volume in a given optic nerve head and to correlate lesional volume with visual function [11]. Importantly, ODD volume correlates with visual field damage, such that larger ODD cause worse visual field defects [11]. The BMO, Fig. 9.2, is used as an anatomical landmark to differentiate between superficial ODD, located above the BMO, and deep ODD, located below. Interestingly, in patients with anterior ischemic optic neuropathy caused by ODD, termed ODD-AION, our group has shown that location matters more than size: specifically, the position of the ODD deep within the nerve head had a greater impact than size of ODD with respect to risk for ODD-AION [12]. In other words, larger ODD contribute to slowly progressing ODD-related visual field defects, whereas deeply located ODD, regardless of size, contribute to sudden visual field defects associated with ischemic optic neuropathy.

9.2.3.2 Other Causes of Pseudopapilledema

Although ODD, especially when deep, are generally considered the main cause of pseudopapilledema, it is well known from a clinical standpoint, that anomalous optic discs often have indistinct optic disc borders. PHOMS may contribute to this observation, as described in detail below. Vitreopapillary traction, due to tractional forces from vitreous adhesion, can cause optic disc elevation, that, when bilateral, can be confused with optic disc edema [13].

9.2.3.3 Peripapillary Hyperreflective Ovoid Mass-Like Structure (PHOMS)

A PHOMS is a newly described marker of nonspecific axoplasmic stasis seen on OCT scans of the optic nerve head, Fig. 9.2. A PHOMS consists of distended axons bulging or herniating laterally, resulting in an upward displacement of the peripapillary retina. A PHOMS can be found in association with multiple disorders affecting the optic nerve head, its etiology being categorized as follows: ODD-associated (type 1), anomalous-disc associated (type 2), and optic disc-edema associated (type 3). Types 1 and 2 are signs of pseudo-papilledema, while type 3—if raised intracranial pressure—is a sign of true papilledema. A PHOMS is the OCT equivalent of the peripapillary axonal distension (PAD) seen on histological specimens [14], and both structures constitute the anatomical substrate for the blurred optic disc margin seen on fundoscopy.

What is now known as PHOMS was first described in a study by Lee et al. in 2011, where the 'hyperreflective, subretinal masses' were thought to represent a specific type of ODD [15]. Later, in 2014 Pichi et al. described 'dome-like hyperreflective structures' peripapillary in children with tilted disc syndrome [16]. In 2018, the Optic Disc Drusen Studies Consortium introduced the term PHOMS and established that this structure is an entity separate from but sometimes seen together with the hyporeflective ODD [10]. With the current knowledge of the origin of a PHOMS, its detection on OCT should prompt the clinician to look for additional signs of raised ICP (see below), ODD, and optic disc anomalies. It should be noted, however, that PHOMS may also occasionally be seen in normal individuals [17].

A PHOMS encircles the optic nerve head in up to 360 degrees, like a torus, or donut [18]. Knowing this, it is possible to calculate the PHOMS volume using the formula for volume of a torus applied on data obtained from the radial circle scan [19]. In patients with ODD the volume of PHOMS decreases with age, the significance of this finding is yet unknown [19].

9.2.3.4 Prelaminar Hyperreflective Lines

In cases with or following axoplasmic flow stasis, such as ODD [10] or idiopathic intracranial hypertension (IIH) [20], prelaminar hyperreflective lines are often seen on OCT scans of the optic nerve head, Fig. 9.2. They are thought to represent ODD precursors, in cases of congenital axonal crowding in the optic nerve head such as in ODD, where longitudinal studies have shown that they can evolve into ODD [21]. In IIH, and likely other syndromes of raised ICP, they are seen to persist after the papilledema has subsided [20]. In these latter cases, they are probably just a crowding phenomenon unrelated to ODD and probably without any pathological relevance.

9.2.3.5 Optic Nerve Head Volume

The optic nerve head volume can be obtained by scanning the manually centered optic nerve head and the surrounding retinal tissues using proprietary software with a high number of axial scans in a 15° × 15° or 20° × 20° cube [22]. In one study of 21 IIH patients the Frisén scale for papilledema grading using funduscopy correlated higher with the OCT-based optic nerve head volume measurement than with the pRNFL thickness [22]. In a large, longitudinal British cohort of women with IIH, OCT-based optic nerve head volume measures, particularly central thickness, reproducibly correlated with ICP [23]. Results from the IIH Treatment Trial (IIHTT) suggested that OCT-based optic nerve head volume measurements could play a role in the monitoring of the longitudinal response to therapy in IIH patients [24].

9.2.3.6 Lamina Cribrosa Position

The lamina cribrosa is a continuation of the inner layer of the posterior sclera. It is a trabecular structure of several layers and pores of different sizes through which the optic nerve fibers pass. The lamina cribrosa separates the ocular cavity with its intraocular pressure (IOP) from the retrolaminar subarachnoid space with its ICP surrounding the optic nerves. The lamina cribrosa is usually visible as a clear hyperreflective, deep band, when performing a transverse, axial optic nerve head scan (Fig. 9.3), deeper and thicker than the prelaminar hyperreflective lines seen in cases of optic nerve head crowding such as ODD (Fig. 9.2). Posterior positioning of the lamina cribrosa is believed to play a role in the pathogenesis of glaucomatous axonal damage, where the so-called translamina cribrosa pressure difference (TLCPD) is increased due to IOP being higher than ICP [25]. An anterior displacement has been observed in a few, small studies of patients with IIH [26, 27] but none have as yet performed a structure–function correlation comparing LC biomechanics with visual function parameters such as visual field.

9.2.3.7 Additional Signs of Optic Disc Edema

Analysis of the *en face* spectral domain OCT provides an opportunity to study in detail the peripapillary wrinkles, folds and creases, well known from funduscopy of patients with raised intracranial pressure. These features (described more in detail in Sect. 9.3) can strengthen suspicion for raised ICP, in the right clinical context. Finally, the transverse axial optic nerve head scan can be used to identify peripapillary fluid leakage, which is unusual in cases of pseudopapilledema such as ODD.

9.2.4 OCT Angiography of the Optic Nerve Head and Macula

OCT angiography is a method for visualizing the retinal vasculature and choroidal vascular layers and provides functional information in a depth-resolved manner on blood flow in these vessels. The technique is based on the concept that the only moving structure in the fundus of the static eye is blood flowing through the vessels. Contrast is generated based on the difference between moving cells in the vasculature and the static surrounding tissue enabling indirect evaluation of retinal blood flow [28]. OCT angiography can provide an alternative quantitative measure of optic nerve head and retinal damage, as atrophied tissue requires less blood supply [29]. It is a suitable method for the diagnosis of neuro-ophthalmic disease in pregnancy, as it does not require intravenous dye injection or pupillary dilation.

OCT angiography of the optic nerve head may be employed in the differentiation between papilledema and pseudopapilledema [30], predict visual outcomes in IIH patients [31] and serve as a clinical marker for detecting early optic nerve damage caused by papilledema [32]. The technique is challenged by the fact that the optic disc edema may induce artefacts that prevent visualization of and darkens the underlying peripapillary network. A careful segmentation of the RNFL may reduce this darkening [33]. OCT angiography of the macula has revealed lower densities of the retinal microvasculature in inflammatory optic neuropathies, when comparing to healthy controls. Qualitative characteristics of retinal microvasculature rendered with OCTA may prove helpful in differentiation between neuroinflammatory disorders [34] and between ischemic optic neuropathies (see below).

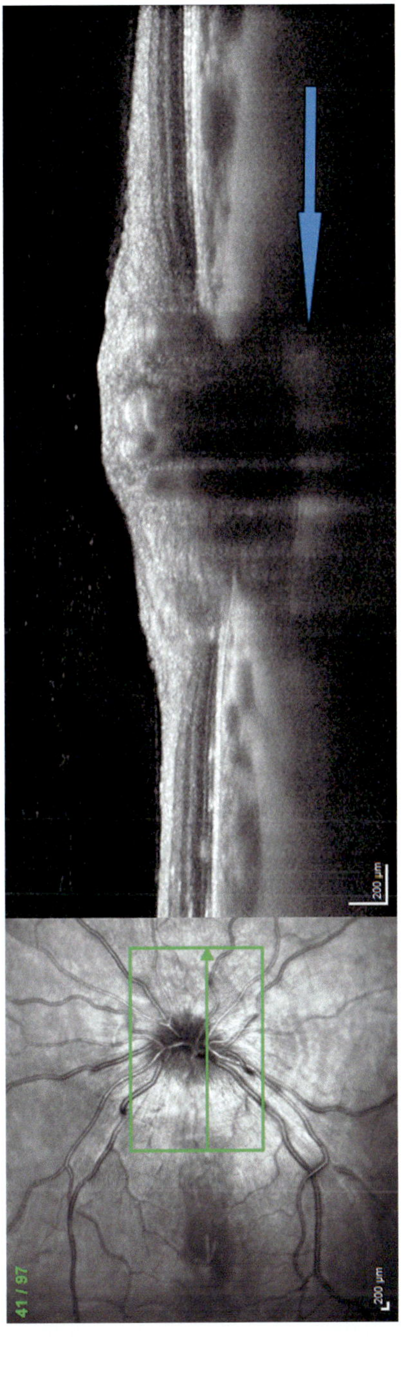

Fig. 9.3 Enhanced depth imaging optical coherence tomography scan of the right eye from a 23-year-old woman, three months after starting medical treatment for an initial massive papilledema as manifestation of idiopathic intracranial hypertension. Initially the disc edema was so massive, that it was impossible to visualize lamina cribrosa, which is now clearly seen as a deep hyperreflective, thick layer in the optic nerve head (blue arrow)

9.3 OCT in Optic Disc Edema from Raised ICP

In cases of papilledema, the main OCT measures used to diagnose and follow the status of the optic nerve head are pRNFL and mGCIPL thicknesses. Importantly, in an era when many clinicians struggle to perform reliable funduscopy [35], OCT can reveal elevations in pRNFL thickness as proof of papilledema, and a structural marker of raised ICP. Gradual regression of pRNFL thickness may indicate resolving papilledema, except in the setting of coincident mGCIPL thinning; the OCT "composite" of dwindling pRNFL and mGCIPL values instead indicates evolving optic disc atrophy. This insight gained from OCT is helpful in the evaluation of papilledema because early signs of neuroaxonal injury cannot be reliably inferred from fundus examination alone. In the long-term management of patients with papilledema, OCT measured pRNFL and mGCIPL thicknesses can be correlated with measures of visual function to gauge the success of ongoing treatment or indicate when to escalate management. Studies have shown that OCT reliably detects manifestations of outer retinal injury that may contribute to vision loss in cases of papilledema including peripapillary wrinkles, subretinal fluid, hyperopic shift, and chorioretinal folds [36, 37]. Knowledge thereof is important in the management of IIH because these outer retinal changes represent mechanisms of vision loss that typically respond well to medical management and do not warrant CSF diversion treatments [36]. One conundrum in the approach to management of patients with papilledema, is that floor effects of the OCT make it difficult to detect progressive neuroaxonal injury with pRNFL and mGCIPL thinning in patients with pre-existing optic atrophy. In this setting, deflections of the retinal pigment epithelium and Bruch's membrane (RPE/BM) towards, and then away from, the vitreous can provide evidence for elevation and regression in ICP, respectively [38]. Peripapillary RPE/BM shape changes can be detected following both acute and chronic IIH treatment, as quickly as 1 h after lumbar puncture intervention [38]. In the OCT sub-study of the Idiopathic Intracranial Hypertension Treatment Trial (IIHTT), RPE/BM shape normalized in patients randomized to receive acetazolamide plus weight management, but did not change in patients treated with placebo plus weight management alone, despite improvements in papilledema in this group [39]. This observation suggests that RPE/BM shape and optic nerve head edema may be independent phenomena.

9.4 OCT in Optic Disc Edema from Ischemia

Anterior ischemic optic neuropathy (AION) manifests with usually unilateral, but occasionally bilateral, sudden visual loss, and funduscopy reveals optic disc edema with or without additional signs of ischemia such as peripapillar hemorrhages and cotton wool spots. AION can be arteritic, A-AION, usually due to giant cell arteritis, but the majority of cases are nonarteritic, NA-AION. Although distinction between the two can be straightforward in case of classical examples—80 year-old with sudden, severe visual loss, jaw claudication, scalp tenderness, elevated sedimentation rate coupled with a uniform, pale optic disc edema in the former, and sudden, moderate painless lower visual field loss in an otherwise asymptomatic 60 year-old, coupled with corresponding segmental optic disc edema and a contralateral disc-at-risk in the latter, clinical scenarios may sometimes be challenging. In these cases, addition of OCT may add value to the diagnostic decision making. In one study of 15 eyes from 15 A-AION patients and 15 eyes from 15 NA-AION patients, quantitative OCT angiography analysis revealed significant differences in vessel density and vessel tortuosity with worse alterations in A-AION than in NA-AION, probably because the more severe optic disc edema occurring in the former [40]. Another retrospective study of 45 patients with AION revealed signs of paracentral acute middle maculopathy (PAMM) on macular OCTs in 4 patients with A-AION but in none of the patients with NA-AION [41]. Recently it was shown, that peripapillary intraretinal and subretinal fluid extending into the macula is a frequent finding in NA-AION but not in A-AION (https://pubmed.ncbi.nlm.nih.gov/39645178/).

In patients aged 40 to 60, it can be more important to distinguish NA-AION from optic neuritis or from AION caused by ODD, so-called ODD-AION. In a retrospective study of 8 patients with NA-AION, 6 patients with papillitis, and 13 patients with papilledema, the morphological analysis of the OCT angiography performed in the acute phase showed promising results separating the three conditions [42]. In a recent study of 45 eyes of 45 NA-AION patients, 32 eyes of 32 optic neuritis patients, and 76 eyes of 76 healthy individuals, machine learning applied to optic nerve head OCT angiography samples provided excellent algorithms to distinguish AION from optic neuritis [43]. A large multicenter study of 127 eyes with NA-AION from 65 patients below the age of 50, who had all been systematically OCT scanned, revealed that more than 50% had underlying ODD [44]. Subsequently Johannesen et al. found, in a study of 34 ODD-AION and 34 patients with NA-AION and no ODD (termed nODD-AION), that ODD-AION patients were significantly younger, had fewer vascular risk factors, significantly more PHOMS and prelaminar hyperreflective lines as well as smaller Bruch's membrane opening diameters, compared to patients with nODD-AION [12]. Based on the results from these studies, it is suggested that a dense EDI-OCT of the optic nerve head is performed in patients with NA-AION under the age of 50 or in older NA-AION patients without apparent vascular risk factors.

9.5 OCT in Optic Disc Edema from Inflammation

Early OCT studies in optic neuritis patients focused on pRNFL thickness as a structural marker of axonal integrity in the retina [45]. Current OCT segmentation techniques allow detailed quantification of different retinal constituents that may reflect evidence of inflammation, axonal degeneration, and neuronal loss in inflammatory optic neuropathies associated with multiple sclerosis (MS) [45] and other central nervous system inflammatory syndromes. In acute optic neuritis, pRNFL values are usually elevated, more so in myelin oligodendrocyte glycoprotein antibody associated disease (MOGAD) optic neuritis than other optic neuritis subtypes because MOGAD optic neuritis tends to be associated with prominent optic disc edema [2, 46, 47]. Within 2 to 3 weeks of symptom onset, early mGCIPL thinning serves as the first sign of neuroaxonal injury for patients with optic neuritis; early and extensive mGCIPL loss may be more evident in neuromyelitis optica spectrum disorder (NMOSD) optic neuritis, because this CNS inflammatory condition is associated with more severe optic nerve injury than, for example, MS optic neuritis [48]. Over a period of several months, pRNFL values regress, and thinning ensues as a marker of optic atrophy after an inflammatory optic nerve injury. The extent of pRNFL and mGCIPL loss observed after optic neuritis parallels the severity of the optic nerve insult and in turn correlates with the extent of functional impairment [2]. Specifically, lower pRNFL and mGCIPL values were associated with worse deficits in visual acuity, visual field, and color vision [2]. Optical coherence tomography measures of inner nuclear layer thickening and microcystic macular edema are believed to reflect more severe optic nerve injury in the setting of inflammation [2], but microcystic macular edema is not a finding unique to inflammatory optic nerve injuries [7].

9.6 Differentiating Optic Disc Edema from Pseudoedema Using OCT

Performing an OCT to rule out pseudo-edema is indicated, when fundoscopy does not reveal a clear-cut disc edema and/or, when the suspected disc edema is discovered incidentally with no symptoms of raised ICP (in papilledema) and no loss of visual function (in ischemic or inflammatory optic neuropathies). In these situations one should perform a dense optic nerve head transverse axial scan with enough slices (at least 97) to rule out ODD [10] and look specifically for auxiliary signs of raised ICP such as peripapillary folds and wrinkles [3], as also described above. Table 9.1 summarizes the OCT features that may be considered when trying to differentiate optic disc edema from various etiologies and to differentiate true disc edema from pseudo-edema.

The use of artificial intelligence and machine learning algorithms is rapidly advancing in the studies of optic neuropathies including those that present with disc edema. Using geometric deep learning it is now possible to assess the robustness of a given optic nerve head from a single OCT volume scan of the optic nerve head, as evidenced from a study of 316 subjects that were OCT scanned before and after acute experimental IOP elevation [49]. In a recent cross-sectional comparative study of 256 imaged optic nerve heads including 105 with ODD, 51 with papilledema, and 100 healthy nerves, a machine learning segmentation algorithm was capable of classifying ODD whenever present with high AUCs for both detection of ODD, detection of papilledema, and detection of healthy optic nerve heads [50]. It is conceivable that future algorithm development will enable a complete automatization of the distinction between papilledema and pseudopapilledema using artificial intelligence. In a recent proof-of-concept study using prediagnostic OCT of 93 patients who subsequently developed papilledema, a trained model was able to predict progression to papilledema with a precision surpassing what would be expected from clinicians [51].

9.7 Conclusions

Optical coherence tomography is an easy-to-use, non-invasive, and widely accessible tool that can be operated for identifying and elucidating an optic disc edema. With the constantly increasing variety in available OCT scanning modalities, it can be demanding in a busy clinic to navigate and choose the relevant and correct imaging techniques and settings. However, with diligent preparation guided by careful neuroophthalmic evaluation, OCT can be of tremendous aid and added value in the diagnosis and subsequent monitoring of optic disc edema arising from any optic neuropathy. To this end, artificial intelligence and deep learning algorithms will soon be valuable partners in the road towards earlier and more accurate diagnoses of disorders affecting the afferent visual pathway.

References

1. Hayreh SS. Pathogenesis of optic disc edema in raised intracranial pressure. Prog Retin Eye Res. 2016;50:108–44.
2. Costello F, Chen JJ. The role of optical coherence tomography in the diagnosis of afferent visual pathway problems: a neuroophthalmic perspective. Handb Clin Neurol. 2021;178:97–113.
3. Sibony PA, Kupersmith MJ, Kardon RH. Optical coherence tomography neuro-toolbox for the diagnosis and management of papilledema, optic disc edema, and pseudopapilledema. J Neuroophthalmol. 2021;41(1):77–92.
4. Petzold A, et al. Diagnosis and classification of optic neuritis. Lancet Neurol. 2022;21(12):1120–34.
5. Bouthour W, Biousse V, Newman NJ. Diagnosis of optic disc oedema: fundus features, ocular imaging findings, and artificial intelligence. Neuroophthalmology. 2023;47(4):177–92.
6. Chapelle AC, Rakic JM, Plant GT. Nonarteritic anterior ischemic optic neuropathy: cystic change in the inner nuclear layer caused by edema and retrograde maculopathy. Ophthalmol Sci. 2023;3(1): 100230.
7. Kessel L, et al. Microcystic macular oedema in optic neuropathy: case series and literature review. Clin Exp Ophthalmol. 2018;46(9):1075–86.
8. Youn S, et al. A comparison of diagnostic accuracy of imaging modalities to detect optic disc drusen: the age of enhanced depth imaging optical coherence tomography. Am J Ophthalmol. 2023;248:137–44.
9. Spaide RF, Koizumi H, Pozzoni MC. Enhanced depth imaging spectral-domain optical coherence tomography. Am J Ophthalmol. 2008;146(4):496–500.
10. Malmqvist L, et al. The optic disc drusen studies consortium recommendations for diagnosis of optic disc drusen using optical coherence tomography. J Neuroophthalmol. 2018;38(3):299–307.

11. Malmqvist L, et al. Quantitatively measured anatomic location and volume of optic disc drusen: an enhanced depth imaging optical coherence tomography study. Invest Ophthalmol Vis Sci. 2017;58(5):2491–7.
12. Johannesen RG, et al. Optic nerve head anatomy and vascular risk factors in patients with optic disc drusen associated anterior ischemic optic neuropathy. Am J Ophthalmol. 2022;242:156–64.
13. Hedges TR, 3rd, Flattem NL, Bagga A. Vitreopapillary traction confirmed by optical coherence tomography. Arch Ophthalmol. 2006;124(2):279–81.
14. Skougaard M, et al. Prevalence and histopathological signatures of optic disc drusen based on microscopy of 1713 enucleated eyes. Acta Ophthalmol. 2020;98(2):195–200.
15. Lee KM, Woo SJ, Hwang JM. Differentiation of optic nerve head drusen and optic disc edema with spectral-domain optical coherence tomography. Ophthalmology. 2011;118(5):971–7.
16. Pichi F, et al. Spectral-domain optical coherence tomography findings in pediatric tilted disc syndrome. Graefes Arch Clin Exp Ophthalmol. 2014;252(10):1661–7.
17. Behrens CM, et al. Peripapillary hyperreflective ovoid mass-like structures (PHOMS) in children: the copenhagen child cohort 2000 eye study. Am J Ophthalmol. 2023;245:212–21.
18. Fraser JA, Hamann S. A 360-degree peripapillary hyper-reflective ovoid mass-like structure (PHOMS). Can J Ophthalmol. 2021;56(2):146.
19. Jorgensen M, et al. Volumetric measurement of peripapillary hyperreflective ovoid masslike structures in patients with optic disc drusen. Ophthalmol Sci. 2022;2(1): 100096.
20. Wibroe EA, Malmqvist L, Hamann S. OCT based interpretation of the optic nerve head anatomy and prevalence of optic disc drusen in patients with idiopathic intracranial hypertension (IIH). Life (Basel). 2021;11(6).
21. Malmqvist L, et al. Progression over 5 years of prelaminar hyperreflective lines to optic disc drusen in the copenhagen child cohort 2000 eye study. J Neuroophthalmol. 2020;40(3):315–21.
22. Dreesbach M, et al. Optic nerve head volumetry by optical coherence tomography in papilledema related to idiopathic intracranial hypertension. Transl Vis Sci Technol. 2020;9(3):24.
23. Vijay V, et al. Using optical coherence tomography as a surrogate of measurements of intracranial pressure in idiopathic intracranial hypertension. JAMA Ophthalmol. 2020;138(12):1264–71.
24. Optical Coherence Tomography Substudy C, Group NIIHS (2015) Papilledema outcomes from the optical coherence tomography substudy of the idiopathic intracranial hypertension treatment trial. Ophthalmology. 2015;122(9):1939–45 e2.
25. Abe RY, et al. Lamina cribrosa in glaucoma: diagnosis and monitoring. Curr Ophthalmol Rep. 2015;3(2):74–84.
26. Villarruel JM, et al. Anterior lamina cribrosa surface position in idiopathic intracranial hypertension and glaucoma. Eur J Ophthalmol. 2017;27(1):55–61.
27. Tatar IT, et al. Morphological assessment of lamina cribrosa in idiopathic intracranial hypertension. Indian J Ophthalmol. 2020;68(1):164–7.
28. Yan Y, Liao YJ. Updates on ophthalmic imaging features of optic disc drusen, papilledema, and optic disc edema. Curr Opin Neurol. 2021;34(1):108–15.
29. Murphy OC, et al. Alterations in the retinal vasculature occur in multiple sclerosis and exhibit novel correlations with disability and visual function measures. Mult Scler. 2020;26(7):815–28.
30. Fard MA, et al. Optical coherence tomography angiography in papilledema compared with pseudopapilledema. Invest Ophthalmol Vis Sci. 2019;60(1):168–75.
31. Pahuja A et al. Evaluation of peripapillary and macular optical coherence tomography angiography characteristics in different stages of papilledema. J Neuroophthalmol. 2023.
32. Rodriguez Torres Y, et al. Correlation between optic disc peripapillary capillary network and papilledema grading in patients with idiopathic intracranial hypertension: a study of optical coherence tomography angiography. J Neuroophthalmol. 2021;41(1):48–53.

33. Rougier MB, et al. OCT angiography analysis in acute non-arteritic anterior ischemic optic neuropathy: the importance of segmentation. Eur J Ophthalmol. 2021;31(6):3471–5.
34. Kleerekooper I, et al. Optical coherence tomography angiography (OCTA) in multiple sclerosis and neuromyelitis optica spectrum disorder. Front Neurol. 2020;11: 604049.
35. Bruce BB, et al. Feasibility of nonmydriatic ocular fundus photography in the emergency department: Phase I of the FOTO-ED study. Acad Emerg Med. 2011;18(9):928–33.
36. Chen JJ, et al. Causes and prognosis of visual acuity loss at the time of initial presentation in idiopathic intracranial hypertension. Invest Ophthalmol Vis Sci. 2015;56(6):3850–9.
37. Sibony PA, et al. Retinal and choroidal folds in papilledema. Invest Ophthalmol Vis Sci. 2015;56(10):5670–80.
38. Malhotra K, Padungkiatsagul T, Moss HE. Optical coherence tomography use in idiopathic intracranial hypertension. Ann Eye Sci. 2020;5.
39. Wall M, et al. Risk factors for poor visual outcome in patients with idiopathic intracranial hypertension. Neurology. 2015;85(9):799–805.
40. Pierro L et al. Vessel density and vessel tortuosity quantitative analysis of arteritic and non-arteritic anterior ischemic optic neuropathies: an optical coherence tomography angiography study. J Clin Med. 2020;9(4).
41. Mairot K, et al. Paracentral acute middle maculopathy as a specific sign of arteritic anterior ischemic optic neuropathy. Am J Ophthalmol. 2023;248:1–7.
42. Rougier MB, Le Goff M, Korobelnik JF. Optical coherence tomography angiography at the acute phase of optic disc edema. Eye Vis (Lond). 2018;5:15.
43. Jalili J et al. Vessel density features of optical coherence tomography angiography for classification of optic neuropathies using machine learning. J Neuroophthalmol. 2023.
44. Hamann S, et al. Young adults with anterior ischemic optic neuropathy: a multicenter optic disc drusen study. Am J Ophthalmol. 2020;217:174–81.
45. Costello F, Burton JM. Retinal imaging with optical coherence tomography: a biomarker in multiple sclerosis? Eye Brain. 2018;10:47–63.
46. Chen JJ, et al. Myelin oligodendrocyte glycoprotein antibody-positive optic neuritis: clinical characteristics, radiologic clues, and outcome. Am J Ophthalmol. 2018;195:8–15.
47. Chen JJ, et al. OCT retinal nerve fiber layer thickness differentiates acute optic neuritis from MOG antibody-associated disease and multiple sclerosis: RNFL thickening in acute optic neuritis from MOGAD vs MS. Mult Scler Relat Disord. 2022;58: 103525.
48. Kraker JA, Chen JJ. An update on optic neuritis. J Neurol. 2023.
49. Braeu FA et al. AI-based clinical assessment of optic nerve head robustness superseding biomechanical testing. Br J Ophthalmol. 2023.
50. Girard MJ et al. Discriminating between papilledema and optic disc drusen using 3D structural analysis of the optic nerve head. Neurology. 2022.
51. Li A et al. Early detection of optic nerve changes on optical coherence tomography using deep learning for risk-stratification of papilledema and glaucoma. J Neuroophthalmol. 2023.

OCT and Compressive Optic Neuropathy

10

Mário Luiz Ribeiro Monteiro

Abstract

Optical coherence tomography (OCT) has emerged as an important tool for quantifying retinal neural loss in many different optic nerve diseases including compressive optic neuropathies. As in other optic neuropathies OCT can be useful for diagnosis and follow-up of both optic nerve and chiasmal compressive diseases. Axonal loss can be assessed both through peripapillary retinal nerve fiber layer measurements as well as using macular thickness measurements, especially when analyzing segmented layers of the retina. By analyzing the amount of axonal loss OCT can also be of help in estimating the possibility of visual improvement in such conditions. Additionally, OCT can provide data to analyze structural optic disc characteristics such as cupping that may occur in compressive optic neuropathies, by evaluating the minimum rim with of the optic disc. Furthermore, OCT angiography enables the assessment of retinal vessel density in these cases. In this chapter, we discuss the main use of OCT in compressive optic neuropathies including primary optic nerve tumors, extrinsic optic nerve compression by tumors or other orbital lesions and the important group of diseases causing chiasmal compression.

Keywords

Optic neuropathy • Optic nerve compression • Optic nerve tumor • Chiasmal syndrome • Pituitary tumors • Band atrophy • Optical coherence tomography • Retinal nerve fiber layer • Macular thickness measurements

M. L. R. Monteiro (✉)
Division of Ophthalmology, Department of Ophthalmology and Otolaryngology, University of São Paulo Medical School, Av. Angélica 1757 Conj. 61, São Paulo, SP 01227-200, Brazil
e-mail: mlrmonteiro2@gmail.com

A. Grzybowski and P. Barboni (eds.), *OCT and Imaging in Central Nervous System Diseases*, https://doi.org/10.1007/978-3-031-72156-4_10

10.1 Introduction

Compressive optic neuropathies are among the most important disorders of the anterior visual pathway, often resulting in significant visual impairment, particularly when an early diagnosis is not obtained. It encompass a wide array of conditions including optic nerve glioma and meningioma, extrinsic optic nerve compression by orbital tumor, enlarged muscles in Graves' orbitopathy, sinus expansive disease or intracranial tumors affecting the optic nerve and chiasm such as occurs in pituitary adenomas, craniopharyngiomas, aneurysms, suprasellar meningioma, glioma, germ cell tumors and metastases [1].

The diagnosis of compressive optic neuropathy usually relies on the history of progressive visual loss and on imaging studies, particularly modern magnetic resonance imaging (MRI) and computed tomography (CT) ophthalmic examination patients with compressive lesions of the anterior visual pathway usually present with visual acuity (VA) and visual field (VF) loss in one or both eyes. Visual loss may occur rapidly in fast growing or hemorrhagic tumors but most of the times visual loss (either central or in the peripheral field) is slow. Optic disc pallor and peripapillary retinal nerve fiber layer (pRNFL) loss is also commonly found in longstanding diseases while proptosis may be present when optic nerve compression occurs at the orbit.

Traditionally evaluation of the visual pathway in such cases was restricted to VA, color vision and VF assessment as well as fundus observation of structural abnormalities in the optic nerve head such as optic disc pallor or edema and pRNFL loss. However, the development of technology that enables to objective measure retinal and optic nerve neuronal integrity has greatly modified our ability to evaluate fundoscopic abnormalities in anterior visual pathway diseases with the introduction of optical coherence tomography (OCT)[2–6]. OCT is the most useful instrument for structural evaluation of the fundus in diseases such as glaucoma and hereditary, demyelinating, degenerative diseases of the central nervous system or compressive lesions affecting the optic pathways [4, 6–10].

OCT became particularly useful in neuro-ophthalmology after the introduction of modern spectral-domain OCT (SD-OCT) and swept-source OCT (SS-OCT) technology that achieved a resolution of 5–7 μm [11, 12]. The current technologies allow for OCT to be of help in the diagnosis and follow-up of compressive optic neuropathies both by quantifying pRNFL and also by measuring retinal thickness in the macular area for estimating particularly macular RNFL and ganglion cell layer (GCL) loss [8, 13–16]. Furthermore, other retinal layers in the macular area, such as the inner nuclear layer (INL) and even outer retinal layers that may also be evaluated and may be affected in optic pathway diseases [17–21]. OCT may also be of help in optic neuropathies associated with optic disc edema by estimating the severity of disc edema and helping analyzing the shape of the peripapillary retinal pigment epithelium layer on linear high-resolution scans passing through the optic disc [22, 23].

Compressive lesions of the anterior visual pathways may go unnoticed by examiners until a significant amount of retinal axonal loss has occurred and clinically detected optic atrophy is present [7, 24]. In such conditions, OCT-measured RNFL and macular thickness measurements may be reduced, indicating retinal neuronal loss. In some cases pRNFL and particularly macular GCL may be reduced even before VF defects are detected [16, 24, 25]. Therefore, by quantifying such structures, the technology can be very useful both in the early diagnosis as well as in the follow-up of compressive diseases of the optic pathway.

Decreased measurements of OCT-assessed pRNFL and macular thickness may help detecting optic neuropathies occurring from intrinsic or extrinsic optic nerve tumors. In cases where visual loss is subtle, characterized by slight decreases in VA, VF, and color vision, the finding of pRNFL thinning offers more concrete evidence of optic neuropathy. Since compressive optic neuropathies usually have an insidious presentation, such finding can be extremely important to raise suspicion and prompting further investigation [26].

In patients with compressive optic neuropathies, OCT serves not only as a diagnostic aid butalso as a valuable tool for estimating the chances of visual improvement after treatment. Ideally such conditions should be detected before retinal axonal loss is present based on history, ophthalmic examination and neuroimaging studies. In such cases, the finding of normal or only mildly reduced OCT measurements in a patient with significant visual loss from compressive optic neuropathy indicates that visual recovery is possible at least to a large extent. Moreover, detailed analysis using high-resolution OCT examinations can assist in evaluating treatment efficacy, particularly in cases where complete lesion removal is not possible. Efficacy of treatment can be estimated with OCT by repeating retinal and optic nerve measurements over time [5].

While OCT has not been extensively studied across all conditions, its potential to offer crucial insights is likely significant in all cases of compressive optic neuropathies. Irrespective of the etiology the most frequent utility of OCT is to assess optic neuropathy through quantification of pRNFL thickness measurements. Additionally, macular thickness measurements, particularly segmented assessments of macular RNFL and GCL (usually measured alongside the inner plexiform layer and labeled as GCL+), as well as the combined measurement of both macular RNFL and GCL+, have also became important tools and are now available in most modern OCT equipments [8, 14, 15, 17].

Additionally, OCT may prove valuable in assessing structural abnormalities at the optic disc, such as deformation of the posterior pole observed in eyes with papilledema or optic nerve tumors, as well as cupping of the optic disc, a common feature of glaucoma that can also manifest in other optic neuropathies, including compressive optic neuropathies[27]. Furthermore, advances in OCT have made it possible to measure peripapillary and macular vessel density (VD) through OCT angiography, which may also be affected in cases of compressive optic neuropathies[28, 29].

In the subsequent paragraphs, we discuss the most important compressive lesions affecting the anterior visual pathway, specifically focusing on those that have undergone prior studies regarding the use of OCT.

10.2 Optic Nerve Tumors

Tumors of the optic nerve constitute approximately 4–10% of all orbital tumors [30–32]. Although rare lesions such as hemangiopericytomas and medulloepitheliomas are occasionally reported, the vast majority are either optic nerve gliomas or optic nerve meningiomas. Gliomas typically manifest in children, whereas optic nerve meningiomas predominantly affect middle-aged individuals, presenting with progressive visual decline, proptosis, disc edema and in some cases optociliary veins on fundus examination [30, 32, 33].

Meningiomas affecting the anterior visual pathway are important compressive lesions of the optic nerve, typically observed in middle-aged patients, resulting in progressive loss of VA and VF, optic atrophy, or optic disc edema, along with abnormalities on imaging studies such as MRI and CT scan. These tumors can arise from either the sheaths of the optic nerve or the meninges adjacent to the nerves [1].

Optic nerve sheath meningiomas (ONSM) are tumors originating from the meninges of the optic nerve and constitute approximately one-third of primary optic nerve tumors[30, 34]. These tumor exhibit a female predominance, with the mean age at diagnosis typically around 40 years [35]. The lesions generally exhibit slow growth and usually lead to gradual visual deterioration. Some tumors are localized to a small segment of the optic nerve, while others surround the entire length of the nerve in the orbit and the optic canal [34]. Patients with ONSM and progressive but recent visual loss or those with long-standing loss but still with useful visual function can be treated with conformational fractioned radiation therapy [36, 37]. By contrast, surgical resection of ONSM leads to significant or complete visual loss and should be restricted to patients with severe irreversible visual loss for correction of disfiguring proptosis or preventing intracranial extension.

One typical manifestation of ONSM involves progressive visual loss, optic atrophy, and the presence of optociliary shunt vessels [33, 35]. In such instances, optic disc edema usually precedes the onset of optic atrophy [33]. However, while optic disc edema or atrophy is frequently observed, in many patients, fundoscopic examination may reveal a normal appearance or only subtle signs of optic atrophy. This can lead to diagnostic challenges, particularly when the tumor is small, as neuroimaging studies may yield inconclusive results. In such cases, OCT can aid in diagnosis by confirming the presence of pRNFL and/or GCL+ loss (Fig. 10.1).

When optic disc edema is present in patients with ONSM the diagnosis is frequently confused with other causes of optic disc edema such as optic neuritis and papilledema. In many patients, subtle optic disc edema may also prevent OCT from detecting axonal loss when evaluating pRNFL. In such cases, careful attention to macular GCL thickness measurements will reveal some degree of neural loss (Fig. 10.2). Another important observation in cases with severe disc edema is that OCT may be of help in the diagnosis by showing indentation of the retinal pigment epithelium (on high-resolution linear scans passing through the nerve) presumably because of lack of compliance of the nerve that exerts pressure on the

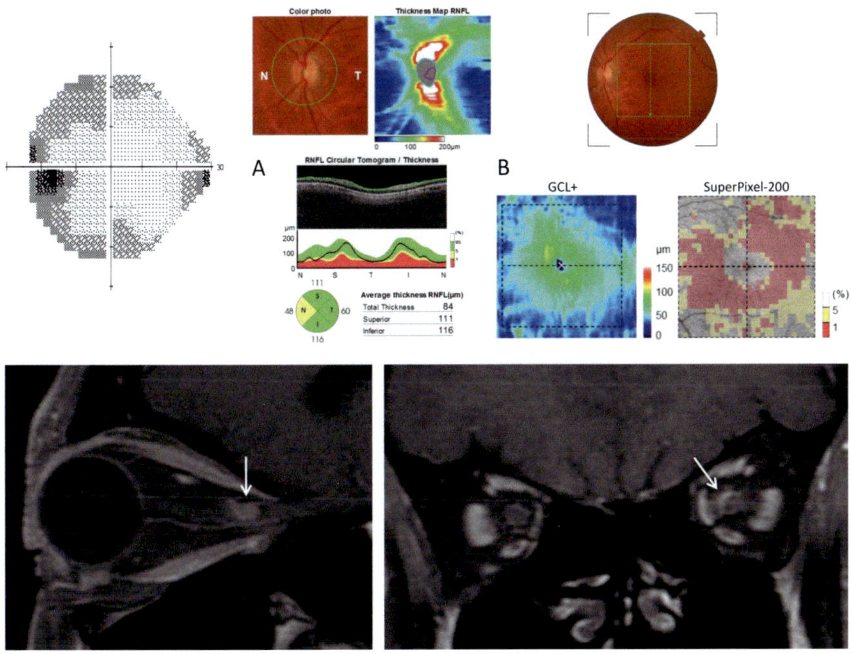

Fig. 10.1 A 72-year-old woman complained of progressive visual loss in the left eye for one year. Visual field showed reduced peripheral sensitivity (upper left) but neuroimaging studies were unrevealing and a diagnosis was not established. Optical coherence tomography (DRI OCT Triton Plus®, Topcon) revealed borderline reduction of the peripapillary retinal nerve fiber layer in the nasal quadrant of the disc (upper middle, A). Segmented macular thickness measurements indicated reduced macular ganglion cell layer (GCL+) volume, significantly reduced compared to normative data (upper right, B). Because of OCT findings a repeat magnetic resonance imaging of the orbit disclosed a small meningioma affecting a segment of the optic nerve on sagittal (lower left, arrow) and coronal cuts (lower right, arrow)

posterior pole (Fig. 10.3) [22]. However, it is important that while such deformation is not encountered in ischemic or inflammatory optic neuropathies it may also occur in papilledema and is not specific for ONSM [23].

OCT can be important not only in diagnosing ONSM but also in predicting the likelihood of visual recovery. If visual loss manifests in a patient with minimal or no retinal neuronal loss, visual improvement can be anticipated (Fig. 10.4). Conversely, when substantial pRNFL and macular GCL loss is evident, signifying established axonal damage, the focus of treatment should shift toward halting further visual decline, and the absence of visual improvement does not necessarily indicate treatment failure (Fig. 10.5). Tang et al. [38] evaluated the outcome of patients with ONSM submitted to radiotherapy treatment and found that out of 39 that performed visual acuity evaluation, 16 (37.2%) had vision improvement. Of the 23 that did not improve, 16 had severe visual loss at diagnosis. Along with

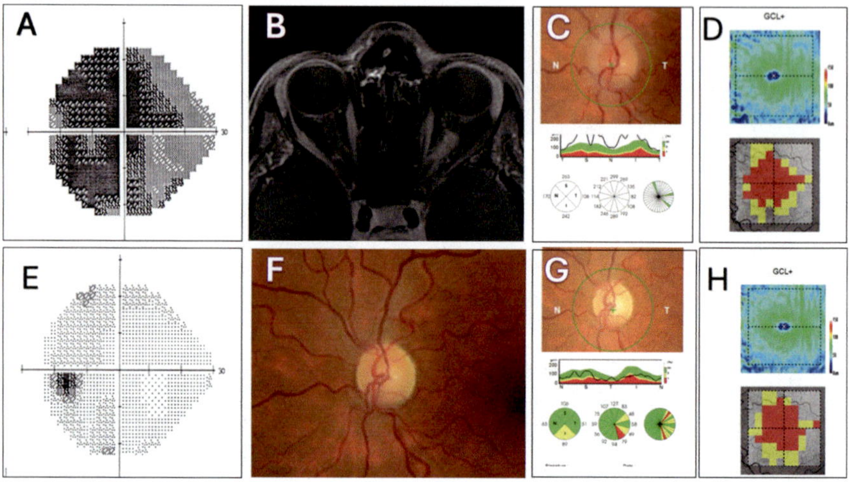

Fig. 10.2 A 47-year-old woman presented with severe visual acuity and field loss (A) and mild optic disc edema in the left eye. Neuroimaging investigation revealed an enhancement of the meninges of the optic nerve compatible with optic nerve sheath meningioma (B). Optical coherence tomography reveals increased peripapillary retinal nerve fibers (C) and reduced macular ganglion cell layer (D) in the affected eye. Radiation therapy resulted in significant improvement of visual acuity and visual field (E). Reduction of disc edema led to disclosure of mild optic disc pallor (F) and peripapillary retinal nerve fiber layer reduction (G) but macular thickness parameters showed stability of retinal neural loss after treatment (H)

visual function measurements, OCT findings may be an important parameter for predicting visual outcome after treatment.

While ONSM are usually treated with radiotherapy, patients with tumors from the skull base meninges but compressing the optic pathway are usually treated with surgery. Visual outcome after decompressive surgery however is variable; while a significant number of patients experience improvement or stability of vision, 20–30% deteriorate [39]. Although several risk factors for poor visual outcomes are known including prolonged duration of symptoms, the presence of disc pallor and incomplete tumor resection, estimating the potential for visual recovery may be difficult based on the clinical exam and imaging finding alone. Loo et al. [20] performed a study to determine the prognostic value of pretreatment OCT measurement of the pRNFL in final visual outcomes of patients with anterior visual pathway meningioma and optic neuropathy. The authors evaluated the outcome of 14 eyes of 12 patients treated in which pretreatment and post-treatment OCT along with clinical examination were performed. After treatment, the group with normal pRNFL experienced significant improvement in the VA, color vision, and VF compared with the group with reduced pRNFL. The findings in this study are a further indication that patients with compressive optic neuropathy due to anterior pathway meningioma are more likely to improve post-treatment if they have a normal pretreatment RNFL.

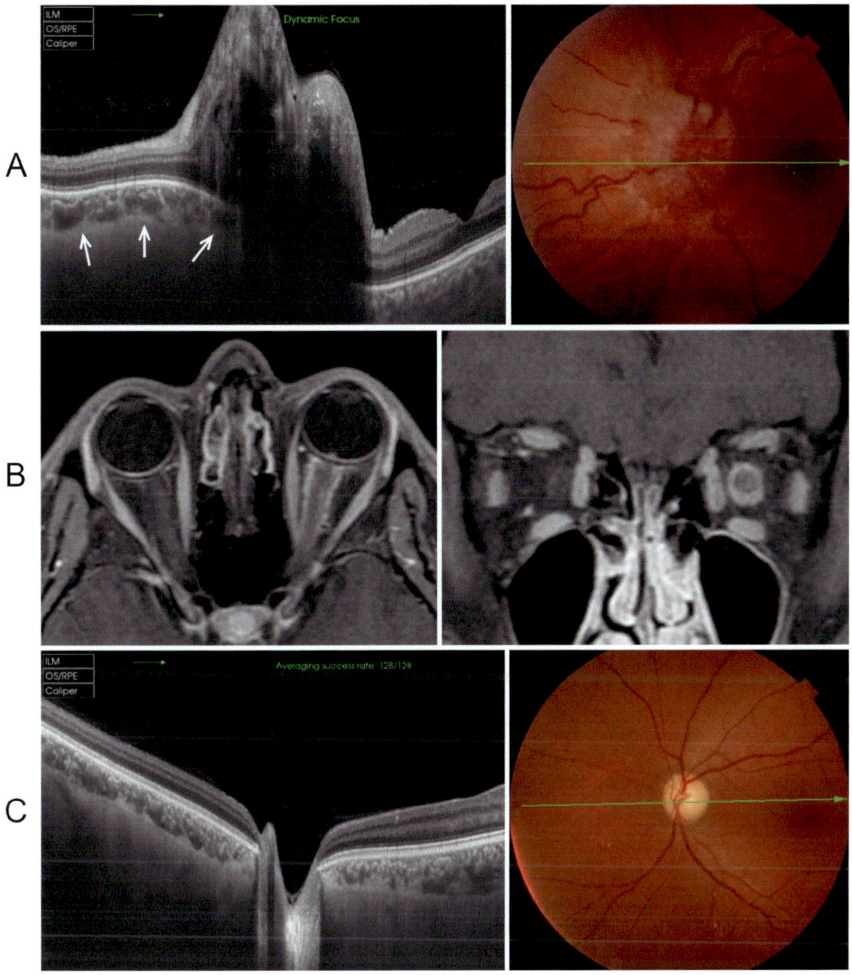

Fig. 10.3 A 26-year-old man presented with blurred vision and optic disc edema in the left eye. Above: swept source optical coherence tomography (DRI OCT Triton Plus®, Topcon) 12-mm linear horizontal scan passing through the optic disc revealing deformation of the peripapillary retinal pigment epithelium layer, with the appearance previously described as an inverted-U shape image (arrows) [22]. Middle: magnetic resonance imaging revealed enhancing lesion around the optic nerve, later confirmed to be an optic nerve sheath meningioma. Below: linear scanning showing the normal V-shape of the peripapillary retinal pigment epithelium layer

Optic nerve gliomas are the most common tumors of the optic nerve but represent only 1% of all intracranial tumors [40]. While malignant gliomas may occur in the adult, the large majority of gliomas are benign juvenile pilocytic astrocytomas that present primarily among children in the first decade of life. The natural history of childhood optic nerve gliomas is almost always benign, and most patients retain stable visual function without treatment. A conservative management is usually

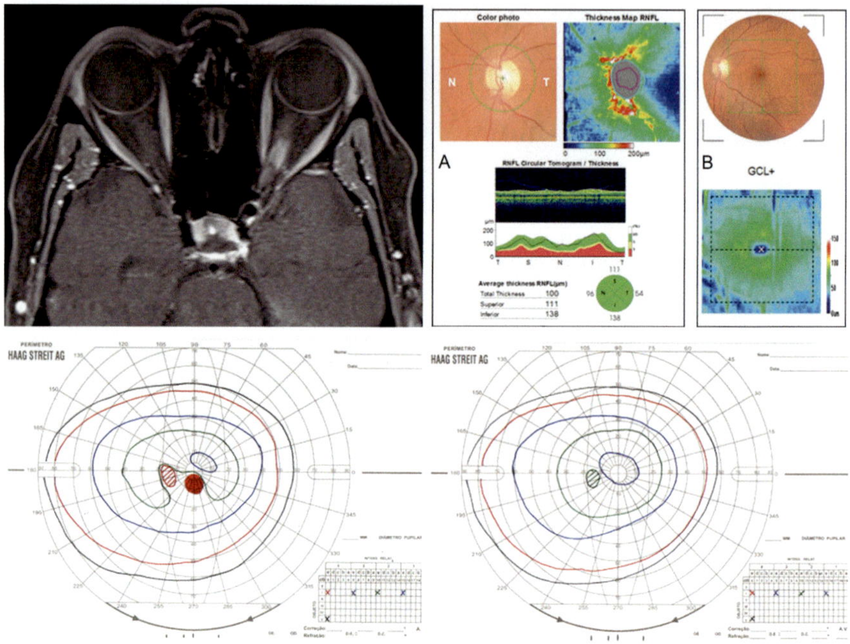

Fig. 10.4 A 51-year-old woman with progressive visual loss in the left eye for one year was found to have an optic nerve sheath meningioma (upper left). Optical coherence tomography (Topcon 3D-OCT 2000™) revealed normal peripapillary retinal nerve fiber layer (upper right, A). Segmented macular thickness measurements indicated normal macular ganglion cell layer (upper right, B). The patient presented with an inferior paracentral scotoma and constricted field (lower left) and showed significant improvement after conformational radiation therapy (lower right)

recommended to patients with unilateral optic nerve gliomas, particularly those with neurofibromatosis type 1 (NF-1) [41]. On the other hand in uncommon cases of more aggressive tumors, particularly those near of affecting the optic chiasm chemotherapy can be used to help stabilize the lesion [42].

Both in patients with optic pathway gliomas (OPG) followed with conservatively without treatment and in those submitted to chemotheraphy, assessment of visual function along with imaging studies is the main parameters used to evaluate disease progression on follow-up examinations. However, monitoring young children with OPGs for visual deterioration can be difficult owing to age-related noncompliance. OCT measures of peripapillary RNFL and macular thickness can be of significant help in monitoring the integrity of the visual pathway and has been proposed as a surrogate marker of vision in previous studies evaluating OCT findings in patients with OPG, as demonstrated in Fig. 10.6.

Chang et al. [43] evaluated both macular and RNFL thickness measurements in patients with NF-1 with or without optic gliomas and controls. The authors found that NF-1 subjects with OPG had average RNFL thickness and macular volume significantly reduced compared to those without gliomas. The study suggests that

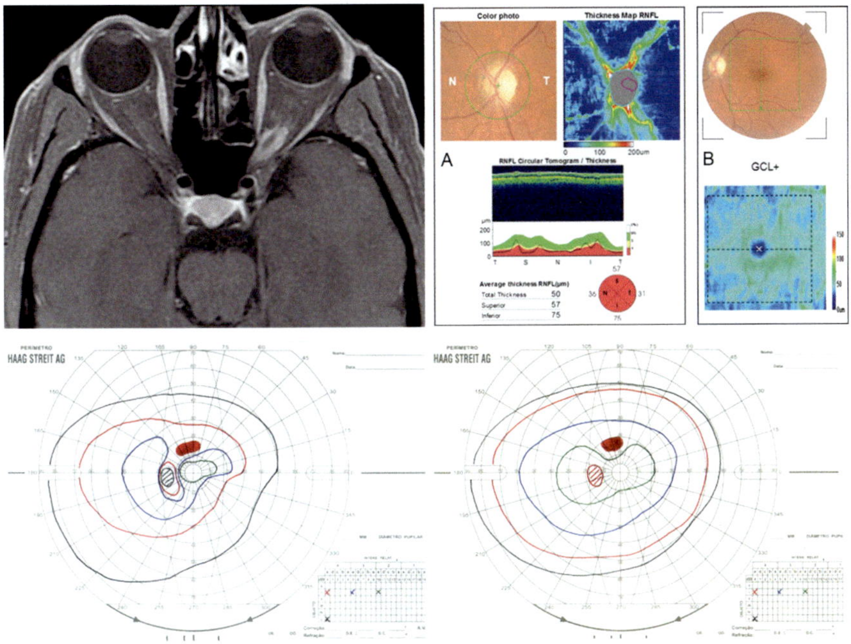

Fig. 10.5 A 49-year-old woman with a 7-year history of visual loss in the left eye from an optic nerve sheath meningioma (upper left). Optical coherence tomography (Topcon 3D-OCT 2000™) revealed severely reduced peripapillary retinal nerve fiber layer (upper right, A). Segmented macular thickness measurements indicated markedly reduced macular ganglion cell layer (upper right, B). The patient presented with a severe constriction, enlarged blind spot and superior paracentral scotoma (lower left). There was only mild visual improvement after conformational radiation therapy (lower right)

OCT can be used to detect RNFL thinning secondary to NF-1 related OPGs and that it may be a useful adjunct to routine clinical ophthalmologic evaluation in children with NF-1.

Avery et al. [44] prospectively evaluated 62 patients with NF-1 and optic nerve gliomas submitted to neuro-ophthalmic examination including TD-OCT of the optic nerve head. Eighty-nine eyes of patients with OPG were included and 41 classified as having abnormal VA or VF loss. Reduced RNFL thickness was associated significantly with reduced VA and contrast sensitivity. The study indicated that reduced OCT-measured RNFL is a sensitive technology to detect visual loss in OPG.

Parrozzoni et al. [45] compared visual function and SD-OCT measured RNFL thickness for the screening of OPG in 57 pediatric patients affected by NF-1. Visual function assessment, RNFL analysis, and optic disc evaluation results correlated with the presence of OPGs, but only RNFL analysis reached statistically significant sensitivity and positive predictive value. The authors concluded that

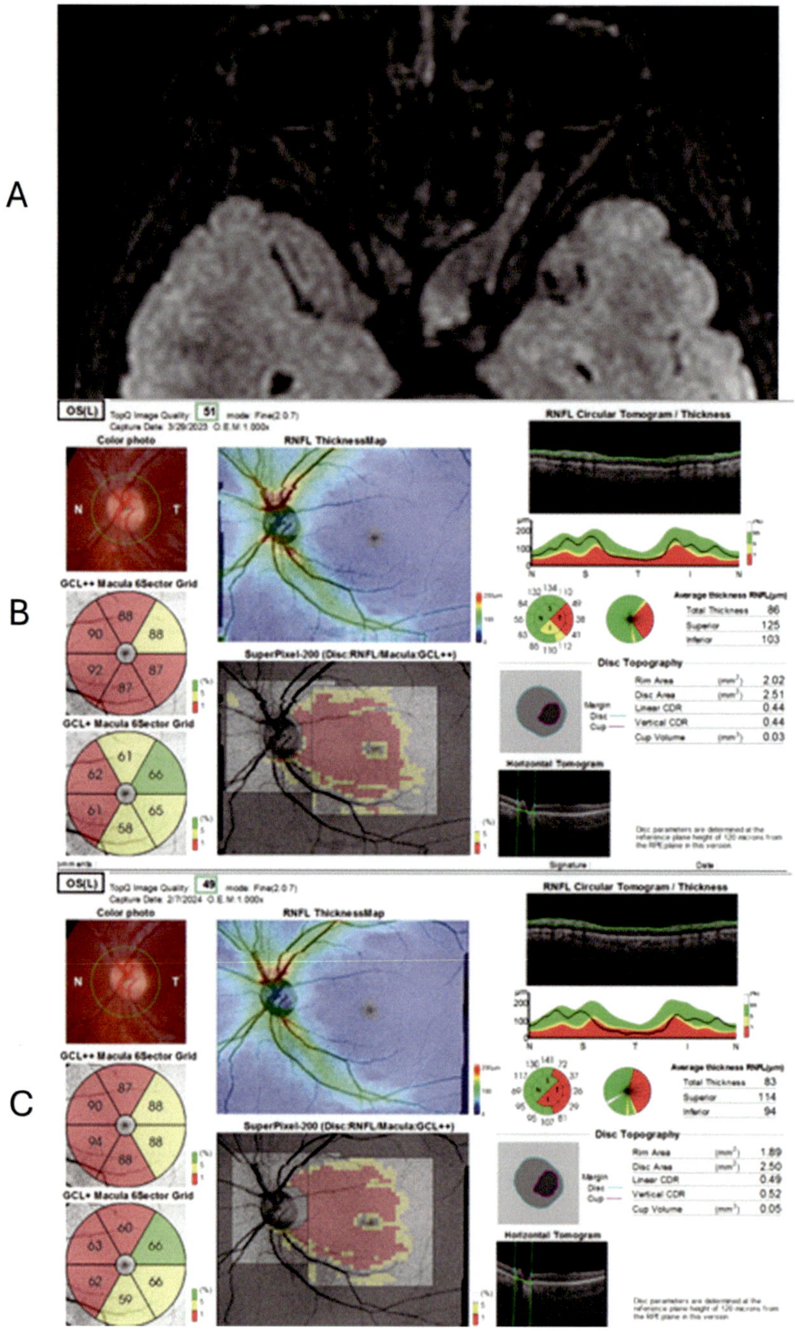
A
B
C
OS(L)
Color photo
RNFL ThicknessMap
RNFL Circular Tomogram / Thickness
GCL++ Macula 6Sector Grid
GCL+ Macula 6Sector Grid
SuperPixel-200 (Disc:RNFL/Macula:GCL++)
Average thickness RNFL(μm)
Total Thickness 86
Superior 125
Inferior 103
Disc Topography
Rim Area (mm²) 2.02
Disc Area (mm²) 2.51
Linear CDR 0.44
Vertical CDR 0.44
Cup Volume (mm³) 0.03
Horizontal Tomogram
Total Thickness 83
Superior 114
Inferior 94
Rim Area (mm²) 1.89
Disc Area (mm²) 2.50
Linear CDR 0.49
Vertical CDR 0.52
Cup Volume (mm³) 0.05

◀**Fig. 10.6** A 6-year-old boy fell down hitting his head and was submitted to a computerized tomography that identified an optic nerve tumor. Magnetic resonance imaging showed fusiform enlargement of the left optic nerve compatible with an optic nerve glioma (A). Clinical examinations disclosed stigmata of neurofibromatosis type 1. Ophthalmic evaluation showed that visual acuity was 20/20 on both eyes but there was mild pallor of the left optic nerve. OCT showed reduced peripapillary retinal nerve fiber layer in the left eye along with reduced macula ganglion cell layer (B). A conservative approach was proposed and a repeat OCT one year later was unchanged (C) showing no axonal deterioration during this period of time

RNFL analysis assessment using SD-OCT is superior to visual function assessment and optic disc evaluation as a clinical screening tool for OPGs. Macular thickness measurements were not investigated.

Fard et al. [46] studied 38 eyes of 23 children with OPG and evaluated the relationship between SD-OCT findings and clinical/radiological changes at diagnosis and on a 24-month follow-up evaluation. Mean changes in average RNFL and macular thickness measurements were significantly higher in patients that had clinical/radiological progression of the gliomas compared to those that did not progressed. OCT measurements were significantly different in patients with tumor progression compared to those that did not progress indicating that OCT measurements may be helpful in monitoring OPG. Gu et al. [47] evaluated the macular GCL-inner plexiform layer (GCL-IPL) thickness in children with or without visual loss from OPG using SD-OCT. Decreased GCL-IPL thickness was able to discriminate between children with and without vision loss from their OPG. The authors concluded that GCL-IPL thickness could be used as a surrogate marker of vision in children with OPGs. Two other reports have also indicated the value of OCT-measured pRNFL and macular thickness parameters in the diagnosis and follow-up of patients with OPG [48, 49].

While the above-mentioned studies have indicated the value of OCT in monitoring visual function in OPG, an important limitation for obtaining OCT measurements in this condition is that gliomas usually occur in young patients, when the technique is also limited by patient cooperation. However, Avery et al. [50] used a hand-held OCT to obtain optic nerve and retinal thickness measurements during sedation in 33 young children with OPGs. The authors concluded that for young children who do not cooperate with vision testing, hand-held OCT measures may be a surrogate marker of vision. More recently, the same authors [51] reported the results of an investigation in 55 eyes of patients with OPG that were followed longitudinally and completed 250 OCT examinations. They concluded that children experiencing visual loss frequently demonstrate a decline $\geq 10\%$ of peripapillary RNFL thickness measurements in one or more sectors of the disc further emphasizing that peripapillary RNFL thickness measurements may be helpful in the follow up of OPG.

10.3 Dysthyroid Optic Neuropathy

Graves' orbitopathy (GO) is an autoimmune inflammatory process affecting the orbital and periorbital tissues, mainly the extraocular muscles but also the retrobulbar fat. GO occurs before, during or after the onset of hyperthyroidism and, less frequently, in euthyroid or hypothyroid patients [52]. The enlargement of the extraocular muscles is responsible for most of the debilitating manifestations of the disease, including proptosis, diplopia, congestive signs and dysthyroid optic neuropathy (DON) [52, 53]

DON is a serious complication of GO occurring in 3.4% of patients, [54] almost always as a result of optic nerve compression at the orbital apex by enlarged extraocular muscles. The diagnosis of DON rests mainly on clinical findings, such as decreased VA, abnormal VF, altered color and brightness perception, delayed visual evoked potentials, afferent pupillary defects and edema or atrophy of the optic nerve head [55]. Nevertheless, DON is often subclinical and in many cases difficult to diagnose due to confounding signs and symptoms, especially significant orbital congestion or decreased corneal transparency due to exposure keratopathy. Establishing a diagnosis may also be difficult because many tests of optic nerve dysfunction, such as VA, color and brightness perception and VF, especially when performed with standard automated perimetry, require full cooperation of an alert and motivated patient and will not infrequently render false positive results, particularly in patients with congestive GO.

Because the prognosis of DON improves significantly with early diagnosis and treatment, much effort has been put into designing objective tests capable of identifying patients at high risk for developing DON. Therefore imaging studies, particularly CT scanning of the orbit are often used to investigate the possibility of DON [56]. Several studies have tested the ability of CT parameters (linear, area and volume measurements of the orbital muscles) to raise suspicion and facilitate the diagnosis of DON [56, 57]. More recently, OCT measurements have been introduced in the management of GO.

In patients with GO, OCT can be of help in the diagnosis and in follow-up of DON. Because DON can present with optic disc edema, OCT can help its detection and measurement to monitor treatment efficacy. While no previous studies have specifically evaluated the use of OCT for monitoring optic disc edema in GO, many studies have documented the ability of the equipment for that purpose in patients with papilledema [58, 59] Presumably the same rationale applies for measuring optic disc edema in patients with DON. On the other hand, many patients with DON present without optic disc edema, either with atrophy or with normal optic disc appearance. As in any other compressive optic neuropathy, OCT thickness measurements can help quantifying axonal loss in patients with DON both help establishing the diagnosis as well as to estimate the chances of reversing visual loss (Fig. 10.7).

Very few studies, however, have critically evaluated OCT in GO and in special those with DON. Forte et al. [60] evaluated the RNFL in patients with GO and ocular hypertension using OCT. The authors found that RNFL loss on OCT was

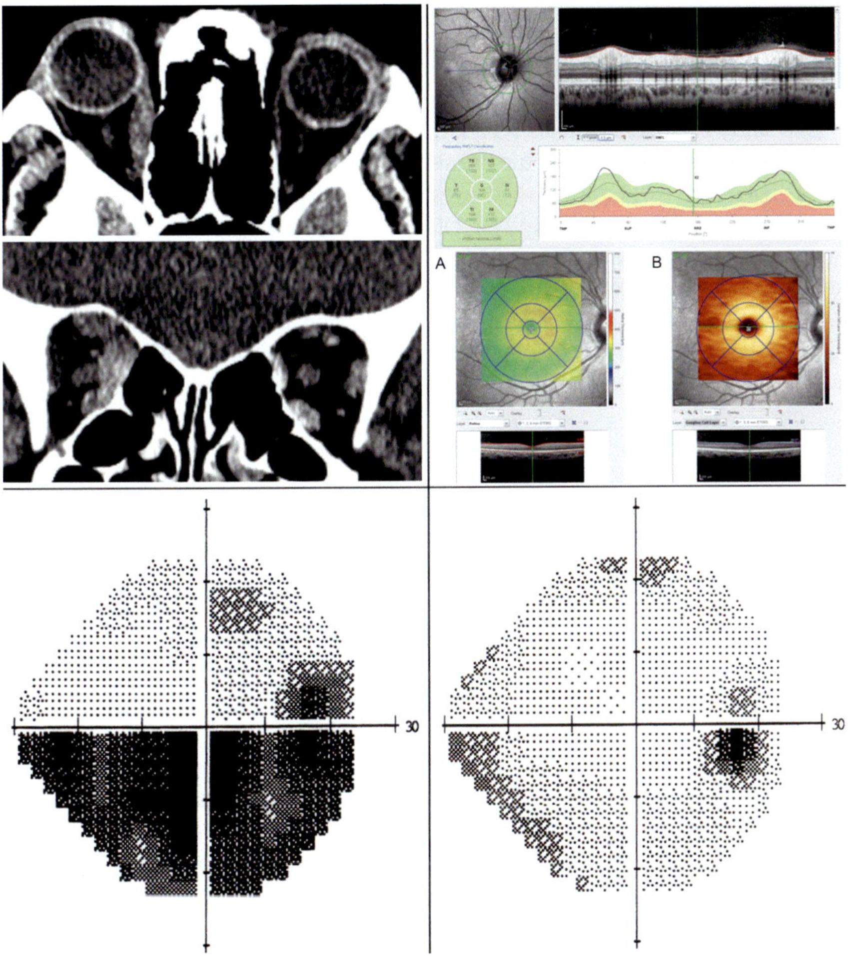

Fig. 10.7 A 50-year-old woman with Graves' orbitopathy presented with double vision, proptosis for 3 months and a 2-week history of visual loss in the right eye (OD). Computerized tomography scan showed enlarged medial and inferior rectus muscles and crowding at the orbital apex (upper left). Visual acuity was 20/200 and there was inferior altitudinal field loss (lower left). Optical coherence tomography (OCT scan (HRA Spectralis™, Heidelberg Engineering) showed normal peripapillary retinal nerve fiber layer (upper right). Macular thickness measurements showed normal full-thickness (A) and normal macular ganglion cell layer (B). There was marked improvement of both visual acuity and visual field after orbital decompressive surgery (lower right) in accordance with the normal retinal neural integrity as assessed by OCT

found in 9 of the 30 patients evaluated. However, apparently the patients did not have well-defined DON and the authors concluded that RNFL loss was important to detect the presence of optic neuropathy but could not differentiate whether the causative effect was DON or the elevated intraocular pressures.

One study evaluated patients with DON using OCT but as a secondary measurement when investigating the value of multifocal visual evoked potentials (mfVEP). Pérez–Rico et al. [61] evaluated 65 eyes of 34 consecutive patients with GO using mfVEP, SAP and OCT (Stratus TD–OCT). The authors found mfVEP abnormalities in 27% of eyes and diffuse VF defects in 20% indicating that a significant number of eyes had DON. OCT-measured RNFL did not differ from normal, and no correlation was found between mfVEP, VF and OCT data. While the study might indicate a poor sensitivity to detect abnormalities on OCT it may also be interpreted as indicating reversibility of visual function abnormalities in the patients.

It is widely known that visual loss in DON can be reversible when properly treated, provided there is no significant permanent optic nerve damage. The finding of normal RNFL in a patient with significant visual loss would therefore be a strong indicator for further treatment to obtain visual recovery (Fig. 10.5).

10.4 Other Compressive Optic Nerve Diseases

Optic nerve compression can also be due to a number of orbital and adnexal conditions including extrinsic tumors of the orbit, osseous diseases leading to optic nerve compression at the canal, sinusal processes invading the orbit, metastases and lymphoproliferative diseases that can lead to optic nerve dysfunction. Very few of these conditions have been evaluated systematically using OCT but the instrument can certainly be an important additional data in the diagnosis by characterizing the presence of an optic neuropathy as well as estimating the chances of visual recovery after treatment (Fig. 10.8).

10.5 Compressive Chiasmal Diseases

Compressive lesions at the optic chiasmal region are among the most important lesions of the anterior visual pathway and can be caused by several lesions including pituitary adenoma, craniopharyngioma, meningioma, Rathke cleft cysts, aneurism and metastatic lesions. Pituitary tumors are the most common cause of chiasmal compression, representing 10–15% of intracranial tumors [62]. Visual loss is a frequent finding and occurs in 32–70% of patients [62]. Functioning tumors can present with clinical symptoms related to hormonal abnormalities, such as impotence, amenorrhea, galactorrhea, acromegaly and Cushing's syndrome, but in many cases visual complaints are the most relevant symptoms at presentation. Conversely, nonfunctioning pituitary adenomas typically present solely with visual

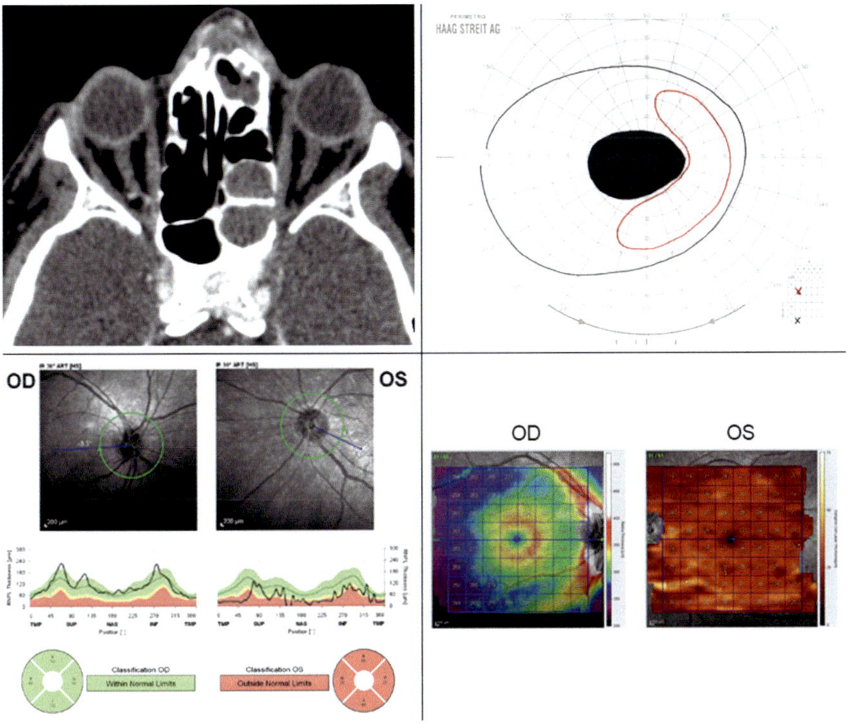

Fig. 10.8 A 52-year-old man had severe visual loss in the left eye (OS) due to a spheno-ethmoidal mucocele compressing the optic nerve at the optic canal and the orbital apex (upper left). Visual field showed a dense central scotoma (upper right) and visual acuity was reduced to finger counting. Optical coherence tomography (OCT) scan (HRA Spectralis™, Heidelberg Engineering) showed severely reduced peripapillary retinal nerve fiber layer in OS and was normal in the right eye (OD) (lower left). Segmented macular scans showed normal macular ganglion cell layer in OD and severely reduced in OS (lower right). There was no significant improvement of vision after surgery in accordance with the severe retinal neural loss observed on OCT

complaints. The lesions produce reduced VA, loss of color vision and particularly VF defects. However, because visual symptoms are usually vague early on the course of the disease, the diagnosis may be delayed until later stages when permanent damage of the visual pathway has already occurred.

Chiasmal lesions can lead to a wide variety of visual and axonal damage to the visual pathway fibers, ranging from mild VF defect and focal peripapillary RNFL and macular GCL loss to severe and diffuse visual loss and optic nerve atrophy and retinal GCL loss. In most cases, however, typical bitemporal VF defect occur and a specific pattern of axonal loss develops. In patients with mid-chiasmal lesions, temporal hemianopia and preserved nasal field, the crossed nerve fibers are lost with preservation of the uncrossed nerve fibers, which originate in the temporal hemiretina and penetrate the optic nerve through the superior and inferior arcuate fiber bundles. Thus, RNFL loss occurs predominantly on the nasal and temporal side of the optic disc, a pattern identified on ophthalmoscopy as band atrophy (BA) of the optic nerve, [63] and the retina may show a clear distinction in the pattern of axonal loss when the temporal hemiretina is compared with the affected nasal hemiretina (Fig. 10.9).

Chiasmal lesions were the first compressive anterior visual pathway diseases to be evaluated using OCT when we and other authors have demonstrated that retinal thickness measurements could detect neural loss in patients with temporal hemianopia caused by suprasellar tumors and that such measurements were able to identify the BA pattern of axonal loss found in this condition, based peripapillary RNFL thickness measurements using early generation time domain-OCT devices [3, 64–66]. Later studies with SD and SS-OCT equipments [14, 17, 67–69] largely confirmed the ability of the technology to detect peripapillary RNFL loss in pituitary tumors, including the characteristic pattern of BA of the optic nerve (Fig. 10.10).

A few years after the initial studies evaluating only peripapillary RFNL thickness parameters, we have demonstrated that full-thickness macular thickness measurements were also able to detect axonal loss in chiasmal compression and correlated well both with peripapillary RNFL and with VF defects [13, 67, 70]. Discrimination ability and the relationship between OCT thickness measurements and VF loss were similar with both sets of measurements although macular thickness measurements allowed a better correlation when quadrantic measurements of the macula were obtained [13]. Because the RNFL of different quadrants and different hemifields enter the optic disc in a way that the fibers from different quadrants superimpose one with the other, specific correlation of RNFL with VF is somewhat cumbersome at the optic disc. With the exception of the nasal area of the disc all other sectors receive retinal nerve fibers from both the nasal and the

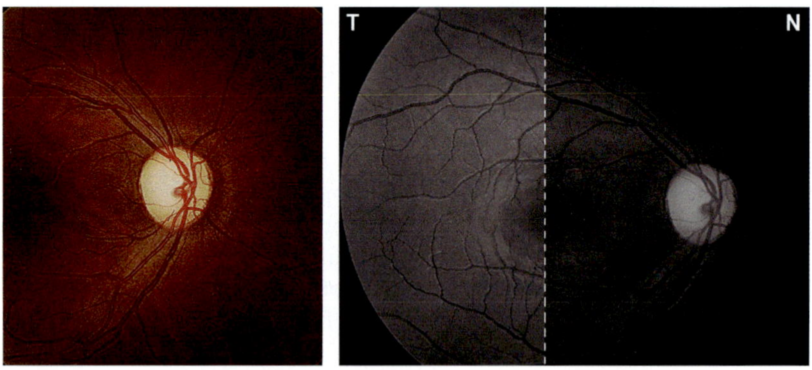

Fig. 10.9 Optic nerve (left) and fundus photograph (right) of a patient complete temporal hemianopia with normal nasal hemifield, band atrophy of the optic nerve and a pattern of retinal nerve fiber layer loss in the temporal and nasal portions of the optic nerve with relative preservation of the superior and inferior arcuate fibers (left) and the demarcation between the retinal area with preserved ganglions cells (temporal) and the ares with atrophic ganglion cells (nasal). T = temporal; N = nasal

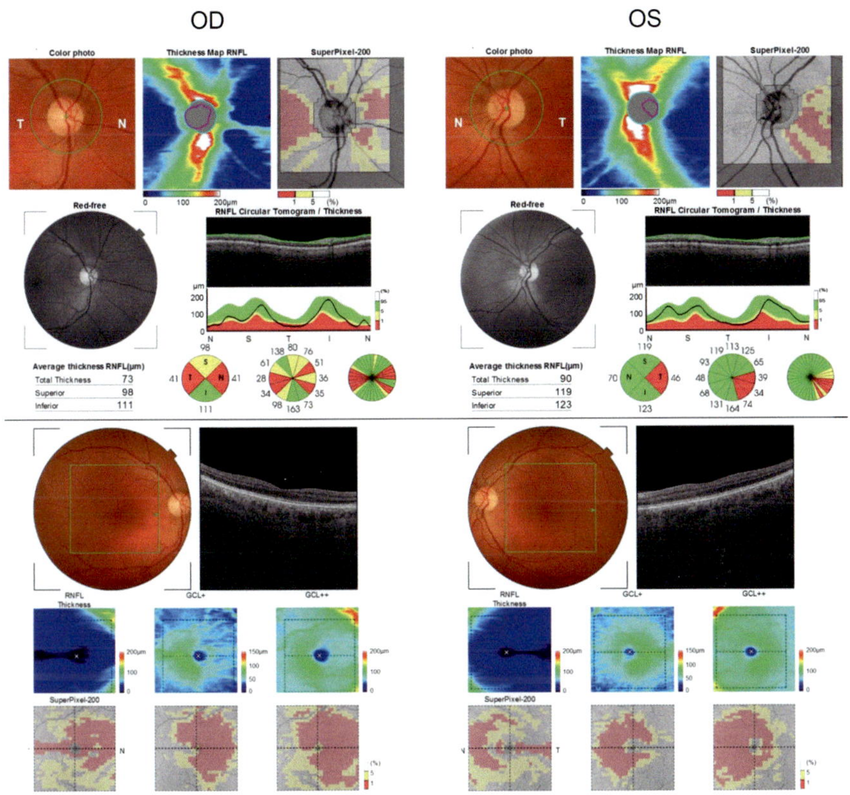

Fig. 10.10 Optical coherence tomography (DRI OCT Triton Plus®, Topcon, Japan) of a 56-year-old woman with a large pituitary adenoma compressing the optic chiasm and bitemporal hemianopia. Above, note significantly reduced peripapillary retinal nerve fiber layer in the nasal and temporal quadrants of the right eye (OD) and in the temporal quadrant in the left eye (OS). Below, scanning of the macular areas shows marked thinning of the ganglion cell layer in the nasal hemiretina of both eyes

temporal hemiretina. The result is a lack of specificity between VF loss and optic disc sectors in patients with lesions of the optic chiasm [13, 14]. For example, when a VF defect affecting the superotemporal quadrant is present, it results in RNFL loss in the nasal, temporal and inferior regions of the optic disc. Since the inferior region of the optic disc also receives nerve fibers from the unaffected nasal VF, there is presumably a lack of specificity in the structure-function relationship.

On the other hand, with macular thickness measurements a superotemporal VF defect may be related to reduced macular thickness below and nasally to the fovea, with a direct correspondence to the quadrantic VF defect. The advantage of macular thickness measurements is even greater in patients with temporal hemianopia, affecting both the superior and the inferior temporal quadrants. Based on the distribution of the RNFL on the optic disc [71], such patients may be expected to have RNFL loss in every quadrant of the optic disc, with a resultant lack of specificity in the structure-function relationship, while macular thickness reduction would be observed almost exclusively nasally to the fovea, probably with a much higher specificity. In previous studies we have demonstrated a closest structure-function relationships observed between macular thickness measurements and VF abnormalities compared to the relationship between peripapillary RNFL thickness measurements and VF defects [13]. The relationship between OCT-measured macular thickness parameters and VF defects were even greater when segmented macular thickness measurements were introduced and separate analysis of the retina GCL became possible (Figs. 10.10 and 10.11), and a number of studies have confirmed the greater sensitivity of inner macular thickness parameters to detect neural loss in chiasmal compression [8, 14, 16, 69, 72–77].

Several studies have evaluated the relationship between OCT findings and VF or electrophysiological testing. In one study, we have also shown that OCT measurements correlated well both with VF and the finding on pattern electroretinogram in patients with chiasmal compression [78]. In another study we have even demonstrated a significant correlation between OCT and multifocal pattern electroretinogram measurements in such patients [79]. Moon et al. [80] showed an important correlation between reduced peripapillary RNFL thickness and decreased b wave on the photopic negative response, both associated with worse VF outcome. We have also documented significant correlation between OCT and multifocal visual evoked potential measurements [68]. Therefore, OCT can also be associated with other electrophysiological methods as prognostic indicator in the preoperative assessment of chiasmal compression.

While in most patients with chiasmal compression treatment is usually necessary, estimating the prognosis for visual recovery is particularly important in patients with recurrent tumors where the need for further surgery is in question. Although it is expected that visual improvement may occur after optic pathway decompression, in many cases such recovery is variable and many times difficult to predict [81–84]. Although other predictive values such as duration of symptoms, age, size of tumor, the severity of VA and VF loss as the presence or absence of optic disc pallor have been used to estimate visual recovery, the results are far from ideal [82–86]. The grading of optic disc pallor is difficult and subjective [85]. Therefore the use of OCT to quantify axonal loss through pRNFL and macular thickness measurements seems to be one of the most important predictor of visual recovery as demonstrated in patients described in Figs. 10.12, 10.13 and 10.14.

While both pRNFL and macular thickness measurements are important for estimating retinal axonal loss in chiasmal compression, studies using high-resolution OCT with segmented analysis of macular thickness measurements demonstrates that GCL+measurements show abnormality before pRNFL loss is detectable (Figs. 10.14 and 10.15) [14, 16, 72–74, 77].

Several studies have evaluated prospectively the ability of OCT in predicting visual improvement in chiasmal compression. Such studies have shown a significant correlation between the depth and thickness of the RNFL measured by OCT

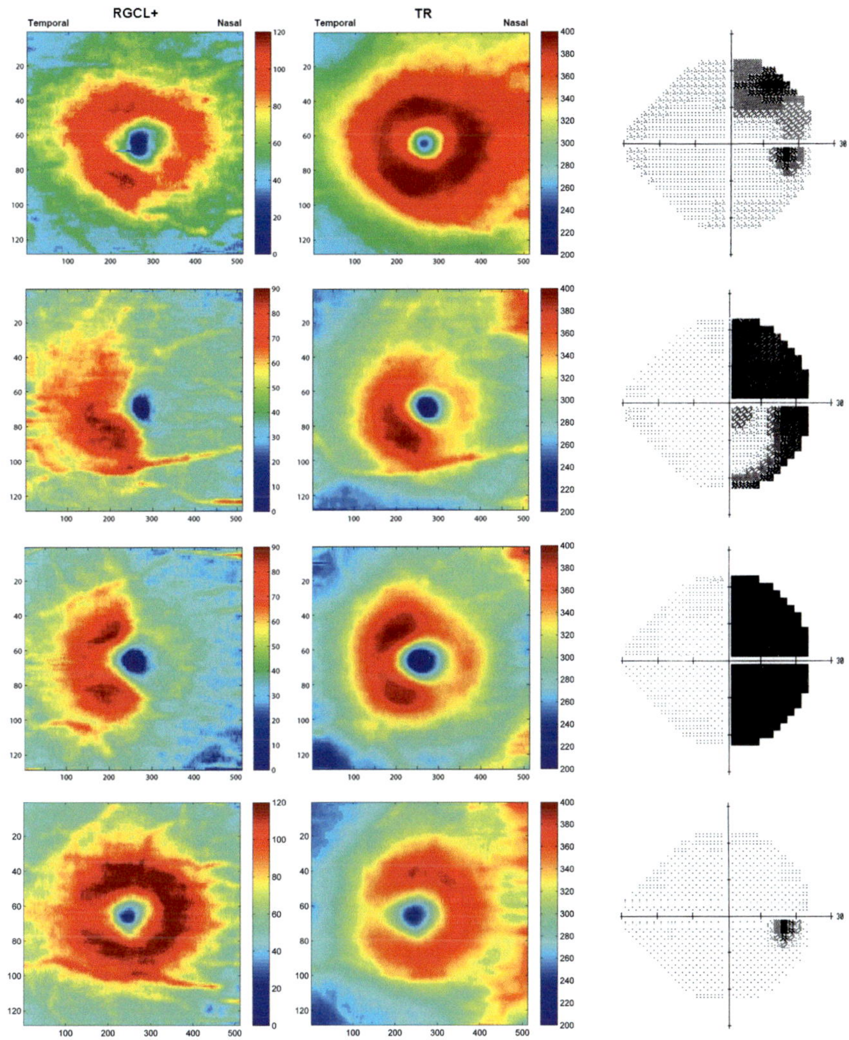

Fig. 10.11 Pseudo-color thickness map generated from cube scan based on the thickness of the macular layers obtained using spectral-domain optical coherence tomography (Topcon 3D-OCT 1000™). First, second and third lines = eyes with band atrophy of the optic nerve and different degrees of visual field loss. Fourth line = a normal control. RGCL+ = retinal ganglion cell layer associated with the inner plexiform layer. TR = total retinal thickness. Notice that thickness reduction in the nasal hemiretinas is more evident in the RGCL+ when compared to TR (modified from Monteiro MLR, et al. Invest Ophthalmol Vis Sci 2014; 55:3328–36)

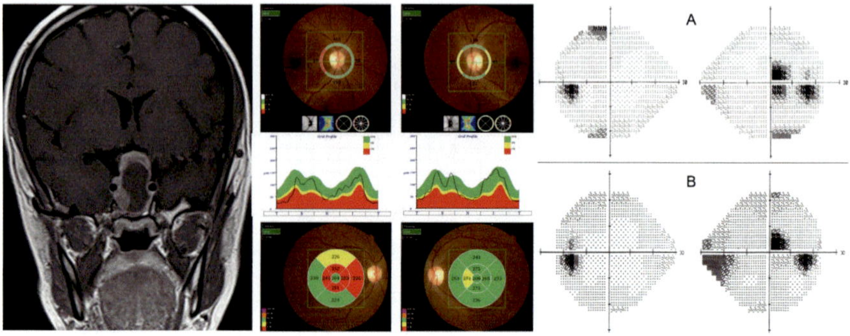

Fig. 10.12 32-year-old woman with a large pituitary adenoma with chiasmal compression (left). Middle: optical coherence tomography (OCT) scan (Topcon 3D-OCT 1000™) revealed reduced peripapillary retinal nerve fiber layer in the temporal portion of the right eye (in red) and in the nasal and temporal portions of the left eye (in yellow). Full-thickness macular measurements showed thinning mostly of the nasal macula (in red or yellow) indicating retinal axonal loss. Right: visual fields showing bilateral defect pre-operatively (A) and no significant improvement after surgery (B) in accordance with the finding of permanent retinal axonal loss on OCT

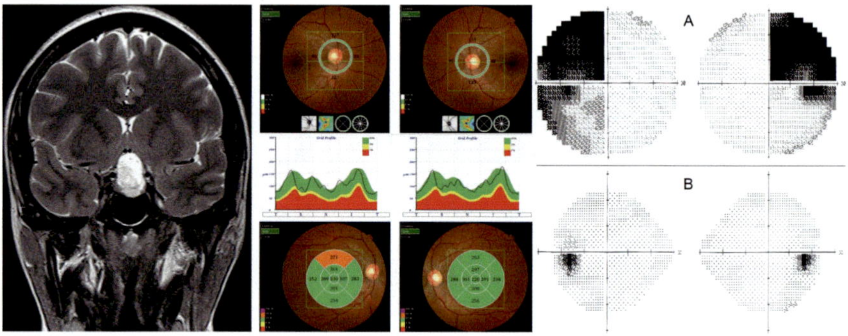

Fig. 10.13 A 24-year-old pregnant woman developed a large pituitary adenoma with chiasmal compression (left). Middle: optical coherence tomography (Topcon 3D-OCT 1000™) revealed normal peripapillary retinal nerve fiber layer in both eyes. Full-thickness macular measurements showed normal measurements indicating retinal axonal normality. Right: visual fields showing bitemporal quadrantic defect pre-operatively (A) and normal visual field after surgery (B) in accordance with normal OCT findings

and the possibility of improvement in patients that undergo surgery for tumors involving the chiamal region [26, 87]. Danesh-Meyer et al. [26] evaluated 40 patients with chiasmal compression with TD-OCT and VF both pre- and post-surgical decompression. Patients with preoperative RNFL below 97.5% of normal values did not demonstrate significant improvement in VA and VF mean deviation in the post-operative period while those with normal RNFL thickness had significant improvement in VA. The authors found that there was an increased likelihood

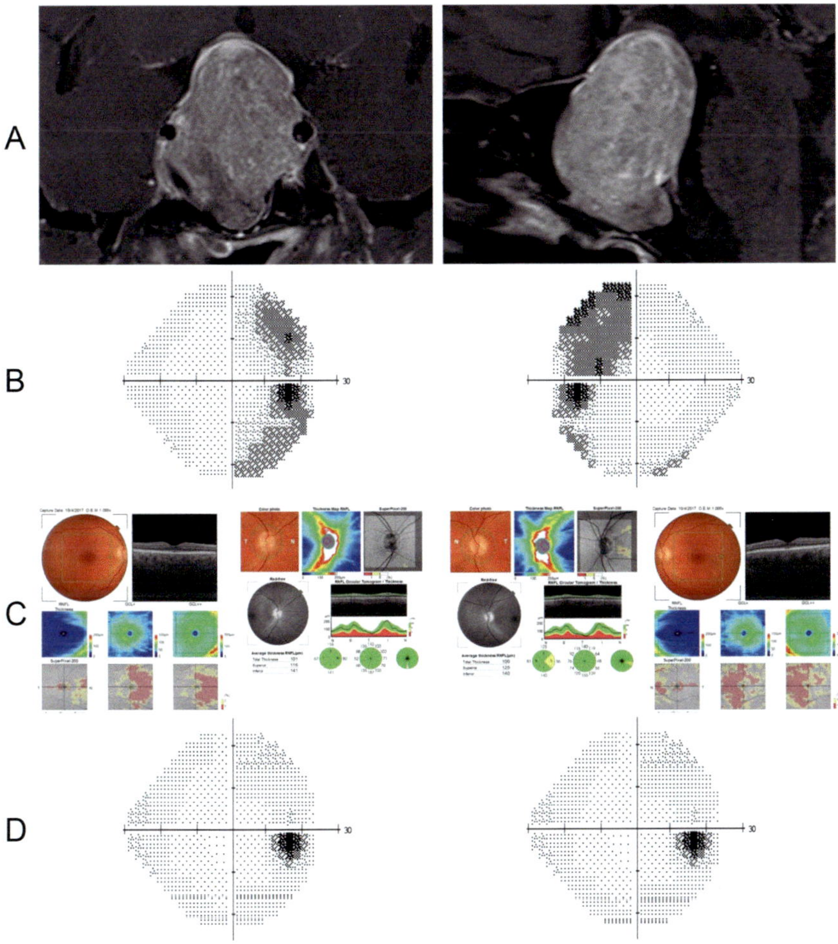

Fig. 10.14 A 45-year-old man underwent neuroimaging studies because of headache. Magnetic resonance imaging on coronal (left) and sagittal (right) cuts showed a large non-secreting pituitary adenoma (A). Standard automated perimetry (24-2 threshold test) revealed bitemporal visual field defects (B). Optical coherence tomography (DRI OCT Triton Plus®, Topcon, Japan) revealed peripapillary retinal nerve fiber layer within normal limits in the right eye and borderline reduction in the temporal quadrant in the left eye (C). Macular thickness measurements revealed significant macular ganglion cell layer loss in the nasal hemiretina of both eyes (C). After surgery, there was significant improvement of visual fields on both eyes. Note that there was significant reduction in macular ganglion cell layer despite only minor abnormalities in the peripapillary retinal nerve fiber (C). Also, note that there was significant improvement in the visual field defect despite the presence of macular ganglion cell layer thinning in both eyes

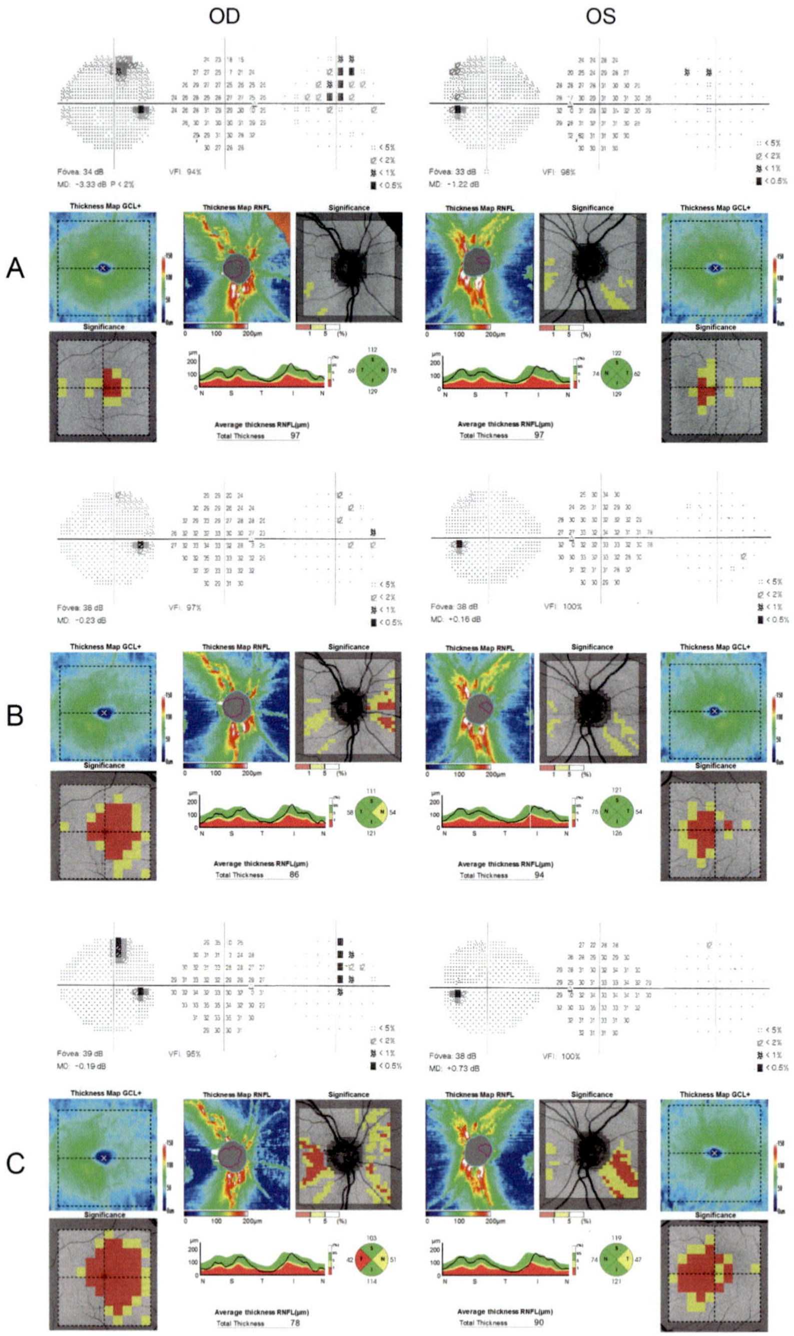
OD
OS
A
B
C
Thickness Map GCL+
Thickness Map RNFL
Significance
Average thickness RNFL(µm)
Total Thickness 97
Total Thickness 86
Total Thickness 94
Total Thickness 78
Total Thickness 90

◀**Fig. 10.15** Data for the right (OD, left row) and left eye (OS, right row) of a patient with a large pituitary tumor compressing the optic chiasm, obtained at three sequential examinations (A: November 2015, B: August 2016, and C: August 2017). The upper row of each point in time shows the visual field (VF) gray scale (left), sensitivity data in decibels (center) and pattern deviation plot (right). The mid and lower rows are optical coherence tomography findings (OCT-2000, Topcon corporation, Tokyo, Japan): pseudo-colored thickness maps of the macular ganglion cell layer + the inner plexiform layer (Thickness Map GCL+) and, immediately below, significance patterns with color-coded grids (no color = within normal limits; yellow = outside the 95% normal limit; red = outside the 99% normal limit); pseudo-colored map of the peripapillary retinal nerve fiber layer (Thickness Map RNFL) and corresponding significance patterns with color-coded grids. Peripapillary global average and quadrantic and RFNL thickness measurements as well as a graphic demonstration of the thickness profile are also presented. Note that retinal GCL+ was abnormal on the first examination although peripapillary RNFL were still within normal limits (A). Also, note definite worsening of peripapillary RNFL thickness profile as well as nasal hemiretina RGC+ layer in both eyes, on the follow-up examinations (B and C) despite only mild worsening of VF defect in the right and none in the left eye (modified from Monteiro MLR. J Neuroophthalmol. 2018; 38:124–127)

of postoperative improvement with thicker preoperative RNFL until approximately 85 μm. In a subsequent study, Danesh-Meyer et al. [88] evaluated the data of 107 patients with pituitary tumor that underwent surgical treatment evaluating pre-operatively peripapillary RNFL and the VF mean deviation (MD). Patients with thin pre-operative RNFL (defined as the fifth percentile of normative values) had more severe VF defects than the group with normal RNFL thickness. Long-term follow up showed that 81% of eyes with normal RNFL, compared to 37.1% with thin RNFL, achieved an MD of 2.00 dB at the final visit. The results showed that long-term visual recovery after surgical decompression of pituitary lesions can be predicted by pre-operative OCT-measured peripapillary RNFL.

Jacob et al. [87] showed that the odds of complete VF recovery in patients with pituitary adenomas compressing the visual pathways that underwent trans-sphenoidal surgery was multiplied by 1.29 for each increase in 1 μm of mean RNFL. The authors concluded that RNFL thinning measured by OCT leads to a decreased chance of recovery of an initial VF defect three months after treatment.

Ohkubo et al. [89] evaluated the relationship between macular GCL and VF parameters in chiasmal compression and the potential for GCL parameters in order to predict the short-term post-surgical VF. Examining the macular GCL was useful for evaluating structural damage in patients with chiasmal compression. Preoperative GCL parameters, especially focal loss of GCL, seemed useful in predicting visual function following surgical decompression of chiasmal compression.

However, while GCL loss certainly indicates that permanent damage exists, it is important to know that presence of GCL+ thinning does not exclude the possibility of significant recovery of VF defect. Tieger et al. [16] reported a series of 23 patients with chiasmal compression evaluated with OCT and standard automated perimetry (SAP) before and after surgical treatment. Because some of their patients showed complete VF recovery despite persistent macular GCL layer thinning on OCT, the authors suggested that RGC loss may precede VF defect, at least when assessed with standard 24-2 or 30-2 threshold strategies with size III target on SAP. I was able to confirm such suggestion in a patient with a pituitary tumor compressing the chiasm that was followed for 21 months with OCT, SAP (using the 24-2 threshold strategy) and manual Goldmann perimetry [90]. Although surgery was indicated, the patient declined it and opted for conservative management. Sequential examinations clearly showed that GCL+ loss preceded the development of peripapillary RNFL reduction (Fig. 10.15). Also, while there was only mild deterioration of the VF over the follow-up period, OCT data (especially GCL+ thickness) displayed significant worsening in both eyes, indicating that in chronic compressive lesions, retinal structures may be impaired prior to clinically detectable VF loss, at least with most commonly used strategies [90].

On the other hand, it is important to consider that axonal loss may appear later in the course of the disease, even after optic pathway decompression has occurred. Moon et al. [76] evaluated 19 patients undergoing chiasmal decompression before and 1 and 3 months after surgery. Visual recovery was significantly correlated with the changes in retinal GCL and RNFL thickness measurements. However, prolonged retrograde degeneration progressed for some period, even after surgical decompression and visual recovery occurred.

More recently OCT angiography was introduced to investigate vessel density (VD) in the retina. While initial interest in the technology was directed to retinal vascular diseases it soon became evident that several optic pathway diseases that cause retinal axonal loss may also show abnormalities in OCT angiography. Suzuki et al. [28] compared peripapillary and macular VD assessed using OCT angiography in patients with BA of the optic nerve from chiasmal compression and normal controls. Compared to controls BA eyes displayed smaller average peripapillary and macular VD values sector measurements. VD reduction was most significant in nasal and temporal peripapillary regions as well as in the nasal hemiretina in the macular area, in direct correspondence with pRFNL and macular GCL loss of the patients (Fig. 10.16). Some recent studies have even suggested that OCT-angiography-measured VD may also be useful for estimating the chances of visual recovery in patients with visual loss from chiasmal compression [29, 91].

10.6 Conclusions

With progressive improvement in technology OCT has become an extremely useful instrument in a number of neuro-ophthalmic diseases. While continued research on the subject is necessary to better understand the precise relationship between OCT and VA, VF and other modalities of visual function evaluation, a large number of previous studies as well as clinical observation clearly indicate the importance of using OCT in diagnosis, treatment as well as follow-up of compressive optic neuropathies. As both technology and interpretation of data continues to advance, the use of OCT in the management of this important group of optic nerve diseases became an extremally useful tool and will certainly continue to increase.

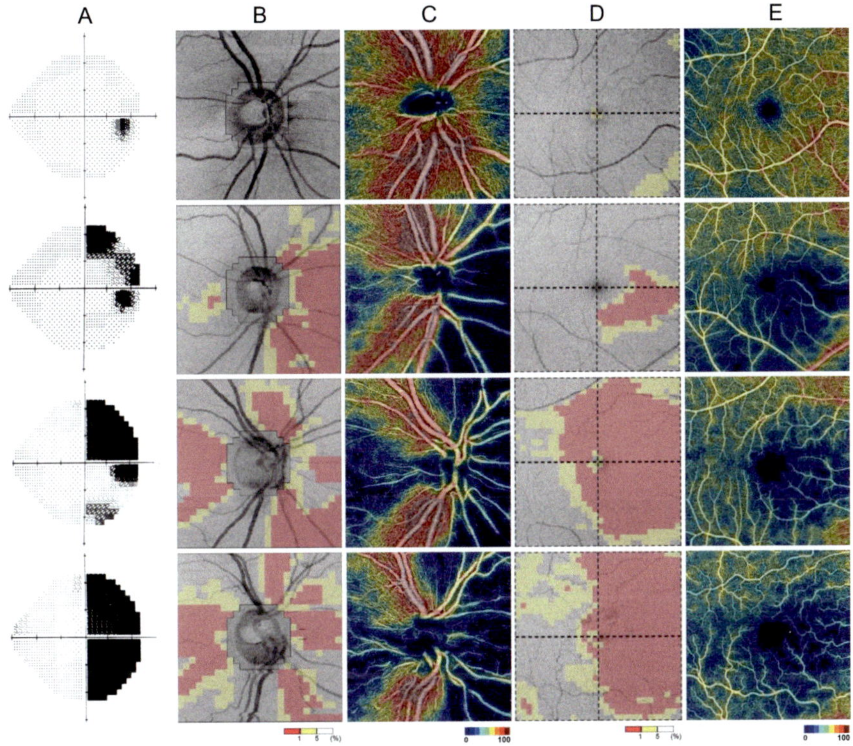

Fig. 10.16 Figure 10.1 findings from a normal subject (first row), two cases with partial temporal visual field defect (second and third rows), and one case with complete temporal visual field defect (bottom row). a. grayscale graphic of 24-2 standard automated perimetry (SAP). b significance pattern deviation of peripapillary RNFL thickness based on the normative range of the DRI OCT Triton Plus® equipment with colour-coded grids (yellow = outside the 95% normal limit; red = outside the 99% normal limit). c pseudo-coloured OCTA peripapillary density map. d significance pattern of macular ganglion cell complex thickness based on the normative range of the equipment with colour-coded grids (yellow = outside the 95% normal limit; red = outside the 99% normal limit). e pseudo-coloured OCTA macular vessel density map. Note that significant reduction of VD shows a direct correspondence with pRNFL and macular ganglion cell layer loss (from Suzuki AC, et al. Eye, 2020; 34:695–703)

References

1. Chan JW. Compressive and infiltrative optic neuropathies. In: Chan JW, editor. Optic nerve disorders diagnosis and management. Springer; 2007. p. 88–129.
2. Sergott RC, Balcer LJ. The latest on optical coherence tomography. J Neuroophthalmol. 2014;34(Suppl):S1-2.
3. Monteiro ML, Leal BC, Rosa AA, Bronstein MD. Optical coherence tomography analysis of axonal loss in band atrophy of the optic nerve. Br J Ophthalmol. 2004;88(7):896–9.

4. Monteiro ML. Optical coherence tomography in neuro-ophthalmology: do we really need it? J Neuroophthalmol. 2016;36(4):353–5.
5. Subei AM, Eggenberger ER. Optical coherence tomography: another useful tool in a neuro-ophthalmologist's armamentarium. Curr Opin Ophthalmol. 2009;20(6):462–6.
6. Chen JJ. Optical coherence tomography and neuro-ophthalmology. J Neuroophthalmol. 2018;38(1):e5–8.
7. Pasol J. Neuro-ophthalmic disease and optical coherence tomography: glaucoma look-alikes. Curr Opin Ophthalmol. 2011;22(2):124–32.
8. Kardon RH. Role of the macular optical coherence tomography scan in neuro-ophthalmology. J Neuroophthalmol. 2011;31(4):353–61.
9. Costello F. Optical coherence tomography in neuro-ophthalmology. Neurol Clin. 2017;35(1):153–63.
10. Mello LGM, Bissoli LB, Saraiva FP, Maia RPD, Monteiro MLR. Retinal layers and choroid measurements in Parkinson's disease with or without pramipexole treatment. Mov Disord. 2020;35(12):2357–9.
11. Adhi M, Duker JS. Optical coherence tomography—current and future applications. Curr Opin Ophthalmol. 2013;24(3):213–21.
12. Mrejen S, Spaide RF. Optical coherence tomography: imaging of the choroid and beyond. Surv Ophthalmol. 2013;58(5):387–429.
13. Monteiro ML, Costa-Cunha LV, Cunha LP, Malta RF. Correlation between macular and retinal nerve fibre layer Fourier-domain OCT measurements and visual field loss in chiasmal compression. Eye. 2010;24(8):1382–90.
14. Monteiro ML, Hokazono K, Fernandes DB, Costa-Cunha LV, Sousa RM, Raza AS, et al. Evaluation of inner retinal layers in eyes with temporal hemianopic visual loss from chiasmal compression using optical coherence tomography. Invest Ophthalmol Vis Sci. 2014;55(5):3328–36.
15. Lam BL. Retinal ganglion cell thickness to assess the optic nerve. J Neuroophthalmol. 2015;35(2):107–8.
16. Tieger MG, Hedges TR 3rd, Ho J, Erlich-Malona NK, Vuong LN, Athappilly GK, et al. Ganglion cell complex loss in chiasmal compression by brain tumors. J Neuroophthalmol. 2017;37(1):7–12.
17. de Araujo RB, Oyamada MK, Zacharias LC, Cunha LP, Preti RC, Monteiro MLR. Morphological and functional inner and outer retinal layer abnormalities in eyes with permanent temporal hemianopia from chiasmal compression. Front Neurol. 2017;8:619.
18. Abegg M, Dysli M, Wolf S, Kowal J, Dufour P, Zinkernagel M. Microcystic macular edema: retrograde maculopathy caused by optic neuropathy. Ophthalmology. 2014;121(1):142–9.
19. Fernandes DB, Raza AS, Nogueira RG, Wang D, Callegaro D, Hood DC, et al. Evaluation of inner retinal layers in patients with multiple sclerosis or neuromyelitis optica using optical coherence tomography. Ophthalmology. 2013;120(2):387–94.
20. Loo JL, Tian J, Miller NR, Subramanian PS. Use of optical coherence tomography in predicting post-treatment visual outcome in anterior visual pathway meningiomas. Br J Ophthalmol. 2013;97(11):1455–8.
21. Monteiro MLR, Sousa RM, Araújo RB, Ferraz D, Sadiq MA, Zacharias LC, et al. Diagnostic ability of confocal near-infrared reflectance fundus imaging to detect retrograde microcystic maculopathy from chiasm compression. A comparative study with OCT findings. PLoS One. 2021;16(6):e0253323.
22. Sibony P, Strachovsky M, Honkanen R, Kupersmith MJ. Optical coherence tomography shape analysis of the peripapillary retinal pigment epithelium layer in presumed optic nerve sheath meningiomas. J Neuroophthalmol. 2014;34(2):130–6.
23. Sibony P, Kupersmith MJ, Rohlf FJ. Shape analysis of the peripapillary RPE layer in papilledema and ischemic optic neuropathy. Invest Ophthalmol Vis Sci. 2011;52(11):7987–95.
24. Ribeiro Monteiro ML. Macular ganglion cell complex reduction preceding visual field loss in a patient with chiasmal compression with a 21-month follow-up. J Neuroophthalmol. 2018;38(1):124–7.

25. Sasagawa Y, Nakahara M, Takemoto D, Nakada M. Optical coherence tomography detects early optic nerve damage before visual field defect in patients with pituitary tumors. Neurosurg Rev. 2023;46(1):85.
26. Danesh-Meyer HV, Papchenko T, Savino PJ, Law A, Evans J, Gamble GD. In vivo retinal nerve fiber layer thickness measured by optical coherence tomography predicts visual recovery after surgery for parachiasmal tumors. Invest Ophthalmol Vis Sci. 2008;49(5):1879–85.
27. Andrade TS, Araújo RB, Rocha AADN, Mello LGM, Cunha LP, Monteiro MLR. Bruch membrane opening minimum rim width and retinal nerve fiber layer helps differentiate compressive optic neuropathy from glaucoma. Am J Ophthalmol. 2022;234:156–65.
28. Suzuki ACF, Zacharias LC, Preti RC, Cunha LP, Monteiro MLR. Circumpapillary and macular vessel density assessment by optical coherence tomography angiography in eyes with temporal hemianopia from chiasmal compression. Correlation with retinal neural and visual field loss. Eye. 2020;34(4):695–703.
29. Ergen A, Kaya Ergen S, Gunduz B, Subasi S, Caklili M, Cabuk B, et al. Retinal vascular and structural recovery analysis by optical coherence tomography angiography after endoscopic decompression in sellar/parasellar tumors. Sci Rep. 2023;13(1):14371.
30. Dutton JJ. Optic nerve sheath meningiomas. Surv Ophthalmol. 1992;37(3):167–83.
31. Spencer WH. Primary neoplasms of the optic nerve and its sheaths: clinical features and current concepts of pathogenetic mechanisms. Trans Am Ophthalmol Soc. 1972;70:490–528.
32. Dutton JJ. Optic nerve gliomas and meningiomas. Neurol Clin. 1991;9(1):163–77.
33. Imes RK, Schatz H, Hoyt WF, Monteiro ML, Narahara M. Evolution of optociliary veins in optic nerve sheath meningioma. Evolution Arch Ophthalmol. 1985;103(1):59–60.
34. Miller NR. New concepts in the diagnosis and management of optic nerve sheath meningioma. J Neuroophthalmol. 2006;26(3):200–8.
35. Parker RT, Ovens CA, Fraser CL, Samarawickrama C. Optic nerve sheath meningiomas: prevalence, impact, and management strategies. Eye Brain. 2018;10:85–99.
36. Saeed P, Blank L, Selva D, Wolbers JG, Nowak PJ, Geskus RB, et al. Primary radiotherapy in progressive optic nerve sheath meningiomas: a long-term follow-up study. Br J Ophthalmol. 2010;94(5):564–8.
37. Solda F, Wharram B, De Ieso PB, Bonner J, Ashley S, Brada M. Long-term efficacy of fractionated radiotherapy for benign meningiomas. Radiother Oncol. 2013;109(2):330–4.
38. Tang T, Wang J, Lin T, Zhai Z, Song X. The treatment efficacy of radiotherapy for optic nerve sheath meningioma. Eye. 2024;38(1):89–94.
39. Rosenberg LF, Miller NR. Visual results after microsurgical removal of meningiomas involving the anterior visual system. Arch Ophthalmol. 1984;102(7):1019–23.
40. Dutton JJ. Gliomas of the anterior visual pathway. Surv Ophthalmol. 1994;38(5):427–52.
41. Miller NR. Primary tumours of the optic nerve and its sheath. Eye. 2004;18(11):1026–37.
42. Kelly JP, Leary S, Khanna P, Weiss AH. Longitudinal measures of visual function, tumor volume, and prediction of visual outcomes after treatment of optic pathway gliomas. Ophthalmology. 2012;119(6):1231–7.
43. Chang L, El-Dairi MA, Frempong TA, Burner EL, Bhatti MT, Young TL, et al. Optical coherence tomography in the evaluation of neurofibromatosis type-1 subjects with optic pathway gliomas. J AAPOS. 2010;14(6):511–7.
44. Avery RA, Liu GT, Fisher MJ, Quinn GE, Belasco JB, Phillips PC, et al. Retinal nerve fiber layer thickness in children with optic pathway gliomas. Am J Ophthalmol. 2011;151(3):542–9 e2.
45. Parrozzani R, Clementi M, Kotsafti O, Miglionico G, Trevisson E, Orlando G, et al. Optical coherence tomography in the diagnosis of optic pathway gliomas. Invest Ophthalmol Vis Sci. 2013;54(13):8112–8.
46. Fard MA, Fakhree S, Eshraghi B. Correlation of optical coherence tomography parameters with clinical and radiological progression in patients with symptomatic optic pathway gliomas. Graefes Arch Clin Exp Ophthalmol. 2013;251(10):2429–36.

47. Gu S, Glaug N, Cnaan A, Packer RJ, Avery RA. Ganglion cell layer-inner plexiform layer thickness and vision loss in young children with optic pathway gliomas. Invest Ophthalmol Vis Sci. 2014;55(3):1402–8.
48. Hepokur M, Sarici AM. Investigation of retinal nerve fiber layer thickness and ganglion cell layer-inner plexiform layer thickness in patients with optic pathway gliomas. Graefes Arch Clin Exp Ophthalmol. 2018;256(9):1757–65.
49. Sahinoglu-Keskek N, Altan-Yaycioglu R, Canan H, Coban-Karatas M, Erbay A, Yazici N, et al. Measurements of retinal nerve fiber thickness and ganglion cell complex in neurofibromatosis type 1, with and without optic pathway gliomas: a case series. Curr Eye Res. 2018;43(3):424–7.
50. Avery RA, Hwang EI, Ishikawa H, Acosta MT, Hutcheson KA, Santos D, et al. Handheld optical coherence tomography during sedation in young children with optic pathway gliomas. JAMA Ophthalmol. 2014;132(3):265–71.
51. Avery RA, Cnaan A, Schuman JS, Trimboli-Heidler C, Chen CL, Packer RJ, et al. Longitudinal change of circumpapillary retinal nerve fiber layer thickness in children with optic pathway gliomas. Am J Ophthalmol. 2015;160(5):944–52 e1.
52. McKeag D, Lane C, Lazarus JH, Baldeschi L, Boboridis K, Dickinson AJ, et al. Clinical features of dysthyroid optic neuropathy: a European Group on Graves' Orbitopathy (EUGOGO) survey. Br J Ophthalmol. 2007;91(4):455–8.
53. Hallin ES, Feldon SE, Luttrell J. Graves' ophthalmopathy: III. Effect of transantral orbital decompression on optic neuropathy. Br J Ophthalmol. 1988;72(9):683–7.
54. Ben Simon GJ, Syed HM, Douglas R, Schwartz R, Goldberg RA, McCann JD. Clinical manifestations and treatment outcome of optic neuropathy in thyroid-related orbitopathy. Ophthalmic Surg Lasers Imaging. 2006;37(4):284–90.
55. Neigel JM, Rootman J, Belkin RI, Nugent RA, Drance SM, Beattie CW, et al. Dysthyroid optic neuropathy. The crowded orbital apex syndrome. Ophthalmology. 1988;95(11):1515–21.
56. Goncalves AC, Gebrim EM, Monteiro ML. Imaging studies for diagnosing Graves' orbitopathy and dysthyroid optic neuropathy. Clinics. 2012;67(11):1327–34.
57. Goncalves AC, Silva LN, Gebrim EM, Monteiro ML. Quantification of orbital apex crowding for screening of dysthyroid optic neuropathy using multidetector CT. AJNR Am J Neuroradiol. 2012;33(8):1602–7.
58. Wang JK, Kardon RH, Kupersmith MJ, Garvin MK. Automated quantification of volumetric optic disc swelling in papilledema using spectral-domain optical coherence tomography. Invest Ophthalmol Vis Sci. 2012;53(7):4069–75.
59. Kupersmith MJ, Sibony P, Mandel G, Durbin M, Kardon RH. Optical coherence tomography of the swollen optic nerve head: deformation of the peripapillary retinal pigment epithelium layer in papilledema. Invest Ophthalmol Vis Sci. 2011;52(9):6558–64.
60. Forte R, Bonavolonta P, Vassallo P. Evaluation of retinal nerve fiber layer with optic nerve tracking optical coherence tomography in thyroid-associated orbitopathy. Ophthalmologica. 2010;224(2):116–21.
61. Perez-Rico C, Rodriguez-Gonzalez N, Arevalo-Serrano J, Blanco R. Evaluation of multifocal visual evoked potentials in patients with Graves' orbitopathy and subclinical optic nerve involvement. Doc Ophthalmol. 2012;125(1):11–9.
62. Anderson D, Faber P, Marcovitz S, Hardy J, Lorenzetti D. Pituitary tumors and the ophthalmologist. Ophthalmology. 1983;90(11):1265–70.
63. Unsold R, Hoyt WF. Band atrophy of the optic nerve. The histology of temporal hemianopsia. Arch Ophthalmol. 1980;98(9):1637–8.
64. Kanamori A, Nakamura M, Matsui N, Nagai A, Nakanishi Y, Kusuhara S, et al. Optical coherence tomography detects characteristic retinal nerve fiber layer thickness corresponding to band atrophy of the optic discs. Ophthalmology. 2004;111(12):2278–83.
65. Danesh-Meyer HV, Carroll SC, Foroozan R, Savino PJ, Fan J, Jiang Y, et al. Relationship between retinal nerve fiber layer and visual field sensitivity as measured by optical coherence tomography in chiasmal compression. Invest Ophthalmol Vis Sci. 2006;47(11):4827–35.

66. Monteiro ML, Leal BC, Moura FC, Vessani RM, Medeiros FA. Comparison of retinal nerve fibre layer measurements using optical coherence tomography versions 1 and 3 in eyes with band atrophy of the optic nerve and normal controls. Eye. 2007;21(1):16–22.
67. Costa-Cunha LV, Cunha LP, Malta RF, Monteiro ML. Comparison of Fourier-domain and time-domain optical coherence tomography in the detection of band atrophy of the optic nerve. Am J Ophthalmol. 2009;147(1):56–63 e2.
68. Sousa RM, Oyamada MK, Cunha LP, Monteiro MLR. Multifocal visual evoked potential in eyes with temporal hemianopia from chiasmal compression: correlation with standard automated perimetry and OCT findings. Invest Ophthalmol Vis Sci. 2017;58(11):4436–49.
69. Al-Louzi O, Prasad S, Mallery RM. Utility of optical coherence tomography in the evaluation of sellar and parasellar mass lesions. Curr Opin Endocrinol Diabetes Obes. 2018;25(4):274–84.
70. Moura FC, Medeiros FA, Monteiro ML. Evaluation of macular thickness measurements for detection of band atrophy of the optic nerve using optical coherence tomography. Ophthalmology. 2007;114(1):175–81.
71. Garway-Heath DF, Poinoosawmy D, Fitzke FW, Hitchings RA. Mapping the visual field to the optic disc in normal tension glaucoma eyes. Ophthalmology. 2000;107(10):1809–15.
72. Shin HY, Park HY, Choi JA, Park CK. Macular ganglion cell-inner plexiform layer thinning in patients with visual field defect that respects the vertical meridian. Graefes Arch Clin Exp Ophthalmol. 2014;252(9):1501–7.
73. Sun M, Zhang Z, Ma C, Chen S, Chen X. Quantitative analysis of retinal layers on three-dimensional spectral-domain optical coherence tomography for pituitary adenoma. PLoS ONE. 2017;12(6):e0179532.
74. Yum HR, Park SH, Park HY, Shin SY. Macular ganglion cell analysis determined by cirrus HD optical coherence tomography for early detecting chiasmal compression. PLoS ONE. 2016;11(4):e0153064.
75. Moon CH, Lee SH, Kim BT, Hwang SC, Ohn YH, Park TK. Diagnostic ability of retinal nerve fiber layer thickness measurements and neurologic hemifield test to detect chiasmal compression. Invest Ophthalmol Vis Sci. 2012;53(9):5410–5.
76. Moon CH, Hwang SC, Ohn YH, Park TK. The time course of visual field recovery and changes of retinal ganglion cells after optic chiasmal decompression. Invest Ophthalmol Vis Sci. 2011;52(11):7966–73.
77. Akashi A, Kanamori A, Ueda K, Matsumoto Y, Yamada Y, Nakamura M. The detection of macular analysis by SD-OCT for optic chiasmal compression neuropathy and nasotemporal overlap. Invest Ophthalmol Vis Sci. 2014;55(7):4667–72.
78. Monteiro ML, Cunha LP, Costa-Cunha LV, Maia OO Jr, Oyamada MK. Relationship between optical coherence tomography, pattern electroretinogram and automated perimetry in eyes with temporal hemianopia from chiasmal compression. Invest Ophthalmol Vis Sci. 2009;50(8):3535–41.
79. Monteiro ML, Hokazono K, Cunha LP, Oyamada MK. Correlation between multifocal pattern electroretinography and Fourier-domain OCT in eyes with temporal hemianopia from chiasmal compression. Graefes Arch Clin Exp Ophthalmol. 2012;251(3):903–15.
80. Moon CH, Hwang SC, Kim BT, Ohn YH, Park TK. Visual prognostic value of optical coherence tomography and photopic negative response in chiasmal compression. Invest Ophthalmol Vis Sci. 2011;52(11):8527–33.
81. Kerrison JB, Lynn MJ, Baer CA, Newman SA, Biousse V, Newman NJ. Stages of improvement in visual fields after pituitary tumor resection. Am J Ophthalmol. 2000;130(6):813–20.
82. Findlay G, McFadzean RM, Teasdale G. Recovery of vision following treatment of pituitary tumours; application of a new system of assessment to patients treated by transsphenoidal operation. Acta Neurochir. 1983;68(3–4):175–86.
83. Gnanalingham KK, Bhattacharjee S, Pennington R, Ng J, Mendoza N. The time course of visual field recovery following transphenoidal surgery for pituitary adenomas: predictive factors for a good outcome. J Neurol Neurosurg Psychiatry. 2005;76(3):415–9.

84. Monteiro ML, Zambon BK, Cunha LP. Predictive factors for the development of visual loss in patients with pituitary macroadenomas and for visual recovery after optic pathway decompression. Can J Ophthalmol. 2010;45(4):404–8.
85. Cohen AR, Cooper PR, Kupersmith MJ, Flamm ES, Ransohoff J. Visual recovery after transsphenoidal removal of pituitary adenomas. Neurosurgery. 1985;17(3):446–52.
86. Barzaghi LR, Medone M, Losa M, Bianchi S, Giovanelli M, Mortini P. Prognostic factors of visual field improvement after trans-sphenoidal approach for pituitary macroadenomas: review of the literature and analysis by quantitative method. Neurosurg Rev. 2012;35(3):369–78; discussion 78–9.
87. Jacob M, Raverot G, Jouanneau E, Borson-Chazot F, Perrin G, Rabilloud M, et al. Predicting visual outcome after treatment of pituitary adenomas with optical coherence tomography. Am J Ophthalmol. 2009;147(1):64–70 e2.
88. Danesh-Meyer HV, Wong A, Papchenko T, Matheos K, Stylli S, Nichols A, et al. Optical coherence tomography predicts visual outcome for pituitary tumors. J Clin Neurosci. 2015;22(7):1098–104.
89. Ohkubo S, Higashide T, Takeda H, Murotani E, Hayashi Y, Sugiyama K. Relationship between macular ganglion cell complex parameters and visual field parameters after tumor resection in chiasmal compression. Jpn J Ophthalmol. 2012;56(1):68–75.
90. Monteiro MLR. Macular ganglion cell complex reduction preceding visual field loss in a patient with chiasmal compression with a 21-month follow-up. J Neuroophthalmol. 2018;38(1):124–7.
91. Yu WJ, Xiao J, Wang GX, Jiang C, Zha W, Liao RF. Predictive visual field outcomes after optic chiasm decompressive surgery by retinal vessels parameters using optical coherence tomography angiography. Int J Ophthalmol. 2024;17(2):365–73.

OCT and Multiple Sclerosis

11

Sezgi Kaçar, Eva M. M. Strijbis, Christina Gerth-Kahlert, Axel Petzold, Sven Schippling, and James V. M. Hanson

Abstract

Multiple sclerosis (MS) is a chronic, currently incurable neurologic disease, which frequently affects the visual system. Optical coherence tomography (OCT) facilitates the viewing of retinal neurons and axons in vivo, and this has enabled researchers and clinicians to better characterise neurodegeneration and inflammation in MS. In this updated review, we discuss the effects of MS on the retinal layers and complexes, and emphasise the importance of optic neuritis (ON) as a confounding variable; the retinal ganglion cells and their axons are particularly vulnerable to damage in patients with MS, a process

S. Kaçar · E. M. M. Strijbis
MS Center Amsterdam, Neurology, Vrije Universiteit Amsterdam, Amsterdam Neuroscience, Amsterdam UMC Location VUmc, Amsterdam, The Netherlands
e-mail: S.Kacar@amsterdamumc.nl

E. M. M. Strijbis
e-mail: E.Strijbis@amsterdamumc.nl

C. Gerth-Kahlert · J. V. M. Hanson (✉)
Department of Ophthalmology, University Hospital Zurich and University of Zurich, Zurich, Switzerland
e-mail: James.Hanson@usz.ch

C. Gerth-Kahlert
e-mail: Christina.Gerth-Kahlert@usz.ch

A. Petzold
The National Hospital for Neurology and Neurosurgery, Queen Square, London, UK
e-mail: A.Petzold@nhs.net

Moorfields Eye Hospital, City Road, London, UK

S. Schippling
Neuroscience and Rare Diseases (NRD), Roche Pharma Research and Early Development (pRED), Basel, Switzerland
e-mail: Sven.Schippling@roche.com

A. Grzybowski and P. Barboni (eds.), *OCT and Imaging in Central Nervous System Diseases*, https://doi.org/10.1007/978-3-031-72156-4_11

that is exacerbated by ON. We also discuss the relationships between OCT parameters and other outcome measures such as clinical rating scales, magnetic resonance imaging (MRI), electrophysiology, and blood-based biomarkers that are increasingly used in clinical care and trials in MS. Finally, we discuss the evidence regarding OCT findings and treatment response, and the use of OCT as an outcome measure in MS clinical trials.

Keywords

Multiple sclerosis (MS) • Optic neuritis (ON) • Optical coherence tomography (OCT) • Retinal nerve fibre layer (RNFL) • Ganglion cell and inner plexiform layer (GCIP) • Inner nuclear layer (INL) • Microcystic macular oedema (MMO) • Magnetic resonance imaging (MRI) • Neurofilament light chain (NfL) • Neurodegeneration • Disease-modifying therapies (DMTs) • Optical coherence tomography angiography (OCTA)

Abbreviations

AI	Artificial intelligence
AQP4	Aquaporin-4 antibodies
Aβ	Beta-amyloid
BM	Bruch's membrane
BMO-MRW	Bruch's membrane opening-minimum rim width
BPF	Brain parenchymal fraction
BVMT-R	Revised Brief Visuospatial Memory Test
CIS	Clinically isolated syndrome
CMO	Cystoid macular oedema
CNS	Central nervous system
CRION	Chronic relapsing inflammatory optic neuropathy
CSF	Cerebrospinal fluid
CVF	Cerebral volume fraction
CVLT-II	California Verbal Learning Test, second edition
DCP	Deep capillary plexus
DMT	Disease-modifying therapy
DVP	Deep vascular plexus
EBV	Epstein-Barr virus
EDSS	Expanded Disability Status Scale
ELM	External limiting membrane
ERG	Electroretinogram
ET-1	Endothelin-1
ETDRS	Early treatment diabetic retinopathy study
EZ	Ellipsoid zone
FAZ	Foveal avascular zone
FLAIR	Fluid-attenuated inversion recovery
GCC	Ganglion cell complex
GCIP	Ganglion cell-inner plexiform layer

GCL	Gangion cell layer
HC	Healthy control subject
HCVA	High-contrast visual acuity
HRF	Hyperrreflective focii
IEAD	Inter-eye absolute difference
IEPD	Inter-eye percentage difference
IgA	Immunoglobulin A
IgG	Immunoglobulin G
INL	Inner nuclear layer
IPL	Inner plexiform layer
LCVA	Low-contrast visual acuity
LHON	Leber's hereditary optic neuropathy
MD	Mean deviation
MF-ERG	Multifocal electroretinogram
MF-VEP	Multifocal visual evoked potential
MMO	Microcystic macular oedema
MOG	Myelin oligodendrocyte glycoprotein
MOGAD	Myelin oligodendrocyte glycoprotein-associated disease
MOGAD-ON	Myelin oligodendrocyte glycoprotein-associated disease optic neuritis
MRI	Magnetic resonance imaging
MS	Multiple sclerosis
MS-ON	Multiple sclerosis optic neuritis
MSSS	Multiple sclerosis severity score
MTP	Macular thinning predominant
NAD	Nicotinamide adenine dinucleotide
NAWM	Normal-appearing white matter
NEDA	No evidence of disease activity
NEI-VFQ-25	National Eye Institute Visual Function Questionnaire 25
NfL	Neurofilament light chain
NMOSD	Neuromyelitis optica spectrum disorder
NMOSD-ON	Neuromyelitis optica spectrum disorder optic neuritis
OCT	Optical coherence tomography
OCTA	Optical coherence tomography angiography
ON	Optic neuritis
ONHC	Optic nerve head component
ONL	Outer nuclear layer
OPL	Outer plexiform layer
PERG	Pattern electroretinogram
PhNR	Photopic negative response
PHOMS	Peripapillary hyper-reflective ovoid mass-like structures
PMB	Papillo-macular bundle
POMS	Paediatric-onset multiple sclerosis
PPMS	Primary progressive multiple sclerosis
PRL	Photoreceptor layer

RAPD	Relative afferent pupil defect
RGC	Retinal ganglion cell
RION	Relapsing isolated optic neuritis
RIS	Radiologically isolated syndrome
RNFL	Retinal nerve fibre layer
RPC	Radial peripapillary capillaries
RRMS	Relapsing-remitting multiple sclerosis
SC	Spinal cord
SCP	Superficial capillary plexus
SDMT	Symbol Digit Modalities Test
SD-OCT	Spectral-domain optical coherence tomography
SPMS	Secondary progressive multiple sclerosis
SPC	Superficial vascular complex
SVP	Superficial vascular plexus
TD-OCT	Time-domain optical coherence tomography
TMV	Total macular volume
VA	Visual acuity
VD	Vessel density
VEP	Visual evoked potential

11.1 Background

11.1.1 Multiple Sclerosis, Optic Neuritis (ON) and Differential Diagnosis

Multiple sclerosis (MS) is a highly heterogeneous autoimmune neurological disorder characterized by inflammation, demyelination, and neuroaxonal degeneration within the central nervous system (CNS). It is the leading cause of neurological disability among young adults worldwide [1]. The precise aetiology remains unknown and may be multifactorial, with a range of environmental factors, including Epstein-Barr virus (EBV) infection, appearing to act against the background of a complex polygenetic trait [2]. It is believed that, initially, the disease is predominantly driven by aberrant peripheral immune cells, including T- and B-cells, that, upon (re)activation, target CNS myelin antigens [2]. MS frequently manifests with an initial inflammatory and demyelinating event affecting the CNS, termed clinically isolated syndrome (CIS) [3]. Current diagnostic criteria require evidence of clinical or radiological disease activity dissemination in both time and space, and allow a diagnosis of MS to be made based on a single clinical event when confirmed by radiological evidence of previous disease activity [4].

Relapsing–remitting MS (RRMS) is the most common form of MS and is characterised by clinical episodes of inflammatory demyelination ('relapses') followed by periods of variable recovery and relatively stable neurological status ('remissions') [3, 4]. Patients initially diagnosed with RRMS may develop a gradual, progressive accumulation of disability independently of relapses, defined as secondary progressive MS (SPMS); alternatively, a minority of patients may exhibit progressive disease activity in the absence of relapses from disease onset, defined as primary progressive MS (PPMS) [3, 4]. In addition to these phenotypical classifications, MS may also be described as clinically or radiologically active, with or without evidence of disease progression [3]. A related condition is radiologically isolated syndrome (RIS), in which asymptomatic patients present with radiological signs of demyelination [3, 5, 6]. The evidence of demyelination is typically an incidental finding when performing brain magnetic resonance imaging (MRI) scans in the evaluation of, for example, headache. There is an approximately 50% risk of conversion to MS in the 5 years after a diagnosis of RIS [3, 5, 6].

Children can also be diagnosed with MS. A small proportion (approximately 2–10%) of MS patients are diagnosed below the age of 16 years, referred to as paediatric-onset MS (POMS) [7]. The relapsing–remitting subtype is by far the most common in POMS patients, and the relapse rate is often higher in comparison to adult MS patients [8].

Despite a highly heterogeneous clinical presentation and disease course, involvement of the visual system is a near-ubiquitous hallmark of MS [9, 10]. The most common manifestation in the afferent visual pathway is optic neuritis (ON), an acute or subacute inflammation of the optic nerve [11, 12], which is the first clinical sign of CIS in over a fifth of patients [13]. Post-mortem evidence of pathological changes to the optic nerve has also been documented in up to 86% of MS eyes, suggesting that ON may also occur asymptomatically [14–17]. It should be noted that ON may also occur idiopathically, in systemic disease, and in immunological conditions other than MS [13] such as myelin oligodendrocyte glycoprotein (MOG)-associated disease (MOGAD) or neuromyelitis optica spectrum disorder (NMOSD); however, for the purpose of this overview, the nomenclature ON should be understood to refer only to that associated with MS and CIS unless stated otherwise. This prevalence of anterior visual pathway involvement, the accessibility of the retina for viewing retinal neurons and their axons in vivo, and the unmyelinated nature of ganglion cell axons within the retina (unique within the CNS), has generated considerable interest in the anterior visual pathway as a model for research in MS [18]. Much of this interest has been facilitated by the development of optical coherence tomography (OCT) and its increasing use in neurological clinics.

Other important entities to be considered in the differential diagnosis of MS are NMOSD and MOGAD [19–23]. Both are specific antibody-mediated diseases with clinical features overlapping with those of MS. Cell-based assays for serologic testing of aquaporin-4 (AQP4) and MOG-antibodies have high specificity [24, 25], but may not always be available in the clinic. Discriminating MS from NMOSD and MOGAD is important because of differences in prognosis and treatment. Differences in ON characteristics between these diseases, as assessed using OCT, may play an important role in aiding accurate diagnosis [19–23]. Differential diagnosis of these conditions using OCT is discussed in more detail in Sect. 11.3.2.

Since the first retinal OCT scans were acquired in 1991 [26], the introduction of spectral-domain OCT (SD-OCT) has offered higher resolution and acquisition speed than previous time-domain OCT (TD-OCT) technology [27]. This has permitted the development of automated or semi-automated software algorithms enabling the definition and delineation of the boundaries separating the retinal layers (Fig. 11.1), in addition to coarse measures of retinal thickness such as total macular volume (TMV). These layers and complexes include the retinal nerve fibre layer (RNFL), which is most commonly measured around the optic nerve head (pRNFL) but may also be measured at the central macular region (mRNFL); the ganglion cell layer (GCL); inner plexiform layer (IPL); the inner nuclear layer (INL); the outer plexiform layer (OPL); the outer nuclear layer (ONL); and the photoreceptor layer (PRL). As the boundary between GCL and IPL may be difficult to visualise and accurately define, these layers are typically combined and described as the ganglion cell and inner plexiform layer (GCIP or GCIPL are equally acceptable abbreviations [28]; throughout this work, GCIP will be used for consistency). However, different proprietary software algorithms and studies may choose to additionally aggregate or otherwise classify layers of the retina (e.g., INL-OPL; outer retinal layers, ORL; ganglion cell complex, GCC). Whichever approach individual laboratories or researchers choose when conducting OCT research in MS patients, transparent and precise definition of the relevant retinal structures is vital [28]. This process of retinal layer delineation, referred to as segmentation, has led to a large and growing body of literature examining the structure of the full range of retinal layers and complexes in the eyes of patients with MS.

11.1.2 OCT Quality Control

Since OCT is increasingly used in neurology clinics as objective evidence for a diagnosis of ON and MS, and there is increasing interest in OCT as a predictor for disability progression and treatment response as an outcome measure in clinical trials [29, 30], it is paramount that measurements and image quality assessments are standardised. The OSCAR-IB consensus criteria [31] are the first OCT quality guidelines validated for use in MS research. These guidelines emphasise the importance of signal strength, scan centration, algorithm performance (i.e., errors of automated segmentation), absence of co-existing retinal pathology (which may affect OCT interpretation), fundus illumination, beam placement, and exclusion of any other obvious acquisition errors when assessing OCT data. Application of the OSCAR-IB criteria has been shown to result in high inter-rater agreement regarding the acceptance or rejection of scans in multi-centre studies [31, 32], and may thus maximise the reproducibility of OCT studies. Recent work analysing the reliability of inter-rater, multi-centre manual correction of automatically segmented OCT scans, utilising the OSCAR-IB criteria, recorded excellent agreement between raters, in particular for the inner retinal layers [33]. The agreement between raters appeared to be greater than in previous work predating the

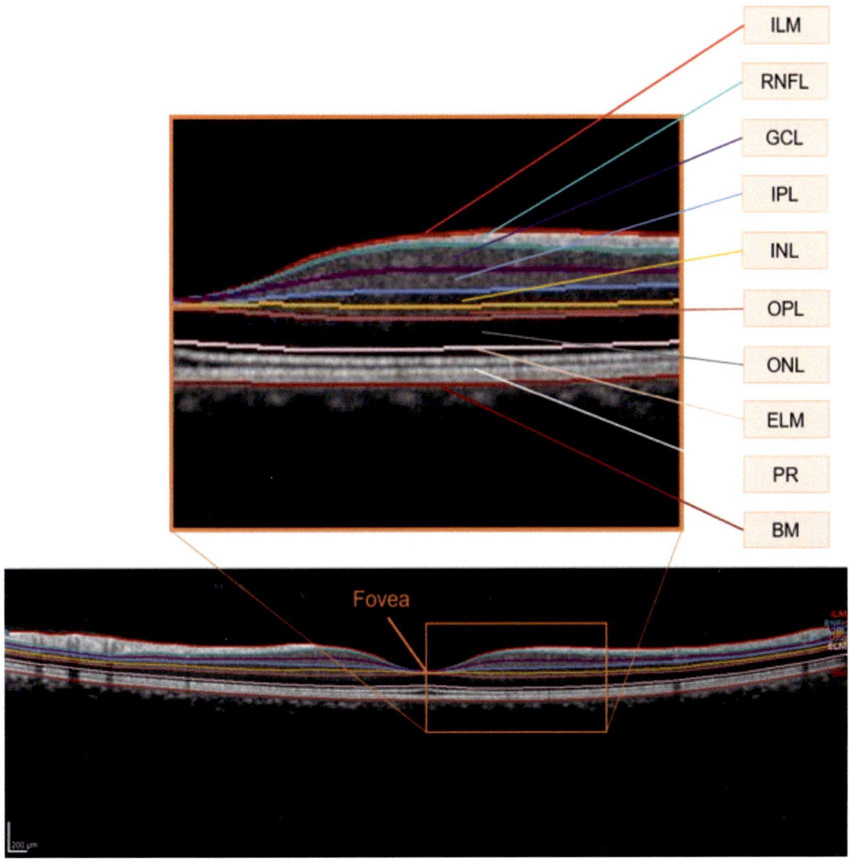

Fig. 11.1 Segmented macula OCT B-scan of a healthy individual, showing the delineation of the retinal layers. ILM: inner limiting membrane; RNFL: retinal nerve fibre layer; GCL: ganglion cell layer; IPL: inner plexiform layer; INL: inner nuclear layer; OPL: outer plexiform layer; ONL: outer nuclear layer; ELM: external limiting membrane; PRL: photoreceptor layer; BM: Bruch's membrane. Note that GCL and IPL are typically aggregated to form the ganglion cell and inner plexiform layer (GCIP), and other layers may also be aggregated, depending on the segmentation software used and/or aims of individual studies

OSCAR-IB criteria [34]. We therefore recommend adherence to the OSCAR-IB criteria at all times when evaluating OCT scans, and to the APOSTEL recommendations for describing OCT scan protocols and analyses [28] (described in detail in Chap. 3), whenever publishing results of OCT studies in MS patients.

We also recommend that all OCT scans for any study are segmented using identical software, as different versions of the same proprietary software have been shown to produce small but significant differences in axonal thickness in patients with MS and control subjects [35]. For large studies or clinical trials, the use of dedicated external staff blinded to patient status to quantify OCT outcome measures may minimise bias and sources of error [36].

11.2 OCT Findings in Patients with MS

11.2.1 Adult MS with ON

Clinically confirmed episodes of ON occur in approximately 70% of MS patients during their disease course, typically during the relapsing–remitting phase [13]. Although presentation is variable, symptoms of ON commonly include reduced vision, periocular or retrobulbar pain (which typically worsens upon eye movements), and altered colour perception [37, 38]. Visual phenomena such as scintillations and/or phosphenes may also be reported [38]. Clinical signs upon examination may include reduced high- and/or low-contrast visual acuity (HCVA; LCVA), a relative afferent pupillary defect (RAPD), perimetric abnormalities (central scotoma [39], centrocecal scotoma, paracentral scotoma, or diffusely reduced sensitivity [40]), and abnormalities on colour vision testing [37] (although note that MS patients without previous ON may display similar abnormalities of colour vision [41]). Swelling of the optic nerve head is visible on fundoscopy in approximately one third of patients [37], with the remainder presenting with a normal fundus appearance due to inflammation being confined to the retrobulbar portion of the optic nerve. Visual function typically recovers spontaneously over a period of weeks to months [42], however many patients experience persistent visual impairment such as reduced LCVA and residual impairment of colour vision perception, with corresponding measures of visual-related quality of life being reduced [43]. The Pulfrich phenomenon, caused by inter-ocular differences in afferent conduction velocity consequent to unilateral demyelination, may be noticed by patients during the recovery phase [38]. These visual findings may be observed even when HCVA returns to normal or near-normal levels [44–46]. Treatment with corticosteroids may accelerate clinical recovery after ON [47] and reduce the risk of progression to MS over approximately two years [48], but has minimal effect on visual outcome [47, 48]. However, hyperacute initiation of steroid treatment may aid preservation of visual acuity (VA) and retinal layers [49], as discussed in Sect. 11.5.2. Given these factors, and the fact that MS patients have been shown to rate vision as their most important bodily function irrespective of disease duration and disability [50], it is clear that ON is of vital importance in the study of MS. Retinal injury is currently believed to occur following inflammatory demyelination and axonal damage of the optic nerve by a process of retrograde degeneration toward the retinal ganglion cells [51].

OCT examination of MS or CIS patients with a history of ON almost invariably reveals reduced pRNFL [52–66]. Meta-analyses have quantified this loss of pRNFL as an average of just over 20 μm relative to healthy control subjects both with SD-OCT and TD-OCT [58, 59]. Considerable inter-individual variation has been documented [57], likely reflecting the heterogeneity both of clinical outcomes after ON and in MS generally. However, this figure of 20 μm refers to the pRNFL averaged over 360° around the optic nerve head; when the superior, inferior, temporal and nasal quadrants are compared, the temporal quadrant may be the most sensitive in visualising and quantifying axonal loss after ON [53,

67–71]. Thickness of the pRNFL in the papillomacular bundle (PMB), comprised of axons from the foveal region and the area between the fovea and optic nerve head which are anatomically separate from the predominating arcuate organisation of RNFL axons, has been reported to be the most sensitive OCT parameter in blinded detection of previous ON despite its inclusion not increasing the overall sensitivity of such analyses [69]. Preferential involvement of the temporal and PMB RNFL would be consistent with the reported predominance of central and centrocecal visual field defects in ON [39, 40]. Thickness of the superior and inferior quadrants is also significantly reduced after ON in MS patients [53, 68, 72, 73], whilst the balance of evidence to date suggests that the nasal quadrant is relatively unaffected [53, 68, 69, 72, 73]. Loss of pRNFL appears to have plateaued by approximately six to 12 months after the first symptoms of ON [53, 56, 57]. An inter-ocular pRNFL thickness difference of more than 5–6 μm is strongly suggestive of a previous unilateral ON [74].

In addition to subacute axonal loss following ON, patients experience ongoing loss of RNFL as a consequence both of MS itself and the normal aging process. The majority of evidence to date suggests that the underlying rate of RNFL loss does not differ between MS eyes with and without previous ON [75, 76]; in other words, the significant insult to RNFL after ON is independent of, and does not affect, the insidious neurodegenerative processes ongoing in the majority of MS patients. In both of these studies, the effect of subacute axonal loss was removed from the analyses by excluding patients with a history of ON within the previous six months [75, 76].

In addition to pRNFL, the thickness of mRNFL is also reduced after ON in MS and CIS patients [59, 63–65] by, on average, just over 6 μm [59]. This loss of thickness is considerably less than that measured in the pRNFL [58, 77], and therefore pRNFL is likely to be a more powerful outcome measure than mRNFL when investigating axonal integrity in ON. pRNFL offers the additional advantages of being quicker to measure and requiring less post-hoc correction (typically one B-scan rather than, e.g., 19).

GCIP thickness has almost universally been found to be reduced following an episode of ON in MS (Fig. 11.2) and CIS patients [43, 55–57, 59, 61, 63–65, 70, 78, 79]. A meta-analysis reported an average GCIP thickness loss of just over 16 μm in MS-ON eyes compared to those of healthy control (HC) subjects [59]. Furthermore, parafoveal and perifoveal GCL thicknesses were found to be lower in MS patients with ON history [80]. When analysing GCIP after ON, a prospective study demonstrated that GCIP thinning was greater in RRMS patients that reported a higher baseline GCIP thickness, consistent with a plateau effect [81]. Focal thickness maps of GCIP, display a characteristic horseshoe-like thickness reduction pattern (U Zone) in MS patients when compared to HCs, which was more pronounced in MS-ON eyes [82, 83].

Despite the subacute loss of GCIP following ON, the underlying rate of GCIP loss does not differ between MS eyes with and without ON [75, 76]. Despite this similarity with pRNFL, GCIP offers important advantages as an outcome measure following ON. One factor already alluded to is that while approximately two

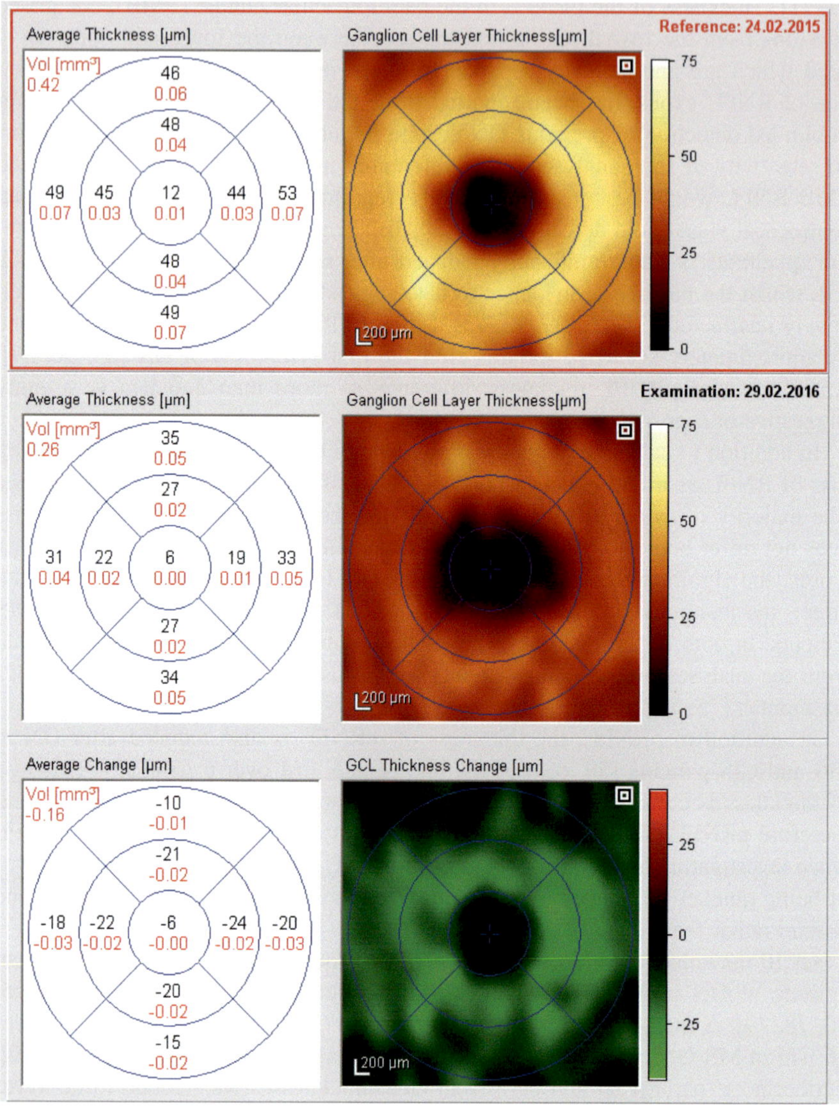

Fig. 11.2 OCT thickness maps of the ganglion cell layer (GCL) of a multiple sclerosis (MS) patient with optic neuritis (ON), showing OCT data acquired in the acute phase of ON (top) and one year later (middle). Atrophy of the GCL has followed ON, reflected in the thinner GCL at follow-up and in the negative thickness change values when the two examinations are compared (bottom). Although GCL is typically aggregated with the inner plexiform layer (IPL) as ganglion cell and inner plexiform layer (GCIP) for quantitative analysis, with this particular proprietary software it is not possible to generate thickness maps for GCIP and so only GCL is shown

thirds of ON patients present with retrobulbar inflammation of the optic nerve, the remaining third present with peripapillary oedema visible on fundoscopy [37]. (In fact, subsequent work employing OCT has suggested that as many as 82% of patients may have increased pRNFL thickness during the acute phase of ON [84], suggesting superior sensitivity of OCT at enabling detection of peripapillary oedema compared to traditional fundoscopy). A consequence of this is that pRNFL thickness during the acute phase of ON, when baseline OCT measurements are ideally acquired, is frequently increased relative to the fellow eye and/or control subjects due to inflammatory oedema [43, 56, 57, 78, 84]. Therefore, it is difficult to ascribe the reduction of pRNFL thickness after the acute phase of ON to either resolution of oedema or axonal loss in isolation, and some authors have suggested that it may be prudent to wait at least three months following an episode of ON before attempting to quantify pRNFL loss (Fig. 11.3) [13, 85].

In contrast, the evidence to date shows that GCIP thickness is not increased relative to that of unaffected contralateral eyes of ON patients [55, 78] or healthy control subjects [78, 86] during the acute phase of ON, and thus assessment of GCIP may enable earlier detection of inner retinal atrophy after ON in MS patients [57]. Supporting this hypothesis, thinning of GCIP appears to have plateaued by approximately three to six months following the clinical onset of ON [56, 57], a considerably shorter period than for pRNFL. Evidence also suggests that analysis of inter-ocular differences in GCIP thickness is more sensitive in detecting a previous ON episode than pRNFL thickness differences [79]. An additional consideration is that GCIP may be less likely to be affected by the presence of non-pathological anatomical variations such as optic disc drusen or ectopically myelinated retinal nerve fibres.

Despite these undoubted advantages of GCIP, pRNFL remains a useful and robust measure of retinal atrophy following ON, with the practical advantage that its segmentation and quantification is quicker and easier than that of GCIP. An understanding of the potential confounding factors described above will assist the clinician when assessing patients with ON using OCT.

With regard to the effects of ON upon the INL, results are more mixed than for the inner retinal layers, with some authors recording some small degree of INL thickening (Fig. 11.4) [61, 65, 78, 87, 88] and others finding INL thickness comparable to normal values [43, 55, 57, 63]. Results may differ even between separate studies from the same laboratory [55, 78], which may reflect differences in sample size and thus statistical power. A meta-analysis including many hundreds of eyes detected an average macular INL thickening in MS eyes with previous ON of 0.77 μm relative to control subjects, and 0.61 μm relative to MS eyes without previous ON [59]. Similarly, a subsequent meta-analysis of data from 11 studies revealed a slight thickening in INL after both ON and non-ON clinical relapses, suggesting that the INL may reflect inflammatory processes in the CNS [89].

An important potential confounding factor associated with INL assessment after ON is the link with microcystic macula oedema (MMO), discussed in detail in Sect. 11.5.1. Interpretation of previous work is made more difficult by the fact

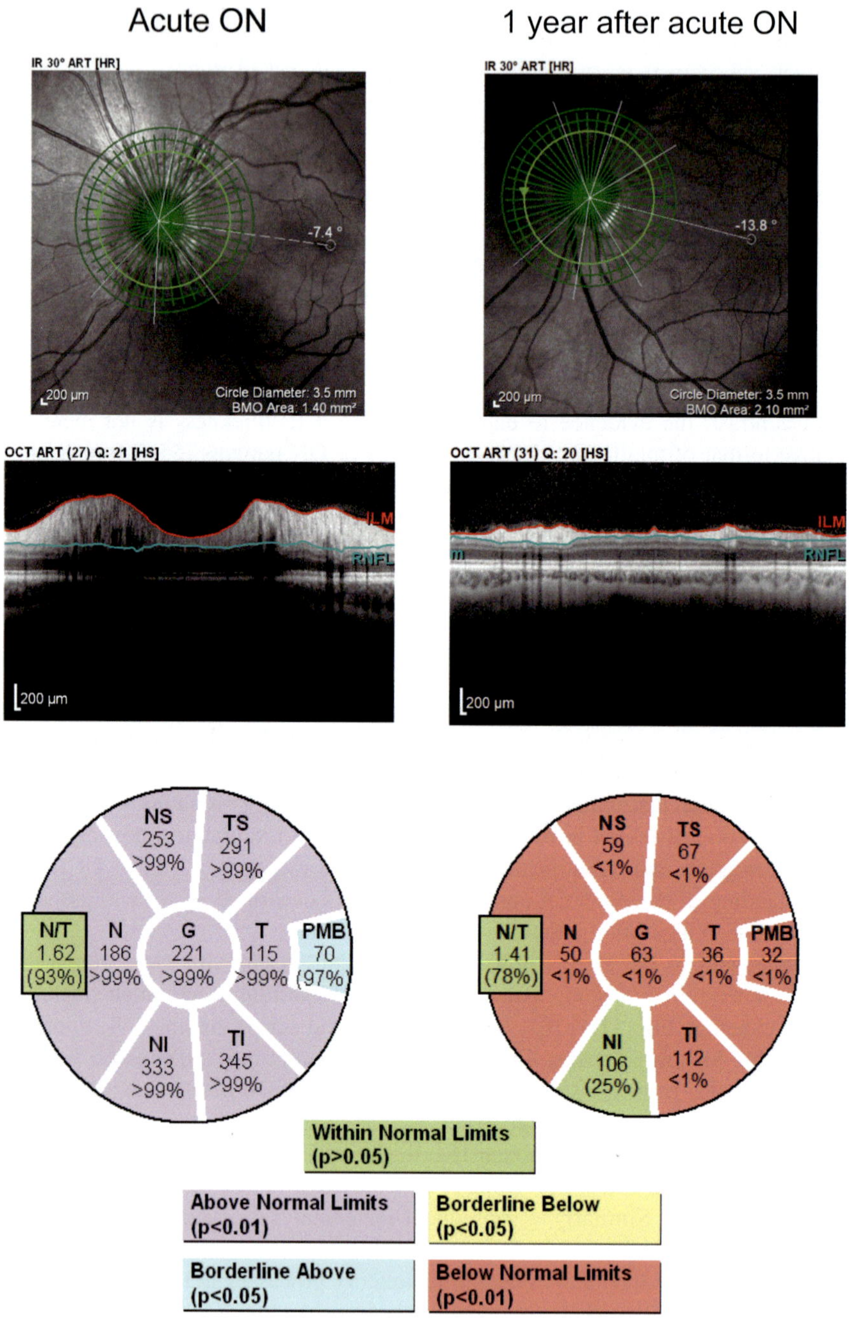

Fig. 11.3 OCT scans of the peripapillary retinal nerve fibre layer (pRNFL) in a patient with acute optic neuritis (ON) (left), and in a different patient one year after ON (right). The patient with acute ON has inflammatory oedema at the optic nerve head, which is reflected in pRNFL thickness measurements significantly thicker than normal values, whereas the patient one year after acute ON shows significant atrophy of the pRNFL, with thickness values reduced compared to normal values

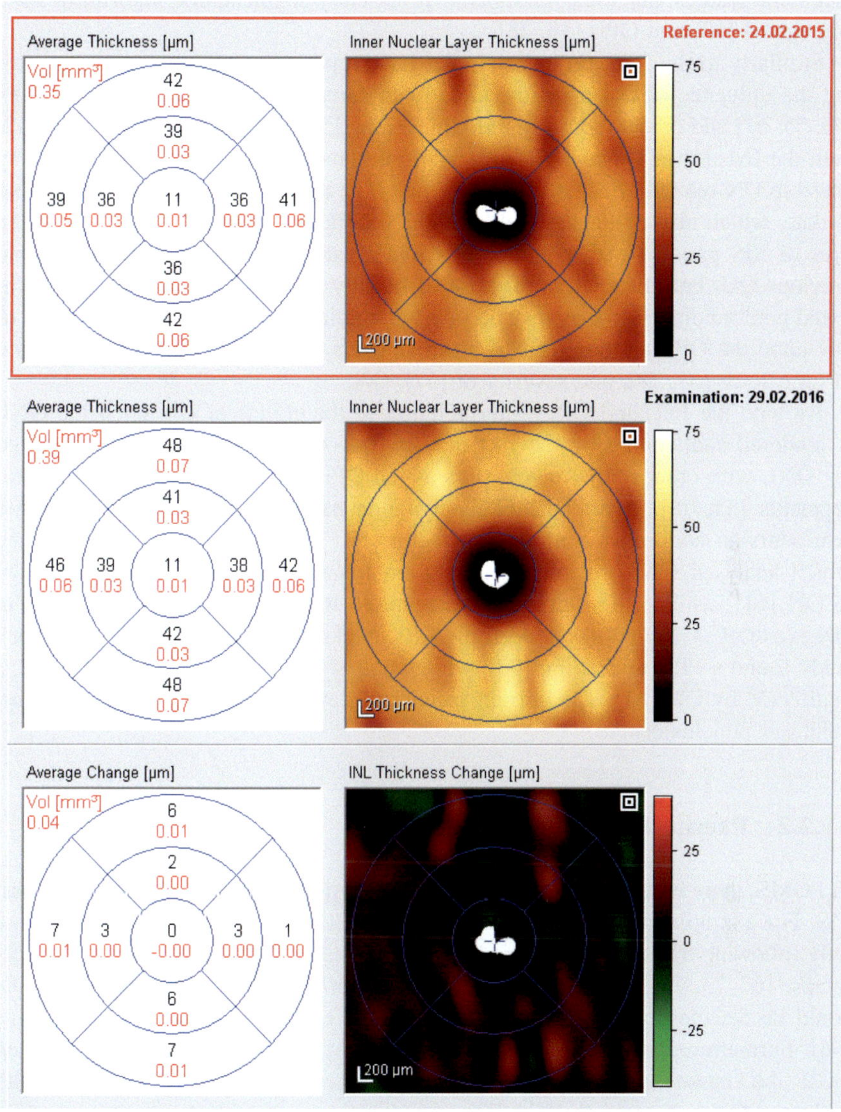

Fig. 11.4 OCT thickness maps of the inner nuclear layer (INL) of a multiple sclerosis (MS) patient with optic neuritis (ON), showing OCT data acquired in the acute phase of ON (top) and one year later (middle). INL is slightly thicker at follow-up, reflected in the small positive thickness change values when the two examinations are compared (bottom)

that some studies and some versions of proprietary segmentation algorithms have aggregated INL and OPL [55, 78].

Similarly to the INL, previous studies have reported conflicting results regarding the influence of ON upon the OPL, with some reporting no influence of ON [43, 55, 61] and others reporting mild thickening [57, 78]. Aggregation of the OPL with the INL [55, 78] and ONL [43, 57] in the majority of studies may mask any possible ON related effect restricted to the OPL; the only meta-analysis available to date, which also aggregated OPL and ONL, showed minimal thickening in the eyes of MS patients with previous ON relative to those of MS patients without previous ON, but not relative to those of healthy control subjects [59]. An additional confounding factor as revealed by longitudinal analyses is that the effect of ON upon the OPL and aggregated layers appears dynamic, varying as a function of time since [57, 78], and severity of [57], ON.

As with the INL and OPL, interpretation of the effects of ON upon the ONL is rendered challenging by the fact that the majority of studies have aggregated the ONL with other retinal layers such as the OPL [43, 57, 59], or photoreceptor segments [55, 78]. Again, the likely dynamic nature of any thickness changes represents an additional confounding factor [57, 78]. One of the studies to date which analysed ONL thickness in isolation found no measurable effect related to ON [61], whilst other authors have reported thickening of the outer retina in ON eyes [59, 90]. Findings concerning PRL thickness differ between studies; one study found a PRL thickening [90], while another demonstrated that the PRL was unaffected by ON [61]. The current paucity of data makes it challenging to draw definitive conclusions.

11.2.2 Paediatric-Onset MS with ON

In POMS, there is similar involvement of the anterior visual pathway to adult-onset MS. For example, a reduction in RNFL and GCIP thicknesses was recorded not only following a first ON episode but also, to a lesser degree, following a non-ON relapse [67, 73, 91–95]. Earlier research also reported that previous subclinical ON could be detected by analyzing interocular RNFL differences in POMS patients [96]. Furthermore, similar to adult-onset MS [95], reduced temporal pRNFL and GCIP thicknesses were recorded in the unaffected eyes of POMS patients with unilateral ON compared to HCs [92].

A growing area of interest is the use of OCT to distinguish between MS and other CNS-related disorders (see also Sect. 11.3.2), which is also relevant to the differential diagnosis of paediatric demyelinating disorders. For instance, recent research has demonstrated that in paediatric MOGAD-ON patients, global atrophy of pRNFL was more pronounced than in POMS-ON patients, while in POMS-ON patients, thinning of the temporal quadrant was found to be more severe [93]. Nasal quadrant pRNFL thickness was the most accurate in differentiating paediatric MOGAD-ON and POMS-ON, followed by global average thickness

[93]. Furthermore, children with MS display less pronounced RNFL swelling in ON-affected eyes compared to children with monophasic demyelination [92].

11.2.3 Adult MS Without ON

pRNFL thickness is reduced in the eyes of CIS, MS and RIS patients without previous ON relative to healthy control subjects [44, 60, 64, 65, 67, 73, 97–105] (Fig. 11.5). Meta-analyses have quantified this loss of thickness in MS patients as being, on average, just over 7 μm whether measured with SD-OCT or TD-OCT technology [58, 59]. Thickness of the temporal quadrant of pRNFL has been suggested to be preferentially affected by MS [73], although other studies failed to observe this pattern in eyes without previous ON [67]. Likewise, sparing of the nasal quadrant has been proposed [73] but not confirmed [67]. Some of these differences may be attributable to subtly different RNFL quantifications obtained by different OCT devices [106]. Longitudinal studies of RNFL atrophy shows that MS eyes without a history of ON undergo an average decline in RNFL thickness of between 0.5–1.5 μm per year [75, 76, 107], approximately 3–10 times faster than in healthy control subjects. This rate of decline is highest in the early stages of the disease (up to approximately 10 years of disease duration) and thereafter declines, consistent with a plateau effect [76]. The inverse relationship between RNFL atrophy rate and disease duration (Fig. 11.6) may explain the different annual RNFL loss rates obtained in different studies in cohorts with varying average disease duration [76]. Supporting this hypothesis, other authors recorded higher annual RNFL atrophy rates in RRMS patients with disease duration < 3 years compared to those with disease duration 3–10 years, suggesting a floor effect in patients with longer-established disease [108].

mRNFL has also been shown to be thinned in MS patients [64, 65, 97], but by an average of just over 2 μm relative to normal individuals [59]; therefore, as in MS eyes with previous ON (Sect. 11.2.1), mRNFL may be of lesser utility as an outcome measure than pRNFL. Additionally, mRNFL has been suggested to be less reliable than pRNFL due to the density of vascular perfusion between the fovea and optic nerve head potentially causing artefact-based segmentation errors [63]. These factors, combined with the relatively recent development of macular segmentation algorithms compared to software able to reliably quantify pRNFL, have ensured that pRNFL remains the more widely studied outcome measure in MS research.

In addition to the RNFL, the thickness of GCIP is also reduced in the eyes of MS and CIS patients without previous ON [55, 64, 65, 97, 98, 100–103, 109–111]. GCIP thinning was found to be, on average, 6.3 μm in MS patients relative to control subjects [59]. Using the 1, 2.22, and 3.45 mm Early Treatment Diabetic Retinopathy Study (ETDRS) grid centred on the fovea, it was shown that average GCIP thickness declined by 0.9 μm over two years in MS patients without previous ON, a rate of loss approximately double that observed in healthy individuals [76]. A similar study also found that MS patients lost GCIP thickness just

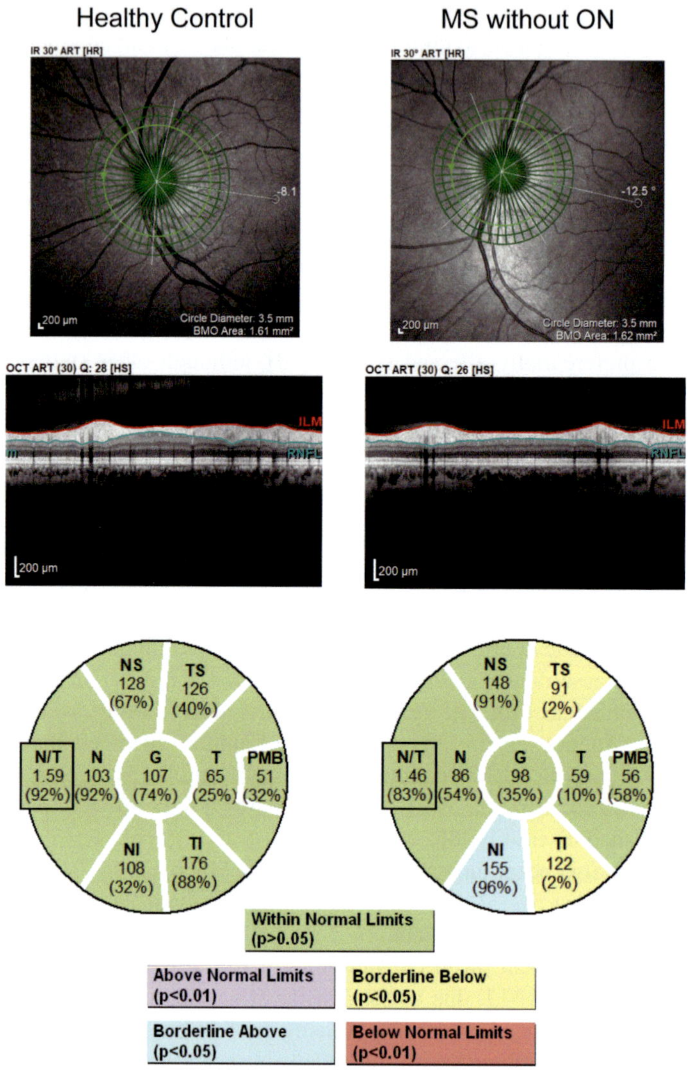

Fig. 11.5 pRNFL analysis from the left eyes of a healthy individual and a patient with multiple sclerosis (MS) without previous optic neuritis (ON), obtained from a Spectralis OCT device (Heidelberg Engineering, Heidelberg, Germany). The global averaged (G) thickness is reduced in the patient with MS relative to the healthy individual, as are the thicknesses of the majority of the individual sectors. In the case of the temporal superior (TS) and temporal inferior (TI) sectors, thickness is below the 95th percentile of age-matched normal values and so is classified as borderline below average (and colour-coded yellow) by the proprietary software. The borderline above average thickness in the nasal inferior (NI) sector in the MS patient is an artefact caused by a retinal blood vessel

over twice as fast as control subjects [107], although quantitative rates of GCIP loss cannot be compared between the two studies due to different OCT devices, acquisition protocols, and retinal areas analysed. As with the RNFL, annual rates of GCIP loss appear to be inversely related to disease duration (Fig. 11.6) [76].

In contrast to the RNFL and GCIP of the inner retina, the INL thickness in MS patients seems to not differ significantly from that of control subjects [65, 66, 101, 110] and appears to remain stable in the eyes of MS patients without ON irrespective of disease duration (Fig. 11.6), at least over a two year period [76]. However, disease activity, treatment status, and (indirectly) disease duration may influence these results [102]. For instance, other authors, using OCT, have suggested that INL (in addition to ONL) may be reduced in thickness in a subset of MS patients exhibiting a severe clinical phenotype [112], and that increased INL thickness is associated with higher levels of disease activity, as evidenced both clinically and through MRI [113]. The INL contains the nuclei of the second-order retinal neurons, bipolar cells, as well as horizontal cells, amacrine cells, and the cell bodies of Müller glia [114]. Interest in the INL amongst MS researchers was initially driven by an influential post-mortem histological study which recorded atrophy of the INL in addition to the ganglion cells [15]. Rather than being a marker for neurodegeneration like the inner retina, the INL currently holds promise as a biomarker for inflammatory disease activity and response to disease-modifying therapy in MS. OCT thus has the potential to objectively capture and quantify the two main hallmarks of MS disease activity, neuronal degeneration and inflammation.

Studies of the structure of the retina distal to the INL are, at the time of writing, challenging to interpret because some studies aggregate two or more of the retinal layers for analyses (e.g., INL & OPL [64]; ONL & PRL [55]). However, published studies to date have consistently found no effects of MS on the thickness of the retinal layers distal to INL [59, 61, 64, 65, 90, 102, 103].

It has been proposed that OCT may be used to define novel MS phenotypes defined by primary retinal pathology (i.e., structural and/or functional changes unrelated to a history of ON) [112]. These authors documented a subset of their MS cohort who exhibited thinning of the macula in the presence of normal RNFL thickness relative to normative data, with segmentation revealing thinning of both the INL and ONL, a phenotype the authors named "macular thinning predominant" (MTP) [112]. No MTP eyes had a prior history of ON, and no significant differences in INL or ONL thickness were observed between non-MTP MS patients and healthy controls [112]. Clinically, MTP-MS patients were found to have reduced HCVA and LCVA and higher Expanded Disability Status Scale (EDSS; the most widely accepted and most broadly applied measure of clinical disability in MS patients) scores when compared to non-MTP MS patients [112]. Subsequent works were unable to confirm the existence of a distinct subset of MS patients consistent with the proposed MTP phenotype [64, 115] and found INL thinning in the absence of ONL changes only in patients with PPMS [103]. Differences in OCT hardware, software, and manufacturer-specific normative databases, as well as in patient populations, doubtless contribute to this apparent dichotomy. However, functional evidence consistent with similarly ON-independent abnormalities of the

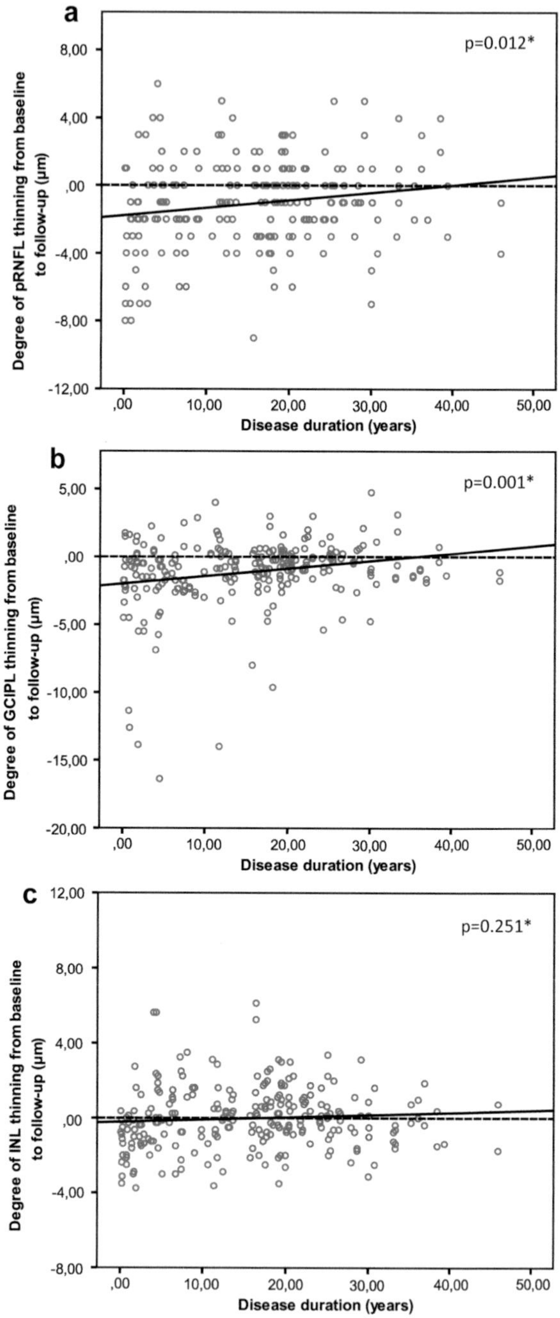

Fig. 11.6 Scatter plots showing the degree of thinning of the peripapillary retinal nerve fibre layer (pRNFL, a), ganglion cell and inner plexiform layer (GCIP; here GCIPL, b), and inner nuclear layer (INL, c) over a two year period in patients with multiple sclerosis (MS). RNFL and GCIP loss was greater in patients with a lower disease duration, whilst INL remained approximately constant over the study period, irrespective of disease duration. Generalised estimating equation (GEE) analyses were corrected for age, sex, history of ON, and inter-eye associations. Reproduced from Balk et al. **Journal of Neurology** 263, 1323–1331 (2016) under the terms of the Creative Commons CC BY license

retinal layers distal to GCIP in patients with MS has been credibly reported by a number of authors working independently [61, 109, 116–119], and INL atrophy in MS eyes has been histologically confirmed post-mortem [15].

11.2.4 Progressive MS

Although the majority of patients with MS exhibit a relapsing–remitting disease course (RRMS), and thus the majority of the studies above relate mainly to RRMS and CIS patients, researchers have also measured differences in OCT parameters between the different MS phenotypes. Patients with progressive forms of MS (PPMS; SPMS) show reduced RNFL thickness compared to patients with RRMS [60, 120], and HCs [103, 120, 121]. As would be expected, GCIP is similarly reduced [103, 120, 121]. INL and, in some [90, 103, 120] but not all [61] studies also ONL, appears thinned in patients with PPMS relative to HCs [103, 120, 122]. In addition, faster rates of retinal thinning were recorded in patients with PPMS compared to those with RRMS and HCs, which were independent of the use of disease-modifying therapies (DMTs) [122]. Findings with regard to the OPL in progressive MS are not unanimous [103, 120], whilst PRL thickness has been reported to be thinner in patients with progressive MS relative to control subjects but comparable to that of patients with RRMS. It should be noted that some OCT parameters are influenced by age [120]. For example, annual rate of GCIP thinning is highest in patients in the youngest quartiles and stabilizes with older age [123], and cross-sectional INL thickness is higher in younger patients [124]. However, pRNFL, GCIP, INL, and ONL thinning rates were found to be independent of aging in progressive MS patients [122].

11.2.5 OCTA Findings in MS

Recent developments in OCT technology have led to the commercial availability of OCT angiography (OCTA), which is able to evaluate both arterial and venous density at the retina and optic nerve head down to the capillary level (Fig. 11.7) [125]. Retinal vascular abnormalities such as periphlebitis have long been known to exist in some patients with MS [73, 126], but precise examination and quantification of the vessels with OCT was not possible until the introduction of OCTA. An important consideration, however, is that some technical limitations remain. First, there is reduced signal strength in the optic nerve head area, making it much more challenging to reliably image the deeper vascular plexuses, particularly in the presence of papillary oedema such as that often occurring in ON. Another known limitation is the presence of imaging artefacts (e.g., due to motion, blinking, and loss of focus), which are more prevalent in MS patients with longer disease duration or a history of ON [127].

Nevertheless, recent work using OCTA has further improved our understanding of retinal pathology in MS. There is a reduction of capillary flow and vessel density

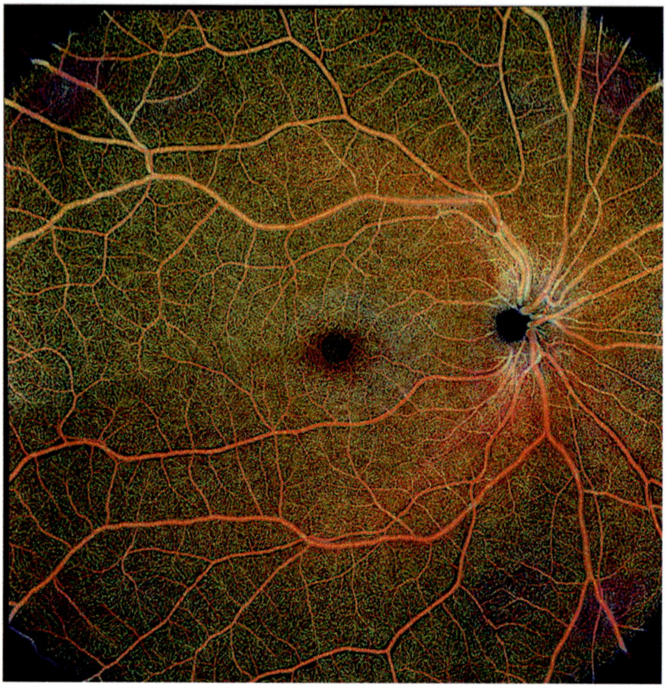

Fig. 11.7 Composite of wide-field OCTA scan in a healthy right eye, performed on a Plex Elite 9000 (Carl Zeiss Meditec). Reproduced from Kleerekooper et al. **Brain** 143, 1999–2008 (2020) with the permission of Oxford University Press and Dr. Iris Kleerekooper

in MS patients compared to healthy control subjects [128–132], which is seen in MS patients with or without a history of ON [128, 129, 133] but is slightly more pronounced in ON eyes [134–137]. Vessel density of both the superficial and deep vascular plexuses (SVP and DVP, respectively) is also found to be lower in MS patients compared to HCs [130–132, 138], as is retinal tissue perfusion [139].

Perfusion of the optic nerve head (as quantified by the density of visible vessels) has also been shown to be reduced in MS eyes compared to control subjects, independent of ON history [140]. Loss of the superficial vascular complex (SVC) was reported to reach a plateau after 180 days after acute ON in RRMS and CIS patients [141]. Additionally, a larger foveal avascular zone (FAZ) area was found in the eyes of RRMS patients [131] and in both CIS and RRMS patients within the first 180 days of an acute ON episode [141]. Furthermore, a larger FAZ was also found in RRMS patients compared to HCs [131], as in MS and NMOSD patients compared to HCs (Fig. 11.8) [142]. Increased vessel density in the choriocapillaris may also be associated with future disease activity in MS [135], via an as-yet-unknown mechanism.

With regard to the relationships between OCTA and disability, results are mixed. Some authors have suggested an association of reduced superficial vascular plexus

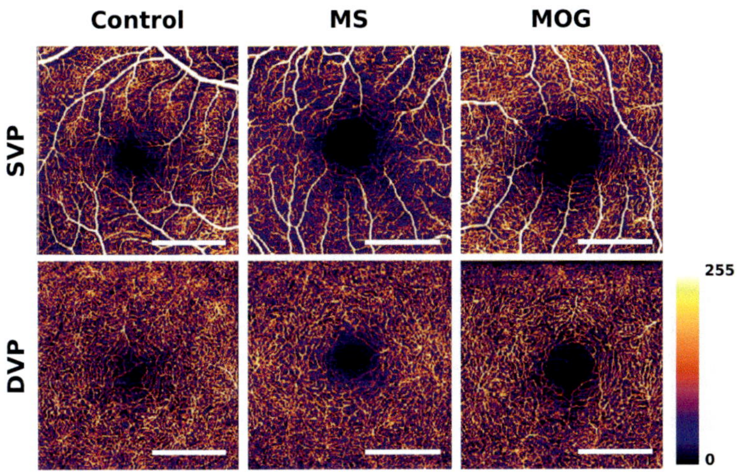

Fig. 11.8 OCTA scans of single eyes of a healthy control subject (HC; 'Control'), a patient with multiple sclerosis (MS), and a patient with myelin oligodendrocyte glycoprotein (MOG) antibody-associated disease, showing the macular superficial vascular plexus (SVP; above) and the deep vascular plexus (DVP; below). These scans were made in eyes without previous optic neuritis (ON). The foveal avascular zone (FAZ) of the HC eye is smaller than those of the MS or MOG patients. Scale bar: 1 mm. Scans are 3 × 3 mm and obtained with the Heidelberg Engineering OCT2 system. Reproduced from Kleerekooper et al. **Frontiers in Neurology** 11, (2020) under the terms of the Creative Commons CC BY license

(SVP) density with disability worsening in general, but also more impaired visual function [137]. However, other authors have recorded a generalised increase in retinal vessel density in RRMS patients, particularly in the SVP, which was related to EDSS worsening, increased disease duration, and reduced LCVA [143]. It is hypothesized that this may occur due to inflammation and related angiogenesis in MS patients [143–145]. Longitudinal and well-controlled studies are needed to resolve this apparent dichotomy.

11.3 Diagnosis and Differential Diagnosis of MS Using OCT

11.3.1 OCT as a Diagnostic Tool for ON or MS

OCT can serve as paraclinical evidence to support a definitive diagnosis of ON in cases where this is clinically suspected [29, 146]. For instance, inter-eye percentage- and absolute differences of the GCIP (IEPD; IEAD) demonstrated a high discriminative power for MS diagnosis in young patients without co-morbidity [147]. The diagnostic accuracy of IEPD and IEAD of the GCIP was also found to be high in patients with longstanding MS [148]. MS patients with asymptomatic optic nerve lesions also have, on average, thinner temporal and global pRNFL thicknesses and GCIP volume, and are likely underdiagnosed [16].

Other studies provide unique class I evidence that the IEPD of pRNFL and GCIP could be utilized for the detection of asymptomatic optic nerve lesions in patients with CIS [17] and MS [149]. IEPD may be a particularly valuable outcome measure due to its dimensionless nature, potentially facilitating easier comparison of data obtained from different OCT devices or locations [149]. A multi-centre study demonstrated that the IEAD of GCIP and pRNFL thickness ($\geq$ 4 or $\geq$ 5 μm, respectively) may aid the identification of unilateral optic nerve lesions [150, 151]. A greater inter-eye difference (IED) in HCVA and LCVA was also found to be correlated with greater intereye RNFL asymmetry [151]. Additionally, IEAD and IEPD measures could also discriminate between bilateral and unilateral ON in MS, thereby implying the possibility of using OCT in the determination of dissemination in space in patients with suspected of having MS and thus aiding MS diagnosis [148]. Another promising line of research is the use of deep learning to accurately detect previous ON in MS patients, which has recently been reported to be feasible using pRNFL ring scans [152].

In addition, inferonasal and mean GCIP and pRNFL thicknesses were reported to predict subsequent development of MS in patients with acute ON [153]. Another study recently demonstrated that the diagnostic accuracy of OCT in MS further improves when pRNFL is adjusted per eye according to individual ocular anatomical (e.g., retinal vessel density, optic disc area) and other (e.g. refractive error, age) factors [154]. Combining compensated pRNFL thickness with macular GCIP thickness further improved diagnostic accuracy [154].

11.3.2 OCT Findings and Differential Diagnosis of Other Causes of ON

As discussed in Sect. 11.1.1, NMOSD and MOGAD have clinical characteristics that frequently overlap with MS but have a different aetiology and prognosis. The likelihood of regaining normal visual acuity after ON is worse in NMOSD and MOGAD than in MS [19, 155], and episodes of ON typically require more aggressive treatment with high dose corticosteroids as early as possible [22, 156]. In the absence of a sufficient response to steroid treatment, plasmapheresis may be indicated [156–158]. Since differentiating between MS and NMOSD/MOGAD is sometimes difficult in the absence of unequivocal serological evidence (for example, not all NMOSD patients are aquaporin-4 antibody [AQP4] seropositive [20, 21]), OCT scans may potentially aid the diagnostic process. Table 11.1 shows the differences in clinical, OCT, MRI and VEP measures between MS-ON, MOGAD-ON and NMOSD-ON patients.

Reduced pRNFL and GCIP thickness was found in NMOSD patients relative to MS patients [159]. Another study also found that definite or "potential" NMOSD patients had significantly lower pRNFL, mRNFL, GCIP, and TMV thicknesses

Table 11.1 Differences in clinical and paraclinical outcome measures between optic neuritis due to multiple sclerosis (MS-ON), myelin-oligodendrocyte glycoprotein antibody-associated disease (MOGAD-ON), and neuromyelitis optica spectrum disorder (NMOSD-ON)

	MS-ON	MOG-ON	NMO-ON
Clinical representation			
Demographics	MS-ON is more often diagnosed in adults than children, is more prevalent in young females in childbearing age	MOG-ON is approximately equally diagnosed between adults and children, has an equivalent male–female prevalence (1:1)	NMOSD-ON is more often diagnosed in adults than in children. NMOSD-ON has a female predominance (9:1), an approximate age of onset of 40 years
Antibody against	Not known	MOG	AQP4
Clinical manifestation			
Symptoms	Subacute (< 2 weeks) monocular loss of vision and pain which worsens on eye movements. Reduced colour and contrast vision, RAPD	Frequently binocular, frequent disc oedema and pain worsening on eye movements. Frequent severe loss of central vision at presentation and profound loss of colour vision with good recovery, better in children than in adults	Unilateral and binocular loss of vision. If binocular frequently without pain worsening with eye movements because of intracranial involvement of the optic nerves/ chiasm. Severe loss of vision with less favorable recovery than in MS-ON and MOG-ON
OCT findings after ~ 3 months			
pRNFL	Diffuse atrophy	Severe atrophy including PMB	Severe atrophy

(continued)

Table 11.1 (continued)

mGCIP	Peri-macular atrophy (doughnut)	Severe doughnut atrophy	Severe atrophy (can be altitudinally pronounced)
OPL	Preserved	Preserved/thickened	Preserved/thickened (MMO)
INL	Preserved	Preserved	Preserved
MRI and pattern-reversal VEP findings after < 8 days			
MRI	Mostly, orbital and canalicular, focal optic nerve signal changes	Mostly anterior, orbital optic nerve signal changes, frequently visualised as perineuritic and diffuse enhancement of the orbital fat	MRI of orbits frequently demonstrates more posterior optic nerve enhancement than in MS-ON, including the optic chiasm
VEP	Occasionally non-recordable, subsequently delayed peak (P100). Amplitudes may be reduced	Frequently non-recordable, subsequently delayed peak (P100). Amplitudes are reduced	Frequently non-recordable, subsequently delayed peak (P100) and reduced amplitudes

AQP4: Aquaporin-4; INL: inner nuclear layer; mGCIP: macular ganglion cell-inner plexiform complex; MMO: microcystic macular oedema; MRI: magnetic resonance imaging; OCT: optical coherence tomography; ON: optic neuritis; OPL: outer plexiform layer; PMB: papillomacular bundle; pRNFL: peripapillary retinal nerve fibre layer; RAPD: relative afferent pupillary defect; VEP: visual evoked potential. Adapted from Bennett et al. **Lancet Neurology** 22, 89–100 (2023)

compared to both HCs and MS patients, independent of a history of ON [160]. IEDs, both absolute and percentages, were found to have high discriminative power for unilateral ON in AQP4-positive NMOSD patients [161]. Furthermore, pRNFL thickness can aid in discriminating MOGAD-ON from MS-ON by showing a greater thickening in the symptomatic eye when compared to the unaffected contralateral eye or a prior baseline in MOGAD-ON patients [162].

Distinctive patterns of neuronal damage across the retina after ON were found in NMOSD and MS patients; in NMOSD, GCIP thinning occurred predominantly from the fovea to the parafovea, while in MS, retinal ganglion cell (RGC) loss was approximately equally distributed across the macula [163]. In addition, ON in MS, NMOSD, and MOGAD causes visual dysfunction of differing severity, with HCVA loss per μm of pRNFL and GCIP thinning greater in NMOSD than in MS and MOGAD patients [164]. Other authors have provided further evidence for poorer visual acuity in NMOSD-ON patients compared to MOGAD-ON [164] or MS-ON patients [164, 165], with GCIP also being thinnest in NMOSD-ON [166].

Furthermore, authors using OCTA have documented reduced macular vessel density and perfusion density in NMOSD eyes relative to MS eyes [159]. Parafoveal and peripapillary vascular changes were also observed in MS and NMOSD patients, which differed in magnitude and pattern between both groups:

in MS, the parafoveal and peripapillary vessel density (VD) was significantly associated with visual acuity and visual field defects, while this association only existed for the peripapillary vessel density in NMOSD patients [167]. Additionally, peripapillary and macular VD and FAZ was decreased in NMOSD-ON eyes compared to MS-ON and HC eyes, and also in AQP4-negative NMOSD-ON patients compared to MS-ON patients [168]. Also, differences in foveal pit morphology were reported in AQP4-positive NMOSD patients compared to MS patients [169].

In summary, OCT and OCTA findings may be of value in distinguishing MOGAD patients, AQP4-positive NMOSD and MS, particularly when serological testing is unavailable or produces ambiguous results [23, 170, 171] The Acute Optic Neuritis Network (ACON) has developed an international multicentre study protocol to increase the understanding of treatment strategies and diagnostic classifications between acute demyelinating ON in AQP4-positive patients, MOG-positive patients, and patients with MS, which will be a valuable aid to clinicians in the future [172].

11.4 Association of OCT Outcomes with Clinical, Structural, and Functional Measures in MS

Despite the manifold benefits of OCT, it remains fundamentally an examination of retinal and optic nerve head structure only; it is currently not possible to perform concurrent measurements of retinal, optic nerve head, or visual function in a manner analogous to (e.g.) functional magnetic resonance imaging (fMRI) of the brain. In MS clinics and research settings, OCT is frequently combined with the quantification of global disability and other structural (e.g., MRI) and/or functional (e.g., visual acuity, retinal or cortical electrophysiology) measures. Here, we examine the relationships between OCT and these different outcome measures.

11.4.1 Visual Function

Clinical tests of visual function have been extensively used in studies in MS. Perhaps the most fundamental and widely-used test of visual function is the measurement of visual acuity (VA), in which the patient must correctly identify letters, numbers or symbols of diminishing size at a pre-defined test distance. In routine ophthalmological or optometric practice, the test is typically performed using black letters on a retro-illuminated white background, with contrast between target and background maximized; this measure is therefore described as high-contrast visual acuity (HCVA). By using grey letters instead of black, the contrast between letter and background is reduced (e.g., to 2.5% or 1.25% contrast rather than close to 100% in HCVA), and thus the measure becomes that of low-contrast visual acuity (LCVA). Examples of charts for measuring HCVA and LCVA can be seen in Fig. 11.9.

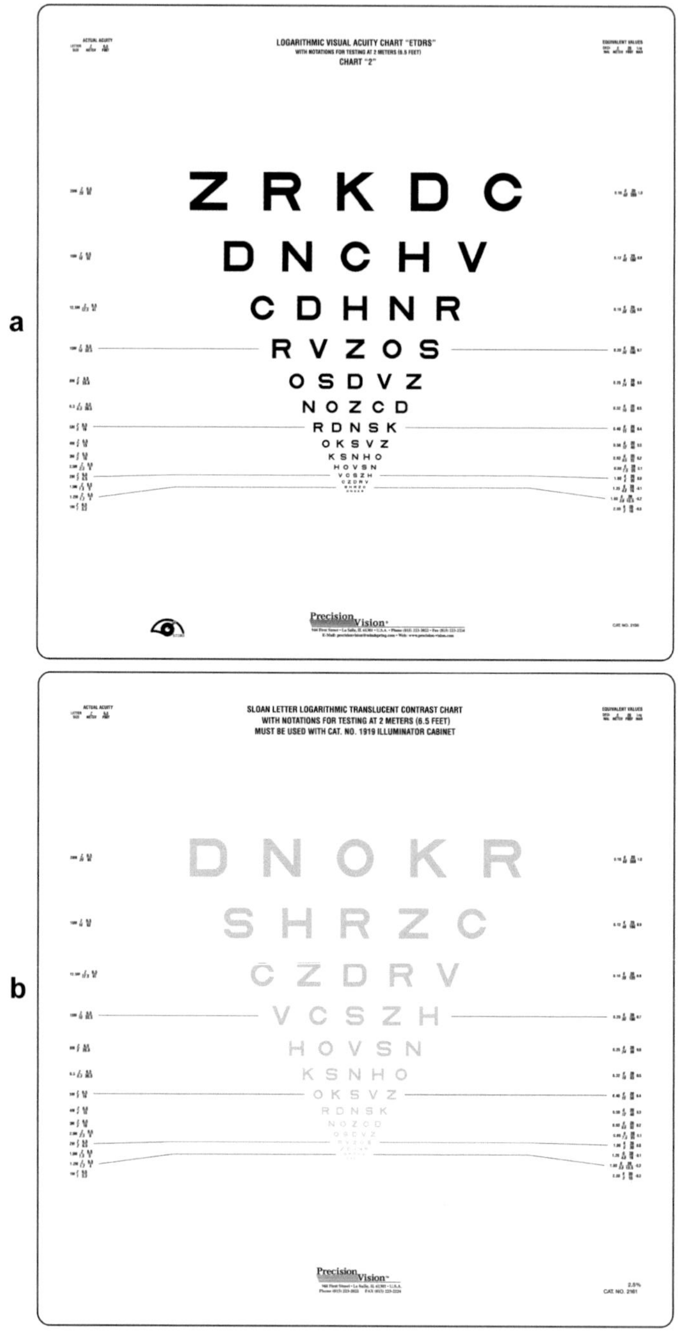

Fig. 11.9 Testing charts for measuring high- and low-contrast visual acuity (HCVA, LCVA). In order to measure HCVA, the contrast between target and background must be as close to 100% as possible, accomplished by using black targets on a white retro-illuminated background (a). Decreasing contrast can be accomplished by altering the colour of the targets from black to grey; the example chart shown here measures 2.5% contrast LCVA (b), but other contrast levels (e.g., 10%) are also possible. Images courtesy of Precision Vision, La Salle IL, U.S.A

Patients with MS are frequently found to have reduced LCVA even when HCVA is normal [16, 173–175], and thus LCVA is considered the more sensitive visual outcome measure in MS [174]. Reduced LCVA is correlated with RNFL thinning cross-sectionally [44, 64, 109, 176–180] and longitudinally [177], although more strongly correlated with thinning of GCIP [64, 176, 180]. LCVA also correlates with PMB thickness, TMV, and foveal volume [179]. Studies have also documented correlations between HCVA and RNFL [44, 64, 176, 177, 179, 180], GCIP [64, 176, 177, 180], and PMB [179] thickness, as well as TMV and foveal volume [179], although some of these relationships are likely to be weaker in comparison to 2.5% contrast LCVA [177] and have not been observed in all studies [109]. A clinically significant decrease in HCVA, 2.5% and 1.25% contrast LCVA is associated with a decrease in peripapillary RNFL thickness of 2.2, 3.3 and 3.3 μm as well as a decrease in GCIP thickness of 1.3, 1.9 and 2.4 μm, respectively [64].

In addition to impaired LCVA, patients with MS are commonly found to have impaired colour vision, in eyes both with and without a history of ON [41, 181], with up to two thirds of patients failing at least one screening test [181]. Studies using OCT have observed that performance in colour vision testing is strongly correlated with thickness of pRNFL [179, 182] and PMB [179, 182], as well as TMV [182], in MS patients. Given that the thicknesses of these retinal layers are reduced in MS eyes with previous ON relative to those without a history of ON [58, 59], it is intuitive that performance in colour vision testing appears worse in those eyes with previous ON [41, 179]. The correlations between OCT and colour vision outcome measures are stronger when using SD-OCT technology than with TD-OCT, likely reflecting the superior resolution and accuracy of the former [179].

A focal thickness reduction of GCIP was also reported to correlate with reduced LCVA in patients without a history of ON [83]; likewise, a positive relationship was found between GCIP and pRNFL thickness and vision-related quality of life [180]. At baseline, GCIP thinning and reduced VA were reported in CIS patients with a history of ON, of which greater baseline GCIP thickness was able to predict improvement of visual function after six months [183]. Poorer VA was also related to elevated levels of B-cell biomarkers in the affected eye of MS patients with an acute ON [184]. Additionally, a reduction in both inner and outer macular volume and layer thicknesses were recorded in MS patients with a history of ON and poor recovery of HCVA, whereas patients in whom HCVA recovered to the equivalent of 1.0 Snellen experienced thinning only of the inner macula layers, similar to patients without previous ON history [185]. Research also demonstrated that a composite score derived from retinal structural and visual functional measurements (GCIP IEDs, GCIP thickness averaged from both eyes, and binocular 2.5% LCVA) enables better discrimination of MS patients and HC than any OCT parameter alone [186].

Perimetry, the subjective measurement of the visual field, may also be employed to ascertain the effects of disease on visual function. The technique is frequently utilized in patients with optic neuropathy, assessing the integrity of the entire visual pathway rather than specifically RGC or optic nerve function [187]. Visual field sensitivity (as measured by the mean deviation [MD] from age-matched normal values in decibels) is reduced in MS patients relative to normal subjects, with the greatest reduction being observed in those eyes with a history of ON [110, 188]. MD was found to be correlated with TD-OCT-derived pRNFL thickness in MS eyes with a history of ON [189, 190], although not with normalised (relative to full retinal thickness) GCIP [191]. At the time of writing, the quantitative relationships between MD and retinal layers distal to GCIP remain unstudied. In addition, the presence of homonymous visual field defects indicative of post-chiasmal lesions has been reported in patients with predominantly RRMS both with and without previous ON [192]. These visual field defects were found to resolve in around 60% of patients but could also recur, and in some patients occurred in the presence of homonymous GCL thinning at the macula. Given the high prevalence of fatigue symptoms in patients with MS [193] and the adverse effects of fatigue on both visual sensitivity and reliability when performing perimetry [187], it is likely that more objective measures of visual function, less dependent on alertness and cognitive performance, may be of greater utility when studying patients with MS.

11.4.2 Disability

Global disability in MS can be assessed using clinical scales such as the EDSS or its variant the multiple sclerosis severity score (MSSS), or using tests for hand function, walking distance and cognition. EDSS scores have been reported as being negatively correlated with RNFL [94, 175, 176, 194–200], although this effect has not consistently been shown in all studies [201, 202]. EDSS also negatively correlates with GCIP thickness [94, 176, 197, 198, 203, 204], although not with TMV [196]. Significant correlations have also been recorded between EDSS and macular thickness in RRMS and SPMS, although not PPMS, patients [176]. The MSSS appears to be unrelated to RNFL thickness [202].

As the majority of MS disability scales may not sufficiently capture all aspects of disability beyond that in the realms of motor function and mobility, and in particular may not adequately reflect visual disability [205], the heterogeneous nature of results regarding the relationships between such scales and OCT is perhaps unsurprising. Despite this, OCT-derived TMV has been found to correlate with ambulatory ability in MS patients [206]. Rating scales focussed on visual function, such as the National Eye Institute Visual Function Questionnaire-25 (NEI-VFQ-25) have been used successfully to capture subjective visual dysfunction in MS patients following ON [43, 207], and this approach may hold promise for future studies in the broader MS population.

Reduced thickness of both RNFL and GCIP are associated with reduced cognitive ability in MS patients [94, 208]. Other studies have confirmed this association with cognition by demonstrating that pRNFL and GCIP thickness seems to be associated with cognitive processing speed, memory, verbal learning and memory, visual learning and memory, and verbal fluency in MS patients regardless of the severity of cognitive impairment [209–211]. Additionally, pRNFL, LCVA, and TMV were reported to be associated with cognitive performance as measured by the revised Brief Visuospatial Memory Test (BVMT-R), Symbol Digit Modalities Test (SDMT), and California Verbal Learning Test, second edition (CVLT-II) [212].

11.4.3 Disability Progression

In addition to cross-sectional associations with disability, OCT has also been shown to predict disability progression in MS patients. Patients with averaged pRNFL thickness of less than 87–88 μm at baseline were approximately twice as likely to show evidence of disability progression (measured by EDSS) over up to three years, and almost four times as likely over five years, as those with an RNFL thickness above this threshold at baseline [213]. Another study also found that an averaged RNFL thickness of 88 μm was associated with a threefold increased risk of disability (EDSS) worsening over three years and a slightly lower, though comparable, risk of accumulating cognitive deficits over the same period [214]. Similarly, a lower TMV at baseline was associated with EDSS progression in MS patients [215] and thinning of the temporal RNFL quadrant was associated with worsening of EDSS and an increased risk of clinical relapses over two years [73]. Furthermore, lower baseline GCIP thickness was associated with long-term worsening of EDSS [216], and lower pRNFL and GCIP thicknesses ($\leq$ 88 and 77 μm, respectively) were found to predict EDSS changes (> 3.0) in early RRMS patients over approximately 5 years [217]. Conversely, another study reported no significant relationships between pRNFL or GCIP thickness and EDSS scores in early CIS and RRMS patients [218]; but it should be noted that the MS cohort in question had little disability (median EDSS 1.0), relatively well-preserved retinal layer thicknesses, and short disease duration.

Using modelling or machine learning approaches, some authors have found that pRNFL thickness may be used to predict MS disease course [217, 219] and MS diagnosis [220], although use of GCIP may enable more accurate prediction of disease course [217].

Annualized rates of RNFL and GCIP loss were reported to be higher in MS patients with EDSS worsening and cognitive deterioration after 6 years [221], with an annual GCIP loss > 1 μm associated with clinical progression and cognitive decline (worsening of EDSS and SDMT, respectively) in RRMS patients [222]. In addition, annualized rates of retinal thinning of the RNFL and GCIP were higher in patients that converted to SPMS than those who remained RRMS, illustrating the potential of OCT to help identify patients that will convert to a progressive disease course [223]. This was also demonstrated by other authors, who recorded that a cut-off rate of annual pRNFL loss of 1.5 μm could discriminate clinically stable from clinically progressing RRMS patients [224]. There is also evidence that measures of GCIP loss may be utilized for early risk stratification of disability accumulation or progression in early CIS and/or RRMS patients [88, 225–227]. Finally, increased baseline INL thickness was associated with a future increase in EDSS in RRMS patients [228].

11.4.4 Magnetic Resonance Imaging (MRI)

MRI remains of vital importance in diagnosis and monitoring of MS patients, with improvements to conventional technology and the development of new imaging techniques increasing sensitivity and permitting measurement of more diffuse CNS pathology [229]. To date, evidence suggests that RNFL thickness in MS patients is related to measures of brain parenchymal fraction (BPF) [230–233] and bicaudate ratio [197], with thinner RNFL being associated with greater brain atrophy, and also positively correlated with volume of both white and grey matter [73, 234–236]. However, the correlation between RNFL and grey matter may only be significant in more advanced MS, rather than at early stages of the disease [237], and some authors have reported that the relationship with white and grey matter may be significant only in eyes without previous ON [204, 236, 238]. Other studies also reported that MS patients with lower pRNFL thicknesses and GCIP volumes were found to have a lower spinal cord (SC) area, which was associated with disease-related disability more than was MRI [230].

RNFL thickness is also associated with MRI lesions in the optic radiations [101, 239–241] and visual cortex [240]. However, RNFL appears not to be associated with non-specific MRI measures of MS disease activity, such as T1 hypo-intense or T2 hyper-intense lesion volumes [73, 237]. GCIP is correlated with brain volume and white matter volume [236], but (as with RNFL) some of these relationships may be significant only in those eyes without previous ON [204, 238]. Faster rates of GCIP loss are associated with correspondingly increased rates of cerebral volume fraction (CVF; a measure of brain volume analogous to BPF) reduction, as well as cortical grey matter and thalamic atrophy, over a four-year period [242]. Another study supports this finding by reporting associations between GCIP thinning and decreased brain parenchymal and myelin volumes in MS and CIS patients [243]. Thinner GCIP and RNFL was also observed in MS patients with leptomeningeal enhancement at baseline [244]. Furthermore, a higher number of paramagnetic rim lesions (PRLs) were associated with lower pRNFL and GCIP thickness in MS patients, thereby suggesting that the presence of PRLs is a sign of a more severe disease course [245]. Finally, INL thickening is associated with prospective T2 hyper-intense and gadolinium-enhancing lesion volume [228].

A particularly interesting aspect of the relationships between OCT and MRI parameters is the finding that different OCT-derived retinal structural measures may be correlated with different MRI outcome measures. For example, in MS eyes RNFL and GCIP thickness were positively correlated with both grey matter and caudate volumes, whilst INL thickness was correlated positively with fluid-attenuated inversion recovery (FLAIR) lesion volume and negatively with normal-appearing white matter (NAWM) volume [204]. The authors reported that whilst these correlations were true of their MS cohort as a whole, they were driven primarily by MS eyes without previous ON [204].

It has been proposed that these differences in the pattern of results between the inner (RNFL; GCIP) and outer (INL) retina may reflect pathologically distinct disease processes in MS [204], a hypothesis supported by subsequent work investigating the relationships between OCT and immune cells and immunoglobulin indices in cerebrospinal fluid (CSF) [228]. This subsequent study found that both GCIP and INL thickness were inversely correlated with CSF $CD19^{+}$ B-cell count, immunoglobulin G (IgG) and immunoglobulin A (IgA) synthesis, but that INL thickness was additionally positively correlated with $CD56^{bright}$ natural killer cell count [228].

Another study provided evidence that patients with active MS, as defined by the presence of new clinical relapse(s), new or enlarging T2 FLAIR lesion, or a new gadolinium-enhancing lesion, demonstrated an increased rate of neuro-axonal loss (decreased GCIP thickness, and whole brain and thalamus volumes) in the first five years after disease onset [246]. After this period, rates of neuro-axonal loss stabilized in both active and stable patients [246]. Lower axonal and myelin volume fractions, in addition to reduced axonal and myelin volume fractions in lesions within the optic radiations and NAWM, were also found in MS patients compared to HCs, and more so in patients with a history of ON [247]. Furthermore, an accelerated decrease in GCIP in the first year after an acute ON was correlated with faster rates of whole-brain, white matter, thalamic, and subcortical grey matter atrophy over 5 years [248].

Whilst all of these results are of interest, it remains challenging to compare the correlation of OCT findings with MRI parameters in MS patients due to the considerable heterogeneity in devices used, acquisition techniques, and analyses and outcome measures employed, particularly in MRI. Additional challenges arise from the fact that it is not currently possible to correlate MRI data from the brain as a whole with OCT data from individual eyes [249], and previous ON appears to affect correlations with MRI parameters in individual eyes considerably [236]. Whether OCT can to some extent replace MRI, along with the relative utilities of each technique, has been the subject of some debate [250, 251]. We suggest that whilst neither OCT nor MRI are without disadvantages as tools for MS research, both will remain vital, complementary investigatory techniques in the future. Robust, long-term longitudinal data may enable better characterisation of the relative merits of both examinations [252].

11.4.5 Biomarkers

In recent years, neurofilament light chain (NfL) has become firmly established as a biomarker for inflammation and degeneration in MS. NfL is a protein that is released in extracellular fluid when axonal damage occurs which can be measured in the blood or CSF, and is known to be increased in level during MS relapses and MRI lesion development [253–257]. One study found that RRMS patients with increased baseline levels of serum NfL (sNfL) experienced faster pRNFL and GCIP thinning independent of a history of ON, a finding not observed in PPMS patients [258]. MS patients with a higher sNfL level at baseline were also found to have an increased risk of disease worsening after 2 years of follow-up; likewise, higher sNfL levels after 2 years were related to increased GCIP atrophy during follow-up [259]. Other authors have proposed combining NfL and OCT measures to obtain a better prediction of future disease activity in early MS patients [260, 261]; for instance, patients with abnormal serum NfL levels in combination with GCIP thinning were reported to have a higher risk of developing new brain lesions and suffering clinical relapses (Fig. 11.10) [262]. Another study proposed that a combination of sNfL levels (i.e., at baseline and over 6 months), RNFL and GCIP thicknesses, and clinical measures were able to accurately predict disability progression in early RRMS patients [263–267].

Other biomarkers have also been studied together with OCT. For instance, lower RNFL thickness was also found in MS patients with reduced levels of cerebrospinal fluid (CSF) β- amyloid$_{1\text{-}42}$ (Aβ), in comparison to the MS subgroup with higher Aβ levels and HCs, thereby giving support to the idea of anterograde retinal neurodegeneration in the early stages of MS [268]. Other authors found that levels of the mitochondrial IV and V complex were associated with brain and retinal atrophy; these levels were measured using neuronal enriched extracellular vesicles from plasma, and could serve as a novel biomarker in the MS clinic [269]. Furthermore, the ellipsoid zone (EZ) integrity was reported to be lesser in SPMS patients compared to RRMS patients; the EZ is visible on OCT scans as a hyperreflective band at the outer retina, with the hyperreflectivity thought to be caused by local mitochondrial accumulation [270].

Ceramide levels have been shown to be elevated in MS patients compared to HCs, higher concentrations of Hex-Cer22:0 and DH-HexCer22:0 associated with a greater amount of GCIP and pRNFL in MS patients [271]. Additionally, alternated levels of molecules implicated in axonal degeneration (decreased nicotinamide adenine dinucleotide [NAD] and increased Aβ) were documented in MS patients during both the chronic and acute phases of ON [272]. Concentrations of these molecules were also found to vary over time in MS patients, potentially implying involvement in progressive neurodegeneration, although further research is necessary for a definitive conclusion [272]. Lastly, elevated levels of endothelin-1 (ET-1) were reported in clinically 'aggressive' compared to non-aggressive MS patients with a diagnosis of ON; ET-1 is a vasoconstrictive peptide released from reactive astrocytes in focal MS lesions [273]. ON patients with 'aggressive' MS were defined in this study using criteria based on visual acuity, perimetry, OCT, MRI, and efferent oculomotor findings [273]. This finding demonstrates that ET-1 levels may be a prognostic marker of ON recovery in MS patients.

11.4.6 Electrophysiological Assessment of the Visual Pathway

Electrophysiological tests such as the visual evoked potential (VEP) and electroretinogram (ERG), quantify the electrical response of the visual cortex and retina, respectively, in response to precisely-defined visual stimuli. Using the ERG, the function of the photoreceptors and bipolar cells over the entire retina can be measured [274]. The multifocal ERG (MF-ERG) also measures the function of the photoreceptors and bipolar cells [275], but from discrete regions of the macula only

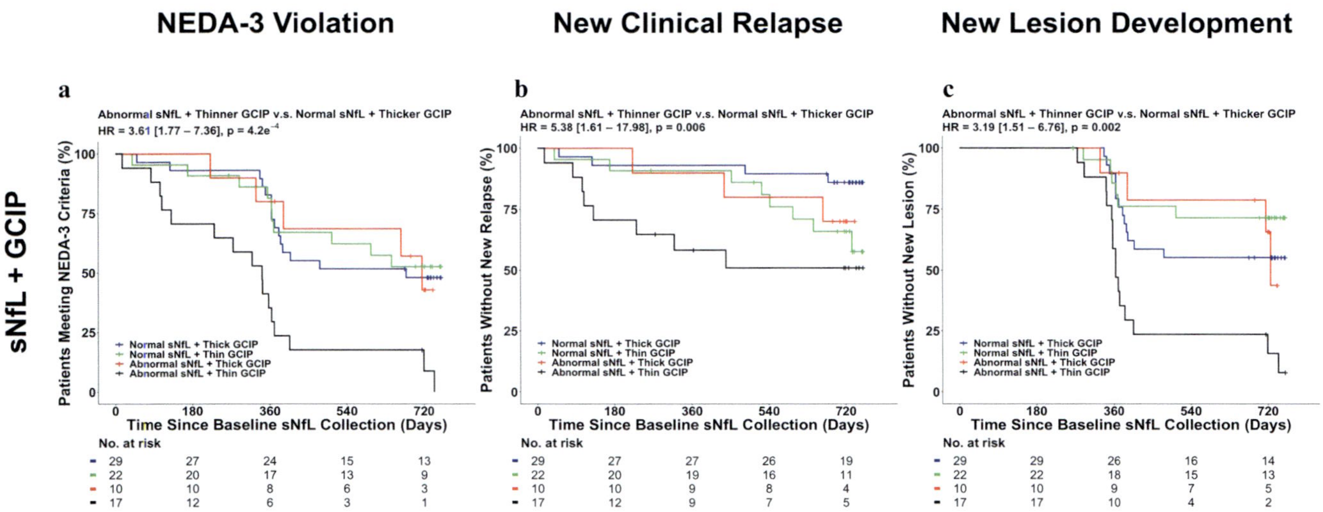

Fig. 11.10 Kaplan–Meier plots for fulfilling three parameter no evidence of disease activity (NEDA-3) criteria or developing new clinical relapses or magnetic resonance imaging (MRI) lesions, with abnormal serum neurofilament (sNfL) and optical coherence tomography (OCT) measurements as risk factors. Cumulative risks for patients with abnormal sNfL and thinner ganglion cell-inner plexiform complex (GCIP) (black), abnormal sNfL and thicker GCIP (red), normal sNfL and thinner GCIP (green), and normal sNfL and thicker GCIP (blue) are shown for violating NEDA-3 criteria (a), experiencing a clinical relapse (b), and developing a new lesion visible on MRI (c). GCIP is categorised as 'thicker' or 'thinner' relative to the group median. Abnormal sNfL combined with thinner GCIP is associated with the greatest risk of NEDA-3 violation, experiencing a clinical relapse, and developing a brain MRI lesion. HR = hazard ratio. Reproduced from Lin et al. **Neurology® Neuroimmunology and Neuroinflammation** 8, (2021) with the permission of Wolters Kluwer Health, Inc. and Junior Prof. Dr. Hanna Zimmermann

[276]. The function of the ganglion cells of the inner retina can be measured using the pattern electroretinogram (PERG) or the photopic negative response (PhNR) of the ERG [277, 278]. The multifocal VEP (MF-VEP), in a manner analogous to the MF-ERG, allows functional assessment of smaller, localized areas of cortex and smaller bundles of axons in the visual pathway [279]. The utility of MF-VEP in clinical routine remains debated by experts in the field for a number of technical reasons, however it remains frequently used within MS research [109, 280–284].

A number of studies have recorded significant correlations between electrophysiological and OCT parameters in MS [285] patients. The response latency of the VEP or MF-VEP is correlated with mean RNFL thickness [109, 195, 286–289], TMV [286], and GCIP thickness [109, 288, 289]. Another study showed that changes in VEP P100 latency over one year were able to predict GCIP atrophy after 3 years in RRMS eyes without a history of ON, and may therefore be a prognostic marker for retinal ganglion cell loss [290]. In SPMS patients, a similar relationship was found between VEP P100 latency and RNFL or GCIP thickness [203].

Furthermore, inter-eye MF-VEP latency was found to be related to inter-eye RNFL thickness asymmetry both at baseline and during follow-up, with baseline latency delay predicted the amount of RNFL thinning in ON eyes during follow-up [288]. MF-VEP amplitude was more significantly associated with GCIP than with RNFL in RRMS patients [289]. MS patients with a delayed VEP or a history of ON were found to have lower RNFL thickness levels [194, 203, 291], with a longer VEP P100 peak time also found to correlate with lower optic nerve head VD [291] and lower VD of the radial peripapillary capillaries (RPCs) [291] and reduced motion perception [292]. Additionally, P100 peak time was also negatively correlated with RNFL and GCIP thicknesses in MS patients, as well as with the VD of the superficial and deep capillary plexuses (SCP and DCP, respectively); VD of both SCP and DCP may aid the detection of damage from previous ON [138]. Finally, P100 peak time was found to be negatively correlated with GCIP in MS patients with previous ON [293] and was associated with RNFL thickness and optic radiation lesion load in non-ON progressive MS patients [294].

Combining OCT measures of RNFL thickness and GCIP thickness [293] with VEP [195] ensures greater sensitivity in detecting anterior visual pathway damage after ON in MS patients than using either test alone [293], in which case OCT is superior to VEP [295]. Another study extended this idea by combining OCT and VEP data into a Z-score-derived OCT-VEP index, finding that differences in ON pathophysiology could aid in distinguishing between NMOSD and MS patients [296]. This study reported a delayed VEP with relatively spared pRNFL in MS patients, while more severe RNFL atrophy was recorded in NMOSD patients, in whom VEP was predominantly non-recordable or delayed [296].

PERG P50 peak time delays and lower amplitudes were reported in MS-ON eyes relative to non-affected eyes, and eyes of MS-NON patients and HCs [297]; likewise, PERG amplitudes were correlated with pRNFL thickness [110, 286, 287, 297], TMV [286], GCIP thickness [110, 297], and total retinal thickness [110]. Normalized PERG amplitudes (the ratio of the amplitudes of the N95 and P50 components) were also correlated with macular volume [286] and RNFL thickness [287]; similarly, PERG P50 latency delays and lower amplitudes were found to be associated with thinning of the mRNFL and GCIP [297].

PhNR is correlated with RNFL thickness in MS eyes without previous ON and with an ON event at least six months previously, but not those with a history of ON less than six months previously [298]; this finding likely reflects the temporal dynamics of RNFL loss after ON as discussed in Sect. 11.2.1. Another study also found that RNFL birefringence in the temporal quadrant was significantly decreased in RRMS patients after 2 years [299]. The cone-driven ERG b-wave response latency has been found to correlate inversely with RNFL and GCIP thickness [109], and increases in EDSS were correlated with a prolongation of the rod-cone ERG b-wave peak time [300]. The predictive power of cone-driven ERG for RNFL and GCIP thickness was significantly weaker than was the MF-VEP latency [109], doubtless reflecting the fact that this ERG component is generated by the bipolar cells and not the ganglion cells or their axons [301]. Subsequent work has documented some degree of negative correlation between ERG a-wave amplitudes and ONL thickness, as well as ERG b-wave amplitudes and INL thickness, in MS patients [61]; however, this study (and others) also recorded that ERG amplitudes are mostly normal in MS patients [61, 109, 118, 302–304]. Conversely, the latency (peak time) of the ERG, particularly those responses driven in whole or in part by the cone system, has been shown to be abnormal to varying degrees in MS patients [61, 109, 118, 119, 302] whilst being uncorrelated with OCT-derived measures of ONL or INL [61]. This lack of correlation would be compatible with dysfunctional, but not atrophic, photoreceptors and bipolar cells in patients with MS. The same study also failed to observe any correlations between MF-ERG parameters and INL structure, despite recording evidence of abnormal MF-ERG P1 latency [61]. However, it may be challenging to reconcile this hypothesis of dysfunction without atrophy with a recent finding of reduced cone photopreceptor density (presumably reflecting some form of atrophy) in patients with MS independent of previous ON [90]. An alternate mechanism could be atrophy-related loss of retinal neurons at a level not detectable with current OCT technology.

With modification of the standard MF-ERG test protocol it is possible to visualize an additional component of the MF-ERG, the optic nerve head component (ONHC), which is generated at the optic nerve head [305]. Abnormalities of the ONHC have been documented [306] in the ipsilateral and (to a lesser extent) contralateral eyes of MS patients with a history of unilateral ON [307]. The number of abnormal ONHC responses correlates strongly with RNFL thickness, so that a 10 μm reduction in pRNFL thickness is associated with 6.8 additional abnormal ONHC responses (from a total of 103 responses) [307]. The relationship between the ONHC and other OCT parameters remains unclear at the time of writing.

11.5 OCT Findings and Treatment Responses

Neuronal and axonal assessment with OCT is of great value within the MS clinic, and of particular significance in the diagnosis and prognosis of MS, choosing the appropriate therapy, differentiation of MS subgroups, and establishing the eligibility of patients for clinical trials. Increasingly, researchers are beginning to use OCT to determine risk profiles for patients with a high risk of future relapses. For example, previous data suggest that CIS patients with lower GCIP thickness are more likely to convert to MS within three years and less likely to remain free of clinical disease activity than those with thicker GCIP [308]. In this section, we provide a current overview of how OCT may be used to guide clinical and treatment decisions in patients with MS.

11.5.1 The Role of INL in Assessment of Treatments Affects and Disease Severity

It has been proposed that the INL responds dynamically to MS disease activity and treatment; untreated MS patients were found to have a greater INL volume than healthy control subjects, and this volume appeared to normalise following successful medical treatment (as evidenced by no clinical relapses or new MRI lesions during the follow-up period) yet remain elevated in patients in whom therapy was unsuccessful (Fig. 11.11) [102]. A particularly noteworthy aspect of this work [102] is that eyes with previous ON were excluded from analysis, ensuring that measures of INL thickness were uncontaminated by potential post-ON thickening [59]. Given that INL does not show atrophy after ON despite the well-documented thinning of the adjacent inner retina [59, 65], it may be that changes to INL thickness reflect inflammatory, rather than neurodegenerative, processes in MS [102].

Microcystic macular oedema (MMO) may also be observed in the INL of patients with MS. MMO was initially described as discrete, cyst-like spaces, visible on at least two adjacent OCT B-scans and predominantly confined to the INL, in 4.7% of MS patients (Fig. 11.12a); these patients on average had higher EDSS and MSSS scores and reduced visual acuity, and were more likely to have previously suffered an episode of ON, in comparison to their cohorts without comparable changes to the INL [309]. These findings appear to be transient in the majority of patients (Fig. 11.12b-c) [310]. The appropriate nomenclature of these findings has been a subject of debate; whilst originally described as microcystic macular oedema [309], the intraretinal spaces appear not to be lined with epithelium and are therefore not truly cystic, but rather cystoid, in nature [311]. When associated with optic atrophy, it has been suggested that INL thickening with or without cystoid lesions in the INL should be termed ‘retrograde maculopathy’ [312]. Nevertheless, the term MMO has persisted and will be used for familiarity here.

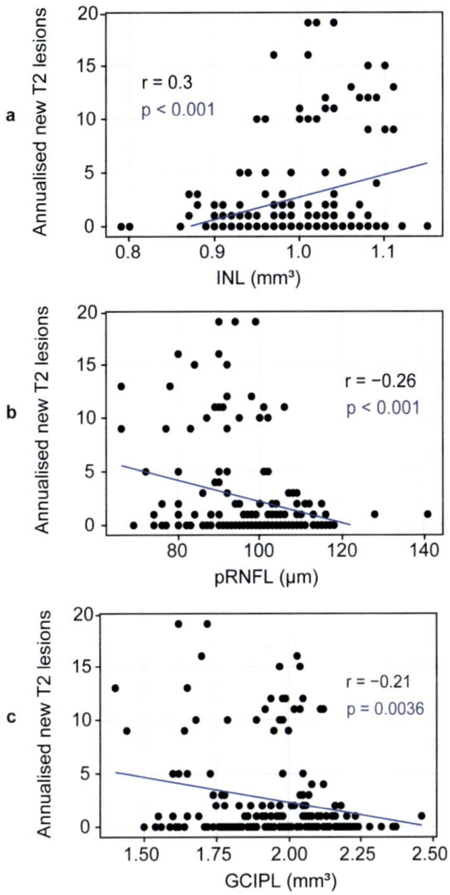

Fig. 11.11 Correlations between baseline inner nuclear layer (INL) volume (a), peripapillary retinal nerve fibre layer (pRNFL) thickness (b), and ganglion cell and inner plexiform layer (GCIP) volume (here named GCIPL; c) and prospective multiple sclerosis (MS) disease activity, as measured by annualised development of new T2 lesions visible using magnetic resonance imaging (MRI). INL volume is positively correlated with the number of new lesions, meaning that higher baseline INL volume is associated with an increased chance of developing new T2 lesions. Conversely, pRNFL thickness and GCIP volume are negatively correlated with the development of new T2 lesions, meaning that higher pRNFL thickness/GCIP volume is associated with a decreased chance of developing new lesions. Reproduced from Knier et al. **Brain** 139, 2855–2863 (2016) with the permission of Oxford University Press and Prof. Thomas Korn

Although MMO was initially described in MS patients [113, 309], particularly in those with a history of ON [113, 309, 313], it rapidly became apparent from subsequent reports that MMO-like OCT findings can be observed in a range of non-MS disease states, including neuromyelitis optica spectrum disease (NMOSD) [313–315], relapsing isolated optic neuritis (RION) [316], chronic relapsing inflammatory optic neuropathy (CRION) [313], glaucoma [317, 318],

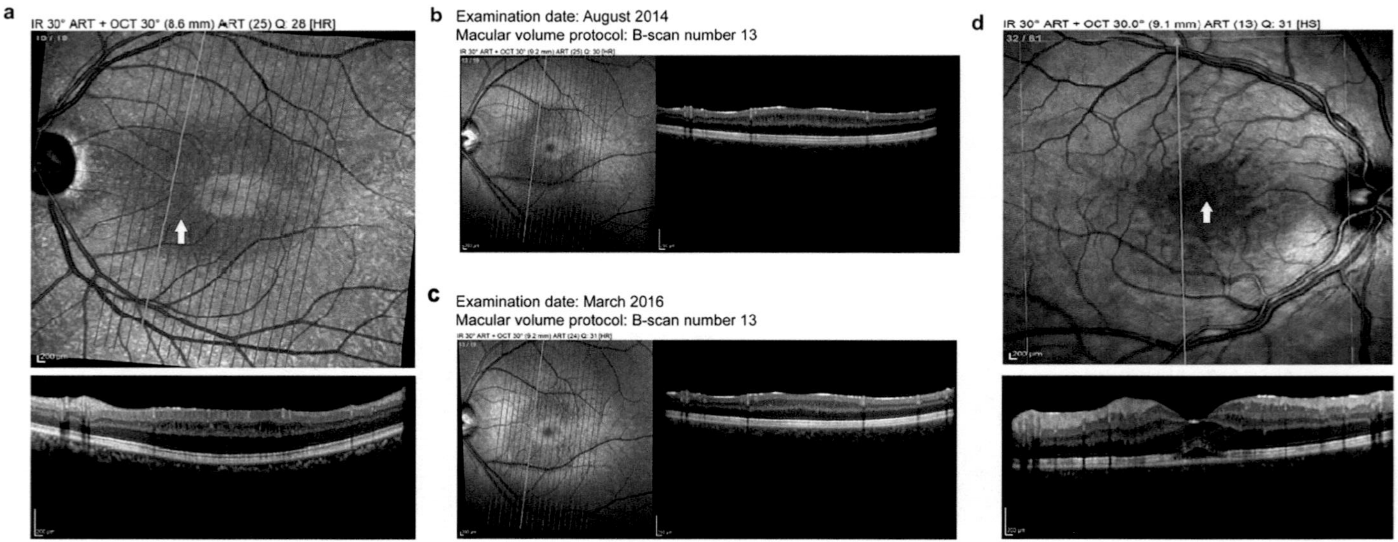

Fig. 11.12 (a) OCT infra-red fundus image (above) and b-scan (below) of a patient with multiple sclerosis (MS) and microcystic macular oedema (MMO). In the fundus image, fluid around the fovea is visible as a ring-shaped darker area of the retina (highlighted with a white arrow). The B-scan shows cystoid lesions confined to the inner nuclear layer (INL), pathognomonic for MMO. (b, c) Illustration of the transient nature of MMO in a patient with MS. The initial OCT scan (b) revealed the presence of microcystoid lesions in the INL, thereby confirming MMO in this patient. At follow-up (c) 19 months later (at the same retinal location, as seen by the identical B-scan numbers), no more cystoid lesions were visible, indicating resolution of MMO. (d) OCT infra-red fundus image (above) and b-scan (below) of a patient with MS who has developed cystoid macula oedema (CMO) consequent to medical treatment with fingolimod (Gilenya®). Fluid at the central retina is visible on the fundus image as a darker-appearing area (highlighted with a white arrow). In the b-scan, cystoid spaces are visible in the outer and (to a lesser extent) inner nuclear layers, as well as a small subfoveal accumulation of subretinal fluid

Leber's hereditary optic neuropathy (LHON) [319], dominant optic atrophy [319, 320], chronic compressive optic neuropathy secondary to glioma in a patient with neurofibromatosis type 1 [321], Tanzanian endemic optic neuropathy [322], traumatic optic neuropathy [317], hydrocephalus [317], tobacco-alcohol optic neuropathy [323], following phacoemulsification [324], and consequent to combined vitrectomy and inner limiting membrane removal [325]. The finding that cystoid changes in INL are observed post-vitrectomy (i.e., following surgical removal of the vitreous body) [325] is particularly relevant, as it provides clear evidence against previous hypotheses [319, 320] that vitreo-retinal traction is necessary for the formation of MMO, but is consistent with the proposal that MMO can occur independently of vitreo-retinal traction [315]. Changes in INL volume such as that seen in MMO have been hypothesised to be mediated by dysfunction, and consequent reduced ability to maintain retinal water homeostasis, of the Müller glial cells (the cell bodies of which are found in the INL) [316], and as potentially representing evidence of a glymphatic system (similar to that found in the brain) within the retina [326].

Despite this considerable lack of specificity, it is important to recognize that MMO in MS patients has to date, without exception, been found to be associated with increased disease severity [113, 309, 313]. This increased severity is observed in OCT scans as decreased RNFL [309] and GCIP [113] thickness, as well as increased INL thickness [113]; currently, there is no unanimity with regard to differences in TMV between MS eyes with and without MMO. [309, 313] Clinical indicators of increased disease severity in MS patients with MMO are reduced HCVA [113, 309, 313] and LCVA [113], higher MSSS values [113, 309, 313], higher EDSS values [309, 313], as well as an increased likelihood of developing gadolinium-enhancing and T2-weighted MRI lesions [113]. African-American MS patients have a higher prevalence of MMO [327], consistent with the more aggressive disease course typically observed in this population [327–330]. Thus, a finding of MMO upon OCT examination may assist clinicians in their decision-making process when considering, for example, whether to recommend medical treatment (or a more efficacious treatment) to a MS patient. It may also lead the clinician to consider the possibility of an earlier insult to the optic nerve and initiate further diagnostic tests, for example VEP.

Whilst the INL may reflect response to medical treatment, as discussed above, a more recent large multi-centre study has also confirmed that clinical relapses are associated with thickening of the INL [89]. However, a number of factors may limit the potential usefulness of INL, at least in a clinical setting. Firstly, OCT-derived measures of INL structure may be confounded both by ON [59, 89] and MMO, as discussed above, in patients with MS. As INL is a relatively thin layer when compared to, for example GCIP or ONL, even small errors of segmentation have the potential to exert a disproportionate influence on thickness measures. An additional potential confound is that the INL contains nuclei of bipolar cells in addition to horizontal cells, amacrine cells, and the cell bodies of the Müller glia [114], meaning that structural changes to INL may be of multiple aetiologies and may not be ascribed to specific cell types (neuronal or glial) or specific types of neuron. Functional tests such as the ERG may measure bipolar integrity in isolation, however abnormal functional parameters appear not to correlate with OCT-derived INL structural measures [61]. More detailed characterisation of the role of the INL in MS, including longitudinal studies, is necessary.

11.5.2 Monitoring of Disease Modifying Treatments in MS

Knowledge of possible responses to disease-modifying therapies (DMTs) in MS patients is of huge importance for clinicians. A prospective study of RRMS patients treated with several DMTs reported no difference in the rate of GCIP atrophy between those treated with high- and low efficacy therapies [81]. Conversely, another study with a larger cohort recorded that GCIP atrophy rates in RRMS patients were slower in patients treated with natalizumab than in those treated with glatiramer acetate or subcutaneous interferon-β-1a [331]. Future research using OCT will be of great benefit in evaluating effects of DMT on neuronal integrity in patients with MS.

Fingolimod (Gilenya®) is a modulator of sphingosine 1-phosphate receptors prescribed as an immunomodulatory therapy in MS. Whilst its high efficacy [332, 333] and oral administration are attractive, a small number of patients (up to 1% of treated RRMS patients [334, 335]) develop cystoid macula oedema (CMO; an accumulation of fluid in the central retina most likely consequent to breakdown of the blood-retinal barrier [336]) as a side-effect of the treatment (Fig. 11.12d). It is therefore recommended that patients undergo ophthalmological examination before commencing therapy, and again 3–4 months afterwards, a time interval in which the majority of CMO cases manifest [337]. OCT has been demonstrated to be significantly more sensitive than fundoscopy in detecting CMO [338], and therefore is of great utility when assessing and monitoring MS patients undergoing treatment with fingolimod. When no CMO occurs in such patients, central foveal thickness and TMV remain stable over a 12 month period [339], although other authors have documented minimal TMV fluctuation over 3–4 months that did not significantly affect VA [340]. Consistent with these findings, subsequent work also recorded no changes to VA over a two-year period after initiation of fingolimod treatment [341]. However, other authors found a slight reduction in contrast sensitivity after six and 12 months of treatment, despite recording stable HCVA, LCVA, and OCT parameters [342]. In summary, adverse effects of fingolimod may be of less concern currently than when the treatment was first used in clinical settings, with one group of authors suggesting that routine ophthalmological monitoring may not be necessary for MS patients without comorbid diabetes or uveitis taking less than 0.5 mg per day [340].

RRMS patients treated with alemtuzumab (a monoclonal antibody binding to CD52 proteins on lymphocytes) were reported to maintain stable RNFL thickness and GCIP volume over a five year period in comparison to patients treated with interferon-β-1a or glatiramer acetate [343]. Therefore, OCT was able to confirm superior neuro-axonal preservation in patients treated with alemtuzumab.

Conversely, another study demonstrated that rituximab-treated RRMS patients experienced faster rates of GCIP atrophy (0.55 μm/year) during their first year than during their second year (0.14 μm/year), with rates of loss during the second year comparable to patients treated with natalizumab and HC subjects [344]. In this case, OCT was used to confirm the neuroprotective effect of rituximab but also to demonstrate that these effects may not be apparent for one year or more. Other studies also demonstrated that rates of GCIP and RNFL thinning could predict disease progression and treatment failure in patients with RRMS [345]. OCT may also aid in prediction of treatment success or failure in progressive MS; in PPMS patients treated with ocrelizumab, INL thinning was slower in patients without evidence of disease progression at one year [346].

Additionally, hyperacute corticosteroid treatment within 2 days of ON minimises loss of GCIP and preserves HCVA in comparison to treatment initiated later than 2 days or when corticosteroids are not used in recurrent ON patients [49]. The use of phenytoin for three months in patients with acute ON also led to 30% less RNFL loss at six months post-ON compared to patients treated with placebo [347]. However, addition of erythropoietin to standard methylprednisone treatment appears to have no significant effects on pRNFL loss over two years post-ON [348]. Research on acute ON is particularly important as the condition may be used as a model to examine neuroprotective and remyelination therapies after acute inflammation [349].

11.6 New Developments in OCT and MS Research

A novel finding recently described in MS is the presence of peripapillary hyperreflective ovoid mass-like structures (PHOMS), which are ovoid structures visible below the nerve fiber layers on OCT scans of the optic nerve head (Fig. 11.13) [350]. The reasons for the presence of PHOMS in MS are currently unclear, but increased levels of intracranial pressure or impaired glymphatic outflow from the eye to the brain have been proposed as possible mechanisms [350]. PHOMS are also found in a range of ophthalmic conditions (e.g., optic disc drusen, papilloedema, and MS-related ON) and could be due to herniating nerve fibers or a consequence of axoplasmic stasis [351–353]. PHOMS were found to be correlated with EDSS worsening and longer disease duration in PPMS patients but not in RRMS patients [354]. Research has also demonstrated that the prevalence of PHOMS seems to be approximately similar between MS-ON, MOGAD-ON, and NMOSD-ON patients [355].

An emerging body of literature has reported the presence of hyperreflective foci (HRF) within the retinae of MS patients, thought to consist primarily of clusters of activated microglia and visible on OCT as roughly round hyperreflective dots up to 30 μm in size [356]. Recent work has reported a higher number of HRF in the INL and a higher INL volume in early RRMS patients [357]. Granular HRF have also been found in the avascular ONL in RRMS patients but not HCs [358]. Given that recent work has reported a positive association between GM lesion volume

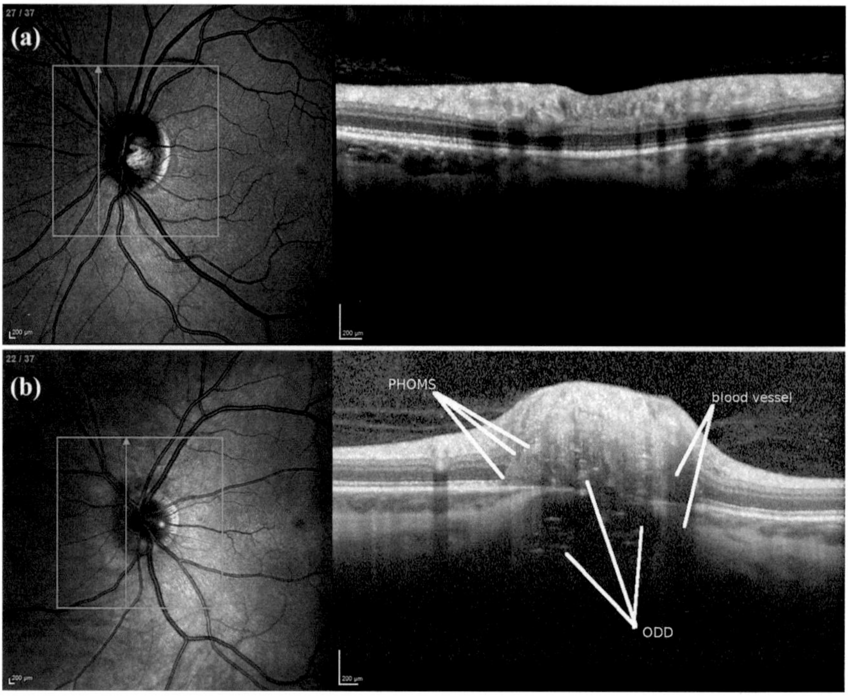

Fig. 11.13 A normal optic disc (a) and an optic disc with peripapillary hyper-reflective ovoid masslike structures (PHOMS) and optic disc drusen (ODD) (b) The hyperintense PHOMS are here visible between the retinal nerve fibre layer (RNFL) and the basal membrane. The ODD are located above and below Bruch's membrane, and were vertically shadowed by blood vessel artefacts. On the left the corresponding infra-red images are shown, on which the vertical green lines illustrate the positions of the OCT B-scans on the right. Reproduced from Petzold et al. **Annals of Neurology** 88, 309–319 (2020) under the terms of the Creative Commons Attribution license

and the amount of HRF in the INL [357], HRF may be associated with disease severity. A greater number of HRF was found in the inner, but not outer, retinae of RRMS patients compared to HCs [359]. Another study found that Bruch's membrane opening-minimum rim width (BMO-MRW) was reduced in MS patients and that BMO-MRW and pRNFL were associated with visual impairment and disability (HCVA, LCVA, and EDSS scores); however, GCIP thickness was the strongest marker of visual impairment [360]. Furthermore, the colour confusion index (CCI) in MS patients with dyschromatopsia correlated with pRNFL, GCL, BPF, SC volume, EDSS, age, and disease duration, implying diffuse chronic neurodegeneration [361].

In recent years, there has also been a growing interest in the question of whether specific blood biomarkers combined with OCT data, or OCT data alone, could serve as a marker in the MS clinic by, for instance, enabling the prediction of disease activity and disease progression, or by providing the ability to define subgroups of MS patients that would benefit the most from specific therapies [49,

343–347, 362–365]. This question has become even more appealing due to the growing interest in using artificial intelligence (AI) for diagnosis, prognosis, and subcategorizing MS. Studies have demonstrated that predictive models of MS diagnosis and monitoring of disease course utilising OCT data (RNFL and GCIP thicknesses) performed well in MS patients [366–372], and so machine learning algorithms that make use of OCT data may ease therapeutic decision making in the future MS clinic. Combining OCT results with other outcome measures is likely to increase diagnostic and/or prognostic accuracy [186, 260–267, 296].

11.7 Summary

Patients with MS and previous ON exhibit significant thinning of the inner retina (RNFL; GCIP), and likely also a small degree of INL thickening. Eyes without previous ON exhibit a lesser degree of inner retinal thinning and no changes to the deeper layers such as INL, OPL, ONL, and PRL. Interpretation of OCT results pertaining to OPL, ONL, and PRL (and, to a lesser extent, the INL) is complicated by inconsistency of aggregation of these layers between different studies and software versions, although it appears that any documented changes to the thickness of these layers occur only after ON, are dynamic in nature and also of considerably lesser magnitude than those observed in the inner retinal layers. With these factors in mind, we suggest that future studies examining outer, rather than inner, retinal structure in MS patients with or without ON may require much larger cohorts in order to achieve sufficient statistical power to detect potentially small differences between patient groups. OCT can be used to identify those patients at risk of a rapid or severely disabling disease course, and initiate timely intervention. In particular, analysis of the INL may in future assist in differentiating degenerative from inflammatory disease activity, and in monitoring treatment efficacy. Although it is unlikely to replace MRI, OCT provides valuable complementary information in patients with MS. The increasing understanding of OCT-derived retinal information may facilitate improvements in diagnosis, monitoring, and treatment outcome prediction in MS patients. In the coming years, it is essential to further evaluate the role of OCT in clinical trials. Another promising line of research involves using AI and machine learning techniques incorporating OCT outcome measures to aid clinical decision making by providing information about prognosis and subcategorizing MS patients. OCTA also holds promise as an outcome measure in MS.

References

1. Kingwell E, Marriott JJ, Jette N, et al. Incidence and prevalence of multiple sclerosis in Europe: a systematic review. BMC Neurol. 2013;13:128. 2013/09/28. https://doi.org/10.1186/1471-2377-13-128
2. Sospedra M, Martin R. Immunology of multiple sclerosis. Seminars in Neurology. 2016;36:115–127. 2016/04/27. https://doi.org/10.1055/s-0036-1579739

3. Lublin FD, Reingold SC, Cohen JA, et al. Defining the clinical course of multiple sclerosis: the 2013 revisions. Neurology. 2014;83:278–286. 2014/05/30. https://doi.org/10.1212/wnl.0000000000000560
4. Thompson AJ, Banwell BL, Barkhof F, et al. Diagnosis of multiple sclerosis: 2017 revisions of the McDonald criteria. Lancet Neurol. 2018;17:162–173. 2017/12/26. https://doi.org/10.1016/s1474-4422(17)30470-2
5. Rival M, Galoppin M, Thouvenot E. Biological markers in early multiple sclerosis: the paved way for radiologically isolated syndrome. Front Immunol. 2022;13(866092):20220427. https://doi.org/10.3389/fimmu.2022.866092.
6. Okuda DT, Siva A, Kantarci O, et al. Radiologically isolated syndrome: 5-year risk for an initial clinical event. PLoS ONE. 2014;9(e90509):20140305. https://doi.org/10.1371/journal.pone.0090509.
7. Alroughani R, Boyko A. Pediatric multiple sclerosis: a review. BMC Neurol. 2018;18(27):20180309. https://doi.org/10.1186/s12883-018-1026-3.
8. Renoux C, Vukusic S, Mikaeloff Y, et al. Natural history of multiple sclerosis with childhood onset. N Engl J Med. 2007; 356: 2603–2613. 2007/06/22. https://doi.org/10.1056/NEJMoa067597
9. McDonald WI, Barnes D. The ocular manifestations of multiple sclerosis. 1. Abnormalities of the afferent visual system. J Neurol Neurosurg Psychiatry. 1992;55:747–752. 1992/09/01.
10. Graham SL, Klistorner A. Afferent visual pathways in multiple sclerosis: a review. Clinical and Experim Ophthalmol. 2017;45:62–72. 2016/03/25. https://doi.org/10.1111/ceo.12751
11. Costello F. Vision disturbances in multiple sclerosis. Seminars in Neurol. 2016;36:185–195. 2016/04/27. https://doi.org/10.1055/s-0036-1579692
12. Pisa M, Pansieri J, Yee S, et al. Anterior optic pathway pathology in CNS demyelinating diseases. Brain. 2022;145:4308–19. https://doi.org/10.1093/brain/awac030.
13. Toosy AT, Mason DF, Miller DH. Optic neuritis. The Lancet Neurol. 2014;13:83–99. https://doi.org/10.1016/s1474-4422(13)70259-x.
14. Ikuta F, Zimmerman HM. Distribution of plaques in seventy autopsy cases of multiple sclerosis in the United States. Neurology. 1976;26:26–28. 1976/06/01.
15. Green AJ, McQuaid S, Hauser SL, et al. Ocular pathology in multiple sclerosis: retinal atrophy and inflammation irrespective of disease duration. Brain. 2010;133:1591–601. https://doi.org/10.1093/brain/awq080.
16. Davion JB, Lopes R, Drumez É, et al. Asymptomatic optic nerve lesions: An underestimated cause of silent retinal atrophy in MS. Neurology. 2020;94:e2468–e2478. 20200520. https://doi.org/10.1212/wnl.0000000000009504
17. Outteryck O, Lopes R, Drumez É, et al. Optical coherence tomography for detection of asymptomatic optic nerve lesions in clinically isolated syndrome. Neurology. 2020;95:e733–e744. 20200728. https://doi.org/10.1212/wnl.0000000000009832
18. Costello F. The afferent visual pathway: designing a structural-functional paradigm of multiple sclerosis. ISRN Neurol. 2013;2013: 134858. https://doi.org/10.1155/2013/134858.
19. Kemchoknatee P, Singhakul C, Arjkongharn N, et al. A 10-year single-center study of the clinical characteristics of optic neuritis-related NMOSD, MS, and double seronegative optic neuritis, together with factors predicting visual outcomes. Vision (Basel). 2023;7:20230228. https://doi.org/10.3390/vision7010016
20. Li X, Zhang C, Jia D, et al. The occurrence of myelin oligodendrocyte glycoprotein antibodies in aquaporin-4-antibody seronegative neuromyelitis optica spectrum disorder: a systematic review and meta-analysis. Mult Scler Relat Disord. 2021;53(103030):20210528. https://doi.org/10.1016/j.msard.2021.103030.
21. Uzawa A, Mori M, Kuwabara S. Neuromyelitis optica: concept, immunology and treatment. J Clin Neurosci. 2014;21(12–21):20130802. https://doi.org/10.1016/j.jocn.2012.12.022.
22. Bennett JL, Costello F, Chen JJ, et al. Optic neuritis and autoimmune optic neuropathies: advances in diagnosis and treatment. Lancet Neurol. 2023;22(89–100):20220922. https://doi.org/10.1016/s1474-4422(22)00187-9.

23. Cortese R, Carrasco FP, Tur C, et al. Differentiating multiple sclerosis from AQP4-neuromyelitis optica spectrum disorder and MOG-antibody disease with imaging. Neurology. 2023;100:e308–23. https://doi.org/10.1212/wnl.0000000000201465.
24. Waters P, McKeon A, Leite MI, et al. Serologic diagnosis of NMO A multicenter comparison of aquaporin-4-IgG assays. Neurology. 2012;78:665–671; discussion 669. https://doi.org/10.1212/WNL.0b013e318248dec1
25. Waters P, Woodhall M, O'Connor KC, et al. MOG cell-based assay detects non-MS patients with inflammatory neurologic disease. Neurol Neuroimmunol Neuroinflamm. 2015;2(e89):20150319. https://doi.org/10.1212/nxi.0000000000000089.
26. Huang D, Swanson EA, Lin CP, et al. Optical coherence tomography. Science (New York, NY) 1991;254:1178–1181. 1991/11/22
27. Cordano C, Nourbakhsh B, Devereux M, et al. PRNFL as a marker of disability worsening in the medium/long term in patients with MS. Neurol Neuroimmunol Neuroinflamm. 2019;6(e533):20181221. https://doi.org/10.1212/nxi.0000000000000533.
28. Cruz-Herranz A, Balk LJ, Oberwahrenbrock T, et al. The APOSTEL recommendations for reporting quantitative optical coherence tomography studies. Neurology. 2016;86:2303–2309. 2016/05/27. https://doi.org/10.1212/wnl.0000000000002774
29. Lambe J, Saidha S, Bermel RA. Optical coherence tomography and multiple sclerosis: update on clinical application and role in clinical trials. Mult Scler. 2020;26(624–639):20190906. https://doi.org/10.1177/1352458519872751.
30. Olbert E, Struhal W. Retinal imaging with optical coherence tomography in multiple sclerosis: novel aspects. Wien Med Wochenschr. 2022;172(329–336):20220328. https://doi.org/10.1007/s10354-022-00925-2.
31. Tewarie P, Balk L, Costello F, et al. The OSCAR-IB consensus criteria for retinal OCT quality assessment. PLoS ONE. 2012;7: e34823. https://doi.org/10.1371/journal.pone.0034823.
32. Schippling S, Balk LJ, Costello F, et al. Quality control for retinal OCT in multiple sclerosis: validation of the OSCAR-IB criteria. Mult Scler. 2015;21:163–170. 2014/06/21. https://doi.org/10.1177/1352458514538110
33. Oberwahrenbrock T, Traber GL, Lukas S, et al. Multicenter reliability of semiautomatic retinal layer segmentation using OCT. Neurol Neuroimmunol Neuroinflamm. 2018;5:e449. 2018/03/20. https://doi.org/10.1212/nxi.0000000000000449
34. Seigo MA, Sotirchos ES, Newsome S, et al. In vivo assessment of retinal neuronal layers in multiple sclerosis with manual and automated optical coherence tomography segmentation techniques. J Neurol. 2012;259:2119–30. https://doi.org/10.1007/s00415-012-6466-x.
35. Coric D, Petzold A, Uitdehaag BMJ, et al. Software updates of OCT segmentation algorithms influence longitudinal assessment of retinal atrophy. J Neurol Sci. 2018;387:16–20. 2018/03/25. https://doi.org/10.1016/j.jns.2018.01.020
36. Sallo FB, Hanson JVM, Lukas S, et al. Role of the OCT reading center. In: Petzold A, editor., et al., Optical coherence tomography in multiple sclerosis: clinical applications. Cham: Springer International Publishing; 2016. p. 185–94.
37. The clinical profile of optic neuritis. Experience of the optic neuritis treatment trial. Optic Neuritis Study Group. Arch Ophthalmol. 1991;109:1673–1678. 1991/12/01
38. Petzold A, Wattjes MP, Costello F, et al. The investigation of acute optic neuritis: a review and proposed protocol. Nature Reviews Neurol. 2014;10:447–458. 2014/07/09. https://doi.org/10.1038/nrneurol.2014.108
39. Gerling J, Meyer JH, Kommerell G. Visual field defects in optic neuritis and anterior ischemic optic neuropathy distinctive features. Graefes Arch Clin Exp Ophthalmol. 1998;236:188–192. 1998/05/09
40. Halilovic EA, Alimanovic I, Suljic E, et al. Optic neuritis as first clinical manifestations the multiple sclerosis. Materia Socio-Medica. 2014;26:246–248. 2014/11/15. https://doi.org/10.5455/msm.2014.246-2481
41. Moura AL, Teixeira RA, Oiwa NN, et al. Chromatic discrimination losses in multiple sclerosis patients with and without optic neuritis using the Cambridge colour test. Vis Neurosci. 2008;25:463–468. 2008/07/05. https://doi.org/10.1017/s0952523808080437

42. Shams PN and Plant GT. Optic neuritis: a review. Int MS J. 2009;16:82–89. 2009/11/03
43. Sanchez-Dalmau B, Martinez-Lapiscina EH, Torres-Torres R, et al. Early retinal atrophy predicts long-term visual impairment after acute optic neuritis. Mult Scler. 2018;24:1196–1204. 2017/07/04. https://doi.org/10.1177/1352458517718628
44. Fisher JB, Jacobs DA, Markowitz CE, et al. Relation of visual function to retinal nerve fiber layer thickness in multiple sclerosis. Ophthalmology. 2006;113:324–32. https://doi.org/10.1016/j.ophtha.2005.10.040.
45. Hickman SJ, Dalton CM, Miller DH, et al. Management of acute optic neuritis. Lancet. 2002;360:1953–1962. 2002/12/21
46. Raz N, Dotan S, Chokron S, et al. Demyelination affects temporal aspects of perception: an optic neuritis study. Ann Neurol. 2012;71:531–538. 2012/03/27. https://doi.org/10.1002/ana.22692
47. Beck RW, Cleary PA, Anderson MM, Jr., et al. A randomized, controlled trial of corticosteroids in the treatment of acute optic neuritis. The optic neuritis study group. N Engl J Med. 1992;326:581–588. 1992/03/08. https://doi.org/10.1056/nejm199202273260901
48. Beck RW, Cleary PA, Trobe JD, et al. The effect of corticosteroids for acute optic neuritis on the subsequent development of multiple sclerosis. The optic neuritis study group. N Engl J Med. 1993;329:1764–1769. 1993/12/09. https://doi.org/10.1056/nejm199312093292403
49. Osinga E, van Oosten B, de Vries-Knoppert W, et al. Time is vision in recurrent optic neuritis. Brain Res. 2017;1673(95–101):20170818. https://doi.org/10.1016/j.brainres.2017.08.012.
50. Heesen C, Haase R, Melzig S, et al. Perceptions on the value of bodily functions in multiple sclerosis. Acta NEurologica Scandinavica 2018;137:356–362. 2017/12/06. https://doi.org/10.1111/ane.12881
51. Shindler KS, Ventura E, Dutt M, et al. Inflammatory demyelination induces axonal injury and retinal ganglion cell apoptosis in experimental optic neuritis. Experimental Eye Research 2008;87:208–213. 2008/07/26. https://doi.org/10.1016/j.exer.2008.05.017
52. Trip SA, Schlottmann PG, Jones SJ, et al. Retinal nerve fiber layer axonal loss and visual dysfunction in optic neuritis. Ann Neurol. 2005;58:383–391. 2005/08/03. https://doi.org/10.1002/ana.20575
53. Costello F, Hodge W, Pan YI, et al. Tracking retinal nerve fiber layer loss after optic neuritis: a prospective study using optical coherence tomography. Mult Scler. 2008;14:893–905. https://doi.org/10.1177/1352458508091367.
54. Henderson AP, Altmann DR, Trip AS, et al. A serial study of retinal changes following optic neuritis with sample size estimates for acute neuroprotection trials. Brain. 2010;133:2592–602. https://doi.org/10.1093/brain/awq146.
55. Syc SB, Saidha S, Newsome SD, et al. Optical coherence tomography segmentation reveals ganglion cell layer pathology after optic neuritis. Brain. 2012;135:521–33. https://doi.org/10.1093/brain/awr264.
56. Costello F, Pan YI, Yeh EA, et al. The temporal evolution of structural and functional measures after acute optic neuritis. J Neurol Neurosurg Psychiatry. 2015. 2015/02/12. https://doi.org/10.1136/jnnp-2014-309704
57. Gabilondo I, Martinez-Lapiscina EH, Fraga-Pumar E, et al. Dynamics of retinal injury after acute optic neuritis. Ann Neurol. 2015;77:517–28. https://doi.org/10.1002/ana.24351.
58. Petzold A, de Boer JF, Schippling S, et al. Optical coherence tomography in multiple sclerosis: a systematic review and meta-analysis. Lancet Neurol. 2010;9:921–932. 2010/08/21. https://doi.org/10.1016/s1474-4422(10)70168-x
59. Petzold A, Balcer LJ, Calabresi PA, et al. Retinal layer segmentation in multiple sclerosis: a systematic review and meta-analysis. Lancet Neurol. 2017;16:797–812. 2017/09/19. https://doi.org/10.1016/s1474-4422(17)30278-8
60. Oberwahrenbrock T, Schippling S, Ringelstein M, et al. Retinal damage in multiple sclerosis disease subtypes measured by high-resolution optical coherence tomography. Mult Scler Int. 2012;2012: 530305. https://doi.org/10.1155/2012/530305.

61. Hanson JVM, Hediger M, Manogaran P, et al. Outer retinal dysfunction in the absence of structural abnormalities in multiple sclerosis. Invest Ophthalmol Vis Sci. 2018;59:549–560. 2018/01/27. https://doi.org/10.1167/iovs.17-22821
62. Parisi V, Manni G, Spadaro M, et al. Correlation between morphological and functional retinal impairment in multiple sclerosis patients. Invest Ophthalmol Vis Sci.1999;40:2520–2527. 1999/10/06.
63. Oberwahrenbrock T, Ringelstein M, Jentschke S, et al. Retinal ganglion cell and inner plexiform layer thinning in clinically isolated syndrome. Mult Scler. 2013;19:1887–95. https://doi.org/10.1177/1352458513489757.
64. Walter SD, Ishikawa H, Galetta KM, et al. Ganglion cell loss in relation to visual disability in multiple sclerosis. Ophthalmology. 2012;119:1250–7. https://doi.org/10.1016/j.ophtha.2011.11.032.
65. Balk LJ, Twisk JW, Steenwijk MD, et al. A dam for retrograde axonal degeneration in multiple sclerosis? J Neurol Neurosurg Psychiatry. 2014;85:782–789. 2014/01/30. https://doi.org/10.1136/jnnp-2013-306902
66. Manogaran P, Vavasour IM, Lange AP, et al. Quantifying visual pathway axonal and myelin loss in multiple sclerosis and neuromyelitis optica. Neuroimage Clin. 2016;11:743–750. 2016/06/23. https://doi.org/10.1016/j.nicl.2016.05.014
67. Bock M, Brandt AU, Dorr J, et al. Patterns of retinal nerve fiber layer loss in multiple sclerosis patients with or without optic neuritis and glaucoma patients. Clin Neurol Neurosurg. 2010;112:647–52. https://doi.org/10.1016/j.clineuro.2010.04.014.
68. Bertuzzi F, Suzani M, Tagliabue E, et al. Diagnostic validity of optic disc and retinal nerve fiber layer evaluations in detecting structural changes after optic neuritis. Ophthalmology. 2010;117:1256–1264.e1251. 2010/04/13. https://doi.org/10.1016/j.ophtha.2010.02.024
69. Laible M, Jarius S, Mackensen F, et al. Adding papillomacular bundle measurements to standard optical coherence tomography does not increase sensitivity to detect prior optic neuritis in patients with multiple sclerosis. PLoS One. 2016;11:e0155322. 2016/05/14. https://doi.org/10.1371/journal.pone.0155322
70. Schneider E, Zimmermann H, Oberwahrenbrock T, et al. Optical coherence tomography reveals distinct patterns of retinal damage in neuromyelitis optica and multiple sclerosis. PLoS One. 2013;8:e66151. 2013/06/28. https://doi.org/10.1371/journal.pone.0066151
71. Neroev VV, Eliseeva EK, Zueva MV, et al. Demyelinating optic neuritis: optical coherence tomography and multifocal electroretinography data correlation. Human Physiol. 2016;42:879–884. journal article. https://doi.org/10.1134/s0362119716080090
72. Loughran-Fjeldstad AS, Carlson NG, Husebye CD, et al. Retinal nerve fiber layer sector-specific compromise in relapsing and remitting multiple sclerosis. eNeurologicalSci. 2015;1:30–37. 2015/10/09. https://doi.org/10.1016/j.ensci.2015.09.004
73. Sepulcre J, Murie-Fernandez M, Salinas-Alaman A, et al. Diagnostic accuracy of retinal abnormalities in predicting disease activity in MS. Neurology. 2007;68:1488–94. https://doi.org/10.1212/01.wnl.0000260612.51849.ed.
74. Nolan RC, Galetta SL, Frohman TC, et al. Optimal intereye difference thresholds in retinal nerve fiber layer thickness for predicting a unilateral optic nerve lesion in multiple sclerosis. J Neuroophthalmol. 2018. 2018/02/01. https://doi.org/10.1097/wno.0000000000000629
75. Narayanan D, Cheng H, Bonem KN, et al. Tracking changes over time in retinal nerve fiber layer and ganglion cell-inner plexiform layer thickness in multiple sclerosis. Mult Scler. 2014;20:1331–41. https://doi.org/10.1177/1352458514523498.
76. Balk LJ, Cruz-Herranz A, Albrecht P, et al. Timing of retinal neuronal and axonal loss in MS: a longitudinal OCT study. J Neurol. 2016;263:1323–1331. 2016/05/05. https://doi.org/10.1007/s00415-016-8127-y
77. Petzold A, Balcer LJ, Calabresi PA, et al. Retinal layer segmentation in multiple sclerosis: a systematic review and meta-analysis. The Lancet Neurol. 2017;16:797–812. https://doi.org/10.1016/S1474-4422(17)30278-8.
78. Al-Louzi OA, Bhargava P, Newsome SD, et al. Outer retinal changes following acute optic neuritis. Mult Scler. 2015. 2015/07/26. https://doi.org/10.1177/1352458515590646

79. Xu SC, Kardon RH, Leavitt JA, et al. Optical coherence tomography is highly sensitive in detecting prior optic neuritis. Neurology. 2019 2019/01/25. https://doi.org/10.1212/wnl.000000000000006873
80. Al-Nosairy KO, Horbrügger M, Schippling S, et al. Structure-Function relationship of retinal ganglion cells in multiple sclerosis. Int J Molecul Sci. 2021;22:20210326. https://doi.org/10.3390/ijms22073419
81. Kabanovski A, Zaslavsky K, Rotstein D, et al. A prospective study of disease modifying therapy and retinal atrophy in relapsing-remitting multiple sclerosis. J Neurol Sci. 2023;446(120552):20230119. https://doi.org/10.1016/j.jns.2023.120552.
82. Hu H, Jiang H, Gameiro GR, et al. Focal thickness reduction of the ganglion cell-inner plexiform layer best discriminates prior optic neuritis in patients with multiple sclerosis. Invest Ophthalmol Vis Sci. 2019;60:4257–69. https://doi.org/10.1167/iovs.19-27574.
83. Shi C, Jiang H, Gameiro GR, et al. Visual function and disability are associated with focal thickness reduction of the ganglion cell-inner plexiform layer in patients with multiple sclerosis. Investigative Ophthalmol Visual Sci. 2019;60:1213–23. https://doi.org/10.1167/iovs.18-25809.
84. Kupersmith MJ, Mandel G, Anderson S, et al. Baseline, one and three month changes in the peripapillary retinal nerve fiber layer in acute optic neuritis: relation to baseline vision and MRI. J Neurol Sci. 2011;308:117–123. 2011/07/19. https://doi.org/10.1016/j.jns.2011.05.039
85. Costello F, Coupland S, Hodge W, et al. Quantifying axonal loss after optic neuritis with optical coherence tomography. Ann Neurol. 2006;59:963–969. 2006/05/24. https://doi.org/10.1002/ana.20851
86. Garas A, Simo M, Hollo G. Nerve fiber layer and macular thinning measured with different imaging methods during the course of acute optic neuritis. Europ J Ophthalmol. 2011;21:473–483. 2010/11/03. https://doi.org/10.5301/ejo.2010.5844
87. Kaushik M, Wang CY, Barnett MH, et al. Inner nuclear layer thickening is inversley proportional to retinal ganglion cell loss in optic neuritis. PLoS ONE. 2013;8: e78341. https://doi.org/10.1371/journal.pone.0078341.
88. Balk LJ, Coric D, Knier B, et al. Retinal inner nuclear layer volume: a potential new outcome measure for optic neuritis treatment trials in MS. Paris: ECTRIMS; 2017.
89. Balk LJ, Coric D, Knier B, et al. Retinal inner nuclear layer volume reflects inflammatory disease activity in multiple sclerosis; a longitudinal OCT study. Mult Scler J Exp Transl Clin. 2019;5:2055217319871582. 2019/09/17. https://doi.org/10.1177/2055217319871582
90. McIlwaine G, Csincsik L, Coey R, et al. Reduced cone density is associated with multiple sclerosis. Ophthalmol Sci. 2023;3: 100308. https://doi.org/10.1016/j.xops.2023.100308.
91. Longoni G, Brown RA, Oyefiade A, et al. Progressive retinal changes in pediatric multiple sclerosis. Mult Scler Relat Disord. 2022;61(103761):20220323. https://doi.org/10.1016/j.msard.2022.103761.
92. Wilbur C, Reginald YA, Longoni G, et al. Early neuroaxonal injury is seen in the acute phase of pediatric optic neuritis. Mult Scler Relat Disord. 2019;36(101387):20190907. https://doi.org/10.1016/j.msard.2019.101387.
93. Pakeerathan T, Havla J, Schwake C, et al. Characteristic retinal atrophy pattern allows differentiation between pediatric MOGAD and MS after a single optic neuritis episode. J Neurol. 2022;269(6366–6376):20220723. https://doi.org/10.1007/s00415-022-11256-y.
94. Birkeldh U, Manouchehrinia A, Hietala MA, et al. The temporal retinal nerve fiber layer thickness is the most important optical coherence tomography estimate in multiple sclerosis. Front Neurol. 2017;8(675):20171213. https://doi.org/10.3389/fneur.2017.00675.
95. Wicki CA, Manogaran P, Simic T, et al. Bilateral retinal pathology following a first-ever clinical episode of autoimmune optic neuritis. Neurol Neuroimmunol Neuroinflamm. 2020;7. 2020/01/24. https://doi.org/10.1212/nxi.0000000000000671
96. Waldman AT, Benson L, Sollee JR, et al. Interocular difference in retinal nerve fiber layer thickness predicts optic neuritis in pediatric-onset multiple sclerosis. J Neuroophthalmol. 2021;41:469–75. https://doi.org/10.1097/wno.0000000000001070.

97. Knier B, Berthele A, Buck D, et al. Optical coherence tomography indicates disease activity prior to clinical onset of central nervous system demyelination. Mult Scler. 2016;22:893–900. 2015/09/13. https://doi.org/10.1177/1352458515604496
98. Pietroboni AM, Dell'Arti L, Caprioli M, et al. The loss of macular ganglion cells begins from the early stages of disease and correlates with brain atrophy in multiple sclerosis patients. Mult Scler. 2017:1352458517740214. 2017/11/11. https://doi.org/10.1177/1352458517740214.
99. Petropoulos IN, Al-Shibani F, Bitirgen G, et al. Corneal axonal loss as an imaging biomarker of neurodegeneration in multiple sclerosis: a longitudinal study. Ther Adv Neurol Disord. 2023;16(17562864221118732):20230206. https://doi.org/10.1177/17562864221118731.
100. Paul F, Calabresi PA, Barkhof F, et al. Optical coherence tomography in multiple sclerosis: a 3-year prospective multicenter study. Ann Clin Transl Neurol. 2021;8(2235–2251):20211118. https://doi.org/10.1002/acn3.51473.
101. Klistorner A, Sriram P, Vootakuru N, et al. Axonal loss of retinal neurons in multiple sclerosis associated with optic radiation lesions. Neurology. 2014;82:2165–72. https://doi.org/10.1212/WNL.0000000000000522.
102. Knier B, Schmidt P, Aly L, et al. Retinal inner nuclear layer volume reflects response to immunotherapy in multiple sclerosis. Brain. 2016. 2016/09/02. https://doi.org/10.1093/brain/aww219
103. Albrecht P, Ringelstein M, Muller AK, et al. Degeneration of retinal layers in multiple sclerosis subtypes quantified by optical coherence tomography. Mult Scler. 2012;18:1422–9. https://doi.org/10.1177/1352458512439237.
104. Pearson T, Chen Y, Dhillon B, et al. Multi-modal retinal scanning to measure retinal thickness and peripheral blood vessels in multiple sclerosis. Sci Rep. 2022;12(20472):20221128. https://doi.org/10.1038/s41598-022-24312-4.
105. Aly L, Havla J, Lepennetier G, et al. Inner retinal layer thinning in radiologically isolated syndrome predicts conversion to multiple sclerosis. Eur J Neurol. 2020;27(2217–2224):20200719. https://doi.org/10.1111/ene.14416.
106. Rebolleda G, Gonzalez-Lopez JJ, Munoz-Negrete FJ, et al. Color-code agreement among stratus, cirrus, and spectralis optical coherence tomography in relapsing-remitting multiple sclerosis with and without prior optic neuritis. Am J Ophthalmol. 2013;155:890–7. https://doi.org/10.1016/j.ajo.2012.11.025.
107. Garcia-Martin E, Ara JR, Martin J, et al. Retinal and optic nerve degeneration in patients with multiple sclerosis followed up for 5 years. Ophthalmology. 2017 2017/02/12. https://doi.org/10.1016/j.ophtha.2017.01.005
108. Cilingir V, Batur M. Axonal Degeneration independent of inflammatory activity: is it more intense in the early stages of relapsing-remitting multiple sclerosis disease? Eur Neurol. 2020;83(508–516):20200921. https://doi.org/10.1159/000510116.
109. Sriram P, Wang C, Yiannikas C, et al. Relationship between optical coherence tomography and electrophysiology of the visual pathway in non-optic neuritis eyes of multiple sclerosis patients. PLoS One. 2014;9:e102546. 2014/08/29. https://doi.org/10.1371/journal.pone.0102546
110. Hokazono K, Raza AS, Oyamada MK, et al. Pattern electroretinogram in neuromyelitis optica and multiple sclerosis with or without optic neuritis and its correlation with FD-OCT and perimetry. Doc Ophthalmol. 2013;127:201–15. https://doi.org/10.1007/s10633-013-9401-2.
111. Albano V, Dammacco R, Manni A, et al. Macular ganglion cell-inner plexiform layer defect patterns in multiple sclerosis patients without optic neuritis: a spectral-domain-optical coherence tomography cross-sectional, case-control, pilot study. Europ J Ophthalmol. 2023;33(546–555):20220707. https://doi.org/10.1177/11206721221112803.
112. Saidha S, Syc SB, Ibrahim MA, et al. Primary retinal pathology in multiple sclerosis as detected by optical coherence tomography. Brain. 2011;134:518–33. https://doi.org/10.1093/brain/awq346.

113. Saidha S, Sotirchos ES, Ibrahim MA, et al. Microcystic macular oedema, thickness of the inner nuclear layer of the retina, and disease characteristics in multiple sclerosis: a retrospective study. The Lancet Neurol. 2012;11:963–72. https://doi.org/10.1016/s1474-4422(12)70213-2.
114. Goldman D. Muller glial cell reprogramming and retina regeneration. Nature Rev Neurosci. 2014;15:431–442. 2014/06/05. https://doi.org/10.1038/nrn3723
115. Brandt AU, Oberwahrenbrock T, Ringelstein M, et al. Primary retinal pathology in multiple sclerosis as detected by optical coherence tomography. Brain. 2011;134:e193. author reply e194. https://doi.org/10.1093/brain/awr095.
116. Gills JP, Jr. Electroretinographic abnormalities and advanced multiple sclerosis. Invest Ophthalmol. 1966;5:555–559. 1966/12/01.
117. Papakostopoulos D, Fotiou F, Hart JC, et al. The electroretinogram in multiple sclerosis and demyelinating optic neuritis. Electroencephalogr Clin Neurophysiol. 1989;74:1–10. 1989/01/01.
118. Forooghian F, Sproule M, Westall C, et al. Electroretinographic abnormalities in multiple sclerosis: possible role for retinal autoantibodies. Doc Ophthalmol. 2006;113:123–32. https://doi.org/10.1007/s10633-006-9022-0.
119. You Y, Graham EC, Shen T, et al. Progressive inner nuclear layer dysfunction in non-optic neuritis eyes in MS. Neurol Neuroimmunol Neuroinflamm. 2018;5:e427. 2017/12/21. https://doi.org/10.1212/nxi.0000000000000427
120. Behbehani R, Abu Al-Hassan A, Al-Salahat A, et al. Optical coherence tomography segmentation analysis in relapsing remitting versus progressive multiple sclerosis. PLoS One. 2017;12:e0172120. 2017/02/14. https://doi.org/10.1371/journal.pone.0172120.
121. Petracca M, Cordano C, Cellerino M, et al. Retinal degeneration in primary-progressive multiple sclerosis: a role for cortical lesions? Mult Scler. 2017;23:43–50. 2016/03/20. https://doi.org/10.1177/1352458516637679
122. Sotirchos ES, Gonzalez Caldito N, Filippatou A, et al. Progressive Multiple sclerosis is associated with faster and specific retinal layer atrophy. Ann Neurol. 2020. 2020/04/15. https://doi.org/10.1002/ana.25738
123. Cordano C, Nourbakhsh B, Yiu HH, et al. Differences in age-related retinal and cortical atrophy rates in multiple sclerosis. Neurology. 2022;99:e1685–e1693. 20220829. https://doi.org/10.1212/wnl.0000000000200977
124. Cellerino M, Cordano C, Boffa G, et al. Relationship between retinal inner nuclear layer, age, and disease activity in progressive MS. Neurol Neuroimmunol Neuroinflamm. 2019;6:20190812. https://doi.org/10.1212/nxi.0000000000000596
125. Kleerekooper I, Petzold A, Trip SA. Anterior visual system imaging to investigate energy failure in multiple sclerosis. Brain. 2020;143:1999–2008. https://doi.org/10.1093/brain/awaa049.
126. Ortiz-Perez S, Martinez-Lapiscina EH, Gabilondo I, et al. Retinal periphlebitis is associated with multiple sclerosis severity. Neurology. 2013;81:877–81. https://doi.org/10.1212/WNL.0b013e3182a3525e.
127. Iftikhar M, Zafar S, Gonzalez N, et al. Image artifacts in optical coherence tomography angiography among patients with multiple sclerosis. Curr Eye Res. 2019;44(558–563):20190128. https://doi.org/10.1080/02713683.2019.1565892.
128. Lanzillo R, Cennamo G, Criscuolo C, et al. Optical coherence tomography angiography retinal vascular network assessment in multiple sclerosis. Mult Scler. 2018;24:1706–1714. 2017/09/22. https://doi.org/10.1177/1352458517729463
129. Farci R, Carta A, Cocco E, et al. Optical coherence tomography angiography in multiple sclerosis: a cross-sectional study. PLoS ONE. 2020;15: e0236090. https://doi.org/10.1371/journal.pone.0236090.
130. Cordon B, Vilades E, Orduna E, et al. Angiography with optical coherence tomography as a biomarker in multiple sclerosis. PLoS ONE. 2020;15(e0243236):20201208. https://doi.org/10.1371/journal.pone.0243236.

131. Montorio D, Cennamo G, Carotenuto A, et al. Correlation analysis between foveal avascular zone and near peripheral retinal hypoperfusion in multiple sclerosis: a wide field optical coherence tomography angiography study. Front Med. 2022;9. Original Research. https://doi.org/10.3389/fmed.2022.1032514
132. Ulusoy MO, Horasanlı B, Işık-Ulusoy S. Optical coherence tomography angiography findings of multiple sclerosis with or without optic neuritis. Neurol Res. 2020;42(319–326):20200212. https://doi.org/10.1080/01616412.2020.1726585.
133. Wang X, Wang X, Chou Y, et al. Significant retinal microvascular impairments in multiple sclerosis assessed through optical coherence tomography angiography. Mult Scler Relat Disord. 2023;70(104505):20230104. https://doi.org/10.1016/j.msard.2023.104505.
134. Wang X, Jia Y, Spain R, et al. Optical coherence tomography angiography of optic nerve head and parafovea in multiple sclerosis. Br J Ophthalmol. 2014;98:1368–1373. 2014/05/17. https://doi.org/10.1136/bjophthalmol-2013-304547
135. Feucht N, Maier M, Lepennetier G, et al. Optical coherence tomography angiography indicates associations of the retinal vascular network and disease activity in multiple sclerosis. Mult Scler. 2018:1352458517750009. 2018/01/06. https://doi.org/10.1177/1352458517750009
136. Liu J, Song S, Gu X, et al. Microvascular impairments detected by optical coherence tomography angiography in multiple sclerosis patients: a systematic review and meta-analysis. Front Neurosci. 2023;16. Systematic Review. https://doi.org/10.3389/fnins.2022.1121899
137. Murphy OC, Kwakyi O, Iftikhar M, et al. Alterations in the retinal vasculature occur in multiple sclerosis and exhibit novel correlations with disability and visual function measures. Mult Scler. 2020;26:815–828. 2019/05/17. https://doi.org/10.1177/1352458519845116
138. Yilmaz H, Ersoy A, Icel E. Assessments of vessel density and foveal avascular zone metrics in multiple sclerosis: an optical coherence tomography angiography study. Eye (Lond). 2020;34(771–778):20191219. https://doi.org/10.1038/s41433-019-0746-y.
139. Liu Y, Delgado S, Jiang H, et al. Retinal tissue perfusion in patients with multiple sclerosis. Curr Eye Res. 2019;44(1091–1097):20190515. https://doi.org/10.1080/02713683.2019.1612444.
140. Spain RI, Liu L, Zhang X, et al. Optical coherence tomography angiography enhances the detection of optic nerve damage in multiple sclerosis. Br J Ophthalmol. 2018;102:520–524. 2017/08/18. https://doi.org/10.1136/bjophthalmol-2017-310477
141. Aly L, Noll C, Wicklein R, et al. Dynamics of retinal vessel loss after acute optic neuritis in patients with relapsing multiple sclerosis. Neurol Neuroimmunol Neuroinflamm. 2022;9:20220317. https://doi.org/10.1212/nxi.0000000000001159
142. Kleerekooper I, Houston S, Dubis AM, et al. Optical Coherence tomography angiography (OCTA) in multiple sclerosis and neuromyelitis optica spectrum disorder. Front Neurol. 2020;11. Review. https://doi.org/10.3389/fneur.2020.604049
143. Jiang H, Gameiro GR, Liu Y, et al. Visual function and disability are associated with increased retinal volumetric vessel density in patients with multiple sclerosis. Am J Ophthalmol. 2020;213(34–45):20200108. https://doi.org/10.1016/j.ajo.2019.12.021.
144. Girolamo F, Coppola C, Ribatti D, et al. Angiogenesis in multiple sclerosis and experimental autoimmune encephalomyelitis. Acta Neuropathol Commun. 2014;2(84):20140722. https://doi.org/10.1186/s40478-014-0084-z.
145. Kirk S, Frank JA, Karlik S. Angiogenesis in multiple sclerosis: is it good, bad or an epiphenomenon? J Neurol Sci. 2004;217:125–30. https://doi.org/10.1016/j.jns.2003.10.016.
146. Petzold A, Fraser CL, Abegg M, et al. Diagnosis and classification of optic neuritis. The Lancet Neurol. 2022;21:1120–34. https://doi.org/10.1016/S1474-4422(22)00200-9.
147. Petzold A, Chua SYL, Khawaja AP, et al. Retinal asymmetry in multiple sclerosis. Brain. 2021;144:224–35. https://doi.org/10.1093/brain/awaa361.
148. Nij Bijvank J, Uitdehaag BMJ, Petzold A. Retinal inter-eye difference and atrophy progression in multiple sclerosis diagnostics. J Neurol Neurosurg Psychiatry. 2022;93(216–219):20211111. https://doi.org/10.1136/jnnp-2021-327468.

149. Coric D, Balk LJ, Uitdehaag BMJ, et al. Diagnostic accuracy of optical coherence tomography inter-eye percentage difference for optic neuritis in multiple sclerosis. Eur J Neurol. 2017;24:1479–1484. 2017/09/10. https://doi.org/10.1111/ene.13443
150. Bsteh G, Hegen H, Altmann P, et al. Validation of inter-eye difference thresholds in optical coherence tomography for identification of optic neuritis in multiple sclerosis. Mult Scler Relat Disord. 2020;45(102403):20200717. https://doi.org/10.1016/j.msard.2020.102403.
151. Nolan-Kenney RC, Liu M, Akhand O, et al. Optimal intereye difference thresholds by optical coherence tomography in multiple sclerosis: an international study. Ann Neurol. 2019;85(618–629):20190410. https://doi.org/10.1002/ana.25462.
152. Motamedi S, Yadav SK, Kenney RC, et al. Prior optic neuritis detection on peripapillary ring scans using deep learning. Ann Clin Transl Neurol. 2022;9(1682–1691):20221025. https://doi.org/10.1002/acn3.51632.
153. Pihl-Jensen G, Wanscher B, Frederiksen JL. Predictive value of optical coherence tomography, multifocal visual evoked potentials, and full-field visual evoked potentials of the fellow, non-symptomatic eye for subsequent multiple sclerosis development in patients with acute optic neuritis. 2021;27:391–400.https://doi.org/10.1177/1352458520917924
154. Chua J, Bostan M, Li C, et al. A multi-regression approach to improve optical coherence tomography diagnostic accuracy in multiple sclerosis patients without previous optic neuritis. NeuroImage: Clinical. 2022;34:103010. https://doi.org/10.1016/j.nicl.2022.103010
155. Akaishi T, Takeshita T, Himori N, et al. Rapid administration of high-dose intravenous methylprednisolone improves visual outcomes after optic neuritis in patients with AQP4-IgG-Positive NMOSD. Front Neurol. 2020;11(932):20200902. https://doi.org/10.3389/fneur.2020.00932.
156. Kleiter I, Gahlen A, Borisow N, et al. Neuromyelitis optica: evaluation of 871 attacks and 1,153 treatment courses. Annals of Neurol. 2016;79:206–16. https://doi.org/10.1002/ana.24554.
157. Levy M. Plasmapheresis for acute attacks in neuromyelitis optica spectrum disorders. Neurol Neuroimmunol Neuroinflamm. 2018;5(e510):20180926. https://doi.org/10.1212/nxi.0000000000000510.
158. Kleiter I, Gahlen A, Borisow N, et al. Apheresis therapies for NMOSD attacks. A retrospective study of 207 therapeutic interventions 2018;5:e504. https://doi.org/10.1212/nxi.0000000000000504.
159. Liu C, Xiao H, Zhang X, et al. Optical coherence tomography angiography helps distinguish multiple sclerosis from AQP4-IgG-seropositive neuromyelitis optica spectrum disorder. Brain Behav. 2021;11(e02125):20210330. https://doi.org/10.1002/brb3.2125.
160. Ayoubi NKE, Moussa H, Younes A, et al. Use of retinal optical coherence tomography to differentiate suspected neuromyelitis optica spectrum disorder from multiple sclerosis: a cross-sectional study. Mult Scler Relat Disord. 2022;68(104160):20220907. https://doi.org/10.1016/j.msard.2022.104160.
161. Oertel FC, Zimmermann HG, Motamedi S, et al. Diagnostic value of intereye difference metrics for optic neuritis in aquaporin-4 antibody seropositive neuromyelitis optica spectrum disorders. J Neurol Neurosurgery and Psychiatry 2023: jnnp-2022–330608. https://doi.org/10.1136/jnnp-2022-330608
162. Chen JJ, Sotirchos ES, Henderson AD, et al. OCT retinal nerve fiber layer thickness differentiates acute optic neuritis from MOG antibody-associated disease and Multiple Sclerosis: RNFL thickening in acute optic neuritis from MOGAD vs MS. Mult Scler Relat Dis. 2022;58. https://doi.org/10.1016/j.msard.2022.103525
163. Shen T, You Y, Arunachalam S, et al. Differing structural and functional patterns of optic nerve damage in multiple sclerosis and neuromyelitis optica spectrum disorder. Ophthalmology. 2019;126(445–453):20180727. https://doi.org/10.1016/j.ophtha.2018.06.022.
164. Gigengack NK, Oertel FC, Motamedi S, et al. Structure-function correlates of vision loss in neuromyelitis optica spectrum disorders. Sci Rep. 2022;12(17545):20221020. https://doi.org/10.1038/s41598-022-19848-4.

165. Bennett JL, de Seze J, Lana-Peixoto M, et al. Neuromyelitis optica and multiple sclerosis: Seeing differences through optical coherence tomography. Mult Scler. 2015;21:678–688. 2015/02/11. https://doi.org/10.1177/1352458514567216
166. Sotirchos ES, Filippatou A, Fitzgerald KC, et al. Aquaporin-4 IgG seropositivity is associated with worse visual outcomes after optic neuritis than MOG-IgG seropositivity and multiple sclerosis, independent of macular ganglion cell layer thinning. Mult Scler. 2020;26(1360–1371):20190731. https://doi.org/10.1177/1352458519864928.
167. Lee GI, Park KA, Oh SY, et al. Differential patterns of parafoveal and peripapillary vessel density in multiple sclerosis and neuromyelitis optica spectrum disorder. Mult Scler Relat Disord. 2021;49(102780):20210119. https://doi.org/10.1016/j.msard.2021.102780.
168. Tiftikcioglu BI, Emre S, Idiman F, et al. Optical coherence tomography angiography (OCTA) in differential diagnosis of aquaporin-4 antibody seronegative NMOSD and multiple sclerosis. Mult Scler Relat Disord. 2022;58(103503):20220110. https://doi.org/10.1016/j.msard.2022.103503.
169. Motamedi S, Oertel FC, Yadav SK, et al. Altered fovea in AQP4-IgG-seropositive neuromyelitis optica spectrum disorders. Neurol Neuroimmunol Neuroinflamm. 2020;7:20200623. https://doi.org/10.1212/nxi.0000000000000805
170. Geraldes R, Ciccarelli O, Barkhof F, et al. The current role of MRI in differentiating multiple sclerosis from its imaging mimics. Nature Rev Neurol. 2018;14:199–213. https://doi.org/10.1038/nrneurol.2018.14.
171. Bartels F, Lu A, Oertel FC, et al. Clinical and neuroimaging findings in MOGAD-MRI and OCT. Clin Exp Immunol. 2021;206(266–281):20210718. https://doi.org/10.1111/cei.13641.
172. Asseyer S, Asgari N, Bennett J, et al. The acute optic neuritis network (ACON): Study protocol of a non-interventional prospective multicenter study on diagnosis and treatment of acute optic neuritis. Front Neurol. 2023;14. Study Protocol. https://doi.org/10.3389/fneur.2023.1102353
173. Balcer LJ, Baier ML, Pelak VS, et al. New low-contrast vision charts: reliability and test characteristics in patients with multiple sclerosis. Multiple Sclerosis. 2000;6:163–171. 2000/06/29.
174. Balcer LJ, Frohman EM. Evaluating loss of visual function in multiple sclerosis as measured by low-contrast letter acuity. Neurology. 2010;74(Suppl 3):S16-23. https://doi.org/10.1212/WNL.0b013e3181dbb664.
175. Garcia-Martin E, Rodriguez-Mena D, Herrero R, et al. Neuro-ophthalmologic evaluation, quality of life, and functional disability in patients with MS. Neurology. 2013;81:76–83. https://doi.org/10.1212/WNL.0b013e318299ccd9.
176. Saidha S, Syc SB, Durbin MK, et al. Visual dysfunction in multiple sclerosis correlates better with optical coherence tomography derived estimates of macular ganglion cell layer thickness than peripapillary retinal nerve fiber layer thickness. Mult Scler. 2011;17:1449–63. https://doi.org/10.1177/1352458511418630.
177. Talman LS, Bisker ER, Sackel DJ, et al. Longitudinal study of vision and retinal nerve fiber layer thickness in multiple sclerosis. Ann Neurol. 2010;67:749–60. https://doi.org/10.1002/ana.22005.
178. Schinzel J, Zimmermann H, Paul F, et al. Relations of low contrast visual acuity, quality of life and multiple sclerosis functional composite: a cross-sectional analysis. BMC Neurol. 2014;14:31. 2014/02/22. https://doi.org/10.1186/1471-2377-14-31
179. Villoslada P, Cuneo A, Gelfand J, et al. Color vision is strongly associated with retinal thinning in multiple sclerosis. Mult Scler. 2012;18:991–999. 2012/02/01. https://doi.org/10.1177/1352458511431972
180. Balk LJ, Coric D, Nij Bijvank JA, et al. Retinal atrophy in relation to visual functioning and vision-related quality of life in patients with multiple sclerosis. Mult Scler. 2018;24:767–776. 2017/05/18. https://doi.org/10.1177/1352458517708463
181. Harrison AC, Becker WJ and Stell WK. Colour vision abnormalities in multiple sclerosis. Can J Neurol Sci. 1987;14:279–285. 1987/08/01.

182. Martinez-Lapiscina EH, Ortiz-Perez S, Fraga-Pumar E, et al. Colour vision impairment is associated with disease severity in multiple sclerosis. Mult Scler. 2014;20:1207–16. https://doi.org/10.1177/1352458513517591.
183. Collorone S, Kanber B, Hashem L, et al. Visual function and brief cognitive assessment for multiple sclerosis in optic neuritis clinically isolated syndrome patients. J Neuroophthalmol. 2022;42:e22–e31. 20210923. https://doi.org/10.1097/wno.0000000000001280
184. Achiron A, Hecht I, Abayev L, et al. B-cell related biomarkers associated with severity of the first demyelinating event of acute optic neuritis. Eye (Lond). 2020;34(954–959):20191010. https://doi.org/10.1038/s41433-019-0614-9.
185. Ziccardi L, Barbano L, Boffa L, et al. Morphological outer retina findings in multiple sclerosis patients with or without optic neuritis. Frontiers in Neurol. 2020;11. https://doi.org/10.3389/fneur.2020.00858
186. Kenney RC, Liu M, Hasanaj L, et al. The role of optical coherence tomography criteria and machine learning in multiple sclerosis and optic neuritis diagnosis. Neurology. 2022;99:e1100-e1112. 20220628. https://doi.org/10.1212/wnl.0000000000200883
187. Henson DB. Visual fields. Oxford, U.K.: Oxford University Press; 1993.
188. Castro SM, Damasceno A, Damasceno BP, et al. Visual pathway abnormalities were found in most multiple sclerosis patients despite history of previous optic neuritis. Arq Neuropsiquiatr. 2013;71:437–441. 2013/07/17. https://doi.org/10.1590/0004-282x20130058
189. Cheng H, Laron M, Schiffman JS, et al. The relationship between visual field and retinal nerve fiber layer measurements in patients with multiple sclerosis. Invest Ophthalmol Vis Sci. 2007;48:5798–805. https://doi.org/10.1167/iovs.07-0738.
190. Merle H, Olindo S, Donnio A, et al. Anatomic and functional correlation of frequency-doubling technology perimetry (FDTP) in multiple sclerosis. Int Ophthalmol. 2011;31:263–270. 2011/06/04. https://doi.org/10.1007/s10792-011-9447-7
191. Vicini R, Brügger D, Abegg M, et al. Differences in morphology and visual function of myelin oligodendrocyte glycoprotein antibody and multiple sclerosis associated optic neuritis. J Neurol. 2021;268:276–84. https://doi.org/10.1007/s00415-020-10097-x.
192. Schmutz L, Borruat FX. Homonymous visual field defects in patients with multiple sclerosis: results of computerised perimetry and optical coherence tomography. Swiss Med Wkly. 2020;150(w20319):20200917. https://doi.org/10.4414/smw.2020.20319.
193. Fisk JD, Pontefract A, Ritvo PG, et al. The impact of fatigue on patients with multiple sclerosis. Can J Neurol Sci. 1994;21:9–14. 1994/02/01.
194. Piedrabuena R, Bittar M. Optical coherence tomography and visual evoked potential and its relationship with neurological disability in patients with relapsing-remitting multiple sclerosis. Mult Scler Relat Disord. 2022;57(103420):20211129. https://doi.org/10.1016/j.msard.2021.103420.
195. Di Maggio G, Santangelo R, Guerrieri S, et al. Optical coherence tomography and visual evoked potentials: which is more sensitive in multiple sclerosis? Mult Scler. 2014;20:1342–7. https://doi.org/10.1177/1352458514524293.
196. Tugcu B, Soysal A, Kilic M, et al. Assessment of structural and functional visual outcomes in relapsing remitting multiple sclerosis with visual evoked potentials and optical coherence tomography. J Neurol Sci. 2013;335:182–185. 2013/10/24. https://doi.org/10.1016/j.jns.2013.09.027
197. Abalo-Lojo JM, Limeres CC, Gomez MA, et al. Retinal nerve fiber layer thickness, brain atrophy, and disability in multiple sclerosis patients. J Neuroophthalmol. 2014;34:23–28. 2013/10/29. https://doi.org/10.1097/wno.0000000000000057
198. Tatrai E, Simo M, Iljicsov A, et al. In vivo evaluation of retinal neurodegeneration in patients with multiple sclerosis. PLoS ONE. 2012;7: e30922. https://doi.org/10.1371/journal.pone.0030922.
199. Soufi G, AitBenhaddou E, Hajji Z, et al. Evaluation of retinal nerve fiber layer thickness measured by optical coherence tomography in Moroccan patients with multiple sclerosis. J Fr Ophtalmol. 2015;38:497–503. 2015/04/22. https://doi.org/10.1016/j.jfo.2014.11.008

200. Spain RI, Maltenfort M, Sergott RC, et al. Thickness of retinal nerve fiber layer correlates with disease duration in parallel with corticospinal tract dysfunction in untreated multiple sclerosis. J Rehabil Res Dev. 2009;46:633–642. 2009/11/03.
201. Jeanjean L, Castelnovo G, Carlander B, et al. [Retinal atrophy using optical coherence tomography (OCT) in 15 patients with multiple sclerosis and comparison with healthy subjects]. Rev Neurol (Paris). 2008;164:927–934. 2008/09/24. https://doi.org/10.1016/j.neurol.2008.03.008
202. Naismith RT, Tutlam NT, Xu J, et al. Optical coherence tomography is less sensitive than visual evoked potentials in optic neuritis. Neurology. 2009;73:46–52. https://doi.org/10.1212/WNL.0b013e3181aaea32.
203. Eklund A, Huang-Link Y, Kovácsovics B, et al. OCT and VEP correlate to disability in secondary progressive multiple sclerosis. Mult Scler Relat Disord. 2022;68(104255):20221019. https://doi.org/10.1016/j.msard.2022.104255.
204. Saidha S, Sotirchos ES, Oh J, et al. Relationships between retinal axonal and neuronal measures and global central nervous system pathology in multiple sclerosis. JAMA Neurol. 2013;70:34–43. https://doi.org/10.1001/jamaneurol.2013.573.
205. Ontaneda D, LaRocca N, Coetzee T, et al. Revisiting the multiple sclerosis functional composite: proceedings from the national multiple sclerosis society (NMSS) task force on clinical disability measures. Multiple Sclerosis. 2012;18:1074–1080. 2012/06/29. https://doi.org/10.1177/1352458512451512
206. Balantrapu S, Sandroff BM, Pula JH, et al. Integrity of the anterior visual pathway and its association with ambulatory performance in multiple sclerosis. Mult Scler Int. 2013;481035. 2013/07/19. https://doi.org/10.1155/2013/481035
207. Sabadia SB, Nolan RC, Galetta KM, et al. 20/40 or better visual acuity after optic neuritis: not as good as we once thought? J Neuroophthalmol. 2016;36:369–376. 2016/07/30. https://doi.org/10.1097/wno.0000000000000421
208. Coric D, Balk LJ, Verrijp M, et al. Cognitive impairment in patients with multiple sclerosis is associated with atrophy of the inner retinal layers. Mult Scler. 2017:1352458517694090. 2017/03/10. https://doi.org/10.1177/1352458517694090
209. Mirmosayyeb O, Zivadinov R, Weinstock-Guttman B, et al. Optical coherence tomography (OCT) measurements and cognitive performance in multiple sclerosis: a systematic review and meta-analysis. J Neurol. 2022;270. https://doi.org/10.1007/s00415-022-11449-5
210. Dreyer-Alster S, Gal A, Achiron A. Optical coherence tomography is associated with cognitive impairment in multiple sclerosis. J Neuroophthalmol. 2022;42:e14–e21. 20210721. https://doi.org/10.1097/wno.0000000000001326
211. Baetge SJ, Dietrich M, Filser M, et al. Association of retinal layer thickness with cognition in patients with multiple sclerosis. Neurol Neuroimmunol Neuroinflamm. 2021;8:20210527. https://doi.org/10.1212/nxi.0000000000001018
212. Jakimovski D, Benedict RHB, Weinstock-Guttman B, et al. Visual deficits and cognitive assessment of multiple sclerosis: confounder, correlate, or both? J Neurol. 2021;268(2578–2588):20210215. https://doi.org/10.1007/s00415-021-10437-5.
213. Martinez-Lapiscina EH, Arnow S, Wilson JA, et al. Retinal thickness measured with optical coherence tomography and risk of disability worsening in multiple sclerosis: a cohort study. Lancet Neurol. 2016;15:574–584. 2016/03/25. https://doi.org/10.1016/s1474-4422(16)00068-5
214. Bsteh G, Hegen H, Teuchner B, et al. Peripapillary retinal nerve fibre layer as measured by optical coherence tomography is a prognostic biomarker not only for physical but also for cognitive disability progression in multiple sclerosis. Mult Scler. 2017:1352458517740216. 2017/11/03. https://doi.org/10.1177/1352458517740216
215. Rothman A, Murphy OC, Fitzgerald KC, et al. Retinal measurements predict 10-year disability in multiple sclerosis. Ann Clin Transl Neurol. 2019;6(222–232):20190119. https://doi.org/10.1002/acn3.674.

216. Lambe J, Fitzgerald KC, Murphy OC, et al. Association of spectral-domain oct with long-term disability worsening in multiple sclerosis. J Neurol. 2021;96:e2058–e2069.https://doi.org/10.1212/WNL.0000000000011788%
217. Bsteh G, Hegen H, Altmann P, et al. Retinal layer thickness predicts disability accumulation in early relapsing multiple sclerosis. Eur J Neurol. 2023;30(1025–1034):20230216. https://doi.org/10.1111/ene.15718.
218. Silva R, Coelho P, Seabra M, et al. Cognitive impairment and markers of optical neurodegeneration in early multiple sclerosis. Neurol Sci. 2022;43(4381–4386):20220212. https://doi.org/10.1007/s10072-022-05945-9.
219. Montolío A, Cegoñino J, Orduna E, et al. A mathematical model to predict the evolution of retinal nerve fiber layer thinning in multiple sclerosis patients. Comput Biol Med. 2019;111:103357. https://doi.org/10.1016/j.compbiomed.2019.103357.
220. Montolío A, Cegoñino J, Garcia-Martin E, et al. Comparison of machine learning methods using spectralis OCT for diagnosis and disability progression prognosis in multiple sclerosis. Ann Biomed Eng. 2022;50(507–528):20220226. https://doi.org/10.1007/s10439-022-02930-3.
221. Berek K, Hegen H, Hocher J, et al. Retinal layer thinning as a biomarker of long-term disability progression in multiple sclerosis. Mult Scler. 2022;28(1871–1880):20220602. https://doi.org/10.1177/13524585221097566.
222. Bsteh G, Berek K, Hegen H, et al. Macular ganglion cell-inner plexiform layer thinning as a biomarker of disability progression in relapsing multiple sclerosis. Mult Scler. 2021;27(684–694):20200702. https://doi.org/10.1177/1352458520935724.
223. El Ayoubi NK, Sabbagh HM, Bou Rjeily N, et al. Rate of retinal layer thinning as a biomarker for conversion to progressive disease in multiple sclerosis. Neurol Neuroimmunol Neuroinflammation. 2022;9: e200030. https://doi.org/10.1212/nxi.0000000000200030.
224. Bsteh G, Hegen H, Teuchner B, et al. Peripapillary retinal nerve fibre layer thinning rate as a biomarker discriminating stable and progressing relapsing-remitting multiple sclerosis. Eur J Neurol. 2019;26(865–871):20190219. https://doi.org/10.1111/ene.13897.
225. Wauschkuhn J, Solorza Buenrostro G, Aly L, et al. Retinal ganglion cell loss is associated with future disability worsening in early relapsing-remitting multiple sclerosis. Eur J Neurol. 2023;30(982–990):20230129. https://doi.org/10.1111/ene.15681.
226. Swinnen S, De Wit D, Van Cleemput L, et al. Optical coherence tomography as a prognostic tool for disability progression in MS: a systematic review. J Neurol. 2023;270(1178–1186):20221113. https://doi.org/10.1007/s00415-022-11474-4.
227. Cellerino M, Priano L, Bruschi N, et al. Relationship between retinal layer thickness and disability worsening in relapsing-remitting and progressive multiple sclerosis. J Neuroophthalmol. 2021;41:329–34. https://doi.org/10.1097/wno.0000000000001165.
228. Knier B, Leppenetier G, Wetzlmair C, et al. Association of retinal architecture, intrathecal immunity, and clinical course in multiple sclerosis. JAMA Neurol. 2017. https://doi.org/10.1001/jamaneurol.2017.0377.
229. Miller TR, Mohan S, Choudhri AF, et al. Advances in multiple sclerosis and its variants: conventional and newer imaging techniques. Radiologic clinics of North America 2014;52:321–336. 2014/03/04. https://doi.org/10.1016/j.rcl.2013.11.011
230. Vidal-Jordana A, Pareto D, Cabello S, et al. Optical coherence tomography measures correlate with brain and spinal cord atrophy and multiple sclerosis disease-related disability. Eur J Neurol. 2020;27(2225–2232):20200728. https://doi.org/10.1111/ene.14421.
231. Dörr J, Wernecke KD, Bock M, et al. Association of retinal and macular damage with brain atrophy in multiple sclerosis. PLoS One. 2011;6:e18132. 2011/04/16. https://doi.org/10.1371/journal.pone.0018132
232. Pfueller CF, Brandt AU, Schubert F, et al. Metabolic changes in the visual cortex are linked to retinal nerve fiber layer thinning in multiple sclerosis. PLoS One 2011;6:e18019. 2011/04/16. https://doi.org/10.1371/journal.pone.0018019

233. Gordon-Lipkin E, Chodkowski B, Reich DS, et al. Retinal nerve fiber layer is associated with brain atrophy in multiple sclerosis. Neurology. 2007;69:1603–9. https://doi.org/10.1212/01.wnl.0000295995.46586.ae.
234. Wang L, Tan H, Yu J, et al. Baseline retinal nerve fiber layer thickness as a predictor of multiple sclerosis progression: new insights from the FREEDOMS II study. Eur J Neurol. 2023;30(443–452):20221115. https://doi.org/10.1111/ene.15612.
235. Pawlitzki M, Horbrügger M, Loewe K, et al. MS optic neuritis-induced long-term structural changes within the visual pathway. Neurol Neuroimmunol Neuroinflamm. 2020;720200122. https://doi.org/10.1212/nxi.0000000000000665
236. Zimmermann H, Freing A, Kaufhold F, et al. Optic neuritis interferes with optical coherence tomography and magnetic resonance imaging correlations. Mult Scler. 2013;19:443–50. https://doi.org/10.1177/1352458512457844.
237. Young KL, Brandt AU, Petzold A, et al. Loss of retinal nerve fibre layer axons indicates white but not grey matter damage in early multiple sclerosis. Eur J Neurol. 2013;20:803–11. https://doi.org/10.1111/ene.12070.
238. Balk LJ, Steenwijk MD, Tewarie P, et al. Bidirectional trans-synaptic axonal degeneration in the visual pathway in multiple sclerosis. J Neurol Neurosurg Psychiatry. 2015;86:419–424. 2014/06/29. https://doi.org/10.1136/jnnp-2014-308189
239. Cagol A, Fuertes NC, Stoessel M, et al. Optical coherence tomography reflects clinically relevant gray matter damage in patients with multiple sclerosis. J Neurol. 2023;270:2139–48. https://doi.org/10.1007/s00415-022-11535-8.
240. Gabilondo I, Martinez-Lapiscina EH, Martinez-Heras E, et al. Trans-synaptic axonal degeneration in the visual pathway in multiple sclerosis. Ann Neurol. 2014;75:98–107. https://doi.org/10.1002/ana.24030.
241. Scheel M, Finke C, Oberwahrenbrock T, et al. Retinal nerve fibre layer thickness correlates with brain white matter damage in multiple sclerosis: a combined optical coherence tomography and diffusion tensor imaging study. Mult Scler. 2014;20:1904–7. https://doi.org/10.1177/1352458514535128.
242. Saidha S, Al-Louzi O, Ratchford JN, et al. Optical coherence tomography reflects brain atrophy in multiple sclerosis: a four-year study. Ann Neurol. 2015;78:801–813. 2015/07/21. https://doi.org/10.1002/ana.24487
243. Borgström M, Tisell A, Link H, et al. Retinal thinning and brain atrophy in early MS and CIS. Acta Neurol Scand. 2020;142(418–427):20200604. https://doi.org/10.1111/ane.13282.
244. Mizell R, Chen H, Lambe J, et al. Association of retinal atrophy with cortical lesions and leptomeningeal enhancement in multiple sclerosis on 7T MRI. Mult Scler. 2022;28(393–405):20210614. https://doi.org/10.1177/13524585211023343.
245. Krajnc N, Dal-Bianco A, Leutmezer F, et al. Association of paramagnetic rim lesions and retinal layer thickness in patients with multiple sclerosis. Mult Scler. 2023;29(374–384):20221220. https://doi.org/10.1177/13524585221138486.
246. Pulido-Valdeolivas I, Andorrà M, Gómez-Andrés D, et al. Retinal and brain damage during multiple sclerosis course: inflammatory activity is a key factor in the first 5 years. Sci Rep. 2020;10:13333. https://doi.org/10.1038/s41598-020-70255-z.
247. Krijnen EA, Ngamsombat C, George IC, et al. Axonal and myelin changes and their interrelationship in the optic radiations in people with multiple sclerosis. Mult Scler J Exp Transl Clin. 2023;9(20552173221147620):20230216. https://doi.org/10.1177/20552173221147620.
248. Murphy OC, Sotirchos ES, Kalaitzidis G, et al. Trans-synaptic degeneration following acute optic neuritis in multiple sclerosis. Ann Neurol. 2023;93(76–87):20221022. https://doi.org/10.1002/ana.26529.
249. Manogaran P, Hanson JV, Olbert ED, et al. Optical coherence tomography and magnetic resonance imaging in multiple sclerosis and neuromyelitis optica spectrum disorder. Int J Molecul Sci. 2016;17. 2016/11/18. https://doi.org/10.3390/ijms17111894
250. Sotirchos ES, Saidha S. OCT is an alternative to MRI for monitoring MS—YES. Multiple Sclerosis J. 2018;24:701–3. https://doi.org/10.1177/1352458517753722.

251. Aboulenein-Djamshidian F, Serbecic N. OCT is an alternative to MRI for monitoring MS—NO. Multiple Sclerosis J. 2018;24:703–5. https://doi.org/10.1177/1352458518754366.
252. Green AJ. OCT is an alternative to MRI for monitoring MS—commentary. Multiple Sclerosis J. 2018;24:705–6. https://doi.org/10.1177/1352458518765673.
253. Ferreira-Atuesta C, Reyes S, Giovanonni G, et al. The evolution of neurofilament light chain in multiple sclerosis. Front Neurosci. 2021;15(642384):20210406. https://doi.org/10.3389/fnins.2021.642384.
254. Barro C, Benkert P, Disanto G, et al. Serum neurofilament as a predictor of disease worsening and brain and spinal cord atrophy in multiple sclerosis. Brain. 2018;141:2382–91. https://doi.org/10.1093/brain/awy154.
255. Disanto G, Adiutori R, Dobson R, et al. Serum neurofilament light chain levels are increased in patients with a clinically isolated syndrome. J Neurol Neurosurg Psychiatry. 2016;87(126–129):20150225. https://doi.org/10.1136/jnnp-2014-309690.
256. Novakova L, Zetterberg H, Sundström P, et al. Monitoring disease activity in multiple sclerosis using serum neurofilament light protein. Neurology. 2017;89:2230–7. https://doi.org/10.1212/wnl.0000000000004683.
257. Lie IA, Kaçar S, Wesnes K, et al. Serum neurofilament as a predictor of 10-year grey matter atrophy and clinical disability in multiple sclerosis: a longitudinal study. J Neurol Neurosurgery and Psychiatry. 2022;93:849–57. https://doi.org/10.1136/jnnp-2021-328568.
258. Sotirchos ES, Vasileiou ES, Filippatou AG, et al. Association of serum neurofilament light chain with inner retinal layer thinning in multiple sclerosis. Neurology. 2022;99:e688–97. https://doi.org/10.1212/wnl.0000000000200778.
259. Brune S, Høgestøl EA, de Rodez Benavent SA, et al. Serum neurofilament light chain concentration predicts disease worsening in multiple sclerosis. Mult Scler. 2022;28(1859–1870):20220604. https://doi.org/10.1177/13524585221097296.
260. Krämer J, Wiendl H, Meuth SG, et al. Combined neurofilament light and optical coherence tomography better predicts multiple sclerosis disease activity than either measure alone. Neurol Neuroimmunol Neuroinflamm. 2021;8:20210804. https://doi.org/10.1212/nxi.0000000000001054
261. Tavazzi E, Jakimovski D, Kuhle J, et al. Serum neurofilament light chain and optical coherence tomography measures in MS: a longitudinal study. Neurol Neuroimmunol Neuroinflamm. 2020;7:20200518. https://doi.org/10.1212/nxi.0000000000000737
262. Lin TY, Vitkova V, Asseyer S, et al. Increased serum neurofilament light and thin ganglion cell-inner plexiform layer are additive risk factors for disease activity in early multiple sclerosis. Neurol Neuroimmunol Neuroinflamm. 2021;8:20210804. https://doi.org/10.1212/nxi.0000000000001051
263. Mallucci G, Patti F, Brescia Morra V, et al. A method to compare prospective and historical cohorts to evaluate drug effects. Application to the analysis of early treatment effectiveness of intramuscular interferon-β1a in multiple sclerosis patients. Mult Scler Relat Dis. 2020;40:101952. https://doi.org/10.1016/j.msard.2020.101952
264. Bergamaschi R, Montomoli C, Mallucci G, et al. BREMSO: a simple score to predict early the natural course of multiple sclerosis. Europ J Neurol. 2015;22:981–9. https://doi.org/10.1111/ene.12696.
265. Cadavid D, Cohen JA, Freedman MS, et al. The EDSS-Plus, an improved endpoint for disability progression in secondary progressive multiple sclerosis. Multiple Sclerosis J. 2017;23:94–105. https://doi.org/10.1177/1352458516638941.
266. Mikol D, Cohen J, Freedman M, et al. Rationale for EDSS-plus, the primary composite endpoint of disability progression in the ASCEND phase 3 study of natalizumab for secondary progressive multiple sclerosis: a post hoc analysis of IMPACT study data. Neurology. 2015;84:P7.240.
267. Tiu VE, Popescu BO, Enache, II, et al. Serum neurofilaments and OCT metrics predict EDSS-plus score progression in early relapse-remitting multiple sclerosis. Biomedicines. 2023;11:20230217. https://doi.org/10.3390/biomedicines11020606

268. Pietroboni AM, Carandini T, Dell'Arti L, et al. Evidence of retinal anterograde neurodegeneration in the very early stages of multiple sclerosis: a longitudinal OCT study. Neurol Sci. 2020;41(3175–3183):20200430. https://doi.org/10.1007/s10072-020-04431-4.
269. Ladakis DC, Yao PJ, Vreones M, et al. Mitochondrial measures in neuronally enriched extracellular vesicles predict brain and retinal atrophy in multiple sclerosis. Mult Scler. 2022;28(2020–2026):20220705. https://doi.org/10.1177/13524585221106290.
270. Yurtogullari S, Erbahceci IE. Inner and outer retina findings determined by optical coherence tomography in different subtypes of multiple sclerosis. Niger J Clin Pract. 2022;25:1069–75. https://doi.org/10.4103/njcp.njcp_1568_21.
271. Filippatou AG, Moniruzzaman M, Sotirchos ES, et al. Serum ceramide levels are altered in multiple sclerosis. Mult Scler. 2021;27(1506–1519):20201214. https://doi.org/10.1177/1352458520971816.
272. Alba-Arbalat S, Andorra M, Sanchez-Dalmau B, et al. In Vivo molecular changes in the retina of patients with multiple sclerosis. Invest Ophthalmol Vis Sci. 2021;62:11. https://doi.org/10.1167/iovs.62.6.11.
273. Castellazzi M, Lamberti G, Resi MV, et al. Increased levels of Endothelin-1 in cerebrospinal fluid are a marker of poor visual recovery after optic neuritis in multiple sclerosis patients. Dis Markers. 2019;2019(9320791):20190910. https://doi.org/10.1155/2019/9320791.
274. McCulloch DL, Marmor MF, Brigell MG, et al. ISCEV standard for full-field clinical electroretinography (2015 update). Doc Ophthalmol. 2015;130:1–12. https://doi.org/10.1007/s10633-014-9473-7.
275. Hood DC, Frishman LJ, Saszik S, et al. Retinal origins of the primate multifocal ERG: implications for the human response. Invest Ophthalmol Vis Sci. 2002;43:1673–1685. 2002/05/01.
276. Bearse MA, Sutter EE. Imaging localized retinal dysfunction with the multifocal electroretinogram. *J* Opt Soc Am A Opt Image Sci Vis. 1996;13:634–640. 1996/03/01.
277. Luo X, Frishman LJ. Retinal pathway origins of the pattern electroretinogram (PERG). Invest Ophthalmol Vis Sci. 2011;52:8571–84. https://doi.org/10.1167/iovs.11-8376.
278. Viswanathan S, Frishman LJ, Robson JG, et al. The photopic negative response of the macaque electroretinogram: reduction by experimental glaucoma. Invest Ophthalmol Vis Sci. 1999;40:1124–1136. 1999/05/11.
279. Klistorner AI, Graham SL, Grigg JR, et al. Multifocal topographic visual evoked potential: improving objective detection of local visual field defects. Invest Ophthalmol Vis Sci. 1998;39:937–950. 1998/05/14.
280. Narayanan D, Cheng H, Tang RA, et al. Reproducibility of multifocal visual evoked potential and traditional visual evoked potential in normal and multiple sclerosis eyes. Doc Ophthalmol. 2015;130:31–41. https://doi.org/10.1007/s10633-014-9467-5.
281. Narayanan D, Cheng H, Tang RA, et al. Longitudinal evaluation of visual function in multiple sclerosis. Optom Vis Sci. 2015;92:976–985. 2015/08/13. https://doi.org/10.1097/opx.0000000000000684
282. Perez-Rico C, Ayuso-Peralta L, Rubio-Perez L, et al. Evaluation of visual structural and functional factors that predict the development of multiple sclerosis in clinically isolated syndrome patients. Invest Ophthalmol Vis Sci. 2014;55:6127–31. https://doi.org/10.1167/iovs.14-14807.
283. Frohman AR, Schnurman Z, Conger A, et al. Multifocal visual evoked potentials are influenced by variable contrast stimulation in MS. Neurology. 2012;79:797–801. https://doi.org/10.1212/WNL.0b013e3182661edc.
284. Blanco R, Perez-Rico C, Puertas-Munoz I, et al. Functional assessment of the visual pathway with multifocal visual evoked potentials, and their relationship with disability in patients with multiple sclerosis. Mult Scler. 2014;20:183–91. https://doi.org/10.1177/1352458513493683.
285. Green AJ, Gelfand JM, Cree BA, et al. Clemastine fumarate as a remyelinating therapy for multiple sclerosis (ReBUILD): a randomised, controlled, double-blind, crossover trial. Lancet. 2017;390:2481–2489. 2017/10/17. https://doi.org/10.1016/s0140-6736(17)32346-2

286. Almarcegui C, Dolz I, Pueyo V, et al. Correlation between functional and structural assessments of the optic nerve and retina in multiple sclerosis patients. Neurophysiol Clin. 2010;40:129–35. https://doi.org/10.1016/j.neucli.2009.12.001.
287. Rodriguez-Mena D, Almarcegui C, Dolz I, et al. Electropysiologic evaluation of the visual pathway in patients with multiple sclerosis. J Clin Neurophysiol. 2013;30:376–381. 2013/08/06. https://doi.org/10.1097/WNP.0b013e31829d75f7
288. Klistorner A, Klistorner S, You Y, et al. Long-term effect of permanent demyelination on axonal survival in multiple sclerosis. Neurol Neuroimmunol Neuroinflammat. 2022;9: e1155. https://doi.org/10.1212/nxi.0000000000001155.
289. Narayanan D, Cheng H, Tang RA, et al. Multifocal visual evoked potentials and contrast sensitivity correlate with ganglion cell-inner plexiform layer thickness in multiple sclerosis. Clin Neurophysiol. 2019;130(180–188):20181113. https://doi.org/10.1016/j.clinph.2018.10.007.
290. Oertel FC, Krämer J, Motamedi S, et al. Visually evoked potential as prognostic biomarker for neuroaxonal damage in multiple sclerosis from a multicenter longitudinal cohort. Neurol Neuroimmunol Neuroinflammat. 2023;10: e200092. https://doi.org/10.1212/nxi.0000000000200092.
291. Ava S, Tamam Y, Hazar L, et al. Relationship between optical coherence tomography angiography and visual evoked potential in patients with multiple sclerosis. Indian J Ophthalmol. 2022;70:873–8. https://doi.org/10.4103/ijo.IJO_431_21.
292. Ayadi N, Oertel FC, Asseyer S, et al. Impaired motion perception is associated with functional and structural visual pathway damage in multiple sclerosis and neuromyelitis optica spectrum disorders. Mult Scler. 2022;28(757–767):20210811. https://doi.org/10.1177/13524585211032801.
293. Moussa H, Sawaya RA, Deeb R, et al. Correlation of pattern reversal and flash visual evoked potential latencies with optical coherence tomography measures in patients with optic neuropathy and patients with multiple sclerosis without optic neuropathy. J Clin Neurophysiol. 2022;39(637–642):20210122. https://doi.org/10.1097/wnp.0000000000000827.
294. Berman S, Backner Y, Krupnik R, et al. Conduction delays in the visual pathways of progressive multiple sclerosis patients covary with brain structure. Neuroimage. 2020;221(117204):20200801. https://doi.org/10.1016/j.neuroimage.2020.117204.
295. Carcelén-Gadea M, Quintanilla-Bordás C, Gracia-García A, et al. Functional and structural changes in the visual pathway in multiple sclerosis. Brain Behav. 2019;9(e01467):20191116. https://doi.org/10.1002/brb3.1467.
296. Vabanesi M, Pisa M, Guerrieri S, et al. In vivo structural and functional assessment of optic nerve damage in neuromyelitis optica spectrum disorders and multiple sclerosis. Sci Rep. 2019;9:10371. https://doi.org/10.1038/s41598-019-46251-3.
297. Jiang H, Gameiro GR, Hu H, et al. Shortened pattern electroretinogram latency and impaired autoregulatory dynamics to steady-state stimuli in patients with multiple sclerosis. 9000; Publish Ahead of Print. https://doi.org/10.1097/wno.0000000000000894
298. Wang J, Cheng H, Hu YS, et al. The photopic negative response of the flash electroretinogram in multiple sclerosis. Invest Ophthalmol Vis Sci. 2012;53:1315–23. https://doi.org/10.1167/iovs.11-8461.
299. Chen Q, Fang M, Miri S, et al. Retinal microvascular and neuronal function in patients with multiple sclerosis: 2-year follow-up. Mult Scler Relat Disord. 2021;56(103314):20211004. https://doi.org/10.1016/j.msard.2021.103314.
300. Hanson JVM, Ng M-Y, Hayward-Koennecke HK, et al. A three-year longitudinal study of retinal function and structure in patients with multiple sclerosis. Doc Ophthalmol. 2022;144:3–16. https://doi.org/10.1007/s10633-021-09855-7.
301. Robson AG, Nilsson J, Li S, et al. ISCEV guide to visual electrodiagnostic procedures. Doc Ophthalmol. 2018;136:1–26. 2018/02/06. https://doi.org/10.1007/s10633-017-9621-y
302. Gundogan FC, Demirkaya S, Sobaci G. Is optical coherence tomography really a new biomarker candidate in multiple sclerosis?—A structural and functional evaluation. Invest Ophthalmol Vis Sci. 2007;48:5773–5781. 2007/12/07. https://doi.org/10.1167/iovs.07-0834

303. Fraser CL, Holder GE. Electroretinogram findings in unilateral optic neuritis. Doc Ophthalmol. 2011;123:173–8. https://doi.org/10.1007/s10633-011-9294-x.
304. Ikeda H, Tremain KE, Sanders MD. Neurophysiological investigation in optic nerve disease: combined assessment of the visual evoked response and electroretinogram. Br J Ophthalmol. 1978;62:227–239. 1978/04/01
305. Sutter EE, Bearse MA, Jr. The optic nerve head component of the human ERG. Vision Res. 1999;39:419–436. 1999/05/26
306. Frohman TC, Beh SC, Saidha S, et al. Optic nerve head component responses of the multifocal electroretinogram in MS. Neurology. 2013;81:545–51. https://doi.org/10.1212/WNL.0b013e31829e6faa.
307. Schnurman ZS, Frohman TC, Beh SC, et al. Retinal architecture and mfERG: optic nerve head component response characteristics in MS. Neurology. 2014;82:1888–96. https://doi.org/10.1212/WNL.0000000000000447.
308. Zimmermann HG, Knier B, Oberwahrenbrock T, et al. Association of retinal ganglion cell layer thickness with future disease activity in patients with clinically isolated syndrome. JAMA Neurol. 2018. https://doi.org/10.1001/jamaneurol.2018.1011.
309. Gelfand JM, Nolan R, Schwartz DM, et al. Microcystic macular oedema in multiple sclerosis is associated with disease severity. Brain. 2012;135:1786–93. https://doi.org/10.1093/brain/aws098.
310. Burggraaff MC, Trieu J, de Vries-Knoppert WA, et al. The clinical spectrum of microcystic macular edema. Invest Ophthalmol Vis Sci. 2014;55:952–961. 2014/01/09. https://doi.org/10.1167/iovs.13-12912
311. Sigler EJ. Microcysts in the inner nuclear layer, a nonspecific SD-OCT sign of cystoid macular edema. Invest Ophthalmol Vis Sci. 2014;55:3282–3284. 2014/05/29. https://doi.org/10.1167/iovs.14-14056
312. Abegg M, Dysli M, Wolf S, et al. Microcystic macular edema: retrograde maculopathy caused by optic neuropathy. Ophthalmology. 2014;121:142–149. 2013/10/22. https://doi.org/10.1016/j.ophtha.2013.08.045
313. Kaufhold F, Zimmermann H, Schneider E, et al. Optic neuritis is associated with inner nuclear layer thickening and microcystic macular edema independently of multiple sclerosis. PLoS ONE. 2013;8: e71145. https://doi.org/10.1371/journal.pone.0071145.
314. Gelfand JM, Cree BA, Nolan R, et al. Microcystic inner nuclear layer abnormalities and neuromyelitis optica. JAMA Neurol. 2013;70:629–633. 2013/03/27. https://doi.org/10.1001/jamaneurol.2013.1832
315. Brandt AU, Oberwahrenbrock T, Kadas EM, et al. Dynamic formation of macular microcysts independent of vitreous traction changes. Neurology. 2014;83:73–7. https://doi.org/10.1212/WNL.0000000000000545.
316. Balk LJ, Killestein J, Polman CH, et al. Microcystic macular oedema confirmed, but not specific for multiple sclerosis. Brain. 2012;135:e226; author reply e227. https://doi.org/10.1093/brain/aws216
317. Wolff B, Basdekidou C, Vasseur V, et al. Retinal inner nuclear layer microcystic changes in optic nerve atrophy: a novel spectral-domain OCT finding. Retina. 2013;33:2133–2138. 2013/05/07. https://doi.org/10.1097/IAE.0b013e31828e68d0
318. Hasegawa T, Akagi T, Yoshikawa M, et al. Microcystic inner nuclear layer changes and retinal nerve fiber layer defects in eyes with glaucoma. PLoS One. 2015;10:e0130175. 2015/06/13. https://doi.org/10.1371/journal.pone.0130175
319. Barboni P, Carelli V, Savini G, et al. Microcystic macular degeneration from optic neuropathy: not inflammatory, not trans-synaptic degeneration. Brain. 2013;136: e239. https://doi.org/10.1093/brain/awt014.
320. Lujan BJ, Horton JC. Microcysts in the inner nuclear layer from optic atrophy are caused by retrograde trans-synaptic degeneration combined with vitreous traction on the retinal surface. Brain. 2013;136: e260. https://doi.org/10.1093/brain/awt154.
321. Abegg M, Zinkernagel M, Wolf S. Microcystic macular degeneration from optic neuropathy. Brain. 2012;135: e225. https://doi.org/10.1093/brain/aws215.

322. Kisimbi J, Shalchi Z, Mahroo OA, et al. Macular spectral domain optical coherence tomography findings in Tanzanian endemic optic neuropathy. Brain. 2013;136:3418–26. https://doi.org/10.1093/brain/awt221.
323. Haldar S, Mukherjee R, Elston J. Microcystic macular edema in a case of tobacco-alcohol optic neuropathy. Canadian J Ophthalmol. J. Canadien d'ophtalmologie 2017;52:e19–e22. 2017/02/27. https://doi.org/10.1016/j.jcjo.2016.07.014
324. Yoon DH, Kang DJ, Kim MJ, et al. New observation of microcystic macular edema as a mild form of cystoid macular lesions after standard phacoemulsification: prevalence and risk factors. Medicine. 2018;97:e0355. 2018/04/12. https://doi.org/10.1097/md.0000000000010355
325. Sigler EJ, Randolph JC, Charles S. Delayed onset inner nuclear layer cystic changes following internal limiting membrane removal for epimacular membrane. Graefes Arch Clin Exp Ophthalmol. 2013;251:1679–1685. 2013/01/12. https://doi.org/10.1007/s00417-012-2253-8
326. Petzold A. Retinal glymphatic system: an explanation for transient retinal layer volume changes? Brain. 2016;139:2816–2819. 2017/11/07. https://doi.org/10.1093/brain/aww239
327. Caldito NG, Saidha S, Sotirchos ES, et al. Brain and retinal atrophy in African-Americans versus Caucasian-Americans with multiple sclerosis: a longitudinal study. Brain 2018;141:3115–3129. 2018/10/13. https://doi.org/10.1093/brain/awy245
328. Kimbrough DJ, Sotirchos ES, Wilson JA, et al. Retinal damage and vision loss in African American multiple sclerosis patients. Ann Neurol. 2015;77:228–36. https://doi.org/10.1002/ana.24308.
329. Naismith RT, Trinkaus K, Cross AH. Phenotype and prognosis in African-Americans with multiple sclerosis: a retrospective chart review. Mult Scler. 2006;12:775–781. 2007/02/01. https://doi.org/10.1177/1352458506070923
330. Kister I, Chamot E, Bacon JH, et al. Rapid disease course in African Americans with multiple sclerosis. Neurology. 2010;75:217–223. 2010/07/21. https://doi.org/10.1212/WNL.0b013e3181e8e72a
331. Button J, Al-Louzi O, Lang A, et al. Disease-modifying therapies modulate retinal atrophy in multiple sclerosis: a retrospective study. Neurology. 2017;88:525–532. 2017/01/13. https://doi.org/10.1212/wnl.0000000000003582
332. Guarnera C, Bramanti P, Mazzon E. Comparison of efficacy and safety of oral agents for the treatment of relapsing-remitting multiple sclerosis. Drug Design, Developm. Therapy. 2017;11:2193–2207. 2017/08/18. https://doi.org/10.2147/dddt.s137572
333. Derfuss T, Bergvall NK, Sfikas N, et al. Efficacy of fingolimod in patients with highly active relapsing-remitting multiple sclerosis. Curr Med Res Opin. 2015;31:1687–1691. 2015/06/30. https://doi.org/10.1185/03007995.2015.1067191
334. Kappos L, Cohen J, Collins W, et al. Fingolimod in relapsing multiple sclerosis: An integrated analysis of safety findings. Mult Scler Relat Disord. 2014;3:494–504. 2015/04/17. https://doi.org/10.1016/j.msard.2014.03.002
335. Calabresi PA, Radue EW, Goodin D, et al. Safety and efficacy of fingolimod in patients with relapsing-remitting multiple sclerosis (FREEDOMS II): a double-blind, randomised, placebo-controlled, phase 3 trial. Lancet Neurol. 2014;13:545–556. 2014/04/02. https://doi.org/10.1016/s1474-4422(14)70049-3
336. Rotsos TG, Moschos MM. Cystoid macular edema. Clin Ophthalmol. 2008;2:919–930. 2009/08/12.
337. Novartis. Gilenya full prescribing information. Novartis;2018.
338. Hajali M, Fishman GA. The prevalence of cystoid macular oedema on optical coherence tomography in retinitis pigmentosa patients without cystic changes on fundus examination. Eye (Lond) 2009;23:915–919. 2008/04/22. https://doi.org/10.1038/eye.2008.110
339. Fruschelli M, Capozzoli M, Gelmi MC, et al. Longitudinal quantitative assessment of macula during therapy with fingolimod in relapsing-remitting multiple sclerosis. Int Ophthalmol. 2019;39(777–781):20180302. https://doi.org/10.1007/s10792-018-0870-x.

340. Nørgaard TL, Andersen CU, Hilt C, et al. Macular oedema and changes in macular thickness in multiple sclerosis patients treated with fingolimod. Basic Clin Pharmacol Toxicol. 2020;126(492–497):20200113. https://doi.org/10.1111/bcpt.13381.
341. d'Ambrosio A, Capuano R, Rossi S, et al. Two-year macular volume assessment in multiple sclerosis patients treated with fingolimod. Neurol Sci. 2021;42(731–733):20201008. https://doi.org/10.1007/s10072-020-04802-x.
342. Garcia-Martin E, Ruiz de Gopegui E, Satue M, et al. Progressive functional and neuroretinal affectation in patients with multiple sclerosis treated with fingolimod. J Neuroophthalmol. 2021;41:e415–e423. https://doi.org/10.1097/wno.0000000000000991
343. Chan JK, Hernandez Martínez de Lapiscina E, Taylor C, et al. Long-term stability of neuroaxonal structure in alemtuzumab-treated relapsing-remitting multiple sclerosis patients. J Neuroophthalmol. 2020;40:37–43. https://doi.org/10.1097/wno.0000000000000802
344. Lambe J, Risher H, Filippatou AG, et al. Modulation of retinal atrophy with rituximab in multiple sclerosis. Neurology. 2021;96:e2525-e2533. 20210407. https://doi.org/10.1212/wnl.0000000000011933
345. Bsteh G, Hegen H, Altmann P, et al. Retinal layer thinning predicts treatment failure in relapsing multiple sclerosis. Eur J Neurol. 2021;28(2037–2045):20210402. https://doi.org/10.1111/ene.14829.
346. Miscioscia A, Puthenparampil M, Miante S, et al. Retinal inner nuclear layer thinning is decreased and associates with the clinical outcome in ocrelizumab-treated primary progressive multiple sclerosis. J Neurol. 2022;269(5436–5442):20220601. https://doi.org/10.1007/s00415-022-11183-y.
347. Raftopoulos R, Hickman SJ, Toosy A, et al. Phenytoin for neuroprotection in patients with acute optic neuritis: a randomised, placebo-controlled, phase 2 trial. Lancet Neurol. 2016;15(259–269):20160126. https://doi.org/10.1016/s1474-4422(16)00004-1.
348. Küchlin S, Ihorst G, Grotejohann B, et al. Treatment with erythropoietin for patients with optic neuritis. Long-term Follow-up. 2023;10: e200067. https://doi.org/10.1212/nxi.0000000000200067.
349. Andorrà M, Alba-Arbalat S, Camos-Carreras A, et al. Using acute optic neuritis trials to assess neuroprotective and remyelinating therapies in multiple sclerosis. JAMA Neurol. 2020;77:234–44. https://doi.org/10.1001/jamaneurol.2019.3283.
350. Petzold A, Coric D, Balk LJ, et al. Longitudinal development of peripapillary hyper-reflective ovoid masslike structures suggests a novel pathological pathway in multiple sclerosis. Ann Neurol. 2020;88(309–319):20200609. https://doi.org/10.1002/ana.25782.
351. Borrelli E, Barboni P, Battista M, et al. Peripapillary hyperreflective ovoid mass-like structures (PHOMS): OCTA may reveal new findings. Eye. 2021;35:528–31. https://doi.org/10.1038/s41433-020-0890-4.
352. Xie X, Liu T, Wang W, et al. Clinical and multi-mode imaging features of eyes with peripapillary hyperreflective ovoid mass-like structures. Front Med. 2022;9. Original Research. https://doi.org/10.3389/fmed.2022.796667
353. Fraser JA, Sibony PA, Petzold A, et al. Peripapillary hyper-reflective ovoid mass-like structure (PHOMS): an optical coherence tomography marker of axoplasmic stasis in the optic nerve head. J Neuroophthalmol. 2021;41:431–41. https://doi.org/10.1097/wno.0000000000001203.
354. Wicklein R, Wauschkuhn J, Giglhuber K, et al. Association of peripapillary hyper-reflective ovoid masslike structures and disease duration in primary progressive multiple sclerosis. Eur J Neurol. 2021;28:20210825. https://doi.org/10.1111/ene.15056
355. Gernert JA, Wicklein R, Hemmer B, et al. Peripapillary hyper-reflective ovoid mass-like structures (PHOMS) in AQP4-IgG-positive neuromyelitis optica spectrum disease (NMOSD) and MOG-IgG-associated disease (MOGAD). J Neurol. 2023;270(1135–1140):20221016. https://doi.org/10.1007/s00415-022-11381-8.

356. Fragiotta S, Abdolrahimzadeh S, Dolz-Marco R, et al. Significance of hyperreflective foci as an optical coherence tomography biomarker in retinal diseases: characterization and clinical implications. J Ophthalmol. 2021;2021(6096017):20211217. https://doi.org/10.1155/2021/6096017.
357. Pengo M, Miante S, Franciotta S, et al. Retinal hyperreflecting foci associate with cortical pathology in multiple sclerosis. Neurol Neuroimmunol Neuroinflamm. 2022;9:20220523. https://doi.org/10.1212/nxi.0000000000001180
358. Schmidt MF, Pihl-Jensen G, Torm MEW, et al. Hyperreflective dots in the avascular outer retina in relapsing-remitting multiple sclerosis. Mult Scler Relat Disord. 2023;72(104617):20230312. https://doi.org/10.1016/j.msard.2023.104617.
359. Pilotto E, Miante S, Torresin T, et al. Hyperreflective foci in the retina of active relapse-onset multiple sclerosis. Ophthalmology. 2020;127(1774–1776):20200329. https://doi.org/10.1016/j.ophtha.2020.03.024.
360. Nguyen J, Rothman A, Gonzalez N, et al. Macular ganglion cell and inner plexiform layer thickness is more strongly associated with visual function in multiple sclerosis than bruch membrane opening-minimum rim width or peripapillary retinal nerve fiber layer thicknesses. J Neuroophthalmol. 2019;39:444–50. https://doi.org/10.1097/wno.0000000000000768.
361. Barreiro-González A, Sanz MT, Carratalà-Boscà S, et al. Dyschromatopsia in multiple sclerosis reflects diffuse chronic neurodegeneration beyond anatomical landmarks. Acta Neurol Belg. 2021;121(1767–1775):20201012. https://doi.org/10.1007/s13760-020-01516-x.
362. Jiang H, Delgado S, Wang J. Advances in ophthalmic structural and functional measures in multiple sclerosis: do the potential ocular biomarkers meet the unmet needs? Current Opinion in Neurol. 2021;34.
363. Chen Y, Larraz J, Wong M, et al. Longitudinal retinal imaging study of newly diagnosed relapsing-remitting multiple sclerosis in Scottish population: baseline and 12 months follow-up profile of FutureMS retinal imaging cohort. BMJ Open Ophthalmol. 2022;7. https://doi.org/10.1136/bmjophth-2022-001024
364. Oertel FC, Zimmermann HG, Brandt AU, et al. Novel uses of retinal imaging with optical coherence tomography in multiple sclerosis. Expert Rev Neurother. 2019;19(31–43):20181227. https://doi.org/10.1080/14737175.2019.1559051.
365. Vujosevic S, Parra MM, Hartnett ME, et al. Optical coherence tomography as retinal imaging biomarker of neuroinflammation/neurodegeneration in systemic disorders in adults and children. Eye. 2023;37:203–19. https://doi.org/10.1038/s41433-022-02056-9.
366. Garcia-Martin E, Ortiz M, Boquete L, et al. Early diagnosis of multiple sclerosis by OCT analysis using Cohen's d method and a neural network as classifier. Comput Biol Med. 2021;129(104165):20201203. https://doi.org/10.1016/j.compbiomed.2020.104165.
367. Cavaliere C, Vilades E, Alonso-Rodríguez MC, et al. Computer-aided diagnosis of multiple sclerosis using a support vector machine and optical coherence tomography features. Sensors. 19. https://doi.org/10.3390/s19235323
368. Tazarjani HD, Amini Z, Kafieh R, et al. Retinal OCT texture analysis for differentiating healthy controls from multiple sclerosis (MS) with/without optic neuritis. Biomed Res Int. 2021;2021(5579018):20210710. https://doi.org/10.1155/2021/5579018.
369. Montolío A, Martín-Gallego A, Cegoñino J, et al. Machine learning in diagnosis and disability prediction of multiple sclerosis using optical coherence tomography. Comput Biol Med. 2021;133(104416):20210426. https://doi.org/10.1016/j.compbiomed.2021.104416.
370. Pérez Del Palomar A, Cegoñino J, Montolío A, et al. Swept source optical coherence tomography to early detect multiple sclerosis disease. The use of machine learning techniques. PLoS One. 2019;14:e0216410. 20190506. https://doi.org/10.1371/journal.pone.0216410
371. Ciftci Kavaklioglu B, Erdman L, Goldenberg A, et al. Machine learning classification of multiple sclerosis in children using optical coherence tomography. Mult Scler. 2022;28(2253–2262):20220809. https://doi.org/10.1177/13524585221112605.

372. Torbus M, Niewiadomska E, Dobrakowski P, et al. The usefulness of optical coherence tomography in disease progression monitoring in younger patients with relapsing-remitting multiple sclerosis: a single-centre study. J Clinical Med. 2022;12:20221222. https://doi.org/10.3390/jcm12010093

OCT in Parkinson's Disease and Related Disorders

12

Jingxin Zhou, Kai Jin, Xiaojun Guan, Juan Ye, and Andrzej Grzybowski

Abstract

Parkinson's disease (PD) is one of predominant degenerative diseases of the central nervous system (CNS), mainly caused by the degeneration of dopaminergic neurons, with the main clinical manifestations being bradykinesia, rest tremor and rigidity. Retina has been regarded as the window towards CNS and contains dopaminergic neurons. Screening, predicting, and assessing the onset, prognosis, and outcome of PD via retina has been a widespread interest in ophthalmology and neuroscience. In recent years, optical coherence tomography (OCT) of the retina, a noninvasive, convenient, and inexpensive retinal imaging technique, has gained broad attention. The significance of OCT in PD has also been widely studied. In this chapter, we first review the histologic, physiologic, and pathologic associations of the retina and PD, followed by a glance of OCT technical features and recent OCT imaging advances, then a demonstration of OCT-based imaging markers in PD, followed by a summary of the

J. Zhou · K. Jin · J. Ye (✉)
School of Medicine, Eye Center, The Second Affiliated Hospital, Zhejiang University, Hangzhou, Zhejiang, China
e-mail: yejuan@zju.edu.cn

J. Zhou
e-mail: zhoujingxin@zju.edu.cn

K. Jin
e-mail: jinkai@zju.edu.cn

X. Guan
Department of Radiology, The Second Affiliated Hospital, Zhejiang University School of Medicine, Hangzhou, Zhejiang, China
e-mail: xiaojunguan1102@zju.edu.cn

A. Grzybowski
Institute for Research in Ophthalmology, Foundation for Ophthalmology Development, Poznan, Poland

A. Grzybowski and P. Barboni (eds.), *OCT and Imaging in Central Nervous System Diseases*, https://doi.org/10.1007/978-3-031-72156-4_12

clinical associations of these markers and PD, then a summarization of OCTA in PD, and finally a brief demonstration of the functional-morphological retinal changes in PD patients. We believe that OCT has a special significance for screening, diagnosis, and efficacy prediction of PD. However, these results need to be examined in large-scale population-based cohorts, and advances in novel image analysis technologies, such as artificial intelligence, will lend fresh impetus into this field.

Keywords

Parkinson's disease • Optical coherence tomography • Retina imaging • Biomarker • Peripapillary retinal nerve fiber layer • Macular thickness • Retinal vasculature • Movement disorder

12.1 Introduction

Parkinson's disease (PD) is a progressive neurodegenerative disease that presents clinically with bradykinesia, rigidity, rest tremor and postural instability [1]. It is estimated to affect more than 10 million people worldwide and is the second most common neurodegenerative disease in the developed world [2]. Lewy bodies, mainly constituted by abnormally deposited α-synuclein (αsyn) protein, and neuronal loss are hallmarks of PD pathology, with substantia nigra as the major affected area. Subsequent dopaminergic degeneration in the substantia nigra is generally considered to be the essential pathological feature of PD [1]. Although PD mainly affects the motor system, there are also non-motor manifestations including alterations in mood and sleep, autonomic nervous system disturbances, and visual hallucinations [3]. Currently, diagnosis of PD is primarily based on clinical symptoms. The presence of bradykinesia, plus rest tremor and/or rigidity is required for documentation of parkinsonism [4]. Further criteria are designed to differentiate PD from atypical parkinsonian syndromes and make the PD diagnosis [4]. PD cannot be completely cured, and supplementation of dopamine using levodopa/carbidopa is currently the most common and effective medication.

Retina is a layered structure, consisting of nerve cells and synapses. The outer nuclear layer (ONL) contains cell bodies of cones and rods photoreceptors; the inner nuclear layer (INL) includes cell bodies of bipolar, horizontal, and dopaminergic amacrine cells; and the ganglion cell layer (GCL) contains ganglion cells and displaced amacrine cells [5]. The fovea is a special area of the retina containing the highest concentration of the cone photoreceptors and essential for visual function. Cone density diminishes with distance from the center of the fovea, while other retinal neurons grow and form a slope at the margin of the foveal pit. The interaction between receptors and their organization into a receptive field structure is responsible for high contrast sensitivity [6]. The foveal region is the thickest part of the retina, mainly due to increased density of photoreceptors (cones) and ganglion cells compared to the peripheral retina. There are abundant synaptic interactions in the central retina leading to a thick inner plexiform layer (IPL) [5]. The retinal nerve fiber layer (RNFL) functions as the retinal output emanating from retinal ganglion cells. The nerve fibers are the axons of retinal ganglion cells and form the optic nerve behind the globe toward the lateral geniculate body and then onto the visual cortex. Further visual processing takes place in visual cortical areas [6].

Years of development have produced multiple retinal assessment methods, from fundus photography to functional assessment of retinal electrical activity. One of the main motivations for investigating the role of retinal pathology in neurodegenerative diseases, including PD, has been this multidimensional form of imaging. In broad terms, these imaging modalities can be divided into those that show structural features of the retina and those that measure some aspect of the function of the retina [2]. Structural features include retinal vessel metrics, retinal pathological lesions and retinal thickness. Functional features of the retina that are quantified by imaging techniques include retinal reaction to light, blood flow and electrical activity, etc. Optical coherence tomography (OCT) is a commonly-used imaging technique able to provide high-resolution images of the cross-sectional retinal structure, including retinal thicknesses, pathologies etc. Because OCT examination is convenient, rapid and non-invasive, retinal OCT imaging is widely used in a variety of medical scenarios, including ocular disorders and CNS degenerative diseases [1].

The relationship between retina and PD is longstanding. On the one hand, visual disorders are common among PD patients, which are generally considered to be the result of dopaminergic deficiency. Reorganization of ganglion cell receptive fields in PD were described decades ago [7, 8], since which many studies put forward functional evidence that foveal vision is impaired in PD, including decreased contrast sensitivity and color vision abnormalities [9]. Psychophysical and electrophysiological functional studies considering the retina imply that impaired retinal electrical signal processing in PD is caused by dopaminergic deficiency [10–12]. On the other hand, with the wide spread of OCT, retinal imaging characteristics are seen as a biomarker for PD screening, differential diagnosis or treatment effect assessment. Peripapillary RNFL (pRNFL) thinning, macular thinning and retinal vasculature rearrangement have all been reported to be correlated with PD [2].

In the present chapter, we first review the histological, physiological, and pathological associations of the retina with PD, followed by an overview of OCT technical features and recent advances in OCT imaging, then a demonstration of OCT-based imaging markers in PD, and finally a summary of the clinical associations of these markers with PD. We believe that OCT has particular relevance in the screening, diagnosis, and efficacy prediction of PD. However, these findings need to be verified in large population-based cohorts, and advances in novel image analysis technologies, such as artificial intelligence, will provide new impetus in this area.

12.2 Retina and PD: Histology, Physiology, and Pathology

As mentioned before, retina is a multilayered structure containing diverse neurons with distinct functions and different neurotransmitters. The retina and optic nerve are derived from the neuroectoderm around 23 days of gestation when they invaginate from the diencephalon [13]. Therefore, the retina shares a common developmental origin and is a part of the central nervous system (CNS). The major cellular components of the retina are the retinal pigment epithelium (RPE) cell, the photoreceptor cells, the interneurons, the ganglion cells, and the glial cells [14]. RPE cells play an important role in maintaining the visual cycle through phagocytosis, protection of the retina structure, working as barrier and substance transporting etc. [15]. The photoreceptors are the sensors of the visual system that convert the capture of photons into a nerve signal in a process called phototransduction [14]. Each photoreceptor consists of an outer segment (OS), inner segment (IS), a nucleus, an inner fiber, and the synaptic terminal [14]. Interneurons in the INL connect the photoreceptor layer with the ganglion cell layer. These interneurons consist of the bipolar, horizontal, amacrine, and inter plexiform cells [14]. The ganglion cells are responsible for visual signal transmission from the retina to the brain. In OCT, the retina is usually segmented as RNFL, ganglion cell layer (GCL), inner plexiform layer (IPL), inner nuclear layer (INL), outer plexiform layer (OPL), outer nuclear layer (ONL), inner segment outer segment (ISOS) and retinal pigment epithelium (RPE) [16]. These layers can be seen and assessed in retinal OCT images, as in Fig. 12.1. In retinal OCT analysis, central macular thickness (CMT) and macular volume (MV) were also commonly utilized to assess retinal neurodegeneration.

Retinal dysfunction in PD patients is multidimensional, including functional, structural, and pathological changes [1]. The functional changes include impaired contrast sensitivity, impaired color discrimination, intermittent double vision, decreased visual acuity, and impaired retinal electronical activity. The structural changes mainly lie in the retinal thinning, nigral dopamine loss, vasculature remodeling. Pathological changes include dopaminergic amacrine cell loss, abnormal coupling of horizontal, amacrine and ganglion cells, reduced density of photosensitive melanopsin-containing retinal ganglion cells, loss of dopaminergic synaptic contacts, circadian dysregulation, phosphorylated α-synuclein aggregation in ganglion cell bodies and dendrites.

The retinopathic changes in PD was generally thought to be the results of dopaminergic deficiency. In 1990, Harnois and Di Paolo described a decrease in dopamine levels in post-mortem retinal tissue from patients with PD [11]. The retinal dopaminergic cells reside at the border of the IPL and INL and they release dopamine in a circadian manner, as in Fig. 12.2 [18, 19]. As is shown in Fig. 12.3a, in normal retina, dopaminergic cells make synaptic contacts with AII amacrine and melanopsin-photosensitive ganglion cells in the IPL. Dopamine uncouples the gap junctions between photoreceptors, horizontal cells, and AII-type amacrine cells. The rod signal is transmitted to ON rod bipolar cells that contact the AII amacrine cells. These amacrine cells transfer information to OFF cone bipolar cells through

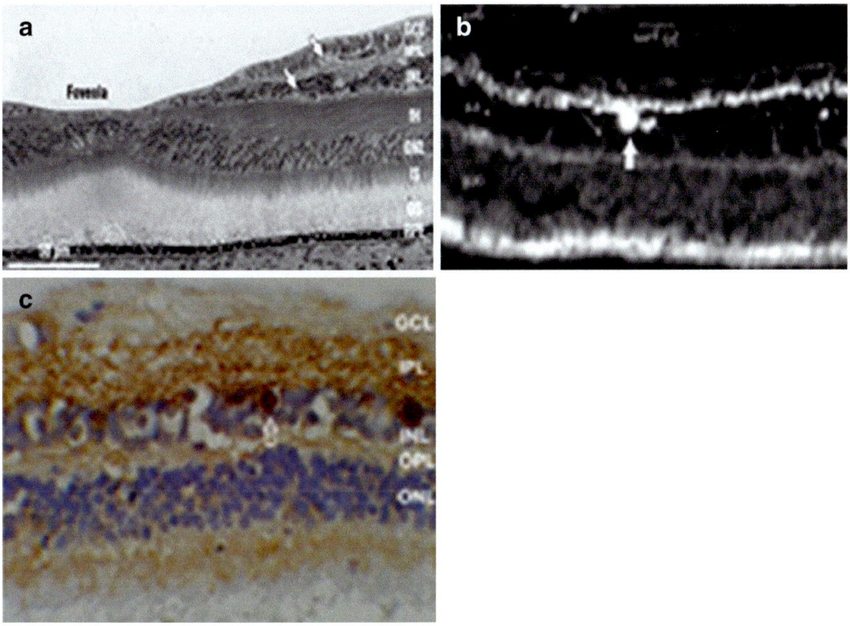

Fig. 12.1 Example of retinal layer segmentation using OCT compared to histology. (A) OCT image depicts retinal layers relative to the corresponding retinal layers on (B) histology in a representative control micrograph stained with hematoxylin and eosin within the macula [17]

chemical synapses and to ON cone bipolar cells via gap junctions, incorporating the rod signal to the cone pathway. In PD retina, as in Fig. 12.3b, the death of dopaminergic cells and loss of their synaptic contacts with AII amacrine cells and melanopsin retinal ganglion cells impair the aforementioned process [1].

12.3 OCT: Equipment and Analysis

OCT technique was first developed and described in 1991 [20] aiming to obtain in-vivo two-dimensional images using low-coherence interferometry to measure the time delay of back-scattered light from different layers of tissue. It was first applied to in-vivo retinal imaging in 1993 [21], and broadly utilized due to its rapid and non-invasive characteristic. Additionally, OCT has been applied to evaluate demyelinating diseases of the CNS including multiple sclerosis, Alzheimer's disease, PD, multiple system atrophy, and Lewy-body disease [22–25].

The original OCT technology was time-domain OCT (TD-OCT) in which retinal thickness data were obtained through successive "slices" through the retina, but the whole process is time-consuming. Third-generation TD-OCT, Stratus OCT (Carl Zeiss Meditec AG, Jena, Germany), has been widely used with the scanning rate of 400 axial scans per second and 10 μm axial resolution [26]. The

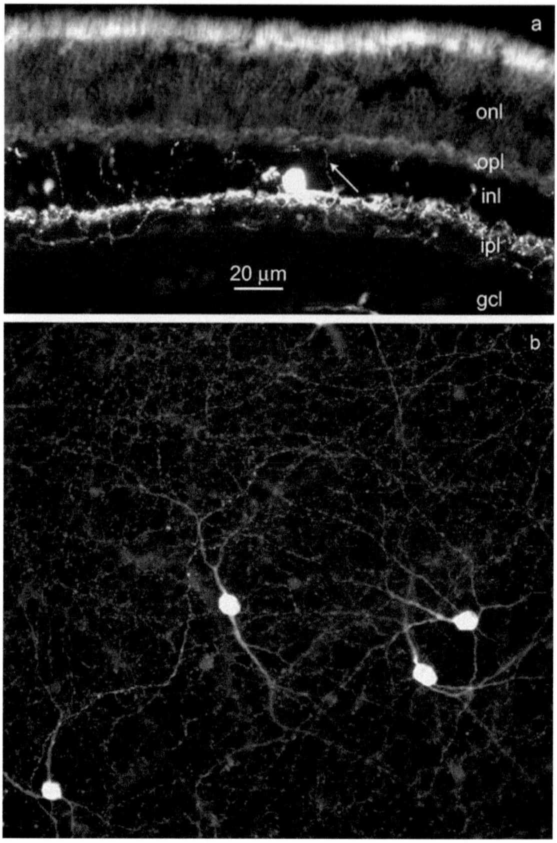

Fig. 12.2 Structural organization of dopaminergic neurons in the rat retina [18]. (a) Vertical section through the rat retina showing a dopaminergic perikaryon and DA processes visualized by immunocytochemical staining with an antibody against tyrosine hydroxylase, marker for dopaminergic neurons. The arrow points to an ascending process which reaches the OPL. (b) A horizontal view showing DA cell bodies, primary dendrites and fine processes disposed in the distal portion of the IPL. The 20 μm marker bar serves for both (a) and (b)

more recent introduction of Fourier-domain or spectral-domain OCT (SD-OCT) provides retinal imaging with faster scan rate and higher resolution, compared to older generation TD-OCT [27]. SD-OCT uses spectral interference and Fourier transform to extract the frequency spectrum of a signal. Fourier domain OCT can measure all light echoes with different delay time simultaneously which increase speed and sensitivity of detection. SD-OCT achieves an axial resolution of 5 μm and a scan velocity of 27,000 axial scans per second [28]. Recently, the maturation of swept-source OCT (SS-OCT) has brought new light into this area. SS-OCT was originally reported in 1995 [29] and recently matured for retinal imaging [30]. Differently from SD-OCT, SS-OCT uses a frequency-swept light source and photodetector. Being able to incorporate longer wavelengths, SS-OCT has shown the ability to simultaneously provide imaging of the vitreous, retina and choroid [31].

Commercially available OCT devices have different scan protocols to evaluate different retina area. The optic nerve head scanning protocol is mostly used in the context of glaucoma or optic nerve diseases, and to measure peripapillary retinal nerve fiber layer (pRNFL). This protocol yields a pRNFL thickness map

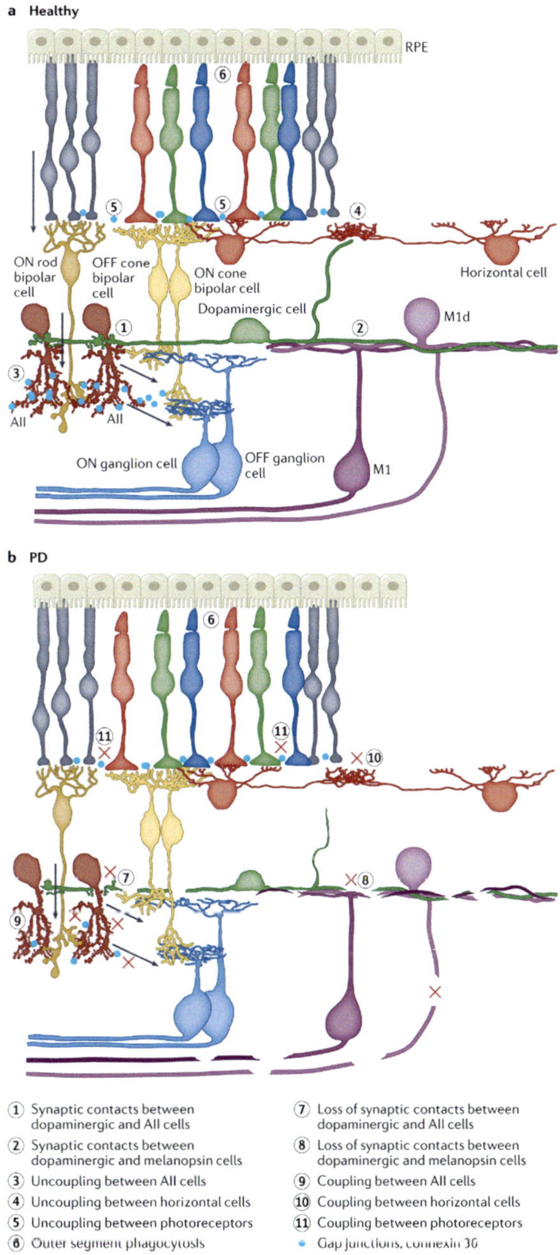

Fig. 12.3 Retinal changes in PD [1]. (a) Structure and circuitry of the healthy retina. (b) Retinopathy in PD patients

in a circle of 3.45 mm in diameter around the optic nerve head. The overall average thickness is separated into different quadrants, including the superior, inferior, temporal, and nasal. Macular scans provide images of the macula with 5–6 mm in diameter, centered at the fovea. Different companies have their own software and protocol with a normative database for statistical comparison of data [32]. This scanning strategy was developed to measure macular thickness according to the 9 map sectors in the Early Treatment Diabetic Retinopathy Study (ETDRS) grid. The inner and outer rings were segmented into 4 quadrants, with radii of 1.5 mm and 3 mm, respectively [33].

OCT image analysis is based on delineating the retinal layers, the so-called retinal image segmentation, and assessing the distances between layers. Image analysis starts with correct detection of the internal limiting membrane (ILM). Commercially available OCT devices use different layer segmentation algorithms based on quantification of the optical properties of the retinal layers. "Segmentation" refers to the establishment of the demarcation of different histological layers. Device dependent algorithm difference affect retinal thickness measures [34]. Accordingly, different sensitivities are reported for different OCT devices when the results are compared in the same subjects [35]. One of the critical variables is the estimation of the borders of different layers. However, the histological borders between layers are not straight line. Hence thickness measurements idealized to straight line approximation of the edges of different layers can suffer various inaccuracies. 3D reconstruction form 2D images is a potential solution towards more precise and comprehensive retinal layer segmentation [36].

With the development of computer technology, artificial intelligence (AI) has become the new star in the field of OCT image analysis. AI has shown great potential in multiple areas including image segmentation, lesion identification and segmentation, disease diagnosis, disease progression prediction, and disease treatment prediction [37]. In OCT image segmentation, many algorithms have been proposed to achieve high accuracy segmentation of the whole retinal layers. In terms of lesion segmentation, disease diagnosis and prediction, retinal diseases are currently the most noticed topic in the field. Artificial intelligence can segment a wide range of lesions including retinal fluid, vitreous drusen, neovascularization and more. At the same time, many neural networks have been trained to perform disease diagnosis and progression prediction, all of which have demonstrated high levels of accuracy that rival human experts. In the field of CNS diseases, there are also studies using artificial intelligence to predict systemic diseases from retina [38, 39].

12.4 OCT-Based Retinal Biomarkers in PD

OCT provides direct in-vivo visualization of retinal structure in the macular area and in the peripapillary area in PD. A potential role for OCT in the prodromal or early stages of the disease is to look for early markers of disease activity that are easily accessible and routinely performed in the clinic, to understand the potential anatomical origin of the functional changes experienced by patients, and to find possible markers that could be used for early detection and monitoring of the disease, as well as for evaluating the efficacy of therapeutic interventions. A good number of OCT studies have shown the effects of PD in the retina. Most reports using OCT describe decreased macular retinal thickness, MV and average pRNFL thickness in patients with Parkinson's disease compared with healthy control (HC) participants. We summarized the results in Table 12.1.

By summarizing the previous results, we have a clearer understanding of the relationship between OCT-based retinal biomarkers and PD. First, it is now generally accepted that retinal thinning is one of the biomarkers of PD. Second, although most studies have reported decreases in retinal layer thickness, there are still generally conflicting results, and there may be complex reasons for this. Third, advances in OCT imaging equipment will provide promise for further investigation into this topic. For example, some studies that were not able to show any OCT changes in PD patients are presented in Table 12.2.

As is mentioned before, the dendrites and cell bodies of RGCs are generally thought to be predominantly located in the mGCC, and pRNFL is mainly composed of the axons of RGCs [100]. Greater reduction in mean pRNFL thickness was also found to be associated with a lower mean mGCC thickness [54]. Therefore, thinner pRNFL and mGCC might indicate fewer RGCs in PD, consistent with the theory of neurodegeneration in the retina of PD patients that a significant loss of cells in the mGCC may be correlated with color vision dysfunction in PD patients [69, 77]. Besides from pRNFL and mGCC, decreased CMT and MV were also shown to be associated with PD, which may partly result from a significant reduction in pRNFL and mGCC. Additionally, INL and IPL have been shown to contain dopaminergic neurons, which is closely related to PD pathogenesis [101].

However, there are notable conflicting findings for the relationship between Parkinson's disease and retinal structure. Some studies found a significant reduction in RNFL thickness when comparing patients to healthy controls [41] correlated to duration and severity of disease [64] and even helping to stratify patients with Parkinson's disease [102]. On the other hand, other studies could not confirm such an effect nor any link with disease duration or severity, although they did note differences between some patient groups [57]. The reasons for the discrepancies are complex and varied. First, it is sometimes clinically difficult to determine the severity of Parkinson's disease in patients due to the presence and fluctuation of drug therapy. Secondly, different OCT hardware and different methods of image analysis may bring about differences.

A recent study by Wagner and his team validated for the first time in a large cohort the predictive power of macular retinal thickness for future Parkinson's disease risk [93]. They used data from two large-scale epidemiologic studies in both cross-sectional and retrospective cohort analyses. The results of the studies showed a significant association between mGCIPL thickness, mINL thickness, and prevalent and incident PD. This study, for the first time, provides evidence from a large cohort study on this topic. It serves as a convincing evidence to support retinal OCT as a biomarker for CNS degenerative diseases.

Table 12.1 Investigations of OCT-based retinal thickness in PD patients

Study	Sample size	Device	Findings
Inzelberg et al. [40]	10 PD, 10 HC	Not mentioned (NM)	pRNFL: ↓mean RNFL thickness, ↓inf, tem quad
Altintaş et al. [41]	17 PD, 11 HC	Stratus	pRNFL: ↓mean RNFL thickness, ↓sup, nasal quad Macula: ↓sup IRL; ↓temp, nasal, inf ORL; no difference in fovea
Hajee et al. [42]	24 PD, 17 HC	Optovue	Macula: ↓IRL in sup and inf quads; no change in ORL
Aaker et al. [34]	9 PD, 16 HC	Spectralis	pRNFL: No RNFL thickness difference Macula: ↓ORL sup; ↑ORL nasal; ↑IRL inf quad
Moschos et al. [43]	16 PD, 20 HC	Stratus	pRNFL: No difference in mean RNFL thickness; ↓thickness in inf, temp quad
Albrecht et al. [44]	40 PD, 35 HC	Spectralis	pRNFL: No RNFL thickness difference Macula: ↓INL especially in temp quad; no difference in other layers
Garcia-Martin et al. [45]	75 PD, 75 HC	Cirrus/ spectralis	pRNFL: ↓RNFL thickness all quads, spectralis more sensitive device than cirrus
Shrier et al. [46]	23 PD, 18 HC	Optovue	Macula: ↓macular volume at 0.5–0.75 mm from the foveola; IOA in IRL
Adam et al. [47]	14 PD, 14 HC	Optovue	Macula: ↓IRL at radial distances (1–1.75 mm) form the foveola, especially sup quadrant
Kirbas et al. [48]	42 PD, 40 HC	Cirrus	pRNFL: ↓mean RNFL thickness, ↓temp quad
La Morgia et al. [49]	43 PD, 86 HC	Stratus	pRNFL: No mean RNFL thickness difference, ↓temp quad, contralateral to d-side
Moreno-Ramos et al. [50]	10 PD, 10 HC	NM	pRNFL: PD with dementia had ↓RNFL thickness compared to HC
Rohani et al. [51]	27 PD, 27 HC	TOPCON	pRNFL: ↓RNFL thickness all quads, ↓inf, nasal quad more in akinetic-rigid PD type
Satue et al. [52]	100 PD, 100 HC	Cirrus/ spectralis	pRNFL: ↓mean RNFL thickness, ↓inf-temp, up-temp quad Macula: ↓mean macular, fovea, ORL inf quad
Spund et al. [53]	30 PD, 27 HC	Optovue	Macula: ↓IRL at 1–2 mm distance from the foveola
Garcia-Martin et al. [54]	129 PD, 129 HC	Spectralis	pRNFL: ↓average RNFL thickness, and ↓RNFL thickness in sup, inf, sup-nasal, inf-nasal, inf-temp, sup-temp Macula: ↓in RNFL, GCL, IPL, OPL; ↑in INL

(continued)

Table 12.1 (continued)

Study	Sample size	Device	Findings
Garcia-Martin et al. [55]	46 PD, 33 HC	Cirrus/ spectralis	pRNFL: ↓mean RNFL thickness, ↓sup, temp, inf quad Macula: ↓fovea, IRL all quad; ↓inf ORL (Cirrus); ↓sup, nasal ORL (Spectralis)
Jiménez et al. [56]	52 PD, 50 HC	Stratus	pRNFL: ↓average RNFL thickness and ↓RNFL thickness in all quads
Lee et al. [57]	56 PD, 30 HC	OPKO/OTI Spectral	Macula: ↓tem parafoveal INL, no difference in other layers; ↓sup outer segment of the total macular thickness
Roth et al. [58]	68 PD, 32 HC	Cirrus	pRNFL: No difference in RNFL thickness Macula: ↓ONL/PRL, no difference in GCIPL, GCC, INL/OPL; no difference in macular volume
Satue et al. [59]	153 PD, 242 HC	Cirrus/ spectralis	pRNFL: ↓average RNFL thickness; ↓RNFL thickness in sup, inf, sup-nasal, inf-nasal, inf-temp, sup-temp Macula: all RNFL quadrants
Sen et al. [60]	18 PD, 11 HC	RTvue	pRNFL: ↓mean RNFL thickness, and ↓inf, sup-temp, inf-temp segment
Bittershol et al. [61]	108 PD, 165 HC	Spectralis	pRNFL: no difference in RNFL thickness Macula: ↓central thickness, ↓central minimum thickness
Kaur et al. [62]	20 PD, 20 HC	Cirrus	pRNFL: ↓average pRNFL, ↓pRNFL sup, temp Macula: ↓average, minimum and all 6 sectors pRNFL
Mailankody et al. [63]	30 PD, 30 HC	Spectralis	Macula: ↓central macular thickness in PD
Sari et al. [64]	54 PD, 54 HC	Cirrus	pRNFL: ↓pRNFL inf, temp Macula: ↓average GCIPL and all sectors
Slotnick et al. [65]	72 PD, 24 HC	Cirrus/ RTVue	Macula: ↓superior/inferior and to a lesser degree nasal-temporal foveal slope in PD
Stemplewitz et al. [66]	108 PD, 165 HC	Cirrus	pRNFL: No difference in RNFL thickness Macula: ↓average macular thickness, ↓macular volume
Eraslan et al. [67]	22 PD, 23 HC	RTVue	Macula: Decreased mean RNFL thickness in PD
Pilat et al. [68]	25 PD, 25 HC	Optopol	RNFL: ↓average pRNFL and all quadrants
Polo et al. [69]	37 PD, 37 HC	Cirrus	RNFL: ↓pRNFL thickness in temp quad Macula: ↓central macular thickness (CMT), ↓in-sup, out-sup, out-inf, out-temp quad macular thickness

(continued)

Table 12.1 (continued)

Study	Sample size	Device	Findings
Ucak et al. [70]	30 PD, 30 HC	Cirrus	RNFL: ↓mean pRNFL, ↓sup, inf quad Macula: ↓GCIPL, no difference in CMT
Statue et al. [71]	30 PD, 30 HC	Spectralis	RNFL: ↓RNFL thickness in sup-temp, inf-temp quad Macula: ↓out-temp MT
Aydin et al. [72]	25 PD, 29 HC	Spectralis	RNFL: ↓mean pRNFL thickness, nas quad
Huang et al. [73]	53 PD, 41 HC	Cirrus	RNFL: ↓mean pRNFL thickness, and inf quad Macula: ↓CMT, MV
Kwapong et al. [74]	38 PD, 28 HC	RTVue	Macula: ↓CMT; thinner in the sup, nasal, and Inf quadrants
Ma et al. [75]	37 PD, 42 HC	Cirrus	RNFL: ↓mean pRNFL thickness Macula: ↓CMT, MV
Matlach et al. [76]	30 PD, 40 HC	Cirrus/ RTVue	RNFL: ↓sup pRNFL thickness Macula: no difference
Marilita et al. [77]	31 PD, 25 HC	Spectralis	RNFL: ↓mean pRNFL thickness and in sup, temp quad Macula: ↓mean GCC thickness and in all quads
Sengupta et al. [78]	34 PD, 50 HC	Spectralis	RNFL: ↓pRNFL in all quads Macula: ↓MV in perifoveal and outer macular regions
Unlu et al. [79]	58 PD, 30 HC	Spectralis	RNFL: ↓pRNFL in tem and sup-tem quads Macula: ↓mRNFL, GCL, IPL, ONL, RPE, PR thickness ↑ OPL thickness
Visser et al. [80]	20 PD, 20 HC	Spectralis	RNFL: ↓pRNFL in tem quad
Gulmez Sevim et al. [81]	41 PD, 35 HC	Spectralis	RNFL: ↓mean pRNFL thickness
Alkabie et al. [82]	12 PD, 12 HC	Spectralis	RNFL: no difference in pRNFL thickness Macula: no difference in MV
Mello et al. [83]	38 PD, 40 HC	NM	Macula: ↓CMT, inf-in mRNFL, GCIPL, GCC, inf-in GCC, IRL, ORL thickness
Rascunà et al. [84]	21 PD, 17 HC	Optovue	RNFL: ↓pRNFL thickness Macula: ↓mRNFL, GCL, IPL, INL thickness
Tugcu et al. [85]	21 PD, 22 HC	Spectralis	RNFL: ↓sup pRNFL thickness Macula: ↓CMT, sup, inf, temp, nas quads foveal thickness
Zou et al. [86]	35 PD, 35 HC	Cirrus	RNFL: ↓temp pRNFL thickness, no difference in mean and other quads pRNFL thickness Macula: ↓MV, macular retinal thickness, GCIPL thickness, no difference in CMT

(continued)

Table 12.1 (continued)

Study	Sample size	Device	Findings
Brown et al. [87]	10 PD, 12 HC	Cirrus/ spectralis	Macula: thicker choroid thickness related to better clinical performance
Kamata et al. [88]	14 PD, 22 HC	Topcon SSOCT	Macula: ↓GCIPL thickness
Mailankody et al. [89]	12 PD	Spectralis	Macula: ↑CMT, ↓outer retinal layer
Wang et al. [90]	397 PD, 427 HC	Cirrus	Macula: ↓pRNFL, macular retinal thickness and MVs
Zhao et al. [91]	30 PD, 20 HC	RTVue	RNFL: ↓mean pRNFL thicknss, and ↓in temp-up, inf-nas, inf-temp, temp-low quads Macula: ↓mean GCC, and sup, inf quads
Gunay et al. [92]	40 PD, 44 HC	Spectralis	Macula: RPE thickening
Wagner et al. [93]	700 PD, 105,770 HC	TOPCON	Macula: GCIPL thinning, INL thinning

Table 12.2 Studies of OCT-based retinal thickness in PD patients showing no changes

Study	Sample size	Device	Findings
Archibald et al. [94]	34 PD, 19 HC	Stratus	Macula: no difference in foveal thickness and macular volume
Tsironi et al. [95]	24 PD, 24 HC	Stratus	pRNFL: no RNFL thickness difference
Cubo et al. [96]	30 PD, 30 HC	Stratus	Macula: no difference in full-thickness macular measures
Quagliato et al. [97]	48 PD, 38 HC	RTvue	pRNFL: no difference in RNFL thickness Macula: no difference in macular thickness
Eraslan et al. [67]	22 PD, 25 HC	RTVue	RNFL: no difference in ONH parameters in PD
Pillai et al. [98]	20 PD, 34 HC	Cirrus	RNFL: no difference in pRNFL thickness Macula: no difference in GCL thickness, MV
Uchida et al. [99]	22 PD, 36 HC	Cirrus	Macula: no difference in outer retinal thickness

Retinal layer thinning can also be correlated with scores on clinical scales (i.e., Hoehn and Yahr scales, the UPDRS (Unified Parkinson's Disease Rating Scale), Mini-Mental State Examination, the Schwab and England Activities of Daily Living scale) or to measured clinical variables, [55] but such a correlation is not universally found [57]. As regards non-motor aspects of PD, some cross-sectional studies have revealed that macular thinning is related to worse visual outcomes [103]. The few studies that have explored the association between retinal parameters and cognitive changes are more consistent, showing decreased cognitive abilities in patients with PD who have reduced pRNFL [45, 50, 70, 104] and macular thickness, especially in the GCIPL [105, 106].

Retinal OCT based imaging biomarkers are also associated with treatment efficacy. Yavas et al. [107] studied the effects of levodopa and dopamine agonists on retinal nerve fiber layer using scanning laser ophthalmoscope, and found that RNFL were significantly thicker in the group treated with levodopa while it was the thinnest in the group receiving dopamine agonists. Therefore, they suggested that levodopa compared to dopamine agonists had a protective effect on the RNFL in PD. Sen et al. [60] described the effects of levodopa on the PD retina using OCT. According to the findings, the average RNFL thickness of PD patients was significantly lower than controls. In addition, retinal thickness of PD patients who underwent dopaminergic treatment was compared with the untreated group. According to this study, although the disease in patients with treated PD was more severe than in the untreated group, no significant difference in the thickness of retina was found between the two groups. Therefore, the authors also proposed a protective effect of L-dopa on the retina in patients with PD.

Advancing in the OCT technology unveils more subtle retinal imaging biomarkers. Recently, the utilization of SS-OCT provides us greater opportunity to simultaneously measure vitreous, retina and choroid [31]. Kamata et al. found that PD patients had significantly thinner choroid area, luminal area, and interstitial compared to those without PD through the analysis of SS-OCT imaging [88].

AI has shown great potential in medical image analysis. Recently, with the help of deep learning (DL), retinal imaging has been proven to be able to be predictors of cardiovascular disease risk [108]. However, the application of deep learning on retinal imaging as a tool for assessing major neurodegenerative disease (including PD) has been rarely used until now. This may be due to the difficulty in obtaining sufficient retinal images from patients with PD, as compared with patients with other systemic diseases. Ahn et al. developed an algorithm that can predict Hoehn and Yahr (H-Y) scale and Unified Parkinson's Disease Rating Scale part III (UPDRS-III) score using fundus photography among patients with PD [39]. This study further confirmed the association between retina and CNS degeneration, as well as demonstrated the huge potential of deep learning in medical image analysis.

12.5 OCT Angiography and PD

OCT angiography (OCTA) is a recent development OCT technology that provides a non-invasive imaging of the microvasculature of the retina and the choroid. It was shown to be used in several neurodegenerative diseases. Although α-synuclein deposition and loss of dopaminergic neurons is the main hallmarks of PD, there is growing evidence showing that vasculature alterations also contribute to the basic pathological process of PD [109]. Researchers have reported reduced vessel length, decreased vessel branching and damaged capillary network in substantia nigra in PD brains. Evidence suggests that α-synuclein accumulation also occurs in the retinal microvasculature, thus resulting in vascular alterations and neuronal loss. This ultimately leads to visual disturbances, as retinal and cerebral vasculature share common origins and features. Furthermore, this also provides us a new oppoturnity of using OCTA as a novel tool in PD monitoring. PD changes in OCTA examination include decreased vessel density (VD) in the superficial capillary plexus (SCP), deep capillary plexus (DCP), radial peripapillary capillaries (RPC), and alterations of the foveal avascular zone (FAZ). However, mixed results still exist concerning this specific topic, possibly due to small sample size, different inclusion criteria and various imaging technique. Revelant studies were summarized in Table 12.3.

Table 12.3 Investigations of OCTA-based retinal vaculature thickness in PD patients

Study	Sample size	Device	Findings
Miri et al. [110]	23 PD 13 HC	RTVue	FAZ inversely correlated with foveal thinning; foveal thinning highly correlated with motor impairment and disease duration
Kwapong et al. [74]	38 PD 28 HC	RTVue	↓SCP VD in total annular zone (TAZ), superior, temporal, inferior, and nasal zones
Rascunà et al. [84]	21 PD 17 HC	RTVue	No VD changes between HC and PD In PD patients, positive correlations were found between the thickness of RNFL, GCL, and INL and the SCP VD
Murueta-Goyena et al. [111]	49 PD 40 HC	Spectralis	↓SCP and DCP FAZ in PD; ↑perfusion density (PFD), skeleton density, FD and lacunarity of capillaries in PD
Robbins et al. [112]	69 PD 137 HC	Cirrus	↓SCP VD and PFD in PD
Zhang et al. [113]	42 PD 75 HC	Svision	↓SCP and DCP VD in PD
Zhou et al. [114]	24 PD 23 HC	Cirrus	↓SCP VD in PD; negative correlation of P100 latency and nasal and superior sectors of macular VD
Li et al. [115]	45 PD 43 HC	RTVue	↓SCP and DCP VD in PD; ↓DCP VD associated with lower executive function
Lin et al. [116]	49 PD 45 HC	RTVue	↓DCP and RPC VD in PD
Statue et al. [117]	42 PD 146 HC	Triton	No differences observed between groups

12.6 Functional-Morphological Correlations in PD

Retinal OCT and OCTA examinations assess the morphological characteristics of the retinal tissue in a holistic manner. On the one hand, as mentioned earlier, this facilitates our assessment of retinal structural changes in PD patients, thus providing more possibilities for the diagnosis and treatment of PD. On the other hand, combined with retinal electrophysical examinations, this also facilitates us to comprehensively understand the retinal functional and morphological changes in PD, providing theoretical bases for the PD visual-related symptoms, which are important non-motor symptoms in PD progression.

Many studies have combined retinal electrophysiological examination and OCT to investigate synergistic changes in retinal function and morphology in patients with PD. In 2014, Garcia-Martin et al. originally reprted the relationship between OCT-based retinal thickness and retinal electrophysiology-based visual function metrics and PD. They found that retinal electrophysiological measures, including pattern electroretinogram (PERG) positive (P) component at 50 ms-P50-, negative (N) component at 95 ms-N95- component amplitude, and PERG P50 component latency, and OCT measurements of RNFL and retinal thickness were decreased in PD patients. However, the complex relationship between retinal morphologic changes, functional changes, and pathologic changes characteristic of PD was still not correlatively elucidated at that time.

In 2015, Kaur et al. reported that subclinical visual dysfunction in PD including impaired color vision and contrast sensitivity, as well as pattern visual evoked response (VER) and multifocal ERG measures correlated with retinal structural changes including ganglion cell layer loss captured on SD-OCT. Based on this, GCL-IPL thinning may be a more reliable parameter than RNFL thickness for structural alterations of the retina in patients with PD. The GC-IPL complex was significantly thinner in PD cases in all 6 sectors. The average and minimum GCL-IPL values were also decreased in PD cases as compared with controls. A weak but significant correlation was also observed between structural changes on OCT (RNFL and GCL-IPL thickness) and functional changes on mfERG (RMS signal and P1 wave amplitude). Pattern VER latency correlated significantly with RNFL thickness but not with GCL-IPL thickness [62]. Later in 2018, Unlu et al., performed topographical assessment of retinal function using multifocal ERG in PD patients. They showed that inner and outer retinal layer and pRNFL were thinned in PD patients [79]. Moreover, multifocal ERG findings suggest that delayed implicit times and decreased amplitudes in PD patients correlate with outer macular volumes and PR thicknesses.

Recently, studies have reported different findings. In 2022, Mello et al. found that in their study, the PD group presented a significantly lower mono- and binocular contrast sensitivity, oscillatory potentials amplitude, b-wave amplitude on full-field ERG, and photopic negative response amplitude. There was no statistically significant difference in OCT measurements between groups. They assumed that functional abnormalities could be detected in PD prior to structural damages. In the future, more multimodal ophthalmic data studies combining visual electrophysiology and retinal OCT data are needed to fully clarify the temporal relationship between changes in visual function and retinal structure during the development of PD disease.

12.7 Concluding Remarks

In this chapter, we first review the histologic, physiologic, and pathologic associations of the retina and PD, followed by a glance of OCT technical features and recent OCT imaging advances, then a demonstration of OCT-based imaging markers in PD, followed by a summary of the clinical associations of these markers and PD, then a summarization of OCTA in PD, and finally a brief demonstration of the functional-morphological retinal changes in PD patients.

Currently, most studies demonstrated pRNFL thinning and macular thickness thinning including GCIPL, GCC, INL etc. Some studies also report correlation between disease severity, clinical scale, treatment efficacy and retinal thinning. OCTA, which allows precise assessment of retinal microvascular status, has given new impetus to this topic. PD, which is primarily characterized by neurodegeneration, also exhibits extensive microvascular abnormalities within the retina. However, there are still contradictory results in the above findings, which can be mainly attributed to the small sample size of the studies in question, different equipment in different studies, and differences in the course/type/treatment regimen of PD. Meanwhile, the specific mechanisms of retinal neurovascular alterations in the pathogenesis of PD need further investigation. What's more, the inclusion of multidimensional visual function assessment metrics allows for broader development of PD-retina studies. Changes in visual function during PD pathogenesis and alterations in retinal structure in relation to disease severity are currently understudied and are a possible future direction.

In conclusion, advances in retinal imaging and visual function assessment techniques have brought new opportunities, as well as new puzzles, to this topic. In this field, it is all the more important for concerned researchers to be cautious and comprehensive when conducting studies and analyzing images. First, accurate OCT retinal thickness measurements are often dependent on the volumetric scanning pattern, alignment and segmentation algorithms of OCT. Second, inclusion of PD patients should fully take into account the duration of disease, morbidity characteristics, nonmotor symptoms, and medication of PD patients. Third, the combination of multimodal ocular data will lead to more comprehensive scientific findings. Fourth, the use of new image analysis and processing techniques, such as artificial intelligence, will bring more possibilities to the field concerned.

References

1. Lee JY, Martin-Bastida A, Murueta-Goyena A, et al. Multimodal brain and retinal imaging of dopaminergic degeneration in Parkinson disease. Nat Rev Neurol. 2022;18(4):203–20.
2. Kashani AH, Asanad S, Chan JW, et al. Past, present and future role of retinal imaging in neurodegenerative disease. Prog Retin Eye Res. 2021;83:100938.
3. Ortuño-Lizarán I, Beach TG, Serrano GE, Walker DG, Adler CH, Cuenca N. Phosphorylated α-synuclein in the retina is a biomarker of Parkinson's disease pathology severity. Movement Disord Official J Movement Disord Soc. 2018;33(8):1315–24.
4. Postuma RB, Berg D, Stern M, et al. MDS clinical diagnostic criteria for Parkinson's disease. Movement Disord Official J Movement Disord Soc. 2015;30(12):1591–601.
5. . Kolb H, Fernandez E, Nelson R, editors. Webvision: the organization of the retina and visual system. Salt Lake City (UT): University of Utah Health Sciences Center. Copyright: © 2023 Webvision; 1995.
6. Bodis-Wollner I. Foveal vision is impaired in Parkinson's disease. Parkinsonism Relat Disord. 2013;19(1):1–14.
7. Bodis-Wollner I, Yahr MD. Measurements of visual evoked potentials in Parkinson's disease. Brain J Neurol. 1978;101(4):661–71.
8. Bodis-Wollner I, Marx MS, Mitra S, Bobak P, Mylin L, Yahr M. Visual dysfunction in Parkinson's disease. Loss in spatiotemporal contrast sensitivity. Brain J Neurol. 1987;110(Pt 6):1675–98.
9. Weil RS, Schrag AE, Warren JD, Crutch SJ, Lees AJ, Morris HR. Visual dysfunction in Parkinson's disease. Brain J Neurol. 2016;139(11):2827–43.
10. Ikeda H, Head GM, Ellis CJ. Electrophysiological signs of retinal dopamine deficiency in recently diagnosed Parkinson's disease and a follow up study. Vision Res. 1994;34(19):2629–38.
11. Harnois C, Di Paolo T. Decreased dopamine in the retinas of patients with Parkinson's disease. Invest Ophthalmol Vis Sci. 1990;31(11):2473–5.
12. Almer Z, Klein KS, Marsh L, Gerstenhaber M, Repka MX. Ocular motor and sensory function in Parkinson's disease. Ophthalmology. 2012;119(1):178–82.
13. Cameron JR, Megaw RD, Tatham AJ, et al. Lateral thinking—interocular symmetry and asymmetry in neurovascular patterning, in health and disease. Prog Retin Eye Res. 2017;59:131–57.
14. Hildebrand GD, Fielder AR. Anatomy and physiology of the retina. In: Reynolds J, Olitsky S, editors. Pediatric retina. Berlin, Heidelberg: Springer Berlin Heidelberg; 2011. p. 39–65.
15. Yang S, Zhou J, Li D. Functions and diseases of the retinal pigment epithelium. Front Pharmacol. 2021;12.
16. Sonka M, Abràmoff MD. Quantitative analysis of retinal OCT. Med Image Anal. 2016;33:165–9.
17. Asanad S, Ross-Cisneros FN, Nassisi M, Barron E, Karanjia R, Sadun AA. The retina in Alzheimer's disease: histomorphometric analysis of an ophthalmologic biomarker. Invest Ophthalmol Vis Sci. 2019;60(5):1491–500.
18. Witkovsky P. Dopamine and retinal function. Documenta ophthalmologica Adv Ophthalmol. 2004;108(1):17–40.
19. Kolb H, Cuenca N, Wang HH, Dekorver L. The synaptic organization of the dopaminergic amacrine cell in the cat retina. J Neurocytol. 1990;19(3):343–66.
20. Huang D, Swanson EA, Lin CP, et al. Optical coherence tomography. Science. 1991;254(5035):1178–81.
21. Swanson EA, Izatt JA, Hee MR, et al. In vivo retinal imaging by optical coherence tomography. Opt Lett. 1993;18(21):1864–6.
22. Bodis-Wollner I, Miri S, Glazman S. Venturing into the no-man's land of the retina in Parkinson's disease. Movement Disord Official J Movement Disord Soc. 2014;29(1):15–22.

23. Cheung CY, Ong YT, Hilal S, et al. Retinal ganglion cell analysis using high-definition optical coherence tomography in patients with mild cognitive impairment and Alzheimer's disease. J Alzheimer's Dis JAD. 2015;45(1):45–56.
24. Petzold A, Balcer LJ, Calabresi PA, et al. Retinal layer segmentation in multiple sclerosis: a systematic review and meta-analysis. Lancet Neurol. 2017;16(10):797–812.
25. Ahn J, Lee JY, Kim TW. Retinal thinning correlates with clinical severity in multiple system atrophy. J Neurol. 2016;263(10):2039–47.
26. Lange AP, Sadjadi R, Saeedi J, Lindley J, Costello F, Traboulsee AL. Time-domain and spectral-domain optical coherence tomography of retinal nerve fiber layer in MS patients and healthy controls. J Ophthalmol. 2012;2012:564627.
27. Sull AC, Vuong LN, Price LL, et al. Comparison of spectral/Fourier domain optical coherence tomography instruments for assessment of normal macular thickness. Retina. 2010;30(2):235–45.
28. Leung CK, Cheung CY, Weinreb RN, et al. Comparison of macular thickness measurements between time domain and spectral domain optical coherence tomography. Invest Ophthalmol Vis Sci. 2008;49(11):4893–7.
29. Fercher AF, Hitzenberger CK, Kamp G, El-Zaiat SY. Measurement of intraocular distances by backscattering spectral interferometry. Opt Commun. 1995;117(1):43–8.
30. Choma MA, Sarunic MV, Yang C, Izatt JA. Sensitivity advantage of swept source and Fourier domain optical coherence tomography. Opt Express. 2003;11(18):2183–9.
31. Laíns I, Wang JC, Cui Y, et al. Retinal applications of swept source optical coherence tomography (OCT) and optical coherence tomography angiography (OCTA). Prog Retin Eye Res. 2021;84:100951.
32. Garas A, Vargha P, Holló G. Diagnostic accuracy of nerve fibre layer, macular thickness and optic disc measurements made with the RTVue-100 optical coherence tomograph to detect glaucoma. Eye. 2011;25(1):57–65.
33. Chan A, Duker JS, Ko TH, Fujimoto JG, Schuman JS. Normal macular thickness measurements in healthy eyes using Stratus optical coherence tomography. Arch Ophthalmol. 2006;124(2):193–8.
34. Aaker GD, Myung JS, Ehrlich JR, Mohammed M, Henchcliffe C, Kiss S. Detection of retinal changes in Parkinson's disease with spectral-domain optical coherence tomography. Clin Ophthalmol. 2010;4:1427–32.
35. Wolf-Schnurrbusch UE, Ceklic L, Brinkmann CK, et al. Macular thickness measurements in healthy eyes using six different optical coherence tomography instruments. Invest Ophthalmol Vis Sci. 2009;50(7):3432–7.
36. Gabriele ML, Wollstein G, Ishikawa H, et al. Three dimensional optical coherence tomography imaging: advantages and advances. Prog Retin Eye Res. 2010;29(6):556–79.
37. Oganov AC, Seddon I, Jabbehdari S, et al. Artificial intelligence in retinal image analysis: Development, advances, and challenges. Survey Ophthalmol. 2023.
38. Wisely CE, Wang D, Henao R, et al. Convolutional neural network to identify symptomatic Alzheimer's disease using multimodal retinal imaging. Br J Ophthalmol. 2022;106(3):388–95.
39. Ahn S, Shin J, Song SJ, et al. Neurologic dysfunction assessment in Parkinson disease based on fundus photographs using deep learning. JAMA Ophthalmol. 2023;141(3):234–40.
40. Inzelberg R, Ramirez JA, Nisipeanu P, Ophir A. Retinal nerve fiber layer thinning in Parkinson disease. Vision Res. 2004;44(24):2793–7.
41. Altıntaş O, Işeri P, Ozkan B, Cağlar Y. Correlation between retinal morphological and functional findings and clinical severity in Parkinson's disease. Documenta ophthalmologica Adv Ophthalmol. 2008;116(2):137–46.
42. Hajee ME, March WF, Lazzaro DR, et al. Inner retinal layer thinning in Parkinson disease. Arch Ophthalmol. 2009;127(6):737–41.
43. Moschos MM, Tagaris G, Markopoulos I, et al. Morphologic changes and functional retinal impairment in patients with Parkinson disease without visual loss. Eur J Ophthalmol. 2011;21(1):24–9.

44. Albrecht P, Müller AK, Südmeyer M, et al. Optical coherence tomography in parkinsonian syndromes. PLoS ONE. 2012;7(4):e34891.
45. Garcia-Martin E, Satue M, Fuertes I, et al. Ability and reproducibility of Fourier-domain optical coherence tomography to detect retinal nerve fiber layer atrophy in Parkinson's disease. Ophthalmology. 2012;119(10):2161–7.
46. Shrier EM, Adam CR, Spund B, Glazman S, Bodis-Wollner I. Interocular asymmetry of foveal thickness in Parkinson disease. J Ophthalmol. 2012;2012:728457.
47. Adam CR, Shrier E, Ding Y, Glazman S, Bodis-Wollner I. Correlation of inner retinal thickness evaluated by spectral-domain optical coherence tomography and contrast sensitivity in Parkinson disease. J Neuro-Ophthalmol Official J North Am Neuro-Ophthalmol Soc. 2013;33(2):137–42.
48. Kirbas S, Turkyilmaz K, Tufekci A, Durmus M. Retinal nerve fiber layer thickness in Parkinson disease. J Neuro-Ophthalmol Official J North Am Neuro-Ophthalmol Soc. 2013;33(1):62–5.
49. La Morgia C, Barboni P, Rizzo G, et al. Loss of temporal retinal nerve fibers in Parkinson disease: a mitochondrial pattern? Eur J Neurol. 2013;20(1):198–201.
50. Moreno-Ramos T, Benito-León J, Villarejo A, Bermejo-Pareja F. Retinal nerve fiber layer thinning in dementia associated with Parkinson's disease, dementia with Lewy bodies, and Alzheimer's disease. J Alzheimer's Dis JAD. 2013;34(3):659–64.
51. Rohani M, Langroodi AS, Ghourchian S, Falavarjani KG, SoUdi R, Shahidi G. Retinal nerve changes in patients with tremor dominant and akinetic rigid Parkinson's disease. Neurol Sci Official J Italian Neurol Soc Italian Soc Clin Neurophysiol. 2013;34(5):689–93.
52. Satue M, Garcia-Martin E, Fuertes I, et al. Use of Fourier-domain OCT to detect retinal nerve fiber layer degeneration in Parkinson's disease patients. Eye. 2013;27(4):507–14.
53. Spund B, Ding Y, Liu T, et al. Remodeling of the fovea in Parkinson disease. J Neural Transmiss. 2013;120(5):745–53.
54. Garcia-Martin E, Larrosa JM, Polo V, et al. Distribution of retinal layer atrophy in patients with Parkinson disease and association with disease severity and duration. Am J Ophthalmol. 2014;157(2):470-8.e2.
55. Garcia-Martin E, Rodriguez-Mena D, Satue M, et al. Electrophysiology and optical coherence tomography to evaluate Parkinson disease severity. Invest Ophthalmol Vis Sci. 2014;55(2):696–705.
56. Jiménez B, Ascaso FJ, Cristóbal JA, López del Val J. Development of a prediction formula of Parkinson disease severity by optical coherence tomography. Movement Disord Official J Movement Disord Soc. 2014;29(1):68–74.
57. Lee JY, Kim JM, Ahn J, Kim HJ, Jeon BS, Kim TW. Retinal nerve fiber layer thickness and visual hallucinations in Parkinson's Disease. Movement Disord Official J Movement Disord Soc. 2014;29(1):61–7.
58. Roth NM, Saidha S, Zimmermann H, et al. Photoreceptor layer thinning in idiopathic Parkinson's disease. Movement Disord Official J Movement Disord Soc. 2014;29(9):1163–70.
59. Satue M, Seral M, Otin S, et al. Retinal thinning and correlation with functional disability in patients with Parkinson's disease. Br J Ophthalmol. 2014;98(3):350–5.
60. Sen A, Tugcu B, Coskun C, Ekinci C, Nacaroglu SA. Effects of levodopa on retina in Parkinson disease. Eur J Ophthalmol. 2014;24(1):114–9.
61. Bittersohl D, Stemplewitz B, Keserü M, Buhmann C, Richard G, Hassenstein A. Detection of retinal changes in idiopathic Parkinson's disease using high-resolution optical coherence tomography and Heidelberg retina tomography. Acta Ophthalmol. 2015;93(7):e578–84.
62. Kaur M, Saxena R, Singh D, Behari M, Sharma P, Menon V. Correlation between structural and functional retinal changes in Parkinson disease. J Neuro-Ophthalmol Official J North Am Neuro-Ophthalmol Soc. 2015;35(3):254–8.
63. Mailankody P, Battu R, Khanna A, Lenka A, Yadav R, Pal PK. Optical coherence tomography as a tool to evaluate retinal changes in Parkinson's disease. Parkinsonism Relat Disord. 2015;21(10):1164–9.

64. Sari ES, Koc R, Yazici A, Sahin G, Ermis SS. Ganglion cell-inner plexiform layer thickness in patients with Parkinson disease and association with disease severity and duration. J Neuro-Ophthalmol Official J North Am Neuro-Ophthalmol Soc. 2015;35(2):117–21.
65. Slotnick S, Ding Y, Glazman S, et al. A novel retinal biomarker for Parkinson's disease: quantifying the foveal pit with optical coherence tomography. Movement Disord Official J Movement Disord Soc. 2015;30(12):1692–5.
66. Stemplewitz B, Keserü M, Bittersohl D, et al. Scanning laser polarimetry and spectral domain optical coherence tomography for the detection of retinal changes in Parkinson's disease. Acta Ophthalmol. 2015;93(8):e672–7.
67. Eraslan M, Balci SY, Cerman E, Temel A, Suer D, Elmaci NT. Comparison of optical coherence tomography findings in patients with primary open-angle glaucoma and Parkinson disease. J Glaucoma. 2016;25(7):e639–46.
68. Pilat A, McLean RJ, Proudlock FA, et al. In vivo morphology of the optic nerve and retina in patients with Parkinson's disease. Invest Ophthalmol Vis Sci. 2016;57(10):4420–7.
69. Polo V, Satue M, Rodrigo MJ, et al. Visual dysfunction and its correlation with retinal changes in patients with Parkinson's disease: an observational cross-sectional study. BMJ Open. 2016;6(5):e009658.
70. Ucak T, Alagoz A, Cakir B, Celik E, Bozkurt E, Alagoz G. Analysis of the retinal nerve fiber and ganglion cell—inner plexiform layer by optical coherence tomography in Parkinson's patients. Parkinsonism Relat Disord. 2016;31:59–64.
71. Satue M, Rodrigo MJ, Obis J, et al. Evaluation of progressive visual dysfunction and retinal degeneration in patients with Parkinson's disease. Invest Ophthalmol Vis Sci. 2017;58(2):1151–7.
72. Aydin TS, Umit D, Nur OM, et al. Optical coherence tomography findings in Parkinson's disease. Kaohsiung J Med Sci. 2018;34(3):166–71.
73. Huang J, Li Y, Xiao J, et al. Combination of multifocal electroretinogram and spectral-domain OCT can increase diagnostic efficacy of Parkinson's disease. Parkinson's Dis. 2018;2018:4163239.
74. Kwapong WR, Ye H, Peng C, et al. Retinal microvascular impairment in the early stages of Parkinson's disease. Invest Ophthalmol Vis Sci. 2018;59(10):4115–22.
75. Ma LJ, Xu LL, Mao CJ, et al. Progressive changes in the retinal structure of patients with Parkinson's disease. J Parkinsons Dis. 2018;8(1):85–92.
76. Matlach J, Wagner M, Malzahn U, et al. Retinal changes in Parkinson's disease and glaucoma. Parkinsonism Relat Disord. 2018;56:41–6.
77. Moschos MM, Chatziralli IP. Evaluation of choroidal and retinal thickness changes in Parkinson's disease using spectral domain optical coherence tomography. Seminars Ophthalmol. 2018;33(4):494–7.
78. Sengupta P, Dutta K, Ghosh S, Mukherjee A, Pal S, Basu D. Optical coherence tomography findings in patients of Parkinson's disease: an Indian perspective. Ann Indian Acad Neurol. 2018;21(2):150–5.
79. Unlu M, Gulmez Sevim D, Gultekin M, Karaca C. Correlations among multifocal electroretinography and optical coherence tomography findings in patients with Parkinson's disease. Neurol Sci Official J Italian Neurol Soc Italian Soc Clin Neurophysiol. 2018;39(3):533–41.
80. Visser F, Vermeer KA, Ghafaryasl B, et al. In vivo exploration of retinal nerve fiber layer morphology in Parkinson's disease patients. J Neural Transm. 2018;125(6):931–6.
81. Gulmez Sevim D, Unlu M, Sonmez S, Gultekin M, Karaca C, Ozturk OA. Retinal vessel diameter obtained by optical coherence tomography is spared in Parkinson's disease. Int Ophthalmol. 2019;39(4):813–9.
82. Alkabie S, Lange A, Manogaran P, Stoessl AJ, Costello F, Barton JJS. Optical coherence tomography of patients with Parkinson's disease and progressive supranuclear palsy. Clin Neurol Neurosurg. 2020;189:105635.

83. Mello LGM, Bissoli LB, Saraiva FP, Maia RPD, Monteiro MLR. Retinal layers and choroid measurements in Parkinson's disease with or without pramipexole treatment. Movement Disord Official J Movement Disord Soc. 2020;35(12):2357–9.
84. Rascunà C, Russo A, Terravecchia C, et al. Retinal thickness and microvascular pattern in early Parkinson's disease. Front Neurol. 2020;11:533375.
85. Tugcu B, Melikov A, Yildiz GB, et al. Evaluation of retinal alterations in Parkinson disease and tremor diseases. Acta Neurol Belg. 2020;120(1):107–13.
86. Zou J, Liu K, Li F, Xu Y, Shen L, Xu H. Combination of optical coherence tomography (OCT) and OCT angiography increases diagnostic efficacy of Parkinson's disease. Quant Imaging Med Surg. 2020;10(10):1930–9.
87. Brown GL, Camacci ML, Kim SD, et al. Choroidal thickness correlates with clinical and imaging metrics of Parkinson's disease: a pilot study. J Parkinsons Dis. 2021;11(4):1857–68.
88. Kamata Y, Hara N, Satou T, Niida T, Mukuno K. Investigation of the pathophysiology of the retina and choroid in Parkinson's disease by optical coherence tomography. Int Ophthalmol. 2022;42(5):1437–45.
89. Mailankody P, Battu R, Lenka A, et al. Retinal changes in parkinson's disease: a longitudinal follow-up study. Neurol India. 2022;70(3):1149–53.
90. Wang X, Jiao B, Jia X, et al. The macular inner plexiform layer thickness as an early diagnostic indicator for Parkinson's disease. NPJ Parkinson's Dis. 2022;8(1):63.
91. Zhao Y, Dai W, Liu D. Quantitative analysis of related parameters of retinal nerve fiber layer and ganglion cell complex thickness in patients with different degrees of Parkinson's disease. Aging Clin Exp Res. 2022;34(10):2355–61.
92. Gunay BO, Usta NC. Retinal pigment epithelial changes in Parkinson's disease: a spectral domain optical coherence tomography study. Photodiagn Photodyn Ther. 2023;41:103213.
93. Wagner SK, Romero-Bascones D, Cortina-Borja M, et al. Retinal optical coherence tomography features associated with incident and prevalent Parkinson disease. 2023. https://doi.org/10.1212/WNL.0000000000207727.
94. Archibald NK, Clarke MP, Mosimann UP, Burn DJ. Retinal thickness in Parkinson's disease. Parkinsonism Relat Disord. 2011;17(6):431–6.
95. Tsironi EE, Dastiridou A, Katsanos A, et al. Perimetric and retinal nerve fiber layer findings in patients with Parkinson's disease. BMC Ophthalmol. 2012;12:54.
96. Cubo E, López Peña MJ, Diez-Feijo Varela E, et al. Lack of association of morphologic and functional retinal changes with motor and non-motor symptoms severity in Parkinson's disease. J Neural Transm. 2014;121(2):139–45.
97. Quagliato LB, Domingues C, Quagliato EM, Abreu EB, Kara-Junior N. Applications of visual evoked potentials and Fourier-domain optical coherence tomography in Parkinson's disease: a controlled study. Arq Bras Oftalmol. 2014;77(4):238–42.
98. Pillai JA, Bermel R, Bonner-Jackson A, et al. Retinal nerve fiber layer thinning in Alzheimer's disease: a case-control study in comparison to normal aging, Parkinson's disease, and Non-Alzheimer's dementia. Am J Alzheimers Dis Other Demen. 2016;31(5):430–6.
99. Uchida A, Pillai JA, Bermel R, et al. Outer retinal assessment using spectral-domain optical coherence tomography in patients with Alzheimer's and Parkinson's disease. Invest Ophthalmol Vis Sci. 2018;59(7):2768–77.
100. Yu DY, Cringle SJ, Balaratnasingam C, Morgan WH, Yu PK, Su EN. Retinal ganglion cells: energetics, compartmentation, axonal transport, cytoskeletons and vulnerability. Prog Retin Eye Res. 2013;36:217–46.
101. Djamgoz MB, Wagner HJ. Localization and function of dopamine in the adult vertebrate retina. Neurochem Int. 1992;20(2):139–91.
102. Cova I, Priori A. Diagnostic biomarkers for Parkinson's disease at a glance: where are we? J Neural Transm. 2018;125(10):1417–32.
103. Murueta-Goyena A, Del Pino R, Reyero P, et al. Parafoveal thinning of inner retina is associated with visual dysfunction in Lewy body diseases. Movement Disord Official J Movement Disord Soc. 2019;34(9):1315–24.

104. Zhang JR, Cao YL, Li K, et al. Correlations between retinal nerve fiber layer thickness and cognitive progression in Parkinson's disease: a longitudinal study. Parkinsonism Relat Disord. 2021;82:92–7.
105. Murueta-Goyena A, Del Pino R, Galdós M, et al. Retinal thickness predicts the risk of cognitive decline in parkinson disease. Ann Neurol. 2021;89(1):165–76.
106. Lee JY, Ahn J, Yoon EJ, Oh S, Kim YK, Jeon B. Macular ganglion-cell-complex layer thinning and optic nerve integrity in drug-naïve Parkinson's disease. J Neural Transm. 2019;126(12):1695–9.
107. Yavas GF, Yilmaz O, Küsbeci T, Oztürk F. The effect of levodopa and dopamine agonists on optic nerve head in Parkinson disease. Eur J Ophthalmol. 2007;17(5):812–6.
108. Cheung CY, Xu D, Cheng CY, et al. A deep-learning system for the assessment of cardiovascular disease risk via the measurement of retinal-vessel calibre. Nat Biomed Eng. 2021;5(6):498–508.
109. Paul G, Elabi OF. Microvascular changes in Parkinson's disease-focus on the neurovascular unit. Front Aging Neurosci. 2022;14:853372.
110. Miri S, Shrier EM, Glazman S, et al. The avascular zone and neuronal remodeling of the fovea in Parkinson disease. Ann Clin Transl Neurol. 2015;2(2):196–201.
111. Murueta-Goyena A, Barrenechea M, Erramuzpe A, et al. Foveal remodeling of retinal microvasculature in Parkinson's disease. Front Neurosci. 2021;15:708700.
112. Robbins CB, Thompson AC, Bhullar PK, et al. Characterization of retinal microvascular and choroidal structural changes in Parkinson disease. JAMA Ophthalmol. 2021;139(2):182–8.
113. Zhang Y, Zhang D, Gao Y, et al. Retinal flow density changes in early-stage Parkinson's disease investigated by swept-source optical coherence tomography angiography. Curr Eye Res. 2021;46(12):1886–91.
114. Zhou M, Wu L, Hu Q, et al. Visual impairments are associated with retinal microvascular density in patients with Parkinson's disease. Front Neurosci. 2021;15:718820.
115. Li Y, Wang X, Zhang Y, et al. Retinal microvascular impairment in Parkinson's disease with cognitive dysfunction. Parkinsonism Relat Disord. 2022;98:27–31.
116. Lin CW, Lai TT, Chen SJ, Lin CH. Elevated α-synuclein and NfL levels in tear fluids and decreased retinal microvascular densities in patients with Parkinson's disease. GeroScience. 2022;44(3):1551–62.
117. Satue M, Castro L, Vilades E, et al. Ability of swept-source OCT and OCT-angiography to detect neuroretinal and vasculature changes in patients with Parkinson disease and essential tremor. Eye. 2023;37(7):1314–9.

Optical Coherence Tomography in Alzheimer's Disease

13

Gianluca Coppola, Vincenzo Parisi, Francesco Casillo, Gianluca Manni, and Alfredo A. Sadun

Abstract

Alzheimer's disease (AD) is a neurodegenerative disorder, which usually starts as mild cognitive impairment (MCI) several years before the full-blown cognitive decline begins. As for other neurodegenerative disorders, optical coherence tomography (OCT) has been used to measure a significant loss in peripapillary retinal nerve fiber layer (RNFL) and in macular thickness and volume in patients affected by a form of mild to severe dementia. These morphological abnormalities correlate to some extent with the severity of the disease as evaluated with neuropsychological tests. Furthermore, these structural measures correlate with electrophysiological parameters of pattern electroretinogram, reflecting integrity of the innermost retinal layers, but not with those of the visual evoked potentials which are deemed to mainly reflect activity of the post-chiasmatic visual pathway. The latter evidence suggests that RNFL thickness reduction is related to neuronal degeneration in the ganglion cell layer and not to a retrograde degeneration from changes in the post-chiasmatic visual pathway. OCT-Angiography (OCT-A) has shown a possible link between retinal vascular parameters and

G. Coppola (✉) · F. Casillo
Department of Medico-Surgical Sciences and Biotechnologies, Sapienza University of Rome Polo Pontino ICOT, Latina, Italy
e-mail: gianluca.coppola@uniroma1.it

V. Parisi
IRCCS—Bietti Foundation, Research Unit of Neurophysiology of Vision and Neuroophthalmology, Rome, Italy
e-mail: vincenzo.parisi@fondazionebietti.it

G. Manni
Department of Clinical Sciences and Translation Medicine, Tor Vergata University of Rome, Rome, Italy

A. A. Sadun
Doheny Eye Institute, David Geffen School of Medicine at UCLA, Pasadena, CA, USA

A. Grzybowski and P. Barboni (eds.), *OCT and Imaging in Central Nervous System Diseases*, https://doi.org/10.1007/978-3-031-72156-4_13

AD perhaps due to the vascular system's role in the disease. These data suggest a possible role of OCT and OCT-A in monitoring the progression of AD and in assessing the effectiveness of purported AD treatments.

Keywords

Alzheimer's disease • Optical coherence tomography • Mild cognitive impairment • Electroretinogram • Psychometric testing • Retina

Abbreviations

AD	Alzheimer's disease
ADAS-Cog	Alzheimer's Disease Assessment Scale
APP	Beta-amyloid precursor protein
aMCI	Amnestic type of mild cognitive impairment
ERG	Electroretinogram
GCL	Ganglion cell layer
HRT	Heidelberg retina tomograph
IPL	Inner plexiform layer
OCT	Optical coherence tomography
ON	Optic nerve
RNFL	Retina nerve fiber layer
PERG	Pattern electroretinogram
PS1	Presenilin 1
RBANS	Repeatable Battery for the Assessment of Neuropsychological Status
VEP	Visual evoked potential

13.1 Introduction

Alzheimer's disease (AD) is the most common cause of dementia with an incidence that increases with age exponentially. According to the World Health Organization the worldwide prevalence of Alzheimer' disease (AD) is increasing yearly and receives growing attention because it affects quality of life, and also because has a significant economic impact, being a major public-health problem [1] and a substantial financial burden on families [2]. The recent publication of the Global Burden of Disease survey 2019 shows that among neurological conditions, the global number of individuals who lives with dementia is approximately 57 million globally in 2019 and is expected to grow to 152 million cases in 2050 [3]. This situation compels us to increase our efforts to identify early disease biomarkers and deepen our understanding of the pathophysiological mechanisms underlying neurodegeneration.

AD is a brain degenerative disorder, where inherited susceptibility and environmental factors are probably interrelated [4, 5]. The clinical evolution of AD includes a slowly progressive and episodic memory loss as the predominant symptom, with various accompanying signs including aphasia, apraxia, and agnosia, and general cognitive symptomology, such as impaired judgement, decision-making, and orientation [4]. Because of the slowness of the disease's progression, the neurodegenerative processes are likely to start 20–30 years before the clinical manifestations of AD. This transitional phase may manifest with mild cognitive impairment (MCI), which has some memory deficit, preservation of general cognitive and functional abilities, and absence of diagnosed dementia as cardinal features [6]. The amnestic type of MCI (aMCI) shows the highest annual incidence of conversion rate to AD [7]. Nonetheless MCI can be comorbid with other neurological disorders, such as nondemented Parkinson's disease (PD) patients and increased risk of progressive cognitive decline and dementia [8].

Despite great advances in the understanding of AD pathophysiology in the last few years, the exact pathogenesis of AD and its precursor MCI is still not comprehensively understood.

At the histopathologic level, neuronal loss, beta-amyloid plaques, neurofibrillary tangles made of hyperphosphorylated tau and neuritic plaques, and granulovacuolar degeneration characterize the brain of AD [4]. These lesions have been seen in the hippocampus and other limbic structures, as well as in the visual associative areas [9, 10], the primary visual cortex [11, 12], and in subcortical structures including the lateral geniculate nuclei and the superior colliculi [13–15], and within the retina [16–18].

Nonetheless, the issue of mixed dementia (AD + cerebrovascular disease) is a topic of ongoing discussion, especially because the pathological processes of AD and cerebrovascular disease may have a synergistic and cumulative effect. Available data suggest that concurrent small cerebrovascular lesions may play a role in cognitive decline, particularly in early stages of AD [19]. Uncertainty surrounds the precise function of beta-amyloid plaques in this neurovascular process, but it is intriguing nonetheless, particularly in light of the pathophysiological similarities between cerebral amyloid angiopathy (CAA) and AD. In fact, both conditions appear to be causally influenced by compromised clearance of Aβ, leading to a self-perpetuating cycle of elevated vascular Aβ levels, which may favor disease progression [20]. Beta-amyloid plaques in the retina were thought to compromise retinal cells and blood vessels, resulting in a reduction in blood flow to the retina. Vascular endothelial growth factors are produced in response to this hypoxic state, but they are unable to bind to the endothelial cells' corresponding receptors and return the retina's blood supply to normal. This may be because the interaction between these growth factors and the endothelial receptors is mechanically hindered by the buildup of amyloid-beta plaques. This results in a situation where vascular damage cannot be repaired and, in fact, can cause pathological phenomena in the process of attempting to repair it [21].

All these evidence and hypotheses suggest that a certain degree of retinal vessel involvement in the progression of the disease, particularly in relation to visual function, can be explained by a specific pathophysiological mechanism, regardless of cognitive status.

AD patients may be affected by various visual disturbances, such as deficits in contrast sensitivity [22–24], motion perception [25, 26], and color discrimination [27–29]. Historically, these visual dysfunctions in AD have been attributed to damage in the primary visual cortex and to degenerative processes in primary and associative visual cortical areas, but cortical dysfunction alone cannot explain the pattern of observed defects. Multiple forms of evidence points toward the involvement of retinal ganglion cells and their axons in the optic nerve as a basis of the visual dysfunction in AD [16, 30]. This peripheral involvement in AD and MCI could be independent from the central one [31].

In the last two decades, several studies have considered the retinal involvement in AD pathophysiology. Sophisticated imaging techniques have been used, such as optical coherence tomography (OCT), optical coherence tomography angiography (OCT-A), scanning laser polarimetry, and pattern electroretinography (PERG), to assess the morphologic and functional changes of the retina in AD [32].

OCT permits the objective quantification in vivo of the retinal nerve fiber layer (RNFL) that consists of axons that form the optic nerve and contributes partially to the retinal thickness. This method employs a non-invasive technology allowing cross-sectional imaging of the eye [33, 34]. The implementation of Spectral-Domain OCT provides advantages in signal-to-noise ratio, permitting faster signal acquisition [35, 36]. Taking in mind that the human eye is an embryological extension of the brain, and the nerves and axons of the retinal nerve fiber layer (RNFL) are similar to those in the brain, it is not surprising that OCT has been widely employed in assessing RNFL thickness in several neurologic as well as neuro-ophthalmologic disorders [37–41].

A novel application of OCT technology is called OCT-A. To find and see blood vessels, it makes use of the variations in OCT reflectance signals brought on by the presence of blood flow that produces a Doppler shift due to the movement of the blood. OCT-A makes it possible to measure the retinal capillaries' size, shape, and blood flow in a live human eye in real time without causing any harm [42].

The intent of this chapter is to provide a comprehensive overview of the results provided by the OCT and OCT-A technique as used to understand morphological retinal changes that occur due to the degenerative processes associated with Alzheimer's disease and other dementing disorders.

13.2 Retina and Alzheimer's Disease

As an integrated part of the nervous system, the retina is physiologically under senescence processes, most of them still under intense scrutiny. Therefore, in order to better evaluating AD patients, it is important to quantify the degree of thinning arising with age in the absence of pathological processes. It is also important to determine whether age-related loss is uniformly distributed across the optic disc and peripapillary retina or has any tendency to be sectorial and might therefore be a confounding factor for a correct evaluation of disease-related processes.

In the quest for understanding the degenerative changes accompanying AD, researchers performed both histological and in-vivo studies on healthy subjects.

Using immunohistochemical techniques, Löffler and colleagues examined the presence and expression of amyloid-related proteins, the same that have been found in specimens of AD patients' brains, in the human retina collected from cadaver eyes at various ages [17]. They did not find any abnormal deposits or immunoreactivity changes in the outer neural retina. On the other hand, they demonstrated the presence of tau proteins and amyloid precursor protein in the inner retina layers, including retinal ganglion cells and nerve fiber layer, of the human retina in older persons. Small amounts of beta-amyloid were detected in the sub-retinal pigment epithelium space [17]. Intracellular and extracellular Aβ deposits were recently detected in immunoreactive melanopsin retinal ganglion cells (mRGC) in AD retinas with abnormal morphology [18].

The analysis of normal in-vivo human retinal nerve fiber layer thickness, as measured by time-domain OCT, has been repeatedly confirmed as an age-related reduction of RNFL thickness in normal subjects [43–46]. This thinning mainly involved the superior and inferior optic disc areas [47–49].

The in vivo analysis of retinal vascularization performed using the OCT-A has also showed that patients with AD can exhibit various vascular alterations, such as a reduction in microvascular density [50, 51].

13.2.1 Animal Model of AD

One of the most recognised theories for the genesis of AD, the "amyloid cascade hypothesis", postulates that APP dysmetabolism and beta-amyloid deposition are the primary events that facilitate the disease process of AD [52].

In the past decade, through the use of genetic engineering techniques, transgenic (Tg) animal models over-expressing mutant forms of amyloid precursor protein (APP) and/or presenilin 1 (PS1) have been generated to mimic various aspects of AD pathology, including Aβ deposition, cognitive deficits, inflammation, and synaptic dysfunction, to test newly proposed therapeutic agents [53]. Recent publications have shown the accumulation of Aβ-plaques within the retina [54–57] and its microvasculature [58], retina ganglion cell death [59], and local neuroinflammation [58] in different Tg animal models. Nevertheless, these transgenic models only mimic part of the pathological features of AD.

An interesting Tg AD rat model, TgF344-AD, expressing mutant human amyloid precursor protein (APPsw) and presenilin 1 genes, seems to more faithfully encapsulate most of the features of AD. This animal model is characterized by an otherwise healthy long lifespan, but the rats suffer from later age cognitive decline, age-dependent cerebral amyloidosis, taupathy, gliosis, and frank neuronal loss that seems to parallel those in humans [60]. Tsai and colleagues investigated a group of TgF344-AD rats and age-matched wild type rats [61]. When compared with age-matched controls, the retinas of Tg rats demonstrated the presence of Aβ plaques, hypertrophic retinal pigment epithelial cells, signs of neuroinflammation, and a significant thinning of retinal choroid [61].

In mice models, non-mutant human Tau (hTau) gene expression may be sufficient to initiate AD and may thus be a more relevant model to study the disease [62]. In hTau mice at 5 and 17 months of age researchers examined functional, histological and molecular changes occurring in the visual system. They unexpectedly observed that hTau expression is not toxic for retinal cells at least in-so-far as the electroretinogram response was not altered in hTau compared with mTKO littermates, but even more pronounced in amplitude in hTau than in KO mice deprived of Tau retinae, suggesting a protective role of hTAU in visual physiology [63].

13.2.2 Histological Studies in Post-mortem AD Eyes

In 1986, histological examination in a human post-mortem study revealed depletion of axons in the optic nerves from AD patients [16]. Sadun and colleagues were the first to demonstrate this primary AD-associated optic neuropathy and further, to characterize, by morphometric analysis, that the predominant effect was on the largest retinal ganglion cells (M-cells) that contribute their large caliber fibers to the optic nerve [30]. Other studies [64, 65] failed to confirm the selective large axon losses. This discrepancy has been attributed, at least in part, to methodological biases such as different *post-mortem* delays, different techniques in axonal counting and/or difficulties in obtaining well-preserved myelinated axons.

Extensive retinal ganglion cell loss in the central retina in AD was also observed in histological studies [16] or by other methods of evaluating the RNFL in vitro. Morphometric analysis of the central retina (fovea/foveola/parafoveal retina) in eyes from 9 AD and 11 age-matched controls revealing an overall decrease of 25% in total numbers of neurons in the ganglion cell layer (GCL) (fovea/parafoveal retina) in AD as compared with control eyes [66]. Moreover, the most severe decrease was observed in the foveal region (− 43%) over the far temporal region. Similar results were obtained in AD patients with the evaluation of the peripheral retina: the neuronal loss was more pronounced in the superior and inferior quadrants (50–59%) and a significantly increased ratio of astrocytes to neurons was detected when compared with control eyes [67]. Moreover, histological signs of degeneration in the retinal ganglion cells (RGCs) were described to include a vacuolated, “frothy” appearance of the cytoplasm in the absence of neurofibrillary tangles within the RGCs, or of neuritic plaques or amyloid angiopathy in the retinas or optic nerves in AD [68].

Koronyo-Hamaoui and colleagues recently identified retinal Aβ plaques in *post-mortem* eyes from 8 AD patients and in 5 suspected early stage cases, but not in five age-matched non-AD individuals [56].

Plaque-like structures were seen in two retinas from two AD patients, with thickening of the retinal choroid and no changes in the retinal pigment epithelial cells [61]. Fibrillar tau or Aβ aggregates were seen in *post-mortem* retinas from the same AD patients that had been previously observed by using an *in-vivo* imaging technique [69].

In a recent post-mortem study [18], researchers identified mRGCs with antibody targeting melanopsin from 14 AD patients with preserved retinal anatomy, and 13 controls. In AD patients, they revealed preserved retinal layers as compared to controls, but smaller RGC somas and thinner dendrites, focal attenuations of melanopsin immunostaining, signs of optic neuropathy with axonal loss predominantly affecting the larger fibers in the superior quadrant. Melanopsin RGC number was significantly correlated with age in controls but not in AD patients, meaning that the degenerative processes at the basis of AD are, at least in part, independent from age related changes. Finally, in a subgroup of subjects, they found evidence of consistent accumulation of Aβ inside immunoreactive mRGCs soma and extracellular/abluminal areas in AD patients, while they were absent in controls [18].

In a recent study, Sci et al. found that Aβ40 was present in all three layers of retinal blood vessels. They used specific antibodies to find Aβ40 in the retinal blood vessels of patients with MCI and AD. In the same patients, the levels of retinal Aβ40 were associated with plaque load in the entorhinal cortex and showed a trend in predicting cognitive decline and cerebral amyloid angiopathy [70].

13.2.3 Clinical Studies Based on the Subjective Evaluation of Fundus Photographs

The RNFL consists of the axons of retinal ganglion cells converging at the optic disc to form the optic nerve.

That retinal ganglion cell degeneration occurs in AD is further evident by means of the use of a boundary-tracking program and RNFL photographs. A higher proportion of AD patients showed signs of optic neuropathy manifesting as optic disc atrophy, pathologic optic disc cupping, and thinning of the neuroretinal rim and of the RNFL [71, 72]. Tsai et al. [72] observed an increased cup-to-disc ratio, cup volume, and decreased optic disc rim area in AD patients by the optic nerve analyser.

Analyzing mild to moderate AD patients with RNFL fundus photographs, Lu and colleagues found that all the AD patients had different types of RNFL abnormalities, including diffuse and wedge shape nerve fiber layer drop-out [73]. These abnormalities in AD patients were associated with a higher cup–disc ratio of 39–43% when compared to that in the control group.

However, these studies required the subjective evaluation of fundus photographs which had an inherent observer bias.

13.3 In-vivo Morphological Analysis in AD and MCI Patients

One confounding factor in analysing MCI and AD -related late-onset progressive changes is that there are anatomical and physiological changes normally found in aging eyes. In animal [74] and human [74, 75] studies, a physiological age-dependent progressive loss of optic nerve fibers, with progressive decrease of mean axonal diameter, has been demonstrated [76–78].

13.3.1 Optical Coherence Tomography (OCT) Studies

OCT is a technique that can also be used for the measurement of the macular thickness and volume in the retina.

OCT can determine RNFL thickness of the peripapillary region reflecting axons and that allows quantification of axonal loss, measurement of macular thickness and volume which reflect retinal neurons, allowing quantification of neuronal loss [33].

Several previous studies using OCT techniques have examined the relationship between age and RNFL measurements. These have consistently shown that optic nerve, RNFL, and macular measurements with OCT all varied with age [45, 79], with the greatest decrease in mean RNFL occurring in the superior [48] and inferior quadrants [46], especially after age 50 years [47]. There was less loss in RNFL thickness in the nasal and temporal quadrants [80, 81]. This age-related decline in normal RNFL measurements needs to be contemplated when considering or monitoring ocular disease.

However, as described below, the reduction in RNFL thickness observed in most studies on AD patients was significantly greater than that observed in the age-matched controls and thus cannot be exclusively ascribed to aging (see some illustrative OCT imaging in Fig. 13.1 and a synopsis of published OCT studies in AD and MCI in Table 13.1).

Parisi and colleagues were the first who used OCT to study a group of 17 AD patients affected from mild severity cognitive impairment and compared them with a group of 14 age-matched controls. In AD patients, OCT results showed thinning of the average peripapillary RNFL and in all quadrants examined, showing the involvement of the neuroretinal tissue in AD [82, 83].

The mean RNFL thickness was corroborated to be reduced in AD patients by several independent groups [18, 73, 84–96]. Patients affected with MCI also showed some RNFL thinning [88, 93, 95–97]. Individual examination of the quadrants was even more revealing. Most studies observed a significant reduction of RNFL thickness in the superior quadrant [18, 73, 82, 83, 86, 87, 90–95, 97–99], but for some also in the inferior quadrant [73, 82, 83, 86, 87, 91–95, 97–99] and, to a lesser extent, also in the nasal [82, 83, 87, 91, 93] and temporal [82–84, 86, 87, 91–93, 95] quadrants. In contradistinction, the preferential involvement of each quadrant is more inconsistent in MCI patients However, some researchers did not

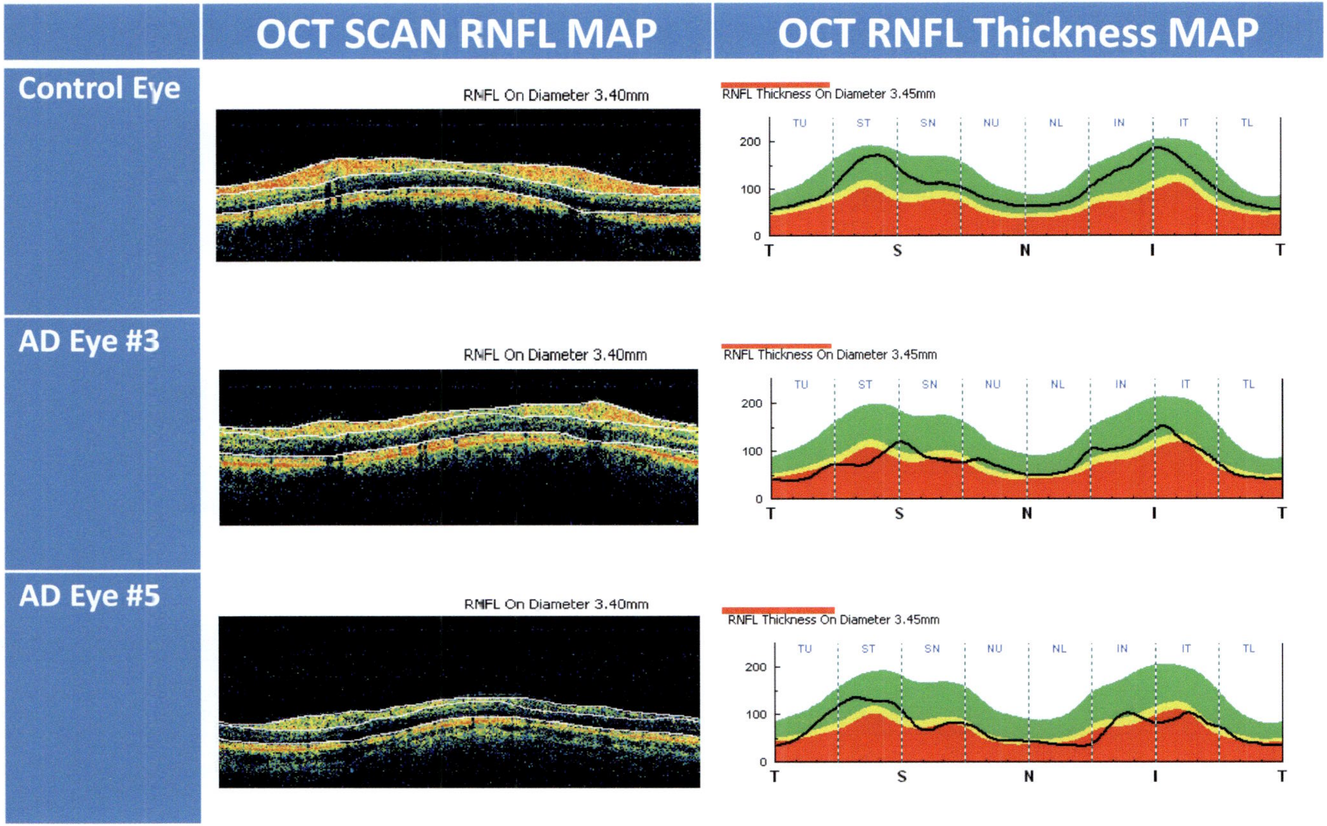

Fig. 13.1 Optical Coherence Tomography (OCT) imaging taken in cylindrical section of tissue surrounding the optic disc of a control eye and of 2 AD patients' eyes. The images in the left panel are raw OCT data, while the maps in the right panel are quantitative data curve. In AD patients' eyes OCT shows a decrease of RNFL reflection (reduced RNFL thickness) in each examined quadrant, with particular prevalence of the temporal ones

Table 13.1 Demographic data and RNFL thickness measurements in patients and controls as determined by OCT

References	No. of subjects and diagnosis	Mean MMSE/ AD stage	Mean age ± SD	OCT machine	Mean RNFL (μm)	Superior quadrant (μm)	Inferior quadrant (μm)	Nasal quadrant (μm)	Temporal quadrant (μm)	Note
Parisi et al. [82, 83]	17 AD 14 controls	/Mild	70.37 ± 6.1	Humphrey	59.5 ± 16.70* 99.9 ± 8.95	72.1 ± 21.4* 104.6 ± 12.1	77.9 ± 26.4* 116.2 ± 9.87	50.4 ± 23.2* 93.4 ± 13.7	37.9 ± 17.60* 85.6 ± 8.21	RNFL overall values correlated with PERG
Iseri et al. [98]	14 AD 15 controls	18.5/ mild to moderate 29.4	70.1 ± 9.7 65.1 ± 9.8	Carl Zeiss Meditec, Model 3000	87.4 ± 23.7* 113.1 ± 6.7	112.6 ± 35.3* 137.1 ± 16.4	103.1 ± 33.6* 141.5 ± 19.1	63.5 ± 19.1* 96.0 ± 34.4	64.9 ± 17.7 72.3 ± 16.4	Decline in both peripapillary and macular thickness and volume in AD eyes
Berisha et al. [143]	9 AD 8 HV	23.8/ mild to moderate 29.5	74.3 ± 3.3 74.3 ± 5.8	Carl Zeiss Meditec, Model 3000		92.2 ± 21.6* 113.6 ± 10.8	117.0 ± 15.3 128.1 ± 11.4	67.0 ± 15.0 69.5 ± 11.1	65.7 ± 15.1 64.1 ± 7.3	Narrowing of the retinal microvasculature
Paquet et al. [89]	23 MCI 14 AD 12 AD 15 controls	28.8 22.6/ mild 16.6/ severe 28.9	78.7 ± 6.2 78.3 ± 5.1 78.8 ± 4.9 75.5 ± 5.1	Carl Zeiss Stratus OCT 3	89.3 ± 2.7* 89.2 ± 2.9* 76.6 ± 3.8* 102.2 ± 1.8					The involvement of retina is an early event in the course of this disorder
Lu et al. [73]	22 AD 22 controls		73 ± 8 68 ± 9	Carl Zeiss Meditec, Model 3000	90 ± 18*(§) 98 ± 12	107 ± 30*(§) 124 ± 16	116 ± 35*(§) 128 ± 18	66 ± 26 70 ± 17	70 ± 20 71 ± 13	Enlarged optic cup to disc ratio in AD
Kesler et al. [97]	24 MCI 30 AD 24 controls	28.1 23.6	71.0 ± 10.0 73.7 ± 9.9 70.9 ± 9.2	Carl Zeiss Stratus OCT 3	85.8 ± 10.0* 84.7 ± 10.6* 94.3 ± 11.3	101.3 ± 15.2 99.0 ± 18.0* 110.0 ± 16.7	111.9 ± 16.1* 110.1 ± 19.1* 127.0 ± 15.5	65.9 ± 15.1 66.8 ± 14.5 76.4 ± 21.8	64.2 ± 13.9 61.7 ± 10.9 67.8 ± 15.1	RNFL thickness not correlated with MMSE

(continued)

Table 13.1 (continued)

References	No. of subjects and diagnosis	Mean MMSE/ AD stage	Mean age ± SD	OCT machine	Mean RNFL (μm)	Superior quadrant (μm)	Inferior quadrant (μm)	Nasal quadrant (μm)	Temporal quadrant (μm)	Note
Kromer et al. [129, 130]	22 AD 22 controls	22.6/ mild to moderate	75.9 ± 6.1 64.0 ± 8.2	Spectralis Heidelberg Engineering	80 (§)(#)	46 (§)(#)		47 (§)(#)		The RNFL of the AD patients did not correlate with pattern VEP latencies
Moreno-Ramos et al. [110]	10 AD 10 LB 10 PD 10 controls	16.4 14.9 16.4 29.2	73.0 ± 6.5 74.2 ± 5.1 74.3 ± 5.0 70.2 ± 5.5	TOPCON 3D OCT-1000	94.5 ± 2.2* 93.3 ± 1.5* 94.8 ± 2.0* 108.0 ± 2.2					Retinal involvement measured by OCT may also be present in non-AD dementias
Marziani et al. [91]	21 AD 21 controls	19.9/ mild to moderate 27.9	79.3 ± 5.7 77.0 ± 4.2	(1) Optovue RTVue-100 & (2) Spectralis Heidelberg Engineering	244.1 ± 17.9^{1} 277.5 ± 21.7^{2} 252.3 ± 19.2^{1} 283.8 ± 27.3^{2} Central sector	274.8^{1}*(+) 304.3^{2}*(+) 288.9^{1}(+) 319.3^{2}(+)	273.25^{1}*(+) 301.7^{2}*(+) 286.25^{1}(+) 314.75^{2}(+)	278.4^{1}*(+) 309.35^{2}*(+) 290.85^{1}(+) 323.55^{2}(+)	271.8^{1}*(+) 291.95^{2}*(+) 286.25^{1}(+) 304.45^{2}(+)	Reduced RNFL in AD patients using 2 different OCT instruments
Kirbas et al. [90]	40 AD 40 controls	21.5	69.3 ± 4.9 68.9 ± 5.1	Spectral domain OCT	65 ± 6.2* 75 ± 3.8	76 ± 6.7* 105 ± 4.8	106 ± 11.5 108 ± 8.7	75 ± 2.8 76 ± 2.7	74 ± 6.7 77 ± 7.3	No correlation between MMSE and OCT results
Larrosa et al. [92]	151 AD 61 controls	18.31	75.29 74.87	(1) Carl Zeiss Meditec Cirrus & (2) Spectralis Heidelberg Engineering	97.5 ± 14.1^{1} 98.2 ± 17.1^{2}* 100.5 ± 13.0^{1} 102.7 ± 6.7^{2}	113.2 ± 18.7^{1}* 117.8 ± 19.0^{1}*	120.4 ± 20.1^{1}* 127.4 ± 21.0^{1}	72.7 ± 17.3^{1} 74.5 ± 17.2^{1}	64.5 ± 21.7^{1}* 67.8 ± 20.0^{1}	RNFL measurements were a very useful and precise tool for AD diagnosis

(continued)

Table 13.1 (continued)

References	No. of subjects and diagnosis	Mean MMSE/ AD stage	Mean age ± SD	OCT machine	Mean RNFL (μm)	Superior quadrant (μm)	Inferior quadrant (μm)	Nasal quadrant (μm)	Temporal quadrant (μm)	Note
Ascaso et al. [93]	21 aMCI 18 AD 41 controls	19.3 28.8	72.1 (AD + aMCI) 72.9	Stratus OCT 3	86.0 ± 7.2* 64.7 ± 15.2* ** 103.6 ± 8.9 (data showed from the right eye only)	96.7 ± 14.6* 73.2 ± 22.0* ** 126.6 ± 13.8	110.1 ± 17.7* 86.2 ± 25.7* ** 135.6 ± 17.6	71.0 ± 16.7 * 43.3 ± 20.4 * ** 77.8 ± 16.7	66.3 ± 12.1 * 56.7 ± 14.9 * ** 75.8 ± 16.6	A significant association between RNFL thickness in superior and nasal quadrants, and MMSE score
Cheung et al. [94]	41 MCI 100 AD 123 controls		70.4 ± 10.2* 73.5 ± 6.23* 65.7 ± 3.77	Carl Zeiss Meditec Cirrus HD-OCT	RNFL 89.21 86.83* 90.37 GC-IPL 73.73* 72.73* 77.79	110.9 105.7* 113.5 73.48* 72.66* 77.65	112.2 108.2* 114.3 70.87* 70.61* 76.83	68.93 68.54 68.10 75.95^* 74.75^* 79.86^	65.10 64.89 65.25 72.99^* 71.88^* 76.31^	In the model adjusted for optic disc areas, hypertension, diabetes and, history of myocardial infarction, only superior quadrant reached the significance level
Feke et al. [100]	21 MCI 10 AD 21 controls		74.3 ± 12.2 74.4 ± 10.5 69.1 ± 6.7	Stratus OCT 3000 (Carl Zeiss Meditec)		118.2 ± 13.4 108.8 ± 13.3 117.7 ± 15.2				No differences between the RNFL thicknesses measured in all retinal quadrants. Solely in AD patients, venous blood flow positively correlated with superior RNFL thickness
Gao et al. [95]	26 MCI 25 AD 21 controls	25.77 19.24 28.57	73.42 ± 1.54 74.72 ± 1.39 72.05 ± 1.02	Cirrus HD-OCT 4000, Carl Zeiss Meditec	92.38* 85.99* 98.60	112.12* 106.10* 122.25	123.87 108.64* 127.59	68.54 66.16 69.71	66.56* 63.14* 74.60	No correlation with MMSE test. AD data still significant after adjusting for age, sex, hypertension and diabetes

(continued)

Table 13.1 (continued)

References	No. of subjects and diagnosis	Mean MMSE/ AD stage	Mean age ± SD	OCT machine	Mean RNFL (µm)	Superior quadrant (µm)	Inferior quadrant (µm)	Nasal quadrant (µm)	Temporal quadrant (µm)	Note
Oktem et al. [96]	35 MCI 35 AD 35 controls	28 18 29	74.1 ± 6.3 75.4 ± 6.9 70.2 ± 8.0	Zeiss Cirrus HD 5000 model OCT device	82.5 ± 7.3* 80.6 ± 9.6* 91.5 ± 7.1					In all study participants, a significant correlation was present between MMSE test and RNFL thickness
Garcia-Martin et al. [84]	150 AD 75 controls	18.35 29.78	75.33 74.79	Spectralis OCT	RNFL 95.67 ± 15.22* 99.23 ± 16.48 GC-IPL 6.27 ± 1.76* 6.45 ± 1.77			RNFL 77.02 ± 16.80 77.54 ± 18.88	RNFL 66.90 ± 15.34* 71.09 ± 15.52	The thickness of the RNFL, ganglion cell and inner plexiform layers were significantly decreased in AD patients with longer disease duration
Cunha et al. [86]	24 AD 24 controls	17.02 29.08	74.8 ± 6.25 72.25 ± 7.31	3D OCT-2000, Topcon Corp	93.75 ± 13.42* 102.96 ± 9.19	110.88 ± 19.76* 122.12 ± 15.55	112.38 ± 23.25* 130.10 ± 12.78	82.64 ± 17.82* 86.46 ± 13.61	66.91 ± 16.66 72.69 ± 9.16	Significant correlation between most OCT parameters and MMSE scores
Pillai et al. [101]	21 aMCI 21 AD 20 non-AD 20 PD 34 controls		68.2 ± 6.7 65.8 ± 11.1 68.7 ± 8.4 62.6 ± 9.5 65.1 ± 8.3	Cirrus 4000 HD-OCT (Zeiss)	89.9 ± 2.1 88.9 ± 2.1 89.9 ± 2.1 88.5 ± 2.1 85.3 ± 1.6	109.3 ± 3.2 107.2 ± 3.3 111.9 ± 3.4 110.1 ± 3.4 106.0 ± 2.6	117.0 ± 3.6 114.4 ± 3.6 114.3 ± 3.7 111.9 ± 3.7 108.7 ± 2.8	69.8 ± 2.5 72.5 ± 2.5 73.8 ± 2.6 72.9 ± 2.5 66.9 ± 2.0	63.4 ± 2.5 61.8 ± 2.5 59.5 ± 2.6 59.2 ± 2.6 59.1 ± 2.0	No retinal involvement in AD and non-AD dementias

(continued)

Table 13.1 (continued)

References	No. of subjects and diagnosis	Mean MMSE/ AD stage	Mean age ± SD	OCT machine	Mean RNFL (μm)	Superior quadrant (μm)	Inferior quadrant (μm)	Nasal quadrant (μm)	Temporal quadrant (μm)	Note
Trebbastoni et al. [102]	36 AD 36 controls	22.7 28.6	72.0 ± 7.3 71.7 ± 6.0	Heidelberg Spectralis (Heidelberg Engineering)	96.7 ± 6.3 97.6 ± 8.3	114.6 ± 11.2 118.5 ± 13.1	126.3 ± 11.7 125.1 ± 11.6	74.1 ± 8.9 76.3 ± 10.9	71.9 ± 9.8 70.9 ± 12.5	After 12 months AD patients had a significant reduction of the total RNFL thickness, as well as the RNFL thickness of the inferior and superior quadrants
Liu et al. [31]	50 CIND 27 AD 47 controls	25.2 16.6 27.4	69.7 ± 8.2 75.2 ± 7.8 67.3 ± 6.2	Cirrus HD-OCT (Carl Zeiss Meditec)	GC-IPL 76.92 ± 6.29* 78.41 ± 5.85 80.19 ± 5.89					Correlation was observed between GC-IPL thickness and WM microstructure and GMV of healthy controls in several brain area. This correlation was absent both in CIND and in AD patients
La Morgia et al. [18]	21 AD 74 controls	18.3	71.2 ± 10.5 69.1 ± 8.1		88.8 ± 8.4* 95.8 ± 12.3	104.4 ± 13.4* 117.1 ± 17.6	116.5 ± 15.5 122.4 ± 18.1	66.6 ± 13.9 74.3 ± 15.3	67.2 ± 10.4 69.3 ± 10.5	Inverse correlation between average RNFL thickness and age
Cunha et al. [87]	50 AD 152 controls		73.1 ± 5.36 71.0 ± 4.62	SD-OCT (Spectralis Heidelberg Engineering)	85.72 ± 14.42* 96.51 ± 9.36	114.44^* 133.14^	96.27^* 106.75^	68.76 ± 16.99* 74.77 ± 13.73	64.22 ± 13.01* 71.38 ± 12.66	AD patients showed thickness reduction in global and temporal quadrants in the peripapillary RNFL and in the superior sector of the macula

(continued)

Table 13.1 (continued)

References	No. of subjects and diagnosis	Mean MMSE/ AD stage	Mean age ± SD	OCT machine	Mean RNFL (μm)	Superior quadrant (μm)	Inferior quadrant (μm)	Nasal quadrant (μm)	Temporal quadrant (μm)	Note
Ferrari et al. [88]	27 MCI 20 mild AD 17 moderate AD 17 FTD 49 controls	26.62 23.0 16.59 21.64	70.45 ± 5.51 69.75 ± 7.51 71.23 ± 6.95 65.59 ± 6.89 68.32 ± 6.96	Fourier-domain OCT Heidelberg Spectralis™	RNFL 92.79 ± 10.31* 94.55 ± 6.84 91.33 ± 13.16* 87.47 ± 7.34* 97.49 ± 8.52 GCL-IPL 55.61 ± 8.17 57.52 ± 0.27 50.07 ± 7.21* 51.83 ± 7.48* 58.18 ± 7.94					GCL-IPL was significantly correlated with raw MMSE in AD
Kwon et al. [99]	30 MCI 30 AD 30 controls	24.17 17.2 27.47	72.17 ± 4.98 73.60 ± 3.67 70.93 ± 4.68	Carl Zeiss Meditec Cirrus HD-OCT	46.31 ± 4.85 42.75 ± 4.53 44.83 ± 4.24	115.0 ± 13.19 106.78 ± 13.5** 115.30 ± 14.78	120.84 ± 17.59 113.82 ± 16.14* 113.70 ± 12.02	68.22 ± 9.40 64.47 ± 7.75 66.40 ± 7.22	68.75 ± 9.79 63.71 ± 9.91 66.23 ± 12.98	
Golzan et al. [103]	23 pre-AD 28 AD 50 controls		80 ± 4 70 ± 9 79 ± 5		RNFL 101.15 99.17 93.18 GLC-IPL 98 ± 9 91 ± 2 96 ± 9* **					The association between RNFL and RGCL thickness and neocortical Aβ standardized uptake value ratio in the grouped control and preclinical cohort

AD, Alzheimer's disease; aMCI, amnestic mild cognitive impairment; CIND, patients with cognitive impairment but no dementia; FTD, frontotemporal dementia; GC-IPL, ganglion cell-Inner plexiform layer; LB, dementia with Lewy bodies; MCI, mild cognitive impairment; MMSE, mini mental state examination; pre-AD, preclinical AD; RNFL, retinal nerve fiber layer; PD, dementia associated with Parkinson's disease; *, significantly different from controls; **, significantly different from MCI; § data extrapolated from the bar chart; #, statistics do not clearly show; + mean of internal plus external sectors; ^ mean of supero-nasal or temporal plus infero-nasal or temporal sectors.

observe reduced RNFL thickness both in AD [100–103] and MCI [94, 99–101, 103] patients in comparison with controls.

When assessed, the mean ganglion cell layer plus inner plexiform layer thickness (GCL-IPL) thickness was found to be reduced in AD eyes by several independent groups [84, 88, 94], and this extended even to some patients affected with MCI [31]. In one study GCL-IPL thickness was reduced in moderate AD and in frontotemporal dementia, but not in MCI and mild AD patients [88].

Some researchers studied optic nerves of AD patients by using confocal scanning laser ophthalmoscopy (cSLO). Ophthalmoscopy in combination with cSLO, revealed an enlargement in the mean vertical cup-to-disc ratio (clinician and instrument derived), rim volume, rim area, and reduced RNFL thickness in patients with AD with respect to controls [104]. Compared with individuals in the lowest quarter of values of cup-to-disc ratios, those with higher values generally had an increased risk of AD [104]. Lu et al. [73] also observed an enlarged cup-to-disc ratio and a thinner RNFL thickness in their 22 mild to moderate AD patients. In contrast, Kergoat et al. [105] found no differences in the regional distribution of RNFL thickness between patients with mild to moderate AD and healthy controls evaluated with scanning laser polarimetry. The same researchers did not observed optic nerve head structural abnormalities in AD by using real-time topographical images obtained with a Heidelberg retina tomograph (HRT) from individuals in the early stages of AD compared with age-matched controls [105]. The same negative results were obtained by Kurna and coworkers in a group of patients with mild to moderate AD [106]. Despite that, Csincsik et al. [107] used ultra-widefield (UWF) scanning laser ophthalmoscope of the retina to determine phenotypic variations in 59 patients with AD and 48 healthy controls and found a significantly higher prevalence of the hard drusen phenotype in the periphery of AD patients compared to controls, as well as changes to the arterial and venular vasculature beyond the posterior pole. The number of optic nerve head drusen increased at the 2 years follow-up measurement in AD patients [107].

In a cross-sectional study on 150 patients with low-to-moderate dementia and 61 controls, researchers compared the parameters provided by two commercially available spectral domain OCT devices, the Cirrus and the Spectralis OCT instruments [92]. With both devices, they confirmed retinal thinning in AD patients, and they found that the best parameter for distinguishing AD patients from healthy controls using OCT measurements was the Spectralis looking at RNFL [92]. Along these lines, Marziani et al. [91] used both Optovue RTVue-100 and Spectralis instruments to evaluate retinal thickness in 21 patients affected by AD in comparison with 21 healthy controls. Both instruments showed a significant difference in full retinal thickness between patients and controls in all the macular sectors except in the central sector and for the superior external sector [91].

In order to verify whether involvement of the retina is an early event in the course of AD, a few studies compared MCI versus AD patients and healthy aged people. Paquet and coworkers [89] enrolled 23 MCI patients, 14 mild AD, 12 moderate to severe AD patients, and 15 healthy subjects. Overall, mean RNFL thickness was reduced in all patient groups in respect to controls. The subgroup analyses revealed no difference between the results observed in MCI and in mild AD patients, whereas RNFL thickness assessed in moderate to severe AD patients was significantly reduced in respect with that assessed in MCI patients [89]. Kesler et al. [97] obtained similar results finding that the mean RNFL was significantly thinner in both AD and MCI patients groups compared to controls, and that the MCI group fell in between the other two groups. This difference was particularly prominent in the inferior quadrant, whereas the AD patients had significantly thinner retinal NFL values also in the superior quadrant [97].

Some investigators attempted to identify individuals who might be at a high risk of developing AD, and observed that, despite the reduction in peripapillary RNFL thickness, central 1-mm foveal thickness and macular volume were significantly increased in MCI patients, but not in AD patients, when compared with age-matched controls. The authors argued that retinal swelling might be the first sign of macular retinal ganglion cell degeneration probably due to inflammation and/or gliosis in the early stages of AD [93]. Other independent research groups found decreased thickness of the RNFL in MCI patients, with values sometime equal to [88, 96] or in between [95] the control and AD groups, sometimes accompanied by a reduced macular volume [95]. However, we noticed that 5 studies were unable to find differences between MCI patients and controls [94, 99–101, 103] challenging the utility of OCT in differentiating MCI from mild-to-moderate AD.

Two studies, relying both on cross-sectional and longitudinal data, recruited individuals in the preclinical stage of the disease to perform a correlation analysis between retinal structural measurements and positron emission tomography (PET) Aβ binding in the neocortex. In adults with preclinical AD, the Aβ positive group of participants showed higher volume in the IPL in comparison with the Aβ negative group [108]. The same research group found that the mean RNFL volume reduction over 27 months was linearly related to neocortical Aβ accumulation, after controlling for normal aging [109].

Finally, it is worth noting that thinning of RNFL is also present in other types of dementia, such as frontotemporal dementia [88], dementia with Lewy bodies, dementia associated with Parkinson's disease [110] and with cerebral autosomal dominant arteriopathy with subcortical infarcts and leuco-encephalopathy (CADASIL) [111] challenging the notion of specificity of OCT findings in AD patients.

13.3.2 Optical Coherence Tomography Angiography (OCT-A) Studies

The introduction of OCT angiography has provided a new drive to the study of the retina and its vessels, offering new research opportunities but also new challenges.

To evaluate a possible correlation between AD and retinal vascular alterations, several authors have used OCT-A techniques to compare values derived from the eyes of AD patients and healthy controls.

Specifically, among the evaluated parameters, retinal vessel density was considered for the whole superficial vascular plexus (SVP), parafoveal SVP, and foveal avascular zone (FAZ).

Using various techniques for mapping retinal vascularization, data on its superficial and deep vascularization were acquired (see Table 13.2). Bulut et al. [50] recruited 26 patients with AD and 26 healthy controls. After undergoing neurological examination and staging with MMSE, all patients underwent OCT-A to assess the parameters of retinal vessel density percentage for the entire retina and for the retina divided into foveal and parafoveal areas. Additionally, the avascular foveal area was calculated for all patients. This study revealed a statistically significant decrease in density throughout the entire macular region, including the foveal and parafoveal zones, in the patient group compared to the control group. Additionally, the area of the foveal avascular zone (FAZ) was significantly larger in the patient group, a datum that was confirmed by other independent research groups [51, 112]. The same OCT-A results regarding the reduction in the percentage of retinal vascularization throughout the examined area, both superficial and deep, were obtained by Zabel et al. [51] on 27 Alzheimer's patients. Partially in agreement with previous results, Lahme et al. [113] found statistically significant results only in relation to superficial, but not deep, vascularization.

Two other studies [114, 115] found statistically significant reduction in the deep layer of foveal vascularization in AD and MCI patients compared to healthy controls.

Notably, Querques et al. [116] observed some evidence for retinal vessel dynamics impairment in a small group of MCI and AD patients. However, they did not find any statistically significant variation in the comparison of OCT-A extracted variables between both patients groups and controls.

13.4 Structural–Functional Correlations

The functional activity of the visual system can be dissected by the use of electrophysiological techniques such as pattern electroretinogram (PERG) and visual evoked potentials (VEPs) that have the capability of assessing, respectively, the bioelectrical activity of retinal ganglion cells and their fibers, and the functional integrity of the entire visual pathways from retina to the visual cortex.

The implicit times were delayed and/or the amplitudes reduced [82, 83, 117–120] in most of the PERG studies performed in AD patients at various stages, reflecting retinal ganglion cell dysfunction. However, in some studies PERG parameters were within the range of normality [121, 122]. In one study luminance pattern ERGs were delayed and amplitudes reduced, whereas isoluminant chromatic ERGs were always within the normal ranges [120].

The implicit time of pattern VEPs was normal in some studies [117, 120, 123, 124] and in others delayed [119, 122, 125, 126], with the amplitudes within the range of normality. A delayed P2 component of the flash VEP was a common

Table 13.2 Demographic data and values of Alzheimer disease patients (AD), Mild Cognitive Impairment (MCI) and controls of: whole retinal vascular density divided in superficial vascular plexus (S) and deep vascular plexus (D) when specified; foveal vascular plexus %; parafoveal vascular plexus %; foveal avascular zone (FAZ) (mm^2)

References	No. of subjects and diagnosis	Mean MMSE	Mean age ± SD	OCTA machine	Whole retinal vascular density %	Foveal %	Parafoveal %	Foveal avascular zone (FAZ) (mm^2)	Note
Bulut et al. [50]	26 AD 26 controls	16.92 ± 7.39	74.23 ± 7.55 72.58 ± 6.28	RTVue XR Avanti spectral-domain OCT system (Optovue, Inc., Fremont, CA, USA)	45.50 ± 3.85* 48.67 ± 3.29*	29.04 ± 7.17* 34.80 ± 6.76*	S 47.96 ± 4.86* S 51.12 ± 4.10*	0.47 ± 0.18* 0.33 ± 0.08*	Vessel density (%) of SVP (whole, fovea and parafovea), outer retina flow rate and FAZ
Lahme et al. [113]	36 AD 38 controls	22.32 ± 4.45	67.97 ± 9.3 66.08 ± 10.11	RTVue XR Avanti spectral-domain OCT system (Optovue, Inc., Fremont, CA, USA)	S 48.77 ± 3.92* D 55.35 ± 3.16 S 51.64 ± 3.28* D 56.72 ± 2.21	29.40 ± 5.72 D 31.21 ± 6.60 31.06 ± 5.35 D 29.32 ± 6.67	S 50.93 ± 4.05 D 57.97 ± 3.30 S 53.55 ± 3.31 D 58.38 ± 4.64		Vessel density (%) of SVP and DVP (whole [2.5-mm diameter circle], fovea [1-mm diameter circle] and parafovea [Ø 1–2.5 mm])

(continued)

Table 13.2 (continued)

References	No. of subjects and diagnosis	Mean MMSE	Mean age ± SD	OCTA machine	Whole retinal vascular density %	Foveal %	Parafoveal %	Foveal avascular zone (FAZ) (mm^2)	Note
Querques et al. [116]	12 AD 32 controls 12 MCI	19.5 ± 3.6 24.9/ 30 ± 2.7	72.90 ± 7.2 71.6 ± 5.9 76.3 ± 6.9	(Zeiss Cirrus HD-5000 with AngioPlex, Carl Zeiss Meditec, Dublin, CA)	S 40.43 ± 1.32 D 44.36 ± 1.63 S 40.31 ± 1.93 D 44.82 ± 1.41 S 40.70 ± 2.76 D 44.49 ± 0.76		S 40.66 ± 2.36 D 43.78 ± 1.00 S 40.92 ± 1.96 D 45.77 ± 1.77 S 42.13 ± 1.26 D 45.05 ± 1.26		Perfusion density (%) of SVP, DVP, choriocapillaris and choroid (3 6 and 3 and 6-mm diameter circle with masked FAZ)
Zabel et al. [51]	39 AD 133 controls	20.55 ± 5.46	74.11 ± 5.87 74.26 ± 7.66	RTVue XR Avanti spectral-domain OCT system (Optovue, Inc., Fremont, CA, USA)	S 47.42 ± 3.04* D 43.95 ± 5.15* S 48.15 ± 3.03* D 49.46 ± 4.27*			0.32 ± 0.09* 0.21 ± 0.07 *	Vessel density (%) of SVP and DVP (whole [6-mm diameter circle], fovea [1-mm diameter circle], parafovea [Ø 1–3 mm] and perifovea [Ø 3–6 mm]) and FAZ

(continued)

Table 13.2 (continued)

References	No. of subjects and diagnosis	Mean MMSE	Mean age ± SD	OCTA machine	Whole retinal vascular density %	Foveal %	Parafoveal %	Foveal avascular zone (FAZ) (mm^2)	Note
Haan et al. [135]	48 AD 38 controls	23 ± 3	65.4 ± 8.1 60.6 ± 5	(Zeiss Cirrus HD-5000 with AngioPlex, Carl Zeiss Meditec, Dublin, CA)		17.3 (±1.5) 17.4 (±1.2)	17.4 (±1.3) 17.8 (±1.1)	0.24 (±0.06) 0.26 (±0.08)	Vessel density of SVP (/mm) (parafovea [Ø 1–3 mm] and perifovea [Ø 3–6 mm]) and FAZ
Li et al. [112]	29 AD 26 controls	24.9 ± 3.61	63.38 ± 8.5 64.81 ± 6.46	(Zeiss Cirrus HD-5000 with AngioPlex, Carl Zeiss Meditec, Dublin, CA)				0.42 ± 0.11* 0.24 ± 0.08*	Vessel density (/mm) of SVP (fovea [1-mm diameter circle], and parafovea [Ø 1–3 mm] and perifovea [Ø 3–6 mm]) and FAZ

(continued)

Table 13.2 (continued)

References	No. of subjects and diagnosis	Mean MMSE	Mean age ± SD	OCTA machine	Whole retinal vascular density %	Foveal %	Parafoveal %	Foveal avascular zone (FAZ) (mm^2)	Note
Wu et al. [114]	18 AD 21 controls	19.67 ± 2.45	69.94 ± 6.39 68.67 ± 5.85	RTVue XR Avanti spectral-domain OCT system (Optovue, Inc., Fremont, CA, USA)		S 49.56 ± 2.81 D 43.1 ± 2.75* S 50.47 ± 2.72 D 52.28 ± 2.89*		0.26 ± 0.07	Vessel density (%) of SVP and DVP (parafovea [Ø 0.6–3 mm] and perifovea [Ø 3–6 mm]) and FAZ
Chua et al. [115]	24 AD 29 controls		74.9 ± 6 76.7 ± 5.3	(Zeiss Cirrus HD-5000 with AngioPlex, Carl Zeiss Meditec, Dublin, CA)		SRCP 14.78 ± 1.14 DRCP 20.42 ± 1.60* SRCP 15.66 ± 0.96 DRCP 21.54 ± 1.55*			Perfusion density (%), vessel density (/mm) SVP and DVP (Ø 1–2.5 mm)

* Significant at $p < 0.05$

finding across studies in AD patients [117, 123, 127, 128], with one exception [125].

Taken as a whole, these electrophysiological results are consistent with the early histological studies showing retinal ganglion cell dysfunction in AD [28, 128] and supports the notion that this damage in AD preferentially affects the larger, faster-conducting retinal ganglion cells and their retinocortical projections.

Parisi and coworkers [82, 83] used OCT and PERG in a group of 17 mild severity AD patients compared with a group of 14 healthy controls. They observed that the general reduction of peripapillary RNFL thickness was accompanied with delayed N35, P50 and N95 implicit times and reduced N35-P50 and P50-N95 amplitudes in their AD patients. More interestingly, in AD eyes, the RNFL overall values were positively correlated to the PERG P50 and N95 implicit times and PERG P50-N95 amplitude. This was not so in controls [82, 83]. However, Iseri et al. [98] did not find significant differences in VEP P100 implicit times and N75-P100 amplitudes recorded at high spatial frequency in a group of 14 mild to moderate AD patients when compared with a group of 15 controls. Moreover, they saw no correlation between any of the abnormalities in RNFL and macular OCT thickness and VEP in AD [98]. This negative correlation, between VEPs parameters recorded at both high and low spatial frequency and OCT peripapillary scans, was later corroborated [129].

Liu et al. [31] observed, for the first time, that thinner macular GC-IPL is associated with lower integrity of the white matter microstructure, as verified using MRI diffusion tension imaging, in healthy controls in fronto-parieto-occipital and cingulate regions, as well as with lower grey matter volumes in occipital pole and cerebellum. These results in controls were contrasted with those obtained in AD and MCI patients where these relationships between macula and brain microstructure and volume were not detectable. The authors suggested that neurodegenerative processes related to the AD and MCI pathology can disrupt the physiological retina-brain coupling [31].

13.5 Correlations with Psychometric Measures

Along with personal history, physical examination and laboratory tests, questionnaires are often used to help test a range of everyday mental skills of persons with symptoms of dementias. Widely used tests include the mini mental state examination (MMSE), the Alzheimer's disease assessment scale- (ADAS-Cog), clinical dementia rating (CDR) score, and the Repeatable Battery for the Assessment of Neuropsychological Status (RBANS).

The previously mentioned parameters of increased cup-to-disc ratio, cup volume, and decreased optic disc rim area, all found in AD patients by optic nerve analyser, positively correlated with ADAS-Cog scores and disease's duration [72]. In AD patients, a significant relationship between inferior RNFL thickness change and ADAS-Cog scores change as well as CDR scores at 12 months follow-up, was observed. Interestingly, the linear regression model revealed that for every 10 μm decrease of RNFL thickness, there was an accompanying ADAS-Cog increase of 5 units [102].

Moreover, the reduced total macular volume in patients with AD was positively correlated with the severity of the disease as assessed by the MMSE [86, 96, 98, 102, 110]. Other studies failed to find the same associations [89, 90, 97, 129, 130]. However, some authors observed that the thinner the RNFL, ganglion cell and inner plexiform layers, the longer the AD disease duration, even if the latter were not significantly related to severity of the disease (assessed with MMSE score) [84]. Nonetheless, RNFL thickness of AD or MCI patients was not associated with other patient demographic features, such as age [89, 92], gender, and AD stage [130]. In another study assessing the association between macular GC-IPL and peripapillary RNFL thicknesses with disease progression in MCI and AD, the CDR scale score exhibited significant negative relationships with the average GC-IPL thickness and GC-IPL thickness in the supero-temporal, supero-nasal, and infero-nasal sectors [131]. Furthermore, the composite memory score exhibited significant positive association with the average GC-IPL thickness and the GCIPL thickness in the supero-temporal, inferonasal, and inferotemporal sectors. A positive association between the central macular thickness and the MMSE score was also observed [131].

More recently, La Morgia et al. [18] with the scope to verify the integrity of a subpopulation of retinal ganglion cells expressing the photopigment melanopsin, observed that clinical parameters (age, age at onset, disease duration, and MMSE score) and OCT data were not correlated to AD patients actigraphic data assessing rest–activity circadian rhythms. There may have been a minimum threshold such that relatively few melanopsin retinal ganglion cells sufficed to maintain circadian rhythms.

In AD patients, but not in MCI, multiple linear regression models showed a strong association between overall RNFL thickness and MMSE score. The same association was found between MMSE and RNFL thickness in superior and nasal quadrants. Macular thickness and volume were not associated with MMSE score either in MCI or in AD patients [93].

A prospective study attempted to determine whether deterioration of patients' cognitive functions, as verified with the RBANS test, correlated to specific OCT findings [132–134]. These investigators followed, for a period of 25 months, two groups of subjects: 82 participants with a normal cognitive status and 22 MCI patients. The participants who completed the observational period were further categorized as 60 participants experiencing a stable cognitive status and 18 participants who experienced a worsening of their cognitive status. The investigators found that in those participants who remained stable, greater attenuation of RNFL in the superior quadrant could predict specific cognitive deteriorations. In contradistinction, in participants who worsened, less attenuation of RNFL in the inferior quadrant could predict greater cognitive deterioration [132–134]. These findings suggest that patients who have less reduction in the thickness of the inferior quadrant of RNFL over time may have a higher risk of developing MCI and dementia, leading the authors to put forward RNFL thickness as a potential biomarker of dementia.

Few studies have been done regarding potential correlations between OCT-A parameter variations and dementia evaluation scales. The FAZ has been found to have a negative correlation with MMSE and MoCA scores thus far [50, 112]. However, this datum was not replicated by others [51, 115, 135].

13.6 Conclusions

The diagnosis of AD is often based on psychometric assessments by a multidisciplinary team (neurologists, psychiatrists, and psychologist) and a neurological examination. Because of inter- and intra-individual variability, neurophysiological and neuroimaging tests have not yet been considered as criteria on which to base a diagnosis. In fact, neurophysiological as well as other paraclinical tests are recommended only on suspicion of secondary causes of dementia as part of the differential diagnosis of AD. The AD diagnosis is confirmed only with *post mortem* histopathology. Nonetheless, the last few decades have seen the use of structural and functional techniques as potential biomarkers that might also identify factors that may predispose individuals to AD. The optical coherence tomography (OCT) technique for the measurement of the peripapillary RNFL, the macular thickness and volume, have been demonstrated as useful for the demonstration of significant retinal changes in patients and these parameters roughly correlate with the severity of the disease (Fig. 13.2). Despite the limited number of studies and partly conflicting results, OCT-A has additionally found a density retinal microvasculature loss in patients with AD and MCI.

Particularly intriguing results of recent experiments include:

- In animal models, expressing mutant forms of amyloid precursors, and histological studies on *post mortem* AD eyes, researchers have observed various retinal pathological changes, such as accumulation of Aβ aggregates within the retina and its microvasculature, retina ganglion cell death and signs of neuroinflammation.
- In evaluations with the optic nerve analyser, a higher proportion of AD patients showed signs of optic neuropathy manifesting as optic disc atrophy, pathologic optic disc cupping, and thinning of the neuroretinal rim and of the RNFL.
- In agreement with *post mortem* studies, OCT data studies indicated a significant decline in peripapillary RNFL and also changes in macular thickness and volume that is progressive from MCI to AD eyes.
- Electrophysiological and OCT studies in AD patients showed RNFL thickness reduction that was related to neuronal degeneration in the retinal ganglion cell layer that was not a consequence of retrograde degeneration from the post-chiasmatic visual pathway.

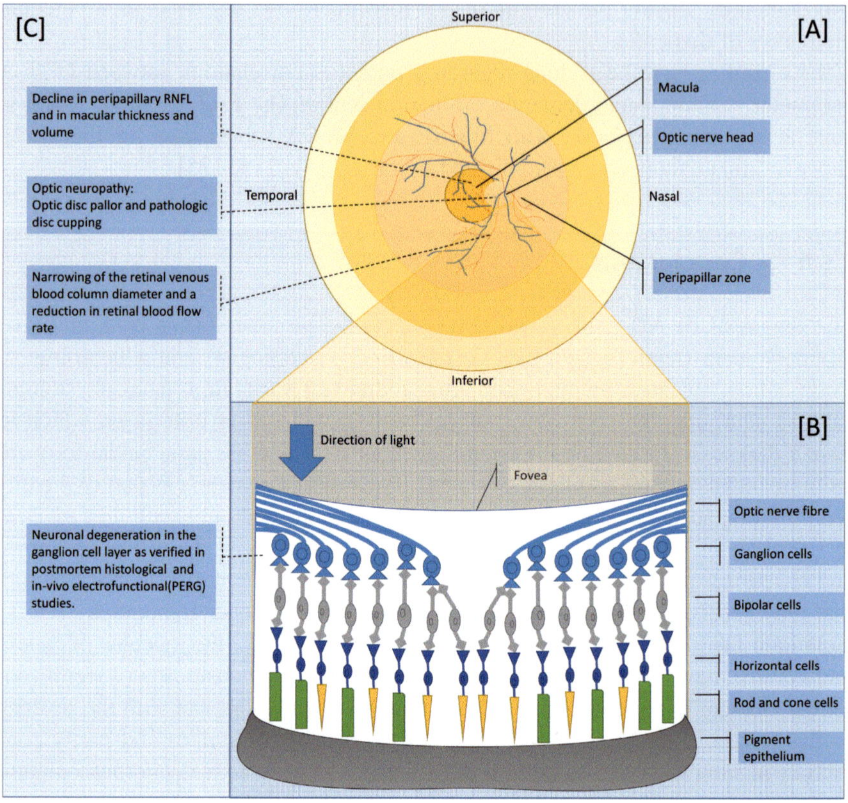

Fig. 13.2 Schematic representation of an entire retina with superimposed anatomic zones (upper panel [A]) and a schematic enlargement of a portion of the retina with the main cell classes (lower panel [B]). Summarized on the left panel [C] are findings from the OCT and electrophysiological studies in AD

- Retinal microvascular density loss was observed in some OCT-A studies, which tends to imply that retinal neural and vascular pathology may interact and have a cumulative effect.
- The acquisition in the same patients of OCT and objective measurements of brain microstructure and volume did not suggest that RNFL could be used as a surrogate for magnetic resonance imaging measurements of the brain.
- The correlations between morphological and clinical features tended to suggest a potential role for the optic nerve head, and to a minor extent, its microvasculature, analysis in monitoring the progression of AD and as outcome measures in the assessment of any purported AD treatments.

Overall, these results suggested that degeneration of the retinal ganglion cells should be added to the constellation of neuropathologic changes found in patients with Alzheimer's disease.

Other neurodegenerative disorders, like Parkinson's disease and glaucoma, may enter in the differential diagnosis of RNFL thinning [136]. There is a controversial association between primary open angle glaucoma (POAG) and AD. This is based on various indirect evidences of some shared genetic, histopathological and functional features [137, 138]. The association of AD and POAG is poorly supported by epidemiological studies [139, 140]. Nonetheless, for some authors, glaucoma could be, in a subgroup of patients, the expression of a neurodegenerative process of the CNS that may be partially influenced by the risk factor of intraocular pressure (IOP) [141, 142]. However, the link between AD and the risk of developing glaucoma persists even without elevated IOP levels [85].

Future research in OCT, and its angiographic counterpart, as a biomarker of AD requires establishing a better specificity of OCT findings in AD. These and similar studies using OCT parameters of retinal changes will be important as objective in vivo outcome measures against which to evaluate new molecules purported to help in the treatment of AD.

References

1. Stefanacci R. The costs of Alzheimer's disease and the value of effective therapies. Am J Manag Care. 2011;13:S356–62.
2. Alzheimer's Association. Alzheimer's disease facts and figures. Alzheimers Dement. 2016;2016(12):459–509.
3. Nichols E, Steinmetz JD, Vollset SE, et al. Estimation of the global prevalence of dementia in 2019 and forecasted prevalence in 2050: an analysis for the Global Burden of Disease Study 2019. Lancet Public Health. 2022;7:e105–25.
4. Blennow K, de Leon MJ, Zetterberg H. Alzheimer's disease. Lancet (London, England). 2006;368:387–403.
5. Waring S, Rosenberg RN. Genome-wide association studies in Alzheimer disease. Arch Neurol. 2008;65:329–34.
6. Morris J, Storandt M, Miller JP, McKeel DW, Price JL, Rubin EH, Berg L. Mild cognitive impairment represents early-stage Alzheimer disease. Arch Neurol. 2001;58:397–405.
7. Winblad B, Palmer K, Kivipelto M, et al. Mild cognitive impairment–beyond controversies, towards a consensus: report of the International Working Group on Mild Cognitive Impairment. J Intern Med. 2004;256:240–6.
8. Litvan I, Goldman JG, Tröster AI, et al. Diagnostic criteria for mild cognitive impairment in Parkinson's disease: Movement Disorder Society Task Force guidelines. Mov Disord. 2012;27:349–56.
9. Whitehouse PJ, Price DL, Clark AW, Coyle JT, DeLong MR. Alzheimer disease: evidence for selective loss of cholinergic neurons in the nucleus basalis. Ann Neurol. 1981;10:122–6.
10. van de Nes JAP, Nafe R, Schlote W. Non-tau based neuronal degeneration in Alzheimer's disease—an immunocytochemical and quantitative study in the supragranular layers of the middle temporal neocortex. Brain Res. 2008;1213:152–65.
11. Leuba G, Kraftsik R. Visual cortex in Alzheimer's disease: occurrence of neuronal death and glial proliferation, and correlation with pathological hallmarks. Neurobiol Aging. 1994;15:29–43.
12. Armstrong RA. Is there a spatial association between senile plaques and neurofibrillary tangles in Alzheimer's disease? Folia Neuropathol. 2005;43:133–8.
13. Leuba G, Saini K. Pathology of subcortical visual centres in relation to cortical degeneration in Alzheimer's disease. Neuropathol Appl Neurobiol. 1995;21:410–22.

14. Baloyannis S, Mauroudis I, Manolides SL, Manolides LS. Synaptic alterations in the medial geniculate bodies and the inferior colliculi in Alzheimer's disease: a Golgi and electron microscope study. Acta Otolaryngol. 2009;129:416–8.
15. Dugger B, Tu M, Murray ME, Dickson DW. Disease specificity and pathologic progression of tau pathology in brainstem nuclei of Alzheimer's disease and progressive supranuclear palsy. Neurosci Lett. 2011;491:122–6.
16. Hinton DR, Sadun AA, Blanks JC, Miller CA. Optic-nerve degeneration in Alzheimer's disease. N Engl J Med. 1986;315:485–7.
17. Löffler K, Edward DP, Tso MO. Immunoreactivity against tau, amyloid precursor protein, and beta-amyloid in the human retina. Invest Ophthalmol Vis Sci. 1995;36:24–31.
18. La Morgia C, Ross-Cisneros FN, Koronyo Y, et al. Melanopsin retinal ganglion cell loss in Alzheimer disease. Ann Neurol. 2016;79:90–109.
19. Jellinger KA. Alzheimer disease and cerebrovascular pathology: an update. J Neural Transm. 2002;109:813–36.
20. Iadecola C, Gottesman RF. Cerebrovascular alterations in Alzheimer disease. Circ Res. 2018;123:406–8.
21. Tsokolas G, Tsaousis KT, Diakonis VF, Matsou A, Tyradellis S. Optical coherence tomography angiography in neurodegenerative diseases: a review. Eye Brain. 2020;12:73–87.
22. Hutton J, Morris JL, Elias JW, Poston JN. Contrast sensitivity dysfunction in Alzheimer's disease. Neurology. 1993;43:2328–30.
23. Gilmore G, Whitehouse PJ. Contrast sensitivity in Alzheimer's disease: a 1-year longitudinal analysis. Optom Vis Sci. 1995;72:83–91.
24. Crow R, Levin LB, LaBree L, Rubin R, Feldon SE. Sweep visual evoked potential evaluation of contrast sensitivity in Alzheimer's dementia. Invest Ophthalmol Vis Sci. 2003;44:875–8.
25. Gilmore G, Wenk HE, Naylor LA, Koss E. Motion perception and Alzheimer's disease. J Gerontol. 1994;49:P52–7.
26. Rizzo M, Nawrot M. Perception of movement and shape in Alzheimer's disease. Brain. 1998;2259–70.
27. Wijk H, Berg S, Sivik L, Steen B. Colour discrimination, colour naming and colour preferences among individuals with Alzheimer's disease. Int J Geriatr Psychiatry. 1999;14:1000–5.
28. Wijk H, Berg S, Bergman B, Hanson AB, Sivik L, Steen B. Colour perception among the very elderly related to visual and cognitive function. Scand J Caring Sci. 2002;16:91–102.
29. Salamone G, Di L, Mosti S, Lupo F, Cravello L, Palmer K, Musicco M, Caltagirone C. Color discrimination performance in patients with Alzheimer's disease. Dement Geriatr Cogn Disord. 2009;27:501–7.
30. Sadun A, Bassi CJ. Optic nerve damage in Alzheimer's disease. Ophthalmology. 1990;97:9–17.
31. Liu S, Ong Y-T, Hilal S, Loke YM, Wong TY, Chen CL-H, Cheung CY, Zhou J. The association between retinal neuronal layer and brain structure is disrupted in patients with cognitive impairment and Alzheimer's disease. J Alzheimers Dis. 2016;54:585–95.
32. Coppola G, Di Renzo A, Ziccardi L, Martelli F, Fadda A, Manni G, Barboni P, Pierelli F, Sadun AA, Parisi V. Optical coherence tomography in Alzheimer's disease: a meta-analysis. PLoS One. https://doi.org/10.1371/journal.pone.0134750
33. Huang D, Swanson EA, Lin CP, et al. Optical coherence tomography. Science (New York, NY). 1991;254:1178–81.
34. Puliafito C, Hee MR, Lin CP, Reichel E, Schuman JS, Duker JS, Izatt JA, Swanson EA, Fujimoto JG. Imaging of macular diseases with optical coherence tomography. Ophthalmology. 1995;102:217–29.
35. Yaqoob Z, Wu J, Yang C. Spectral domain optical coherence tomography: a better OCT imaging strategy. Biotechniques. 2005;39:S6-13.
36. Kiernan D, Mieler WF, Hariprasad SM. Spectral-domain optical coherence tomography: a comparison of modern high-resolution retinal imaging systems. Am J Ophthalmol. 2010;149:18–31.

37. Schuman JS, Hee MR, Puliafito CA, Wong C, Pedut-Kloizman T, Lin CP, Hertzmark E, Izatt JA, Swanson EA, Fujimoto JG. Quantification of nerve fiber layer thickness in normal and glaucomatous eyes using optical coherence tomography. Arch Ophthalmol. 1995;113:586–96.
38. Parisi V, Manni G, Gandolfi SA, Centofanti M, Colacino G, Bucci MG. Visual function correlates with nerve fiber layer thickness in eyes affected by ocular hypertension. Invest Ophthalmol Vis Sci. 1999;40:1828–33.
39. Parisi V, Manni G, Spadaro M, Colacino G, Restuccia R, Marchi S, Bucci MG, Pierelli F. Correlation between morphological and functional retinal impairment in multiple sclerosis patients. Invest Ophthalmol Vis Sci. 1999;40:2520–7.
40. Parisi V, Manni G, Centofanti M, Gandolfi SA, Olzi D, Bucci MG. Correlation between optical coherence tomography, pattern electroretinogram, and visual evoked potentials in open-angle glaucoma patients. Ophthalmology. 2001;108:905–12.
41. Kardon RH. Role of the macular optical coherence tomography scan in neuro-ophthalmology. J Neuroophthalmol. 2011;31:353–61.
42. Hagag AM, Gao SS, Jia Y, Huang D. Optical coherence tomography angiography: technical principles and clinical applications in ophthalmology. Taiwan J Ophthalmol. 2017;7:115–29.
43. Sung K, Wollstein G, Bilonick RA, Townsend KA, Ishikawa H, Kagemann L, Noecker RJ, Fujimoto JG, Schuman JS. Effects of age on optical coherence tomography measurements of healthy retinal nerve fiber layer, macula, and optic nerve head. Ophthalmology. 2009;116:1119–24.
44. Mwanza J, Durbin MK, Budenz DL, Girkin CA, Leung CK, Liebmann JM, Peace JH, Werner JS, Wollstein G. Profile and predictors of normal ganglion cell-inner plexiform layer thickness measured with frequency-domain optical coherence tomography. Invest Ophthalmol Vis Sci. 2011;52:7872–9.
45. Girkin C, McGwin G, Sinai MJ, et al. Variation in optic nerve and macular structure with age and race with spectral-domain optical coherence tomography. Ophthalmology. 2011;118:2403–8.
46. Alasil T, Wang K, Keane PA, Lee H, Baniasadi N, de B, Chen TC. Analysis of normal retinal nerve fiber layer thickness by age, sex, and race using spectral domain optical coherence tomography. J Glaucoma. 2013;22:532–41.
47. Parikh R, Parikh SR, Sekhar GC, Prabakaran S, Babu JG, Thomas R. Normal age-related decay of retinal nerve fiber layer thickness. Ophthalmology. 2007;114:921–6.
48. Feuer W, Budenz DL, Anderson DR, Cantor L, Greenfield DS, Savell J, Schuman JS, Varma R. Topographic differences in the age-related changes in the retinal nerve fiber layer of normal eyes measured by Stratus optical coherence tomography. J Glaucoma. 2011;20:133–8.
49. Lee J, Hwang YH, Lee SM, Kim YY. Age and retinal nerve fiber layer thickness measured by spectral domain optical coherence tomography. Korean J Ophthalmol. 2012;26:163–8.
50. Bulut M, Kurtuluş F, Gözkaya O, Erol MK, Cengiz A, Akldan M, Yaman A. Evaluation of optical coherence tomography angiographic findings in Alzheimer's type dementia. Br J Ophthalmol. 2018;102:233–7.
51. Zabel P, Kaluzny JJ, Wilkosc-Debczynska M, Gebska-Toloczko M, Suwala K, Zabel K, Zaron A, Kucharski R, Araszkiewicz A. Comparison of retinal microvasculature in patients with Alzheimer's disease and primary open-angle glaucoma by optical coherence tomography angiography. Invest Ophthalmol Vis Sci. 2019;60:3447–55.
52. Hardy J, Allsop D. Amyloid deposition as the central event in the aetiology of Alzheimer's disease. Trends Pharmacol Sci. 1991;12:383–8.
53. Braidy N, Muñoz P, Palacios AG, Castellano-Gonzalez G, Inestrosa NC, Chung RS, Sachdev P, Guillemin GJ. Recent rodent models for Alzheimer's disease: clinical implications and basic research. J Neural Transm. 2012;119:173–95.
54. Ning A, Cui J, To E, Ashe KH, Matsubara J. Amyloid-beta deposits lead to retinal degeneration in a mouse model of Alzheimer disease. Invest Ophthalmol Vis Sci. 2008;49:5136–43.

55. Perez S, Lumayag S, Kovacs B, Mufson EJ, Xu S. Beta-amyloid deposition and functional impairment in the retina of the APPswe/PS1DeltaE9 transgenic mouse model of Alzheimer's disease. Invest Ophthalmol Vis Sci. 2009;50:793–800.
56. Koronyo-Hamaoui M, Koronyo Y, Ljubimov AV, Miller CA, Ko MK, Black KL, Schwartz M, Farkas DL. Identification of amyloid plaques in retinas from Alzheimer's patients and noninvasive in vivo optical imaging of retinal plaques in a mouse model. Neuroimage. 2011;1:S204–17.
57. Koronyo Y, Salumbides BC, Black KL, Koronyo-Hamaoui M. Alzheimer's disease in the retina: imaging retinal Aß plaques for early diagnosis and therapy assessment. Neurodegener Dis. 2012;10:285–93.
58. Liu B, Rasool S, Yang Z, Glabe CG, Schreiber SS, Ge J, Tan Z. Amyloid-peptide vaccinations reduce {beta}-amyloid plaques but exacerbate vascular deposition and inflammation in the retina of Alzheimer's transgenic mice. Am J Pathol. 2009;175:2099–110.
59. Cordeiro M, Guo L, Coxon KM, et al. Imaging multiple phases of neurodegeneration: a novel approach to assessing cell death in vivo. Cell Death Dis. 2010;1:10.
60. Cohen R, Rezai-Zadeh K, Weitz TM, et al. A transgenic Alzheimer rat with plaques, tau pathology, behavioral impairment, oligomeric aβ, and frank neuronal loss. J Neurosci. 2013;33:6245–56.
61. Tsai Y, Lu B, Ljubimov AV, Girman S, Ross-Cisneros FN, Sadun AA, Svendsen CN, Cohen RM, Wang S. Ocular changes in TgF344-AD rat model of Alzheimer's disease. Invest Ophthalmol Vis Sci. 2014;55:523–34.
62. Andorfer C, Acker CM, Kress Y, Hof PR, Duff K, Davies P. Cell-cycle reentry and cell death in transgenic mice expressing nonmutant human tau isoforms. J Neurosci. 2005;25:5446–54.
63. Rodriguez L, Mdzomba JB, Joly S, Boudreau-Laprise M, Planel E, Pernet V. Human tau expression does not induce mouse retina neurodegeneration, suggesting differential toxicity of tau in brain vs. retinal neurons. Front Mol Neurosci. 2018;11:293.
64. Curcio C, Drucker DN. Retinal ganglion cells in Alzheimer's disease and aging. Ann Neurol. 1993;33:248–57.
65. Davies D, McCoubrie P, McDonald B, Jobst KA. Myelinated axon number in the optic nerve is unaffected by Alzheimer's disease. Br J Ophthalmol. 1995;79:596–600.
66. Blanks J, Torigoe Y, Hinton DR, Blanks RH. Retinal pathology in Alzheimer's disease. I. Ganglion cell loss in foveal/parafoveal retina. Neurobiol Aging. 1996;17:377–84.
67. Blanks JC, Schmidt SY, Torigoe Y, Porrello KV, Hinton DR, Blanks RHI. Retinal pathology in Alzheimer's disease. II. Regional neuron loss and glial changes in GCL. Neurobiol Aging. 1996;17:385–95.
68. Blanks J, Hinton DR, Sadun AA, Miller CA. Retinal ganglion cell degeneration in Alzheimer's disease. Brain Res. 1989;501:364–72.
69. Schön C, Hoffmann NA, Ochs SM, et al. Long-term in vivo imaging of fibrillar tau in the retina of P301S transgenic mice. PLoS ONE. 2012;7:10.
70. Shi H, Koronyo Y, Rentsendorj A, et al. Identification of early pericyte loss and vascular amyloidosis in Alzheimer's disease retina. Acta Neuropathol. 2020;139:813–36.
71. Hedges TR, Perez G, Speigelman D, Barbas NR, Peli E, Yardley CJ. Retinal nerve fiber layer abnormalities in Alzheimer's disease. Acta Ophthalmol Scand. 1996;74:271–5.
72. Tsai C, Ritch R, Schwartz B, Lee SS, Miller NR, Chi T, Hsieh FY. Optic nerve head and nerve fiber layer in Alzheimer's disease. Arch Ophthalmol. 1991;109:199–204.
73. Lu Y, Li Z, Zhang X, Ming B, Jia J, Wang R, Ma D. Retinal nerve fiber layer structure abnormalities in early Alzheimer's disease: evidence in optical coherence tomography. Neurosci Lett. 2010;480:69–72.
74. Balazsi AG, Rootman J, Drance SM, Schulzer M, Douglas GR. The effect of age on the nerve fiber population of the human optic nerve. Am J Ophthalmol. 1984;97:760–6.
75. Fortune B, Reynaud J, Cull G, Burgoyne CF, Wang L. The effect of age on optic nerve axon counts, SDOCT scan quality, and peripapillary retinal nerve fiber layer thickness measurements in rhesus monkeys. Transl Vis Sci Technol. 2014;3:2.

76. Johnson BM, Miao M, Sadun AA. Age-related decline of human optic nerve axon populations. Age (Omaha). 1987;10:5–9.
77. Repka M, Quigley HA. The effect of age on normal human optic nerve fiber number and diameter. Ophthalmology. 1989;96:26–32.
78. Sadun AA. Discussion of the Effect of Age on normal human optic nerve fiber number and diameter. Ophthalmology. 1989;96:31–2.
79. Bowd C, Zangwill LM, Blumenthal EZ, Vasile C, Boehm AG, Gokhale PA, Mohammadi K, Amini P, Sankary TM, Weinreb RN. Imaging of the optic disc and retinal nerve fiber layer: the effects of age, optic disc area, refractive error, and gender. J Opt Soc Am Opt image Sci vision. 2002;19:197–207.
80. Leung C, Yu M, Weinreb RN, Ye C, Liu S, Lai G, Lam DS. Retinal nerve fiber layer imaging with spectral-domain optical coherence tomography: a prospective analysis of age-related loss. Ophthalmology. 2012;119:731–7.
81. Celebi A, Mirza GE. Age-related change in retinal nerve fiber layer thickness measured with spectral domain optical coherence tomography. Invest Ophthalmol Vis Sci. 2013;54:8095–103.
82. Parisi V, Restuccia R, Fattapposta F, Mina C, Bucci MG, Pierelli F. Morphological and functional retinal impairment in Alzheimer's disease patients. Clin Neurophysiol. 2001;112:1860–7.
83. Parisi V. Correlation between morphological and functional retinal impairment in patients affected by ocular hypertension, glaucoma, demyelinating optic neuritis and Alzheimer's disease. Semin Ophthalmol. 2003;18:50–7.
84. Garcia-Martin E, Bambo MP, Marques ML, Satue M, Otin S, Larrosa JM, Polo V, Pablo LE. Ganglion cell layer measurements correlate with disease severity in patients with Alzheimer's disease. Acta Ophthalmol. 2016;94:e454–9.
85. Cesareo M, Martucci A, Ciuffoletti E, Mancino R, Cerulli A, Sorge RP, Martorana A, Sancesario G, Nucci C. Association between Alzheimer's disease and glaucoma: a study based on Heidelberg retinal tomography and frequency doubling technology perimetry. Front Neurosci. 2015;9:479.
86. Cunha LP, Lopes LC, Costa-Cunha LVF, Costa CF, Pires LA, Almeida ALM, Monteiro MLR. Macular thickness measurements with frequency domain-OCT for quantification of retinal neural loss and its correlation with cognitive impairment in Alzheimer's disease. PLoS ONE. 2016;11: e0153830.
87. Cunha JP, Proença R, Dias-Santos A, Almeida R, Águas H, Alves M, Papoila AL, Louro C, Castanheira-Dinis A. OCT in Alzheimer's disease: thinning of the RNFL and superior hemiretina. Graefe's Arch Clin Exp Ophthalmol. 2017;255:1827–35.
88. Ferrari L, Huang S-C, Magnani G, Ambrosi A, Comi G, Leocani L. Optical coherence tomography reveals retinal neuroaxonal thinning in frontotemporal dementia as in Alzheimer's disease. J Alzheimer's Dis. 2017;56:1101–7.
89. Paquet C, Boissonnot M, Roger F, Dighiero P, Gil R, Hugon J. Abnormal retinal thickness in patients with mild cognitive impairment and Alzheimer's disease. Neurosci Lett. 2007;420:97–9.
90. Kirbas S, Turkyilmaz K, Anlar O, Tufekci A, Durmus M. Retinal nerve fiber layer thickness in patients with Alzheimer disease. J Neuroophthalmol. 2013;33:58–61.
91. Marziani E, Pomati S, Ramolfo P, Cigada M, Giani A, Mariani C, Staurenghi G. Evaluation of retinal nerve fiber layer and ganglion cell layer thickness in Alzheimer's disease using spectral-domain optical coherence tomography. Invest Ophthalmol Vis Sci. 2013;54:5953–8.
92. Larrosa J, Garcia-Martin E, Bambo MP, Pinilla J, Polo V, Otin S, Satue M, Herrero R, Pablo LE. Potential new diagnostic tool for Alzheimer's disease using a linear discriminant function for Fourier domain optical coherence tomography. Invest Ophthalmol Vis Sci. 2014;55:3043–51.
93. Ascaso F, Cruz N, Modrego PJ, Lopez-Anton R, Santabárbara J, Pascual LF, Lobo A, Cristóbal JA. Retinal alterations in mild cognitive impairment and Alzheimer's disease: an optical coherence tomography study. J Neurol. 2014;261:1522–30.

94. Cheung C, Ong Y, Hilal S, et al. Retinal ganglion cell analysis using high-definition optical coherence tomography in patients with mild cognitive impairment and Alzheimer's disease. J Alzheimers Dis. 2015;45:45–56.
95. Gao L, Liu Y, Li X, Bai Q, Liu P. Abnormal retinal nerve fiber layer thickness and macula lutea in patients with mild cognitive impairment and Alzheimer's disease. Arch Gerontol Geriatr. 2015;60:162–7.
96. Oktem EO, Derle E, Kibaroglu S, Oktem C, Akkoyun I, Can U. The relationship between the degree of cognitive impairment and retinal nerve fiber layer thickness. Neurol Sci. 2015;36:1141–6.
97. Kesler A, Vakhapova V, Korczyn AD, Naftaliev E, Neudorfer M. Retinal thickness in patients with mild cognitive impairment and Alzheimer's disease. Clin Neurol Neurosurg. 2011;113:523–6.
98. Iseri P, Altinaş O, Tokay T, Yüksel N. Relationship between cognitive impairment and retinal morphological and visual functional abnormalities in Alzheimer disease. J Neuroophthalmol. 2006;26:18–24.
99. Kwon JY, Yang JH, Han JS, Kim DG. Analysis of the retinal nerve fiber layer thickness in Alzheimer disease and mild cognitive impairment. Korean J Ophthalmol. 2017;31:548.
100. Feke GT, Hyman BT, Stern RA, Pasquale LR. Retinal blood flow in mild cognitive impairment and Alzheimer's disease. Alzheimer's Dement (Amsterdam, Netherlands). 2015;1:144–51.
101. Pillai JA, Bermel R, Bonner-Jackson A, Rae-Grant A, Fernandez H, Bena J, Jones SE, Ehlers JP, Leverenz JB. Retinal nerve fiber layer thinning in Alzheimer's disease. Am J Alzheimer's Dis Other Dementiasr. 2016;31:430–6.
102. Trebbastoni A, D'Antonio F, Bruscolini A, Marcelli M, Cecere M, Campanelli A, Imbriano L, de Lena C, Gharbiya M. Retinal nerve fibre layer thickness changes in Alzheimer's disease: results from a 12-month prospective case series. Neurosci Lett. 2016;629:165–70.
103. Golzan SM, Goozee K, Georgevsky D, et al. Retinal vascular and structural changes are associated with amyloid burden in the elderly: ophthalmic biomarkers of preclinical Alzheimer's disease. Alzheimers Res Ther. 2017;9:13.
104. Danesh-Meyer H, Birch H, Ku JY, Carroll S, Gamble G. Reduction of optic nerve fibers in patients with Alzheimer disease identified by laser imaging. Neurology. 2006;67:1852–4.
105. Kergoat H, Kergoat MJ, Justino L, Chertkow H, Robillard A, Bergman H. An evaluation of the retinal nerve fiber layer thickness by scanning laser polarimetry in individuals with dementia of the Alzheimer type. Acta Ophthalmol Scand. 2001;79:187–91.
106. Kurna SA, Akar G, Altun A, Agirman Y, Gozke E, Sengor T. Confocal scanning laser tomography of the optic nerve head on the patients with Alzheimer's disease compared to glaucoma and control. Int Ophthalmol. 2014;34:1203–11.
107. Csincsik L, MacGillivray TJ, Flynn E, et al. Peripheral retinal imaging biomarkers for Alzheimer's disease: a pilot study. Ophthalmic Res. 2018;59:182–92.
108. Snyder PJ, Johnson LN, Lim YY, Santos CY, Alber J, Maruff P, Fernández B. Nonvascular retinal imaging markers of preclinical Alzheimer's disease. Alzheimer's Dement Diagnosis Assess Dis Monit. 2016;4:169–78.
109. Santos CY, Johnson LN, Sinoff SE, Festa EK, Heindel WC, Snyder PJ. Change in retinal structural anatomy during the preclinical stage of Alzheimer's disease. Alzheimer's Dement Diagnosis Assess Dis Monit. 2018;10:196–209.
110. Moreno-Ramos T, Benito-León J, Villarejo A. Bermejo-Pareja F Retinal nerve fiber layer thinning in dementia associated with Parkinson's disease, dementia with Lewy bodies, and Alzheimer's disease. J Alzheimers Dis. 2013;34:659–64.
111. Parisi V, Pierelli F, Coppola G, Restuccia R, Ferrazzoli D, Scassa C, Bianco F, Parisi L, Fattapposta F. Reduction of optic nerve fiber layer thickness in CADASIL. Eur J Neurol. 2007;14:627–31.
112. Li ZB, Lin ZJ, Li N, Yu H, Wu YL, Shen X. Evaluation of retinal and choroidal changes in patients with Alzheimer's type dementia using optical coherence tomography angiography. Int J Ophthalmol. 2021;14:860–8.

113. Lahme L, Esser EL, Mihailovic N, Schubert F, Lauermann J, Johnen A, Eter N, Duning T, Alnawaiseh M. Evaluation of ocular perfusion in Alzheimer's disease using optical coherence tomography angiography. J Alzheimers Dis. 2018;66:1745–52.
114. Wu J, Zhang X, Azhati G, Li T, Xu G, Liu F. Retinal microvascular attenuation in mental cognitive impairment and Alzheimer's disease by optical coherence tomography angiography. Acta Ophthalmol. 2020;98:e781–7.
115. Chua J, Hu Q, Ke M, et al. Retinal microvasculature dysfunction is associated with Alzheimer's disease and mild cognitive impairment. Alzheimers Res Ther. https://doi.org/10.1186/S13195-020-00724-0
116. Querques G, Borrelli E, Sacconi R, De Vitis L, Leocani L, Santangelo R, et al. Functional and morphological changes of the retinal vessels in Alzheimer's disease and mild cognitive impairment. Sci Rep. https://doi.org/10.1038/S41598-018-37271-6
117. Katz B, Rimmer S, Iragui V, Katzman R. Abnormal pattern electroretinogram in Alzheimer's disease: evidence for retinal ganglion cell degeneration? Ann Neurol. 1989;26:221–5.
118. Trick G, Barris MC, Bickler-Bluth M. Abnormal pattern electroretinograms in patients with senile dementia of the Alzheimer type. Ann Neurol. 1989;26:226–31.
119. Krasodomska K, Lubiński W, Potemkowski A, Honczarenko K. Pattern electroretinogram (PERG) and pattern visual evoked potential (PVEP) in the early stages of Alzheimer's disease. Doc Ophthalmol Ophthalmol. 2010;121:111–21.
120. Sartucci F, Borghetti D, Bocci T, Murri L, Orsini P, Porciatti V, Origlia N, Domenici L. Dysfunction of the magnocellular stream in Alzheimer's disease evaluated by pattern electroretinograms and visual evoked potentials. Brain Res Bull. 2010;82:169–76.
121. Strenn K, Dal-Bianco P, Weghaupt H, Koch G, Vass C, Gottlob I. Pattern electroretinogram and luminance electroretinogram in Alzheimer's disease. J Neural Transm. 1991;33:73–80.
122. Kergoat H, Kergoat MJ, Justino L, Chertkow H, Robillard A, Bergman H. Visual retinocortical function in dementia of the Alzheimer type. Gerontology. 2002;48:197–203.
123. Philpot M, Amin D, Levy R. Visual evoked potentials in Alzheimer's disease: correlations with age and severity. Electroencephalogr Clin Neurophysiol. 1990;77:323–9.
124. Justino L, Kergoat M, Bergman H, Chertkow H, Robillard A, Kergoat H. Neuroretinal function is normal in early dementia of the Alzheimer type. Neurobiol Aging. 2001;22:691–5.
125. Pollock V, Schneider LS, Chui HC, Henderson V, Zemansky M, Sloane RB. Visual evoked potentials in dementia: a meta-analysis and empirical study of Alzheimer's disease patients. Biol Psychiatry. 1989;25:1003–13.
126. Partanen J, Hartikainen P, Könönen M, Jousmäki V, Soininen H, Riekkinen P. Prolonged latencies of pattern reversal visual evoked early potentials in Alzheimer disease. Alzheimer Dis Assoc Disord. 1994;8:250–8.
127. Coburn K, Ashford JW, Moreno MA. Visual evoked potentials in dementia: selective delay of flash P2 in probable Alzheimer's disease. J Neuropsychiatry Clin Neurosci. 1991;3:431–5.
128. Moore N, Tucker KA, Jann MW, Hostetler RM, Coburn KL. Flash P2 delay in primary degenerative dementia of the Alzheimer type. Prog Neuropsychopharmacol Biol Psychiatry. 1995;19:403–10.
129. Kromer R, Serbecic N, Hausner L, Froelich L, Beutelspacher S. Comparison of visual evoked potentials and retinal nerve fiber layer thickness in Alzheimer's disease. Front Neurol. 2013;4:203.
130. Kromer R, Serbecic N, Hausner L, Froelich L, Aboul-Enein F, Beutelspacher S. Detection of retinal nerve fiber layer defects in Alzheimer's disease using SD-OCT. Front Psychiatry. 2014,5.22.
131. Choi SH, Park SJ, Kim NR. Macular ganglion cell-inner plexiform layer thickness is associated with clinical progression in mild cognitive impairment and Alzheimers disease. PLoS ONE. 2016;11: e0162202.
132. Shen Y, Shi Z, Jia R, Zhu Y, Cheng Y, Feng W, Li C. The attenuation of retinal nerve fiber layer thickness and cognitive deterioration. Front Cell Neurosci. 2013;7:142.

133. Shen Y, Liu L, Cheng Y, Feng W, Shi Z, Zhu Y, Wu W, Li C. Retinal nerve fiber layer thickness is associated with episodic memory deficit in mild cognitive impairment patients. Curr Alzheimer Res. 2014;11:259–66.
134. Shi Z, Wu Y, Wang M, Cao J, Feng W, Cheng Y, Li C, Shen Y. Greater attenuation of retinal nerve fiber layer thickness in Alzheimer's disease patients. J Alzheimers Dis. 2014;40:277–83.
135. den Haan J, van de Kreeke JA, van Berckel BN, Barkhof F, Teunissen CE, Scheltens P, Verbraak FD, Bouwman FH. Is retinal vasculature a biomarker in amyloid proven Alzheimer's disease? Alzheimer's Dement (Amsterdam, Netherlands). 2019;11:383–91.
136. Yu J, Feng Y, Xiang Y, Huang J, Savini G, Parisi V, Yang W, Fu X. Retinal nerve fiber layer thickness changes in Parkinson disease: a meta-analysis. PLoS ONE. 2014;9:10.
137. Janssen S, Gorgels TG, Ramdas WD, Klaver CC, van D, Jansonius NM, Bergen AA. The vast complexity of primary open angle glaucoma: disease genes, risks, molecular mechanisms and pathobiology. Prog Retin Eye Res. 2013;37:31–67.
138. Ghiso JA, Doudevski I, Ritch R, Rostagno AA. Alzheimer's disease and glaucoma: mechanistic similarities and differences. J Glaucoma. 2013;22(Suppl 5):S36–8.
139. Tamura H, Kawakami H, Kanamoto T, Kato T, Yokoyama T, Sasaki K, Izumi Y, Matsumoto M, Mishima HK. High frequency of open-angle glaucoma in Japanese patients with Alzheimer's disease. J Neurol Sci. 2006;246:79–83.
140. Ou Y, Grossman DS, Lee PP, Sloan FA. Glaucoma, Alzheimer disease and other dementia: a longitudinal analysis. Ophthalmic Epidemiol. 2012;19:285–92.
141. Nucci C, Martucci A, Cesareo M, Mancino R, Russo R, Bagetta G, Cerulli L, Garaci FG. Brain involvement in glaucoma: advanced neuroimaging for understanding and monitoring a new target for therapy. Curr Opin Pharmacol. 2013;13:128–33.
142. Nucci C, Martucci A, Cesareo M, Garaci F, Morrone LA, Russo R, Corasaniti MT, Bagetta G, Mancino R. Links among glaucoma, neurodegenerative, and vascular diseases of the central nervous system. Prog Brain Res. 2015;221:49–65.
143. Berisha F, Feke GT, Trempe CL, McMeel JW, Schepens CL. Retinal abnormalities in early Alzheimer's disease. Invest Ophthalmol Vis Sci. 2007;48:2285–9.

Optical Coherence Tomography Findings in Rare Syndromic Optic Neuropathies

14

Chiara La Morgia and Michele Carbonelli

Abstract

Optic nerve and retinal involvement are a frequent finding in many neurodegenerative disorders. Optic atrophy can be severe and diffuse or sectorial and can be associated with visual complaints and reduction of visual acuity. We here report the main optical coherence tomography (OCT) findings in rare neurological syndromes for which OCT data are available. In Friedreich's ataxia, which is an autosomal recessive disease, there is evidence of subclinical optic neuropathy. OCT studies describe a diffuse and progressive thinning of the retinal nerve fiber layer (RNFL) thickness with a relative sparing of the papillo-macular bundle. In rare case also the presence of a Leber's hereditary optic Neuropathy (LHON)-like presentation has been reported. DNA (cytosine-5)-methyltransferase 1 (DNMT1) disease is an autosomal dominant multisystem disorder characterized by the association of narcolepsy, deafness, sensory neuropathy and optic atrophy. The presence of subclinical optic atrophy more evident in the temporal quadrant has been reported in both the autosomal dominant cerebellar ataxia, deafness and narcolepsy (ADCA-DN) associated with mutations in exon 21 of the *DNMT1* gene and the hereditary sensory autonomic neuropathy with dementia and hearing loss type IE (HSAN IE) associated with mutations in exon 20 of the *DNMT1* gene. Hereditary spastic paraplegias (HSP) are a heterogeneous group of inherited neurological disorders characterized by spastic paraparesis. RNFL thinning and pigmentary retinopathy are frequent findings in these diseases. We here report ophthalmological findings of SPG7, SPG11 and SPG45-related spastic paraplegia. Cerebral autosomal dominant arteriopathy with subcortical infarcts and leukoencephalopathy (CADASIL) is an autosomal dominant disorder in which retinal vascular changes and neurodegeneration

C. La Morgia (✉) · M. Carbonelli
UOC Clinica Neurologica, IRCCS Istituto delle Scienze Neurologiche di Bologna, Bologna, Italy
e-mail: chiara.lamorgia@unibo.it

Dipartimento di Scienze Biomediche e Neuromotorie, Università di Bologna, Bologna, Italy

A. Grzybowski and P. Barboni (eds.), *OCT and Imaging in Central Nervous System Diseases*, https://doi.org/10.1007/978-3-031-72156-4_14

of the neuroretina are frequent findings. Moreover, OCT-angiography studies demonstrated in CADASIL patients the presence of a reduced retinal vessel density. Wolfram's syndrome is rare genetic condition, typically characterized by the occurrence of diabetes and optic atrophy in childhood. OCT studies demonstrated the presence of a pattern of diffuse and severe optic atrophy, not strictly selective for the temporal fibers of the papillomacular bundle, at difference with mitochondrial optic neuropathies, with a fast deterioration of visual function and structural OCT parameters since early age and with RGC axonal degeneration preceding cellular body atrophy by about a decade, at difference with Dominant Optica Atrophy in which a more stable visual function is evident with predominant early loss of GCL. Autosomal recessive spastic ataxia of Charlevoix-Saguenay (ARSACS) is a hereditary spastic ataxia due to progressive degeneration of the cerebellum and spinal cord, characterized by retinal nerve fiber hypertrophy detected by OCT. Spinocerebellar ataxias (SCAs) are heterogeneous genetically determined disorders for which OCT studies available show variable findings ranging from isolated thinning of the temporal RNFL to retinal photoreceptor abnormalities.

Keywords

Optical coherence tomography • Optic nerve • Retina • Macula • Fundus • Friedreich's ataxia • DNMT1 • SPG • Cadasil • Wolfram syndrome • Autosomal recessive spastic ataxia of Charlevoix-Saguenay • Spinocerebellar ataxias

14.1 Friedreich's Ataxia

Friedreich's ataxia (FA) is an autosomal recessive slowly progressive neurodegenerative disorder starting usually in young adulthood or childhood [1]. FA is characterized by spinocerebellar and sensory ataxia with absence of deep tendon reflexes, dysarthria, hypertrophic cardiomyopathy and scoliosis [2]. FA is due to a GAA triplet expansion in the first intron of the frataxin gene (FXN) on chromosome 9q13-q21.1. A minority of FRDA patients are compound heterozygotes for the GAA triplet expansion and a point mutation [3].

Frataxin is a mitochondrial protein with a crucial role in the insertion of Fe-S cluster in different enzymes of the mitochondrial respiratory chain and in particular complex I, II and III and aconitase [4, 5]. The abnormal function of FXN leads to dysregulation of cellular iron metabolism with mitochondrial accumulation [6]. Evidence of mitochondrial defective respiration has been demonstrated in the heart and muscle of FA patients [7, 8]. Recent studies demonstrated that mitochondrial dysfunction induced by frataxin is also related to abnormal calcium handling in the mitochondria leading to increased autophagy [9]. Overall, frataxin deficiency leads to abnormal iron homeostasis [10] and increased oxidative stress [11, 12].

Visual system involvement is well characterized in FA [13, 14]. In particular, abnormalities of the visual efferent system such as fixation instability (square wave jerks), saccadic dysmetria, disrupted pursuit, and vestibular abnormalities have been reported [13]. Moreover, optic neuropathy, optic radiation abnormalities and retinitis pigmentosa have been described in FA patients [14–20].

The optic neuropathy described in FA is usually asymptomatic and does not affect central vision [16]. The most severe visual phenotype has been associated with large GAA expansion of the FTX gene and with compound heterozygous mutations [17]. Visual evoked potentials demonstrated delayed latency and reduced amplitude of the cortical responses [16, 17]. Visual field defects may vary from small paracentral or arcuate to diffuse and generalized defects [17]. Only rarely FA patients present an acute loss of visual acuity, which resembles Leber's hereditary optic neuropathy (LHON) [17].

A few optical coherence tomography (OCT) studies are available for FA. These described a diffuse reduction of the retinal nerve fiber layer (RNFL) thickness without a preferential involvement of the temporal quadrant, [14, 17–21] unlike mitochondrial optic neuropathies [22]. The severity of optic atrophy can be variable and usually is not associated with a subjective visual complaint [16, 17]. Specifically, time-domain OCT studies reported a generalized RNFL thinning in FA patients [17–19]. Interestingly, in the largest OCT series (63 FA patients) available to now, the only sector with a significant RNFL thinning was the superior [19] (Table 14.1).

Retinal nerve fiber layer thinning significantly correlated with age at onset and International Cooperative Ataxia Rating Scale (ICARS) in the series (n = 26) by Fortuna and coauthors [17]; with ICARS score, disease duration, visual acuity (VA) and low-contrast letter VA in the series (n = 23) by Noval and coauthors [18] and with VA, GAA repeat length, Friedreich's Ataxia Rating Scale (FARS) and age at onset in the series (n = 63) by Seyer and coauthors [19] (Table 14.1).

Similarly, spectral domain OCT studies documented a generalized RNFL thinning in FA patients with a relative sparing of the temporal sector [14, 20, 21], as well as of the ganglion cell layer which was more pronounced in the superior and inferior macula [20] (Table 14.1). Furthermore, a recent longitudinal study using swept-source OCT, evaluating the presence of OCT measurement changes over time, demonstrated the presence of a progressive RNFL thinning which was correlated with disease severity and visual acuity, again supporting the concept of an ongoing and progressive neurodegeneration [21].

Interestingly, in a recent study evaluating the entire visual pathway in 62 genetically-confirmed FA patients, a significant correlation between the RNFL thinning and frataxin levels was reported. This result points to the possibility of using OCT findings as potential biomarker for future clinical trials, especially gene therapy trials aimed at increasing the frataxin levels [14]. Moreover, in this report the authors reported that again the superior and inferior sectors are those most severely affected with a relative sparing oh the temporal sector and papillo-macular bundle (PMB) [14].

Table 14.1 OCT findings and clinical correlates in Friedreich ataxia

	OCT	No. of pts	Main findings	Correlations
Fortuna et al. [17]	TD-Stratus	26	↓avg RNFL ↓RNFL in all 4 sectors	ICARS, age at onset
Noval et al. [18]	TD-Stratus	17	↓avg RNFL in 75% Temporal RNFL thickness normal Normal Macular morphology and thickness	ICARS, disease duration, VA, low-contrast VA
Seyer et al. [19]	TD-Stratus	63	↓RNFL (52.7% of eyes below 5th percentile of controls) Only superior thickness significantly lower	VA, GAA expansion, age at onset, FARS
Seyer et al. [19]	SD-Cirrus	23	Macular thickness below the 1st percentile of controls in 20.7%	Not significant
Dağ et al. [20]	SD	10	↓avg RNFL ↓RNFL in all 4 quadrants ↓Peripapillary and foveal retinal thickness Choroidal thickness not significant ↓GCL thickness in superior and inferior macula	VA, ICARS (RNFL thickness) Disease duration (foveal thickness)
Bogdanova-Mihaylova et al. [21]	Swept-source	48	↓RNFL more pronounced in the superior sector of the optic nerve Decline of RNFL over time	Significant correlation between disease severity, visual acuity and OCT measurements
Thomas-Black et al. [14]	SD	62	↓RNFL more pronounced in the superior and inferior sectors ↓GCL and IPL thickness	Significant correlation between the RNFL thinning and frataxin levels

Legend OCT = Optical Coherence Tomography; TD = Temporal Domain; SD = Spectral Domain; RNFL = retinal nerve fiber layer; avg = average; ICARS = International Cooperative Ataxia Rating Scale; FARS = Friedreich's Ataxia Rating Scale; VA = visual acuity

Macular thickness has been reported as normal in one study [18], significantly reduced [20] and below the 1st percentile of controls in 20.7% of the FA patients examined in another series [19] (Table 14.1).

Correlation of OCT measurement with VA is not consistent across the studies and the degree of VA loss is reported as variable, but usually not clinically significant [17, 18]. Differently, low contrast visual acuity is significantly reduced in FA patients [18]. Fundus oculi abnormalities are detected only in a variable percentage of the FA subjects with loss of retinal nerve fibers documented by OCT [18, 21].

Overall, OCT measurements in FA are able to detect subclinical optic neuropathy in the large majority of FA cases (about 70%) being a more sensible measure of optic nerve degeneration than other metrics (visual acuity, visual fields and/or fundus examination). It is not clear yet why the PMB is not primarily affected in FA, even if a mitochondrial dysfunction is well known in FA.

In line with OCT data, visual evoked potentials (VEPs) documented an increased P100 latency and reduced amplitude of cortical responses [16, 17] in the large majority of patients. These electrophysiological and anatomical data suggest a slowly progressive degeneration of the anterior and posterior optic pathway, as proved also by the increased diffusion in optic radiations demonstrated in FA patients by magnetic resonance imaging studies [17].

Examples of swept-source (Triton, Topcon) OCT images and fundus oculi pictures are provided for two FA patients presenting different degrees of optic atrophy (Fig. 14.1).

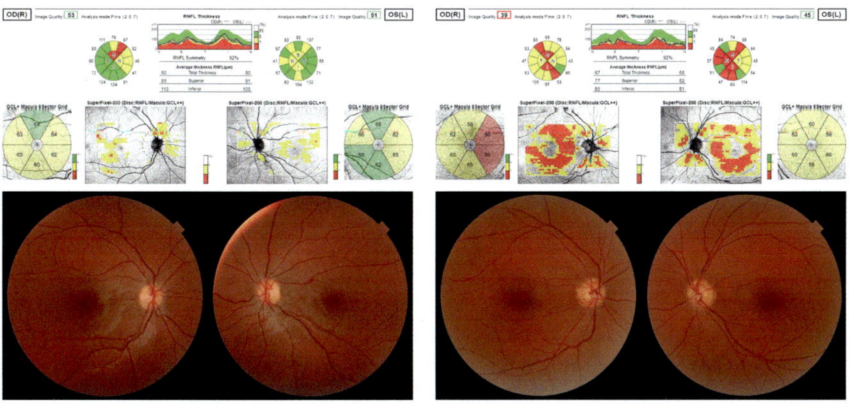

Fig. 14.1 **OCT findings in Friedreich's ataxia**. On the left (**a**) OCT and fundus images are shown for a 24 year female patient (disease onset with ataxia at 15 years). Visual acuity is 12/10 bilaterally. OCT shows a mild superior RNFL thinning and a small GCC defect. Fundus oculi showed mild temporal pallor bilaterally. On the right (**b**) OCT and fundus images are shown for a 42 year-old male patient (disease onset at 16 years of age). Visual acuity is 10/10 bilaterally. OCT shows generalized mild RNFL thinning; GCL analysis reveals a mild defect relatively relatively sparing the PMB

14.2 DNMT1 Disease

DNA (cytosine-5)-methyltransferase 1 (DNMT1) disease is a complex neurodegenerative disorder due to autosomal dominant mutations in the *DNMT1* gene (DNA-methyltransferase 1) [23].

Two distinct phenotypes have been described in association with mutations in the *DNMT1* gene: the autosomal dominant cerebellar ataxia, deafness and narcolepsy (ADCA-DN) [24] associated with mutations in exon 21 of the *DNMT1* gene and the hereditary sensory autonomic neuropathy with dementia and hearing loss type IE (HSAN IE), described in association with mutations in exon 20 [23]. Our group demonstrated that the boundaries between these two distinct entities are less pronounced [25]. In fact, both diseases share the presence of narcolepsy as a prominent feature [25]. Moreover, we demonstrated that subclinical optic atrophy is a common finding to both phenotypes [25]. Visual acuity was normal in all five DNMT1 patients included in the study (two with the ADCA-DN and three with the HSAN IE phenotype). Fundus oculi disclosed temporal pallor in one ADCA-DN case, diffuse pallor in the other ADCA-DN and mild temporal pallor of the optic disc in all three HSAN IE subjects. Pattern VEPs were abnormal in both ADCA-DN probands, showing increased latency and decreased amplitude of cortical responses, whereas they were normal in HSAN IE patients [25]. OCT showed RNFL thinning more evident in the temporal than in the superior and inferior quadrants with nasal sparing in one ADCA-DN patient, more diffuse in the other ADCA-DN patient with nasal sparing. In the HSAN IE cases OCT disclosed a diffuse RNFL thinning in one case, a diffuse thinning with nasal sparing in the second case, and temporal and less evident superior/inferior quadrants thinning in the third case.

Macular ganglion cell layer (GCL) analysis disclosed diffuse atrophy in both ADCA-DN probands and diffuse thinning in all three HSAN IE subjects [25].

Examples of swept-source OCT (RNFL and macular GCL) (Triton, Topcon) and fundus oculi image are reported for two DNMT1 patients carrying respectively the p.Pro507Arg mutation at exon 20 and the c.1709C > T (p.Ala507Val) at exon 21 [25] (Fig. 14.2).

Interestingly, optic atrophy was previously reported in the ADCA-DN phenotype [26, 27] but never described in the HSAN IE phenotype. OCT investigation in our DNMT1 case series revealed a subclinical optic nerve involvement in all cases with a prevalent involvement of the temporal sector and relative nasal sparing that resembles the pattern observed in mitochondrial optic neuropathies [22]. The mitochondrial pattern of optic nerve degeneration may be explained by the possible effect of defective methylation of nuclear DNA on nuclear encoded mitochondrial proteins [28] or a direct effect on DNA methylation of the mitochondrial-targeted isoform of DNMT1 [29, 30]. DNMTs including DNMT1, through epigenetic regulation may play a role in the development and homeostasis of photoreceptors and other retinal neurons within the mammalian retina [31]. Furthermore, the presence of optic atrophy has been reported also in a case with a complex phenotype including epilepsy, cataplexia, REM behavior disorder, developmental regression

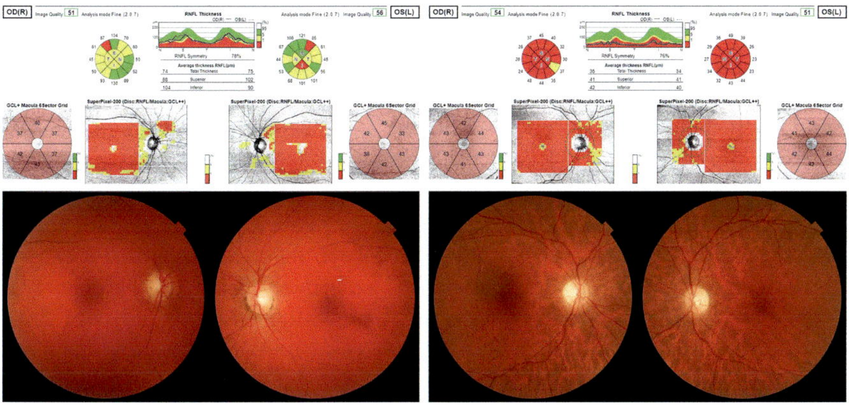

Fig. 14.2 **OCT findings in DNMT1 patients**. On the left OCT and fundus images are shown for a 45 years old female with disease onset at with deafness at 26 years and neuropathy since 30 years of age and ataxia. Visual acuity is 12/10 bilaterally; OCT shows mild generalized RNFL thinning more prominent on the temporal sector with evidence of mild temporal pallor in the LE. A diffuse defect was evident at GCC analysis. Genetic analysis revealed the presence of the p.Pro507Arg mutation in DNMT1 gene. On the right OCT and fundus images are shown for a 48 year-old female with 1st evidence of optic atrophy at 42 years of age and deafness from 45 years. Visual acuity is 6.3/10 bilaterally with generalized severe RNFL thinning and diffuse optic disc pallor at fundus oculi. A diffuse defect was evident at GCC analysis. Genetic analysis revealed the presence of heterozygous c.1709C > T (p.Ala507Val)-exon 20

and myoclonus carrying a novel mutation outside the targeting sequence domain of the *DNMT1* gene at difference with previously reported cases [32].

14.3 Hereditary Spastic Paraplegia

Hereditary spastic paraplegia (HSP) is a group of inherited neurological disorders characterized by progressive spastic weakness of the lower limbs due to degeneration of the corticospinal tracts. HSP are a heterogeneous group of neurodegenerative disorders characterized by a variable phenotypic expression, which includes a pure spastic paraparesis or "uncomplicated" and a "complicated" form. The genetic basis of HSP is heterogeneous including autosomal dominant, autosomal recessive, X-linked, or maternally inherited (mitochondrial) inheritance [33].

More than 56 HSP loci and 41HSP-related genes have been identified [33].

14.3.1 Hereditary Spastic Paraplegia Due to *SPG7* Mutations

Mutations in the *SPG7* gene are responsible for autosomal recessive SPG7-HSP. The first *SPG7* mutation was identified in 1998 [34, 35]. *SPG7* gene encodes for paraplegin, which is a metalloprotease protein belonging to the AAA (ATPase associated with various cellular activities) proteins. Paraplegin is a mitochondrial protein localized to the inner mitochondrial membrane and it assembles with the paralogous AFG3L2 protein in the mAAA protease complex [36–39]. Mitochondrial dysfunction has been described in SPG7 pedigrees including OXPHOS defects in muscle biopsy [34, 35]. Interestingly, mAAA protease like paraplegin plays also a role in the processing of the OPA1 protein [40]. Given the mitochondrial pathogenesis of SPG7 HSP the presence of optic atrophy is expected, but not systematically investigated. Optic atrophy has been reported in the first identified pedigrees [34, 35, 39]. Klebe and coauthors extensively described the phenotype of 23 SPG7 families. In a subgroup (n = 10) investigated by OCT, RNFL thinning was detected in 100% of cases even if it was symptomatic only in one case, associated with reduced visual acuity in 40% and with optic disc pallor at fundus examination in 50% of cases. These data suggest that the OCT investigation may detect subtle abnormalities in SPG7 patients and the presence of optic atrophy in the context of an autosomal recessive spastic paraplegia should point to the *SPG7* gene. In this case series one French pedigree positive for the SPG7 mutation presented with an isolated autosomal dominant early onset (1st decade of life) progressive optic atrophy. Electroneurography disclosed in this pedigree also the presence of mixed peripheral polyneuropathy [41].

On the basis of the clinical findings of this cohort the authors proposed that *SPG7* gene should be screened in autosomal recessive or sporadic HSP patients with middle-age onset particularly if spastic paraplegia is associated with cerebellar atrophy/signs and/or optic neuropathy (also if detected only with OCT).

Van Gassen and coauthors, in another large SPG7 Dutch case-series (n = 49), demonstrated the presence of a severe optic atrophy with childhood onset in two siblings carrying a homozygous missense mutation (p.Arg470Gln, exon 10) *SPG7* mutation and in one case with compound heterozygous (p.Arg485_Glu487 and p.Leu706fs) *SPG7* mutation. For one of the p.Arg470Gln mutation carriers, postmortem tissues including the optic nerve were available. In this case a severe optic atrophy was documented. Interestingly, the p.Arg470Gln mutation was located in the ATPase AAA core domain and the authors hypothesized that the severe optic nerve involvement can be explained by a possible deleterious interaction of SPG7 with OPA1. Unfortunately, for these patients OCT data were not available [42].

Moreover, Marcotulli and coauthors have described a 43-year-old male SPG7 case presenting with severe congenital optic atrophy. This patient developed spastic paraparesis at 30 years of age. OCT documented reduced RNFL and macular thickness [43].

Overall, these data suggest that optic neuropathy is a common finding in SPG7-related HSP and the use of OCT screening in large cohort of HSP patients might be a useful tool to reveal subclinical optic atrophy and guide the diagnostic process.

In this context, Wiethoff and coauthors conducted an OCT study on 28 HSP patients including "pure" (n = 22) and "complicated" (n = 6) HSP demonstrating a significant RNFL thinning only in the "complicated" group. The case series included also 3 SPG7 cases and two of them, presenting a complicated phenotype, manifested a global RNFL thinning, especially in the temporal quadrant [44].

We had the opportunity to diagnose the presence of compound heterozygous *SPG7* mutations in a 24 year-old female who presented ophthalmological features (Fig. 14.3) indistinguishable from *OPA1* patients. Neurological examination was unremarkable except for the presence of optic nerve temporal pallor and specifically did not reveal any sign of spastic paraparesis. This case highlights the possibility that SPG7 mutations might be associated with pure optic atrophy cases.

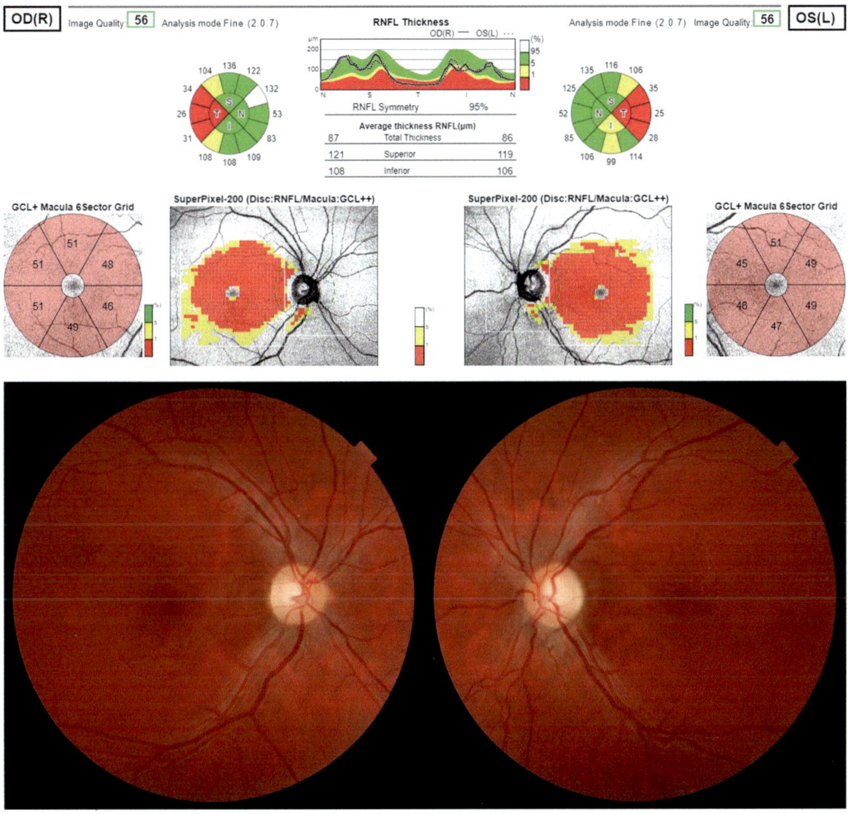

Fig. 14.3 OCT findings in a SPG7 patient. Ophtalmological findings in a 24-year-old female carrying compound heterozygous mutations—c.524 T > C (p.LI75P) + c1968_69 ins A (p.165NfsX22) in the *SPG7* gene. Visual acuity is 0.63. Fundus oculi reveals bilateral temporal optic nerve pallor. OCT (Triton, Topcon) demonstrates a temporal RNFL thinning bilaterally. Brain MRI, somatosensory and motor evoked potentials were normal. Neurological examination excluded the presence of pyramidal signs and spastic paraparesis

14.3.2 Hereditary Spastic Paraplegia Due to *SPG11* Mutations (SPG11)

SPG11-associated spastic paraplegia is a rare disease accounting for 19–31% of autosomal recessive HSP [45]. SPG11 is characterized by progressive spasticity and weakness of the lower limbs, frequently associated with mild intellectual disability and/or progressive cognitive decline, peripheral neuropathy, pseudobulbar involvement, and increased reflexes in the upper limbs.

Less frequent findings include: cerebellar signs, retinal degeneration (Kjellin's syndrome), clubfoot, scoliosis and parkinsonism with thinning of the corpus callosum. Onset occurs mainly during infancy or adolescence (range: age 1–30 years) [46].

SPG11 encodes spatacsin, a protein that interacts with the SPG15 and SPG48 protein products [47] and is an accessory protein of the adaptor protein 5 complex [48]. It is involved in the regulation of vesicle endocytosis and intracellular trafficking [49]. The loss of spatacsin function is associated with reduced clearance of lipids from lysosomes with accumulation of gangliosides and cholesterol on membranes and consequently calcium homeostasis alteration [50].

Patients may exhibit, during the course of the disease, a pigmentary retinopathy (classically described as part of Kjellin syndrome) with a clinical manifestation ranging from a mild dark adaptation defect and/or color vision loss, up to the loss of central vision [51].

Here, we report ophthalmological including OCT findings of two patients carrying biallelic mutations in the *SPG11* gene, showing variable degrees of retinopathy (Figs. 14.4 and 14.5).

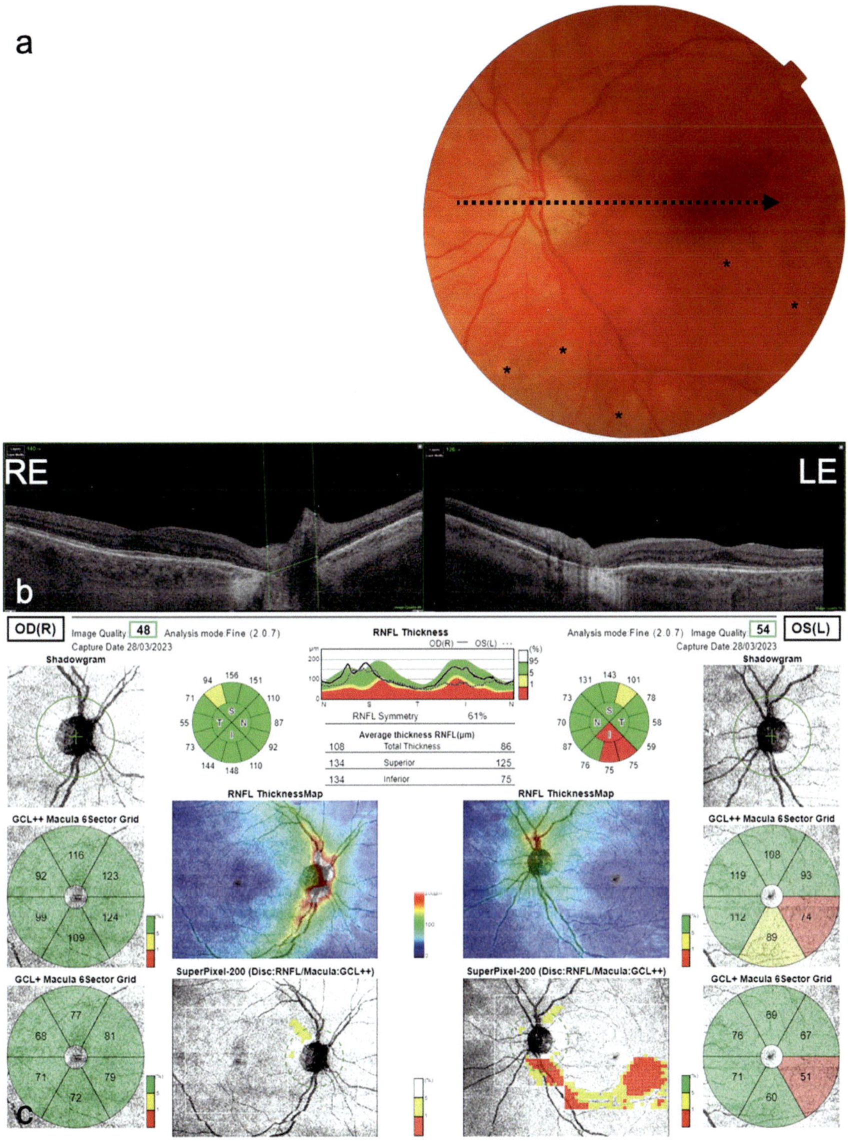

Fig. 14.4 **OCT findings in SPG11 patient**. Ophtalmological findings in a 61-years old man with visual acuity (VA) of 20/20 in his right eye and 20/32 in his left eye, low grade of bilateral cataract, normal IOP and some pale-yellow demarcated spots in the posterior pole with macular pigmentary anomalies (best visualized in the left eye) (a). The OCT scans through the fovea, reveal irregularities of the retinal pigment epithelium (RPE)/Bruch complex with discontinuance of the ellipsoid zone (EZ) and preservation of the external limiting membrane (ELM) (b). RNFL and GCC analyses show an inferior arciform RNFL defect in the left eye, consistent with a misunderstood glaucomatous damage (c)

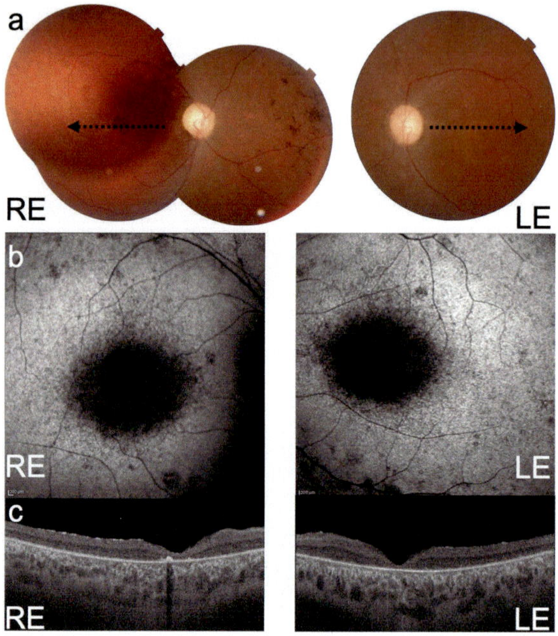

Fig. 14.5 **OCT findings in SPG11 patient**. A 28-years patient with bilateral VA counting fingers and ophthalmoscopically a bilateral pallid optic nerve, attenuated blood vessels, and peripheric bone spicule pigmentation (visible in this figure only in the right eye) (a). The fundus photograph shows a maculopathy with central RPE hyperplasia in the right eye and a pale-yellow maculopathy with superficial wrinkles in the left eye (a). OCT line scans through the macula reveal the almost total preservation of the inner retina (i.e. nerve fiber layer, ganglion cell layer, inner plexiform and inner nuclear layer) and the thinning of the outer retina (c). Furthermore, it is evident the disappearance of the EZ and the ELM all along the line scan and the complete atrophy of the RPE/Bruch complex and the outer nuclear layer in the foveal region (c). The fundus autofluorescence (FAF) imaging reveal a background hyperfluorescence with patchy areas of decreased FAF and central hypofluorescence, corresponding to RPE atrophy (b)

14.3.3 Hereditary Spastic Paraplegia Due to *NT5C2* Mutations (SPG45)

SPG45-spastic paraplegia is a form of spastic paraplegia characterized by a slow, gradual, progressive weakness and spasticity of the lower limbs. Rate of progression and the severity of symptoms are quite variable. Initial symptoms may include difficulty with balance, weakness and stiffness in the legs, muscle spasms, and spastic paraparesis. In some patients, bladder symptoms (such as incontinence) may appear, and spasticity may affect also upper limbs. Some SPG45 patients manifest intellectual disability, contractures, learning disability and thinning of the corpus callosum [52].

SPG45 is caused by homozygous mutation in the *NT5C2* gene on chromosome 10q24. This gene (part of nucleotide metabolism related genes) encodes a hydrolase that serves to maintain the normal balance of purines' pool in the brain, which seems to play a pivotal role in the normal development of central white matter structures [53].

A few case reports of SPG45 families (18 affected individuals of 7 pedigrees) have been published in literature and only sporadic ophthalmologic signs are reported such as strabismus, optic atrophy [54] and pendular nystagmus [52].

Here, we report the OCT findings of a 66-year-old male patient affected by SPG45 with unremarkable ophthalmologic findings except for the presence of macular RPE abnormalities most prominent in the left eye, and a mild cataract in right eye (Fig. 14.6). Ophthalmoscopically, the patient showed a spotted yellow-appearing change of the macula with RPE mottling and a normal appearance of

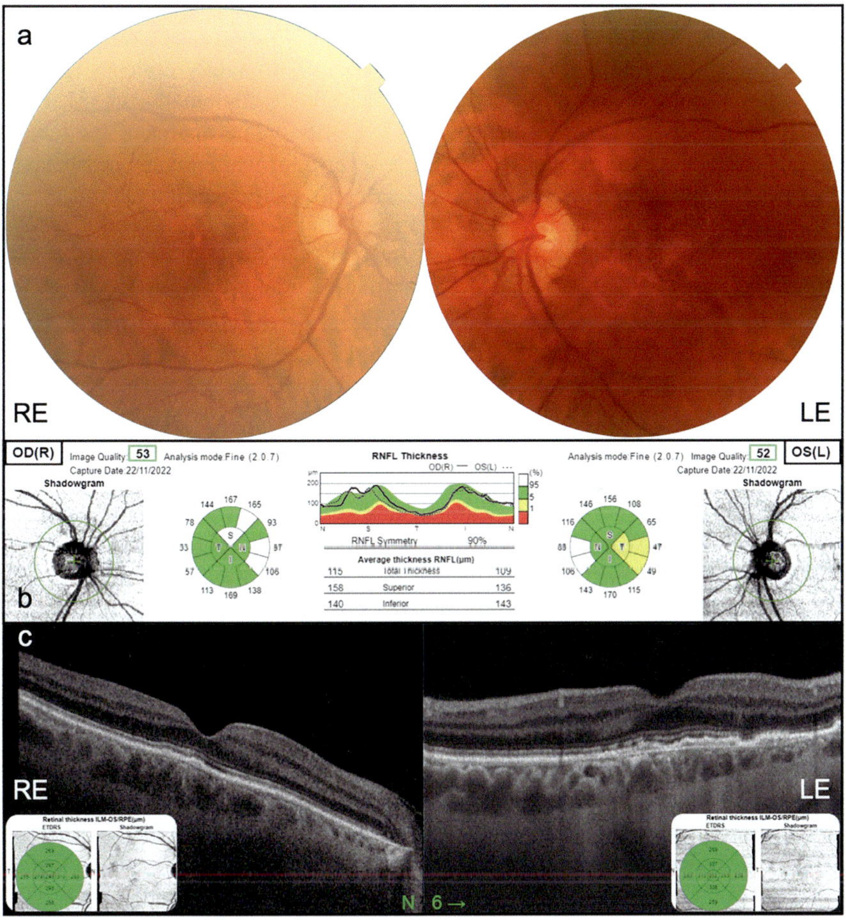

Fig. 14.6 OCT findings in SPG45 patient. Ophthalmological findings in a 66-years male patient carrying homozygous mutation in the NT5C2 gene on chromosome 10q24 for SPG45 disease. The Fundus photographs show a spotted yellow-appearing change of the macula with RPE mottling and a normal appearance of the optic disk bilaterally (a). OCT revealed normal thickness of both the peripapillary RNFL and the macula (b–c) and only the linear scan detect RPE/Bruch complex irregularities with drusenoid deposits in both eyes and some EZ discontinuities only in the left eye (c)

the optic disk bilaterally. OCT revealed normal thickness of both the peripapillary RNFL and the macula and only the linear scan detected RPE/Bruch complex irregularities with drusenoid deposits in both eyes and some EZ discontinuities in the left eye.

Overall, these data support the use of OCT in the diagnostic framework of HSP patients and in the follow-up of patients to establish the monitor the progression of the disease.

14.4 CADASIL

Cerebral autosomal dominant arteriopathy with subcortical infarcts and leukoencephalopathy (CADASIL) is an autosomal dominant disorder characterized by the occurrence of juvenile subcortical ischemic events, migraine, epilepsy, psychiatric disturbances and cognitive impairment in variable combinations [55]. Brain MRI typically shows T2 hyperintensity involving the white matter of the temporal pole and/or the external capsulae, but the severity of white matter involvement can be highly variable evolving into most cases to a diffuse bilateral subcortical leukoencephalopathy [56].

CADASIL is due to mutations of the *NOTCH3 (Neurogenic locus notch homolog protein 3)* gene, located on chromosome 19 [57]. Notch3 is a protein mainly expressed in vascular smooth cells with a crucial role in the control of vascular tone [58]. Cerebral vasculopathy is the main hallmark of the disease, due to the degeneration of the vascular smooth muscle cells with deposition of granular osmiophilic material, but also retinal vascular changes have been described in CADASIL [59–61]. These changes include retinal arteriolar narrowing, arteriovenous nicking and arteriolar sheating [60, 62]. Moreover, electrophysiological [63], histological [64] and OCT studies [62, 65, 66] documented a specific neurodegeneration of the neuroretina in CADASIL. In particular, Parisi and coauthors demonstrated by time-domain OCT a diffuse reduction of the RNFL thickness involving all the quadrants in 6 CADASIL patients (three asymptomatic mutation carriers) [65]. The authors interpreted these findings as secondary to the chronic vascular changes characterizing the disease. Similarly, Rufa and coauthors demonstrated with time-domain OCT a diffuse RNFL thinning in all optic nerve quadrants except the nasal one in 17 CADASIL patients. In particular, this thinning was more evident in the superior sector [66]. Furthermore, fundus oculi examination revealed neuroretinal rim pallor in 41% and a crowded optic disc in 18% of the 34 CADASIL patients described by Pretegiani and coauthors. The optic nerve involvement in CADASIL is also confirmed by histological findings in a postmortem study, which demonstrated diffuse demyelination in the optic nerve and chiasm with loss of nerve fibers [64]. The loss of fibers in the optic nerve is usually not associated with a reduction of the visual acuity and can be associated with variable visual field defects [62].

OCT studies are also particularly relevant for highlighting the vascular component of retinal changes in CADASIL patients. In particular, OCT-angiography (OCT-A) studies demonstrated reduced vessel density in the deep retinal plexus

(DRP) of CADASIL patients [67]. These abnormalities may reflect pericyte dysfunction in retinal capillaries secondary to NOTCH3 mutations and hypoperfusion in the DRP may cause nutritional deficiency in the synaptic connections of the retinal elements. In this case series choroidal vessels are affected in CADASIL patients [67]. These results are in line with previous OCT studies demonstrating increased wall thicknesses and outer diameters of arterial and venous retinal vessels [68]. Interestingly, retinal vessel changes may be correlated to brain MRI findings, highlighting the possible role of retinal changes as biomarker of the disease [69]. These results pointing to a reduced retinal vessel density in CADASIL are a confirmation of previous studies demonstrating by fractal analysis a reduced retinal vessel branching in CADASIL [70]. Furthermore, more recent OCT-A studies further support the presence of retinal vessel abnormalities in CADASIL. Specifically, Krivosic and colleagues, reported in case series of 104 CADASIL patients, the presence of an early and significant reduction of VD related to age in the superficial and deep vascular plexus of the whole foveal or parafoveal retinal area. These findings were not correlated with the severity of clinical or imaging findings in these patients [71]. Differently, Lin and colleagues evaluated by OCT-A 35 patients with CADASIL demonstrating no significant difference compared to controls in terms of vessel density, but they found that the vessel density in the superficial retinal plexus in the macula and the inner retinal thickness was significantly lower in the CADASIL patients presenting with stroke than in the group without stroke [72].

14.5 Wolfram Syndrome

Wolfram syndrome (WS) was first described in 1938 [73]. It is a rare neurodegenerative disorder characterized by the occurrence of diabetes mellitus and optic atrophy starting in childhood and a variable association of diabetes insipidus, other endocrinopathies, deafness, cerebellar ataxia, neurogenic bladder, cardiomyopathy and psychiatric disturbances [74]. In fact, it is also known as DIDMOAD (Diabetes Insipidus, Diabetes Mellitus, Optic Atrophy) [75, 76]. Usually diabetes is the first sign of the disease. Optic atrophy appears in the first–second decade of life and it is in most cases severe [75, 77]. Wolfram's disease is due to mutations in the wolframin gene (*WFS1*) [78] and in the large majority of cases is inherited in an autosomal recessive fashion, but autosomal dominant inheritance has also been reported [78]. In these latter cases optic atrophy can be milder [79] and can be associated with deafness without diabetes [80]. Autosomal dominant mutations in the *WFS1* gene have been associated also with non-syndromic deafness [81], diabetes [82] and cataract [83]. Neuropathological studies reported atrophy of the optic nerve, chiasm, lateral geniculate nucleus, optic tracts and occipital cortex in WS [84–88].

A few OCT studies are available for WS. In a case report [89], spectral domain OCT documented a diffuse optic atrophy more evident in the superior and inferior quadrants in a 21 year-old male. Bucca and coauthors reported OCT time-domain findings in a 13 year-old female showing loss of retinal nerve fibers in the temporal quadrant [90]. More recently, Grenier and coauthors reported OCT findings in a case series of 15 WS cases carrying both autosomal recessive-ar (11 cases, 8 with diabetes and 3 without diabetes) and 4 autosomal dominant-ad *WFS1* mutations with hearing loss. Using SD-OCT, the authors showed that RNFL loss was more profound in the group with syndromic ar-WS compared to the WS cases without diabetes, especially in the inferior sectors. The comparison of ar-WS cases with ad-WS cases by time-domain OCT revealed a more severe RNFL thinning in the ar-WS group in both the superior and inferior quadrants [91].

In a pediatric case series of 12 genetically confirmed WS cases, the authors reported a significant reduction in the WS cases compared with individual with type 1 diabetes and controls of OCT parameters (including average and single quadrants RNFL thickness, macular full-thickness and macular ganglion cell layer/inner plexiform layer) especially in the superior and inferior sectors and brain MRI visual pathway measurements (intraorbital and intracranial thickness of the optical nerve, as well as the optic chiasm and visual tracts). Interestingly, in this case series some optic nerve parameters measured by MRI such as the thickness of the intraorbital parts of the optic nerves in WS cases correlated with superior RNFL thickness of the optic nerve evaluated by OCT [92].

Another interesting OCT finding in 8 ad-WS cases compared to 6 ar-WS cases is the presence of an abnormal reflectivity (lamination) of the outer plexiform layer, which may be related to the high wolframin expression in the retinal Müller cells [93].

Moreover, OCT parameters can be used as a marker of disease progression, as showed by a recent paper evaluating OCT changes over time in a group of 12 WS cases compared to type 1 diabetes patients. In this paper the WS cases were re-evaluated after a follow-up period of about 2 years and OCT measurements, including total thickness of the RNFL, average retinal thickness and total retinal volume, significantly decreased compared to the baseline investigation [94].

Interestingly, a postmortem study documented a specific pattern of optic atrophy predominantly involving the temporal and inferior quadrants, i.e. the papillomacular bundle of the optic nerve, in a WS case. This pattern resembles that described in mitochondrial optic neuropathies [88].

Furthermore, we reported OCT (time-domain and spectral-domain) findings in a cohort of 13 ar WS cases compared to a cohort of OPA1-DOA patients (n = 16) and controls (n = 70) demonstrating a diffuse and severe RNFL thinning in all cases examined. Average RNFL was thinner in both DOA and WS compared to controls and was lower in WS compared to DOA, at difference of visual acuity (VA), which was not significantly different between DOA and WS. Moreover, looking at the single quadrants, a significant difference between WS and DOA was evident for all quadrants, except for temporal and nasal quadrants. Analysis of ganglion cell layer (GCL) thickness in a subgroup of patients (n = 6) showed a significant reduction in both WS and DOA compared to controls for all nine sectors, whereas the difference between WS and DOA was not significant for all sectors [95]. Overall, these results suggest that in WS there is a pattern of more diffuse and severe optic atrophy, not strictly selective for the temporal fibers of the papillomacular bundle, which is instead typical for DOA suggesting that in WS the mitochondrial dysfunction is not primary.

These results are further reinforced by our recent findings demonstrating that the pattern of RGC loss in WS is distinct from DOA [96]. In fact, we demonstrated in a cohort of 25 ar WS patients and 33 age-matched *OPA1*-DOA cases, that VA, MD, and RNFL thickness loss were worse in WS with a faster decline since early age as compared with DOA, who displayed a more stable visual function over the years. Conversely, GCL sectors were overall thinner in patients with DOA since early age compared to patients with WS, in which GCL thickness started to decline later in life. Interestingly, the analysis of brain MRI in 11 WS patients revealed the presence of a bilateral thinning of the anterior optic pathway, especially of the prechiasmatic optic nerves and optic tracts which significantly correlated with GCL but not with RNFL parameters [96]. Overall, these findings support the presence of a generally more severe and diffuse degeneration of both anterior and posterior visual pathways in patients with WS, with fast deterioration of visual function and structural OCT parameters since early age and that the RGC axonal degeneration precedes cellular body atrophy by about a decade, at difference with DOA in which a more stable visual function is evident with predominant early loss of GCL. These findings again point to a lack of a primary mitochondrial dysfunction in patients with WS, as previously suggested [95, 96].

More recently, O'Bryhim and colleagues reported the long-term (mean follow-up of 6.44 years) ophthalmological findings in a cohort of 38 WS patients (3 with autosomal dominant mutations) including rates of visual decline, macular thinning, RNFL thinning, and outer plexiform layer (OPL) lamination. They found that visual acuity declined over time in all participants, with a mean slope of 0.059 logMAR/year, which was more rapid in 25% of cases. RNFL thickness decreased in superior, inferior, and nasal quadrants ($\beta = -0.5$ μm/y, -0.98 μm/y, -0.28 μm/y, respectively). Finally, these authors documented the presence of OPL lamination in 3 patients, 2 of whom had autosomal dominant mutations [97].

We here show the OCT findings of two WS patients (Fig. 14.7). A brief summary of their clinical history is reported below and ophthalmological findings are illustrated in Fig. 14.7 legend.

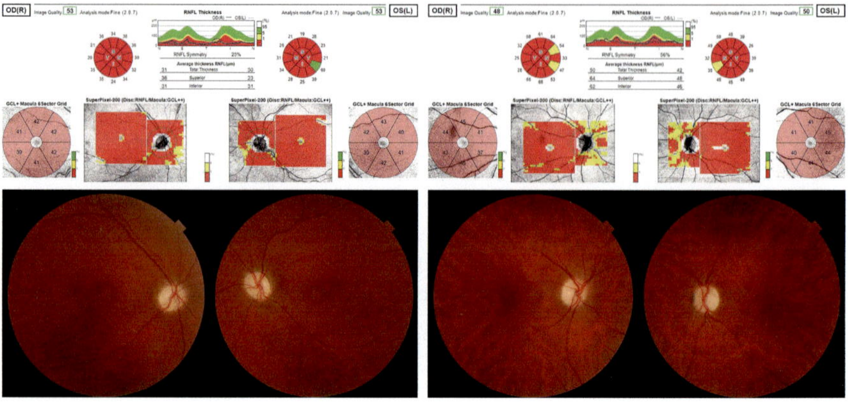

Fig. 14.7 **OCT findings in Wolfram's disease**. On the left OCT and fundus images are shown for a 32-year-old female (mozygous for the c.1620_1622delGTG deletion in *WFS1* gene). She presented, since 21 years of age, optic atrophy and diabetes. Visual acuity is 6.3/100 in OD and CF at 30 cm in OS. OCT shows severe optic atrophy with generalized GCC damage. Fundus oculi examination revealed a diffuse optic nerve pallor. On the right OCT and fundus images are shown for a 29 year-old female (compound heterozygous 1381A > C + 2099G > A in *WFS1* gene). She had diabetes from 6 years of age, deafness from 17 years. Optic atrophy was recognized at 20 years. Visual acuity is 5/10 in OD and 3.2/10 in OS. OCT shows severe optic atrophy with generalized GCC damage. Fundus examination showed diffuse optic nerve pallor

14.6 Autosomal Recessive Spastic Ataxia of Charlevoix-Saguenay (ARSACS)

Autosomal recessive spastic ataxia of Charlevoix-Saguenay (ARSACS) is a complex hereditary neurodegenerative disorder characterized by early childhood-onset cerebellar ataxia [98], peripheral neuropathy [99] and pyramidal tract signs [100, 101].

The name of the disease derives from its high prevalence in the French-Canadian population of the Charlevoix-Saguenay region in the northeast of Quebec, as a result of a founder effect. After these initial reports ARSACS was also described in other countries and ethnic groups worldwide [102, 103].

ARSACS is due to mutations in the *SACS* gene, which were first identified by Engert and coauthors in 2000, and more than 200 different mutations have now been described [104]. The *SACS* gene is located on chromosome 13q12.12 and encodes the protein sacsin with a chaperone activity [105–107]. Sacsin is required for normal mitochondrial dynamics, and loss of function of this protein can result in an altered balance between mitochondrial fusion and fission [108]. Furthermore, a recent study on a sacsin-knockout mouse model described a disruption of mitochondrial fission/fusion dynamics [108].

The majority of ARSACS patients show early ocular signs including the alteration of smooth ocular pursuit (horizontal gaze-evoked nystagmus) and the presence of prominent myelinated fibers radiating from the optic disc. These myelinated fibers are visible ophthalmoscopically and were considered the main clinical manifestations of ARSACS. However, there is phenotypic variability, and the presence of myelinated fibers was rarely described in non-Quebec patients [109–116].

In the original characterization of ARSACS the authors described yellow streaks of hypermyelinated fibers that focally embed the retinal vessels, emanating radially from the edges of the optic disc [102]. In recent years, with the advent of new and more sophisticated quantitative retinal imaging technologies, the nature of the myelinated fibers in ARSACS has been debated.

In 2011, different OCT studies demonstrated that the typical ophthalmoscopic appearance in ARSACS patients is due to the increased hyper-reflectivity and thickness of the peripapillar RNFL and not to the presence of myelinated fibers [117–119]. Vingolo and coauthors [117] showed that the absence of shadowing behind the fibers in the OCT of ARSACS patients differentiates them from subjects with persistent myelinated fibers. In the latter, in fact, OCT clearly revealed a posterior shadowing, due to the hyper-reflectivity and consequent "shield-effect" of the myelinated areas, which does not allow the OCT infrared laser to enter into the retina (Fig. 14.8).

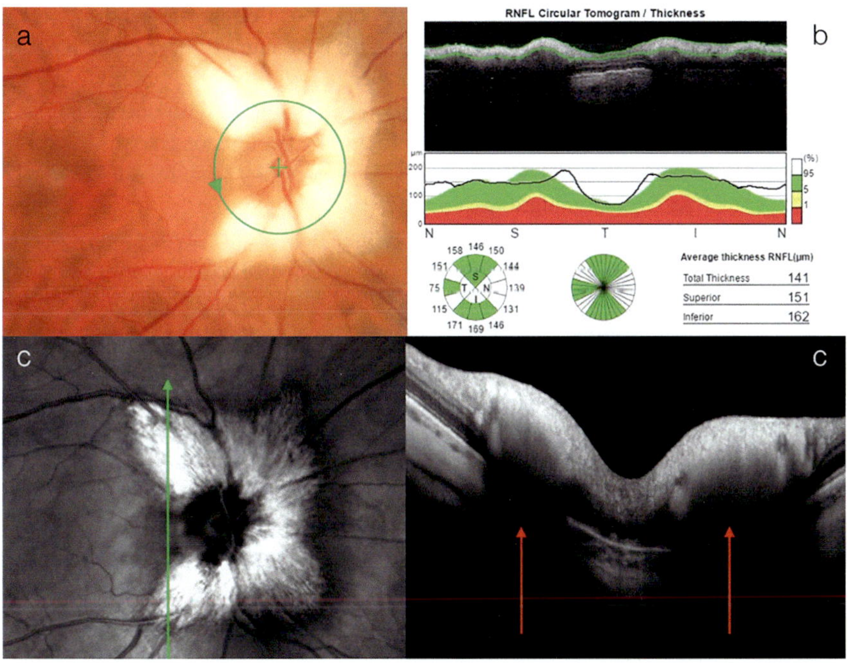

Fig. 14.8 **OCT findings in persistent myelinated fibers**. a) Fundus photography of peripapillary myelinated fibers. b, c) Thickening of the peripapillar retinal fibers hiding the deep layers of retina (red arrow)

The thickening of the retinal fibers, appearing ophthalmoscopically as peripapillary retinal striations, can overcome the peripapillary region and reach the macula. Thus, the average macular thickness (mainly in nasal quadrant) and the average foveolar thickness may be increased in ARSACS patients [119].

Moreover, with the advent of Spectral Domain-OCT (SD-OCT), it has also been possible to visualize changes in the innermost retinal layers in addition to the fiber layer. In 2016, Shah and coauthors describing the characteristics of the fovea in an ARSAC patient, detected the incursion of inner retinal layers upon the foveal region leading to the loss of pit, exactly resembling the abnormality of development as seen in grade 2 foveal hypoplasia [120]. Recently, Rezende and coauthors reported distinct structural abnormalities such as that may provide new insights in the pathogenesis of the disease such as macular microcysts in the inner nuclear layer (INL), a dentate appearance of the inner retina and papillo-macular folds [121].

Parkinson and coauthor, studying a large cohort of ARSACS patients found an inverse correlation between peripapillary RNFL thickness and both age at examination and age at onset; however, without a significant correlation between the average peripapillary RNFL thickness and disease duration [122].

Typically, visual acuity is normal or rarely slightly reduced, without any central visual field defects (only mild and peripheral visual defects are reported). These findings overall support the absence of myelin deposition in the retina of these patients, given that the presence of myelin, would have caused more evident visual field defects (such as blind spot enlargement) [123].

Concerning the ARSACS asymptomatic carriers (subjects with only one abnormal gene copy), the results of two recent studies have been inconsistent so that is it unclear whether there is some degree of RNFL hypertophy in individuals carrying heterozygous SACS gene mutations [122, 124].

Thus, it is preferable to use the term “retinal nerve fiber hypertrophy” [118] to define the retinal aspect of patients with ARSACS. In fact, the new OCT findings, at least among non-Quebec patients, suggest that retinal hypermyelination has been used inappropriately to describe the striated appearance of a thickened RNFL around the optic discs in ARSACS patients [125]. Yu-Wai-Man and coauthors in 2013 have proposed the speculative hypothesis that the RNFL thickening in ARSACS could be related to the axoplasmic stasis within the long axons of the RGCs as they converge to form the optic nerve in the anatomically tight region of the lamina cribrosa [125]. We here show OCT, Angio -OCT and fundus findings in our Charlevoix-Saguenay patient demonstrating also that the nerve fiber hypertrophy appeared to remain stable over the years, as shown in Figs. 14.9, 14.10 and 14.11.

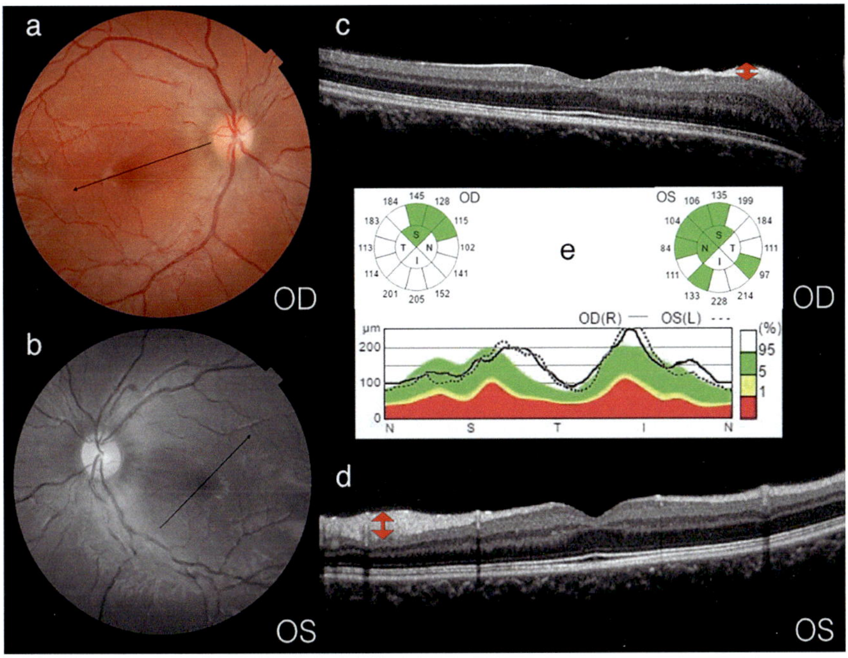

Fig. 14.9 **OCT findings in ARSACS patient**. This is a 25-year old female carrying the mutations in the *SACS* gene located on chromosome 13q12.12p. Visual acuity is 10/10 bilaterally. a, b) Color and red-free fundus photograph. c–d) OCT scans through the fovea reveal the hypertrophy of the nerve fiber layer (red arrows) and the incursion of inner retinal layers upon the foveal region as seen in grade 2 foveal hypoplasia e) Increased thickness of peripapillar RNFL predominant in upper and lower temporal sectors

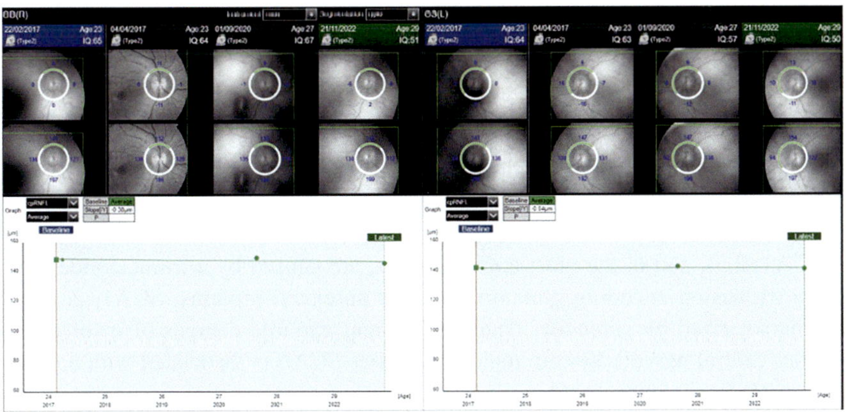

Fig. 14.10 **OCT findings follow-up in ARSACS patient**. The figure shows the pRNFL average thickness trend over time of the same patient shown in Fig. 14.8. The pRNFL average thickness remains unchanged in both eyes over a period of almost 3 years

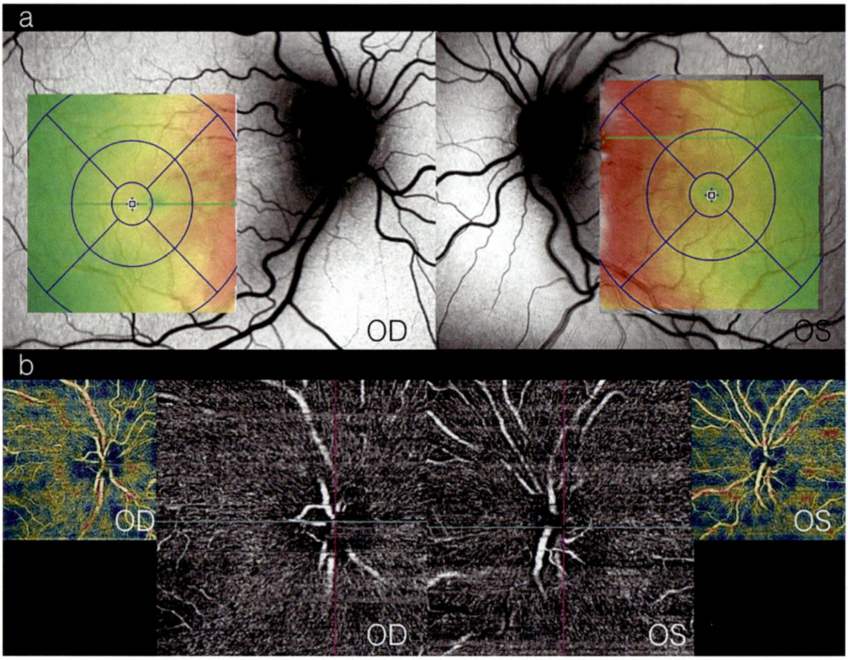

Fig. 14.11 **AF and Angio-OCT findings in ARSACS patient**. Same patient as in Fig. 14.9. a) Fundus autofluorescence with superimposed the ETDR thickness map shows a shadowing of the AF signal and a thickening in the OCT map in the area of the RNFL hypertrophy. b) Angio-OCT of the ONH shows an increase of the numbers of the radial peripapillary capillaries (RPC), probably due to the increased metabolic demand of the hypertrophic fibers

14.7 Spinocerebellar Ataxias (SCAs)

Spinocerebellar ataxias (SCAs) are a genetically heterogeneous group of autosomal dominant neurodegenerative disorders characterized by ataxia, ocular motor abnormalities, and variable other neurological features, such as pyramidal tract, basal ganglia or brainstem dysfunction [126, 127]. The SCAs are classified on the basis of the genotype and currently include more than 40 genetically distinct entities [128, 129].

SCA1, 2, 3, and 6, the most common ones, are caused by a trinucleotide CAG repeat expansion encoding glutamine in four unrelated proteins. SCA1, 2, and 3 are characterized by cerebellar degeneration and variable degrees of involvement of other central nervous system regions, whereas SCA6 is associated with a nearly pure cerebellar atrophy [126].

Abnormal afferent visual testing and optic atrophy have been described as a feature of SC1, SCA2 and SCA3 [130, 131]. Rarely, SCA2 is also associated with retinitis pigmentosa, most notably in the infantile form with extremely expanded

CAG repeats, [132] and pigmentary retinopathy has been reported in a patient homozygous for a pathological repeat expansion in the SCA6 gene [133].

Unlike other SCAs, patients with SCA7 exhibit a spectrum of severity of retinal disease from mild to severe dysfunction. Early functional abnormalities occur in both cones and rods, but greater centrally than peripherally [134, 135].

14.7.1 Spinocerebellar Ataxia Type 2-3-6 (SCA2-3-6)

Pula et al. [136] in a spectral-domain OCT study reported in 29 SCA and cerebellar multisystem atrophy patients (SCA1-2-3-6 and MSA-C) a significant RNFL thinning for SCA2 and SCA3 patients only. This RNFL thinning correlated with the severity of the disease (Scale for the Assessment and Rating of Ataxia, SARA score).

Another study by Alvarez and colleagues [137] demonstrated a significant RNFL thinning in 9 SCA3 patients compared to age- and sex-matched controls. The authors reported RNFL thinning in all quadrants except the temporal one, preserved in all eyes. Therefore, papillomacular bundle probably is not primarily involved in SCA-3 and consequently visual acuity is preserved in these patients (mean BCVA 20/25 and normal colour vision in all patients, except for the one with congenital dyscromatopsia). RNFL thickness was inversely correlated to SARA score. The mean macular thickness was lower compared to the control group only in two eyes (11.11%). In four patients, (eight eyes) OCT studies were performed with an average follow-up of 14.25 months, and in five eyes (62.50%) there was a trend towards a RNFL thickness reduction. Thus, the authors concluded that the pattern of the optic nerve involvement in SCA-3 is more similar to that observed in Alzheimer's and Parkinson's disease than to SCA-1 and toxic or mitochondrial optic nerve diseases where there is a preferential involvement of the papillo-macular bundle [137].

14.7.2 Spinocerebellar Ataxia Type 1 (SCA1)

Spinocerebellar ataxia type 1 (SCA1) is an autosomal dominantly inherited, late-onset neurodegenerative disease primarily affecting the cerebellar cortex and brainstem. Affected patients suffer from disturbed motor coordination, slurred speech, dysphagia, spasticity, extrapyramidal movements such as dystonia or chorea, cerebellar oculomotor disturbances, ophthalmoparesis, saccade slowing and cognitive impairment [138].

SCA1 is due to a CAG-repeat expansion of variable length reaching between 39 and 83 repeats encoding for a prolonged polyglutamine chain in the *ATXN1* gene on chromosome 6p23 encoding for the ataxin1 protein [138].

In SCA1 patients, besides the well-described cerebellar oculomotor abnormalities, there is also evidence of ocular pathology. There is evidence of visual acuity reduction, color vision impairment and central scotoma or contraction of visual fields [139, 140]. In some case series there is evidence of worsening of ocular symptoms with disease duration [141, 142]. The reduced visual acuity in SCA1 has been attributed to optic atrophy, which was first described at fundus examination [142]. Optic nerve involvement was also suggested by abnormal VEP findings in SCA1 patients [143, 144]. However, VEPs were normal in 40–50% of SCA1 patients and retinal or optic nerve pathology was not consistently reported in SCA1 [145].

Stricker et al. [146], in a series of 9 SCA1 subjects compared to age- and sex-matched controls, demonstrated with OCT a pattern of temporal atrophy of the RNFL in most of the patients, suggesting a preferential involvement of the papillo-macular bundle. Segmentation analysis of the retina confirmed temporal RNFL thickness reduction whereas there was no significant difference in the average ganglion cell layer, inner and outer plexiform layer, photoreceptor layer and pigment epithelium. SCA1 patients showed a reduction in visual acuity and average RNFL thickness compared to healthy controls (84.0 μm vs. 97.2 μm). RNFL thinning was predominant and significant in temporal sectors ($p < 0.001$,) and was not found in nasal sectors. OCT findings were correlated with disease duration and disease severity measured by SARA score. The patient with the longest disease duration and highest SARA score showed additional severe macular atrophy, indicating that, at a later disease stage, nerve fiber atrophy could lead to ganglion cell degeneration and consecutively to macular volume reduction. Differently, VEP P100 latencies were not significantly different between SCA1 patients and controls [146]. The authors speculated that the selective temporal RNFL involvement could be explained by a differential vulnerability of the parvocellular axons to mutated ataxin1. In fact, the pattern of temporal RNFL thinning seen in these SCA1 patients could be due to localized oxidative dysfunction, which does not involve the magnocellular ganglion cell axons and the photoreceptors [146].

In 2013, two different groups [139, 140] simultaneously described a case series of six SCA1 patients presenting with progressive maculopathy and retinal dysfunction. The patients exhibited bilateral, progressive painless visual loss with macular drusen and mild pigmentary alterations at fundus examination.

In particular, Vaclavik and coauthors [140] showed two genetically confirmed SCA1 patients with bilateral areas of hypopigmented retinal pigment epithelium within the macula. Autofluorescence imaging revealed a central macular hyperautofluorescence surrounded by a ring of hypoautofluorescence. Spectral-domain OCT disclosed bilateral hyporeflective "foveal cavitation" corresponding to loss of the highly reflective inner segment/outer segment junction, as well as thinning of the outer nuclear layer. Outside the macula, the retina was within normal range. Fluorescein angiography showed small areas of patchy hyperfluorescence in the macula, corresponding to areas of depigmented retinal pigment epithelium without any leakage at later stages. Goldmann kinetic manual perimetry revealed a relative central scotoma bilaterally. The retinal function was tested using full-field ERG which was within normal limits under photopic and scotopic conditions. Multifocal electroretinography (mfERG) was not performed [140].

Two other patients with bilateral foveal cavities had OCT features similar to those reported previously in achromatopsia [147], and cone dystrophy [148], whereas RNFL thickness was not evaluated. Similarly, Lebranchu and coauthors reported a SCA1 family with maculopathy [139]. Four SCA1 patients showed central scotoma in most of the eyes at visual field examination and visual acuities ranged between 20/20 and 20/200. Central retinal thinning with disorganized photoreceptor layers or foveal cavitation were found at OCT. Two patients showed mild temporal optic disc pallor at fundoscopy and thinning of the temporal RNFL at OCT, confirming the involvement of the papillomacular bundle [139]. In one patient, multifocal electroretinography (mfERG) revealed central retinal dysfunction. In these patients, OCT demonstrated alterations of the external layers of the fovea, suggesting a loss of structural integrity of the photoreceptors. The authors suggested that foveolar cavitation associated with the thinning of the whole macular area (including the surrounding perifoveolar retina) could be related to a cone dystrophy, as supported by the fact that a cluster of genes (*GUCA1A, PRPH2*) involved in macular diseases is located in a chromosome region (6p21.1) near the SCA1 gene [139].

More recently, Oertel and colleagues in 2020 [149] investigated neurodegeneration of retina and optic nerve, macula, and their functional relevance in a cross-sectional cohort of 20 cases with SCA-*ATXN1* mutation. They found that a 25% of patients showed a distinct macular pathology with a disruption of the ellipsoid zone (EZ) and confirmed previous reports on optic nerve atrophy as part of the clinical picture of SCA1 showing peripapillary RNFL and GCIP (ganglion cell and inner plexiform layer) thinning.

In contrast, inner nuclear layer (INL) and outer retinal layers at the macula level were similar between SCA-1 patients and healthy controls.

14.7.3 Spinocerebellar Ataxia Type 7 (SCA7)

Spinocerebellar ataxia type 7 (SCA7) is a progressive ataxia that is characterized by a high prevalence of retinal photoreceptor abnormalities. Recent studies suggest that the retinopathy of SCA7 is a cone-rod dystrophy [134, 135]. This degenerative retinopathy initially affects cones, and then progresses to cone–rod dystrophy [134]. Fundus examination demonstrates macular pigmentary changes, sometimes associated with mild temporal optic disc pallor [150, 151]. The gene encodes for a protein (ataxin-7) widely expressed in the human retina [152]. This protein may interact with the function of CRX (cone–rod homeobox), a known transcription factor implicated in human cone–rod dystrophy [153].

In the last 10 years, with the advent of high-resolution spectral domain optical coherence tomography (SD-OCT), many studies demonstrated the presence of different grade of outer retinal atrophy with loss of the outer nuclear layer and ellipsoid zone in the central macula in SCA7 patients (Fig. 14.12). Thus, the loss of the subfoveal ellipsoid zone corresponds to loss of cone photoreceptor

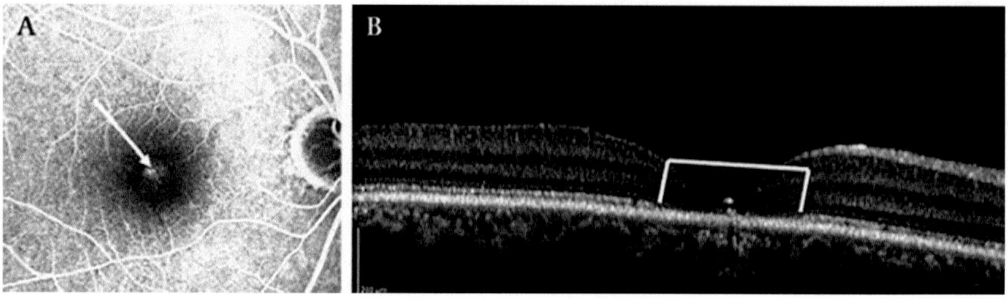

Fig. 14.12 **OCT findings in SCA7 maculopathy**. Optical coherence tomography image shows foveal photoreceptor loss between the outer nuclear layer and retinal pigment epithelium in a patient with SCA7 maculopathy (from Kumar N, Pulido JS. High-definition spectral domain optical coherence tomography in the evaluation of ataxia with visual impairment. Br J Ophthalmol. 2011;95(4):591–598; with kind permissions of Springer Science + Business Media) [154]

cells which may be the earliest clinical sign of cone-rod dystrophy associated with SCA7 [153–157].

Manrique et al. [155] have described a case series of 7 patients with SCA7 in which the subjects with mild disease showed retinal thinning only at the fovea and subjects with more advanced disease tended to present retinal thinning also in the outer zone of the macula. Mean peripapillary RNFL thickness was decreased in all patients with sparing of the temporal quadrant until the advanced phases of the disease.

Furthermore, another study by Ahn et al. [156], using OCT and mfERG, revealed that retinal thinning extended outside the visible atrophic lesions and that the areas of functional deficits were greater than those of anatomic deficits. Additionally, at a later stage of disease the maculopathy can evolve into a "bull's eye" pattern [154]. The sparing of the temporal sector has been discussed as a possible result of the relative sparing of the inner macula around the central fovea associated with normal ganglion cell layer thickness at an earlier disease stage [156–158].

14.7.4 Spinocerebellar Ataxia Type 10 (SCA10)

SCA 10 is caused by a pentanucleotide (ATTCT) repeat expansion on chromosome 22q13-qter. The SCA10 patients can present a purely cerebellar syndrome or a cerebellar syndrome concomitantly with epilepsy, polyneuropathy, and hematologic heart and liver conditions [159]. SCA10 shows a less aggressive clinical course than SCA3.

In 2017, Spina Tensini e coauthors used OCT to compare peripapillary RNFL and macular GCL thickness in patients with SCA3 and those with SCA10. They confirmed the reduction of the RNFL thickness in all quadrants but the temporal one in SCA3 patients and moreover they found RNFL thicker in SCA10 ($p > 0.05$) without any correlation between size of expansion, SARA, and RNFL or GCL thickness in SCA10 patients. These OCT structural findings result in accordance with the clinical course of SCA10, less aggressive than other SCAs [160].

Acknowledgment Chiara La Morgia is a member of the European Reference Network for Neuromuscular Diseases ERN EURO-NMD.

References

1. Collins A. Clinical neurogenetics: friedreich ataxia. Neurol Clin. 2013;31:1095–120.
2. Parkinson MH, Boesch S, Nachbauer W, Mariotti C, Giunti P. Clinical features of Friedreich's ataxia: classical and atypical phenotypes. J Neurochem. 2013;126(Suppl 1):103–17.
3. Campuzano V, Montermini L, Moltò MD, Pianese L, Cossée M, Cavalcanti F, et al. Friedreich's ataxia: autosomal recessive disease caused by an intronic GAA triplet repeat expansion. Science. 1996;271:1423–7.
4. Tan G, Napoli E, Taroni F, Cortopassi G. Decreased expression of genes involved in sulfur amino acid metabolism in frataxin-deficient cells. Hum Mol Genet. 2003;12:1699–711.
5. Shan Y, Napoli E, Cortopassi G. Mitochondrial frataxin interacts with ISD11 of the NFS1/ISCU complex and multiple mitochondrial chaperones. Hum Mol Genet. 2007;16:929–41.
6. Martelli A, Puccio H. Dysregulation of cellular iron metabolism in Friedreich ataxia: from primary iron-sulfur cluster deficit to mitochondrial iron accumulation. Front Pharmacol. 2014;5:130.
7. Rötig A, de Lonlay P, Chretien D, Foury F, Koenig M, Sidi D, et al. Aconitase and mitochondrial iron-sulphur protein deficiency in Friedreich ataxia. Nat Genet. 1997;17:215–7.
8. Lodi R, Cooper JM, Bradley JL, Manners D, Styles P, Taylor DJ, et al. Deficit of in vivo mitochondrial ATP production in patients with Friedreich ataxia. Proc Natl Acad Sci USA. 1999;96:11492–5.
9. Bolinches-Amorós A, Mollá B, Pla-Martín D, Palau F, González-Cabo P. Mitochondrial dysfunction induced by frataxin deficiency is associated with cellular senescence and abnormal calcium metabolism. Front Cell Neurosci. 2014;8:124.
10. Babcock M, de Silva D, Oaks R, Davis-Kaplan S, Jiralerspong S, Montermini L, et al. Regulation of mitochondrial iron accumulation by Yfh1p, a putative homolog of frataxin. Science. 1997;276:1709–12.
11. Wong A, Yang J, Cavadini P, Gellera C, Lonnerdal B, Taroni F, et al. The Friedreich's ataxia mutation confers cellular sensitivity to oxidant stress which is rescued by chelators of iron and calcium and inhibitors of apoptosis. Hum Mol Genet. 1999;8:425–30.
12. Gomes CM, Santos R. Neurodegeneration in Friedreich's ataxia: from defective frataxin to oxidative stress. Oxid Med Cell Longev. 2013;2013:487534.
13. Kersten HM, Roxburgh RH, Danesh-Meyer HV. Ophthalmic manifestations of inherited neurodegenerative disorders. Nat Rev Neurol. 2014;10:349–62.
14. Thomas-Black G, Altmann DR, Crook H, Solanky N, Carrasco FP, Battiston M, et al. Multimodal analysis of the visual pathways in Friedreich's ataxia reveals novel biomarkers. Mov Disord. 2022.
15. Andermann E, Remillard GM, Goyer C, Blitzer L, Andermann F, Barbeau A. Genetic and family studies in Friedreich's ataxia. Can J Neurol Sci. 1976;3:287–301.
16. Carroll WM, Kriss A, Baraitser M, Barrett G, Halliday AM. The incidence and nature of visual pathway involvement in Friedreich's ataxia. A clinical and visual evoked potential study of 22 patients. Brain. 1980;103:413–34.
17. Fortuna F, Barboni P, Liguori R, Valentino ML, Savini G, Gellera C, et al. Visual system involvement in patients with Friedreich's ataxia. Brain. 2009;132:116–23.
18. Noval S, Contreras I, Sanz-Gallego I, Manrique RK, Arpa J. Ophthalmic features of Friedreich ataxia. Eye 2012;26:315–20.

19. Seyer LA, Galetta K, Wilson J, Sakai R, Perlman S, Mathews K, et al. Analysis of the visual system in Friedreich ataxia. J Neurol. 2013;260:2362–9.
20. Dağ E, Örnek N, Örnek K, Erbahçeci-Timur IE. Optical coherence tomography and visual field findings in patients with Friedreich ataxia. J Neuroophthalmol. 2014;34:118–21.
21. Bogdanova-Mihaylova P, Plapp HM, Chen H, Early A, Cassidy L, Walsh RA, et al. Longitudinal assessment using optical coherence tomography in patients with Friedreich's ataxia. Tomography. 2021;7:915–31.
22. Barboni P, Carbonelli M, Savini G, Ramos Cdo V, Carta A, Berezovsky A, et al. Natural history of Leber's hereditary optic neuropathy:longitudinal analysis of the retinal nerve fiber layer by optical coherence tomography. Ophthalmology. 2010;117:623–7.
23. Klein CJ, Botuyan MV, Wu Y, Ward CJ, Nicholson GA, Hammans S, et al. Mutations in DNMT1 cause hereditary sensory neuropathy with dementia and hearing loss. Nat Genet. 2011;43:595–600.
24. Winkelmann J, Lin L, Schormair B, Kornum BR, Faraco J, Plazzi G, et al. Mutations in DNMT1 cause autosomal dominant cerebellar ataxia, deafness and narcolepsy. Hum Mol Genet. 2012;21:2205–10.
25. Moghadam KK, Pizza F, La Morgia C, Franceschini C, Tonon C, Lodi R, et al. Narcolepsy is a common phenotype in HSAN IE and ADCA-DN. Brain. 2014;137:1643–55.
26. Melberg A, Hetta J, Dahl N, Nennesmo I, Bengtsson M, Wibom R, et al. Autosomal dominant cerebellar ataxia deafness and narcolepsy. J Neurol Sci. 1995;134:119–29.
27. Lundberg PO, Wranne I, Brun A. Family with optic atrophy and neurological symptoms. Acta Neurol Scand. 1967;43:87–105.
28. Takasugi M, Yagi S, Hirabayashi K, Shiota K. DNA methylation status of nuclear-encoded mitochondrial genes underlies the tissue-dependent mitochondrial functions. BMC Genom. 2010;11:481.
29. Shock LS, Thakkar PV, Peterson EJ, Moran RG, Taylor SM. DNA methyltransferase 1, cytosine methylation, and cytosine hydroxymethylation in mammalian mitochondria. Proc Natl Acad Sci USA. 2011;108:3630–5.
30. Bellizzi D, D'Aquila P, Scafone T, Giordano M, Riso V, Riccio A, et al. The control region of mitochondrial DNA shows an unusual CpG and non-CpG methylation pattern. DNA Res. 2013;20:537–47.
31. Singh RK, Mallela RK, Hayes A, Dunham NR, Hedden ME, Enke RA, Fariss RN, Sternberg H, West MD, Nasonkin IO. Dnmt1, Dnmt3a and Dnmt3b cooperate in photoreceptor and outer plexiform layer development in the mammalian retina. Exp Eye Res. 2017;159:132–146.
32. Bi H, Hojo K, Watanabe M, Yee C, Maski K, Saba S, Graff-Radford J, et al. Expanded genetic insight and clinical experience of DNMT1-complex disorder. Neurol Genet. 2020;6:e456.
33. Lo Giudice T, Lombardi F, Santorelli FM, Kawarai T, Orlacchio A. Hereditary spastic paraplegia: clinical-genetic characteristics and evolving molecular mechanisms. Exp Neurol. 2014;261C:518–39.
34. Casari G, De Fusco M, Ciarmatori S, Zeviani M, Mora M, Fernandez P, et al. Spastic paraplegia and OXPHOS impairment caused by mutations in paraplegin, a nuclear-encoded mitochondrial metalloprotease. Cell. 1998;93:973–83.
35. De Michele G, De Fusco M, Cavalcanti F, Filla A, Marconi R, Volpe G, et al. A new locus for autosomal recessive hereditary spastic paraplegia maps to chromosome 16q24.3. Am J Hum Genet. 1998;63:135–9.
36. Rugarli EI, Langer T. Translating m-AAA protease function in mitochondria to hereditary spastic paraplegia. Trends Mol Med. 2006;12:262–9.
37. Nolden M, Ehses S, Koppen M, Bernacchia A, Rugarli EI, Langer T. The m-AAA protease defective in hereditary spastic paraplegia controls ribosome assembly in mitochondria. Cell. 2005;123:277–89.
38. Atorino L, Silvestri L, Koppen M, Cassina L, Ballabio A, Marconi R, et al. Loss of m-AAA protease in mitochondria causes complex I deficiency and increased sensitivity to oxidative stress in hereditary spastic paraplegia. J Cell Biol. 2003;163:777–87.

39. McDermott CJ, Dayaratne RK, Tomkins J, Lusher ME, Lindsey JC, Johnson MA, et al. Paraplegin gene analysis in hereditary spastic paraparesis (HSP) pedigrees in northeast England. Neurology. 2001;56:467–71.
40. Ehses S, Raschke I, Mancuso G, Bernacchia A, Geimer S, Tondera D, et al. Regulation of OPA1 processing and mitochondrial fusion by m-AAA protease isoenzymes and OMA1. J Cell Biol. 2009;187:1023–36.
41. Klebe S, Depienne C, Gerber S, Challe G, Anheim M, Charles P, et al. Spastic paraplegia gene 7 in patients with spasticity and/or optic neuropathy. Brain. 2012;135:2980–93.
42. van Gassen KL, van der Heijden CD, de Bot ST, den Dunnen WF, van den Berg LH, Verschuuren-Bemelmans CC, et al. Genotype-phenotype correlations in spastic paraplegia type 7: a study in a large Dutch cohort. Brain. 2012;135:2994–3004.
43. Marcotulli C, Leonardi L, Tessa A, De Negris AM, Cornia R, Pierallini A, et al. Early-onset optic neuropathy as initial clinical presentation in SPG7. J Neurol. 2014;261:1820–1.
44. Wiethoff S, Zhour A, Schöls L, Fischer MD. Retinal nerve fibre layer loss in hereditary spastic paraplegias is restricted to complex phenotypes. BMC Neurol. 2012;12:143.
45. Vander Stichele G, Durr A, Yoon G, Schüle R, Blackstone C, Esposito G, et al. An integrated modelling methodology for estimating global incidence and prevalence of hereditary spastic paraplegia subtypes SPG4, SPG7, SPG11, and SPG15. BMC Neurol. 2022;22:115.
46. Stevanin G, Azzedine H, Denora P et all on behalf of the SPATAX Consortium. 2008. Mutations in SPG11 are frequent in autosomal recessive spastic paraplegia with thin corpus callosum, cognitive decline and lower motor neuron degeneration. Brain 131:772–784.
47. Słabicki M, Theis M, Krastev DB, Samsonov S, Mundwiller E, Junqueira M, et al. A genome-scale DNA repair RNAi screen identifies SPG48 as a novel gene associated with hereditary spastic paraplegia. PLoS Biol. 2010;8:e1000408.
48. Hirst J, Barlow LD, Francisco GC, Sahlender DA, Seaman MN, Dacks JB, Robinson MS. The fifth adaptor protein complex. PLoS Biol. 2011;9:e1001170.
49. Chang J, Lee S, Blackstone C. Spastic paraplegia proteins spastizin and spatacsin mediate autophagic lysosome reformation. J Clin Invest. 2014;124:5249–62.
50. Boutry M, Pierga A, Matusiak R, Branchu J, Houllegatte M, Ibrahim Y, Balse E, El Hachimi KH, Brice A, Stevanin G, Darios F. Loss of spatacsin impairs cholesterol trafficking and calcium homeostasis. Commun Biol. 2019;2:380.
51. Frisch IB, Haag P, Steffen H, et al. Kjellin's syndrome: fundus autofluorescence, angiographic, and electrophysiologic findings. Ophthalmology. 2002;109:1484–91.
52. Dursun U, Koroglu C, Orhan EK, Ugur SA, Tolun A. Autosomal recessive spastic paraplegia (SPG45) with mental retardation maps to 10q24.3-q25.1. Neurogenetics 2009; 10:325–31.
53. Elsaid MF, Ibrahim K, Chalhoub N, Elsotouhy A, El Mudehki N, Abdel AA. NT5C2 novel splicing variant expands the phenotypic spectrum of Spastic Paraplegia (SPG45): case report of a new member of thin corpus callosum SPG-Subgroup. BMC Med Genet. 2017;18:33.
54. Novarino G, Fenstermaker A, Zaki M, et al. Exome sequencing links corticospinal motor neuron disease to common neurodegenerative disorders. Science. 2014;343:506–11.
55. Chabriat H, Joutel A, Dichgans M, Tournier-Lasserve E, Bousser MG. Cadasil. Lancet Neurol. 2009;8:643–53.
56. O'Sullivan M, Jarosz JM, Martin RJ, Deasy N, Powell JF, Markus HS. MRI hyperintensities of the temporal lobe and external capsule in patients with CADASIL. Neurology. 2001;56:628–34.
57. Joutel A, Corpechot C, Ducros A, Vahedi K, Chabriat H, Mouton P, et al. Notch3 mutations in cerebral autosomal dominant arteriopathy with subcortical infarcts and leukoencephalopathy (CADASIL), a mendelian condition causing stroke and vascular dementia. Ann NY Acad Sci. 1997;826:213–7.
58. Belin de Chantemèle EJ, Retailleau K, Pinaud F, Vessières E, Bocquet A, Guihot AL, et al. Notch3 is a major regulator of vascular tone in cerebral and tail resistance arteries. Arterioscler Thromb Vasc Biol. 2008;28:2216–24.

59. Robinson W, Galetta SL, McCluskey L, Forman MS, Balcer LJ. Retinal findings in cerebral autosomal dominant arteriopathy with subcortical infarcts and leukoencephalopathy (CADASIL). Surv Ophthalmol. 2001;45:445–8.
60. Roine S, Harju M, Kivelä TT, Pöyhönen M, Nikoskelainen E, Tuisku S, et al. Ophthalmologic findings in cerebral autosomal dominant arteriopathy with subcortical infarcts and leukoencephalopathy: a cross-sectional study. Ophthalmology. 2006;113:1411–7.
61. Haritoglou C, Rudolph G, Hoops JP, Opherk C, Kampik A, Dichgans M. Retinal vascular abnormalities in CADASIL. Neurology. 2004;62:1202–5.
62. Pretegiani E, Rosini F, Dotti MT, Bianchi S, Federico A, Rufa A. Visual system involvement in CADASIL. J Stroke Cerebrovasc Dis. 2013;22:1377–84.
63. Parisi V, Pierelli F, Fattapposta F, Bianco F, Parisi L, Restuccia R, et al. Early visual function impairment in CADASIL. Neurology. 2003;60:2008–10.
64. Rufa A, Malandrini A, Dotti MT, Berti G, Salvadori C, Federico A. Typical pathological changes of CADASIL in the optic nerve. Neurol Sci. 2005;26:271–4.
65. Parisi V, Pierelli F, Coppola G, Restuccia R, Ferrazzoli D, Scassa C, et al. Reduction of optic nerve fiber layer thickness in CADASIL. Eur J Neurol. 2007;14:627–31.
66. Rufa A, Pretegiani E, Frezzotti P, De Stefano N, Cevenini G, Dotti MT, et al. Retinal nerve fiber layer thinning in CADASIL: an optical coherence tomography and MRI study. Cerebrovasc Dis. 2011;31:77–82.
67. Nelis P, Kleffner I, Burg MC, Clemens CR, Alnawaiseh M, Motte J, ET AL. OCT-Angiography reveals reduced vessel density in the deep retinal plexus of CADASIL patients. Sci Rep. 2018;8:8148.
68. Alten F, Motte J, Ewering C, Osada N, Clemens CR, Kadas EM, et al. Multimodal retinal vessel analysis in CADASIL patients. PLoS One. 2014;9:e112311.
69. Fang XJ, Yu M, Wu Y, Zhang ZH, Wang WW, Wang ZX, Yuan Y. Study of enhanced depth imaging optical coherence tomography in cerebral autosomal dominant arteriopathy with subcortical infarcts and leukoencephalopathy. Chin Med J. 2017;130(9):1042–8.
70. Cavallari M, Falco T, Frontali M, Romano S, Bagnato F, Orzi F. Fractal analysis reveals reduced complexity of retinal vessels in CADASIL. PLoS One. 2011 Apr 27;6(4):e19150.
71. Krivosic V, Paques M, Hervé D, Duliére C, Taleb A, Gastellier N, et al. Retinal vascular density in CADASIL (cerebral autosomal dominant arteriopathy with subcortical infarcts and leukoencephalopathy). BMJ Neurol Open. 2023;5(1):e000417.
72. Lin CW, Yang ZW, Chen CH, Cheng YW, Tang SC, Jeng JS. Reduced macular vessel density and inner retinal thickness correlate with the severity of cerebral autosomal dominant arteriopathy with subcortical infarcts and leukoencephalopathy (CADASIL). PLoS ONE. 2022;17(5):e0268572.
73. Wolfram D, Wagener HP. Diabetes mellitus and simple optic atrophy among siblings: report of four cases. Proc Staff Meet Mayo Clin. 1938;13: 715–18.
74. Rigoli L, Di Bella C. Wolfram syndrome 1 and Wolfram syndrome 2. Curr Opin Pediatr. 2012;24:512–7.
75. Barrett TG, Poulton K, Bundey S. DIDMOAD syndrome; further studies and muscle biochemistry. J Inherit Metab Dis. 1995;18:218–20.
76. Barrett TG, Bundey SE. Wolfram (DIDMOAD) syndrome. J Med Genet. 1997;34:838–41.
77. Barrett TG, Bundey SE, Fielder AR, Good PA. Optic atrophy in Wolfram (DIDMOAD) syndrome. Eye. 1997;11:882–8.
78. Inoue H, Tanizawa Y, Wasson J, Behn P, Kalidas K, Bernal-Mizrachi E, et al. A gene encoding a transmembrane protein is mutated in patients with diabetes mellitus and optic atrophy (Wolfram syndrome). Nat Genet. 1998;20:143–8.
79. Eiberg H, Hansen L, Kjer B, Hansen T, Pedersen O, Bille M, et al. Autosomal dominant optic atrophy associated with hearing impairment and impaired glucose regulation caused by a missense mutation in the WFS1 gene. J Med Genet. 2006;43:435–40.
80. Rendtorff ND, Lodahl M, Boulahbel H, Johansen IR, Pandya A, Welch KO, et al. Identification of p.A684V missense mutation in the WFS1 gene as a frequent cause of autosomal dominant optic atrophy and hearing impairment. Am J Med Genet A. 2011;155A:1298–313.

81. Bai X, Lv H, Zhang F, Liu J, Fan Z, Xu L, et al. Identification of a novel missense mutation in the WFS1 gene as a cause of autosomal dominant nonsyndromic sensorineural hearing loss in all-frequencies. Am J Med Genet A. 2014;164:3052–60.
82. Bonnycastle LL, Chines PS, Hara T, Huyghe JR, Swift AJ, Heikinheimo P, et al. Autosomal dominant diabetes arising from a Wolfram syndrome 1 mutation. Diabetes. 2013;62:3943–50.
83. Berry V, Gregory-Evans C, Emmett W, Waseem N, Raby J, Prescott D, et al. Wolfram gene (WFS1) mutation causes autosomal dominant congenital nuclear cataract in humans. Eur J Hum Genet. 2013;21:1356–60.
84. Carson MJ, Slager UT, Steinberg RM. Simultaneous occurrence of diabetes mellitus, diabetes insipidus, and optic atrophy in a brother and sister. Am J Dis Child. 1977;131:1382–5.
85. Jackson MJ, Bindoff LA, Weber K, Wilson JN, Ince P, Alberti KG, et al. Biochemical and molecular studies of mitochondrial function in diabetes insipidus, diabetes mellitus, optic atrophy, and deafness. Diabetes Care. 1994;17:728–33.
86. Shannon P, Becker L, Deck J. Evidence of widespread axonal pathology in Wolfram syndrome. Acta Neuropathol. 1999;98:304–8.
87. Hilson JB, Merchant SN, Adams JC, Joseph JT. Wolfram syndrome: a clinicopathologic correlation. Acta Neuropathol. 2009;118:415–28.
88. Ross-Cisneros FN, Pan BX, Silva RA, Miller NR, Albini TA, Tranebjaerg L, et al. Optic nerve histopathology in a case of Wolfram Syndrome: a mitochondrial pattern of axonal loss. Mitochondrion. 2013;13:841–5.
89. Bababeygy SR, Wang MY, Khaderi KR, Sadun AA. Visual improvement with the use of idebenone in the treatment of Wolfram syndrome. J Neuroophthalmol. 2012;32:386–9.
90. Bucca BC, Klingensmith G, Bennett JL. Wolfram syndrome: a rare optic neuropathy in youth with type 1 diabetes. Optom Vis Sci. 2011;88:E1383–90.
91. Grenier J, Meunier I, Daien V, Baudoin C, Halloy F, Bocquet B, Blanchet C, Delettre C, Esmenjaud E, Roubertie A, Lenaers G, Hamel CP. WFS1 in optic neuropathies: mutation findings in nonsyndromic optic atrophy and assessment of clinical severity. Ophthalmology. 2016;123(9):1989–98.
92. Zmyslowska A, Waszczykowska A, Baranska D, Stawiski K, Borowiec M, Jurowski P, Fendler W, Mlynarski W. Optical coherence tomography and magnetic resonance imaging visual pathway evaluation in Wolfram syndrome. Dev Med Child Neurol. 2018.
93. Majander A, Bitner-Glindzicz M, Chan CM, Duncan HJ, Chinnery PF, Subash M, Keane PA, Webster AR, Moore AT, Michaelides M, Yu-Wai-Man P. Lamination of the outer plexiform layer in optic atrophy caused by dominant WFS1 mutations. Ophthalmology. 2016;123(7):1624–6.
94. Zmyslowska A, Fendler W, Waszczykowska A, Niwald A, Borowiec M, Jurowski P, Mlynarski W. Retinal thickness as a marker of disease progression in longitudinal observation of patients with Wolfram syndrome. Acta Diabetol. 2017;54(11):1019–24.
95. La Morgia C, Maresca A, Amore G, Gramegna LL, Carbonelli M, Scimonelli E, et al. Calcium mishandling in absence of primary mitochondrial dysfunction drives cellular pathology in Wolfram syndrome. Sci Rep. 2020;10:4785.
96. Barboni P, Amore G, Cascavilla ML, Battista M, Frontino G, Romagnoli M, et al. The pattern of retinal ganglion cell loss in Wolfram syndrome is distinct from mitochondrial optic neuropathies. Am J Ophthalmol. 2022;241:206–16.
97. O'Bryhim BE, Samara A, Chen L, Hershey T, Tychsen L, Hoekel J. Longitudinal changes in vision and retinal morphology in Wolfram syndrome. Am J Ophthalmol. 2022;243:10–8.
98. Bouhlal Y, Amouri R, El Euch-Fayeche G, Hentati F. Autosomal recessive spastic ataxia of Charlevoix-Saguenay: an overview. Parkinsonism Relat Disord. 2011;17:418–22.
99. Berciano J, García A, Infante J. Peripheral nerve involvement in hereditary cerebellar and multisystem degenerative disorders. Handb Clin Neurol. 2013;115:907–32.
100. Duquette A, Brais B, Bouchard JP, Mathieu J. Clinical presentation and early evolution of spastic ataxia of Charlevoix-Saguenay. Mov Disord. 2013;28:2011–4.
101. Baets J, Deconinck T, Smets K, Goossens D, Van den Bergh P, Dahan K, et al. Mutations in SACS cause atypical and late-onset forms of ARSACS. Neurology. 2010;28(75):1181–8.

102. Bouchard JP, Barbeau A, Bouchard R, Bouchard RW. Autosomal recessive spastic ataxia of Charlevoix-Saguenay. Can J Neurol Sci 1978;5:61e9.
103. De Braekeleer M, Giasson F, Mathieu J, Roy M, Bouchard JP, Morgan K. Genetic epidemiology of autosomal recessive spastic ataxia of CharlevoixeSaguenay in northeastern Quebec. Genet Epidemiol 1993;10:17–25.
104. Thiffault I, Dicaire MJ, Tetreault M, Huang KN, Demers-Lamarche J, Bernard G, et al. Diversity of ARSACS mutations in French-Canadians. Can J Neurol Sci. 2013;40:61–6.
105. Engert JC1, Bérubé P, Mercier J, Doré C, Lepage P, Ge B, Bouchard JP, Mathieu J, et al. ARSACS, a spastic ataxia common in northeastern Québec, is caused by mutations in a new gene encoding an 11.5-kb ORF. Nat Genet 2000;24:120–5.
106. Cheetham ME, Caplan AJ. Structure, function and evolution of DnaJ: conservation and adaptation of chaperone function. Cell Stress Chaperones 1998;3:28–36.
107. Parfitt DA, Michael GJ, Vermeulen EG, Prodromou NV, Webb TR, Gallo JM, et al. The ataxia protein sacsin is a functional co-chaperone that protects against polyglutamine-expanded ataxin-1. Hum Mol Genet 2009;18:1556–65.
108. Girard M, Larivière R, Parfitt DA, Deane EC, Gaudet R, Nossova N, et al. Mitochondrial dysfunction and Purkinje cell loss in autosomal recessive spastic ataxia of Charlevoix-Saguenay (ARSACS). Proc Natl Acad Sci USA. 2012;109:1661–6.
109. El Euch-Fayache G, Lalani I, Amouri R, Turki I, Ouahchi K, Hung WY, et al. Phenotypic features and genetic findings in sacsin-related autosomal recessive ataxia in Tunisia. Arch Neurol. 2003;60:982–8.
110. Grieco GS, Malandrini A, Comanducci G, Leuzzi V, Valoppi M, Tessa A, et al. Novel SACS mutations in autosomal recessive spastic ataxia of charlevoixe-saguenay type. Neurology 2004;62:103–6.
111. Criscuolo C, Banfi S, Orio M, Gasparini P, Monticelli A, Scarano V, et al. A novel mutation in SACS gene in a family from southern Italy. Neurology 2004;62:100–2.
112. Takiyama Y. Autosomal recessive spastic ataxia of CharlevoixeSaguenay. Neuropathology 2006;26:368–75.
113. Bouhlal Y, Zouari M, Kefi M, Ben Hamida C, Hentati F, Amouri R. Autosomal recessive ataxia caused by three distinct gene defects in a single consanguineous family. J Neurogenet 2008;22:139–48.
114. Vermeer S, Meijer RP, Pijl BJ, Timmermans J, Cruysberg JR, Bos MM, et al. ARSACS in the Dutch population: a frequent cause of early-onset cerebellar ataxia. Neurogenetics 2008;10:87.
115. Bouhlal Y, El Euch-Fayeche G, Hentati F, Amouri R. A novel SACS gene mutation in a Tunisian family. J Mol Neurosci. 2009;39:333–6.
116. Takiyama Y. Sacsinopathies: sacsin-related ataxia. Cerebellum. 2007;6:353–9.
117. Vingolo EM, Di Fabio R, Salvatore S, Greco G, Bertini E, Lezzi V, et al. Myelinated retinal fibers in autosomal recessive spastic ataxia of Charlevoix-Saguenay. Eur J Neurol. 2011;18:1187–90.
118. Pablo LE, Garcia-Martin E, Gazulla J, Larrosa JM, Ferreras A, Santorelli FM, et al. Retinal nerve fiber hypertrophy in ataxia of Charlevoix-Saguenay patients. Mol Vis. 2011;17:1871–6.
119. Desserre J, Devos D, Sautière BG, Debruyne P, Santorelli FM, Vuillaume I, et al. Thickening of peripapillar retinal fibers for the diagnosis of autosomal recessive spastic ataxia of Charlevoix-Saguenay. Cerebellum. 2011;10:758–62.
120. Shah CT, Ward TS, Matsumoto JA, et al. Foveal hypoplasia in autosomal recessive spastic ataxia of Charlevoix-Saguenay. J AAPOS. 2016;20(1):81–3.
121. Rezende Filho FM, Bremner F, Pedroso JL, de Andrade JBC, Marianelli BF, Lourenço CM, et al. Retinal architecture in autosomal recessive spastic ataxia of Charlevoix-Saguenay (ARSACS): insights into disease pathogenesis and biomarkers. Mov Disord. 2021;36:2027–35.
122. Parkinson MH, Bartmann AP, Clayton LMS, et al. Optical coherence tomography in autosomal recessive spastic ataxia of Charlevoix-Saguenay. Brain. 2018;141(4):989–99.

123. Gazulla J, Benavente I, Vela AC, Marín MA, Pablo LE, Tessa A, Barrena MR, et al. New findings in the ataxia of Charlevoix-Saguenay. J Neurol. 2012;259:869–78.
124. Van Lint M, Hoornaert K, Ten Tusscher MPM. Retinal nerve fiber layer thickening in ARSACS carriers. J Neurol Sci 2016;370:119–122.
125. Yu-Wai-Man P, Pyle A, Griffin H, Santibanez-Korev M, Chinnery PF. Abnormal retinal thickening is a common feature among patients with ARSACS-related phenotypes. Br J Ophthalmol. 2014;98:711–3.
126. Koeppen AH. The pathogenesis of spinocerebellar ataxia. Cerebellum. 2005;4:62–73.
127. Durr A. Autosomal dominant cerebellar ataxias: polyglutamine expansions and beyond. Lancet Neurol. 2010;9:885–94.
128. Mudwiler A, Shakkottai VG. Autosomal-dominant cerebellar ataxias. Handb Clin Neurol. 2018;147:173–85.
129. Coarelli G, Coutelier M, Durr A. Autosomal dominant cerebellar ataxias: new genes and progress towards treatments. Lancet Neurol. 2023;22:735–49.
130. Pula JH, Gomez CM, Kattah JC. Ophthalmologic features of the common spinocerebellar ataxias. Curr Opin Ophthalmol. 2010;21:447–53.
131. Newman NJ, Biousse V. Hereditary optic neuropathies. Eye. 2004;18(11):1144–60.
132. Rufa A, Dotti MT, Galli L, Orrico A, Sicurelli F, Federico A. Spinocerebellar ataxia type 2 (SCA2) associated with retinal pigmentary degeneration. Eur Neurol. 2002;47:128–9.
133. Fukutake T, Kamitsukasa I, Arai K, Hattori T, Nakajima T. A patient homozygous for the SCA6 gene with retinitis pigmentosa. Clin Genet. 2002;61:375–9.
134. Aleman TS, Cideciyan AV, Volpe NJ, Stevanin G, Brice A, Jacobson SG. Spinocerebellar ataxia type 7 (SCA7) shows a cone-rod dystrophy phenotype. Exp Eye Res. 2002;74:737–45.
135. Abe T, Tsuda T, Yoshida M, Wada Y, Kano T, Itoyama Y, et al. Macular degeneration associated with aberrant expansion of trinucleotide repeat of the SCA7 gene in 2 Japanese families. Arch Ophthalmol. 2000;118:1415–21.
136. Pula JH, Towle VL, Staszak VM, Cao D, Bernard JT, Gomez CM. Retinal nerve fibre layer and macular thinning in spinocerebellar ataxia and cerebellar multisystem atrophy. Neuroophthalmology. 2011;35(3):108–14.
137. Alvarez G, Rey A, Sanchez-Dalmau FB, Muñoz E, Ríos J, Adán A. Optical coherence tomography findings in spinocerebellar ataxia-3. Eye. 2013;27:1376–81.
138. Schöls L, Bauer P, Schmidt T, Schulte T, Riess O. Autosomal dominant cerebellar ataxias: clinical features, genetics, and pathogenesis. Lancet Neurol. 2004;3:291–304.
139. Lebranchu P, Le Meur G, Magot A, David A, Verny C, Weber M, et al. Maculopathy and spinocerebellar ataxia type 1: a new association? J Neuroophthalmol. 2013;33:225–31.
140. Vaclavik V, Borruat FX, Ambresin A, Munier FL. Novel maculopathy in patients with spinocerebellar ataxia type 1 autofluorescence findings and functional characteristics. JAMA Ophthalmol. 2013;131:536–8.
141. Abe T, Abe K, Tsuda T, Itoyama Y, Tamai M. Ophthalmological findings in patients with spinocerebellar ataxia type 1 are not correlated with neurological anticipation. Graefes Arch Clin Exp Ophthalmol. 2001;239:722–8.
142. Abe T, Abe K, Aoki M, Itoyama Y, Tamai M. Ocular changes in patients with spinocerebellar degeneration and repeated trinucleotide expansion of spinocerebellar ataxia type 1 gene. Arch Ophthalmol. 1997;115:231–6.
143. Abele M, Bürk K, Andres F, Topka H, Laccone F, Bösch S et al. Autosomal dominant cerebellar ataxia type I. Nerve conduction and evoked potential studies in families with SCA1, SCA2 and SCA3. Brain 1997;120: 2141–8.
144. Perretti A, Santoro L, Lanzillo B, Filla A, De Michele G, Barbieri F, et al. Autosomal dominant cerebellar ataxia type I: multimodal electrophysiological study and comparison between SCA1 and SCA2 patients. J Neurol Sci. 1996;142:45–53.
145. Robitaille Y, Schut L, Kish SJ. Structural and immunocytochemical features of olivopontocerebellar atrophy caused by the spinocerebellar ataxia type 1 (SCA-1) mutation define a unique phenotype. Acta Neuropathol. 1995;90:572–81.

146. Stricker S, Oberwahrenbrock T, Zimmermann H, Schroeter J, Endres M, Brandt AU, et al. Temporal retinal nerve fiber loss in patients with spinocerebellar ataxia type 1. PLoS ONE. 2011;6:e23024.
147. Varsányi B, Somfai GM, Lesch B, Vámos R, Farkas A, et al. Optical coherence tomography of the macula in congenital achromatopsia. Invest Ophthalmol Vis Sci. 2007;48:2249–53.
148. Birch DG, Wen Y, Locke K, Hood DC. Rod sensitivity, cone sensitivity, and photoreceptor layer thickness in retinal degenerative diseases. Invest Ophthalmol Vis Sci. 2011;52:7141–7.
149. Oertel FC, Zeitz O, Rönnefarth M, et al. Functionally relevant maculopathy and optic atrophy in spinocerebellar ataxia type 1. Mov Disord Clin Pract. 2020;7:502–8.
150. Aleman TS, Cideciyan AV, Volpe NJ, Stevanin G, Brice A, Jacobson SG. Spinocerebellar ataxia type 7 (SCA7) shows a cone-rod dystrophy phenotype. Exp Eye Res. 2002;74:737–45.
151. Gouw LG, Digre KB, Harris CP, Haines JH, Ptacek LJ. Autosomal dominant cerebellar ataxia with retinal degeneration: clinical, neuropathologic, and genetic analysis of a large kindred. Neurology. 1994;44:1441–7.
152. Cancel G, Duyckaerts C, Holmberg M, Zander C, Yvert G, Lebre AS, et al. Distribution of ataxin-7 in normal human brain and retina. Brain. 2000;123:2519–30.
153. La Spada AR, Fu Y, Sopher BL, Libby RT, Wang X, Li LY, et al. Polyglutamine-expanded ataxin-7 antagonizes CRX function and induces cone-rod dystrophy in a mouse model of SCA7. Neuron. 2001;31:913–27.
154. Kumar N, Pulido JS. High-definition spectral domain optical coherence tomography in the evaluation of ataxia with visual impairment. Br J Ophthalmol. 2011;95:591–8.
155. Manrique RK, Noval S, Aguilar-Amat MJ, Arpa J, Rosa I, Contreras I. Ophthalmic features of spinocerebellar ataxia type 7. J Neuroophthalmol. 2009;29:174–9.
156. Ahn JK, Seo JM, Chung H, Yu HG. Anatomical and functional characteristics in atrophic maculopathy associated with spinocerebellar ataxia type 7. Am J Ophthalmol. 2005;139:923–5.
157. McLaughlin ME. Dryja TP Ocular findings in spinocerebellar ataxia 7. Arch Ophthalmol. 2002;120:655–9.
158. Levinson JD, Yan J, Lambert SR, Shankar SP. Multimodal imaging of a family with spinocerebellar ataxia type 7 demonstrating phenotypic variation and progression of retinal degeneration. Retin Cases Brief Rep. 2016;10(3):267–72.
159. Teive HAG, Munhoz RP, Arruda WO, et al. Spinocerebellar ataxia type 10-a review. Park Relat Disord. 2011;17:655–61.
160. Spina Tensini F, Sato MT, Shiokawa N, Ashizawa T, Teive HAG. A comparative optical coherence tomography study of spinocerebellar ataxia types 3 and 10. Cerebellum. 2017;16(4):797–801.

Other Neurological Disorders: Migraine, Neurosarcoidosis, Schizophrenia, Obstructive Sleep Apnea-Hypopnea Syndrome and Bipolar Disorder

15

Francisco J. Ascaso, Javier Mateo, Laura Cabezon, Paula Casas, and Andrzej Grzybowski

Abstract

Optical coherence tomography (OCT) is a common, objective, rapid, reproducible, non-invasive and economical, transpupillary diagnostic imaging technique that enables quantitative in vivo high-resolution measurement of peripapillary retinal nerve fiber layer (RNFL), ganglion cell layer (GCL), and choroid layer thickness. Since the official commercialization of OCT technology in 2002, an increasing number of studies have used OCT technology to analyze certain neurological disorders. In this chapter we report the changes in structural OCT and OCT angiography (OCTA) in migraine, neurosarcoidosis, schizophrenia, Obstructive Sleep Apnea-Hypopnea syndrome and bipolar disorder.

F. J. Ascaso (✉) · J. Mateo · P. Casas
Department of Ophthalmology, Hospital Clínico Universitario, Zaragoza, Spain
e-mail: jascaso@gmail.com

Aragon Health Research Institute (IIS Aragón), Zaragoza, Spain

F. J. Ascaso
Department of Surgery, School of Medicine, University of Zaragoza, Zaragoza, Spain

L. Cabezon
Hospital Quirón, Malaga, Spain

A. Grzybowski
Institute for Research in Ophthalmology, Foundation for Ophthalmology Development, Poznan, Poland

A. Grzybowski and P. Barboni (eds.), *OCT and Imaging in Central Nervous System Diseases*, https://doi.org/10.1007/978-3-031-72156-4_15

Keywords

Optical coherence tomography (OCT) • OCT angiography (OCTA) • Migraine • Neurosarcoidosis • Schizophrenia • Obstructive sleep apnea síndrome (OSAS) • Bipolar disorder

15.1 OCT and Migraine

15.1.1 Introduction

Migraine is a chronic disorder characterized by unilateral, pulsating, and often moderate-to-severe repetitive episodes of headache [1]. It may be accompanied by vegetative symptoms such as nausea, vomiting, sensitivity to light (photophobia) and sound (phonophobia), and other neurological symptoms [2–5]. People with migraine may also experience premonitory [6] and postdromal [7] symptoms, such as fatigue and mood changes, in the hours or days leading up to and after an attack. Episodic migraine is defined as 0–14 headache days per month, whereas chronic migraine is defined as 15 or more headache days per month. Episodic migraine is classified into two major groups: migraine with aura (MwA, or classic migraine) and migraine without aura (MwoA, or common migraine) [8]. Aura, which manifests as transient ocular and neurological disturbances, including flashes of light, blind spots, periorbital pain, and photophobia, affects about 25% of patients, usually immediately before but sometimes following the headache [9, 10].

This condition, which affects approximately 15% of the general population, is the third most frequent global disorder in both genders [11] and the most common episodic neurological disease [12–14] According to the Global Burden of Disease Project, migraine ranks second only to stroke in terms of disability-adjusted life years across all ages. When considering the life period of peak productivity (15–49 years), migraine is the leading cause of years lived with disability [15] It mainly affects women aged 20–45 years [16, 17], and symptoms typically last 4–72 h [18–20]. Migraine has generally increased in incidence worldwide in the last years, mainly in developing countries, possibly with adverse lifestyle changes brought about by rapid urbanization in these regions [21–23].

There is no consensus on the pathogenesis of migraine, but it is generally accepted that activation and sensitisation occurs episodically in the trigeminal vascular system [5, 24, 25], which is also found in extracranial structures, such as retina and choroid [26]. Its activation causes inflammation, in addition to vasodilation and subsequent vasoconstriction in both structures, and finally induces pain [24, 25]. Both neuronal and vascular mechanisms would be critically involved [24, 27–29]. Although migraine is a transient phenomenon of cerebral and ocular vasoconstriction, its chronic nature may be the cause of permanent structural and functional retinal alterations [30–34]. There is evidence that ganglion cell death in migraine patients may be secondary to alterations in the microcirculation of the optic nerve head or even in the quality of retinal perfusion [35, 36].

All these retinal changes can be measured by optical coherence tomography (OCT). This technique is a common, objective, rapid, reproducible, non-invasive, and economical, transpupillary diagnostic imaging technique that enables quantitative in vivo high-resolution measurement of peripapillary retinal nerve fiber layer (RNFL), ganglion cell layer (GCL), and choroid layer thickness [36–42]. Similar to intravascular ultrasonography, OCT uses near-infrared light to generate cross-sectional vascular images and it has been shown to be reliable and reproducible. Since the official commercialization of OCT technology in 2002, an increasing number of studies have used OCT technology to study optic neuropathy [5]. OCT has been developed to help diagnose neuro-ophthalmic diseases and detect disease development [43, 44]. It continues to evolve, and spectral domain OCT (SD-OCT) and swept source OCT (SS-OCT) have replaced time-domain OCT (TD-OCT) as the first choice for ocular OCT devices [45], showing faster scanning speed, higher sensitivity, deeper penetration, and superior high resolution, especially for more accurate segmentation of the retinal layer [46–48].

15.1.2 Optic Nerve Structural Changes in Migraine

In the last years, numerous authors have studied the changes of RNFL thickness in people with migraine compared with healthy controls. However, results have not been very consistent. In fact, whereas some studies observed that mean peripapillary RNFL thickness was thinner in migraneurs than in controls, others reported only a thinner RNFL in a specific quadrant [33, 49–58] and even a few articles yielded an increase of RNFL thickness [59, 60]. The most recent systematic review and meta-analysis combined data from 26 studies, to investigate outcomes in a total population of 1530 people with migraine versus 1105 healthy controls [61]. The conclusion was that RNFL is, on average, thinner in patients with migraine, particularly those with MwA. Nevertheless, all studies included in this review were cross-sectional, which means that we cannot demonstrate a cause-and-effect relationship between RNFL thinning and migraine episodes. Likewise, no significant associations were found between RNFL thickness and the following factors: age, sex, disease duration, attack frequency and intraocular pressure. The absence of an association with age, and disease duration, could mean that any RNFL thinning is not accumulative [27]. For the first time, Rego et al. [62] have recently evaluated RNFL thickness looking for differences between MwA and MwoA in the pediatric population. They have found that children with MwA may present a reduction in RNFL thickness, which is associated with the number of attacks per month. RNFL thickness measurement might be useful as an objective biomarker to follow the evolution of migraine and to evaluate the efficacy of prophylactic treatments. Furthermore, RNFL evaluation in these patients may also improve our comprehension of migraine pathophysiology.

15.1.3 Macular Changes in Migraine

Retrograde transsynaptic neuronal degeneration of the retinal ganglion cells (RGCs) secondary to damage to structures in the posterior visual pathway has been demonstrated in various settings. Segmentation of retinal layers by spectral-domain OCT has enabled a detailed study of functional areas. This is most useful at the macula, where the density of RGCs is maximal and where other anatomical structures are absent [63, 64]. Some authors have also included measures of macular parameters, typically as part of protocols primarily focused on the exploration of inner retinal alterations. Their results are contradictory because, in the context of structural investigation of the macula in patients with migraine [59, 65, 66], there is no consistent protocol that has been used, with measurements being reported for whole retinal thickness in the macular area, ganglion cell complex, or other measures such as macular cube volume. The lack of common methodology and the small samples lead to an inability to make strong conclusions. However, there appears to be little evidence for consistent structural changes to macular thickness in those with migraine. Future studies using more sensitive imaging protocols may reveal thinning consistent with reported RNFL thinning outside of the macula, or that can be spatially directly associated to purported macular vascular nonperfusion [27].

15.1.4 Choroidal Changes in Migraine

Migraine has been shown to decrease posterior ciliary artery blood supply [67] hence is predicted to potentially produce dysregulation of choroidal vascular flow. Several authors that have structurally investigated choroidal thickness by means of OCT suggest choroidal thinning [55, 68] particularly in patients with chronic migraine; nevertheless, these studies used OCT technology with limited ability to accurately visualize the posterior choroid. In 2018, Gunes et al. [66] used Enhanced Depth Imaging (EDI) OCT to enable better depth sensitivity for the demarcation of posterior structures. EDI-OCT has demonstrated a choroidal thickening during the immediate migraine attack event, alongside choroidal thinning interictally.

Thicker choroidal measurements immediately during the episode have been proposed to detect acute changes in vascular regulation of the eye in response to the migrainous neurovascular attack [27]. In between episodes, nevertheless, choroidal thinning was proposed to be potentially representative of chronic vascular dysregulation or more permanent vascular damage due to repeated migraine events. It is not possible to establish if this observation serves as evidence for a vascular ocular susceptibility that might contribute to retinal neural degeneration without longitudinal study [27]. Recently, Gouravani et al. [69] found in a meta-analysis that the mean choroidal thickness was significantly thinner in migraineurs than in healthy controls. In addition, the subfoveal choroid was significantly thinner in the MwA than those MwoA. They stated that the alterations of choroidal thickness in migraineurs may be the result of recurrent transient vasospasms supporting the theory of a neurovascular pathophysiology in migraine.

15.1.5 Vascular Perfusion as Measured by OCT Angiography in Migraine

OCT angiography (OCTA), as a functional extension of structural OCT, detects motion contrast with depth resolution and enables an algorithmically derived reconstruction of perfused blood vessels at different retinal layers. OCTA has evolved to be able to image the different capillary plexuses (the radial peripapillary capillary plexus, as well as the superficial, intermediate, and deep capillary plexuses), although known difficulties exist in reliably assessing the deeper vasculature due to projection artefacts, particularly in earlier versions of the technology [27]. Due to the similarities between the microvascular networks, blood-neural barriers and vascular responses of the retina and the brain, there has been growing interest in using OCTA to diagnose potential retinal involvement in brain conditions where cerebrovascular variations may be mirrored in retinal vascular changes [70, 71], including certain studies in migraineurs. Chang et al. [72] used OCTA to assess the macular and peripapillary region in patients with migraine with and without aura, and nonheadache healthy individuals. They found an enlarged foveal avascular zone and reduced superior peripapillary vessel density in the MwA group, but not MwoA group, relative to non-headache controls. The underlying mechanisms and clinical significance of these findings are not well understood. Although it is speculative, increased foveal avascularity could indicate capillary remodelling or be a consequence of microvascular ischemic episodes, whereas reduced vessel density at the optic nerve head could lead to chronic peripapillary hypoperfusion, thereby increasing the risk of glaucoma [27]. Furthermore, the reported decrease in superior peripapillary vessel density was associated by a slight reduction in superior peripapillary RNFL thickness in the MwA individuals. This might indicate that decreased local vascular perfusion in migraineurs may increase susceptibility to local structural damage at the optic disc, corroborating other findings of increased vasospastic tendencies and migraine prevalence in glaucomatous patients [73] and focal ischemic glaucomatous damage to the optic disc [74]. While an attractive hypothesis, the current evidence in the literature for a causal relationship between localised vascular and neural alteration at the optic disc in migraine is very limited, and once again requires longitudinal studies of progression to be established. Since the research of Chang et al. [72], other authors using OCTA in migraineurs have shown contradictory results. Thus, while some studies reported increased size of the foveal avascular zone in patients with migraine compared to non-migraine healthy subjects [72, 75], others found decreased vessel density at different areas of interest (at the macula only [75], at the macula and optic disc [72, 76], or at the superior peripapillary sector only [72]. These differences are due to the absence of systematic protocols for analysis that are robust across imaging platforms.

A possibly critical factor to take into account in the interpretation of OCTA in the context of migraine is age. Older people are more likely to have suffered more migraines over a lifetime and may, therefore, be more susceptible to damage over time due to cumulative episodes [27]. Moreover, ageing is associated with an increased prevalence of vascular co-morbidities (e.g. diabetes), which may lead to greater susceptibility of eyes to neurovascular migrainous events. There are still insufficient OCTA data to conclude the existence of an effect of age in migraine patients.

15.1.6 Clinical Meaning of OCT Findings in Migraine

Given the cross-sectional nature of studies to date, the predictive power of current OCT observations in migraine (e.g., RNFL thinning, decreased retinal vascular perfusion) is not possible to evaluate. While there are reasonable data to suspect that these findings point to neural damage and vascular insufficiency that would increase the risk of glaucoma, in the absence of a carefully constructed longitudinal trial, the positive and negative predictive value of these findings cannot be established. Therefore, the results do not tell us if the reported differences are a result of ischemia over recurrent migraine episodes, or a systemic factor (vasculopathy, vascular dysregulation) that predisposes to retinal microvascular disorders. If due to repeated ischemic attacks, then better management of migraines to reduce event frequency may help to maintain retinal health and decrease the risk of associated ocular disease such as glaucoma. Nevertheless, if a systemic issue, then identifying people with key risk profiles might assist in glaucoma risk appraisal and suggest which patients with glaucoma and a history of migraine are at a greater risk of quick progression [27]. Likewise, longitudinal trials could demonstrate if retinal vascular dysregulation in some patients with migraine is able to predict concurrent development of cortical vascular disorder.

The aim of this update was to review the published data on the etiological and pathogenic mechanisms of migraine. We analyze evidence on the role of OCT for measurement of peripapillary RNFL thickness and macular and choroidal changes in migraineurs. We conclude that there is abundant evidence on cerebral and retrobulbar vascular involvement in the etiology of migraine.

15.2 OCT and Neurosarcoidosis

15.2.1 Introduction

Sarcoidosis is a granulomatous disease of unknown origin that can affect most of the organs of the body, although the lungs, skin, lymph nodes—mainly thoracic—liver and the eyes, are more frequently affected. The non-caseating granulomas are formed by macrophages, epithelioid cells and lymphocytes, and can be found in different organs after an abnormal immune response [77, 78].

Its incidence is low in people from countries such as Japan or Spain (0.2–2 out of 100,000) but is very high in Scandinavian and African origin patients (5–82 out of 100,000). It usually appears before 50 years of age; however, the incidence is higher between 20 and 39 years [77–80].

Sarcoidosis is diagnosed after radiologic, clinical and histologic findings. Differential diagnosis includes other granulomatous diseases, lymphoma, adverse reactions to certain drugs or infections such as tuberculosis or fungal infections [79].

Although often asymptomatic, sarcoidosis can show various clinical signs, depending on the organs that are affected. Common symptoms include fatigue, weakness, asthenia, dry cough, dyspnea, weight loss, fever, erythema nodosum, joint pain, as well as the presence of lymph nodes and night sweating [78, 79].

Sarcoidosis can affect the CNS in 5–16% of cases, thus being called neurosarcoidosis [67, 81–84]. Basal leptomeninges are usually affected, causing cranial polyneuropathies, aseptic meningitis, hydrocephalus and polyradiculopathy. Cranial neuropathies are also frequently present, mainly showing facial palsy, but also alteration of the cranial nerve VIII and, less commonly, nerves V, VI, IX and X. Other possible neurologic symptoms are seizures, fever, headaches or dysfunction of the hypothalamic-pituitary axis [81–85].

The most frequent ophthalmologic finding in sarcoidosis is anterior granulomatous uveitis with mutton-fat endothelial precipitates. Less common ocular manifestations include conjunctival nodules, dry eye, iris nodules, cataract, vitritis, intermediate uveitis with aggregates of inflammatory cells in the vitreous (snowballs), posterior segment uveitis with associated macular edema, epiretinal membrane, branch retinal vein occlusion, choroiditis and perivascular sheathing [77, 79, 86–88].

Nevertheless, in neurosarcoidosis, even though anterior uveitis is still the most common alteration, other important signs that can be found include optic neuropathy, followed by cranial nerve involvement (mainly diplopia caused by common ocular motor nerve palsy) [89–92].

15.2.2 Optic Nerve Changes in Neurosarcoidosis

OCT, and especially SD-OCT, is an excellent noninvasive and noncontact technique, which can be very useful for studying the optic neuropathy present in some cases of neurosarcoidosis. As well as in other neurologic disorders, the measurement of the RNFL thickness can be used to detect structural damage of the optic nerve [49, 93].

Other way of studying the optic neuropathy would be the segmentation of the GCL in the macular area [94–96]. Some articles have studied choroidal, retinal and optic nerve granulomas in sarcoidosis. They are described as hypo or hypereflective homogeneous choroidal thickening with thinning of the overlying choriocapillaris and intrarretinal hyperreflective inflammatory lesions, which can be accompanied by subretinal fluid. Following treatment with corticosteroids, the granulomas significantly decreased their size or even disappeared and, sometimes, subretinal fibrosis and alterations of outer retina and choroid appeared [83, 88, 97–109].

As in other neurologic diseases, OCT can demonstrate alteration of the optic nerve in sarcoidosis. Peripapillary abnormalities of the RNFL could be detected and, even when the patients showed no ophthalmologic clinical signs, the RNFL was thinner when compared with healthy controls, likely being a consequence of previous optic neuropathy. Macular thickness had decreased in numerous patients, probably as a result of neuropathy and/or repeated CME in uveitis. Increased RNFL thickness was found in some patients, probably as a manifestation of optic neuritis [110].

15.2.3 Macular Changes in Neurosarcoidosis

Macular thickness study is also important to evaluate the cystoid macular edema (CME), present in patients with sarcoidosis who develop posterior segment uveitis [77–79].

A few case reports of CME in patients with posterior uveitis or panuveitis and sarcoidosis can also be found. In these cases, OCT helped to make the diagnosis of sarcoidosis and to make a detailed study of the macular edema and its favorable evolution following therapy [88, 110–112].

15.2.4 Choroidal Changes in Neurosarcoidosis

OCT, EDI-OCT and OCTA have proved to be very useful in the assessment of choroid changes in neurosarcoidosis.

Choroidal structure can be studied with EDI-OCT, showing a thickening of the choroid during active posterior uveitis or posterior scleritis, mainly involving Sattler's medium-sized vessel layer, and a thinning of it during inactive phases. Serous retinal detachment can also be present during active inflammation, in the presence of large granulomas or due to secondary choroidal neovascularization [88, 113–115].

Choroidal granulomas are seen as clearly limited, homogeneous hyporeflective lesions with a thinner choriocapillary. Occasionally, choroidal neovascularization can develop at its edge and exudative retinal detachment can be found [88].

15.2.5 Vascular Perfusion as Measured by OCT Angiography in Neurosarcoidosis

OCTA has shown to be a very useful complementary examination to fluorescein angiography (FA) in patients with ocular sarcoidosis. It is even better than FA for the disclosure of macular ischemia.

This technique evaluates the superficial and deep capillary plexuses in the fovea, as well as the choriocapillaris. It shows that the capillary vessels density in the fovea is below normal or event absent in some areas in eyes affected by sarcoidosis. Other alterations found include capillary dropout and hypoperfusion usually in the superficial plexus, and capillary abnormalities most frequently in the deep plexus [88, 116–118].

15.2.6 Clinical Meaning of OCT Findings in Neurosarcoidosis

OCT and its features, including OCTA, EDI-OCT and GCL segmentation, has become an essential part of the ophthalmological examination in disorders like sarcoidosis, that can affect the optic nerve, the retina and the choroid.

It can detect abnormalities in these structures, even if the patient has shown no ophthalmologic symptoms, being also very useful for the follow-up of the disease and its response to the treatment.

15.3 OCT and Schizophrenia

15.3.1 Introduction

Schizophrenia is a devastating mental condition which involves one of the most important psychiatric disorders from the viewpoint of public health [119]. The course of the disease is often chronic and highly variable, causing a great loss of quality of life of patients and their families, as well as a high cost to society. Only in the US up to 2 million people are affected by this disease [120].

Schizophrenia is a clinical syndrome with a variable psychopathology that affects cognition, emotion, perception, and other aspects of human behavior. The expression of these manifestations is different in each patient and varies with time [121, 122]. However, schizophrenia lacks a clearly defined or diagnostic neuropathological signature, and its etiology remains poorly understood. The diagnosis of schizophrenia is still based on clinical history and symptoms observed and reported by the patient [123, 124].

The best validated neuropathological abnormalities include possible reductions of neuronal density in the thalamus, reductions in the number of some interneurons and in the number and function of oligodendrocytes [124]. Neuroimaging techniques such as structural magnetic resonance imaging (sMRI) and functional magnetic resonance imaging (fMRI) have been extensively studied in recent years aiming at developing new diagnostic biomarkers for schizophrenia.

These studies have been very important to try to understand the biological substrate of the disease. The most striking abnormal findings include white and gray matter abnormalities [125–127]. Nevertheless, it is difficult to establish solid conclusions regarding the precise neuropathological changes that underlie these neuroimaging findings [128, 129].

15.3.2 Optic Nerve Changes in Schizophrenia

One of the difficulties in measuring brain volumes in schizophrenic patients with MRI is that the volumetric loss is less than 4% per year, which may be near the limit of detection by MRI, known the precision of the volumetric methods [130, 131]. In the search for new biomarkers in schizophrenia, which may be obtained quickly, non-invasively and with less cost than MRI, lie the observable changes in the retina, as this through the optic nerve is not more than a projection of CNS.

In 2010, we published the first preliminary study relating the schizophrenic disease with RNFL thickness changes measured by OCT [132]. This study showed that patients with schizophrenia have a decreased peripapillary RNFL thickness. This reduction was statistically significant, both in terms of value average (in all four quadrants) RNFL thickness as in relation to nasal quadrant. Posterior studies have supported these findings, Yilmaz et al. reported a reduction in average and nasal RNFL thicknesses in schizophrenic patients [133].

Similar research has been carried out by Chu et al. in patients with schizophrenia [133]. In this study, which included 38 patients with schizophrenia and 11 patients with schizo-affective disorder, no statistically significant differences were found in the RNFL thickness globally and individually in each of its quadrants between healthy controls and patients. However, it was observed that patients with schizo-affective disorder had RNFL nasal quadrant thickness of the right eye statistically decreased than those patients with schizophrenia. This difference from the previous study may be due to these authors recruited patients with first episode of psychosis and included in their sample not only patients with schizophrenia, but also patients with schizo-affective disorder.

Lee et al. reported that schizophrenic patients showed a statistically significant reduction in overall peripapillary RNFL thickness [134]. Furthermore, the degree of thinning and reduction was more significant in the chronic phase of the disease and correlated with the duration of illness [134]. This correlation between illness duration and retinal measurements was not supported by Ascaso et al. [135]. However, they found reduced RNFL measurements only in patients with non-recent illness episodes.

Subsequently, Komatsu et al. observed thinning of the RNFL in schizophrenia spectrum disorders and they suggest that the retinal abnormalities may be applicable as state/trait markers in this disease [136].

15.3.3 Macular Changes in Schizophrenia

Yilmaz et al. also reported a reduction in macular thicknesses of nasal outer and inferior outer quadrants [133].

Moreover, Chu et al. observed an inverse and significant association between the values of macular volume in patients with schizophrenia and schizo-affective disorder and the severity of positive symptomatology. Also, if the analysis considered only the patients with schizophrenia this association between macular volume and severity of positive symptoms was stronger [133].

A posterior study that uses SD-OCT for retina segmentation reports that the GCL and IPL volumes were decreased in the patients with schizophrenia compared with the controls. In addition, the GCL and IPL volumes were lower in the treatment-refractory patients with schizophrenia compared to the treatment responsive patients. They found higher correlations of these two measurements with disease parameters than RNFL thickness [137].

LEE et al. reported that schizophrenic patients also showed a statistically significant reduction in, macular thickness, as well as macular volume [134]. Other study concludes that macular thinning rather than reduced RNFL is an early manifestation in acute schizophrenia patients and can be considered as a potential early biomarker of neurodegeneration in schizophrenia [137].

15.3.4 Choroidal Changes in Schizophrenia

Respect to choroidal thickness, there is a study in which six psychotic patients showed a decreased choroidal thickness compared to age- and sex-matched healthy controls [138].

Given evidence of microvascular disruption in psychosis patients, Chloe Y Li et al. suggested that the pathogenesis of psychotic illness affects choroidal microvasculature in a sex-specific manner [139].

15.3.5 Vascular Perfusion as Measured by OCT Angiography in Schizophrenia

As the human retina and retinal imaging technologies continue to increasingly gain the attention of schizophrenia researchers, Kyle M Green et al. have proposed that the OCT Angiography Offer New Insights and Opportunities in Schizophrenia Research and Treatment [140].

Koman-Wierdak et al. observed the retinal microvascular dysfunction occurs in the macula in patients with schizophrenia but not around optic disc and they suggest that the OCTA can become an essential additional diagnostic tool in detection of psychiatric disorders [141].

Other studies have quantified the retinal microvascular morphology in Schizophrenia Using Swept-Source Optical Coherence Tomography Angiography, and they suggest the presence of microvascular dysfunction associated with early-stage in schizophrenia. Clinical associations with microvascular alterations further implicate this hypothesis, with higher measures being associated with worse symptom severity and functioning in early stages and with lower symptom severity and better functioning in later stages [142, 143].

15.3.6 Clinical Meaning of OCT Findings in Schizophrenia

There is still the controversy in schizophrenia in relation to neurodegenerative model, that begins at about the time of symptoms onset and manifests as progressive volumetric loss thereafter, and neurodevelopmental model that results in abnormal brain volume beginning at an early age [144], so that only longitudinal studies using OCT may help to clarify the underlying neurobiological processes in both models [145, 146].

According to all this studies we could say the retina provides an indirect assessment of inflammation and degeneration in the brain.

15.4 Optical Coherence Tomography in Obstructive Sleep Apnea–Hypopnea Patients

Obstructive sleep apnea-hypopnea syndrome (OSAHS) is part of a broad group of disorders known as "sleep-related breathing disorders". OSAHS is characterized by brief episodes of complete or partial upper airway collapse during sleep, causing an increased thoraco-abdominal effort and decreased arterial oxygen saturation, leading to an arousal response which takes the form of apneas and periodic hypopneas during sleep [147]. This fact produces an excessive daytime sleepiness. Local and systemic inflammation play an important role in the pathogenesis of OSAHS, contributing to anatomic narrowing of the upper airway, increased collapsibility of the airway tissues, and abnormalities in reflexes that affect upper respiratory tract caliber and pharyngeal inspiratory muscle function [148]. In OSAHS, balance between vasodilators, such as nitric oxide, and vasoconstrictors such as endothelin, is disturbed [149]. As well as hypoxia-reoxygenation pattern contributes to the activation of sympathetic system [150]. Moreover, there is some evidence that OSAHS is a risk factor for neurovascular and cardiovascular diseases. Arterial hypertension, cardiac arrhythmia and/or ischemia, congestive heart failure, and cerebrovascular disease are events more likely in the presence of the obstructive sleep disturbance [151, 152].

Clinical features of OSAHS have inspired studies about brain structural abnormalities in this disease [153–156]. Magnetic resonance imaging (MRI) studies have reported two different patterns of cerebral impairment. The first would indicates tissue loss and cellular damage, with gray matter atrophy, cortical thinning and higher white matter diffusivities, it is characteristic of patients with functional daytime impairments such as cognitive dysfunction or sleepiness. The opposite pattern would be characterized by gray matter hypertrophy and lack of white matter hyperintensities, mainly in minimally symptomatic apneic cohorts [157]. Disturbed brain activity in functional MRI studies also show a functional impairment [158, 159] even a persistent impact of sleep apnea on daytime brain resting-state dynamics has been reported [160].

In the last few years, multiple investigators have stablished the relationship between the apneic syndrome and some ophthalmological disorders such as floppy eyelid syndrome [161–168], retinal vein occlusion [169–171], diabetic macular edema [172–175] and non-arteritic anterior ischaemic optic neuropathy [176–178]. Other pathologies as central serous chorioretinopathy [179–184] or certain optic nerve dysfunctions as papilledema [185–187] or glaucoma remain unclear.

Although historically the presence of certain neuropathies such as normotensive and open-angle glaucoma had been associated with obstructive sleep apnea [188–195], the most recent meta-analyses, which consider other confounding factors as obesity, hypertension and diabetes, still cannot establish a causal relationship [196, 197]. Lee et al. [197] proposes as a more relevant research question the value or detriment that the treatment of obstructive sleep apnea with positive pressure devices could exert on the risk of producing glaucoma or its progression.

15.5 Peripapillary RNFL Findings in Apneic Disorder

The latest research reveals a diffuse loss of ganglion cells in the optic nerve of patients with apnea, without the characteristics of glaucomatous neuropathy, including generalized/focal enlargement of the cup, usually at superior and inferior poles, accompanied of visual field defects as nasal step, paracentral or arcuate scotomas, or arcuate blind spot enlargement [198]. Kargi et al. [199] published a diffuse loss of RNFL thickness measured with GDx polarimetry. Sagiv et al. [200] and Lin et al. [201] detected a decreased RNFL thickness in the superior, inferior and temporal quadrants compared with a control group. Reduction in the peripapillary RNFL thickness was also confirmed by Moghimi et al. [202] (with laser polarimetry GDX®), Lin [203], Xin [194] and Gutierrez-Díaz [204]. Nevertheless, they did not exclude patients with glaucoma, what could have influenced their results. Other studies, which eliminated the confounding factor of glaucoma from the study sample, reaffirmed the idea of a diffuse loss in the RNFL without any preferential location [205–207] Zengin et al. [208] described in OSAHS patients a progressive thinning of RNFL thickness, over 1 year-follow up, in spite using CPAP device. In addition, severe OSAHS patients showed a greater decrease of RNFL thickness compared with mild-moderate OSAHS and controls [201, 209]. Furthermore, certain studies have found a significant negative correlation between the RNFL thickness and apnea–hypopnea index (AHI) [199, 208–210].

On the other hand, Casas et al. [211] reported a localized RNFL reduction in nasal sector of optic nerve in OSAHS patients once glaucoma criteria were excluded. Recently, Bussan et al. [212] notice a RNFL thinning focused in the superior and inferior regions of the optic disc and peripapillary region, twenty percent of the study group had to be referred to a glaucoma unit, with a high percentage of diagnosis after study.

Despite these promising impressions, opposing results have also been published. Thus, several authors have found no significant difference between OSAHS and controls regarding the average RNFL thickness [213–217]. Salzgeber et al. [218] found no differences in RNFL and optic nerve morphological parameters in their study with laser polarimetry GDX® and confocal laser scanning HRT II®.

Yuvaci et al. [219] did not report any differences between OSAHS and controls, but they detected a reduction in RNFL after CPAP treatment in patients with severe OSAHS. Therefore, there is no consensus about whether the severity of OSAHS reflects the RNFL thickness.

Although several theories have been proposed, the pathogenesis of optic nerve damage is complex and remains still unknown. Thus, recurrent episodes of nocturnal hypoxia during apnea may result in direct anoxic damage, or in an indirect effect on optic nerve head blood flow, vascular dysregulation of the optic nerve by OSAHS could result from hypoxia-induced imbalance between nitric oxide and endothelin [220]. Another presumption is the recurrent papilledema, which would be secondary to a hypoxemic cerebral vasodilation phenomenon. The perpetuation of RNFL swelling could lead to a cellular loss, with the consequent thinning of RNFL as the disease progresses [211]. Based on this idea, Huseyinoglu et al. [209] do not approve OCT to demonstrate neurodegeneration in OSAHS patients, considering that different confusing data such as normal or increased RNFL thickness as a result of optic nerve subtle edema, could mask possible peripapillary axonal loss (Fig. 15.1).

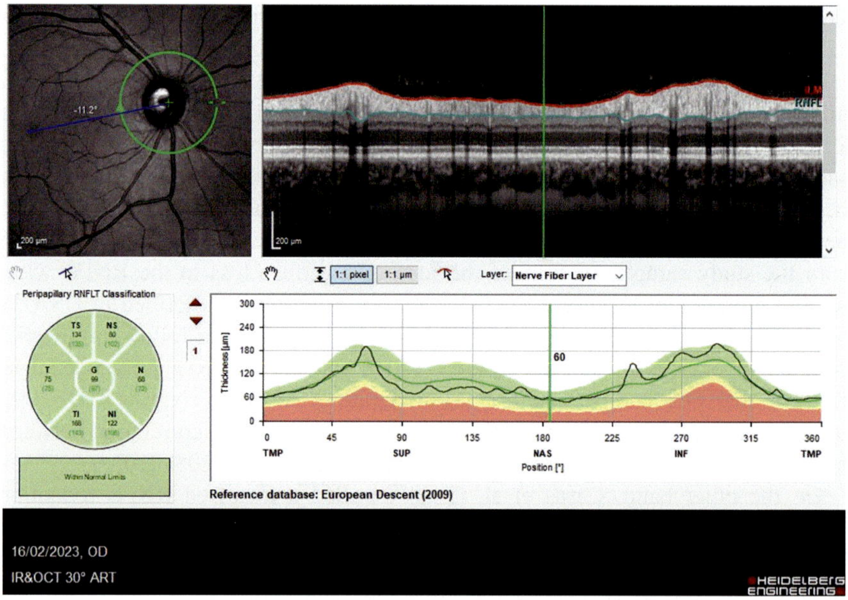

Fig. 15.1 Heidelberg Spectralis® Optical Coherence tomography for RNFL examination in an OSAHS patient

15.5.1 Macular and Choroidal Findings in Apneic Disorder

Regarding macular thickness, Casas et al. [211] reported that temporal inner macular thickness was significantly higher in mild–moderate OSAHS compared to severe patients and controls. When SD-OCT segmentation was applied, Ferrández et al. [221] not described any difference between controls and OSAHS in macular GCL and ganglion cell-inner plexiform layer (GC-IPL) thicknesses. Nevertheless, Kara et al. [216] reported that average GC-IPL and minimum GC-IPL thicknesses were significantly lower in severe OSAHS group than in healthy controls. Moreover, there was a significant negative correlation between AHI and both average GCL and IPL. Guven et al. [222] found a macular layer thinning including both the inner and outer retina with photoreceptor and ganglion cell layers in OSAHS patients, unrelated to the disease severity. Unlike previous studies described, Chalkiadaki et al. [223] described a positive correlation between the mean apnea–hypopnea duration (MAD) and GC-IPL thickness, patients with MAD > 30 s have significantly thicker GC-IPL.

Xin et al. [224] found that foveal and macular thickness in nasal area of healthy individuals were significantly thinner than those in OSAHS patients with severe disorder, whereas subfoveal and nasal choroid were thinner in severe OSAHS comparing to controls. They suggested that a sympathetic nervous regulation disorder exists in OSAHS patients because of chronic intermittent hypoxia, which is followed by changes in the structure of the normal retina and choroid. However, the authors did not exclude the subjects having systemic diseases, such as arterial hypertension, that could be a possible error source. Bahyan et al. [225] and Yazgan et al. [206] confirm the difference in choroidal thickness between severe OSAHS versus moderate-controls in a group of patients without systemic pathologies. Uslu et al. [226] found an increase in choroidal thicknesses after 12 month of CPAP therapy. On the other hand, Yuvaci et al. [227] and Naranjo-Bonilla et al. [228] observed a thinning in OSAHS choroidal thickness after treatment was administered.

The proposed hypothesis for these findings is in relation with the double retinal blood supply from the central retinal artery and the choroid. The inner retina is provided by retinal blood vessels and is sensitive to tissue oxygen partial pressure changes. Thus, anoxia may result in an increased blood flow to the retina [229]. On the other hand, outer retina and choroid is supplied by choroidal system. The adaptation of choroidal resistance is achieved through the sympathetic nervous system [230]. The hypoxia-reoxygenation pattern and sleep fragmentation associated with OSAHS contribute to the activation of sympathetic system. Thus, expecting choroidal structural changes is reasonable.

There are also studies presenting no macular and choroidal disturbances in apneic patients [201, 231–233]. Zengin et al. [231] and Karaca et al. [232] compared choroidal thickness in patients recently diagnosed with OSAHS and healthy controls and found that the difference in mean choroidal thickness was not statistically significant. Furthermore, choroidal thickness did not significantly differ among the mild, moderate, and severe OSAHS groups and no correlation between

AHI and choroidal thickness was found [231, 232, 234]. Khayi et al. [233] did not found any differences in choroidal vascular responses to posture and exercise between healthy control subjects and healthy OSAHS patients. Similar results were reported by Lin et al. [201] regarding to macular thickness in OSAHS patients and controls.

Tonini et al. [235] studied vascular choroidal reactivity during hyperoxia and hypercapnia with choroidal laser Doppler flowmetry. Patients with OSAHS without comorbidities and control subjects exhibited similar choroidal reactivity during hyperoxia and hypercapnia. The authors suggested that other microvascular comorbidities as atherosclerosis or arterial hypertension have an important role in the choroidal vascular regulation and healthy individuals with OSAHS have long-term adaptive mechanisms active in ocular microcirculation.

With the recent arrival of the OCTA some articles have been published on the peripapillary and macular microvasculature in patients with OSAHS. Apparently, a decreased vessel density in peripapillary and parafoveal areas with a larger foveal avascular zone could be found in patients with apneic disorder, moreover OCTA could be negatively correlated with AHI [236–240]. These results are controversial, Moyal et al. [241], in a sample of 53 eyes with OSAHS, did not find differences when the macular, optic nerve head and radial peripapillary capillaries vessel density were compared to healthy control eyes. Cai et al. found no differences regarding the foveal avascular area in a population of twenty-six OSAHS patients [242].

15.6 OCT in Bipolar Disorder

Bipolar disorder (BD) is a chronic psychiatric disease that alternates episodes of mania with episodes of depression. It is a major public health problem, with an estimated prevalence ranging from 1 to 6% of the general population [243, 244]. There are many published articles on morphological (mostly OCT, and recently also OCTA), morphological-functional correlations, published in recent years reporting retinal axonal loss in these patients.

15.7 Morphological Studies

Kalenderoglu et al. [245] compared the GCL volume and RNFL thickness in 43 BD patients and 43 healthy subjects by using SD-OCT. Patients showed a lower RNFL thickness com- pared with controls at all measured regions, and this reduction was statistically significant for the global RNFL value. The GCL volume was also significantly lower in the patient group. A negative correlation between some disorder parameters, such as duration of the disease and number of hospitalizations, and GCL volume. According to the authors, these findings would reflect that neurodegeneration occurs during the course of BD. This degeneration may be demonstrated by reduced GCL at early phases, and as the disorder progresses, involvement of other retinal layers, such as the RNFL and IPL, may be observed.

Khalil et al. [246] compared 40 inpatients with BD to 40 matched healthy controls. BD patients showed thinning of RNFL and reduced GCC in comparison with control individuals. Age at onset, number of episodes, and disease severity did not significantly correlate with SD-OCT measurements. Furthermore, Mehraban et al. [247], by using SD-OCT, compared the peripapillary RNFL thickness in 60 eyes corresponding to 30 patients with BD and 60 eyes of 30 age-matched controls. Reduction of peripapillary RNFL thickness was reported in BD patients and is related to the duration of disorder. They conclude that RNFL thickness might be a beneficial biomarker for studying neurodegenerative changes over time to detect the severity and duration of the disease. Finally, Polo et al. [248] have used the recent swept source (SS) technology for OCT in the study of retinal changes in 23 patients with BD and 23 healthy subjects. They reported that BD patients were shown to have significant thinning of full retinal thickness and the GCL in the macular area, as well as a peripapillary reduction of the RNFL and GCL thickness. The authors state that the analysis of the retinal sublayers with SS-OCT might be a useful marker to demonstrate degeneration and monitor disease progression in BD.

Kilicarslan et al. [249] evaluated the OCT findings and oxidative stress parameters in patients with BD and their unaffected first-degree relatives (FDRs). They found that total oxidant status (TOS) was higher in patients with BD and FDRs than healthy controls (HCs) ($p < 0.001$ and $p = 0.012$, respectively). Disulfide (DIS), oxidative stress index (OSI), and 4-hydroxy-2-none-nal (HNE) levels were higher in patients with BD and FDRs than HCs ($p < 0.001$). Total thiol (TT), native thiol (NT), and total antioxidant status (TAS) levels were lower in patients and FDRs than HCs ($p < 0.001$). Minimum foveal thicknesses (MFT) and central macular thicknesses (CMT) of patients with BD was thinner than HCs ($p = 0.001$ and $p = 0.006$, respectively). The groups did not differ on RNFL and choroidal thickness or GCL and IPL volume.

Ayık et al. [250] investigated the retinal changes in BD patients and their healthy siblings (HS) by comparing them with the healthy control (HC) group and to explore these findings as potential endophenotype candidates. They found that the mean RNFL thicknesses did not differ between groups. All GCL+IPL thicknesses were found to be significantly lower in the patient and sibling groups compared to the HCs. GCL+IPL thicknesses were significantly correlated with functionality of patients and severity of the disorder.

Onur et al. [251] evaluated the relationship between OCT findings and suicidal behavior (SB) in patients with bipolar disorder type 1 (BPD1) in comparison to healthy controls.

They analyzed forty-five euthymic BPD1 patients with previous suicide attempts (BPD1+), 46 euthymic BPD1 patients without previous suicide attempts (BPD1−) and 63 healthy controls. All OCT measures were lower in patients with BPD1 than healthy controls ($p < 0.001$). No significant differences were found between (BPD1+) and (BPD1−) in all GCC levels and inferior RNFL values (p

> 0.05), however the superior RNFL and global RNFL values were found to be lower in the (BPD1+) than in the (BPD1−) ($p = 0.037$, $p = 0.028$, respectively). Moreover, global RNFL predicted suicide risk in a multivariate logistic regression model ($p = 0.024$ Exp(B):0.930).

Liu et al. [252] analyzed the correlation of the clinical data with retinal nerve fiber layer (RNFL) thickness and macular thickness in bipolar disorder patients and major depression patients. The aim of this study is to explore factors that affect RNFL thickness in BD patients and major depression (MDD) patients, with a view to providing a new diagnostic strategy. They found that RNFL and macula lutea in BD and MDD patients were thinner than control. Triglyceride and uric acid (UA) levels were the highest in the BD group, while alanine aminotransferase (ALT) and glutamic oxalacetic transaminase (AST) levels in the MDD group. Age onset and ALT were positively while UA was negatively correlated with RNFL thickness in BD patients. Cholesterol level was positively correlated with RNFL thickness while the duration of illness was correlated with RNFL thickness of left eye in MDD patients.

Khalil and Said [253] evaluated changes in OCT parameters including peripapillary RNFL thickness and GCC thickness in Egyptian patients with BD, and correlated them with disease severity and clinical characteristics. They reported thinning of average (RNFL) and average (GCC) thickness of right and left eye in patients with BPD (whether received electroconvulsive therapy or not) compared to control, but the number of episodes, age at onset and severity of disease showed insignificant correlation with OCT parameters.

Cokunlu et al. [254] investigated the possible differences in OCT parameters during euthymic, manic, and depressive episodes in patients diagnosed with BD. Ganglion cell complex thicknesses were increased in in perifoveal superior and perifoveal inferior quadrants in BD patient group vs control ($p < 0.001$, $p < 0.001$).

Gokcinar et al. [255] compared the retinal changes between patients with BD and healthy individuals. They found that BD was significantly associated with a decrease in the average peripapillary RNFL, with the average peripapillary total retinal (TR), and with the average ganglion cell complexes (GCC) thickness ($P = 0.033$, $P = 0.008$, and $P = 0.009$, respectively). The peripapillary RNFL and TR thinnings were prominent in the superior ($P = 0.039$, $P = 0.033$, respectively) and inferior quadrants ($P = 0.031$, $P = 0.018$, respectively). The BD effects on GCC thinning was prominent in the superior half ($P = 0.001$) and in the nasal sectors (except in the inner superonasal sector; all $P < 0.05$). BD was associated with a decrease in macular TR thickness only at the inner superior sector ($P = 0.014$). Moreover, disease duration was inversely correlated with the peripapillary RNFL, TR, and macular GCC thicknesses ($P < 0.05$).

Altun et al. investigated the effects of drugs used in bipolar disorder (BD) on retinal nerve fiber layer (RNFL) and macular thickness. Serum valproate level was a significant positive predictor of thickness in the right macular inferior outer, left macular nasal outer region, right RNFL inferotemporal, left temporal and inferotemporal regions, what implies that valproate has neuroprotective effects on the optic nerve and macula.

Koman-Wierdak et al. [141] measured RNFL and vasculature around the optic disc and in the macula in with BD using OCTA. They found that the macular thickness in the whole vascular complex and in the fovea was significantly lower in BD than in the control group, but the radiant peripapillary vascular density and RNFL thickness were similar.

Bannai et al. [256] analyzed retinal layer topography in psychosis and its correlation with clinical and imaging parameters. No thinning was noted for the retinal nerve fiber, ganglion cell or inner plexiform layers. On the other hand, they found significant thinning in the right inner temporal, right central, and left inner superior quadrants of the outer nuclear layer (ONL) in probands compared to control. Thickening of the outer plexiform layer (OPL) was observed in the right inner temporal, left inner superior, and left inner temporal quadrants. The right inner temporal and left inner superior quadrants of both the OPL and ONL showed significant inverse correlations. Retinal pigment epithelium thinning correlated with worse mania symptoms and thinning in the ONL was associated with worse cognitive function. ONL thinning was also associated with smaller total brain and white matter volume.

Orduna et al. [257] assessed the ability of the new Spectralis OCT Posterior Pole protocol to detect degeneration of the inner retinal layers in patients with BD and evaluated the correlation between the neuroretinal thickness and disease duration.

They found differences ($p < 0.05$) in RNFL and GCL thickness between BD patients and healthy controls, in parafoveal and perifoveal cells respectively. Significant inverse correlations were found between RNFL and GCL thinning at their thickest location and the duration of bipolar disorder. Several predictive variables were observed with a binary logistic regression for the presence/absence of BD: cell 1.3 RNFL ($p = 0.028$) and GCL in cells 7.8 ($p = 0.012$), 2.7 ($p = 0.043$) and 1.3 ($p = 0.047$).

Polo et al. [248] evaluated the ability of SS-OCT to detect retinal changes in patients with BD. Patients with BD were shown to have significant thinning of the macular full retinal thickness in the center ($p = 0.049$), inner temporal ($p = 0.045$), inner nasal ($p = 0.016$), and inner inferior ($p = 0.016$) of the ETDRS areas. The macular GCL layer was reduced in patients compared with controls (average, $p = 0.002$; superior, $p = 0.009$; superonasal, $p = 0.009$; inferonasal, $p = 0.003$; and inferior, $p = 0.009$). Peripapillary reduction of full retinal thickness (average, $p < 0.001$; superotemporal, $p < 0.001$; superonasal, $p = 0.003$; nasal, $p = 0.005$; and inferotemporal, $p = 0.033$), GCL (nasal, $p = 0.025$), and RNFL thickness (average, $p = 0.002$; superotemporal, $p < 0.001$; and superonasal, $p = 0.045$) was observed in patients compared with controls. No significant differences were observed in choroidal thickness measurements.

15.7.1 Morphological-Functional Correlations

Satue et al. [258] assessed the visual and retinal changes in patients with BD over 5 years, compared with controls. Visual function parameters, including visual acuity, contrast sensitivity vision with the Pelli Robson and CSV 1000E tests in BD patients remained unchanged during the follow-up period. A progressive decrease affecting macular and peripapillary RNFL thickness ($p < 0.050$) was observed in patients. Progressive changes in BD were more pronounced when compared with healthy controls ($p < 0.050$). A significant correlation between GCL thickness changes and disease duration was found (GCL outer temporal, $r = -0.680$, $p = 0.016$; GCL central, $r = -0.540$, $p = 0.038$).

García-Martín et al. [259] evaluated visual and retinal changes in patients with bipolar disorder and analyzed the correlation between structural changes and visual function parameters. Patients with BD presented worse color vision compared with controls (Lanthony's index, $P = 0.002$). Full macular thickness, the retinal nerve fiber layer (RNFL), ganglion cell layer, and inner plexiform layer were reduced in patients compared with healthy individuals ($P < 0.005$). The inner nuclear layer was significantly thickened in patients ($P < 0.005$). Peripapillary RNFL thickness was reduced in all temporal sectors ($P < 0.005$). Significant correlations were found between visual acuity and the RNFL thickness, the Pelli-Robson score and the inner plexiform layer, and between the Lanthony's color index and the ganglion cell layer thickness.

15.7.2 Retinal Microvascularity Studies

Mustafa and Turgay [260] evaluated vascular changes by OCTA in patients with BD. In the multivariate regression model, such variables as nasal quadrant of retinal nerve fiber layer, inferior and nasal quadrants of radial peripapillary capillary plexus and superficial vessel density variables were determined to have a significant and independent effect in differentiating patients with BD from the participants in the healthy control group.

Li et al. [261] sought to determine evidence of microvascular disruption in the choroids in patients with psychosis by swept-source optical coherence tomography angiography. Male patients had significantly lower choroid vascular density, whereas female patients had significantly lower maximum choroid thickness with correspondingly decreased choroid vascular volume vs controls, after adjusting for age. When all psychiatric patients were compared with controls, no significant differences in CT, CVD, or CVV were noted.

15.7.3 AI-Based Studies

Sánchez-Morla et al. [262] explored the diagnosis of BD based on OCT data which are analyzed using artificial intelligence. BD patients presented retinal thinning affecting most layers, compared to controls. The retinal thickness of the parafoveolar area showed a high capacity to discriminate BD subjects from healthy individuals, specifically for the ganglion cell (area under the curve (AUC) = 0.82) and internal plexiform (AUC = 0.83) layers. The best classifier showed an accuracy of 0.95 for classifying BD versus controls, using as variables of the feature vector the IPL (inner nasal region) and the INL (outer nasal and inner inferior regions) thickness.

15.8 Conclusions

The accumulation of different studies in this field led to the recent few review articles [263–265]. Moreover, Lizano et al. [266] conducted a meta-analysis of the retinal layers' abnormalities in patients with BD. The peripapillary retinal nerve fiber layer (RNFL) showed significant thinning in BD eyes compared to control eyes ($n = 12$, SMD = $-$ 0.74, $-$ 0.51, $-$ 1.06, respectively). RNFL thinning was greatest in the nasal, temporal, and superior regions. The combined peripapillary ganglion cell layer and inner plexiform layer (GCL-IPL) showed significant thinning in BD eyes compared to control eyes ($n = 4$, SMD = $-$ 0.39, $-$ 0.44, $-$ 0.28, respectively). No statistically significant differences were identified in other retinal or choroidal regions. Clinical variables were unrelated to the RNFL or GCL-IPL thickness by meta- regression.

Among all the retinal parameters evaluated, RNFL thickness is undoubtedly the one that has provided the most significant findings in the BD. Great majority of the studies conducted on patients BD showed significant thinning compared with the healthy controls. Other retinal layers, GCL (ganglion cell layer) and IPL (inner plexiform layer), were also proposed as potential markers for neurodegenerative progression and prognosis. The RNFL may indicate axonal damage in the chronic phase. Differences between changes in GCL and RNFL could help evaluate inflammatory symptoms and reactive gliosis in axons. These parameters may also indicate disease progression and stage. The RNFL might be a marker of inflammation in the active phase, while the INL (inner nuclear layer) could be explored as a marker of chronic inflammation. These markers could be useful for assessing the efficacy of new neuroprotective or anti-inflammatory treatments. Additionally, GCL and INL could aid in the differential diagnosis between unipolar and bipolar disorder. Several measurements associated with familial psychiatric history might serve as potential biomarkers for an at-risk mental state. However, further research is required to confirm and clarify these findings. Investigating mood disorders at different stages and assessing all retinal layers could determine whether these values are reliable biomarkers in a clinical setting. Incorporating different approaches, such as combining structural and functional parameters with biological values, could lead to specific profiles for mood disorders like major depressive disorder (MDD) and bipolar disorder (BD). This research could improve understanding of the variability in their pathophysiology and enhance treatment strategies [265].

References

1. Ascaso FJ, Marco S, Mateo J, Martínez M, Esteban O, Grzybowski A. Optical coherence tomography in patients with chronic migraine: literature review and update. Front Neurol. 2017;8:684.
2. Giffin NJ, Ruggiero L, Lipton RB, et al. Premonitory symptoms in migraine: an electronic diary study. Neurology. 2003;60:935–40.
3. Vecchia D, Pietrobon D. Migraine: a disorder of brain excitatoryinhibitory balance? Trends Neurosci. 2012;35:507–20.
4. Dinkin M. Trans-synaptic retrograde degeneration in the human visual system: slow, silent, and real. Curr Neurol Neurosci Rep. 2017;17:16.
5. Lin X, Yi Z, Zhang X, Liu Q, Cai R, Chen C, Zhang H, Zhao P, Pan P. Retinal nerve fiber layer changes in migraine: a protocol for systematic review and meta-analysis. Medicine. 2020;99:33.
6. Karsan N, Goadsby PJ. Biological insights from the premonitory symptoms of migraine. Nat Rev Neuro. 2018;14:699–710.
7. Bose P, Goadsby PJ. The migraine postdrome. Curr Opin Neurol. 2016;29:299–301.
8. The International Classification of Headache Disorders. 2nd edition. Headache Classification Subcommittee of the International Headache Society. Cephalalgia 2004; 24:9–160.
9. Sharma P, Sridhar J, Mehta S. Flashes and floaters. Prim Care. 2015;42:425–35.
10. Charles A, Hansen JM. Migraine-aura: new ideas about cause, classification and clinical significance. Curr Opin Neurol. 2015;28:255–60.
11. Ripa P, Ornello R, Degan D, Tiseo C, Stewart J, Pistoia F, et al. Migraine in menopausal women: a systematic review. Int J Womens Health. 2015;20:773–82.
12. Buse DC, Silberstein SD, Manack AN, et al. Psychiatric comorbidities of episodic and chronic migraine. J Neurol. 2013;260:1960–9.
13. Wang SJ, Chen PK, Fuh JL. Comorbidities of migraine. Front Neurol. 2010;1:16.
14. Jacobs B, Dussor G. Neurovascular contributions to migraine: moving beyond vasodilation. Neurosci. 2016;338:133–44.
15. GBD Neurology Collaborators. Global, regional, and national burden of neurological disorders, 1990–2016: a systematic analysis for the Global Burden of Disease Study 2016. Lancet Neurol. 2019;18:459–80.
16. Pietrobon D, Striessnig J. Neurobiology of migraine. Nat Rev Neurosci. 2003;4:386–98.
17. Waters WE, O'Connor PJ. Prevalence of migraine. J Neurol Neurosurg Psychiatry. 1975;38:613–6.
18. Friberg L, Olesen J, Lassen NA, Olsen TS, Karle A. Cerebral oxygen extraction, oxygen consumption, and regional cerebral blood flow during the aura phase of migraine. Stroke. 1994;25:974–9.
19. Steiner TJ, Stovner LJ, Birbeck GL. Migraine: the seventh disabler. Headache. 2013;53:227–9.
20. Malone CD, Bhowmick A, Wachholtz AB. Migraine: treatments, comorbidities, and quality of life, in the USA. J Pain Res. 2015;12:537–47.
21. Global, regional, and national incidence, prevalence, and years lived with disability for 328 diseases and injuries for 195 countries, 1990–2016: a systematic analysis for the Global Burden of Disease Study 2016. Lancet 2017; 390:1211–59.

22. Global, regional, and national incidence, prevalence, and years lived with disability for 310 diseases and injuries, 1990–2015: a systematic análisis for the Global Burden of Disease Study 2015. Lancet 2016; 388:1545–602.
23. Woldeamanuel YW, Cowan RP. Migraine affects 1 in 10 people worldwide featuring recent rise: a systematic review and meta-analysis of community-based studies involving 6 million participants. J Neurol Sci. 2017;372:307–15.
24. Goadsby P, Charbit A, Andreou A, Akerman S, Holland P. Neurobiology of migraine. Neurosci. 2009;161:327–41.
25. Ayata C. Cortical spreading depression triggers migraine attack: pro. Headache J Head Face Pain. 2010;50:725–30.
26. Raga I, Povedano FJ, Hernández J, López F. Decrease retinal thickness in patients with chronic migraine evaluated by optical coherence tomography. Diagnostics. 2023;13:5.
27. McKendrick AM, Nguyen BN. The eye in migraine: a review of retinal imaging findings in migraine. Clin Exp Optom. 2022;105:186–93.
28. Burstein R, Noseda R, Borsook D. Migraine: multiple processes, complex pathophysiology. J Neurosci. 2015;35:6619–29.
29. Cutrer FM. Pathophysiology of migraine. Semin Neurol. 2010;30:120–30.
30. Karalezli A, Simsek C, Celik G, Eroglu FC. Evaluation of choroidal thickness using spectral-domain optical coherence tomography in migraine patients during acute migraine attacks: a comparative study. Eye. 2014;28:1477–81.
31. Demircan S, Atas M, Yüksel SA, Ulusoy MD, Yuvacı I, Arifoglu HB, Baskan B, Zararsız G. The impact of migraine on posterior ocular structures. J Ophthalmol. 2015;2015: 868967.
32. Abdul-Rahman AM, Gilhotra JS, Selva D. Dynamic focal retinal arteriolar vasospasm in migraine. Indian J Ophthalmol. 2011;59:51–3.
33. Gipponi S, Scaroni N, Venturelli E, et al. Reduction in retinal nerve fiber layer thickness in migraine patients. Neurol Sci. 2013;34:841–5.
34. Zengin MO, Elmas Z, Cinar E, et al. Choroidal thickness changes in patients with migraine. Acta Neurol Belg. 2015;115:33–7.
35. Gabriele ML, Wollstein G, Ishikawa H, Kagemann L, Xu J, Folio LS, Schuman JS. Optical coherence tomography: history, current status, and laboratory work. Investig Ophthalmol Vis Sci. 2011;52:2425–36.
36. Huang D, Swanson EA, Lin CP, Schuman JS, Stinson WG, Chang W, Hee MR, Flotte T, Gregory K, Puliafito CA, et al. Optical coherence tomography. Science. 1991;254:1178–81.
37. Drexler W, Sattmann H, Hermann B, Ko TH, Stur M, Unterhuber A, et al. Enhanced visualization of macular pathology with the use of ultrahigh-resolution optical coherence tomography. Arch Ophthalmol. 2003;121:695–706.
38. Fercher AF. Optical coherence tomography—development, principles, applications. Z Med Phys. 2010;20:251–76.
39. McCabe JM, Croce KJ. Optical coherence tomography. Circulation. 2012;126:2140–3.
40. Mwanza J-C, Oakley JD, Budenz DL, et al. Macular ganglion cell-inner plexiform layer: automated detection and thickness reproducibility with spectral domain-optical coherence tomography in glaucoma. Invest Ophthalmol Vis Sci. 2011;52:8323–9.
41. Kim KE, Yoo BW, Jeoung JW, et al. Long-term reproducibility of macular ganglion cell analysis in clinically stable glaucoma patients. Invest Ophthalmol Vis Sci. 2015;56:4857–64.
42. Tatham AJ, Medeiros FA. Detecting structural progression in glaucoma with optical coherence tomography. Ophthalmology. 2017;124:S57-65.
43. Chen JJ. Optical coherence tomography and neuro-ophthalmology. J Neuroophthalmol. 2018;38:e5-8.
44. Trick GL, Calotti FY, Skarf B. Advances in imaging of the optic disc and retinal nerve fiber layer. J Neuroophthalmol. 2006;26:284–95.
45. Fujimoto J, Swanson E. The development, commercialization, and impact of optical coherence tomography. Invest Ophthalmol Vis Sci. 2016;57:1–3.
46. Sergott RC, Balcer LJ. The latest on optical coherence tomography. J Neuroophthalmol. 2014;34:S1–2.

47. Savino PJ. Evaluation of the retinal nerve fiber layer: descriptive or predictive? J Neuroophthalmol. 2009;29:245–9.
48. Costello FE. Optical coherence tomography technologies: which machine do you want to own? J Neuroophthalmol. 2014;34:S3–9.
49. Galetta KM, Calabresi PA, Frohman EM, Balcer LJ. Optical coherence tomog-raphy (OCT): imaging the visual pathway as a model for neurodegeneration. Neurother. 2011;8:117–32.
50. Monterio ML, Fermandes DB, Apóstolos-Pereira SL, Callegaro D. Quantification of retinal neural loss in patients with neuromyelitis optica and multiple sclerosis with or without optic neuritis using Fourier-domain optical coherence tomography. Invest Ophthalmol Vis Sci. 2012;53:3959–66.
51. Martinez A, Proupim N, Sanchez M. Retinal nerve fibre layer thickness measurements using optical coherence tomography in migraine patients. Br J Ophthalmol. 2008;92:1069–75.
52. Martínez A, Proupim N, Sanchez M. Scanning laser polarimetry with variable corneal compensation in migraine patients. Acta Ophthalmol. 2009;87:746–53.
53. Sorkhabi R, Mostafaei S, Ahoor M, Talebi M. Evaluation of retinal nerve fiber layer thickness in migraine. Iran J Neurol. 2013;12:51–5.
54. Yülek F, Dirik EB, Eren Y, Simavlı H, Ugurlu N, Cagil N, et al. Macula and retinal nerve fiber layer in migraine patients: analysis by spectral domain optic coherence tomography. Semin Ophthalmol. 2015;30:124–8.
55. Reggio E, Chisari CG, Ferrigno G, Patti F, Donzuso G, Sciacca G, et al. Migraine causes retinal and choroidal structural changes: evaluation with ocular coherence tomography. J Neurol. 2017;264:494–502.
56. Simsek IB. Retinal nerve fibre layer thickness of migraine patients with or with-out white matter lesions. Neuroophthalmol. 2016;41:7–11.
57. Abdellatif MK, Fouad MM. Effect of duration and severity of migraine on retinal nerve fiber layer, ganglion cell layer, and choroidal thickness. Eur J Ophthalmol. 2018;28:714–21.
58. Ao R, Wang R, Yang M, et al. Altered retinal nerve fiber layer thickness and choroid thickness in patients with migraine. Eur Neurol. 2018;80:130–7.
59. Yener AÜ, Korucu O. Quantitative analysis of the retinal nerve fiber layer, ganglion cell layer and optic disc parameters by the swept source optical coherence tomography in patients with migraine and patients with tension-type headache. Acta Neurol Belg. 2019;119:541–8.
60. Simsek IB, Aygun D, Yildiz S. Retinal nerve fibre layer thickness in migraine patients with or without aura. Neuroophthalmol. 2015;39:17–21.
61. Lin X, Yi Z, Zhang X, et al. Retinal nerve fiber layer changes in migraine: a systematic review and meta-analysis. Neurol Sci. 2021;42:871–81.
62. Rego D, Burgos B, Ginés C, Carrasco M, De Santos MT, Santos E. Retinal nerve fiber layer analysis in children with migraine with and without aura using optical coherence tomography: a case-control study. J Pediatr Ophthalmol Strabismus. 2022;1:7.
63. Keller J, Sánchez-Dalmau BF, Villoslada P. Lesions in the posterior visual pathway promote trans-synaptic degeneration of retinal ganglion cells. PLoS One. 2014;9: e97444.
64. Gupta S, Zivadinov R, Ramanathan M, Weinstock-Guttman B. Optical coherence tomography and neurodegeneration: are eyes the windows to the brain? Expert Rev Neurother. 2016;16:765–75.
65. Cankaya C, Tecellioglu M. Foveal thickness alterations in patients with migraine. Med Arch. 2016;70:123–6.
66. Gunes A, Karadag AS, Yazgan S, et al. Evaluation of retinal nerve fibre layer, ganglion cell layer and choroidal thickness with optical coherence tomography in migraine patients: a case-control study. Clin Exp Optom. 2018;101:109–15.
67. Kara SA, Erdemoglu AK, Karadeniz MY, et al. Color Doppler sonography of orbital and vertebral arteries in migraineurs without aura. J Clin Ultrasound. 2003;31:308–14.
68. Ekinci M, Ceylan E, Cagatay HH, et al. Retinal nerve fibre layer, ganglion cell layer and choroid thinning in migraine with aura. BMC Ophthalmol. 2014;14:75.

69. Gouravani M, Salehi MA, Mohammadi S, et al. Choroidal thickness in eyes of migraine patients measured using spectral domain-optical coherence tomography: a meta-analysis. Surv Ophthalmol. 2023;68:67–77.
70. Tsokolas G, Tsaousis KT, Diakonis VF, et al. Optical coherence tomography angiography in neurodegenerative diseases: a review. Eye Brain. 2020;12:73–87.
71. Pellegrini M, Vagge A, Ferro Desideri LF, et al. Optical coherence tomography angiography in neurodegenerative disorders. J Clin Med. 2020;9(6):1706.
72. Chang MY, Phasukkijwatana N, Garrity S, et al. Foveal and peripapillary vascular decrement in migraine with aura demonstrated by optical coherence tomography angiography. Invest Ophthalmol Vis Sci. 2017;58:5477–84.
73. Alizadeh R, Vickers L, Hirunpatravong P, et al. A phenotype of primary open-angle glaucoma with systemic vasospasm. J Glaucoma. 2018;27:987–92.
74. Broadway DC, Drance SM. Glaucoma and vasospasm. Br J Ophthalmol. 1998;82:862–70.
75. Tasli NG, Ersoy A. Altered macular vasculature in migraine patients without aura: is it associated with ocular vasculature and White matter hyperintensities? J Ophthalmol. 2020;2020:3412490.
76. Ulusoy MO, Horasanli B, Kal A. Retinal vascular density evaluation of migraine patients with and without aura and association with White matter hyperintensities. Acta Neurol Belg. 2019;119:411–7.
77. Whitcup SM. Sarcoidosis. In: Nussenblatt RB, Whitcup SM, editors. Uveitis. Fundamentals and clinical practice. 3rd ed. Philadelphia: Mosby; 2004. p. 301–10.
78. Ianuzzi MC, Rybicki BA, Teirstein AS. Sarcoidosis. N Eng J Med. 2007;357:2153–65.
79. Nunes H, Bouvry D, Valeyre D. Sarcoidosis. Orphanet J Rare Dis. 2007;2:46.
80. Reich JM. A critical analysis of sarcoidosis incidence assessment. Multidiscip Respir Med. 2013;8:57.
81. Hoyle JC, Jablonski C, Newton HB. Neurosarcoidosis: clinical review of a disorder with challenging inpatient presentations and diagnostic considerations. Neurohospitalist. 2014;4:94–101.
82. Nowak DA, Widenka DC. Neurosarcoidosis: a review of its intracranial manifestation. J Neurol. 2001;248:363–72.
83. Desai A, Chaon B, Berkenstock M. Neurosarcoidosis and ocular inflammation: a case series and literature review. J Neuro-Ophthalmol. 2021;41:e259–66.
84. Hendersosn A, Tian J, Carey AR. Neuro-ophthalmic manifestations of sarcoidosis. J Neuro-Ophthalmol. 2021;41(4):e591–7.
85. Titlic M, Bradic-Hammoud M, Miric L, Punda A. Clinical manifestations of neurosarcoidosis. Bratisl Lev Listy. 2009;110:576–9.
86. Bezo C, Majzoub S, Nochez Y, Leruez S, Charlin JF, Milea D, Pisella PJ. Sarcoïdose oculaire et neuro-ophtalmologique: étude retrospective sur 30 cas. J Fr Ophtalmol. 2013;36:473–80.
87. Hickman SJ, Quhill F, Pepper M. The evolution of an optic nerve head granuloma due to sarcoidosis. Neuro-ophthalmology. 2016;40:59–68.
88. Allegri P, Olivari S, Rissotto F, Rissotto R. Sarcoid uveitis: an intriguing challenger. Medicina (Kaunas). 2022;58:898.
89. Koczman JJ, Rouleau J, Gaunt M, Kardon RH, Wall M, Lee AG. Neuro-ophthalmic sarcoidosis: the University of Iowa experience. Semin Ophthalmol. 2008;23:157–68.
90. Menezo V, Lobo A, Yeo TK, du Bois RM, Lightman S. Ocular features in neurosarcoidosis. Ocul Immunol Inflamm. 2009;17:170–8.
91. Frohman LP, Guirgis M, Turbin RE, Bielory L. Sarcoidosis of the anterior visual pathway. 24 new cases. J Neuroophthalmol. 2003;23:190–7.
92. Beardsley TL, Brown SV, Sydnor CF, Grimson BS, Klintworth GK. Eleven cases of sarcoidosis of the optic nerve. Am J Ophthalmol. 1984;97:62–77.
93. Frohman EM, Fujimoto JG, Frohman TC, Calabresi PA, Cutter G, Balcer LJ. Optical coherence tomography: a window into the mechanisms of multiple sclerosis. Nat Clin Pract Neurol. 2008;4:664–75.

94. Rebolleda G, Muñoz-Negrete FJ. ¿Macular segmentation in Neuroophthalmology: descriptive or predictive? Arch Soc Esp Oft. 2013;88:289–90.
95. Syc SB, Saidha S, Newsome SD, Ratchford JN, Levy M, Ford E, Crainiceanu CM, Durbin MK, Oakley JD, Meyer SA, Frohman EM, Calabresi PA. Optical coherence tomography segmentation reveals ganglion cell layer pathology after optic neuritis. Brain. 2012;135:521–33.
96. Kardon R. The role of the macula OCT scan in neuro-ophthalmology. J Neuroophthalmol. 2011;31:353–61.
97. Modi YS, Epstein A, Bhaleeya S, Harbour JW, Albini T. Multimodal imaging of sarcoid choroidal granulomas. J Ophthalmic Inflamm Infect. 2013;3:58.
98. Wong M, Javowicz M, Tessler HH, Goldstein DA. Hight-resolution optical coherence tomography of presumed sarcoid retinal granulomas. Retina. 2009;29:1545–6.
99. Rostaqui O, Querques G, Haymann P, Fardeau C, Coscas G, Souied EH. Visualization of sarcoid choroidal granuloma by enhanced depth imaging optical coherence tomography. Ocul Immunol Inflamm. 2014;22:239–41.
100. Papavasileiou E, Miller JB, Sobrin L. Swept-source optical coherence tomography findings in convalescent phase of treated sarcoid choroidal granulomas. Retin Cases Brief Rep. 2016;10:32–6.
101. Pichi F. Vascularized sarcoid granuloma complicated by placoid disease in a pediatric patient. Retin Cases Brief Rep. 2021;15:426–30.
102. Turkoglu EB, Lally SE, Shields CL. Choroidal sarcoid granuloma simulating prostate carcinoma metastasis. Retin Cases Brief Rep. 2017;11:S226–8.
103. Inverzzini A, Agarwal A, Mapelli C, Nguyen QD, Staurenghi G, Viola F. Longitudinal follow-up of choroidal granulomas using enhanced depth imaging optical coherence tomography. Retina. 2017;37:144–53.
104. Qu-Knafo L, Auregan-Giocanti A. Granulome papillair sarcoïdosique. J Fr Ophtalmol. 2017;40:115–7.
105. Goldberg NR, Jabs DA, Busingye J. Optical coherence tomography image of presumed sarcoid retinal and optic nerve nodules. Ocul Immunol Inflamm. 2016;24:293–6.
106. Inverzzini A, Mapelli C, Viola F, Cigada M, Cimino L, Ratiglia R, Staurenghi G, Gupta A. Choroidal granulomas visualized by enhanced depth imaging optical coherence tomography. Retina. 2015;35:525–31.
107. Isihara M, Shibuya E, Tanaka S, Mizuki N. Diagnostic and therapeutic evaluation of multiple choroidal granulomas in a patient with confirmed sarcoidosis using enhanced depth imaging optic coherence tomography. Int Ophthalmol. 2018;38:2603–8.
108. Ferchaud MA, Amari F, Vignal-Clermont C, Bodaghi B, Fajnkuchen F, Giocanti-Auregan A. Oedeme papillaire bilateral isolé révélant une neurosarcoïdose. J Fr Ophtalmol. 2021;44:e629–32.
109. McMahon JF, Adam MK, Dunn JP. Optical coherence tomography and management of retinal granuloma in presumed ocular sarcoidosis. Ocul Immunol Inflamm. 2018. https://doi.org/10.1080/09273948.2018.1497662.
110. Eckstein C, Saidha S, Sotirchos ES, Byraiah G, Seigo M, Stankiewicz A, Syc SB, Ford E, Sharma S, Calabresi PA, Pardo CA. Detection of clinical and subclinical retinal abnormalities in neurosarcoidosis with optical coherence tomography. J Neurol. 2012;259:1390–8.
111. Cabrillo-Estévez L, Juan-Marcos L, Kyriakou D, Hernández-Galilea E. Cistoid macular edema as first manifestation of sarcoidosis. Int Ophthalmol. 2014;34:961–5.
112. Simmons-Rear A, Yeh S, Chan-Kai BT, Lauer AK, Flaxel CJ, Smith JR, Rosenbaum JT, Suhler EB. Characterization of serous retinal detachments in uveitis patients with optical coherence tomography. J Ophthalm Inflamm Infect. 2012;2:191–7.
113. Baltmr A, Lightman S, Tomkins-Netzer O. Examining the choroid in ocular inflammation: a focus on enhanced depth imaging. J Ophthalmol. 2014;2014: 459136.
114. Mehta H, Sim DA, Keane PA, Zarranz-Ventura J, Gallagher K, Egan CA, Westcott M, Lee RWJ, Tufail A, Pavesio CE. Structural changes of the choroid in sarcoid and tuberculosis related granulomatous uveitis. Eye. 2015;29:1060–8.

115. Güngör SG, Akkoyun I, Reyhan HN, Yesilirmak N, Yilmaz G. Choroidal thickness in ocular sarcoidosis during quiescent phase using enhanced depth imaging optical coherence tomography. Ocul Immunol Inflamm. 2014;22:287.
116. Cerquaglia A, Iaccheri B, Fiore T, Fruttini D, Belli FB, Khairallah M, Lupidi M, Cagini C. New insights on ocular sarcoidosis: an optical coherence tomography angiography study. Ocul Immunol Inflamm. 2019;27:1057–66.
117. Hassan LM, Asaad A, ElSanabary Z, Yousef MM. Evaluation of the retinal and choroidal microvasculature changes in cases of sarcoid and tuberculosis-associated porterior uveitis using OCT angiography. Int Ophthalmol. 2022. https://doi.org/10.1007/s10792-022-02464-6.
118. Abucham-Neto JZ, Miranda Torriceli AA, Fioravanti Lui AC, Napoli Guimaraes S, Nascimento H, Regatieri CV. Comparison between optical coherence tomography angiography and fluorescein angiography findings in retinal vasculitis. Int J Ret Vit. 2018;4:15.
119. Mueser KT, McGurk SR. Schizophrenia. Lancet. 2004;363:2063–72.
120. Wu EQ, Birnbaum HG, Shi L, et al. The economic burden of schizophrenia in the United States in 2002. J Clin Psychiatry. 2005;66:1122–9.
121. Sadock B, Sadock V. Sinopsis de Psiquiatría. Kaplan & Sadock, 10th ed. Madrid: Wolters Kluwer; 2008.
122. Svensson AC, Lichtenstein P, Sandin S, Öberg S, Sullivan PF, Hultman CM. Familial aggregation of schizophrenia: the moderating effect of age at onset, parental immigration, paternal age and season of birth. Scand J Public Health. 2012;40:43–50.
123. Siever LJ, Davis KL. The pathophysiology of schizophrenia disorders: perspectives from the spectrum. Am J Psychiatry. 2004;161:398–413.
124. Harrison PJ, Weinberger DR. Schizophrenia genes, gene expression, and neuropathology: on the matter of their convergence. Mol Psychiatry. 2005;10:40–68.
125. Bracht T, Horn H, Strik W, et al. White matter pathway organization of the reward system is related to positive and negative symptoms in schizophrenia. Schizophr Res. 2014;153:136–42.
126. Takayanagi M, Wentz J, Takayanagi Y, et al. Reduced anterior cingulate gray matter volume and thickness in subjects with deficit schizophrenia. Schizophr Res. 2013;150:484–90.
127. Glahn DC, Laird AR, Ellison-Wright I, et al. Meta-analysis of gray matter anomalies in schizophrenia: application of anatomic likelihood estimation and network analysis. Biol Psychiatry. 2008;64:774–81.
128. Arnone D, Cavanagh J, Gerber D, Lawrie SM, Ebmeier KP, Mcintosh AM. Magnetic resonance imaging studies in bipolar and schizophrenia: meta-analysis. Br J Psychiatry. 2009;195:194–201.
129. Fornito A, Yücel M, Dean B, Wood SJ, Pantelis C. Anatomical abnormalities of the anterior cingulate cortex in schizophrenia: bridging the gap between neuroimaging and neuropathology. Schizophr Bull. 2009;35:973–93.
130. Howard MA, Roberts N, García-Fiñana M, Cowell PE. Volume estimation of prefrontal cortical subfields using MRI and stereology. Brain Res Brain Res Protoc. 2003;10:125–38.
131. MacFall JR, Payne ME, Krishnan KRR. MR scanner geometry changes: phantom measurements compared to intracranial contents calculations. Proc Int Soc Magnetic Resonance Med. 2004;11:2182.
132. Yılmaz U, Küçük E, Ülgen A, Özköse A, Demircan S, Ulusoy DM, Zararsız G. Retinal nerve fiber layer and macular thickness measurement in patients with schizophrenia. Eur J Ophthalmol. 2016;26:375–8.
133. Chu EM, Kolappan M, Barnes TR, Joyce EM, Ron MA. A window into the brain: an in vivo study of the retina in schizophrenia using optical coherence tomography. Psychiatry Res. 2012;203:89–94.
134. Lee WW, Tajunisah I, Sharmilla K, Peyman M, Subrayan V. Retinal nerve fiber layer structure abnormalities in schizophrenia and its relationship to disease state: evidence from optical coherence tomography. Invest Ophthalmol Vis Sci. 2013;54:7785–92.

135. Ascaso FJ, Rodriguez-Jimenez R, Cabezón L, López-Antón R, Santabárbara J, De la Cámara C, Modrego PJ, Quintanilla MA, Bagney A, Gutierrez L, Cruz N, Cristóbal JA, Lobo A. Retinal nerve fiber layer and macular thickness in patients with schizophrenia: influence of recent illness episodes. Psychiatry Res. 2015;229:230–6.
136. Komatsu H, Onoguchi G, Jerotic S, Kanahara N, Kakuto Y, Ono T, Funakoshi S, Yabana T, Nakazawa T, Tomita H. Retinal layers and associated clinical factors in schizophrenia spectrum disorders: a systematic review and meta-analysis. Mol Psychiatry. 2022;27(9):3592–616. https://doi.org/10.1038/s41380-022-01591-x.
137. Sarkar S, Rajalakshmi AR, Avudaiappan S, Eswaran S. Exploring the role of macular thickness as a potential early biomarker of neurodegeneration in acute schizophrenia. Int Ophthalmol. 2021;41(8):2737–46. https://doi.org/10.1007/s10792-021-01831-z.
138. Joe P, Ahmad M, Riley G, Weissman J, Smith RT, Malaspina D. A pilot study assessing retinal pathology in psychosis using optical coherence tomography: choroidal and macular thickness. Psychiatry Res. 2018;263:158–61.
139. Li CY, Garg I, Bannai D, Kasetty M, Katz R, Adhan I, Douglas KAA, Wang JC, Kim LA, Keshavan M, Lizano P, Miller JB. Sex-specific changes in choroid vasculature among patients with schizophrenia and bipolar disorder. Clin Ophthalmol. 2022;28(16):2363–71. https://doi.org/10.2147/OPTH.S352731.
140. Green KM, Choi JJ, Ramchandran RS, Silverstein SM. OCT and OCT angiography offer new insights and opportunities in schizophrenia research and treatment. Front Digit Health. 2022;18(4): 836851. https://doi.org/10.3389/fdgth.2022.836851.
141. Koman-Wierdak E, Róg J, Brzozowska A, Toro MD, Bonfiglio V, Załuska-Ogryzek K, Karakuła-Juchnowicz H, Rejdak R, Nowomiejska K. Analysis of the peripapillary and macular regions using OCT angiography in patients with schizophrenia and bipolar disorder. J Clin Med. 2021;10(18):4131. https://doi.org/10.3390/jcm10184131.
142. Bannai D, Adhan I, Katz R, Kim LA, Keshavan M, Miller JB, Lizano P. Quantifying retinal microvascular morphology in schizophrenia using swept-source optical coherence tomography angiography. Schizophr Bull. 2022;48(1):80–9. https://doi.org/10.1093/schbul/sbab111.
143. Boudriot E, Schworm B, Slapakova L, Hanken K, Jäger I, Stephan M, Gabriel V, Ioannou G, Melcher J, Hasanaj G, Campana M, Moussiopoulou J, Löhrs L, Hasan A, Falkai P, Pogarell O, Priglinger S, Keeser D, Kern C, Wagner E, Raabe FJ. Optical coherence tomography reveals retinal thinning in schizophrenia spectrum disorders. Eur Arch Psychiatry Clin Neurosci. 2022. https://doi.org/10.1007/s00406-022-01455-z.
144. Maynard TM, Sikich L, Lieberman JA, LaMantia AS. Neural development, cell-cell signaling, and the 'two-hit' hypothesis of schizophrenia. Schizophr Bull. 2001;27:457–76.
145. Kochunov P, Hong LE. Neurodevelopmental and neurodegenerative models of schizophrenia: white matter at the center stage. Schizophr Bull. 2014;40:721–8.
146. Pantelis C, Yücel M, Wood SJ, et al. Structural brain imaging evidence for multiple pathological processes at different stages of brain development in schizophrenia. Schizophr Bull. 2005;31:672–96.
147. Guilleminault C. Clinical features and evaluation of obstructive sleep apnea syndrome. In: Kryger MH, Roth T, Dement WC, editors. Principles and practice of sleep medicine. Philadelphia: WB Saunders; 1994. p. 667–77.
148. Hatipoğlu U, Rubinstein I. Inflammation and obstructive sleep apnea syndrome pathogenesis: a working hypothesis. Respiration. 2003;70:665–71.
149. Lavie L, Hefetz A, Luboshitzky R, Lavie P. Plasma levels of nitric oxide and L-arginine in sleep apnea patients: effects of nCPAP treatment. J Mol Neurosci. 2003;21:57–63.
150. Grover DP. Obstructive sleep apnea and ocular disorders. Curr Opin Ophthalmol. 2010;21:454–8.
151. Shahar E, Whitney CW, Redline S, Lee ET, Newman AB, Javier Nieto F, O'Connor GT, Boland LL, Schwartz JE, Samet JM. Sleep-disordered breathing and cardiovascular disease: cross sectional results of the Sleep Heart Health Study. Am J Respir Crit Care Med. 2001;163:19–25.

152. Rudnicka A, Pływaczewski R, Jończak L, Górecka D, Sliwiński P. Prevalence of stroke in patients with obstructive sleep apnoea. Pneumonol Alergol Pol. 2010;78:121–5.
153. Macey PM, Henderson LA, Macey KE, Alger JR, Frysinger RC, Woo MA, Harper RK, Yan-Go FL, Harper RM. Brain morphology associated with obstructive sleep apnea. Am J Respir Crit Care Med. 2002;166:1382–7.
154. Kumar R, Birrer BV, Macey PM, Woo MA, Gupta RK, Yan-Go FL, Harper RM. Reduced mammillary body volume in patients with obstructive sleep apnea. Neurosci Lett. 2008;438:330–4.
155. Chokesuwattanaskul A, Chirakalwasan N, Jaimchariyatam N, Pitakvej N, Sarutikriangkri Y, Chunharas C, Phanthumchinda K, Likitjaroen Y. Associations between hypoxia parameters in obstructive sleep apnea and cognition, cortical thickness, and white matter integrity in middle-aged and older adults. Sleep Breath. 2021;25(3):1559–70.
156. Ho BL, Tseng PT, Lai CL, Wu MN, Tsai MJ, Hsieh CF, Chen TY, Hsu CY. Obstructive sleep apnea and cerebral white matter change: a systematic review and meta-analysis. J Neurol. 2018;265(7):1643–53.
157. Baril AA, Martineau-Dussault MÈ, Sanchez E, André C, Thompson C, Legault J, Gosselin N. Obstructive sleep apnea and the brain: a focus on gray and white matter structure. Curr Neurol Neurosci Rep. 2021;21(3):11.
158. Khazaie H, Veronese M, Noori K, et al. Functional reorganization in obstructive sleep apnoea and insomnia: a systematic review of the resting-state fMRI. Neurosci Biobehav Rev. 2017;77:219–31.
159. Tahmasian M, Rosenzweig I, Eickhoff SB, et al. Structural and functional neural adaptations in obstructive sleep apnea: an activation likelihood estimation meta-analysis. Neurosci Biobehav Rev. 2016;65:142–56.
160. Santarnecchi E, Sprugnoli G, Sicilia I, Dukart J, Neri F, Romanella SM, Cerase A, Vatti G, Rocchi R, Rossi A. Thalamic altered spontaneous activity and connectivity in obstructive sleep apnea syndrome. J Neuroimaging. 2022;32(2):314–27.
161. McNab AA. Floppy eyelid syndrome and obstructive sleep apnea. Ophthal Plast Reconstr Surg. 1997;13:98–114.
162. Woog JJ. Obstructive sleep apnea and the floppy eyelid syndrome. Am J Ophthalmol. 1990;110:314–5.
163. Karger RA, White WA, Park WC, et al. Prevalence of floppy eyelid syndrome in obstructive sleep apnea-hypopnea syndrome. Ophthalmology. 2006;113:1669–74.
164. Muniesa M, Sánchez-de-la-Torre M, Huerva V, Lumbierres M, Barbé F. Floppy eyelid syndrome as an indicator of the presence of glaucoma in patients with obstructive sleep apnea. J Glaucoma. 2014;23:81–5.
165. Pedrotti E, Demasi CL, Bruni E, Bosello F, Di Sarro PP, Passilongo M, Fasolo A, Gennaro N, De Gregorio A, Ferrari M, Marchini G. Prevalence and risk factors of eye diseases in adult patients with obstructive sleep apnoea: results from the SLE.E.P.Y cohort study. BMJ Open. 2017;7:e016142.
166. Aiello F, Gallo Afflitto G, Alessandri Bonetti M, Ceccarelli F, Cesareo M, Nucci C. Lax eyelid condition (LEC) and floppy eyelid syndrome (FES) prevalence in obstructive sleep apnea syndrome (OSA) patients: a systematic review and meta-analysis. Graefes Arch Clin Exp Ophthalmol. 2022;261(6):1505–14.
167. Bulloch G, Seth I, Alphonse S, Sathe A, Jennings M, Sultan D, Rahmeh R, McNab AA. Prevalence of obstructive sleep apnea with floppy eyelid syndrome: a systematic review and meta-analysis. Ophthalmic Plast Reconstr Surg. 2022;39(3):243–53.
168. Cheong AJY, Ho OTW, Wang SKX, Woon CY, Yap K, Ng KJY, Xu FWX, See A, Ng ACW, Loh SRH, Chee SP, Toh ST. Association between obstructive sleep apnea and floppy eyelid syndrome: a systematic review and metaanalysis. Surv Ophthalmol. 2023;68(2):257–64.
169. Leroux les Jardins G, Glacet-Bernard A, Lasry S, Housset B, Coscas G, Soubrane G. Retinal vein occlusion and obstructive sleep apnea syndrome. J Fr Ophtalmol. 2009;32:420–4.
170. Wan W, Wu Z, Lu J, Wan W, Gao J, Su H, Zhu W. Obstructive sleep apnea is related with the risk of retinal vein occlusion. Nat Sci Sleep. 2021;2(13):273–81.

171. Qin Z, Xiang L, Ren H, Song W, Su L, Gao X. The correlation between obstructive sleep apnea and retinal vein obstruction: a meta-analysis and systematic review. Contrast Media Mol Imaging. 2022;2022:8065629.
172. Chang AC, Fox TP, Wang S, Wu AY. Relationship between obstructive sleep apnea and the presence and severity of diabetic retinopathy. Retina. 2018;38(11):2197–206.
173. Vié AL, Kodjikian L, Agard E, Voirin N, El Chehab H, Denis P, Coste O, Dot C. Evaluation of obstructive sleep apnea syndrome as a risk factor for diabetic macular edema in patients with type II diabetes. Retina. 2019;39(2):274–80.
174. Nakayama LF, Tempaku PF, Bergamo VC, Polizelli MU, Santos da Cruz NF, Bittencourt LRA, Regatieri CVS. Obstructive sleep apnea and the retina: a review. J Clin Sleep Med. 2021;17(9):1947–52.
175. Wei DYW, Chew M, Sabanayagam C. Obstructive sleep apnoea, other sleep parameters and diabetic retinopathy. Curr Diab Rep. 2021;21(12):58.
176. Hayreh SS, Zimmerman MB, Podhajsky P, Alward WL. Nocturnal arterial hypotension and its role in optic nerve head and ocular ischemic disorders. Am J Ophthalmol. 1994;17:603–24.
177. Yang HK, Park SJ, Byun SJ, Park KH, Kim JW, Hwang JM. Obstructive sleep apnoea and increased risk of non-arteritic anterior ischaemic optic neuropathy. Br J Ophthalmol. 2019;103(8):1123–8.
178. Raizada K, Margolin E. Non-arteritic Anterior Ischemic Optic Neuropathy. 2022 Oct 31. In: StatPearls [Internet]. Treasure Island (FL): StatPearls Publishing; 2023 Jan.
179. Kloos P, Laube I, Thoelen A. Obstructive sleep apnea in patients with central serous chorioretinopathy. Graefes Arch Clin Exp Ophthalmol. 2008;246:1225–8.
180. Jain AK, Kaines A, Schwartz S. Bilateral central serous chorioretinopathy resolving rapidly with treatment for obstructive sleep apnea. Graefes Arch Clin Exp Ophthalmol. 2010;248:1037–9.
181. Chatziralli I, Kabanarou SA, Parikakis E, Chatzirallis A, Xirou T, Mitropoulos P. Risk factors for central serous chorioretinopathy: multivariate approach in a case-control study. Curr Eye Res. 2017;42:1069–73.
182. Wu CY, Riangwiwat T, Rattanawong P, Nesmith BLW, Deobhakta A. Association of obstructive sleep apnea with central serous chorioretinopathy and choroidal thickness: a systematic review and meta-analysis. Retina. 2018;38(9):1642–51.
183. Pan CK, Vail D, Bhattacharya J, Cao M, Mruthyunjaya P. The effect of obstructive sleep apnea on absolute risk of central serous chorioretinopathy. Am J Ophthalmol. 2020;218:148–55.
184. Lee CY, Yeung L, Kuan Jen C, Sun MH, Sun CC. Relationship between obstructive sleep apnea and central serous chorioretinopathy: a health insurance database study. Ophthalmic Epidemiol. 2022;29(3):302–9.
185. Purvin VA, Kawasaki A, Yee RD. Papilledema and obstructive sleep apnea syndrome. Arch Ophthalmol. 2000;118:1626–30.
186. Franklin KA. Cerebral haemodynamics in obstructive sleep apnoea and Cheyne-Stokes respiration. Sleep Med Rev. 2002;6:429–41.
187. Stein JD, Kim DS, Mundy KM, Talwar N, Nan B, Chervin RD, Much DC. The association between glaucomatous and other causes of optic neuropathy and sleep apnea. Am J Ophthalmol. 2011;152(6):989–98.
188. Mojon DS, Hess CW, Goldblum D, Fleischhauer J, Koerner F, Bassetti C, Mathis J. High prevalence of glaucoma in patients with sleep apnea syndrome. Ophthalmology. 1999;106:1009–12.
189. Mojon DS, Hess CW, Goldblum D, Böhnke M, Körner F, Mathis J. Primary open-angle glaucoma is associated with sleep apnea syndrome. Ophthalmologica. 2000;214:115–8.
190. Bendel RE, Kaplan J, Heckman M, Fredrickson PA, Lin SC. Prevalence of glaucoma in patients with obstructive sleep apnoea—a cross-sectional case-series. Eye (Lond). 2008;22:1105–9.

191. Faridi O, Park SC, Liebmann JM, Ritch R. Glaucoma and obstructive sleep apnoea syndrome. Clin Exp Ophthalmol. 2012;40:408–19.
192. Sergi M, Salerno DE, Rizzi M, Blini M, Andreoli A, Messenio D, Pecis M, Bertoni G. Prevalence of normal tension glaucoma in obstructive sleep apnea syndrome patients. J Glaucoma. 2007;16:42–6.
193. Bilgin G. Normal-tension glaucoma and obstructive sleep apnea syndrome: a prospective study. BMC Ophthalmol. 2014;14:27.
194. Xin C, Zhang W, Wang L, Yang D, Wang J. Changes of visual field and optic nerve fiber layer in patients with OSAS. Sleep Breath. 2015;19:129–34.
195. Friedlander AH, Graves LL, Chang TI, Kawakami KK, Lee UK, Grabich SC, Fang ZT, Zeidler MR, Giaconi JA. Prevalence of primary open-angle glaucoma among patients with obstructive sleep apnea. Oral Surg Oral Med Oral Pathol Oral Radiol. 2018;126(3):226–30.
196. García-Sánchez A, Villalaín I, Asencio M, García J, García-Rio F. Sleep apnea and eye diseases: evidence of association and potential pathogenic mechanisms. J Clin Sleep Med. 2022;18(1):265–78.
197. Lee SSY, Nilagiri VK, Mackey DA. Sleep and eye disease: a review. Clin Exp Ophthalmol. 2022;50(3):334–44.
198. Examen del paciente. Campo visual. In: European glaucoma society, editor. Terminología y pautas para el glaucoma. 3rd ed. Savona: Dogma; 2009.p. 61–89.
199. Kargi SH, Altin R, Koksal M, Kart L, Cinar F, Ugurbas SH, Ayoglu F. Retinal nerve fibre layer measurements are reduced in patients with obstructive sleep apnoea syndrome. Eye (Lond). 2005;19:575–9.
200. Sagiv O, Fishelson-Arev T, Buckman G, Mathalone N, Wolfson J, Segev E, Peled R, Lavi I, Geyer O. Retinal nerve fiber layer thickness measurements by optical coherence tomography in patients with sleep apnea syndrome. Clin Experiment Ophthalmol. 2014;42:132–8.
201. Lin PW, Friedman M, Lin HC, Chang HW, Pulver TM, Chin CH. Decreased retinal nerve fiber layer thickness in patients with obstructive sleep apnea/hypopnea syndrome. Graefes Arch Clin Exp Ophthalmol. 2011;249:585–93.
202. Moghimi S, Ahmadraji A, Sotoodeh H, Sadeghniat K, Maghsoudipour M, Fakhraie G, Latifi G, Nassiri N, Giaconi JA. Retinal nerve fiber thickness is reduced in sleep apnea syndrome. Sleep Med. 2013;14:53–7.
203. Lin PW, Friedman M, Lin HC, Chang HW, Wilson M, Lin MC. Normal tension glaucoma in patients with obstructive sleep apnea/hypopnea syndrome. J Glaucoma. 2011;20:553–8.
204. Gutiérrez-Díaz E, Pérez-Rico C, de Atauri MJ, Mencía-Gutiérrez E, Blanco R. Evaluation of the visual function in obstructive sleep apnea syndrome patients and normal-tension glaucoma by means of the multifocal visual evoked potentials. Graefes Arch Clin Exp Ophthalmol. 2012;250:1681–8.
205. Ozge G, Dogan D, Koylu MT, Ayyildiz O, Akincioglu D, Mumcuoglu T, Mutlu FM. Retina nerve fiber layer and choroidal thickness changes in obstructive sleep apnea syndrome. Postgrad Med. 2016;128:317–22.
206. Yazgan S, Erboy F, Celik HU, Ornek T, Ugurbas SH, Kokturk F, Ayar O, Akdemir MO, Celik E. Peripapillary choroidal thickness and retinal nerve fiber layer in untreated patients with obstructive sleep apnea-hypopnea syndrome: a case-control study. Curr Eye Res. 2017;42:1552–60.
207. Uslu H, Kanra AY, Sarac S. Structural assessment of the optic nerve in patients with obstructive sleep apnea syndrome: case-control study. Eur J Ophthalmol. 2021;31(4):1741–8.
208. Zengin MO, Tuncer I, Karahan E. Retinal nerve fiber layer thickness changes in obstructive sleep apnea syndrome: one year follow-up results. Int J Ophthalmol. 2014;7:704–8.
209. Huseyinoglu N, Ekinci M, Ozben S, Buyukuysal C, Kale MY, Sanivar HS. Optic disc and retinal nerve fiber layer parameters as indicators of neurodegenerative brain changes in patients with obstructive sleep apnea syndrome. Sleep Breath. 2014;18:95–102.
210. Shiba T, Takahashi M, Sato Y, Onoda Y, Hori Y, Sugiyama T, Bujo H, Maeno T. Relationship between severity of obstructive sleep apnea syndrome and retinal nerve fiber layer thickness. Am J Ophthalmols. 2014;157:1202–8.

211. Casas P, Ascaso FJ, Vicente E, Tejero-Garcés G, Adiego MI, Cristóbal JA. Retinal and optic nerve evaluation by optical coherence tomography in adults with obstructive sleep apnea-hypopnea syndrome (OSAHS). Graefes Arch Clin Exp Ophthalmol. 2013;251:1625–34.
212. Bussan KA, Stuard WL, Mussi N, Lee W, Whitson JT, Issioui Y, Rowe AA, Wert KJ, Robertson DM. Differential effects of obstructive sleep apnea on the corneal subbasal nerve plexus and retinal nerve fiber layer. PLoS One. 2022;17(6):e0266483.
213. Nowak MS, Jurowski P, Gos R, Prost ME, Smigielski J. Pulsatile ocular blood flow in subjects with sleep apnoea syndrome. Arch Med Sci. 2011;7:332–6.
214. Adam M, Okka M, Yosunkaya S, Bozkurt B, Kerimoğlu H, Turan M. The evaluation of retinal nerve fiber layer thickness in patients with obstructive sleep apnea syndrome. J Ophthalmol. 2013;2013: 292158.
215. Ferrandez B, Ferreras A, Calvo P, Abadia B, Marin JM, Pajarin AB. Assessment of the retinal nerve fiber layer in individuals with obstructive sleep apnea. BMC Ophthalmol. 2016;16:40.
216. Kara N, Sayin N, Bayramoglu SE, Savas AU. Peripapillary retina nerve fiber layer thickness and macular ganglion cell layer thickness in patients with obstructive sleep apnea syndrome. Eye (Lond). 2018;32:701–6.
217. Teberik K, Eski MT, Balbay EG, Kaya M. Evaluation of intraocular pressure, corneal thickness, and retinal nerve fiber layer thickness in patients with obstructive sleep apnea syndrome. Pak J Med Sci. 2018;34(4):817–22.
218. Salzgeber R, Iliev ME, Mathis J. Do optic nerve head and visual field parameters in patients with obstructive sleep apnea syndrome differ from those in control individuals? Klin Monbl Augenheilkd. 2014;231:340–3.
219. Yuvacı İ, Pangal E, Bayram N, Yüksel SA, Alabay B, Ağadayı A, Sırakaya E, Gülhan A. Evaluation of posterior ocular changes using enhanced depth imaging-optical coherence tomography in patients with obstructive sleep apnea syndrome. Arq Bras Oftalmol. 2016;79:247–52.
220. Kato M, Roberts-Thomson P, Phillips BG, Haynes WG, Winnicki M, Accurso V, Somers VK. Impairment of endothelium dependent vasodilation of resistance vessels in patients withobstructive sleep apnea. Circulation. 2000;102:2607–10.
221. Ferrandez B, Ferreras A, Calvo P, Abadia B, Pajarin AB, Marin JM, Iester M. Macular retinal ganglion cell layer thickness is not reduced in patients with obstructive sleep apnea. Ophthalmic Res. 2016;56:85–91.
222. Guven S, Kilic D, Bolatturk OF. Thinning of the inner and outer retinal layers, including the ganglion cell layer and photoreceptor layers, in obstructive sleep apnea and hypopnea syndrome unrelated to the disease severity. Int Ophthalmol. 2021;41(11):3559–69.
223. Chalkiadaki E, Andreanos K, Karmiris E, Florou C, Tsiafaki X, Amfilochiou A, Georgalas I, Koutsandrea C, Papaconstantinou D. Ganglion cell layer thickening in patients suffering from obstructive sleep apnea-hypopnea syndrome with long mean apnea-hypopnea duration during sleep. Int Ophthalmol. 2021;41(3):923–35.
224. Xin C, Wang J, Zhang W, Wang L, Peng X. Retinal and choroidal thickness evaluation by SD-OCT in aduls with obstructive sleep apnea-hypopnea syndrome (OSAS). Eye (Lond). 2014;28:415–21.
225. Bayhan HA, Bayhan SA, Intepe YS, Muhafız E, Gurdal C. Evaluation of the macular choroidal thickness using spectral optical coherence tomography in patients with obstructive sleep apnea syndrome. Clin Exp Ophthalmol. 2015;43(2):139–44.
226. Uslu H, Kanra AY, Cetintas G, Tatar MG. Effect of therapy on choroidal thickness in patients with obstructive sleep apnea syndrome. Ophthalmic Surg Lasers Imaging Retina. 2018;49(11):846–51.
227. Yuvaci İ, Pangal E, Bayram N, Yüksel SA, Alabay B, Ağadayı A, Sırakaya E, Gülhan A. Evaluation of posterior ocular changes using enhanced depth imaging-optical coherence tomography in patients with obstructive sleep apnea syndrome. Arq Bras Oftalmol. 2016;79:247–52.
228. Naranjo-Bonilla P, Muñoz-Villanueva MC, Giménez-Gómez R, Jurado-Gámez B. Retinal and choroidal thickness measurements in obstructive sleep apnea: impacts of continuous positive airway pressure treatment. Graefes Arch Clin Exp Ophthalmol. 2021;259(11):3381–93.

229. Frayser R, Gray GW, Houston CS. Control of the retinal circulation at altitude. J Appl Physiol. 1974;37:302–4.
230. Delaey C, Van De Voorde J. Regulatory mechanisms in the retinal and choroidal circulation. Ophthalmic Res. 2000;32:249–56.
231. Zengin MÖ, Oz T, Baysak A, Cinar E, Küçükerdönmez C. Changes in choroidal thickness in patients with obstructive sleep apnea syndrome. Ophthalmic Surg Lasers Imaging Retina. 2014;45:298–304.
232. Karaca EE, Ekici F, Yalçin NG, Ciftçi TU, Ozdek S. Macular choroidal thickness measurements in patients with obstructive sleep apnea syndrome. Sleep Breath. 2015;19:335–41.
233. Khayi H, Pepin JL, Geiser MH, Tonini M, Tamisier R, Renard E, Baguet JP, Levy P, Romanet JP, Chiquet C. Choroidal blood flow regulation after posture change or isometric exercise in men with obstructive sleep apnea syndrome. Invest Ophthalmol Vis Sci. 2011;52:9489–96.
234. Davanian A, Williamson L, Taylor C, Harrover A, Bollinger K, Chaudhary B, Taskar V, Lee TJ, Liu Y, Chen Q, Marcus DM. Optical coherence tomography angiography and Humphrey visual field in patients with obstructive sleep apnea. J Clin Sleep Med. 2022;18(9):2133–42.
235. Tonini M, Khayi H, Pepin JL, Renard E, Baguet JP, Lévy P, Romanet JP, Geiser MH, Chiquet C. Choroidal blood-flow responses to hyperoxia and hypercapnia in men with obstructive sleep apnea. Sleep. 2010;33:811–8.
236. Yu J, Xiao K, Huang J, Sun X, Jiang C. Reduced retinal vessel density in obstructive sleep apnea syndrome patients: an optical coherence tomography angiography study. Invest Ophthalmol Vis Sci. 2017;58:3506–12.
237. Ucak T, Unver E. Alterations in parafoveal and optic disc vessel densities in patients with obstructive sleep apnea syndrome. J Ophthalmol. 2020;10(2020):4034382.
238. Lin PW, Lin HC, Chang CT, Lin MC, Friedman M, Salapatas AM. Decreased peripapillary and macular vascular densities in patients with moderate/severe obstructive sleep apnea/hypopnea syndrome. Nat Sci Sleep. 2023;12(15):1–12.
239. Ava S, Erdem S, Karahan M, Dursun ME, Hazar L, Sen HS, Keklikci U. Evaluation of the effect of obstructive sleep apnea syndrome on retinal microvascularity by optical coherence tomography angiography. Photodiagnosis Photodyn Ther. 2022;38: 102761.
240. Loureiro T, Rodrigues-Barros S, Lopes D, Carreira AR, Gomes R, Marques N, Telles P, Vide Escada A, Campos N. Retinal vascular impairment in patients newly diagnosed with obstructive sleep apnea syndrome. Multidiscip Respir Med. 2021;16(1):773.
241. Moyal L, Blumen-Ohana E, Blumen M, Blatrix C, Chabolle F, Nordmann JP. Parafoveal and optic disc vessel density in patients with obstructive sleep apnea syndrome: an optical coherence tomography angiography study. Graefes Arch Clin Exp Ophthalmol. 2018;256:1235–43.
242. Cai Y, Liu WB, Zhou M, Jin YT, Sun GS, Zhao L, Han F, Qu JF, Shi X, Zhao MW. Diurnal changes of retinal microvascular circulation and RNFL thickness measured by optical coherence tomography angiography in patients with obstructive sleep apnea-hypopnea. Front Endocrinol (Lausanne). 2022;9(13): 947586.
243. Kessler RC, Bergland P, Demler O, et al. Lifetime prevalence and age-of-onset distributions of DSM-IV disorders in the National Comorbidity Survey Replication. Arch Gen Psychiatry. 2005;62:593–602.
244. Akiskal HS, Bourgeois ML, Angst J, Post R, Möller H, Hirschfeld R. Re-evaluating the prevalence of and diagnostic composition within the broad clinical spectrum of bipolar disorders. J Affect Disord. 2000;59:S5-30.
245. Kalenderoglu A, Sevgi-Karadag A, Celik M, Egilmez OB, Han-Almis B, Ozen ME. Can the retinal ganglion cell layer (GCL) volume be a new marker to detect neurodegeneration in bipolar disorder? Compr Psychiatry. 2016;67:66–72.
246. Khalil MA, Saleh AA, Gohar SM, Khalil DH, Said M. Optical coherence tomography findings in patients with bipolar disorder. J Affect Disord. 2017;218:115–22.
247. Mehraban A, Samimi SM, Entezari M, Seifi MH, Nazari M, Yaseri M. Peripapillary retinal nerve fiber layer thickness in bipolar disorder. Graefes Arch Clin Exp Ophthalmol. 2016;254:365–71.

248. Polo V, Satue M, Gavin A, Vilades E, Orduna E, Cipres M, Garcia-Campayo J, Navarro-Gil M, Larrosa JM, Pablo LE, Garcia-Martin E. Ability of swept source OCT to detect retinal changes in patients with bipolar disorder. Eye (Lond). 2019;33(4):549–56.
249. Kilicarslan T, Sahan E, Kirik F, Guler EM, Kurtulmus A, Yildiz FBP, Ozdemir MH, Kocyigit A, Kirpinar I. The relation of optical coherence tomography findings with oxidative stress parameters in patients with bipolar disorder and unaffected first-degree relatives. J Affect Disord. 2022;1(296):283–90.
250. Ayık B, Kaya H, Tasdelen R, Sevimli N. Retinal changes in bipolar disorder as an endophenotype candidate: comparison of OCT-detected retinal changes in patients, siblings, and healthy controls. Psychiatry Res. 2022;313: 114606.
251. Onur ÖŞ, Yeşilkaya ÜH, Subaş E, Açar ÖPA, Onur İU, Karamustafalioğlu N, Eriş E. Can optical coherence tomography findings be related with suicide attempt in bipolar disorder? Photodiagnosis Photodyn Ther. 2023;41: 103268.
252. Liu Y, Tong Y, Huang L, Chen J, Yan S, Yang F. Factors related to retinal nerve fiber layer thickness in bipolar disorder patients and major depression patients. BMC Psychiatry. 2021;21(1):301.
253. Khalil DH, Said MM. Peripapillary retinal nerve fiber layer and ganglion cell complex degeneration in Egyptian patients with bipolar disorder. Eye (Lond). 2019;33(12):1852–8.
254. Cokunlu Y, Mirza E, Caliskan AM, Inanli I, Cicek IE, Ozcimen M, Eren I. Ganglion cell complex thickness changes in patients with different states of bipolar disorder. Eye (Lond). 2022;36(5):1034–41.
255. Gokcinar NB, Buturak SV, Ozkal F, Ozcicek G, Yumusak ME, Turgal E. Optical coherence tomography neurodegenerative findings in patients with bipolar disorder. Asia Pac Psychiatry. 2020;12(4): e12394.
256. Bannai D, Lizano P, Kasetty M, Lutz O, Zeng V, Sarvode S, Kim LA, Hill S, Tamminga C, Clementz B, Gershon E, Pearlson G, Miller JB, Keshavan M. Retinal layer abnormalities and their association with clinical and brain measures in psychotic disorders: a preliminary study. Psychiatry Res Neuroimaging. 2020;30(299): 111061.
257. Orduna E, Cordón B, Vilades E, García-Martín E, García-Campayo J, López-Del-Hoyo Y, Polo V, Larrosa JM, Pablo LE, Satue M. Ganglion cell and retinal nerve fiver layers correlated with time disease of bipolar disorder using 64 cell grid OCT tool. Curr Eye Res. 2021;46(8):1214–22.
258. Satue M, Fuentes JL, Vilades E, Orduna E, Vicente MJ, Cordon B, Perez-Velilla J, Garcia-Campayo J, Garcia-Martin E. Evaluation of progressive retinal degeneration in bipolar disorder patients over a period of 5 years. Curr Eye Res. 2022;47(7):1061–7.
259. García-Martín E, Gavín A, García-Campayo J, Vilades E, Orduna E, Polo V, Larrosa JM, Pablo LE, Satue M. Visual function and retinal changes in patients with bipolar disorder. Retina. 2019;39(10):2012–21.
260. Mustafa A, Turgay U. Optical coherence tomography angiography in patients with euthymic bipolar disorder. J Affect Disord. 2022;15(317):15–21. https://doi.org/10.1016/j.jad.2022.08.036.
261. Li CY, Garg I, Bannai D, Kasetty M, Katz R, Adhan I, Douglas KAA, Wang JC, Kim LA, Keshavan M, Lizano P, Miller JB. Sex-specific changes in choroid vasculature among patients with schizophrenia and bipolar disorder. Clin Ophthalmol. 2022;28(16):2363–71.
262. Sánchez-Morla EM, Fuentes JL, Miguel-Jiménez JM, Boquete L, Ortiz M, Orduna E, Satue M, Garcia-Martin E. Automatic diagnosis of bipolar disorder using optical coherence tomography data and artificial intelligence. J Pers Med. 2021;11(8):803.
263. García-Portilla MP, García-Álvarez L, de la Fuente-Tomás L, Velasco-Iglesias Á, Sáiz PA, González-Blanco L, Bobes Bascarán MT, Baamonde B, Alcalde I, Merayo-Lloves J, Bobes J. Could structural changes in the retinal layers be a new biomarker of mental disorders? A systematic review and thematic synthesis. Rev Psiquiatr Salud Ment (Engl Ed). 2019;12(2):116–29.

264. Gavín A, Garcia-Martin E, Garcia-Campayo J, Viladés E, Orduna E, Satué M. The use of optical coherence tomography in the evaluation of patients with bipolar disorder. Arch Soc Esp Oftalmol (Engl Ed). 2021;96(3):141–51.
265. Clémence-Fau M, Schwan R, Angioi-Duprez K, Laprévote V, Schwitzer T. Retinal structural changes in mood disorders: the optical coherence tomography to better understand physiopathology? Prog Neuropsychopharmacol Biol Psychiatry. 2021;8(108): 110080.
266. Lizano P, Bannai D, Lutz O, Kim LA, Miller J, Keshavan M. A meta-analysis of retinal cytoarchitectural abnormalities in schizophrenia and bipolar disorder. Schizophr Bull. 2020;46(1):43–53.
267. Ascaso FJ, Cabezón L, Quintanilla MA, Gutiérrez-Galve L, López-Antón R, Cristóbal JA, Lobo A. Retinal nerve fiber layer thickness measured by optical coherence tomography in patients with schizophrenia: a short report. Eur J Psychiat. 2010;24:227–35.
268. Celik M, Kalenderoglu A, Sevgi Karadag A, Bekir Egilmez O, Han-Almis B, Şimşek A. Decreases in ganglion cell layer and inner plexiform layer volumes correlate better with disease severity in schizophrenia patients than retinal nerve fiber layer thickness: findings from spectral optic coherence tomography. Eur Psychiatry. 2016;32:9–15.
269. Altun IK, Turedi N, Aras N, Atagun MI. Psychopharmacological signatures in the retina in schizophrenia and bipolar disorder: an optic coherence tomography study. Psychiatr Danub. 2020;32(3–4):351–8.

Isolated Hereditary Optic Neuropathies

16

Piero Barboni, Nicole Balducci, and Alfredo A. Sadun

Abstract

Optical coherence tomography (OCT) has improved our understanding of hereditary mitochondrial optic neuropathies like Leber's hereditary optic neuropathy (LHON) and dominant optic atrophy (DOA). In LHON mutation carriers and in subacute stage, OCT shows a thickening of the temporal peripapillary retinal nerve fiber layer (RNFL), due to a preferential involvement of the papillomacular bundle (PMB). In the early pre-symptomatic stage and in subacute stage, an early and progressive thinning of the ganglion cells layer (GCL) is also detectable, following a centrifugal and spiral pattern, reflecting the anatomic distribution of the PMB. A simultaneous thickening takes place in the inferior RNFL sectors for the first 3 months, after which these fibers begin to thin. The superior and nasal sectors are involved later. Once the optic nerve is atrophic, all RNFL and GCL sectors are thinner. Analysis of the optic nerve head (ONH) reveals that larger optic discs are associated with a better prognosis. In DOA, the RNFL and GCL analysis reveals diffuse atrophy in all the sectors. The RNFL thinning is more pronounced in the temporal and inferior quadrants and less evident in the superior and nasal ones. Analysis of the macular GCL suggests an earlier involvement of the macular area. The analysis of choroidal thickness and the introduction of the optical coherence tomography angiography (OCT-A), studying the retinal, optic nerve head and choroidal

P. Barboni (✉)
Scientific Institute San Raffaele, Milan, Italy
e-mail: p.barboni@studiodazeglio.it

P. Barboni · N. Balducci
Studio Oculistico d'Azeglio, Bologna, Italy

N. Balducci
IRCCS-Policlinico Sant'Orsola Malpighi, Bologna, Italy

A. A. Sadun
Doheny Eye Institute, UCLA, Los Angeles, CA, USA

A. Grzybowski and P. Barboni (eds.), *OCT and Imaging in Central Nervous System Diseases*, https://doi.org/10.1007/978-3-031-72156-4_16

microvascular circulations, show microvascular changes in LHON and DOA and could became useful biomarkers to monitor the disease process, evaluate therapeutic efficacy and elucidate pathophysiology.

Keywords

Hereditary optic neuropathy • Leber's hereditary optic neuropathy • Dominant optic atrophy • Mitochondrial optic neuropathy • LHON • DOA • Optic disc size • Microcystic macular edema

Hereditary optic neuropathies are diseases affecting the optic nerve due to genetic causes. They may occur as isolated optic neuropathies or in association with systemic diseases. The minimum point prevalence of hereditary optic neuropathies is 1 per 10,000 subjects [1]. The most common isolated optic neuropathies are: Leber's Hereditary Optic Neuropathy (LHON) and Dominant Optic Atrophy (DOA) [2] They are also known as mitochondrial optic neuropathies as they both share a defect of the mitochondria function that leads to the selective loss of retinal ganglion cells (RGC) and axons, in particular of the papillo-macular bundle (PMB), which requires great energy for its highly demanding activity. Consequent to the PMB involvement, the main symptoms are related to loss of central vision and color vision defects. Over the last decades optical coherence tomography (OCT) has been extensively used to investigate the changes occurring in optic nerve and macular areas in these diseases.

16.1 Leber's Hereditary Optic Neuropathy

LHON is a maternally inherited genetic disorder due to mitochondrial DNA (mtDNA) mutations and predominantly affects men. The three most frequent pathogenic mutations affect nucleotide positions 11,778, 3460, and 14,484, respectively, in ND4, ND1, and ND6 subunit genes of complex I [2–4]. The mtDNA mutation is necessary but not sufficient to induce the blindness. Other, still poorly defined, genetic or environmental factors may be implicated [5]. Thus, penetrance in LHON is not complete and may vary even in different sub-branches of the same family harboring a homoplasmic mtDNA mutation [5].

LHON usually leads to large bilateral centrocecal scotomas in otherwise healthy young adults [3, 4]. The smaller-caliber fibers of the PMB are selectively lost at a very early stage of the pathologic process, which eventually extends to the rest of the nerve, leading to optic atrophy [6–9].

Clinically, most patients with LHON go through pre-symptomatic ophthalmoscopic and OCT changes before the acute phase, characterized by visual loss, develops.

Four clinical stages of LHON have been defined by an International LHON consensus statement [10], according to time from onset and clinical investigations:

0. Asymptomatic (mutation carriers)
1. Subacute (< 6 months from onset)
2. Dynamic (6–12 months)
3. Chronic (> 12 months)

Ophthalmoscopic features, already present at the **asymptomatic stage**, include peripapillary microangiopathy, small vessel tortuosity, mild swelling of the retinal nerve fiber layer (RNFL) and lack of vessel leakage at fluorescein angiography [11, 12]. These characteristics may wax and wane throughout life in many carrier subjects. Once the disease becomes symptomatic and the patient experiences loss of central vision during the **subacute stage**, the vascular changes increase with swelling of the superior and inferior fiber arcades and rapid loss of the papillomacular bundle [12, 13]. As the pathologic process progresses, temporal pallor of the optic disc may become evident. Then nerve fiber swelling decreases concomitantly with the extension of optic disc pallor toward complete atrophy during the **dynamic stage**. By 6 months after onset, optic atrophy is usually evident, and visual loss stabilizes, having reached the nadir [14, 15]. The **chronic stage** is universally reached by 1 year after onset. Rare reports described a stepwise worsening of visual acuity, whereas some individuals may recover different degrees of visual acuity [3, 4, 15].

16.1.1 Retinal Nerve Fiber Layer Analysis

OCT has been used to investigate the RNFL of LHON asymptomatic carriers [16, 17], as well as LHON affected patients in the different stages of the disease [17–19].

As regards LHON asymptomatic carriers, a significant thickening has been observed in the temporal RNFL quadrant and, in males, also in the inferior quadrant (Fig. 16.1) [16], and more specifically in the inferotemporal sector (clock hour 8 for a right eye) [17].

This finding confirms that in asymptomatic LHON, the PMB is selectively involved. This preferential involvement of the PMB has been linked to the disadvantageous energetic conditions of small axons that constitute the macular parvocellular retinal ganglion cells. These small fibers have a high firing rate, and are thought to be very energy dependent as they have the greatest surface area to volume ratio [8]. RNFL thickening seems mostly related to axonal swelling, which has been proposed to be a sign of impaired axonal transport, with redistribution of mitochondria within the dysfunctional retinal ganglion cells, particularly affecting the prelaminar, unmyelinated portion of the axons at the optic nerve head [8, 20]. Moreover, the peripapillary RNFL in LHON carriers showed higher thickness variability compared to controls, when measured at different time points [21].

The explanation of the RNFL variability could be either a compensatory mechanism (due to increased mitochondrial biogenesis) or an axonal stasis preceding the RGCs loss [8]. Another subclinical factor, which may cause RNFL variability, is LHON microangiopathy [21]. It is important to note that OCT measures the fiber layers that contain both retinal ganglion cell axons and vessels, so it cannot quantitatively differentiate fiber swelling from microangiopathy.

The beginning of the conversion coincided with an increase in the thickness of the sectors bordering the PMB (6 and 7 for the inferior sectors, 10 and 11 for the superior sectors in a right eye) synchronous with the thinning of sectors 8 and then 9 in a right eye [17].

Then, more generally, in the subacute phase, RNFL analysis shows thickening in the superior and inferior quadrants, whereas the temporal quadrant shows no

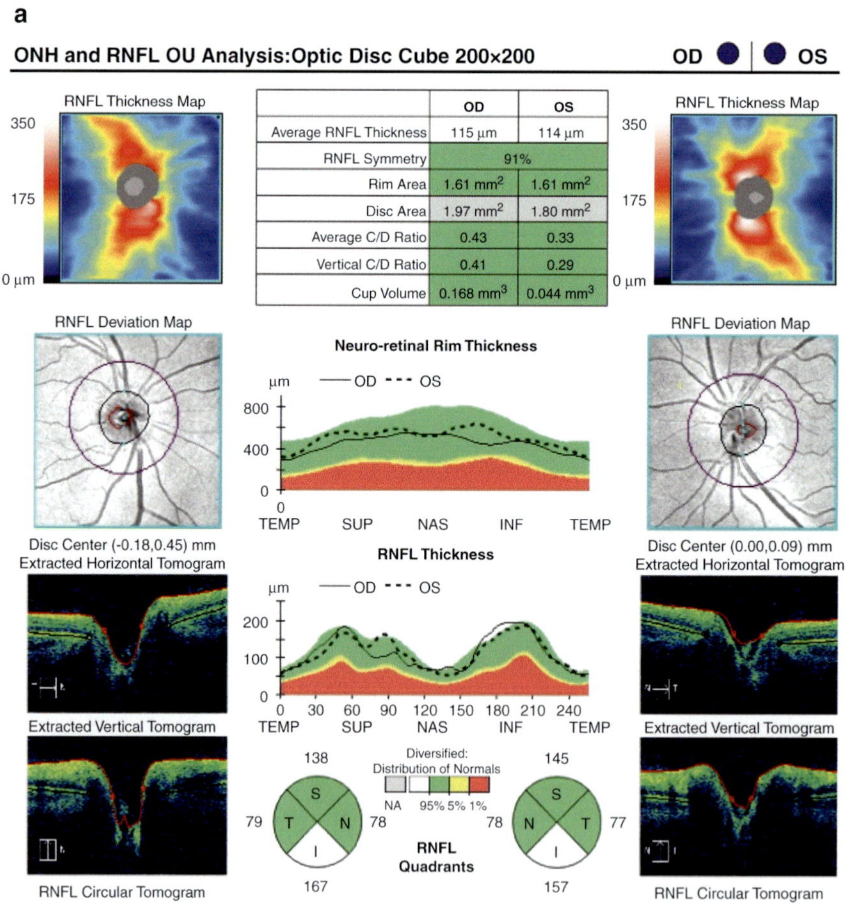

Fig. 16.1 (A) Peripapillary RNFL thickening more evident in the inferior quadrant of an unaffected LHON-carrier; (B) The left eye optic disc of the same patient

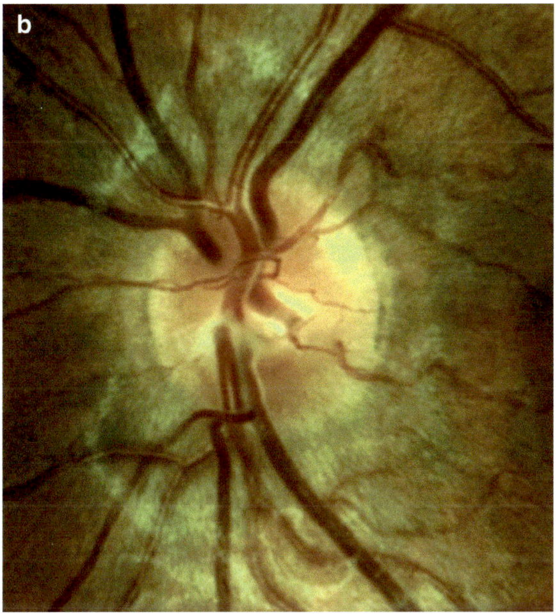

Fig. 16.1 (continued)

significant differences or reduction compared to the controls (Fig. 16.2a, b) [18, 22–24]. In fact, the PMB shows marked swelling at the time of visual loss, but its thickness starts decreasing soon due to early atrophy. A simultaneous thickening takes place in the inferior RNFL sectors for the first 3 months, after which the fibers begin to thin [22]. The superior and nasal sector are involved in a subsequent stage and show thickening after 3 months, when the other sectors are already in the atrophic phase [22]. The subacute phase of LHON has proven to be a progressive phase, being characterized by a series of events lasting at least 3 months (Fig. 16.3a, b) [22].

A study of the swelling and subsequent atrophy RNFL pattern hypothesized a different natural course between patients carrying 11,778 versus 14,484 mutations [25]. The RNFL thickening in the subacute stage and thinning in the dynamic stage was significant greater in 11,778 patients than in 14,484 [25]. These results could explain the different visual prognosis between these mutations and establish a correlation between the initial swelling of RNFL and the visual prognosis [25].

Finally, once the optic nerve is atrophic, all quadrants of the peripapillary RNFL show a thinning of the fibers. In the chronic stage, patients with visual recovery maintain a thicker RNFL than the subgroup without visual recovery in all quadrants, but the temporal one [18]. The three primary mtDNA mutations have different visual prognoses: worst for 3460/ND1, intermediate for 11778/ND4, and better for 14484/ND6 [14]. OCT studies did not show any differences in RNFL thickness between chronic patients without visual recovery carrying 11,778 and 3460 mutations [18] The rare LHON mtDNA 3890/ND1 mutation is associated with a bad visual prognosis and a severe thinning of the peripapillary RNFL [26].

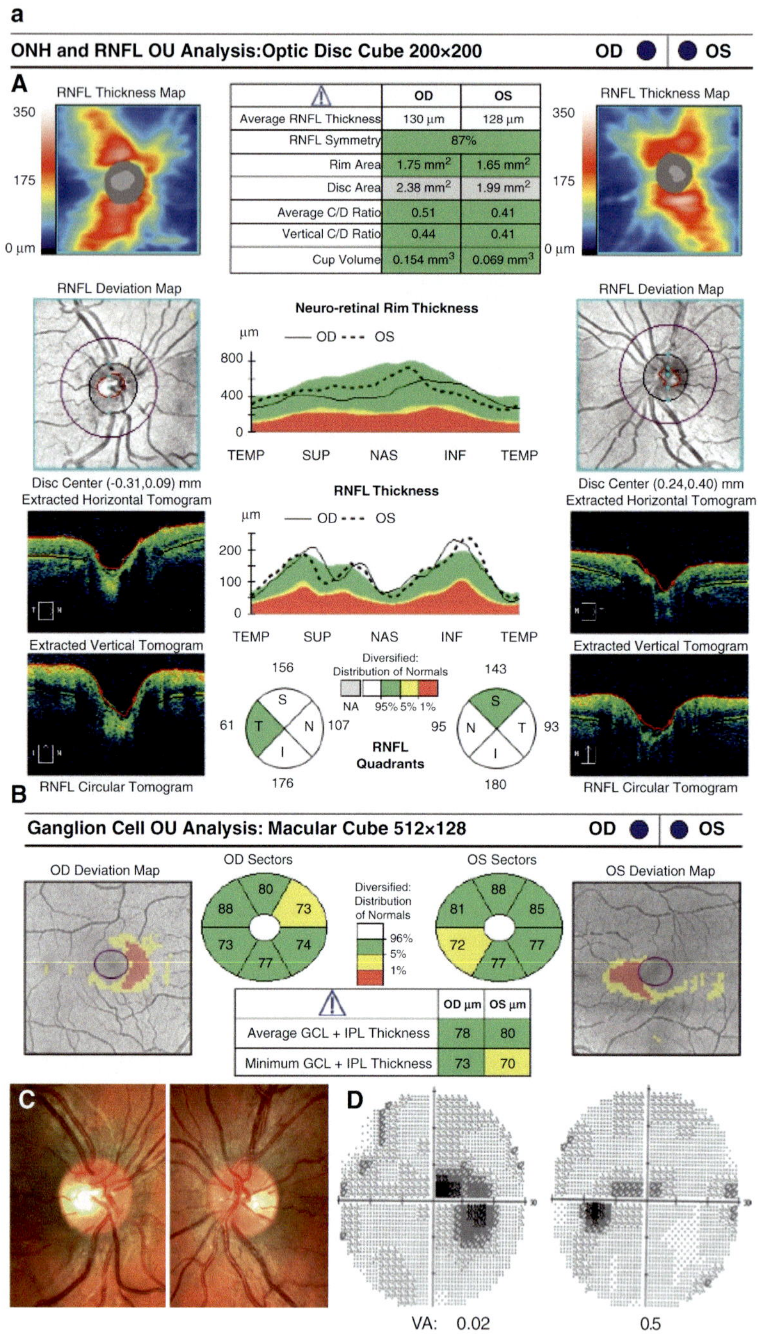

Fig. 16.2 (a) Acute stage of LHON with (A) peripapillary RNFL thickening, (B) early ganglion cell thinning, (C) temporal pallor of the optic disc and (D), central scotoma in the visual field. (B) (a) RNFL thickness and deviation maps (top) RNFL progression analysis (bottom); (b) Progressive RNFL thinning in LHON from acute (top) to the chronic (bottom) stage; (c) RNFL thickness profile

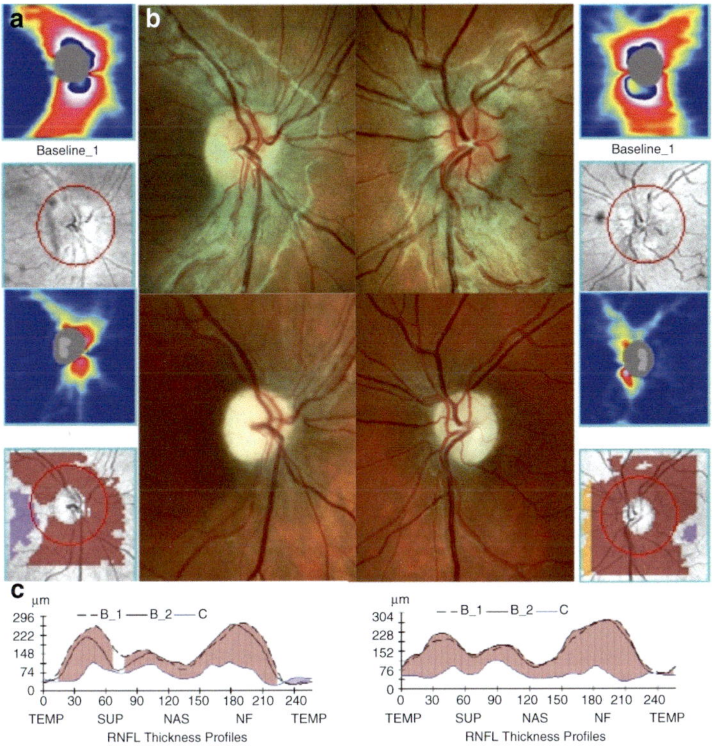

Fig. 16.2 (continued)

A study in a large cohort of Korean LHON patients demonstrated a similar pattern of RNFL thinning in patients carrying primary and secondary mtDNA mutations, despite the better visual prognosis in patients with secondary mutation [27].

OCT analysis of the RNFL in **childhood LHON** (defined as children with disease presentation before the age of 12 years) [10] showed diffuse fiber atrophy affecting all quadrants (Fig. 16.4) [28]. The common presentation is the *subacute bilateral* one that does not differ from the adult-onset presentation [29].

In children, other presentations can be more frequently found like *insidious bilateral, unilateral, subclinical bilateral, and slowly progressive.* No significant differences in RNFL thickness are found in the different groups or based on age of presentation [29].

Insidious, subclinical and slowly progressive forms show a significant fiber reduction in the temporal quadrant, which extends, albeit mildly, to the inferior quadrant, with relative preservation of fibers in the other sectors [28, 29].

16.1.2 Retinal Ganglion Cell Analysis

The macular retinal ganglion cell layer (GCL) is diffusely thinner in LHON affected patients [30, 31]. The early and preferential involvement of macular RGCs, which precedes RNFL thinning, has been demonstrated by OCT in the subacute stage of the disease [19, 24, 30–32].

In the presymptomatic stage, about 4 weeks before the onset of visual loss, topographical analysis of the macular region demonstrated an early involvement of the inner ring of the nasal sectors, where the RGC bodies, that contribute to the PMB fibers, are located (Fig. 16.5) [33–35]. In this phase the macular GCL deviation map is more sensitive than the sector analysis provided by OCT (Fig. 16.5).

Subsequently, the macular GCL thinning progresses, following a centrifugal and spiral pattern (sequential pattern: inner ring of inferior sector, outer ring of the nasal sector, inner ring of the temporal and the superior sectors, outer ring of the temporal sector, outer ring of the superior and inferior sectors) [35].

A correlation between GCL thickness and worsening vision was found [32].

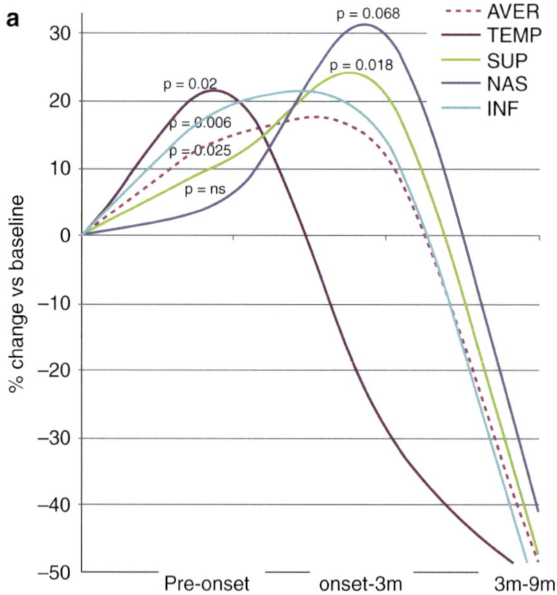

Fig. 16.3 (a) Longitudinal RNFL changes from the onset of visual symptoms to the chronic stage of LHON. The temporal quadrant reveals early thickening, whereas the remaining quadrants undergo later thickening up to 3 months. The RNFL thickness changes are expressed as percent with respect to baseline (asymptomatic stage). *AVER* average, *INF* inferior, *NAS* nasal, *SUP* superior, *TEMP* temporal (reproduced with permission from: Barboni et al. [19]) (b) Example of progressive RNFL thinning in a patient with LHON from the subacute stage to the chronic stage. Note that the OCT software fails to detect temporal thinning in the late stages as the RNFL thickness is too low, producing a floor effect

b

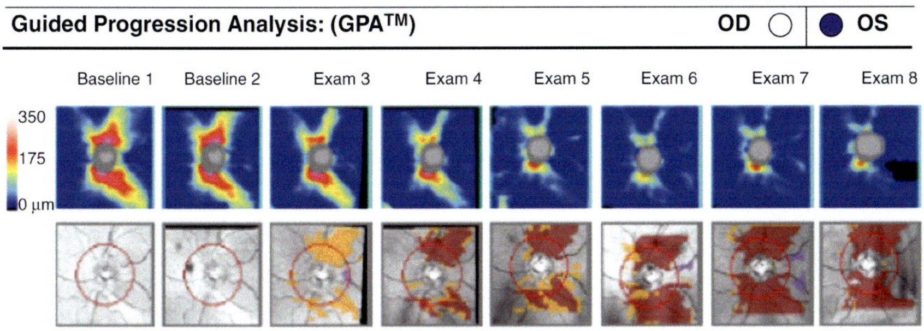

RNFL and ONH Summary Parameters

		Exam Date/Time	Serial Number	Registration Method	SS	Avg RNFL Thickness (µm)	Inf Quadrant RNFL (µm)	Sup Quadrant RNFL (µm)	Rim Area (mm²)	Average Cup-to-Disc Ratio	Vertical Cup-to-Disc Ratio	Cup Volume (mm³)
Baseline 1:	1	12/16/2010 1:16:30 PM	4000-2487		9/10	105	144	130	1.76	0.46	0.37	0.136
Baseline 2:	2	1/20/2011 12:40:56 PM	4000-2487	R2	7/10	96	136	125	1.86	0.46	0.37	0.142
	3	6/27/2011 1:38:32 PM	4000-2487	R2	8/10	80	116	91	1.54	0.54	0.45	0.193
	4	9/29/2011 1:31:33 PM	4000-2487	R2	7/10	70	99	79	1.36	0.60	0.50	0.231
	5	3/16/2012 3:06:54 PM	4000-2487	R1	7/10	61	76	66	1.23	0.67	0.56	0.273
	6	11/26/2012 1:31:48 PM	4000-2487	R1	7/10	59	69	64	1.18	0.69	0.60	0.304
	7	4/16/2013 1:18:51 PM	4000-2487	R1	8/10	58	68	57	1.18	0.69	0.60	0.287
Current:	8	11/25/2013 1:09:17 PM	4000-2487	R1	6/10	55	66	58	1.31	0.72	0.63	0.350

Fig. 16.3 (continued)

In childhood LHON, a significant GCL thinning was found only in insidious unilateral patients compared with insidious bilateral patients [29].

OCT was also used to assess the presence of clinical biomarkers predicting the response to Idebenone therapy in patients with LHON and the thinning of the GCL in the superior and temporal parafoveal regions was associated with worse long-term visual outcomes in these patients [36].

Another study showed that visual acuity gain after Idebenone treatment was weakly associated with GCL volume at baseline, but not with RNFL thickness, patients age or diseases duration [37].

16.1.3 Optic Nerve Head Analysis

OCT also enabled the investigation of the size of the optic nerve head (ONH). Asymptomatic LHON carriers showed a larger ONH than symptomatic patients and even healthy controls (Fig. 16.6) [38]. Moreover, the LHON-affected subgroup

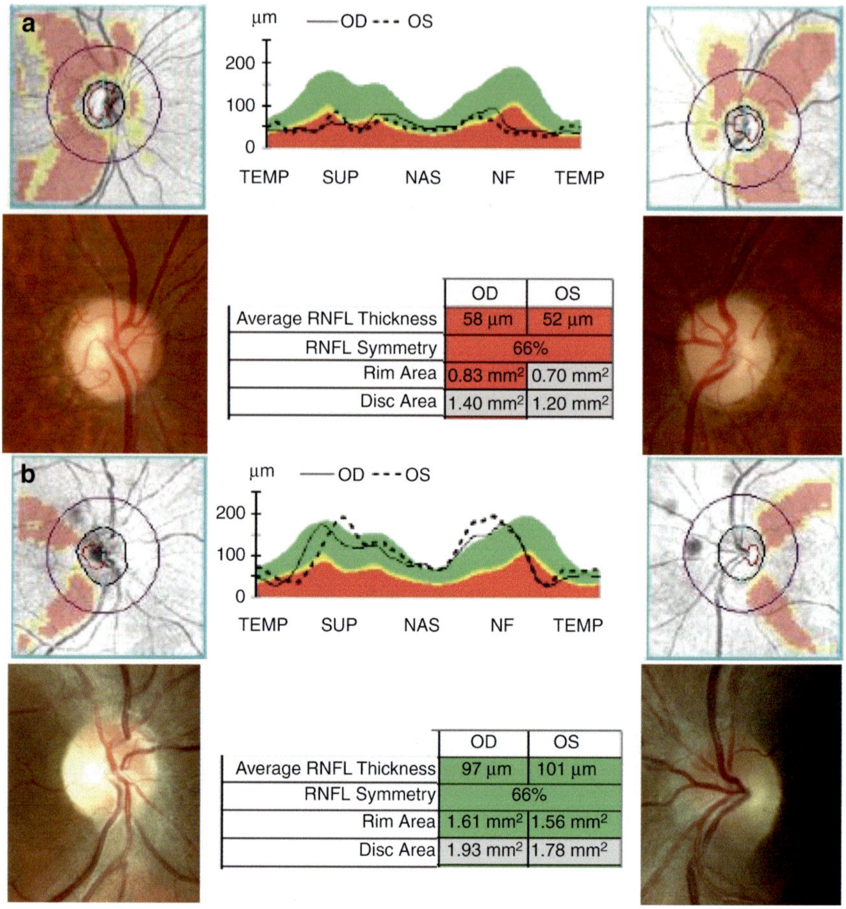

Fig. 16.4 OCT and color fundus pictures of the right and left optic nerve head in (A) a child with subacute LHON presentation: note the small optic disc size, the diffuse RNFL thinning and the temporal optic disc pallor; (B) a child with uncategorized early onset before the age of 6: note the medium optic disc size, the temporal RNFL thinning and the nasal RNFL swelling. The OCT software fails to detect the RNFL thinning in the temporal sector due to the floor effect

of patients with visual recovery also had a significantly larger ONH. Therefore, it has been suggested that a larger ONH size, probably associated with less crowding of RGC axons, may represent a favorable prognostic factor and be a protective factor preserving LHON carriers from developing the acute phase of the disease, improving the visual prognosis and influencing the final visual outcome in those individuals who develop optic neuropathy. The role of the ONH size may be related to the mechanical compression of the PMB fibers: the greater space for nerve fibers may reduce the risk of focal compression of swelling axons.

After stratifying LHON affected and carrier patients by mtDNA mutations, 11,778, 3460 and 3733 carriers had larger optic nerve discs than affected [27].

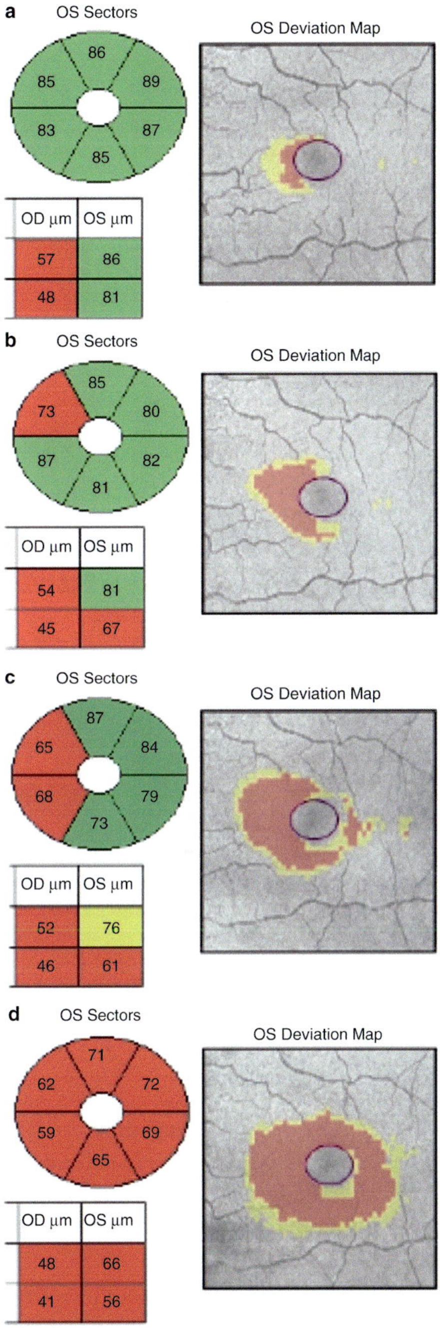

Fig. 16.5 Progressive retinal ganglion cells atrophy in a patient followed from the presymptomatic stage (about 4 weeks before visual loss). Ganglion cell layer sectors and deviation map in pre-symptomatic stage (a), at 1 month (b), 2 months (c) and 5 months (d) from disease onset

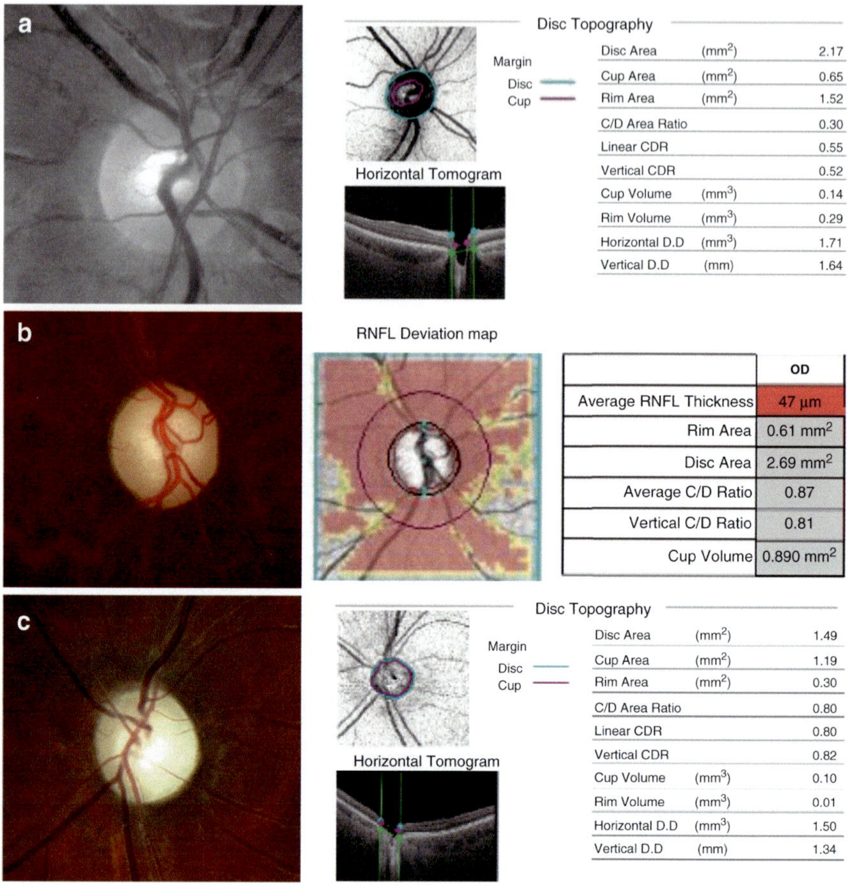

Fig. 16.6 Representative optic nerve head color pictures and OCT analysis: (A) asymptomatic LHON mutation carrier with large optic disc area; (B): chronic LHON patient with large optic disc area and partial visual recovery; (**C**): chronic LHON patient with small optic disc area and without visual recovery

14,484 affected and carrier patients had the same disc size and that was larger than for the other mutations [38].

Moreover, ONH analysis in subacute childhood LHON patients (subacute bilateral LHON) showed smaller optic disc areas compared with patients with slowly progressive and subclinical courses of the disease and controls (Fig. 16.4) [28].

16.2 Dominant Optic Atrophy (DOA)

DOA hereditary degenerative optic neuropathy with similarities to LHON. It too preferentially involves the PMB. However, DOA is due to a mutation in the nuclear genome and is transmitted in an autosomal dominant manner. Most cases of DOA have been associated with mutations in the OPA1 gene on the long arm of chromosome 3q28–q29, which encodes a dynamin-related GTPase targeted to mitochondria [39]. Seventy-five percent of DOA patients have a mutation in OPA1 gene; two loci, OPA4 and OPA5, are associated to pure DOA, one X-linked, OPA2, and two autosomal recessive ones, at OPA6 and OPA7, and two syndromic recessive or dominant ones, at OPA3 and OPA8 [40–42].

DOA patients with OPA1 mutation can be also defined by the mutation type: OPA1 mutation causing haploinsufficiency and an OPA1 missense mutation [43].

DOA has a clinical picture more insidious than that of LHON, as it is characterized by very slowly progressive bilateral visual loss starting in childhood and ultimately leading to moderate or severe optic atrophy [44–47]. The disease has incomplete penetrance and variable expression between and within families; it ranges from subclinical manifestations to legal blindness. Twenty percent of DOA patients with OPA1 mutations have a more severe disease with neuromuscular features (DOA plus) [48, 49].

16.2.1 Retinal Nerve Fiber Layer Analysis

OCT analysis of the RNFL in DOA reveals fiber atrophy affecting all quadrants [50–52]. The retinal thinning involves the RNFL and GCL, whereas the photoreceptors are morphologically unaffected (Fig. 16.7).

The RNFL thinning is more pronounced in the temporal and inferior quadrants and less evident in the superior and nasal ones [50–52], confirming the vulnerability of the small fibers of the PMB and the subsequent wedge defect as a pathognomonic sign of mitochondrial optic neuropathies. Patients with DOA plus disease show a more severe thinning of RNFL in all quadrants compared with simple DOA patients [52].

The progressive fiber loss in affected patients (0.19–0.20 μm/year for the 360° average measurement) is similar to that occurring with age in healthy subjects, where the loss ranges between 0.16 and 0.25 μm/year [53–55]. This observation, in combination with the smaller ONH of DOA patients (see the next paragraph), suggests that visual loss in DOA patients is related to progressive fiber loss in eyes with already lower congenital or neonatal fiber counts.

The pattern of fiber loss, studied by OCT, in OPA8 patients did not differ from that found in OPA1 patients [56]. A genotype/phenotype correlation, stratifying OCT measurement by OPA1 mutation type, shows that missense mutations had the most severe reductions in both RNFL and macular GCL thickness [33].

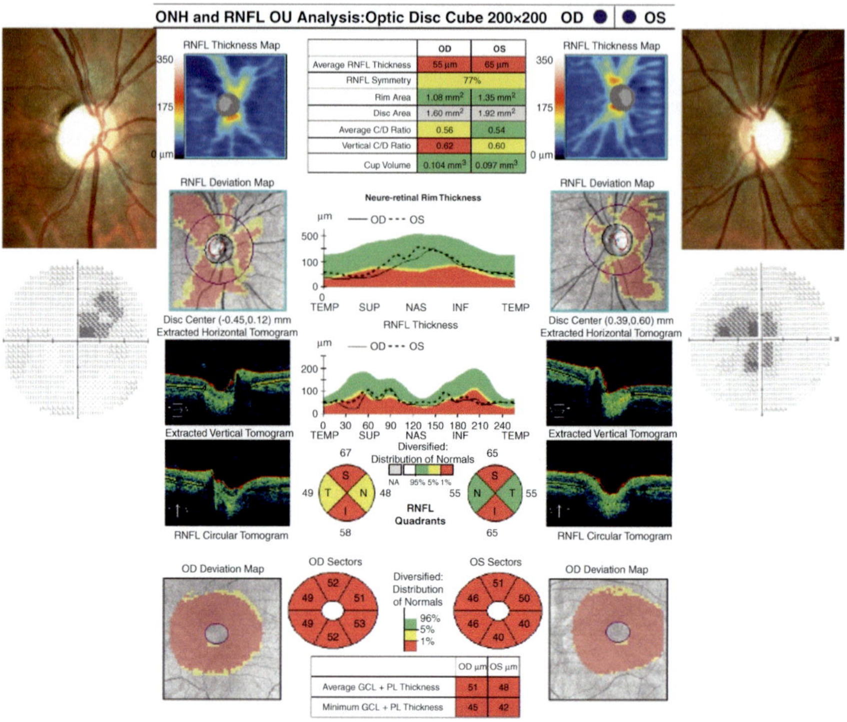

Fig. 16.7 Peripapillary RNFL, macular ganglion cell layer analysis, color fundus image and visual fields in a patient with DOA

16.2.2 Retinal Ganglion Cell Analysis

OCT of DOA patients showed an earlier involvement of the macular RGCs, whose thickness is reduced in all macular sectors and the thinner sectors were the nasal and inferior ones [33, 57, 58]. As the disease progresses and visual acuity worsened, the macular RGCs measurements correlated with visual acuity losses better than measures of RNFL thinning (Fig. 16.7) [33, 58]. GCL thickness also declined with age [33].

GCL sectors were overall thinner in patients with DOA since early age compared to patients with Wolfram Syndrome (WS), in which GCL thickness started to decline later in life. Conversely, RNFL thickness loss were worse in patients with WS with a faster decline from early age as compared with patients with DOA, who displayed a more stable visual function over the years. The early loss of GCL indirectly support the presence of a primary mitochondrial dysfunction in patients with DOA [59]

16.2.3 Optic Nerve Head Analysis

Patients affected with DOA and carrying OPA1 gene mutations reveal a smaller ONH (both optic disc area and ONH diameters) than controls [60]. By stratifying these results according to OPA1 mutation, it is possible to identify different degrees of optic disc size, where the mutations range from those associated with a normal optic disc size to those associated with much smaller sizes and more severe clinical features of DOA. The proposed hypothesis is that OPA1 expression regulates apoptosis, thereby playing an important role in the embryonic development of the eye and contributing to the determination of optic disc size and conformation. DOA patients with the poorest visual acuity have a smaller optic disc area, as measured by OCT, compared to controls [61].

OCT analysis showed that DOA patients who do not recover vision on Idebenone therapy have thinner RNFL and smaller ONH than patients with visual recovery [60]. This result adds further evidence for the prognostic value of OCT in therapeutic protocols.

16.3 Other OCT Macular Findings

OCT analysis of the macular region shows, in addition, that a minority (about 6%) of LHON and DOA patients have microcystic changes in the inner nuclear layer (Fig. 16.8) [62, 63]. Microcystic macular edema (MME) is present in the absence of any leakage of fluorescein.

MME could be related to focal retinal (RNFL) atrophy that leads to granular schisis by vitreous traction [62], or to retrograde transsynaptic degeneration in the visual pathways [64, 65], Muller cells dysfunction [66] or inflammation [67].

16.4 OCT and Vascular Supply Analysis

Advances in OCT allowed the study of the choroidal thickness and choroidal vascular index, using enhanced depth imaging (EDI) technique or the swept source OCT (SS-OCT). Moreover, the vascular supply of the optic nerve head, the macula and the choriocapillaris is displayable using the optical coherence tomography angiography (OCT-A).

Those exams were performed in hereditary optic neuropathies and could elucidate the role of the vasculature in the disease process.

Changes of the choroidal thickness have been documented in LHON patients during disease conversion. Specifically, both macular and peripapillary choroidal thickness increase in the subacute stage and then decrease in the chronic stage, following the same trend of peripapillary RNFL (increased thickness, followed by thinning), but RNFL changes preceded those affecting the choroid [68]. The evidence that increased thickness of axons precedes the increase of choroidal thickness suggests that the first event leads to the second one. The choroidal thickening

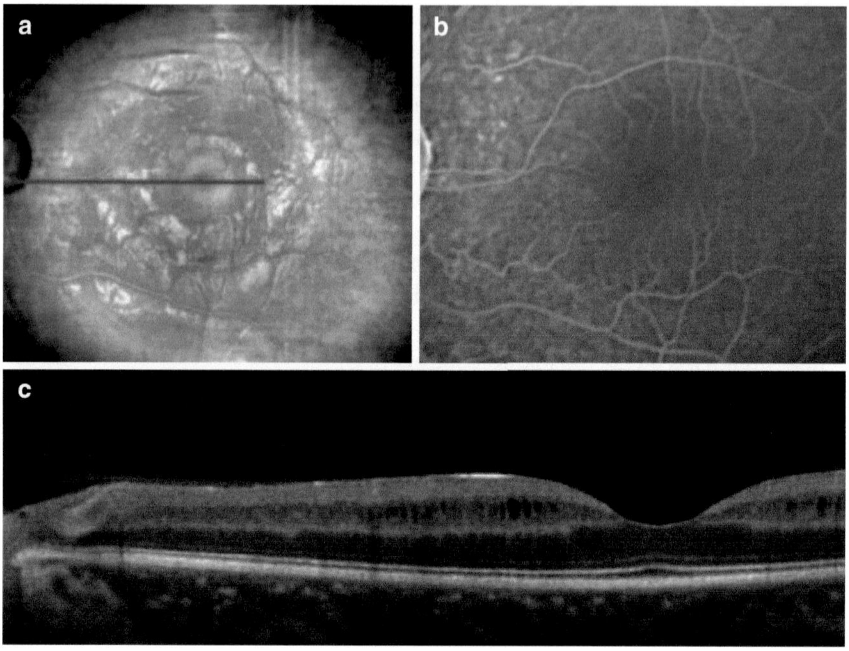

Fig. 16.8 Microcystic macular edema in a patient with LHON. (a) Red free fundus picture, (b) fluorescein angiography and (c) corresponding HD-OCT line of the macula

seen during the LHON subacute stage may be due to a compensatory response to hypoxia and increased oxygen demand. In the chronic stage, the choroid was thicker in LHON than in DOA (whereas the RNFL thickness followed an opposite trend being thinner in LHON as compared to DOA) [68]. Moreover, in chronic LHON the choroidal thinning correlated strongly with both RNFL and GCC thicknesses [69]

The choroidal vascularity index (CVI, obtained as the ratio of luminal choroidal area and total choroidal area) is preserved in chronic LHON and DOA, suggesting that even in the chronic phase the choroidal structure is not irreversibly compromised [70].

However, peripapillary choroidal vascularity seems to remain stable after gene therapy in LHON [71].

Using OCT-A, peripapillary telangiectatic blood vessels have been documented in the LHON subacute stage [72–75]. Subsequently, a progressive peripapillary vascular reduction was detected starting from the temporal and inferior sectors as the disease progressed [76], then spreading to all the other peripapillary vessels in the chronic phase (Fig. 16.9) [76, 77]. Studying the vascular network separately from fibers revealed that microvascular changes in the temporal sector preceded the changes of RNFL and mirrored the GCL changes [76]. A reduction of the vessel density in the parafoveal region in LHON, mainly confined to the nasal

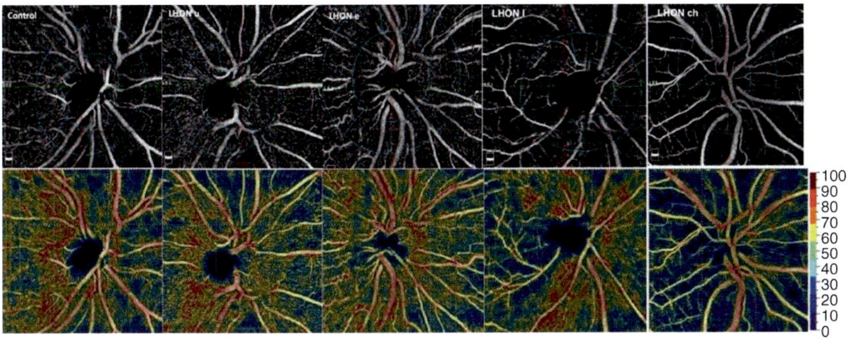

Fig. 16.9 Example of OCT-A in the different LHON stages. Example of vascular visualization of Radial Peripapillary Capillaries (RPC, top images) layer and density maps (bottom images) in 5 groups (control; LHON u: unaffected carrier; LHON e: early subacute stage; LHON l: late subacute stage; LHON ch: chronic stage). Note the progressive vessel density reduction as the disease advances, starting from the temporal sector (Reproduced with the permission from: Balducci et al. [73])

and inferior sectors, corresponding to the PMB, was documented [78]. Moreover, an association between the visual loss and the superficial capillary plexus flow impairment was detected [78].

In DOA a reduction of optic nerve head and peripapillary vessel density was detected [79–81].

Moreover, vessel densities of the superficial and deep macular vascular plexi were significantly decreased in DOA patients [81] and showed correlation with GCC thickness and with visual acuity [81]

16.5 Expanding Phenotype

In the field of hereditary optic neuropathies, advancements in genetic techniques have led to the discovery of new mutations and an expanded understanding of the phenotypic manifestations associated with these conditions. With the advent of next-generation sequencing and other molecular diagnostic approaches, we are able to identify previously unknown genetic variations responsible for hereditary optic neuropathies [82, 83].

In the past, the genotype-phenotype correlation in hereditary optic neuropathies was thought to be relatively straightforward, with specific mutations leading to consistent clinical manifestations. However, recent studies have revealed a more complex picture. It is now recognized that there can be considerable variability in the isolated or syndromic form of optic atrophy, even among individuals carrying the same genetic mutation.

The clinical picture of LHON is primarily caused by mutations in mtDNA; whereas, LHON-like disease is also associated with mutations in nuclear genes

[84]. The identification of recessive mutations in *DNAJC30, NDUFS2, MCAT* genes in LHON-like disease has significantly expanded our understanding of mitochondrial disorders and their phenotypic variability. While the underlying genetic causes differ between these conditions, both LHON and LHON-like disease exhibit distinctive clinical and optical coherence tomography (OCT) patterns that aid in their diagnosis and management [85–87].

Even if the most common causes of DOA are mutations in the *OPA1* gene, which accounts for the majority of cases, it is important to note that several other genes, both recessive and dominant, can also present with a similar phenotype of isolated, slowly progressive visual loss [2, 88]. While optic atrophy can be a feature of various syndromic disorders, it is important to recognize that genetic variants associated with syndromic patterns can also manifest as isolated optic atrophy with no other systemic manifestations. Conditions such as Wolfram syndrome, ACO2, AFG3L2 and SSBP1-related optic atrophy exemplify this phenomenon, where a clinical isolated pattern of optic atrophy is observed despite the underlying genetic association with syndromic disorders [89–91]. There is limited information available on the specific OCT patterns in optic atrophy associated with these conditions. OCT findings have been described primarily in isolated case reports and need better understanding and potential differences compared to typical DOA [89–91].

16.6 Conclusions

Over the last decades, OCT enabled us to better understand the diagnosis and follow-up of optic neuropathies. Moreover, the additional information achieved by OCT and OCT-A about the pathophysiology of these related diseases have improved our knowledge on the disease conversion and progression. We hope that soon OCT and OCT-A can be used as a biomarker with which to assess purported new therapeutic approaches.

References

1. Yu-Wai-Man P, Griffiths PG, Chinnery PF. Mitochondrial optic neuropathies disease mechanisms and therapeutic strategies. Prog Retin Eye Res. 2011;30:81–114.
2. Rocatcher A, Desquiret-Dumas V, Charif M, Ferré M, Gohier P, Mirebeau-Prunier D, Verny C, Milea M, Lenaers G, HON Collaborators Group, Bonneau D, Reynier P, Amati-Bonneau P. The top 10 most frequently involved genes in hereditary optic neuropathies in 2186 probands. Brain. 2013;146(2):455–60.
3. Newman NJ. Hereditary optic neuropathies. In: Miller NR, Newman NJ, editors. Walsh and Hoyt's clinical neuro-ophthalmology. 5th ed. Baltimore: Williams & Wilkins; 1998. p. 742–53.
4. Carelli V. Leber's hereditary optic neuropathy. In: Schapira AHV, DiMauro S, editors. Mitochondrial Disorders in Neurology. 2nd ed. Blue Books of Practical Neurology. Vol. 26. Boston: Butterworth-Heinemann; 2002. p. 115–42.
5. Carelli V, Giordano C, d'Amati G. Pathogenic expression of homoplasmic mtDNA mutations needs a complex nuclear-mitochondrial interaction. Trends Genet. 2003;19:257–62.

6. Sadun AA, Kashima Y, Wurdeman AE, et al. Morphological findings in the visual system in a case of Leber's hereditary optic neuropathy. Clin Neurosci. 1994;2:165–72.
7. Kerrison JB, Howell N, Miller NR, et al. Leber hereditary optic neuropathy. Electron microscopy and molecular genetic analysis of a case. Ophthalmology. 1995;102:1509–16.
8. Sadun AA, Win PH, Ross-Cisneros FN, et al. Leber's hereditary optic neuropathy differentially affects smaller axons in the optic nerve. Trans Am Ophthalmol Soc. 2000;98:223–32.
9. Pan BX, Ross-Cisneros FN, Carelli V, Rue KS, Salomao SR, Moraes-Filho MN, Moraes MN, Berezovsky A, Belfort R Jr, Sadun AA. Mathematically modeling the involvement of axons in Leber's hereditary optic neuropathy. Invest Ophthalmol Vis Sci. 2012;53:7608–17.
10. Carelli V, Carbonelli M, de Coo IF, Kawasaki A, Klopstock T, Lagrèze WA, La Morgia C, Newman NJ, Orssaud C, Pott JWR, Sadun AA, van Everdingen J, Vignal-Clermont C, Votruba M, Yu-Wai-Man P, Barboni P. International consensus statement on the clinical and therapeutic management of Leber hereditary optic neuropathy. J Neuroophthalmol. 2017;37:371–81.
11. Nikoskelainen E, Hoyt WF, Nummelin K. Ophthalmoscopic findings in Leber's hereditary optic neuropathy. I. Fundus findings in asymptomatic family members. Arch Ophthalmol. 1982;100:1597–602.
12. Nikoskelainen E, Hoyt WF, Nummelin K. Ophthalmoscopic findings in Leber's hereditary optic neuropathy. II. The fundus findings in affected family members. Arch Ophthalmol. 1983;101:1059–68.
13. Smith JL, Hoyt WF, Susac JO. Ocular fundus in acute Leber optic neuropathy. Arch Ophthalmol. 1973;90:349–54.
14. Riordan-Eva P, Sanders D, Govan GG, et al. The clinical features of Leber's hereditary optic neuropathy defined by the presence of a pathogenic mitochondrial DNA mutation. Brain. 1995;118:319–37.
15. Nikoskelainen EK, Huoponen K, Juvonen V, et al. Ophthalmologic findings in Leber hereditary optic neuropathy, with special reference to mtDNA mutations. Ophthalmology. 1996;103:504–14.
16. Savini G, Barboni P, Valentino ML, Montagna P, Cortelli P, De Negri AM, Sadun F, Bianchi S, Longanesi L, Zanini M, Carelli V. Retinal nerve fiber layer evaluation by optical coherence tomography in unaffected carriers with Leber's hereditary optic neuropathy mutations. Ophthalmology. 2005;112:127–31.
17. Carbonelli M, La Morgia C, Romagnoli M, Amore G, D'agati P, Valentino ML, Caporali L, Cascavilla ML, Battista M, Borrelli E, Di Renzo A, Parisi V, Balducci N, Carelli V, Barboni P. Capturing the pattern of transition from carrier to affected in Leber hereditary optic neuropathy. Am J Ophthalmol. 2022;241:71–9.
18. Barboni P, Savini G, Valentino ML, Montagna P, Cortelli P, De Negri AM, et al. Retinal nerve fiber layer evaluation by optical coherence tomography in Leber's hereditary optic neuropathy. Ophthalmology. 2005;112:120–6.
19. Hedges TR, Gobuty M, Manfready RA, Erlich-Malona N, Monaco C, Mendoza-Santiesteban CE. The optical coherence tomographic profile of Leber hereditary optic neuropathy. Neuroophthalmology. 2016;40:107–12.
20. Carelli V, Ross-Cisneros FN, Sadun AA. Mitochondrial dysfunction as a cause of optic neuropathies. Prog Retin Eye Res. 2004;23:53–89.
21. Barboni P, Savini G, Feuer WJ, Budenz DL, Carbonelli M, Chicani F, Ramos CD, Salomao SR, De Negri A, Parisi V, Carelli V, Sadun AA. Retinal nerve fiber layer thickness variability in Leber hereditary optic neuropathy carriers. Eur J Ophthalmol. 2012;4(22):985–91.
22. Barboni P, Carbonelli M, Savini G, et al. Natural history of Leber's hereditary optic neuropathy: longitudinal analysis of the retinal nerve fiber layer by optical coherence tomography. Ophthalmology. 2010;117:623–7.
23. Zhang Y, Huang H, Wei S, Qiu H, Gong Y, Li H, Dai Y, Jiang Z, Liu Z. Characterization of retinal nerve fiber layer thickness changes associated with Leber's hereditary optic neuropathy by optical coherence tomography. Exp Ther Med. 2014;7:483–7.

24. Teng D, Peng CX, Qian HY, Li L, Wang W, Wang JQ, Chen B, Zhou HF, Wei SH. Structural impairment patterns in peripapillary retinal fiber layer and retinal ganglion cell layer in mitochondrial optic neuropathies. Int J Ophthalmol. 2018;11:1643–8.
25. Seo JH, Hwang JM, Park SS. Comparison of retinal nerve fibre layers between 11778 and 14484 mutations in Leber's hereditary optic neuropathy. Eye. 2010;24:107–11.
26. Caporali L, Ghelli AM, Iommarini L, Maresca A, Valentino ML, La Morgia C, Liguori R, Zanna C, Barboni P, De Nardo V, Martinuzzi A, Rizzo G, Tonon C, Lodi R, Calvaruso MA, Cappelletti M, Porcelli AM, Achilli A, Pala M, Torroni A, Carelli V. Cybrid studies establish the causal link between the mtDNA m.3890G>A/MT-ND1 mutation and optic atrophy with bilateral brainstem lesions. Biochim Biophys Acta 2013;1832:445–52.
27. Yum HR, Chae H, Shin SY, Kim Y, Kim M, Park SH. Pathogenic mitochondrial DNA mutations and associated clinical features in Korean patients with Leber's hereditary optic neuropathy. Invest Ophthalmol Vis Sci. 2014;55:8095–101.
28. Barboni P, Savini G, Valentino ML, La Morgia C, Bellusci C, De Negri AM, Sadun F, Carta A, Carbonelli M, Sadun AA, Carelli V. Leber's hereditary optic neuropathy with childhood onset. Invest Ophthalmol Vis Sci. 2006;47:5303–9.
29. Barboni P, La Morgia C, Cascavilla ML, Hee Hong E, Battista M, AMajander A, Caporali L, Starace V, Amore G, Di Renzo A, Carbonelli M, Nucci P, Jurkute N, Chen BS, Panebianco R, De Negri AM, Sadun F, Parisi V, Bandello F, Sadun AA, Carelli V, Yu-Wai-Man P. Childhood-onset Leber hereditary optic neuropathy—clinical and prognostic insights. Am J Ophthalmol 2023;249: 99–107.
30. Akiyama H, Kashima T, Li D, Shimoda Y, Mukai R, Kishi S. Retinal ganglion cell analysis in Leber's hereditary optic neuropathy. Ophthalmology. 2013;120:1943-1944e5.
31. Mizoguchi A, Hashimoto Y, Shinmei Y, Nozaki M, Ishijima K, Tagawa Y, et al. Macular thickness changes in a patient with Leber's hereditary optic neuropathy. BMC Ophthalmol. 2015;15:27.
32. Moster SJ, Moster ML, Scannell, Bryan M, Sergott RC. Retinal ganglion cell and inner plexiform layer loss correlate with visual acuity loss in LHON: a longitudinal, segmentation OCT analysis. Invest Ophthalmol Vis Sci. 2016;57:3872–83.
33. Barboni P, Savini G, Cascavilla M, Caporali L, Milesi J, Borrelli E, et al. Early macular retinal ganglion cell loss in dominant optic atrophy: genotype-phenotype correlation. Am J Ophthalmol. 2014;158:628–36.
34. Zhang Y, Huang H, Wei S, Gong Y, Li H, Dai Y, Zhao S, Wang Y, Yan H. Characterization of macular thickness changes in Leber's hereditary optic neuropathy by optical coherence tomography. BMC Ophthalmol. 2014;14:105.
35. Balducci N, Savini G, Cascavilla ML, La Morgia C, Triolo G, Giglio R, Carbonelli M, Parisi V, Sadun AA, Bandello F, Carelli V, Barboni P. Macular nerve fibre and ganglion cell layer changes in acute Leber's hereditary optic neuropathy. Br J Ophthalmol. 2016;100:1232–7.
36. Borrelli E, Berni A, Cascavilla ML, Barresi C, Battista M, Lari G, Reibaldi M, Bandello F, Barboni P. Visual outcomes and optical coherence tomography biomarkers of vision improvement in patients with leber hereditary optic neuropathy treated with idebenone. Am J Ophthalmol. 2023;247:35–41.
37. Pemp B, Mitsch C, Kircher K, Reitner A. Changes in visual function and correlations with inner retinal structure in acute and chronic Leber's hereditary optic neuropathy patients after treatment with idebenone. J Clin Med. 2021;10:151.
38. Ramos C do V, Bellusci C, Savini G, et al. Association of optic disc size with development and prognosis of Leber's Hereditary Optic Neuropathy. Invest Ophthalmol Vis Sci. 2009;50:1666–74.
39. Alexander C, Votruba M, Pesch UE, et al. OPA1, encoding a dynamin-related GTPase, is mutated in autosomal dominant optic atrophy linked to chromosome 3q28. Nat Genet. 2000;26:211–5.
40. Ferre M, Amati-Bonneau P, Tourmen Y, Malthièry Y, Reynier P. eOPA1: an online database for OPA1 mutations: Hum Mutat. 2005;25:423–8. PubMed: 15832306.

41. Ferre M, Bonneau D, Milea D, Chevrollier A, Verny C, Dullfus H, et al. Molecular screening of 980 cases of suspected hereditary optic neuropathy with a report on 77 novel OPA1 mutations. Hum Mutat. 2009;30:E692-705.
42. Yu-Wai-Man P, Shankar SP, Biousse V, Miller NR, Bean LJ, Coffee B, et al. Genetic screening for OPA1 and OPA3 mutations in patients with suspected inherited optic neuropathies. Ophthalmology. 2010;118:558–63.
43. Amati-Bonneau P, Valentino ML, Reynier P, Gallardo ME, Bornstein B, Boissière A, et al. OPA1 mutations induce mitochondrial DNA instability and optic atrophy "plus" phenotypes. Brain. 2008;131:338–51.
44. Kjer P. Infantile optic atrophy with dominant mode of inheritance: a clinical and genetic study of 19 Danish families. Acta Ophthalmol Suppl. 1959;164(suppl):1–147.
45. Newman NJ. Hereditary optic neuropathies. In: Miller NR, Newman NJ, editors; Biousse V, Kerrison JB, associate editors. Walsh and Hoyt's Clinical Neuro-Ophthalmology. 6th ed. vol 1. Philadelphia: Lippincott Williams & Wilkins; 2005. p. 465–501.
46. Cohn AC, Toomes C, Hewitt AW, Kearns LS, Inglehearn CF, Craig JE, et al. The natural history of OPA1-related autosomal dominant optic atrophy. Br J Ophthalmol. 2008;92:1333–6.
47. Yu-Wai-Man P, Griffiths PG, Burke A, Sellar PW, Clarke MP, Gnanaraj L, et al. The prevalence and natural history of dominant optic atrophy due to OPA1 mutations. Ophthalmology. 2010;117:1538–46.
48. Amati-Bonneau P, Guichet A, Olichon A, Chevrollier A, Viala F, Miot S, Ayuso C, et al. OPA1 R445H mutation in optic atrophy associated with sensorineural deafness. Ann Neurol. 2005;58:958–63.
49. Hudson G, Amati-Bonneau P, Blakely EL, Stewart JD, He L, Schaefer AM, et al. Mutation of OPA1 causes dominant optic atrophy with external ophthalmoplegia, ataxia, deafness and multiple mitochondrial DNA deletions: a novel disorder of mtDNA maintenance. Brain. 2008;131:329–37.
50. Milea D, Sander B, Wegener M, et al. Axonal loss occurs early in dominant optic atrophy. Acta Ophthalmol. 2010;88:342–6.
51. Barboni P, Savini G, Parisi V, et al. Retinal nerve fiber layer thickness in dominant optic atrophy measurements by optical coherence tomography and correlation with age. Ophthalmology. 2011;118:2076–80.
52. Yu-Wai-Man P, Bailie M, Atawan A, Chinnery PF, Griffiths PG. Pattern of retinal ganglion cell loss in dominant optic atrophy due to OPA1 mutations. Eye. 2011;25:596–602.
53. Parikh RS, Parikh SR, Sekhar GC, et al. Normal age-related decay of retinal nerve fiber layer thickness. Ophthalmology. 2007;114:921–6.
54. Sung KR, Wollstein G, Bilonick RA, et al. Effects of age on optical coherence tomography measurements of healthy retinal nerve fiber layer, macula and optic nerve head. Ophthalmology. 2009;116:1119–24.
55. Budenz DL, Anderson DR, Varma R, et al. Determinants of normal retinal nerve fiber layer thickness measured by Stratus OCT. Ophthalmology. 2007;114:1046–52.
56. Carelli V, Schimpf S, Fuhrmann N, Valentino ML, Zanna C, Iommarini L, Papke M, Schaich S, Tippmann S, Baumann B, Barboni P, Longanesi L, Rugolo M, Ghelli A, Alavi MV, Youle RJ, Bucchi L, Carroccia R, Giannoccaro MP, Tonon C, Lodi R, Cenacchi G, Montagna P, Liguori R, Wissinger B. A clinically complex form of dominant optic atrophy (OPA8) maps on chromosome 16. Hum Mol Genet. 2011;20:1893–905.
57. Ito Y, Nakamura M, Yamakoshi T, Lin J, Yatsuya H, Terasaki H. Reduction of inner retinal thickness in patients with autosomal dominant optic atrophy associated with OPA1 mutations. Invest Ophthalmol Vis Sci. 2007;48:4079–86.
58. Rönnbäck C, Milea D, Larsen M. Imaging of the macula indicates early completion of structural deficit in autosomal-dominant optic atrophy. Ophthalmology. 2013;120:2672–7.
59. Barboni P, Amore G, Cascavilla ML, Battista M, Frontino G, Romagnoli M, Caporali L, Baldoli C, Gramegna LL, Sessagesimi E, Bonfanti R, Romagnoli A, Scotti R, Brambati M, Carbonelli M, Starace V, Fiorini C, Panebianco R, Parisi V, Tonon C, Bandello F, Carelli V,

La Morgia C. The pattern of retinal ganglion cell loss in wolfram syndrome is distinct from mitochondrial optic neuropathies. Am J Ophthalmol. 2022;241:206–16.

60. Barboni P, Valentino ML, La Morgia C, Carbonelli M, Savini G, De Negri A, Simonelli F, Sadun F, Caporali L, Maresca A, Liguori R, Baruzzi A, Zeviani M, Carelli V. Idebenone treatment in patients with OPA1-mutant dominant optic atrophy. Brain. 2013;136(Pt2): e231.
61. Barboni P, Carbonelli M, Savini G, Foscarini B, Parisi V, Valentino ML, Carta A, De Negri AM, Sadun F, Zeviani M, Sadun AA, Schimpf S, Wissinger B, Carelli V. OPA1 mutations associated with dominant optic atrophy influence optic nerve head size. Ophthalmology. 2010;117:1547–53.
62. Barboni P, Carelli V, Savini G, Carbonelli M, La Morgia C, Sadun AA. Microcystic macular degeneration from optic neuropathy: not inflammatory, not trans-synaptic degeneration. Brain. 2013;136(Pt 7): e239.
63. Carbonelli M, La Morgia C, Savini G, Cascavilla ML, Borrelli E, Chicani F, Ramos CdVF, Salomao SR, Parisi V, Sebag J, Bandello F, Sadun AA, Carelli V, Barboni P. Macular microcysts in mitochondrial optic neuropathies: prevalence and retinal layer thickness measurements. Plos One. 2015;10:e0127906.
64. Abegg M, Zinkernagel M, Wolf S. Microcystic macular degeneration from optic neuropathy. Brain. 2012;135: e225.
65. Jindahra P, Petrie A, Plant GT. The time course of retrograde trans-synaptic degeneration following occipital lobe damage in humans. Brain. 2012;135:534–41.
66. Bhargava P, Calabresi PA. The expanding spectrum of aetiologies causing retinal microcystic macular change. Brain 2013;136:3212–4.
67. Gelfand JM, Nolan R, Schwatz DM, Graves J, Green AJ. Microcystic macular oedema in multiple sclerosis is associated with disease severity. Brain. 2012;135:1786–93.
68. Borrelli E, Triolo G, Cascavilla ML, La Morgia C, Rizzo G, Savini G, Balducci N, Nucci P, Giglio R, Darvizeh F, Parisi V, Bandello F, Sadun AA, Carelli V, Barboni P. Changes in choroidal thickness follow the RNFL changes in Leber's hereditary optic neuropathy. Sci Rep. 2016;6:37332.
69. Darvizeh F, Asanad S, Ghasemi Falavarjani K, Wu J, Tian JJ, Bandello F, Ross-Cisneros FN, Barboni P, Borrelli E, Sadun AA. Choroidal thickness and the retinal ganglion cell complex in chronic Leber's hereditary optic neuropathy: a prospective study using swept-source optical coherence tomography. Eye. 2020;34:1624–30.
70. Battista M, Cascavilla ML, Borrelli E, Barresi C, Lari G, Caporali L, Viganò C, Berni A, Carelli V, Bandello F, Barboni P. Choroidal vascularity index in hereditary optic neuropathies. Eye. https://doi.org/10.1038/s41433-023-02383-5
71. Jiang J, Sun G, Miao Q, Li B, Wang D, Yuan J, Chen C. Observation of peripapillary choroidal vascularity in natural disease course and after gene therapy for Leber's hereditary optic neuropathy. Front Med. 2021;8: 770069.
72. Ghasemi Falavarjani K, Tian JJ, Akil H, Garcia GA, Sadda SR, Sadun AA. Swept-source optical coherence tomography angiography of the optic disk in optic neuropathy. Retina. 2016;36:S168–77.
73. De Rojas JO, Rasool N, Chen RW, Horowitz J, Odel JG. Optical coherence tomography angiography in Leber hereditary optic neuropathy. Neurology. 2016;87:2065–6.
74. Takayama K, Ito Y, Kaneko H, Kataoka K, Ra E, Terasaki H. Optical coherence tomography angiography in Leber hereditary optic neuropathy. Acta Ophthalmol. 2017;95:e344–5.
75. Akil H, Ghasemi Falavarjani K, Sadda SS, Sadun AA. Optical coherence tomography angiography of the optic disc; an overview. J Ophthalmic Vis Res. 2017;12:98–105.
76. Balducci N, Cascavilla ML, Ciardella A, La Morgia C, Triolo G, Parisi V, Bandello F, Sadun AA, Carelli V, Barboni P. Peripapillary vessel density changes in Leber's hereditary optic neuropathy: a new biomarker. Clin Exp Ophthalmol. 2018. https://doi.org/10.1111/ceo.13326. Epub ahead of print.
77. Kousal B, Kolarova H, Meliska M, Bydzovsky J, Diblik P, Kulhanek J, Votruba M, Honzik T. Peripapillary microcirculation in Leber hereditaryoptic neuropathy. Acta Opthalmol. 2019;97:e71–6.

78. Borrelli E, Balasubruman S, Triolo G, Barboni P, Sadda SS, Sadun AA. Topographic macular microvascular changes and correlation with visual loss in chronic Leber hereditary optic neuropathy. Am J Ophthalmol. 2018;192:217–28.
79. Balducci N, Ciardella A, Gattegna R, Zhou Q, Cascavilla ML, La Morgia C, Savini G, Parisi V, Bandello F, Carelli V, Barboni P. Optical coherence tomography angiography of the peripapillary retina and optic nerve head in dominant optic atrophy. Mitochondrion. 2017;36:60–5.
80. Martins A, Rodrigues TM, Soares M, Dolan M, Murta JN, Silva R, Marques JP. Peripapillary and macular morpho-vascular changes in patients with genetic or clinical diagnosis of autosomal dominant optic atrophy: a case-control study. Graefes Arch Clin Exp Ophthalmol. 2019;257(5):1019–27.
81. Cesareo M, Giannini C, Di Marino M, Aloe G, Martucci A, Francesco F, Cusumano A, Mancino R, Ricci R, Sorge RP, Nucci C. Optical coherence tomography angiography in the multimodal assessment of the retinal posterior pole in autosomal dominant optic atrophy. Acta Ophthalmol. 2022;100:e798–806.
82. Yu-Wai-Man P, Votruba M, Burté F, La Morgia C, Barboni P, Carelli V. A neurodegenerative perspective on mitochondrial optic neuropathies. Acta Neuropathol. 2016;132(6):789–806. https://doi.org/10.1007/s00401-016-1625-2. Epub 2016 Sep 30. PMID: 27696015; PMCID: PMC5106504.
83. Newman NJ, Yu-Wai-Man P, Biousse V, Carelli V. Understanding the molecular basis and pathogenesis of hereditary optic neuropathies: towards improved diagnosis and management. Lancet Neurol. 2023;22(2):172–188. https://doi.org/10.1016/S1474-4422(22)00174-0. Epub 2022 Sep 22. PMID: 36155660.
84. Lenaers G, Beaulieu C, Charif M, Gerber S, Kaplan J, Rozet JM. Autosomal recessive Leber hereditary optic neuropathy, a new neuro-ophthalmo-genetic paradigm. Brain. 2023;18:awad131. https://doi.org/10.1093/brain/awad131. Epub ahead of print. PMID: 37071596.
85. Gerber S, Ding MG, Gérard X, Zwicker K, Zanlonghi X, Rio M, Serre V, Hanein S, Munnich A, Rotig A, Bianchi L, Amati-Bonneau P, Elpeleg O, Kaplan J, Brandt U, Rozet JM. Compound heterozygosity for severe and hypomorphic NDUFS2 mutations cause non-syndromic LHON-like optic neuropathy. J Med Genet. 2017;54(5):346–56.
86. Stenton SL, Sheremet NL, Catarino CB, Andreeva NA, Assouline Z, Barboni P, Barel O, Berutti R, Bychkov I, Caporali L, Capristo M, Carbonelli M, Cascavilla ML, Charbel Issa P, Freisinger P, Gerber S, Ghezzi D, Graf E, Heidler J, Hempel M, Heon E, Itkis YS, Javasky E, Kaplan J, Kopajtich R, Kornblum C, Kovacs-Nagy R, Krylova TD, Kunz WS, La Morgia C, Lamperti C, Ludwig C, Malacarne PF, Maresca A, Mayr JA, Meisterknecht J, Nevinitsyna TA, Palombo F, Pode-Shakked B, Shmelkova MS, Strom TM, Tagliavini F, Tzadok M, van der Ven AT, Vignal-Clermont C, Wagner M, Zakharova EY, Zhorzholadze NV, Rozet JM, Carelli V, Tsygankova PG, Klopstock T, Wittig I, Prokisch H. Impaired complex I repair causes recessive Leber's hereditary optic neuropathy. J Clin Invest. 2021;131(6): e138267.
87. Gerber S, Orssaud C, Kaplan J, Johansson C, Rozet JM. MCAT mutations cause nuclear LHON-like optic neuropathy. Genes (Basel). 2021;12(4):521. https://doi.org/10.3390/genes12040521. PMID: 33918393; PMCID: PMC8067165.
88. Fiorini C, Ormanbekova D, Palombo F, Carbonelli M, Amore G, Romagnoli M, d'Agati P, Valentino ML, Barboni P, Cascavilla ML, De Negri A, Sadun F, Carta A, Testa F, Petruzzella V, Guerriero S, Bianchi Marzoli S, Carelli V, La Morgia C, Caporali L. The Italian reappraisal on the most frequent genetic defects in hereditary optic neuropathies and the global top 10. Brain. 2023;13:awad080.
89. Caporali L, Magri S, Legati A, Del Dotto V, Tagliavini F, Balistreri F, Nasca A, La Morgia C, Carbonelli M, Valentino ML, Lamantea E, Baratta S, Schöls L, Schüle R, Barboni P, Cascavilla ML, Maresca A, Capristo M, Ardissone A, Pareyson D, Cammarata G, Melzi L, Zeviani M, Peverelli L, Lamperti C, Marzoli SB, Fang M, Synofzik M, Ghezzi D, Carelli V, Taroni F. ATPase domain AFG3L2 mutations alter OPA1 processing and cause optic neuropathy. Ann Neurol. 2020;88(1):18–32.

90. Charif M, Gueguen N, Ferré M, Elkarhat Z, Khiati S, LeMao M, Chevrollier A, Desquiret-Dumas V, Goudenège D, Bris C, Kane S, Alban J, Chupin S, Wetterwald C, Caporali L, Tagliavini F, LaMorgia C, Carbonelli M, Jurkute N, Barakat A, Gohier P, Verny C, Barth M, Procaccio V, Bonneau D, Zanlonghi X, Meunier I, Weisschuh N, Schimpf-Linzenbold S, Tonagel F, Kellner U, Yu-Wai-Man P, Carelli V, Wissinger B, Amati-Bonneau P, Reynier P; European ION Group; Lenaers G. Dominant ACO2 mutations are a frequent cause of isolated optic atrophy. Brain Commun. 2021;3(2):fcab063.
91. Del Dotto V, Ullah F, Di Meo I, Magini P, Gusic M, Maresca A, Caporali L, Palombo F, Tagliavini F, Baugh EH, Macao B, Szilagyi Z, Peron C, Gustafson MA, Khan K, La Morgia C, Barboni P, Carbonelli M, Valentino ML, Liguori R, Shashi V, Sullivan J, Nagaraj S, El-Dairi M, Iannaccone A, Cutcutache I, Bertini E, Carrozzo R, Emma F, Diomedi-Camassei F, Zanna C, Armstrong M, Page M, Stong N, Boesch S, Kopajtich R, Wortmann S, Sperl W, Davis EE, Copeland WC, Seri M, Falkenberg M, Prokisch H, Katsanis N, Tiranti V, Pippucci T, Carelli V. SSBP1 mutations cause mtDNA depletion underlying a complex optic atrophy disorder. J Clin Invest. 2020;130(1):108–25.

Trans-synaptic Retrograde Degeneration in the Visual Pathway in Central Nervous System Diseases

17

Bernardo F. Sanchez-Dalmau, Elena Brotons, Anna Camos-Carreras, Rafel Alcubierre, and Pablo Villoslada

Abstract

Retrograde trans-synaptic retinal degeneration may occur in patients with post-geniculate optic radiations lesions and can be showed in congenital/long standing homonymous hemianopia, acquired homonymous hemianopia and neurodegenerative diseases like multiple sclerosis or Alzheimer's disease. This trans-synaptic retinal degeneration has been reported using spectral-domain optical coherence tomography (SD-OCT) of the macula, ganglion cell complex (GCC) and retinal nerve fiber layer (RNFL). OCT-angiography can also show decrease of vascular density in macular and peripapillary area.

Keywords

Transsynaptic degeneration • OCT • OCT-A • Retinal ganglion cell layer • Retinal nerve fiber layer • Homonymous hemianopia • Multiple sclerosis • Alzheimer disease • Parkinson disease

17.1 Introduction

The anterior visual pathway comprises axons from retinal ganglion cells, which form the optic nerve, optic chiasm, and optic tract, and synapse in the lateral geniculate nucleus. The posterior visual pathway comprises axons from the lateral

B. F. Sanchez-Dalmau (✉) · B. F. Sanchez-Dalmau (✉) · E. Brotons · A. Camos-Carreras · R. Alcubierre
Neuroophthalmology Unit, Ophthalmology Department, Hospital Clínic, Barcelona, Spain
e-mail: BSANCHEZ@clinic.cat

P. Villoslada (✉) · P. Villoslada (✉)
Department of Neurology, Hospital del Mar—Pompeu Fabra University, Barcelona, Spain
e-mail: pablo.villoslada@upf.edu

A. Grzybowski and P. Barboni (eds.), *OCT and Imaging in Central Nervous System Diseases*, https://doi.org/10.1007/978-3-031-72156-4_17

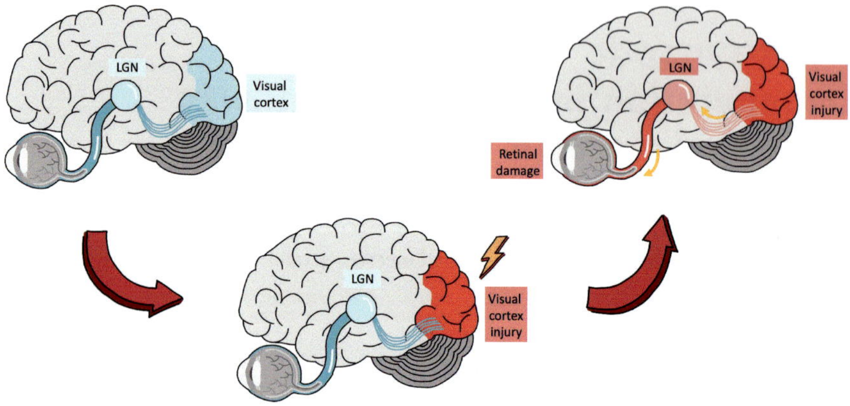

Fig. 17.1 The visual pathway as a model to study trans-synaptic neuronal degeneration

geniculate nucleus that form the optic radiations and project into the visual cortex. About 90% of retinal axons synapse in the lateral geniculate nucleus and travel with the optic radiations to the occipital cortex. The remaining 10% is projected into the pretectal region of the midbrain.

Damage from the posterior to anterior visual pathway requires transmission through the synapses in the lateral geniculate nucleus by retrograde trans-synaptic degeneration or trans-neuronal degeneration (Fig. 17.1). Trans-synaptic retrograde degeneration in humans is well known. It has been demonstrated from the early twentieth century [1], but clinical evidence of TRD has been controversial for many years. In 1982, Beatty et al. [2] reported histological evidence in a case 40 years after occipital lobectomy. The reasons for this controversy were mainly three:

(a) The presence of retinal degeneration is not related to brain injury
(b) The possibility of direct damage to the optic tracts in patients with occipital-temporal lesions and
(c) The lack of good retinal neurohistology in humans.

The indirect analysis with different techniques like pattern electroretinogram [3–6], fundus photography, and ophthalmic examination [7] was used, but the results were contradictory.

In this condition, the advent of Optical Coherence Tomography (OCT) and its subsequent use in neuro-ophthalmology allowed the first reliable and reproducible analysis of retinal anatomy in humans. Since that moment, it has been possible to understand the trans-synaptic retrograde degeneration following damage to the central nervous system (CNS) pathways.

Levin suggested in 2005 that retrograde trans-synaptic degeneration of neurons of retinal ganglion cells and their axons in the optic nerve and the optic tract occurred only following prenatal (not post-natal) acquired damage to the posterior visual pathway [8]. More recent studies demonstrated thinning of the retinal nerve fiber layer (RNFL) [9], or in the ganglion cell layer [10], using OCT or thinning of the optic tract using MRI [11, 12] in acquired damage. The use of OCT to evaluate trans-synaptic retrograde degeneration has been described in different clinical settings, such as congenital/long-standing homonymous hemianopia, acquired homonymous hemianopia, and neurodegenerative diseases like multiple sclerosis (MS) or Alzheimer's disease (AD).

17.2 Trans-synaptic Retrograde Degeneration in Congenital/Long-Standing Homonymous Hemianopia

The first description of using OCT to evidence the presence of trans-synaptic retrograde degenerating retinal nerve fiber layer thinning was reported by Cowey [13]. One year later, another group published a report with two female patients with no visual symptoms and homonymous hemianopia secondary to an old occipital infarction showing an RNFL thinning in nasal and temporal regions compatible with the visual field deficit [14]. These results were subsequently confirmed by the same group with more patients (seven cases) [9]. Both studies showed a strong correlation between the size of brain lesions, visual fields, and thinning of the retinal nerve fiber layer. Still, it was impossible to determine an appropriate temporal sequence between the occipital damage and thinning of the RNFL due to the lack of the exact timing of occipital damage and no follow-up of patients in these series.

17.3 Trans-synaptic Retrograde Degeneration by OCT in Acquired Homonymous Hemianopia

Jindahra et al. described the first retinal nerve fiber layer thinning in 19 cases with acquired homonymous hemianopia in 2009 [9]. The observed thinning had the same characteristics and magnitude as previously described in patients with congenital disabilities. In 2012, 15 patients with homonymous hemianopia or smaller homonymous visual field defects with occipital cerebral infarction were studied by OCT after the onset of stroke and follow-up in the following years. All patients with homonymous hemianopia showed a retinal nerve fiber layer thinning with a decreasing trend during the measurement period [15], maximal in the first year after the occipital injury, followed by a much slower rate in the following years. Similar results were observed in another study comparing 46 patients with occipital infarction and 46 healthy controls [16]. The RNFL thickness was significantly reduced as early as 3.6 months in the superior, inferior, and nasal quadrants in the contralateral and superior, inferior, and temporal quadrants in the ipsilateral eyes.

The change from time-domain optical coherence tomography to spectral-domain OCT and the development of better segmentation software allowed the measurement of all the retinal layers. Evaluating the ganglion cell layer appeared more effective and reliable than the retina's nerve fiber layer in quantifying trans-synaptic degeneration. We can quantify each inner layer (RNFL, ganglion cells, or inner plexiform). However, there is a tendency to group them into two forms, GC complex (GCC) including the 3 layers described or including only the ganglion cell plus the inner plexiform layers (GCIPL). Yamashita et al. used this technology in three unilateral posterior cerebral artery infarction patients. These patients showed a GCC thinning in the hemi-retinae corresponding to the affected hemi-fields without fundoscopic evidence of optic atrophy [17]. This study showed that transsynaptic degeneration of GCL likely begins much earlier.

Our study [18] showed macular GCL atrophy in patients with a retrogeniculate lesion with at least 1-year evolution. Therefore, the finding of sector macular GCL atrophy proves retrograde transsynaptic degeneration of neurons in the visual pathway in cases without other ophthalmic or neurological disease. The functional correlation between sector thinning of the GCL and the sensitivity loss of the visual field in the corresponding field indicates that this may occur in lesions regardless of their size, as shown in quadrantanopic cases [15]. However, we found a significantly stronger correlation between the visual field defect and GCL thickness than the peripapillary RNFL. This is probably because, at the macula, the bodies of the neurons are more numerous and topographically organized to correspond to the visual fields. In contrast, the anatomical distribution of fibers in the peripapillary RNFL is more complex, making a correlation with the visual field more difficult to establish.

Retrograde transsynaptic degeneration was observed in the GCL 15 of 22 patients with homonymous visual field loss due to varying etiologies [19]. Still, in some cases, RNFL thinning was absent and confirmed that the retrograde transsynaptic degeneration must begin earlier than 1 year. Remarkably, retrograde transsynaptic degeneration did not occur in some cases with quadrantanopia with a follow-up over 10 years or more. In 22 cases with significant GCL thinning, RFNL thinning was only observed in 75% of the cases [20] and in 9 patients with GCL thinning without RNFL loss [21].

An essential element is the presence or absence of blood vessels or other structures that may interfere with the OCT image acquisition. The higher resolution of spectral-domain OCT also allows for studying the segmentation of the retina in layers in more detail [17]. It is noteworthy that cases with macular sparing hemi- and quadrantanopia also showed macular GCL atrophy away from the fovea, perhaps explained by the representation of 15–20° of the visual field in the area scanned by the OCT instrument used and the absence of ganglion cells on the fovea. Similar findings can be observed in patients with homonymous visual field defects after epilepsy surgery (Fig. 17.2).

OCT-Angiography is a noninvasive technique used to study the blood flow in the retinal vessels that have revealed a significant decrease of peripapillary and

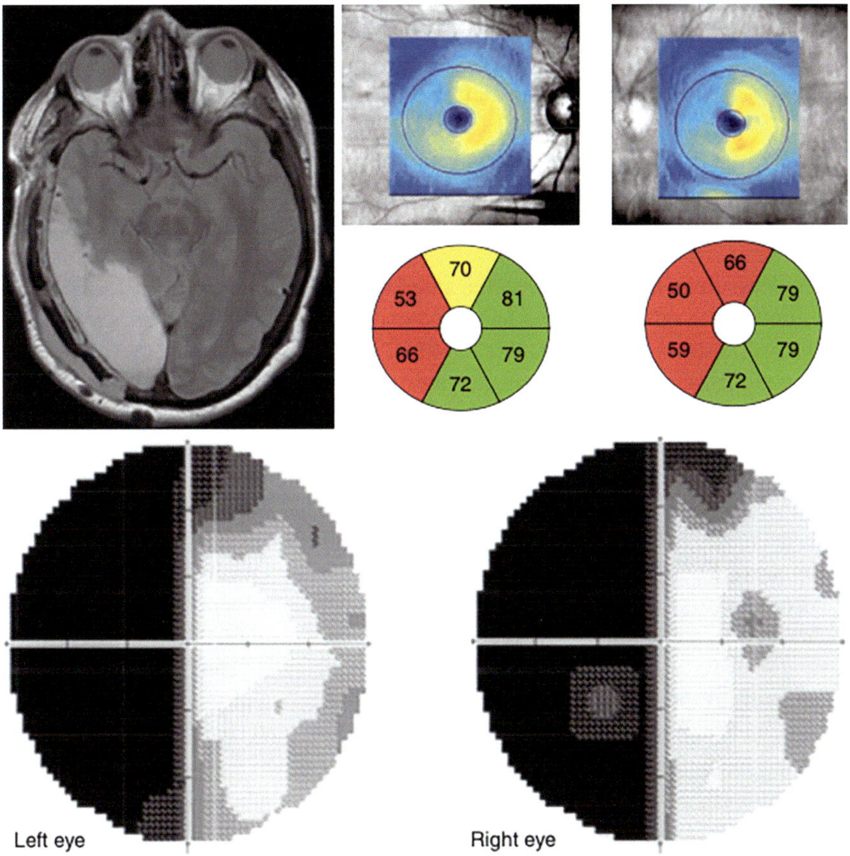

Fig. 17.2 Sectorial ganglion cells layer thinning secondary to an epilepsy surgery, 6 months after surgery. Visual field shows a complete left homonymous hemianopia

macular vascular density in patients with homonymous visual field defect and retrograde trans-synaptic degeneration and correlation with RNFL and GCC thinning [22]. Our data confirm similar results. This technique is improving day by day, and new methods of quantification are appearing.

17.4 Trans-synaptic Axonal Degeneration by OCT in Multiple Sclerosis

There is evidence of postmortem atrophy of retinal layers after long-standing MS [23]. However, due to the multiple CNS lesions that may develop in patients with multiple sclerosis, establishing the presence of trans-synaptic degeneration is difficult. Because patients with multiple sclerosis lesions can have both the anterior visual pathway and the posterior visual pathway anterograde trans-synaptic degeneration in patients with a history of optic neuritis, trans-synaptic retrograde degeneration in patients with lesions of the posterior visual pathway, this is important to assess retrograde trans-synaptic degeneration. Patients with previous optic neuritis should be differentiated and excluded from the analysis because trans-synaptic RGC degeneration could be masked by the pronounced loss caused by damage to the anterior visual pathway in multiple sclerosis optic neuritis. Previous optic neuritis may generate residual impairment of RNFL and CGL, distorting the quantification of trans-synaptic degeneration on the anterior visual pathway [24].

The measurement of damage to the anterior visual pathway by OCT [25] and its association with other variables have improved the understanding of neurodegenerative processes in Multiple Sclerosis (MS). By studying a cohort of 100 patients with multiple sclerosis, we evaluated the influence of the damage to the posterior visual pathway on retinal atrophy by linear regression analysis [26]. Retinal atrophy was used as the dependent variable, and measures of posterior visual pathway damage and other relevant clinical measures (sex, age at study inclusion, and EDSS score) were used as independent variables. The regression model indicated that a decrease of 1 cm^3 in visual cortex volume predicts a reduction of 0.6 μm in retinal nerve fiber layer thickness independent of other variables.

After this first description of the presence of trans-synaptic neuronal degeneration in MS by using the high resolution of OCT combined with MRI, many more studies have found evidence of the process [27, 28]. The effects of posterior visual pathway pathology on the retina in MS patients and vice versa, reveals an association between MRI measures of optic radiation integrity and retinal integrity measured by temporal quadrant RNFL thickness using OCT [29–34]. RNFL thickness correlated with thalamic, lateral geniculate nucleus and cortical volume, confirming the retrograde trans-synaptic degeneration [32, 35, 36]. Indeed, in a series of six cases with homonymous, hemi-macular GCIPL thickness reduction in MS lesions of the thalamus (2 cases) and occipital (4 cases) with homonymous hemianopia was found [37]. In a recent study during the acute damage of the visual pathway in acute optic neuritis, authors found accelerated atrophy of the occipital grey matter, calcarine cortex, and thalamus [38]. More, the atrophy rate of the cortex correlated with the atrophy rate of the retina thereafter, supporting the presence of anterograde trans-synaptic degeneration in MS. It has been suggested that neural plasticity existed in the inner nuclear layer due to the interaction between bipolar, amacrine, and horizontal cells that blocked the posterior trans-synaptic degeneration, allowing the affectation of ganglion cells only [39, 40].

17.5 Trans-synaptic Axonal Degeneration by OCT in Alzheimer's Disease

Visual impairment is often one of the earliest complaints in patients with Alzheimer's Disease (AD) [41]. Several researchers attribute this impairment to damage in the primary visual cortex with degeneration of cortical areas and, secondarily, retrograde loss of nerve fibers in the retina and optic nerve. However, it has been reported the presence of beta-amyloid and tau deposits in the retina [42], its presence in the GCIPL induces neuroinflammation that could cause retinal degeneration [43]. Accordingly, the visual damage is determined by direct toxicity of beta-amyloid and its derivatives in the retina and the retrograde degeneration of retinal nerve fibers. Thinning of the retinal nerve fiber layer and ganglion cells layer has been described in patients with AD and mild cognitive impairment [44–47] and correlates well with the Mini-Mental State Examination and the disease stage.

It has been postulated that the RNFL thinning may be the earliest sign of AD, even before the hippocampal region damage that affects memory [48]. A linear discriminant function based on OCT was described for AD diagnosis. According to their results, the most reliable tool for diagnosing Alzheimer's disease was the OCT-based linear discriminant function with an area under the ROC curves of 96%, sensitivity of 94%, and specificity of 88% [49]. Indeed, areas of thickening and thinning in RNFL and GCIPL in mild cognitive impairment and AD patients, suggest dynamic changes in the evolution of the disease [50]. A systematic review and meta-analysis of 30 studies, including 1,257 patients, confirmed the associations between retinal measurements of OCT and AD, highlighting the potential usefulness of OCT measurements as biomarkers of AD [51]. Despite these promising preliminary studies [52], whether AD affects the retina directly, secondarily by trans-synaptic degeneration, remains to be determined.

17.6 Trans-synaptic Axonal Degeneration in Parkinson

A study revealed RNFL thinning in patients with PD and visual hallucinations as compared to PD patients without hallucinations and controls. With the assumption that patients with PD and hallucinations have dysfunction of the primary visual cortex or visual association cortex, the authors concluded that the RNFL thinning might be the product of retrograde transsynaptic degeneration [53]. In another way, PD can directly affect retinal cells, generating anterograde transsynaptic degeneration in the optic tracts and optic radiations [54].

17.7 Summary

The visual pathway comprises four neuron chains that transfer visual information from the retina to the primary visual cortex. Acute or chronic damage on the posterior visual pathway induces trans-neuronal retrograde degeneration. Measuring the degeneration of the anterior visual pathway was difficult before the OCT imaging technology. With this technology, trans-neuronal retrograde degeneration has been well described in several CNS diseases like MS, stroke, PD, AD, or homonymous hemianopia. OCT allows the reliable and noninvasive measurement of the macular RNFL and GCC, and these measurements have a high correlation with the CNS lesions and the visual system's function [55, 56]. Indeed, OCT helps evaluate the magnitude and timing of damage, supporting our understanding of the pathophysiology of the diseases, and can be used as a reliable biomarker of axonal loss in neurological diseases.

References

1. Campbell AW. Histological studies on the localization of cerebral function. C. U. Press, Ed.; 1905.
2. Beatty RM, Sadun AA, Smith L, Vonsattel JP, Richardson EP Jr. Direct demonstration of transsynaptic degeneration in the human visual system: a comparison of retrograde and anterograde changes. J Neurol Neurosurg Psychiatry. 1982;45:143–6.
3. Stoerig P, Zrenner E. A pattern ERG study of transneuronal retrograde degeneration in the human retina after a post-geniculate lesion. In: Kulikowski JJ, Dickinson C, Murray JJ, editors. Seeing contour and colour. Oxford: Pergamon Press; 1993.
4. Porrello G, Falsini B. Retinal ganglion cell dysfunction in humans following post-geniculate lesions: specific spatio-temporal losses revealed by pattern ERG. Vision Res. 1999;39:1739–45.
5. Azzopardi P, King SM, Cowey A. Pattern electroretinograms after cerebral hemispherectomy. Brain. 2001;124:1228–40.
6. Skrandies W, Leipert KP. Visual field defects are not accompanied by electrophysiological evidence of transsynaptic retrograde degeneration. Clin Vis Sci. 1988;3:45–57.
7. Hoyt WF, Rios-Montenegro EN, Behrens MM, Eckelhoff RJ. Homonymous hemioptic hypoplasia. Fundoscopic features in standard and red-free illumination in three patients with congenital hemiplegia. Br J Ophthalmol. 1972;56:537–45.
8. Levin LA. Optical diagnosis of chiasmal and retrochiasmal disorders. In: Miller NR, Newman NJ, editors. Walsh and Hoyt's clinical neuro-ophthalmology. Lippincott, Williams & Wilkins, Baltimore; 2005.
9. Jindahra P, Petrie A, Plant GT. Retrograde trans-synaptic retinal ganglion cell loss identified by optical coherence tomography. Brain. 2009;132:628–34.
10. Meier PG, Maeder P, Kardon RH, Borruat FX. Homonymous ganglion cell layer thinning after isolated occipital lesion: macular OCT demonstrates transsynaptic retrograde retinal degeneration. J Neuroophthalmol. 2015;35:112–6.
11. Bridge H, Jindahra P, Barbur J, Plant GT. Imaging reveals optic tract degeneration in hemianopia. Invest Ophthalmol Vis Sci. 2011;52:382–8.
12. Millington RS, et al. Quantifying the pattern of optic tract degeneration in human hemianopia. J Neurol Neurosurg Psychiatry. 2014;85:379–86.
13. Cowey A. The 30th Sir Frederick Bartlett lecture. Fact, artefact, and myth about blindsight. Q J Exp Psychol A. 2004;57:577–609.

14. Mehta JS, Plant GT. Optical coherence tomography (OCT) findings in congenital/long-standing homonymous hemianopia. Am J Ophthalmol. 2005;140:727–9.
15. Jindahra P, Petrie A, Plant GT. The time course of retrograde trans-synaptic degeneration following occipital lobe damage in humans. Brain. 2012;135:534–41.
16. Park HY, Park YG, Cho AH, Park CK. Transneuronal retrograde degeneration of the retinal ganglion cells in patients with cerebral infarction. Ophthalmology. 2013;120:1292–9.
17. Yamashita T, et al. Reduced retinal ganglion cell complex thickness in patients with posterior cerebral artery infarction detected using spectral-domain optical coherence tomography. Jpn J Ophthalmol. 2012;56:502–10.
18. Keller J, Sanchez-Dalmau BF, Villoslada P. Lesions in the posterior visual pathway promote trans-synaptic degeneration of retinal ganglion cells. PLoS ONE. 2014;9: e97444.
19. Mitchell JR, Oliveira C, Tsiouris AJ, Dinkin MJ. Corresponding ganglion cell atrophy in patients with postgeniculate homonymous visual field loss. J Neuroophthalmol. 2015;35:353–9.
20. Shin HY, Park HY, Choi JA, Park CK. Macular ganglion cell-inner plexiform layer thinning in patients with visual field defect that respects the vertical meridian. Graefes Arch Clin Exp Ophthalmol. 2014;252:1501–7.
21. Herro AM, Lam BL. Retrograde degeneration of retinal ganglion cells in homonymous hemianopsia. Clin Ophthalmol. 2015;9:1057–64.
22. Rebolleda G, Diez-Alvarez L, Garcia Marin Y, de Juan V, Munoz-Negrete FJ. Reduction of peripapillary vessel density by optical coherence tomography angiography from the acute to the atrophic stage in non-arteritic anterior ischaemic optic neuropathy. Ophthalmologica. 2018;240:191–9.
23. Green AJ, McQuaid S, Hauser SL, Allen IV, Lyness R. Ocular pathology in multiple sclerosis: retinal atrophy and inflammation irrespective of disease duration. Brain. 2010;133:1591–601.
24. Balk LJ, et al. A dam for retrograde axonal degeneration in multiple sclerosis? J Neurol Neurosurg Psychiatry. 2014;85:782–9.
25. Galetta KM, Calabresi PA, Frohman EM, Balcer LJ. Optical coherence tomography (OCT): imaging the visual pathway as a model for neurodegeneration. Neurotherapeutics. 2011;8:117–32.
26. Gabilondo I, et al. Trans-synaptic axonal degeneration in the visual pathway in multiple sclerosis. Ann Neurol. 2014;75:98–107.
27. Filippatou AG, Calabresi PA, Saidha S, Murphy OC. Spotlight on trans-synaptic degeneration in the visual pathway in multiple sclerosis. Eye Brain. 2023;15:153–60.
28. Murphy OC, Calabresi PA, Saidha S. Trans-synaptic degeneration as a mechanism of neurodegeneration in multiple sclerosis. Neural Regen Res. 2023;18:2682–4.
29. Klistorner A, et al. Axonal loss of retinal neurons in multiple sclerosis associated with optic radiation lesions. Neurology. 2014;82:2165–72.
30. Sriram P, et al. Relationship between optical coherence tomography and electrophysiology of the visual pathway in non-optic neuritis eyes of multiple sclerosis patients. PLoS ONE. 2014;9: e102546.
31. Lin TY, et al. Interactions of optic radiation lesions with retinal and brain atrophy in early multiple sclerosis. Ann Clin Transl Neurol. 2024;11:45–56.
32. Miante S, et al. Trans-synaptic degeneration in the optic pathway: exploring the role of lateral geniculate nucleus in early stages of relapsing-remitting multiple sclerosis. Multiple Sclerosis Relat Disord. 2023;77: 104877.
33. Ngamsombat C, et al. Axonal damage in the optic radiation assessed by white matter tract integrity metrics is associated with retinal thinning in multiple sclerosis. Neuroimage Clin. 2020;27: 102293.
34. Pawlitzki M et al. MS optic neuritis-induced long-term structural changes within the visual pathway. Neurol Neuroimmunol Neuroinflammation. 2020; 7.
35. Petracca M, et al. Retinal degeneration in primary-progressive multiple sclerosis: a role for cortical lesions? Mult Scler. 2017;23:43–50.

36. Ganapathy Subramanian R, et al. Multiple sclerosis optic neuritis and trans-synaptic pathology on cortical thinning in people with multiple sclerosis. J Neurol. 2023;270:3758–769.
37. Al-Louzi O, Button J, Newsome SD, Calabresi PA, Saidha S. Retrograde trans-synaptic visual pathway degeneration in multiple sclerosis: a case series. Mult Scler. 2017;23:1035–9.
38. Murphy OC, et al. Trans-synaptic degeneration following acute optic neuritis in multiple sclerosis. Ann Neurol. 2023;93:76–87.
39. Balk LJ, et al. Bidirectional trans-synaptic axonal degeneration in the visual pathway in multiple sclerosis. J Neurol Neurosurg Psychiatry. 2015;86:419–24.
40. Panneman EL, Coric D, Tran LMD, de Vries-Knoppert W, Petzold A. Progression of anterograde trans-synaptic degeneration in the human retina is modulated by axonal convergence and divergence. Neuroophthalmology. 2019;43:382–90.
41. Berisha F, Feke GT, Trempe CL, McMeel JW, Schepens CL. Retinal abnormalities in early Alzheimer's disease. Invest Ophthalmol Vis Sci. 2007;48:2285–9.
42. Koronyo Y, Salumbides BC, Black KL, Koronyo-Hamaoui M. Alzheimer's disease in the retina: imaging retinal abeta plaques for early diagnosis and therapy assessment. Neurodegener Dis. 2012;10:285–93.
43. Garcia-Martin ES, et al. Macular thickness as a potential biomarker of mild Alzheimer's disease. Ophthalmology. 2014;121:1149–51 e1143.
44. Iseri PK, Altinas O, Tokay T, Yuksel N. Relationship between cognitive impairment and retinal morphological and visual functional abnormalities in Alzheimer disease. J Neuroophthalmol. 2006;26:18–24.
45. Kesler A, Vakhapova V, Korczyn AD, Naftaliev E, Neudorfer M. Retinal thickness in patients with mild cognitive impairment and Alzheimer's disease. Clin Neurol Neurosurg. 2011;113:523–6.
46. Kirbas S, Turkyilmaz K, Anlar O, Tufekci A, Durmus M. Retinal nerve fiber layer thickness in patients with Alzheimer disease. J Neuroophthalmol. 2013;33:58–61.
47. Marziani E, et al. Evaluation of retinal nerve fiber layer and ganglion cell layer thickness in Alzheimer's disease using spectral-domain optical coherence tomography. Invest Ophthalmol Vis Sci. 2013;54:5953–8.
48. He XF, et al. Optical coherence tomography assessed retinal nerve fiber layer thickness in patients with Alzheimer's disease: a meta-analysis. Int J Ophthalmol. 2012;5:401–5.
49. Larrosa JM, et al. Potential new diagnostic tool for Alzheimer's disease using a linear discriminant function for Fourier domain optical coherence tomography. Invest Ophthalmol Vis Sci. 2014;55:3043–51.
50. Lad EM, et al. Evaluation of inner retinal layers as biomarkers in mild cognitive impairment to moderate Alzheimer's disease. PLoS ONE. 2018;13: e0192646.
51. Chan VTT, et al. Spectral-domain OCT measurements in Alzheimer's disease: a systematic review and meta-analysis. Ophthalmology. 2019;126:497–510.
52. Alves C, et al. Interplay between macular retinal changes and white matter integrity in early Alzheimer's disease. J Alzheimers Dis. 2019;70:723–32.
53. Lee JY, et al. Retinal nerve fiber layer thickness and visual hallucinations in Parkinson's disease. Mov Disord. 2014;29:61–7.
54. Bodis-Wollner I, Kozlowski PB, Glazman S, Miri S. Alpha-Synuclein in the inner retina in Parkinson disease. Ann Neurol. 2014;75:964–6.
55. Moon H, Yoon JY, Lim HT, Sung KR. Ganglion cell and inner plexiform layer thickness determined by spectral domain optical coherence tomography in patients with brain lesions. Br J Ophthalmol. 2015;99:329–35.
56. Dinkin M. Trans-synaptic retrograde degeneration in the human visual system: slow, silent, and real. Curr Neurol Neurosci Rep. 2017;17:16.

18 OCT in Toxic and Nutritional Optic Neuropathies

Andrzej Grzybowski, Iwona Obuchowska, and Carl Arndt

Abstract

Despite the recent developments of OCT in neuro-ophthalmology, its use for diagnosing and monitoring nutritional and toxic optic neuropathies is still limited, due to the lack of powered, longitudinal studies. Small series have suggested that OCT may be useful in various toxic optic neuropathies in the acute stage, disclosing subtle retinal nerve fibre layer thickening, ophthalmoscopically undetectable. At later stages, retinal nerve fibre layer thinning affects the papillomacular bundle, and then, all quadrants, but only rarely before visual loss. Macular volume OCT studies have suggested that in toxic optic neuropathies, the primary site of injury may involve the retinal ganglion cells layers. Retinal nerve fibre layer thinning in the nasal quadrant in patients treated with vigabatrin appears to be predictive of visual field constriction.

Keywords

Toxic optic neuropathy • Ethambutol • Methanol • Amiodarone • Nutritional optic neuropathy • Mitochondria • Malabsorption • Vitamin B deficiency • Bariatric surgery • Vigabatrin

A. Grzybowski (✉)
University of Warmia and Mazury, Olsztyn, Poland
e-mail: ae.grzybowski@gmail.com

A. Grzybowski · A. Grzybowski
Institute for Research in Ophthalmology, Poznań, Poland

I. Obuchowska
Department of Ophthalmology, Medical University of Białystok, Białystok, Poland
e-mail: iwonaobu@wp.pl

C. Arndt
Department of Ophthalmology, CHU Reims, Reims, France

A. Grzybowski and P. Barboni (eds.), *OCT and Imaging in Central Nervous System Diseases*, https://doi.org/10.1007/978-3-031-72156-4_18

18.1 OCT and Toxic Optic Neuropathies

The anterior visual pathways are susceptible to damage from numerous toxic agents [1]. Toxic optic neuropathies can classically be caused by ingestion of numerous substances, including alcohol (methanol, ethylene glycol), anti-tubercular drugs (ethambutol, isoniazid), antibiotics (linezolid, sulphonamides, chloramphenicol), antimalarials (chloroquine, quinine), anti-cancer drugs (vincristine, methotrexate), antiarrhythmic (digitalis, amiodarone). Although this list of potentially toxic agents for the optic nerves is constantly increasing, due to the current exponential development of new therapies, only few drugs exhibit a firm evidence of causal relationship.

Toxic optic neuropathies, which are clinically often undistinguishable from nutritional optic neuropathies, typically present as painless, progressive, symmetric and bilateral visual impairment due to central or centrocecal scotoma, dyschromatopsia often being the initial symptom. The site of the primary injury can be very variable, including the retina, retinal ganglion cells, intraocular nerve fibre axons, or chiasm. The majority of clinical findings are caused by selective damage to the papillomacular bundle, which fibres are most susceptible due to their long unmyelinated part in the retina and their relatively small calibre. Preferential involvement of the papillomacular bundle is a common feature to many acquired and genetic optic neuropathies. On the cellular level they also share the similar pathophysiology mechanism based on disruption of oxidative phosphorylation in mitochondria, esp. in retinal ganglion cells, and this is the reason to name them mitochondrial optic neuropathies. Drugs shown to cause mitochondrial optic neuropathy by blocking oxidative phosphorylation include ethambutol, chloramphenicol, linezolid, erythromycin, streptomycin, and antiretroviral drugs [2].

Other drugs provoking optic neuropathy, less strongly related to mitochondrial dysfunction include amiodarone, infliximab, quinine, dapsone, pheniprazine, suramin, and isoniazid [2].

It was suggested that since axonal transport is highly energy dependent and mitochondria need to be transported from the neuron body to the distal synaptic terminals, retinal ganglion cells (RGC) with their long axons are particularly vulnerable [2]. In early drug toxicity mitochondria accumulate within RGC axons, and this is detectable as axonal swelling by OCT [3]. In subacute and chronic stages of mitochondrial optic neuropathies OCT demonstrates RNFL thinning of the papillomacular bundle, esp. in the inferotemporal sector. In the later stages, OCT reveals thinning of RNFL in all layers [2]. Early diagnosis is crucial for intervention, i.e. discontinuation of the drug, which may allow clinical recovery. However, early clinical diagnosis may be difficult, due to the normal ophthalmoscopic appearance of the optic disc pallor. Only at later stages is optic disc pallor or atrophy is clinically visible. For this reason, optical coherence tomography (OCT), has been initially considered as a potential method for early diagnosis and possibly monitoring drug toxicity affecting the retina, the retinal ganglion cells complex or the retinal nerve fiber layer (RNFL). Indeed, beyond its extensive use in glaucoma

[4], OCT is now commonly used for the evaluation of various optic neuropathies including optic neuritis, ischemic optic neuropathies, papilledema, traumatic optic neuropathy [5–7]. However, interestingly, the number of OCT studies dedicated to toxic optic neuropathies remains relatively small and no OCT guidelines exist to monitor optic nerve drug toxicities.

18.1.1 Ethambutol

Ethambutol hydrochloride is a bacteriostatic antitubercular agent and probably the most common therapy implicated in toxic optic neuropathy. Ethambutol and its metabolite ethylenediaminodibutyric acid chelates several metal-containing enzyme systems like copper and zinc in the nucleic acid structures of mycobacteria leading to decreased levels of metalloproteins [8, 9]. Similar disruption is seen within the cytochromes of the human mitochondria, leading to apoptosis of retinal ganglion cells [8, 9] and subsequent optic neuropathy [10]. Early animal experiments have also demonstrated ethambutol toxicity affecting the retinal ganglion cells, the optic nerve, chiasm and optic tracts [11, 12].

Ethambutol induced optic neuropathy, which may become clinically patent at any time from 2 to 12 months after the initial treatment, is often reversible, if the condition is early recognized, However, permanent damage may occur at toxic or even standard doses (15–25 mg/kg/day), especially in debilitated patients, i.e. with associated renal failure. The ethambutol induced optic neuropathy has a predilection for the papillo-macular bundle of the retinal nerve fibre layer. Therefore, ophthalmoscopic changes of the optic nerve head are often subtle at the early stages, making OCT a good candidate for early ethambutol optic nerve toxicity detection.

The most common OCT finding in advanced optic nerve ethambutol toxicity is thinning of the retinal nerve fibre layer, especially in the infero-temporal quadrant, corresponding to the papillo-macular bundle [9, 12, 13]. Patients with thinner temporal quadrants display lower visual acuity and significantly reduced colour vision. These OCT findings may also correspond well with the visual field defects on Humphrey visual field analysis. Limited case series have suggested that at early stages, the ethambutol induced optic neuropathy might be associated with increased RNFL thickness [14]. In addition, after cessation of ethambutol, reversible RNFL changes, detectable by OCT may occur [14]. Apart from RML, significant decreases in retinal have been observed at various levels including ganglion cell layer and inner plexiform layer [15, 16].

The up-to-date study, included a group of 21 patients (42 eyes) treated with ethambutol for 2–12 months, showed that early ethambutol-induced optic neuropathy was associated with edema and thickening of peripapillary retinal nerve fiber layer (pRNFL) which persisted for up to 3 months after the onset of symptoms [17]. Also, an initial decrease in the ganglion cell layer plus inner plexus layer (GCIPL) was observed, more remarkable in inner locations (inner ring) than in outer locations. On follow-up OCT, conducted after 6 months, mean thickness of the pRNFL at the temporal, nasal and inferior locations, mean thickness of the inner GCIPL at the temporal, nasal and inferior locations, and mean thickness of the outer GCIPL at the superior and inferior locations were significantly lower than during the baseline examination. The relative decrease in the thickness of the analyzed layers between the first and the second OCT turned out to be markedly more evident for pRNFL than for GCIPL.

The analysis of correlation between the GCIPL thickness and vision recovery after the withdrawal of ethambutol demonstrated a significant positive association between the thickness of the temporal inner GCIPL and the degree of visual acuity improvement within 12 months of the agent discontinuation. A 10-μm loss in the inner GCIPL thickness turned out to be associated with a 0.5 decrease in the amount of logMAR visual acuity recovery at 12 months. No similar relationships were observed at 1, 3 and 6 months after the ethambutol withdrawal, except the temporal inner GCIPL, the thickness of which showed a significant correlation with visual recovery [17]. Taken altogether, these findings imply that temporal GCIPL may serve as an anatomic marker to predict visual acuity improvement both in early-phase neuropathy and at later period, i.e. 12 months after cessation of ethambutol.

Furthermore, the results of this study suggest that the toxic effect of ethambutol is not limited only to the papillomacular bundle, as the damage was observed in both nasal and temporal GCIPL.

An OCT study of patients who received ethambutol at a dose of 15–19 mg/kg/day for approximately 5 months demonstrated that the treatment contributed to an increase in RNFL thickness. The thickness of RNFL returned to its baseline level within 12 months of ethambutol discontinuation. This implies that OCT may be a useful test for early detection of subclinical ethambutol-induced optic neuropathy [18].

Another OCT study of two patients with ethambutol-induced optic neuropathy (developed within 8 and 12 months of the treatment) demonstrated a significant decrease in retinal thickness (especially at the inner ring) when combined RNFL, GCL and IPL map was subjected to the analysis. However, when only the thickness of RNFL was considered, no abnormalities were found in 1 out of the 2 patients. These results suggest that ethambutol may affect both RNFL and retinal GCL [19].

The OCT analysis of pre- and post-treatment RNFL thickness of 38 patients with ethambutol-induced optic neuropathy, who received combined therapy with Boqihuoxue Formula + Methycobal, demonstrated increase of this parameter in all quadrants, especially in the lower and temporal quadrant. These findings imply that OCT may be a useful instrument for the monitoring of treatment effects, and perhaps also recovery after ethambutol discontinuation [20].

In summary, OCT is a potentially interesting tool to assess the degree of optic nerve damage in the ethambutol induced optic neuropathy, especially in the early stages of the condition, when the optic disc has a normal ophthalmoscopic appearance. However, large studies are missing to confirm these preliminary findings, especially regarding early localized temporal RNFL thickening, as an early sign of the disease. Therefore, OCT is not recommended as the sole method for monitoring potential ethambutol optic nerve toxicity.

18.1.2 Methanol

Methanol is a common cause of toxic optic neuropathy especially in the developing world. It is also the most dreaded cause, due to its systemic consequences, potentially leading to metabolic acidosis, visual loss, coma and death. These adverse effects are due to indirect toxicity related to formic acid, catabolised from methyl alcohol via formaldehyde by the enzyme alcohol dehydrogenase in the liver and red blood cells.

The changes in the optic nerves are mostly due to cytotoxic oedema within the retina and the optic nerve, occurring during the first 48 h after methanol ingestion. The retinal ganglion cells and the retrolaminar myelin sheath are also affected due to degeneration of optic nerve axons. Several animal studies also supported these findings by identifying demyelination of optic nerve sheath [21]. The treatment of methanol intoxication is based on ethanol, B-group vitamins, and systemic steroids; however, the prognosis is usually poor and the final visual acuity is counting fingers or worse [22]. It was shown that fomepizole is safe and effective in the treatment of methanol poisoning [23], but high costs limits its availability. The visual improvement after treatment of 2 patients with a combination of intravenous erythropoietin, systemic corticosteroids, vitamins, and folic acid was reported [24]. OCT has been used for exploring macula and peripapillary retina in methanol-induced retinal toxicity, showing peripapillary nerve fibre swelling and accumulation of intraretinal fluid in the acute phase, with subsequent thinning in the chronic phase (Fig. 18.1). Therefore, OCT could he a useful tool in this setting, for evaluation of the severity of retinal edema and the temporal changes in the retinal profile [25].

18.1.2.1 Methanol Toxicity in a 19-Year-Old Female Student: A Case Report

Examination of the patient's right eye revealed inferonasal colobomatous defect of the iris, inferonasal chorioretinal coloboma and tilting and mild peripapillary atrophy of the optic nerve. In the left eye, trace segmental pallor of the temporal optic nerve head was observed during the examination conducted 4 weeks after the methanol ingestion. OCT conducted 4 weeks after the methanol intoxication revealed right ocular changes that corresponded to the coloboma. Neither thinning nor thickening of the RNFL were found in the left eye, other than a mild thinning in the nasal macula. OCT of the macula conducted 8 months after the acute intoxication with methanol revealed multiple retinal microcysts in nasal segments of both eyes. The microcysts appeared highly uniform and localized to the inner nuclear layer. OCT scan of the RNFL was normal, but bilateral wedge-shaped segmental defects of the papillomacular bundles were found during the assessment of ganglion cell layer [26].

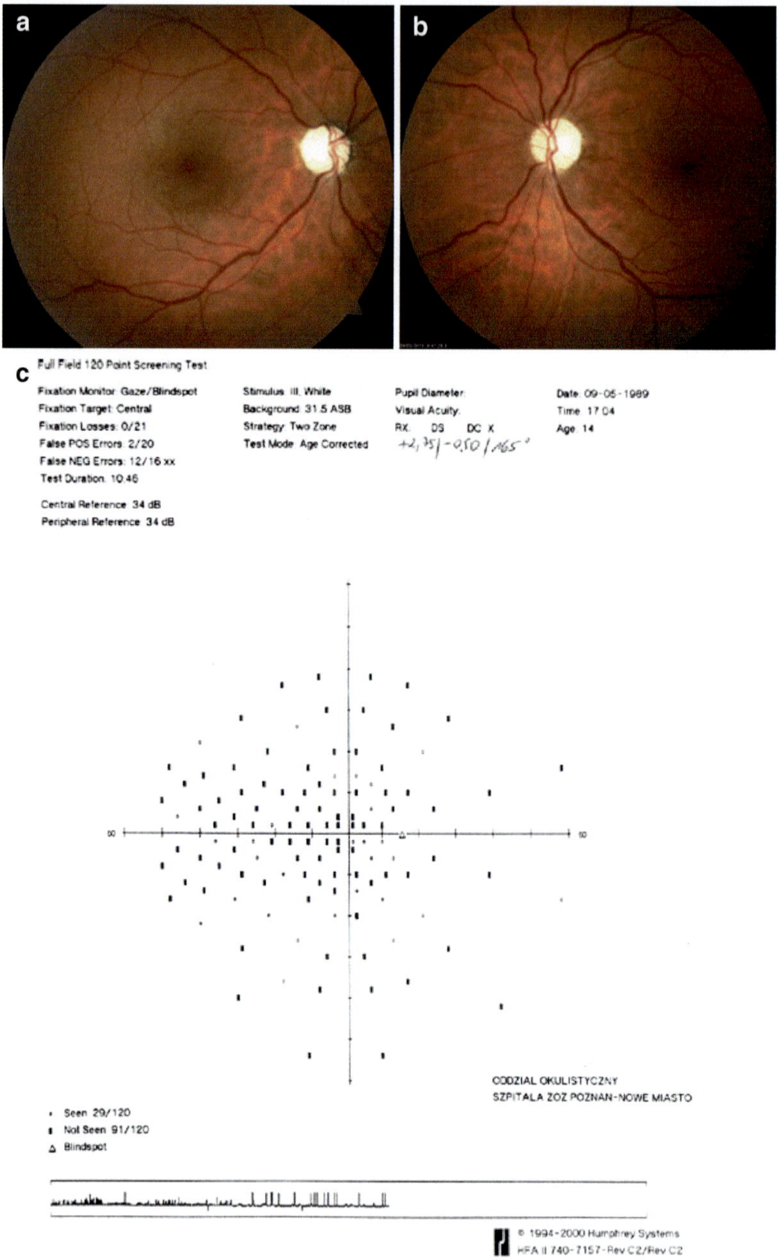

Fig. 18.1 Case report of Methanol Optic Neuropathy. A 40 year old patient with no light perception in both eyes and dilated non-responsive pupils transferred from Toxicology Department after accidental methanol intoxication. After 1-month follow up patient presented improvement of VA in both eyes (counting fingers in right eye and 0.16 in left eye) and kept stable. After 3 months optic nerve atrophy was clearly recognized with pale optic discs in fundoscopy (**a**, **b**), centrocecal scotoma in both eyes (**c**, **d**), decrease in RNFL thickness in both eyes (**e**), and decreased volume of ganglion cells in both eyes (**f**, **g**)

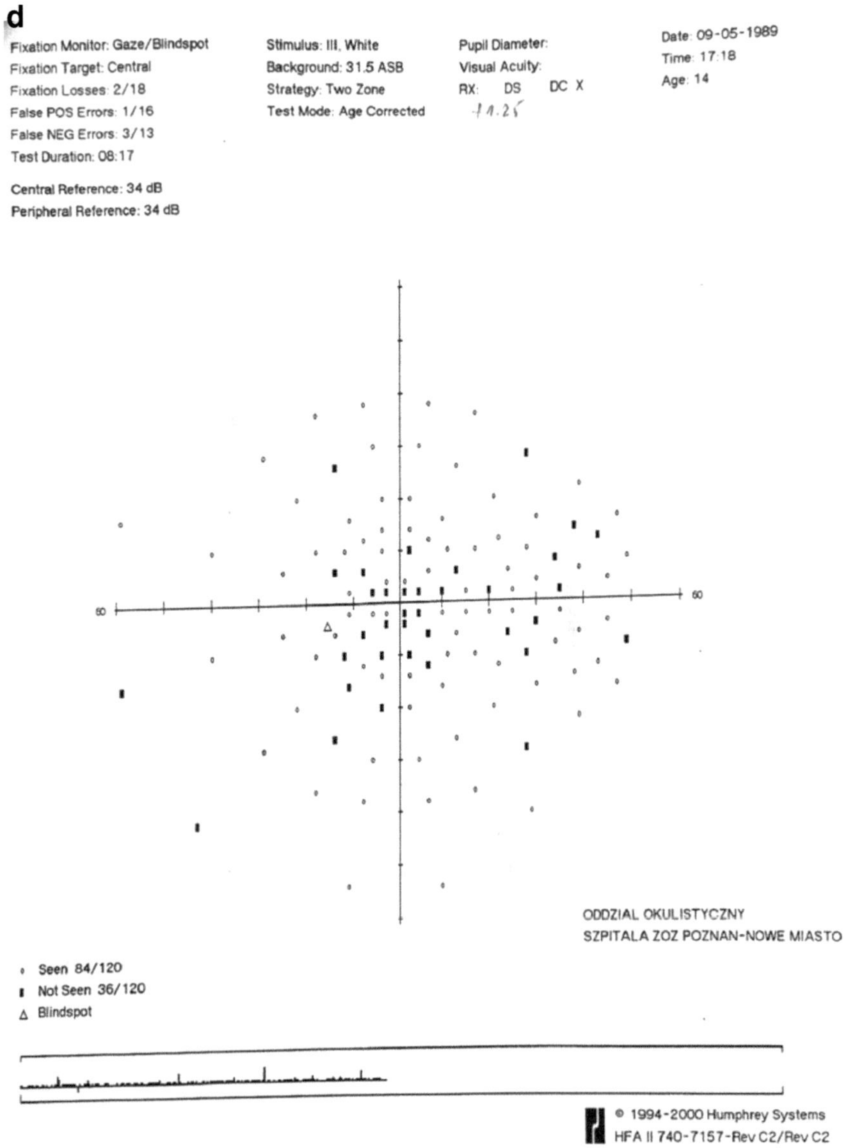

Fig. 18.1 (continued)

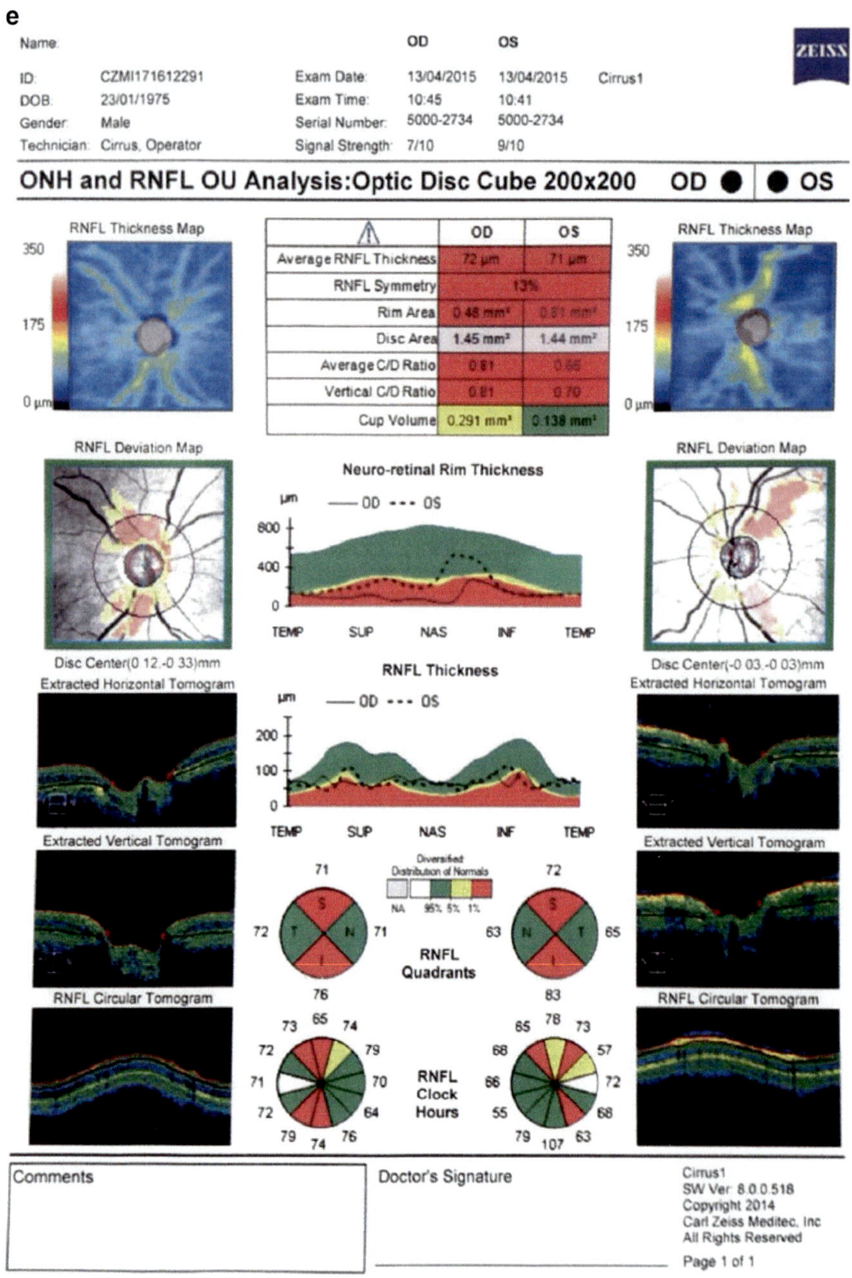

Fig. 18.1 (continued)

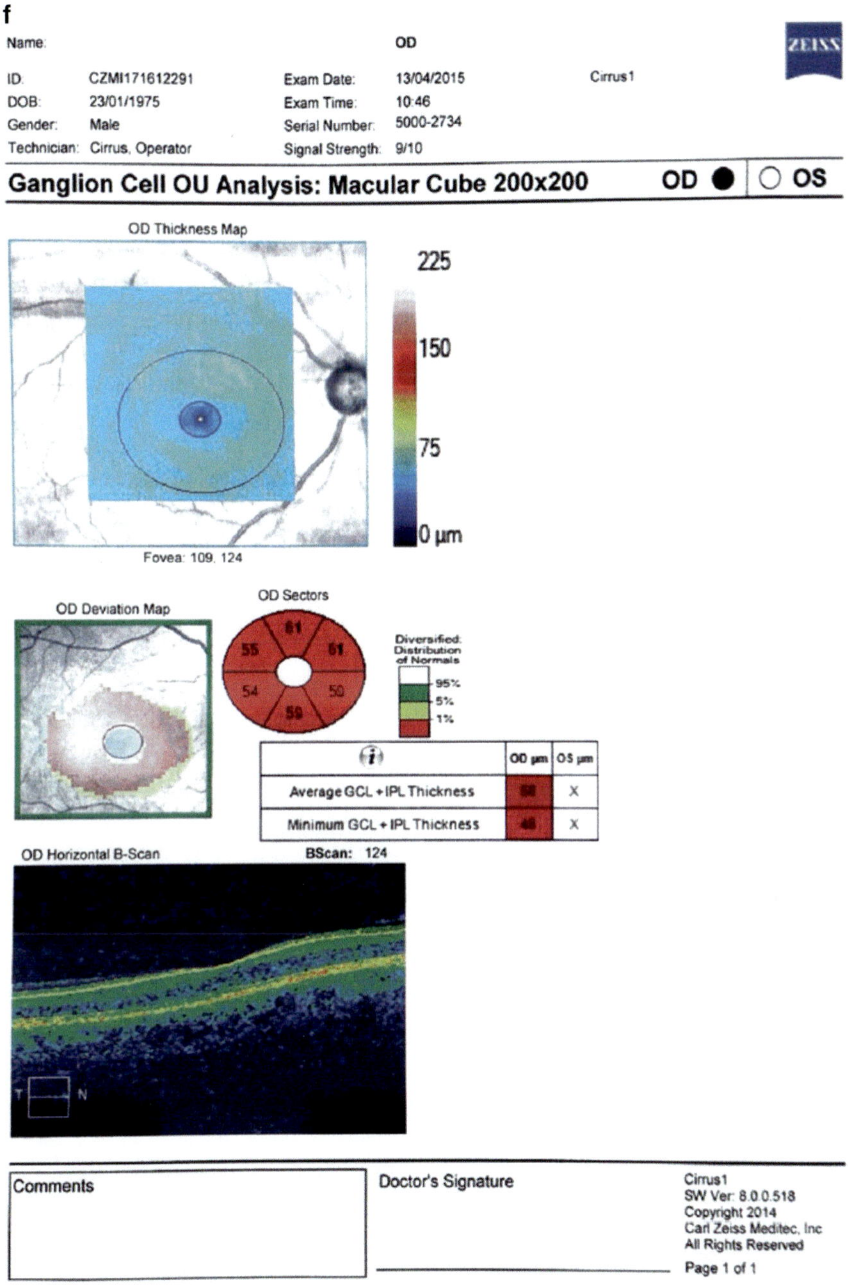

Fig. 18.1 (continued)

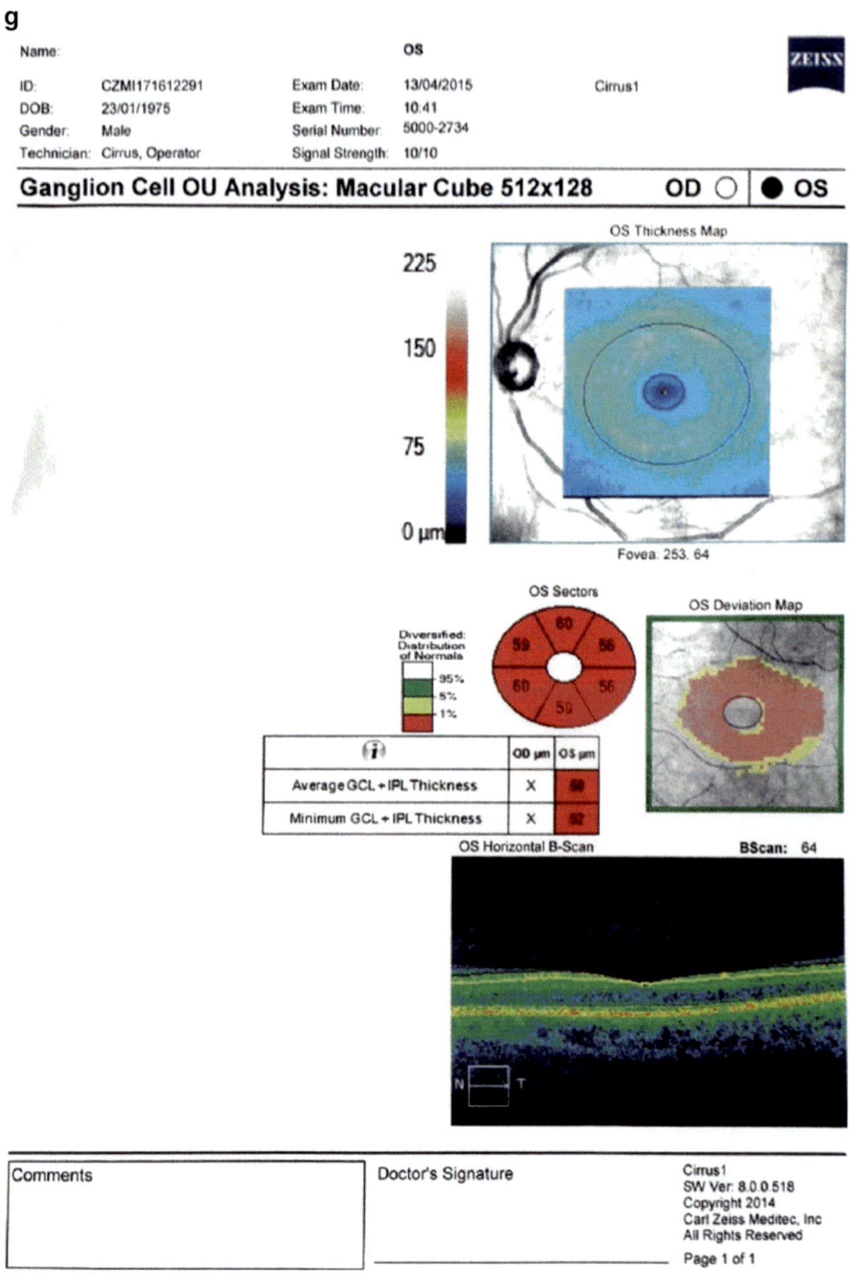

Fig. 18.1 (continued)

The microcysts found on OCT in patients with methanol intoxication are characteristic and unlikely to be confused with those observed in cystoid macular edema. They are highly uniform, small, have characteristic shape and are located in the inner nuclear layer. The microcysts are found in both eyes, occur symmetrically and are not accompanied by macular thickening. In contrast, the cysts observed in cystoid macular edema are larger, more irregular and can also be found in the outer plexiform layer. The lesions are either unilateral or bilateral, asymmetrical.

Several mechanisms of microcyst formation have been proposed thus far, including trans-synaptic retrograde degeneration, glial cell activation and mitochondrial dysfunction. Fluorescein angiography suggests that the lesions have nonvascular etiology. Presence of microcysts in the inner nuclear layer might correspond to retinal ganglion cell loss, and represent a damage to small caliber axons rich in mitochondria in the papillomacular bundle [26].

The OCT study of patients with methanol-induced optic neuropathy demonstrated significant decrease of global RNFL thickness during the following years. The most remarkable loss was detectable in the temporal segments. The highest rate of thickness was seen in the most severely poisoned patients [27]. Therefore, OCT could be a potentially interesting tool to assess the degree of chronic retinal axonal loss in patients with acute methanol-induced optic neuropathy.

18.1.3 Tobacco

The toxic optic neuropathy caused by tobacco seems to be mysterious entity since all confirmed cases were reported many years ago, in the era before OCT and genetic studies. It was shown that at least part of this disorder in fact was Leber's Hereditary Optic Neuropathy (LHON) [28–30]. It was proposed that smoking, especially in genetically susceptible individuals might affect sulphur metabolism, leading to chronic cyanide intoxication [31, 32]. The disorder was characterized by slowly progressive papillomacular bundle damage, centrocecal scotoma and visual loss. The appearance of the optic nerve is usually normal at the initial stages, with occasional peripapillary dilated vessels and haemorrhages, while pallor ensues only in the later stages [32]. Since the clinical picture of TON is similar to other optic neuropathies, the diagnosis of TON is by exclusion only of other toxic, nutritional and hereditary optic neuropathies. A few new articles [33–35] claimed that they presented patients with tobacco optic neuropathy, but they were undermined as they did not convincingly proofed the diagnosis [36–40].

18.1.4 Amiodarone

Amiodarone is a very efficient antiarrhythmic agent primarily used to treat atrial or ventricular tachyarrhythmias and fibrillation. The clinical presentation of amiodarone induced optic neuropathy may be sometimes indistinguishable from that of non-arteritic anterior ischaemic optic neuropathy (NAION) [41]. Amiodarone induced optic neuropathy has typically an insidious onset with a milder degree of visual loss, a longer duration of disc edema, and is more commonly bilateral than typical NAION, though there can be a considerable overlapping between these two conditions. Furthermore, disc edema and optic neuropathy may continue to progress even after cessation of the drug [41]. The mechanism of amiodarone-induced optic neuropathy is possibly due to the accumulation of cytoplasmic lamellar inclusions in the lysosomes due to binding of amiodarone with phospholipids. These complexes are not degraded by phospholipase enzymes leading to deposition of amiodarone deposits in the optic nerve as well as in other ocular tissues, including cornea and lens.

OCT has shown that in amiodarone-related optic neuropathy, there is transient RNFL thickening, during the initial months of therapy, followed by subsequent axonal loss and optic nerve atrophy [42]. OCT has been proposed as follow-up method for documenting edema or RNFL thinning in this setting.

18.1.5 Linezolid

Linezolid is a widely used broad-spectrum antibiotic. OCT studies demonstrated that patients with the signs of linezolid-induced optic neuropathy presented with microcystic spaces in the retinal nerve fiber layer and at the border of the RNFL and the retinal ganglion cell layer. The microcystic spaces in the RNFL resolved within 6 weeks of linezolid discontinuation. The degree of changes documented on OCT was shown to be proportional to deterioration of visual acuity [43, 44].

18.1.6 Chemotherapy

There is a published case report of neuropathy induced by intravenous chemotherapy (cytarabine and daunorubicin) in a patient with acute myeloid leukemia. OCT, conducted 6 weeks after the onset of symptoms, demonstrated thinning of the retinal nerve fiber layer in both eyes. Moreover, thinning and alteration of the foveal contour were observed in both eyes on OCT of the macula. The progression of changes documented on OCT was no longer observed when the patient was switched to another chemotherapy regimen [45].

18.2 OCT and Nutritional Optic Neuropathies

Nutritional optic neuropathy is more common among alcohol abusers and those who are undernourished [46]. Isolated nutritional optic neuropathies are rare, they are more frequent in regions of famine, where they may be epidemic. Nutritional optic neuropathies may be associated with various causes, including unbalanced diet, bariatric surgery, hunger strike, anorexia nervosa, absorption deficiency of vitamin B [47].

As in toxic neuropathies, the anterior visual pathways are susceptible to nutritional deficiency associating papillomacular bundle damage, central or cecocentral scotoma and reduction of color vision. The primary lesion is not necessarily localized into the optic nerve itself; it may be located at various levels, such as the retinal ganglion cells, nerve fiber layers, chiasm, or the optic tracts [48].

The exact mechanism by which nutritional deficits damage the optic nerve remains largely unknown. Specific deficiencies of vitamin B-12 (cyanocobalamin), thiamine (vitamin B-1) [49], other vitamins (riboflavin, niacin, and pyridoxine), folic acid, copper [50, 51] and other proteins with sulfur-containing amino acids have been associated with optic neuropathies [52]. It has been postulated that these deficiencies affect mitochondrial oxidative phosphorylation, and therefore nutritional optic neuropathies may be part of the acquired mitochondrial optic neuropathies spectrum [53]. The visual prognosis depends on multiple factors, including the cause and the duration of symptoms. At advanced stages of the condition, associated with optic atrophy, recovery is less likely to occur than at early stages [50]. Nutritional optic neuropathies are very rare in children.

Nutritional and toxic optic neuropathies have similar clinical presentations, i.e. bilateral, painless visual loss associated with colour vision disturbances and central scotoma. When an optic neuropathy is suspected, a thorough history should cover diet, drug/toxin exposure, social history (including alcohol consumption) and the professional environment. Treatment of any chronic disease such as pernicious anemia should be elucidated. Sensory symptoms and gait disturbance may be associated, due to either peripheral neuropathy or cerebellar dysfunction. A family history should be taken, to identify environmental factors or predisposition for hereditary optic neuropathies.

Clinically, patients with nutritional optic neuropathies complain of gradual blurring of vision, at far and near. Often, the slow progression of the symptoms delays diagnosis and treatment. Rarely, the visual symptoms may be asymmetric, but almost never strictly unilateral. Dyschromatopsia can be the initial symptom in nutritional optic neuropathies. In case of orbital pain, pain on ocular movement, unilateral vision loss, other diagnoses should be considered.

In nutritional optic neuropathies, visual acuity may vary from minimal reduction of vision to no light perception (NLP). However, most patients have 20/200 vision or better. Both pupils are sluggish to light, and there is no relative afferent pupillary defect due to the bilateral involvement. The optic disc may be normal or slightly hyperemic (Fig. 18.2) in the early stages, with small peripapillary hemorrhages. After several weeks to months, a papillomacular bundle dropout and temporal disc pallor may occur, followed by optic atrophy (Fig. 18.2). Isolated, purely nutritional optic neuropathies have been rarely explored with OCT, which might be able to closely monitor subtle RNFL changes, i.e. thickening at initial stages, followed at later stages by RML thinning, predominantly encountered in the temporal sector [51] (Figs. 18.3 and 18.4).

A recent OCT study conducted in chronic alcohol and tobacco users demonstrated substantial thinning of the RNFL in all quadrants except the nasal quadrant. The severity of axonal loss in ganglion cells was shown to be proportional to the degree of nicotine dependence. In the case of alcohol abuse, however, the relationship was not as straightforward [54]. These findings suggest that OCT may be a useful screening instrument to predict visual morbidities in persons with nutritional optic neuropathies.

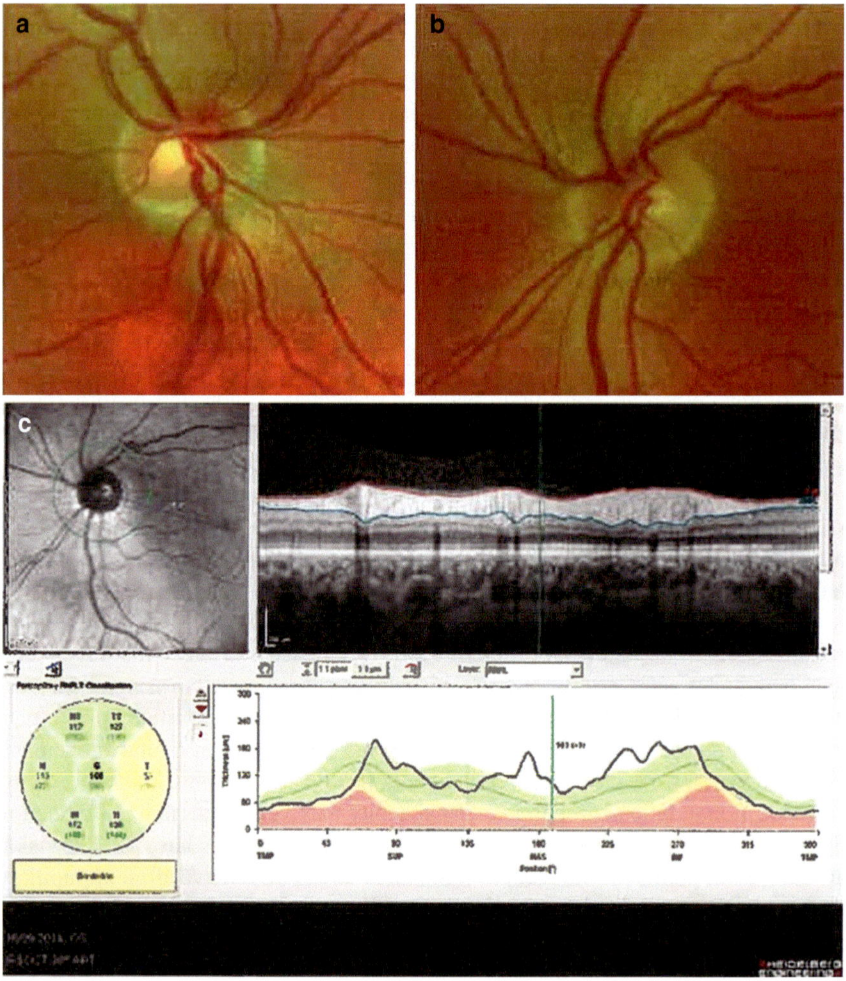

Fig. 18.2 Nutritional optic neuropathy, associated with reduced serum thiamine (Vitamin B 1), in a 30-year-old male patient presenting with blurred vision, painful dysesthesia in both legs and gait instability. Visual acuity was 20/200 in both eyes. Bilateral temporal pallor of the optic discs (**a**, **b**) and moderate reduction of the temporal retinal nerve fibre layer, visible on OCT (**c**, **d**). Vision recovered after intramuscular vitamin Bl administration

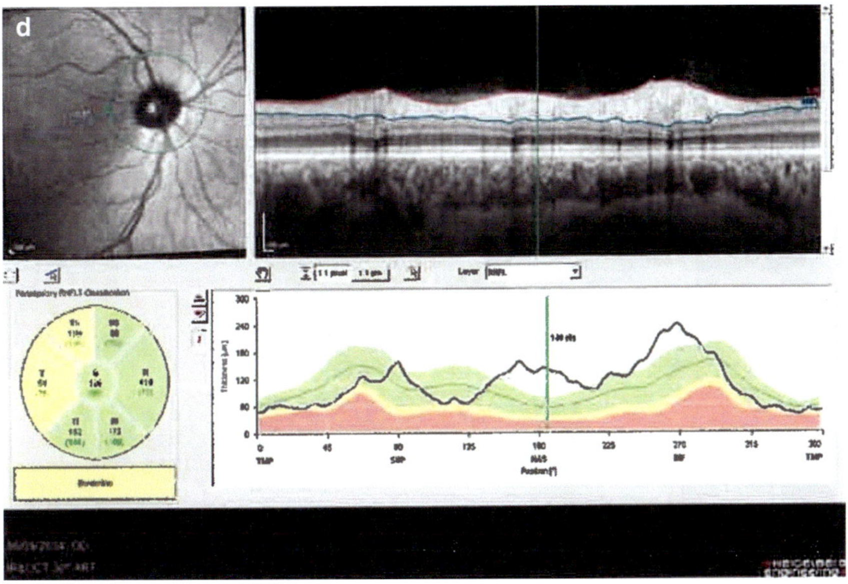

Fig. 18.2 (continued)

18.2.1 Copper Deficiency

Copper deficiency is an extremely rare finding in patients after bariatric surgeries. According to one published case report, a woman subjected to Roux-en-Y bypass surgery and partial gastrectomy, approximately 3 years after the procedure showed the signs of progressive binocular loss of visual acuity and disorders of color vision with central visual field scotoma in both eyes. OCT conducted 2 months after the onset of the symptoms revealed binocular thinning of the retinal ganglion cell-inner plexiform layer in the macula. However, the average peripapillary retinal nerve fiber layer thickness was normal. The authors of the report did not provide an explanation for such result of the OCT [55].

18.3 OCT and Antiepileptic Drug Toxic Maculopathy

Vigabatrin (Sabril) is a second-line anti-epileptic drug prescribed in partial epilepsy, with or without secondary generalization (mainly after failure of other drugs). As a first-line/monotherapy, Vigabatrin is licensed only for the treatment of infantile spasms (West's syndrome). Vigabatrin acts as a selective irreversible inhibitor of GABA-transaminase. Treatment therefore causes an increase in the concentration of GABA (gamma aminobutyric acid), the major inhibitory neurotransmitter in the brain but also in the retina. Maximal efficacy in adults is usually

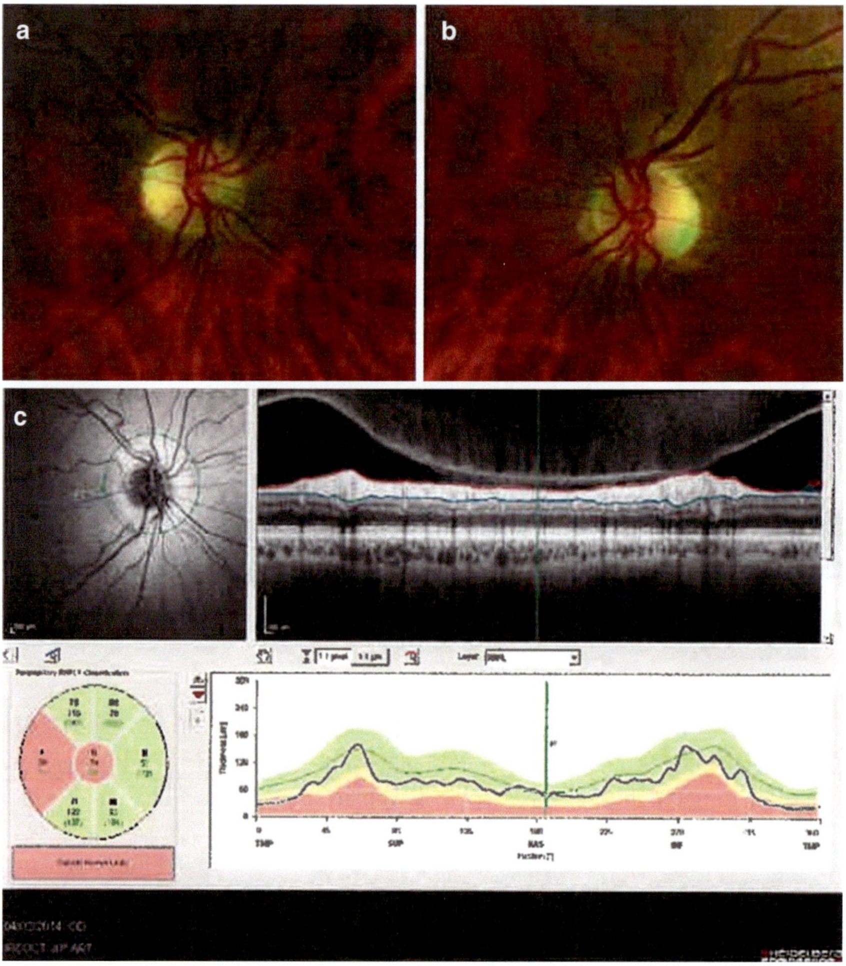

Fig. 18.3 A 60-ycar-old patient presented with bilateral visual loss ongoing for 6 months, (visual acuity was 20/200 in the right eye and 20/400 in the left eye), temporal disc pallor (**a**, **b**) and severe weight loss. There was no history of smoking or alcohol abuse. Decreased RNFL thickness was selectively located in the temporal area (**c**, **d**). Bilateral centrocaecal scotomas were encountered on Goldmann perimetry in both eyes (**e**, **f**). A megaloblastic anemia and folate deficiency was found on the blood test. Eventually a glucagonoma was discovered on abdominal MRI. Malabsorption responsible for malnutrition and particularly for folate deficiency was the suspected mechanism, After successful surgery and folate supplementation, visual acuity improved to 20/30 in the right eye and 20/80 in the left eye

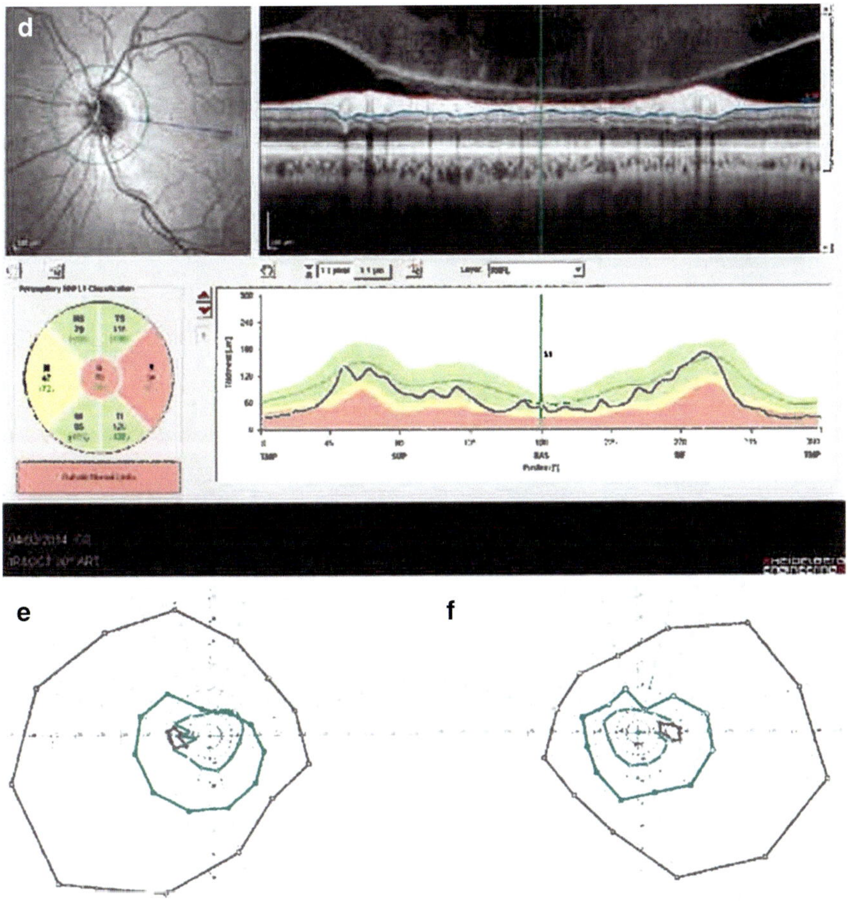

Fig. 18.3 (continued)

seen in the 2–3 g/day range. The recommended maintenance dose in children is 50–100 mg/kg/day.

During its clinical development, vigabatrin has rarely been associated with symptomatic visual field constriction and retinal disorders. In 1997, 3 cases of severe, symptomatic, persistent visual field constriction attributed to vigabatrin (VAVFC) were described by Eke [56].

Vigabatrin toxicity is typically associated with bilateral, concentric, predominantly nasal constriction of visual fields. However, patients with perimetric loss due to vigabatrin exhibit normal visual acuity and are unaware of the visual field constriction unless it extends into the central field [57]. The prevalence of VAVFC varies widely between studies, but is generally estimated to be 30–40% [58, 59].

The precise site of toxicity is controversial, but retina is involved in this condition.

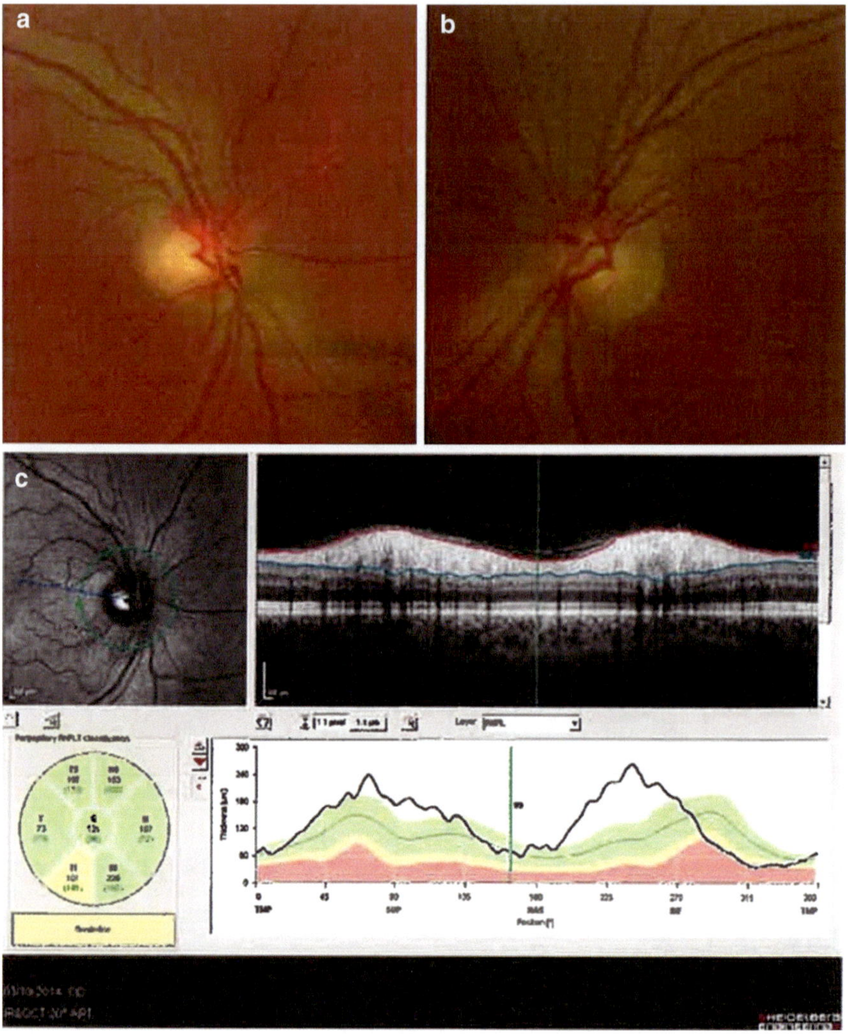

Fig. 18.4 A 40-year-old female patient presented with isolated severe visual loss and a history of mental anorexia in her teens. She stated being well aware of her irregular and unbalanced food intake. Visual acuity was 20/200 in both eyes. The optic disc are slightly hyperaemic with telangiectasia in the peripapillar retina (**a**, **b**). RNFL thickness was at higher normal limit in both eyes (**c**, **d**). The ganglion cell layer was normal in both eyes (**e**, **f**). Leber's hereditary optic neuropathy was ruled out, and the work-up disclosed low vitamin pp and carnitine levels. Six months after supplementation, visual acuity dramatically improved to 20/30 in the right eye and 20/40 in the left eye, although bilateral optic disc pallor had developed and temporal RNFL loss (**g**, **h**) and central ganglion cell loss in both eyes had occurred (**i**, **j**)

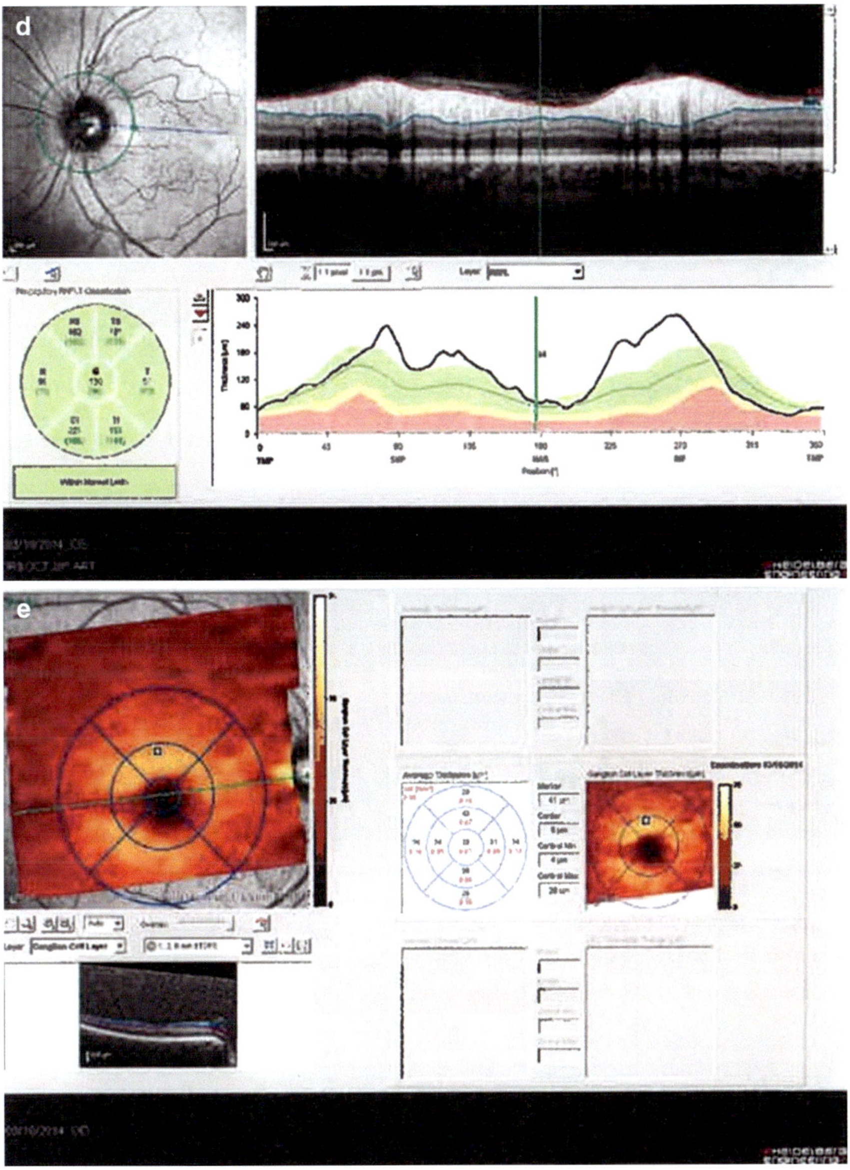

Fig. 18.4 (continued)

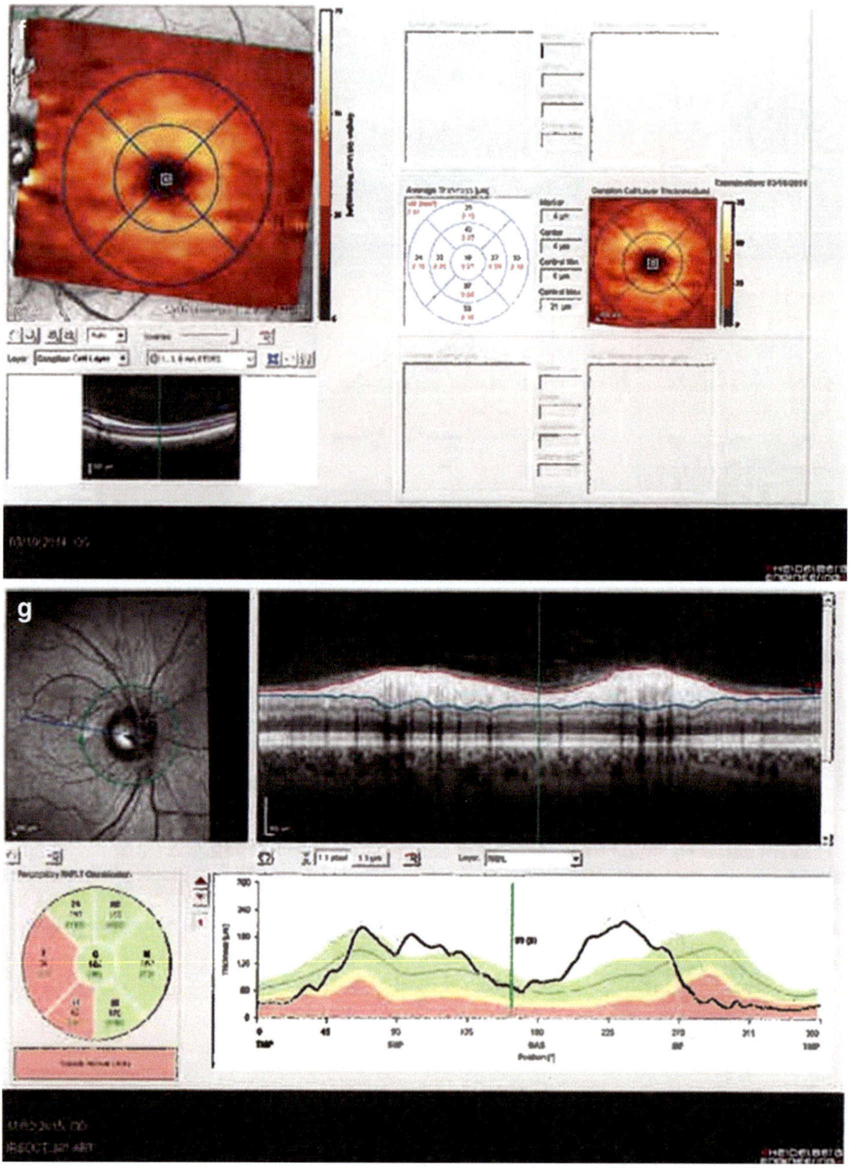

Fig. 18.4 (continued)

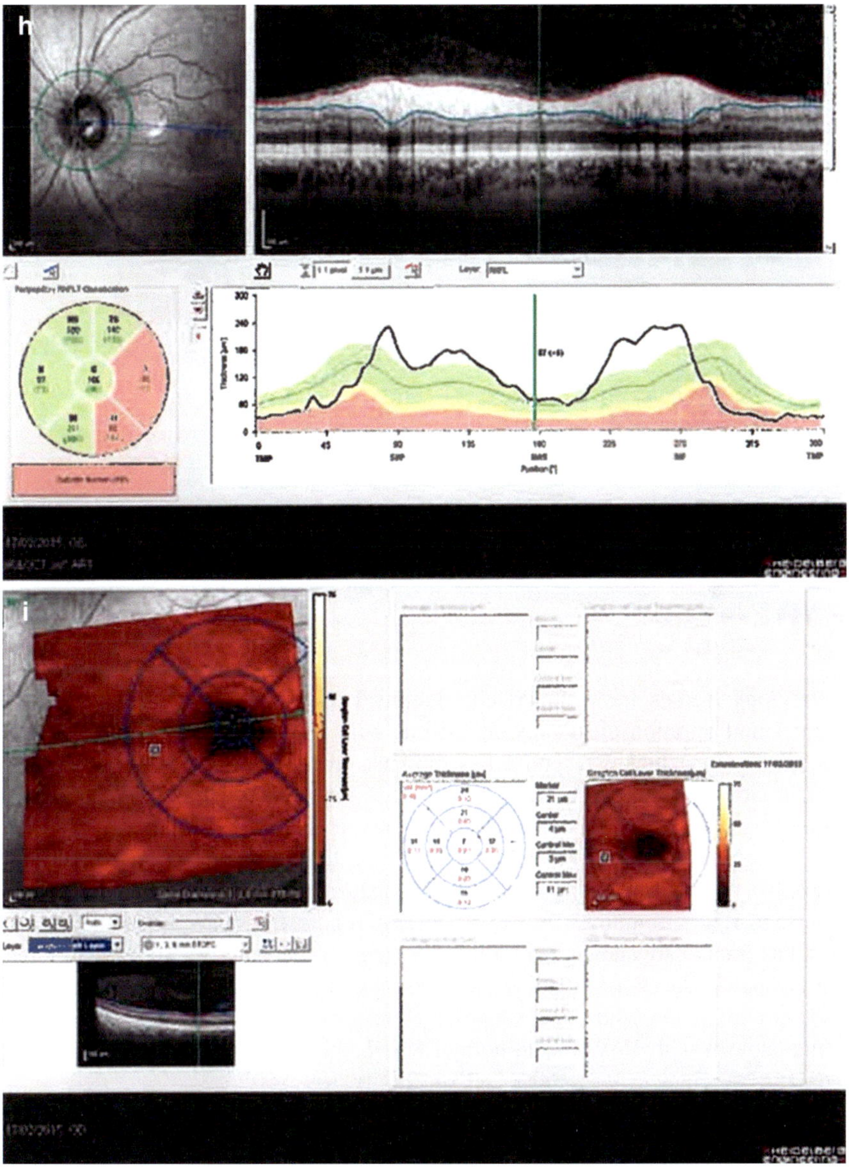

Fig. 18.4 (continued)

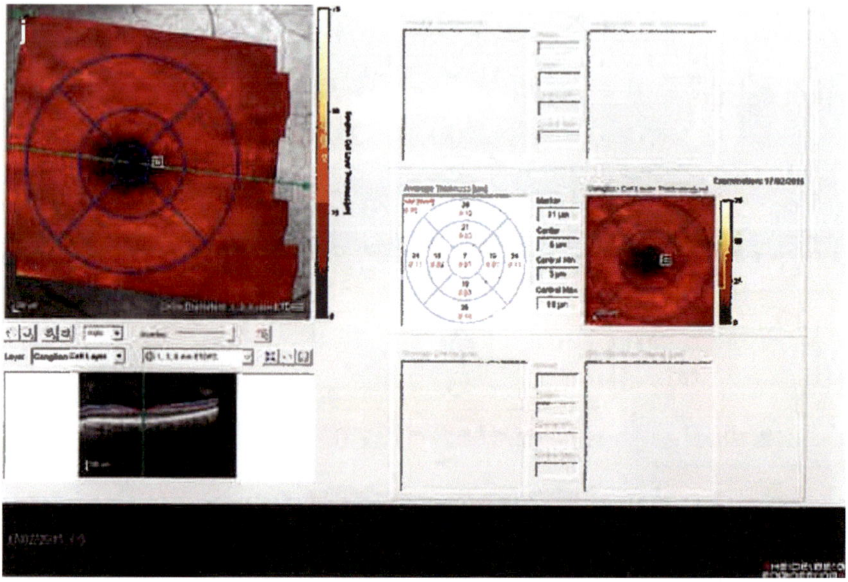

Fig. 18.4 (continued)

Previous studies have shown correlations between the severity of the ERG changes and duration of therapy, as well as with severity of VAVFC. The amplitude of the cone flicker response has the best predictive value for VAVFC, with a sensitivity of 100% and a specificity of 75% [59]. Therefore, ERG screening is currently used for toxicity detection in patients unable to perform perimetry.

Although visual field (VF) loss may occur in this setting despite any clinically detectable retinal changes, patients on Vigabatrin may exhibit optic nerve head pallor and RNFL thinning (Fig. 18.5) [60]. RNFL loss displayed on time domain OCT has previously shown a significant correlation between VAVFC and cumulative vigabatrin doses [61]. Patients with VAVFC displayed a reduced mean RNFL thickness compared with those under Vigabatrin but without field loss. Since none of the patients with VAVFC had normal RNFL thickness, the OCT sensitivity for detecting VF changes was 100% and specificity 70% [60].

Thickness of the nasal quadrant of RNFL appears to be particularly interesting in predicting vigabatrin associated visual filed constriction, with comparable results in terms of sensitivity (67–100%) and specificity (66–73%) [61, 62]. On the opposite, the temporal RNFL sector was not significantly different from control patients with epilepsy (not treated with gabaergic medications) and healthy volunteers [61, 62].

Thus, time domain and spectral domain optical coherence tomography seem to be reliable, in terms of sensitivity, for detecting RNFL thinning associated with

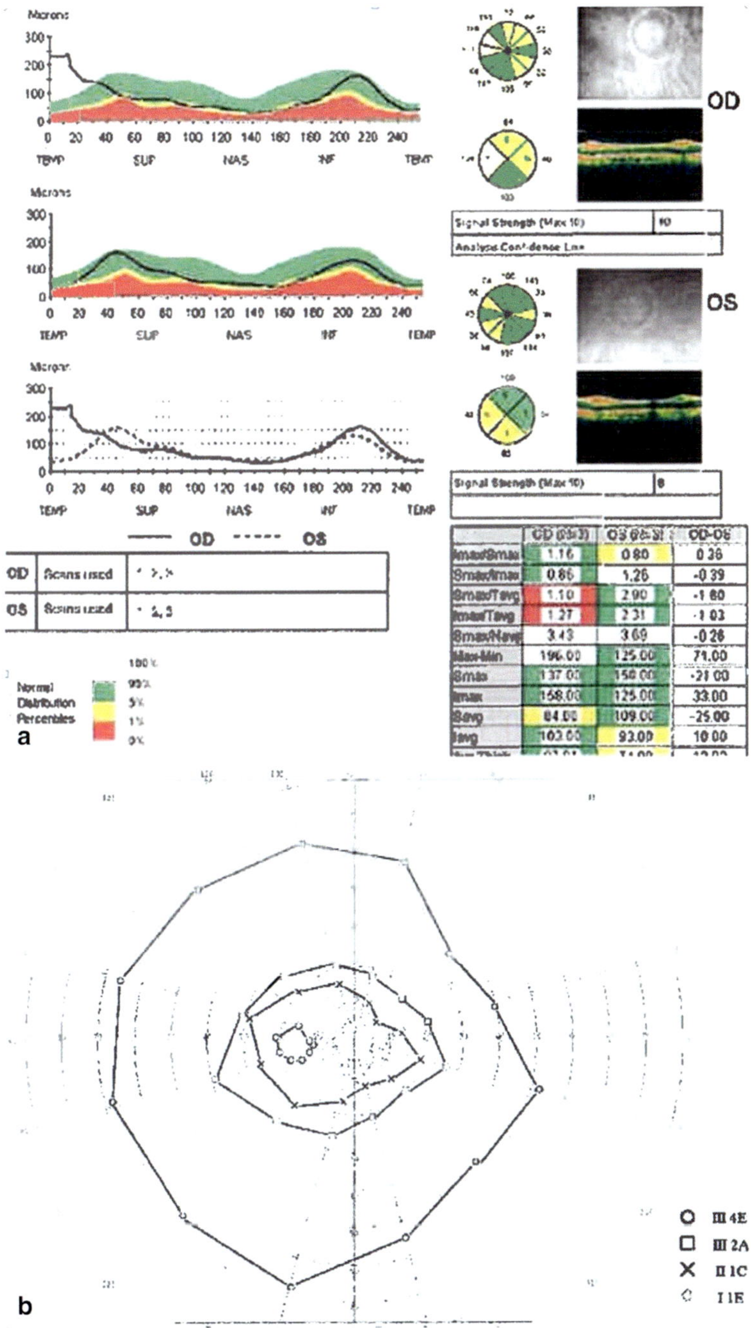

Fig. 18.5 Reduced nasal thickness on time domain OCT (**a**) in a patient treated with vigabatrin and presenting with vigabatrin associated visual field constriction in the nasal hemifield of the left eye (**b**)

vigabatrin-related visual field loss. It appears that both time domain and spectral domain OCT screening for vigabatrin treated patients may accurately monitor those at risk for VAVFC, especially when they are unable to perform perimetry.

In conclusion, OCT may be useful for quantifying the RNFL and retinal ganglion cells complex parameters in toxic and nutritional optic neuropathies [63]. Several studies have suggested that at early stages, localized, subtle RNFL thickening may be detected with OCT, prior to ophthalmoscopically visible changes. In the long term, localized, followed by diffuse RNFL thinning may occur, witnessing global axonal death.

References

1. Grzybowski A, Zulsdorff M, Wilhelm H, Tonagel F. Toxic optic neuropathies: an updated review. Acta Ophthalmol. 2015;93:402–10. https://doi.org/10.1111/aos.12515.
2. Wang MY, Sadun AA. Drug-related mitochondrial optic neuropathies. J Neuroophthalmol. 2013;33:172–8.
3. Zoumalan CI, Agarwal M, Sadun AA. Optical coherence tomography can measure axonal loss in patients with ethambutol-induced optic neuropathy. Graefes Arch Clin Exp Ophthalmol. 2005;243:410–6.
4. Sihota R, Sony P, Gupta V, et al. Diagnostic capability of optical coherence tomography in evaluating the degree of glaucomatous retinal nerve fiber damage. Invest Ophthalmol Vis Sci. 2006;47:2006–10.
5. Rebolleda G, Noval S, Contreras I, et al. Optic disc cupping after optic neuritis evaluated with optic coherence tomography. Eye (Lond). 2008;23:890–4.
6. Medeiros FA, Moura FC, Vessani RM, Susanna R. Axonal loss after traumatic optic neuropathy documented by optical coherence tomography. Am J Ophthalmol. 2003;135:406–8.
7. Fisher JB, Jacobs DA, Markowitz CF, et al. Relation of visual function to retinal nerve fiber layer thickness in multiple sclerosis. Ophthalmology. 2006;113:324–32.
8. Kozak SF, Inderlied CB, Hsu HY, et al. The role of copper on ethambutol's antimicrobial action and implications for ethambutol-induced optic neuropathy. Mycobacteriology. 1998;30:83–7.
9. Masvidal D, Parrish RK II, Lam BL. Structural-functional dissociation in presumed ethambutol optic neuropathy. J Neuroophthalmol. 2010;30:305–10.
10. Sadun AA, Wang MY. Ethambutol optic neuropathy: how we can prevent 100,000 new cases of blindness each year. J Neuroophthalmol. 2008;28:265–8.
11. Sivakumaran P, Harrisson AC, Marschner J. Ocular toxicity from ethambutol: a review of four cases and recommended precautions. N Z Med J. 1998;13:428–30.
12. Kinoshita J, Iwata N, Maejima T, Kimotsuki T, Yasuda M. Retinal function and morphology in monkeys with ethambutol-induced optic neuropathy. Invest Ophthalmol Vis Sci. 2012;53:7052–62.
13. Chai SJ, Foroozan R. Decreased retinal nerve fibre layer thickness detected by optical coherence tomography in patients with ethambutol-induced optic neuropathy. Br J Ophthalmol. 2007;91:895–7.
14. Kim U, Hwang JM. Early stage ethambutol optic neuropathy: retinal nerve fiber layer and optical coherence tomography. Eur J Ophthalmol. 2009;19:466–9.
15. Han J, Byun MK, Lee J, Han SY, Lee JB, Han SH. Longitudinal analysis of retinal nerve fiber layer and ganglion cell-inner plexiform layer thickness in ethambutol-induced optic neuropathy. Graefes Arch Clin Exp Ophthalmol. 2015;253:2293–9.
16. Vieira LM, Silva NF, et al. Retinal ganglion cell layer analysis by optical coherence tomography in toxic and nutritional optic neuropathy. J Neuroophthalmol. 2015;35(3):242–5.

17. Lee JY, Choi JH, Park KA, Oh SY. Ganglion cell layer and inner plexiform layer as predictors of vision recovery in ethambutol-induced optic neuropathy: a longitudinal OCT analysis. Invest Ophthalmol Vis Sci. 2018;59:2104–9.
18. Kim KL, Park SP. Visual function test for early detection of ethambutol induced ocular toxicity at the subclinical level. Cutan Ocul Toxicol. 2016;35:228–32.
19. Makino S. Utility of optical coherence tomography in the evaluation of patients with ethambutol-induced optic neuropathy. Int J Ophthalmol Vis Sci. 2014;12(1).
20. Junli X, Qi D, Shuangqing W, Wenyan S, Shanping Z, Liangyu Z. Treatment of ethambutol-induced optic neuropathy by buqihuoxue formula combined with methycobal. Int J Clin Exp Med. 2017;10:7100–15.
21. Fanta H, Mayer-Obcrditsch L. Ein Bcitrag zur Pathologie im Schncrven bci Methylalkoholvergiftung (Tierversuche). Klin Monatsbl Augenheilkd. 1953;122:288–394.
22. Sanaei-zadeh H, Zamani N, Shadnia SH. Outcomes of visual disturbances after methanol poisoning. Clin Toxicol (Phila). 2011;49:102–7.
23. Brent J, McMartin K, Phillips S, Aaron C, Kulig K. Fomepizole for the treatment of methanol poisoning. N Engl J Med. 2001;344:424–9.
24. Pakravan M, Sanjari N. Erythropoietin treatment for methanol optic neuropathy. J Neuroophthalmol. 2012;32:325–8.
25. Fujihara M, Kikuchi M, Kurimoto Y. Methanol-induced retinal toxicity patient examined by optical coherence tomography. Jpn J Ophthalmol. 2006;50:239–41.
26. Klein KA, Warren AK, Baumal CR, Hedges TR III. Optical coherence tomography findings in methanol toxicity. Int J Retina Vitreous. 2017;3:36.
27. Nurieva O, Diblik P, Kuthan P, Sklenka P, Meliska M, Bydzovsky J, Heissigerova J, Urban P, Kotikova K, Navratil T, Komarc M, Seidl Z, Vaneckova M, Pelclova D, Zakharov S. Progressive chronic retinal axonal loss following acute methanol-induced optic neuropathy: four-year prospective cohort study. Am J Ophthalmol. 2018;191:100–15.
28. Cullom ME, Heher KL, Miller NR, Savino PJ, Johns DR. Leber's hereditary optic neuropathy masquerading as tobacco-alcohol amblyopia. Arch Ophthalmol. 1993;111:1482–5.
29. Mackey D, Howell N. Tobacco amblyopia. Am J Ophthalmol. 1994;117:817–9.
30. Johns DR, Heher KL, Miller NR, Smith KH. Leber's hereditary optic neuropathy. Clinical manifestations of the 14484 mutation. Arch Ophthalmol. 1993;111:495–8.
31. Freeman AG. Optic neuropathy and chronic cyanide intoxication: a review. J R Soc Med. 1988;81:103–6.
32. Grzybowski A, Holder GE. Tobacco optic neuropathy (TON)—the historical and present concept of the disease. Acta Ophthalmol. 2011;89:495–9.
33. Behbehani R, Sergott RC, Savino PJ. Tobacco-alcohol amblyopia: a maculopathy? Br J Ophthalmol. 2005;89:1543–4.
34. Kee C, Hwang J-M. Optical coherence tomography in a patient with tobacco-alcohol amblyopia. Eye (Lond). 2008;22:469–70.
35. Moura FC, Monteiro ML. Evaluation of retinal nerve fiber layer thickness measurements using optical coherence tomography in patients with tobacco-alcohol-induced toxic optic neuropathy. Indian J Ophthalmol. 2010;58:143–6.
36. Grzybowski A. Tobacco amblyopia: does it really exist? Eye (Lond). 2007;21:1448–9.
37. Grzybowski A, Pieniazek M. Tobacco-alcohol amblyopia: nonexistent entity. Ind Psychiatry J. 2012;21:79.
38. Grzybowski A, Pieniążek M. Tobacco-alcohol amblyopia does not exist. Acta Ophthalmol. 2014;92:e77–8.
39. Grzybowski A. Mitochondrial optic neuropathies: additional facts and concepts. Clin Exp Ophthalmol. 2013. https://doi.org/10.1111/ceo.12148.
40. Grzybowski A, Pieniazek M. Tobacco-alcohol amblyopia—nonexistent entity cannot be diagnosed. J Neurol Sci. 2013;332:156.
41. Macaluso DC, Shults WT, Fraunfelder FT. Features of amiodarone-induced optic neuropathy. Am J Ophthalmol. 1999;127:610–2.

42. Martínez-López-Portillo A, Martínez-Gamero BO, Mohamed-Noriega J, Cavazos-Adame H, Mohamed-Hamsho J. Behaviour of disc oedema during and after amiodarone optic neuropathy: case report. J Clin Diagn Res. 2014;8:VD04–5.
43. Pilania RK, Arora A, Agarwal A, Jindal AK, Aggarwal K, Krishnan G, Suri D, Gupta A, Singh S, Gupta V. Linezolid-induced mitochondrial toxicity presenting as retinal nerve fiber layer microcysts and optic and peripheral neuropathy in a patient with chronic granulomatous disease. Retin Cases Brief Rep. 2018;25. https://doi.org/10.1097/ICB.0000000000000777
44. Ishii N, Kinouchi R, Inoue M, Yoshida A. Linezolid-induced optic neuropathy with a rare pathological change in the inner retina. Int Ophthalmol. 2016;36:761–6.
45. David JM, Anupriya A, Sheeja SJ. Presumed chemotherapy-induced optic neuropathy and maculopathy: a case report. Open Ophthalmol J. 2017;11:298–304.
46. Orssaud C, Roche O, Dufier JL. Nutritional optic neuropathies. J Neurol Sci. 2007;262:158–64.
47. Sawicka-Pierko A, Obuchowska I, Hady RH, Mariak Z, Dadan J. Nutritional optic neuropathy following bariatric surgery. Wideochir Inne Tech Maloinwazyjne. 2014;9(4):662–6.
48. Becker M, Masterson K, Delavelle J, Viallon M, Vargas ML, Becker CD. Imaging of the optic nerve. Eur J Radiol. 2010;74:299–313.
49. Gratton SM, Lam BL. Visual loss and optic nerve head swelling in thiamine deficiency without prolonged dietary deficiency. Clin Ophthalmol. 2014;8:1021–4.
50. Pineles SL. Combined optic neuropathy and myelopathy secondary to copper deficiency. Surv Ophthalmol. 2010;55:386–92.
51. Naismith RT, Shepherd JB, Weihl CC, Tutlam NT, Cross AH. Acute and bilateral blindness due to optic neuropathy associated with copper deficiency. Arch Neurol. 2009;66:1025–7.
52. Spinazzi M, De Lazzari F, Tavolato B, Angelini C, Manara R, Armani M. Myelo-opticoneuropathy in copper deficiency occurring after partial gastrectomy: do small bowel bacterial overgrowth syndrome and occult zinc ingestion tip the balance? J Neurol. 2007;254:1012–7.
53. Woon C, Tang RA, Pardo G. Nutrition and optic nerve disease. Semin Ophthalmol. 1995;10:195–202.
54. Ahuja S, Kumar PS, Kumar VP, Kattimani S, Akkilagunta S. Effect of chronic alcohol and tobacco use on retinal nerve fiber layer thickness: a case-control study. BMJ Open Ophthalmol. 2016;1: e000003. https://doi.org/10.1136/bmjophth-2016-000003.
55. Rapoprt Y, Lavin PJM. Nutritional optic neuropathy caused by copper deficiency after bariatric surgery. J Neuroophthalmol. 2016;36:178–81.
56. Eke T, Talbot JF, Lawden MC. Severe persistent visual field constriction associated with vigabatrin. BMJ. 1997;314:180–1.
57. Daneshvar H, Racette L, Coupland SG, Kertes PJ, Guberman A, Zackon D. Symptomatic and asymptomatic visual loss in patients taking vigabatrin. Ophthalmology. 1999;106:1792–8.
58. Lawden MC, Eke T, Degg C, Harding GF, Wild JM. Visual field defects associated with vigabatrin therapy. J Neurol Neurosurg Psychiatry. 1999;67:716–22.
59. Miller NR, Johnson MA, Paul SR, Girkin CA, Perry JD, Endres M, et al. Visual dysfunction in patients receiving vigabatrin: clinical and electrophysiologic findings. Neurology. 1999;53:2082–7.
60. Wild JM, Ahn HS, Baulac M, Bursztyn J, Chiron C, Gandolfo E, et al. Vigabatrin and epilepsy: lessons learned. Epilepsia. 2007;48:1318–27.
61. Versino M, Veggiotti P. Reversibility of vigabratin-induced visual-field defect. Lancet. 1999;354:486.
62. Frisen L, Malmgren K. Characterization of vigabatrin-associated optic atrophy. Acta Ophthalmol Scand. 2003;81:466–73.
63. Iorga RE, Moraru A, Ozturk MR, Costin D. The role of optical coherence tomography in optic neuropathies. Rom J Ophthalmol. 2018;62:3–14.

Animal Models in Neuro Ophthalmology

19

Eduardo M. Normando, Azeem Sher, Radhika Pooja Patel, Navya Arora, and M. Francesca Cordeiro

Abstract

Neuro-ophthalmology is the branch of ophthalmology dedicated to the study of neurological conditions which affect the visual system. An adequate understanding of the aetiology and pathophysiology of neuro-ophthalmic conditions is fundamental for establishing successful therapeutic strategies. Animal models are therefore considered crucial for understanding and investigating pathological events. Several animal models have been developed for studying neuro-ophthalmic disorders. However, their validity is closely related to the level of similarity with human pathology. Rodent models are extensively used due to their accessibility and cost efficiency. In particular, mouse models are recognised as among the best genetic models due to the ability to alter their genomes easily. Rats are easy to breed and are mainly used for toxic/pharmacological and surgical models. Nevertheless, rodent models are still suboptimal for human neuro-ophthalmic conditions because of anatomical differences between species. Primate models have the advantage of sharing vast anatomical and genomic similarities with humans. However, monkeys are expensive, difficult to breed and can only be handled by qualified personnel, limiting their suitability. Hence, there is no perfect species for studying neuro-ophthalmic conditions. This chapter will focus on the most common animal models of neuro-ophthalmic conditions.

E. M. Normando · A. Sher · R. P. Patel · N. Arora · M. F. Cordeiro (✉)
Imperial College Ophthalmology Research Group (ICORG), Department of Surgery and Cancer, Imperial College London, London, UK
e-mail: m.cordeiro@imperial.ac.uk

E. M. Normando · R. P. Patel · M. F. Cordeiro
Western Eye Hospital, Imperial College Healthcare NHS Trust, London, UK

M. F. Cordeiro
Glaucoma and Retinal Neurodegeneration Research, Visual Neuroscience, UCL Institute of Ophthalmology, London, UK

A. Grzybowski and P. Barboni (eds.), *OCT and Imaging in Central Nervous System Diseases*, https://doi.org/10.1007/978-3-031-72156-4_19

Keywords

Neuro-ophthalmology • Multiple sclerosis • Ischemic optic neuropathy • Leber hereditary optic neuropathy • Alzheimer's disease • Parkinson's disease

19.1 Animal Models of Demyelinating Conditions

Demyelinating conditions such as multiple sclerosis (MS) are a major cause of disability, and appropriate neuroprotective strategies have not been successfully developed yet [1]. MS is the most common type of human idiopathic inflammatory demyelinating disease (IIDD) [2]. It can affect the visual system, most commonly manifesting as optic neuritis. Patients can often present with a subacute, unilateral loss of vision associated with periorbital pain. Therefore, the eye can be used as a surrogate in assessing the disease's natural history and possible neuroprotective treatments. Although MS is a human specific condition, animal models of similar diseases have been developed, such as Experimental autoimmune encephalomyelitis (EAE), viral induced models (mainly mediated by Theiler's Murine Encephalomyelitis Virus), and toxicity-induced models such as the cuprizone model and lysolecithin-induced focal demyelination [3] (Table 19.1). These endeavour to mimic histological changes seen in MS and clinical phenotypes.

19.1.1 Experimental Autoimmune Encephalomyelitis (EAE)

EAE is an animal model of neuro-inflammation and is the most commonly used model of MS [4]. It is based on both antigen–antibody and cell-mediated response. It can be induced in several animal species (rat, mouse, rabbit, guinea pig and monkey) by spinal cord homogenate inoculation or by injecting different emulsified proteins or peptides in the animal CNS [5]. The proteins/peptides commonly used to induce EAE are myelin constituent peptides such as myelin basic protein (MBP), myelin proteolipid protein (PLP), and myelin oligodendrocyte glycoprotein (MOG) [6]. EAE is primarily mediated by specific T cells (CD4+), which migrate to the CNS and cause the autoimmune inflammatory response. The natural history of EAE can be variable, similarly to human MS, and it is both species and agent dependent [7]. Hallmark signs include weight loss, ataxia, spastic/flaccid paralysis, and incontinence. The lesions in the EAE model are characterised mainly by spinal inflammation and demyelination, while in human MS, lesions are more commonly seen in the brain [8]. Literature reviews have shown that in recent decades, several possible MS therapeutic strategies were successfully tested in animal models of EAE and that it was possible to control the disease in these immune-induced models [9–11]. This has led to the development of successful immunomodulatory therapies such as interferon-beta and glatiramer acetate, both initially demonstrated in EAE models in mice [12, 13]. However, it is essential

Table 19.1 Animal models in neuro ophthalmology

Disease	Animal model	Method	Benefits	Limitations	References
MS	EAE (rat, mouse, monkey) Cuprizone, lysolecithin (mouse)	Induced	Similar variation in natural history Simplicity; rapid	Limited brain involvement Reversible	[2, 4, 8, 9, 15–18]
AD	PS-1 and / or PS-2 APP transgenic Mutation mouse P301L tau mutation mouse 5xFAD mouse 3xTg-AD mouse	Genetic	Progressive development of senile plaques Robust model of NFT pathology Rapid deposition of large amounts of Aβ Follows natural history of AD	Difficult connection between injuries and increased deposition of Aβ oligomers 1st generation model No NFT formation	[54, 63–65, 68, 71]
NA-AION	Rat, primate	Rose Bengal injection	Resembles human AION pathology	Does not reflect pathogenesis of NA-AION	[31]
LHON	CBA/J mice Mice, Rats Mice	Rotenone-induced Mitochondrial ND4 mutation Mitochondrial ND6 mutation	Quick and simple, reproduce the pathophysiologic phenotype-reduced RGC layer thickness, increased apoptosis, decreased retinal metabolic capacity, increased superoxide Mechanistic resemblance to LHON Clinical, biochemical and anatomical hallmarks of human LHON when induced in animal at 14 and 24 months	The causal role of toxins in human LHON has not been demonstrated The mutation can be fatal (ND4 mutation), it is technically demanding	[40–42]

(continued)

Table 19.1 (continued)

Disease	Animal model	Method	Benefits	Limitations	References
NOM	EAE 'passive transfer' mouse Mice	Passive transfer of IgG Injection of IgG	Very similar pathology to human NMO Similar pathology with myelin involvement also	No injury to myelin Dependent on co-injection of human complement	[20]
	"2D2" EAE mouse	Genetic	Similar clinical picture to human NMO	No histological changes in keeping with NMO	[23]

to note that on several occasions, successes in animal studies did not translate into successful therapies when it came to human clinical trials [14]. For example, roquinimex, a synthetic immunomodulator, showed promising results in some animal models [15]. Through inhibition of IFNγ and TNFα, roquinimex prevented symptom manifestation and acute EAE development up to a week after disease induction. However, in multicentre phase III studies, the trial was terminated swiftly following detrimental adverse effects such as cardiopulmonary toxicities in patients [16].

Alterations in the optic nerve and retina have been described in EAE, where optical coherence tomography (OCT) detected GCC changes, which may be similar to what is observed in MS [17]. EAE not only promotes apoptosis in the retina, but also promotes apoptosis in the retina and causes glial response [18, 19]. B-cell dependent EAE has also been observed to affect the M-cone pathway more than the S-cone pathway, evident from photopic ERGs and M-opsin upregulation [20]. As the retina lacks myelin, it is most likely affected by a secondary reaction from myeline-reactive T cells and antibodies [21].

The central nervous system infection with the Theiler's virus induces an immune-mediated demyelinating disease and provides an important model for the study of MS [22]. The demyelinating disease induced by Theiler's Murine Encephalomyelitis Virus (TMEV) is similar to chronic-progressive MS. It is characterised by demyelination of the CNS mediated by a Th1 response with manifestation of spastic paralysis of the lower limbs. Further research has shown that TMEV exposure results in excess cytokine production of molecules such as IFN-α/β, IL-6, IL-1, and prostaglandin E2. This results in viral persistence by reducing Th1 responses [23]. In particular, in the mouse model of TMEV, the damage to myelin is closely dependent on the CD8 mediated antiviral action, demonstrating how brain inflammation could result in demyelination and axonal damage [17–19].

Intracerebral infection of TMEV to the SJL/L mouse strain causes a persistent viral infection of the mouse CNS. This results in a chronic progressive biphasic disease called TMEV-IDD and is an experimental model for progressive MS. The acute phase occurs one week post infection whilst the chronic phase happens one month post TMEV infection [24, 25]. Hind limb weakness that progresses to spastic paralysis is the hallmark of the chronic phase [26]. The persisting viral infection results in demyelination of the mouse CNS. This persistence is partly related to the innate immune response. Activation of the innate immune response results in the secretion of pro-inflammatory chemicals, which, in turn, activate the adaptive immune response [27]. Cytokines of the type 1 interferon (IFN) type are induced by viral infections causing an antiviral effect. The SJL/J model has low interferon stimulated gene (ISG) expression [28], unlike the C57BL/6J mouse strain that clears TMV and does not develop an MS-type disease. Further, lower levels of IFN-γ are associated with increased virus persistence in TMEV-infected mice [29] and C57BL/6J IFN-γ knock out mice cannot clear TMEV either, resulting in CNS demyelination [30].

Regulatory T-cells (Tregs) are implicated in the decreased anti-viral $CD8^+$ T cell response to viral infections. There is an inverse relationship between Tregs depletion and increased viral clearance by CD8+ T cells [31–34]. TMEV infection results in high Treg recruitment in the acute phase with a ratio of 1:4 ($CD8^+$ T-effector: Treg) in the SJL/J mouse, compared to 1:1.2 in the C57BL/6J model [35]. The depressed $CD8^+$ T-effector activity leads to a persistent viral infection and reduced viral clearance [27]. In the acute phase, the virus targets neurons and grey matter structures such as the hippocampus and cerebral cortex [36]. Recruitment of pro-inflammatory cells such as $CD4^+$ and $CD8^+$ T cells to the grey matter structures causes CNS inflammation [37–39]. Whilst the viral load decreases, ineffective clearance leads to a chronic infection. In this phase, inflammation continues in the white matter and demyelination of the spinal cord and axonal damage occur [25]. Unlike the acute phase, TMEV is only found in glial cells and macrophages, not in neurones, as per immunohistochemical and in situ hybridisation studies [37, 40–44]. $CD4^+$ and $CD8^+$ T cells are the primary infiltrating cells during this stage, demonstrating that whilst TMEV induces demyelination, the resulting immune response is the causal mechanism involved [27].

19.1.2 Toxic Models of Demyelinating Conditions

Toxic models of demyelination have also been developed. Cuprizone, a copper chelating agent, can induce rapid oligodendrocyte apoptosis with subsequent demyelination. The most important advantage of the cuprizone model is its simplicity. Mice orally exposed to cuprizone express a rapid onset of MS like symptoms, including ataxia and spastic paralysis. Histological features of this model are oligodendrocyte apoptosis, microglial infiltration, disruption of myelin sheets and macrophage activation, which are in keeping with Human MS. Particularly, this model affects specific brain structures, more in keeping with MS in humans [45]. Cuprizone impairs visual function, as demonstrated by multifocal electroretinography [46]. However, this is a reversible model; when cuprizone is eliminated from the mouse diet, remyelination occurs followed by complete restitutio-ad-integrum [47, 48]. Lysolecithin, an activator of phospholipase A2, can also induce demyelination when injected into the spinal cord of experimental animals. It generates rapid demyelination due to the activation of lymphocytes B and T, followed by macrophage infiltration with subsequent disruption of myelin sheets. Like the cuprizone model, remyelinization occurs 6–8 weeks after Lysolecithin injection. Hence, this model also does not entirely represent human MS [49, 50].

Ethidium bromide (EB) is a planar molecule that can intercalate between base pairs in double stranded DNA, inhibiting transcription and replication [51]. EB is cytotoxic to any cell, provided a cell body exists in the target area [52, 53]. Axons with cell bodies not in the lesion area are spared unless very high doses of EB are administered [54]. Lesions due to EB are large, with remyelination occurring more slowly than lysolecithin lesions. This is likely due to an impaired immune response and death of progenitor and glial cells [54, 55]. Astrocyte cell death results in increased Schwann cell contribution towards remyelination as astrocytes prevent the oligodendrocyte progenitor cells from differentiating into Schwann cells [56, 57]. However, as with the above models, this is not representative of human MS as remyelination happens. In conclusion, none of the currently available animal models of MS can replicate the human disease and further research is needed in the field.

19.1.3 Animal Models of Neuromyelitis Optica

Neuromyelitis Optica (NMO) is a neuroinflammatory disorder that preferentially targets the optic nerves and spinal cord, causing recurrent and simultaneous inflammation and demyelination of these structures, leading to blindness and paralysis [58]. Once thought to be a subtype of MS, the discovery that NMO is associated with the NMO-IgG biomarker, an antibody which targets the aquaporin-4 (AQP4) water channel on the end feet of astrocytes, has seen it recognised as a spectrum of disorders distinct from MS [59]. Classical presentation is with an episode of optic neuritis causing a loss of vision, or visual field defects and dyschomatopsia occurring in isolation, accompanied by acute spinal cord dysfunction such as paraparesis or quadriparesis with sensory signs, or loss of bladder control.

There is circumstantial evidence from studies which suggests that NMO-IgG is pathogenic in humans, with the presence of the antibodies in patients with transverse myelitis or optic neuritis conferring a strong likelihood that these patients will develop NMO in the future compared to patients who test negative for the antibodies [60]. One animal model of NMO involves the passive transfer of NMO-IgG via intraperitoneal injection into the EAE rat model. The IgG appears to exacerbate inflammation and modulate the immune response in the context of this model, resulting in complement activation, immunoglobulin deposition, and granulocyte influx in perivascular areas of the spinal cord [61]. These changes represent very similar pathology to that seen in human NMO lesions. However, the major limitation of this model is the lack of injury to the myelin. Another model of NMO involves direct injection of NMO-IgG into the brain of mice. Lesion development was dependent on the co-injection of human complement, resulting in similar pathological changes to those seen in human NMO lesions, and in contrast to the rat NMO models also demonstrated damage to the myelin [62]. A genetic animal model of NMO which does not involve IgG has also been developed. The "2D2" EAE model was developed in which mice born with T cells directed against myelin oligodendrocyte glycoprotein (MOG35–55) were crossed with mice that have a transgenic B cell receptor to MOG. The resultant progeny spontaneously developed a clinical picture involving optic neuritis and severe inflammatory spinal cord lesions, with sparing of the brain, as seen in human NMO patients [63]. In this model, the drawback was that histological changes such as complement deposition and granulocyte recruitment were not seen.

In another study, an intrathecal injection of NMO-IgG was injected at L5-L6 [64, 65]. Whilst wild-type mice were only mildly affected, CD59-knockouts developed considerable white matter damage. By day 2, there was loss of AQP4 and glial fibrillary acidic protein with extensive inflammation, demyelination, and associated hindlimb weakness. However, partial remyelination had occurred with observable motor recovery by day five. In a study where patient-derived NMO-IgG was administered via intraventricular infusion for seven days [65, 66], human IgG was seen in the brain, spinal cord and optic nerve. This was associated with a loss of AQP4 and reactive astrocytes in the spinal cord and optic nerve. In the spinal cord, axonal injury and demyelination were also apparent.

As yet, no single animal model has recreated all of the clinical and pathological features of NMO, but a combination of active immunisation, passive transfer, and genetic models is helping to elucidate individual pathological events in NMO. Retinal involvement is a feature of NMO. However, effective animal models of optic neuritis in NMO (NMO-ON) are lacking. Asavapanumas N. et al. have generated a mouse model of NMO-ON by continuous infusion near the optic chiasm of NMO-IgG [67]. Zeka B et al. have shown Aquaporin 4-specific T cells and NMO-IgG cause primary retinal damage in a mouse model of NMO [68].

19.2 Animal Models of Ischemic Optic Neuropathy

Ischemic optic neuropathy (ION) is caused by an ischaemia of the optic nerve head and is the most frequent cause of sudden visual loss in patients older than 50 years. ION is characterised by a severe reduction in visual acuity associated with visual field defect, oedema of the optic nerve head and disc haemorrhages. Ischemic optic neuropathy is differentiated into two different clinical forms: non-arteritic (NAION), which is caused by an infarct of the short posterior ciliary arteries associated with anatomical risk factors such as small optic disc; and the arteritic form (AION), which is part of a generalised disease (e.g. giant cells arteritis), caused by an inflammatory reaction. The ischaemic outcome of either event will result in nerve fibre atrophy and often gives rise to a pale optic disc on clinical examination [69, 70].

The major problem regarding animal models of ION lies in the anatomical differences between the optic nerve head (ONH) in humans and small animals. The ONH in rodents lacks a lamina cribrosa, and the connective tissue surrounding the axon bundles has different collagen components and hysteresis compared to what is found in humans [71]. The vascular structure of the rodent ONH is also different. While rats have a vascular ring around the ONH, which is somewhat similar to primates, mice often lack this anatomical feature [72]. Therefore, this intrinsic inter-species variability translates into entirely different manifestations of an ischaemic event.

Furthermore, the number of axons constituting the optic nerve differs between species. Human and non-human primates have 1–1.2 million axons, rats 100,000 and mice 50,000 [73–75]. Again, this crucial anatomical difference results in contrasting manifestations of ONH ischaemia. However, the ONH in non-human primates is almost identical to humans.

The most diffuse model of ION is found in an induced model where a dye (Rose Bengal—RB) is injected intravenously and then locally activated by a focal laser beam (532 nμ) projected onto the ONH of the animal [76]. The activation of the RB provokes reactive oxygen species formation, which subsequently triggers platelet activation and capillary endothelial disruption [77]. Repeatability, which was the major problem of this model, has been overcome recently by introducing custom-made rodent contact lenses, enabling constant and reproducible insults [78]. The generated damage has similar features to human ION; however, the ischaemia resolves rapidly, and the disc oedema disappears after a maximum of 5 days post insult. However, Retinal Ganglion Cell (RGCs) apoptosis occurs, and reduction in retinal fibres is clearly visible one month after laser exposure using both direct visualisation and computerised techniques. The hallmark of the disease, RGC apoptosis, is also clearly assessable histologically, alongside structural changes to vessels, ONH oligodendrocytes apoptosis and ONH fibrosis [79, 80]. The same method generates similar results when applied to mice and non-human primates, making this technique a straightforward model of ION [81, 82] (Table 19.1). Recent studies have shown that overexpression of Dedicator of cytokinesis 3 (Dock3), which is part of the guanine nucleotide exchange factors family, protects myelin in the corpus callosum in a rodent model of ION [83].

19.3 Animal Models of Leber Hereditary Optic Neuropathy

Leber's hereditary optic neuropathy (LHON) is a rare disorder caused by mitochondrial DNA point mutations in genes coding for specific protein subunits of the respiratory chain complex I (G3460A, T14484C, G11778A) [84, 85]; it is characterised by severe, painless acute unilateral visual loss which becomes bilateral within days or weeks. LHON predominantly affects young men (20 years) and, less frequently, women. However, few paediatric and elderly cases have been reported [86]. The classic manifestation of LHON is accompanied by dyschromatopsia, followed by the involvement of the fellow eye within days or weeks. The evolution of the visual field defect is generally represented by progressive enlargement of the blind spot with rapid progress towards the central vision. LHON diagnosis should always be considered in young male patients with bilateral optic neuritis, regardless of age [86].

Genetic studies of LHON began over two decades ago. However, the pathogenic mechanisms that produce the specific RGCs degeneration are still not fully understood, and aetiological therapeutic strategies are still under development. This is mainly due to the need for better animal models of LHON. The first animal model was generated by intravitreal administration of rotenone, a mitochondrial complex I inhibitor, directly into the mouse eye, where histological analysis showed a significant decrease in RGC layer thickness one day after rotenone injection [87]. Another experimental mouse model consists of an intravitreal injection of a genetically-engineered ribozyme. This procedure is responsible for a specific degradation of nuclear mRNA, resulting in the onset of optic neuropathy with reduced superoxide dismutase activity and similar histological features observed in patients with LHON [88]. Another model of rodent LHON can be generated by injecting rotenone microspheres directly into the rat's superior colliculus [89]. These animal models showed the most common signs of LHON: visual loss within two weeks of injection, and absence of early RGCs loss with subsequent apoptosis. Intravitreal injections of yeast NADH dehydrogenase (Ndi1) in these models produce restoration of normal vision. This has opened a window of opportunity for novel therapeutic strategies [89].

Another such example is Idebenone (6-[10-hydroxydecil]-2,3-dymethoxy-5-methyl-1,4-benzoquinone), which has been shown in LHON mouse models to protect against RCG loss and prevent retinal thinning [90]. Although this is the primary, disease-specific pharmacological treatment for LHON in the EU, the main clinical trial for the drug found no statistically best-corrected visual acuity (BCVA) and change in visual acuity (VA) of the best eye in humans and treatment remains challenging [91]. Genetic models of LHON are also available [92]. A mouse with a G14600A mutation has been developed, resulting in mouse optic atrophy with synaptosomes, electron transport chain dysfunction, and increased ROS production, eventually leading to RGC death [93].

Two other models involving human pathologic complex 1 subunit expression have been developed. In the first model, allotopic expression of mutated human ND4 was induced by injecting a viral vector intraocularly, resulting in optic neuropathy in mice [94, 95]. Then, a transgenic mouse model expressing mutant human ND4 was created via germline mitochondrial gene transfer and using a mitochondrial-targeting viral vector [96]. The potential for gene therapy in treating LHON was tested by injecting wild-type human ND4 into these mice, which reversed the optic atrophy. A small study involving 9 LHON patients with the G11778A mutation was injected with wild-type ND4 in humans. Six patients had a visual acuity improvement by at least 0.3 log MAR at nine months [97], demonstrating the potential of gene therapy in these patients. Phase 3 trials [98–100] have shown evidence of bilateral improvement in visual acuity despite only one eye being injected with wild-type ND4. However, they missed their target of improving visual acuity in treated eyes alone.

19.4 Animal Models of Alzheimer's Disease

Alzheimer's disease (AD), the most common cause of dementia, is characterised by the insidious onset of a progressive decline in cognitive function due to the loss of neurons in the brain [101]. The pathology underlying the degeneration of neurons in AD brain is the formation of extracellular senile plaques via amyloid-beta (Aβ) deposition and intracellular neurofibrillary tangles (NFTs) via hyperphosphorylation of tau protein [102]. Although much progress has been made in our understanding of AD, early and more accurate diagnosis is currently unavailable, and a definitive diagnosis of AD can still only be made by neuropathology after the patient has died [103]. This prevents effective treatment in the early stages of the disease. Perhaps the main problem in the early diagnosis of AD is the inability to visualise changes in the brain directly.

However, increasing evidence has shown that the retina is also affected in AD, along with the changes in the brain [104, 105]. Studies have shown significant anatomical changes such as RNFL thinning during stages of early cognitive impairment as well as those with severe AD compared to controls [106, 107]. More significantly, the hallmarks of Alzheimer's in the brain have also been identified in the retina in both animal models and human subjects. Recent studies have demonstrated that RGCs, the RNFL and inner plexiform of the transgenic mice exhibit a significant rise in the immunoreactivity of Aβ and APP when compared to wild-type mice, with the changes being age-dependent [108, 109]. Histological studies in transgenic AD mouse models have demonstrated the presence of Aβ in the retina. Using a single transgenic Tg2576 mouse model which contains the APP double Swedish mutation, Liu et al. have shown increased Aβ immunoreaction occurring predominantly in the retinal ganglion cell layer and the outer retina [110]. Retinal Aβ deposition, along with increased APP, has also been found in double transgenic mouse models expressing APP and presenilin (PS) mutations, a finding which increased with age [108, 109, 111]. Using a triple transgenic AD mouse model that harbours three mutations of APP, tau and PS, a recent study has also demonstrated increased Aβ deposition and tau hyperphosphorylation in the RGC layer compared to age-matched controls.

A fascinating finding is that retinal Aβ plaques in AD mice can be stained with curcumin and imaged in vivo; more significantly, the retinal plaques occurred before the development of plaques in the brain [112]. This is hugely relevant as it suggests that retinal changes could potentially be used to make an early diagnosis of AD. Similar to the findings in mice, APP immunoreaction has also been demonstrated in the human retina, being prominent in RGCs and the RNFL, and again found in increased abundance with age [113]. In AD patients, Aβ specific plaques have been identified in the retina and increased with the severity of the disease by histological analysis of post-mortem eyes [112] (Fig. 19.1).

Transgenic rat models of AD have also been developed but to a lesser degree than mouse models [114]. Transgenic rats have larger brains, allowing for more accessible CSF collection and imaging [115]. Nevertheless, as with transgenic mice, expression of multiple familial AD mutations accelerates disease development, and all models develop amyloid plaques. The TgF344-AD rat model also develops neurofibrillary tangles despite only expressing endogenous rat tau, probably due to the similarity between rat and human tau protein [114].

The TgF344-AD rat model also shows evidence of amyloid plaque deposition in the brain and retina [116]. There is evidence of choroidal thinning, choroid inflammation, and hypertrophy of the retinal pigmented epithelium (RPE). The study showed increased levels of RPE hypertrophy in 14- and 19-month-old TgF344-AD rats compared to their age-matched wild-type counterparts, highlighting the retinal damage caused by amyloid deposition [116]. The clinical endpoint for AD

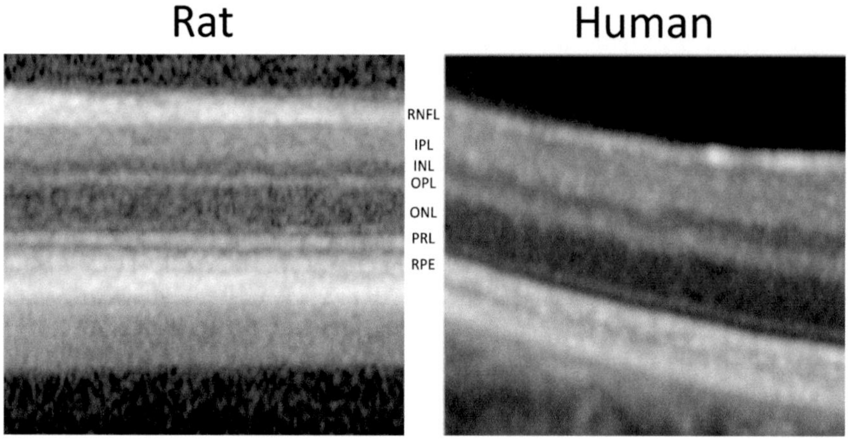

Fig. 19.1 OCT differences between rat retina and human retina. RNFL: retinal nerve fibre layer. IPL: inner plexiform layer. INL: inner nuclear layer. OPL: outer plexiform layer. ONL: outer nuclear layer. PRL: photoreceptor layer. RPE: retinal pigmented epithelium

pathology is neuronal loss and tissue atrophy in the brain, in which both apoptosis and necrosis play a crucial role [117].

19.4.1 PS-1 and/or PS-2 APP Transgenic Mutation

Copies of human APP and PS1-2, which are implicated in familial AD, have been used to create models of transgenic AD mice [118]. Transgenic models generated APP mutation with amyloid peptide deposition, which is similar but not identical to the one found in human senile plaques and commonly associated with amyloid angiopathy. Deposit of amyloid peptides is observed with associated dystrophic alterations in axons and dendrites. These models have often been used to understand the natural history of senile plaques [119], to study the plaque removing action of microglia [120], and to study protein interactions [121]. The double APP + PS1 mutant transgenic models show a progressive and rapid development of senile plaques at three months of age with maximum expression at 12 months [122].

Since the development of this model, several questions have been raised regarding the mechanism of neuronal loss, the accumulation of Aβ in the cell body, inflammation, and gliosis. This model has also been used to determine the involvement of oxidative stress in AD [123, 124]. The biggest drawback of this model is the difficulty to draw a connection between symptoms, injuries and increased deposition of Aβ oligomers [125]. Another problem of this mouse model is that neurofibrillary tangles (NFTs) are present only in mouse lines that overexpress mutated tau protein [125, 126].

19.4.2 Transgenic Tauopathies

Tauopathies are a group of degenerative diseases characterised histologically by the presence of filamentous inclusions in neurons (neurofibrillary pathology) and occasionally in the glial cells. These filaments are composed of hyperphosphorylated forms of tau protein, which together generate NFT. The discovery of the tau gene mutation on chromosome 17 in frontotemporal dementia has facilitated the development of tau-transgenic mice [127–129].

There has been significant progress in the development of models of this group of diseases. In particular, mice expressing P301L tau mutation demonstrated that it is possible to generate robust animal models of neurofibrillary pathology [130], which can be assessed in vivo. However, this transgenic model only represents a first generation of mice affected by human tauopathies [131].

19.5 Mutations Model

This model, developed by Oakley et al., is based on 5 mutations that occur in APP and presenilins (PS-1 and PS-2), leading to an increased production of Aβ-42. This model is known as 5xFAD, which represents the five mutations that occur in familial AD. In this model, a rapid production of Aβ-42 leads to the formation of senile plaques similar to those found in patients with AD [132]. Aβ deposits begin at two months of age in the neuronal soma and dendrites, especially in deep cortical layers, well before the formation of senile plaques.

In this model, synaptic dysfunction occurs with ageing, showing a marked decrease in synaptophysin, syntaxin and PDS95 and loss of pyramidal cortical neurons [132] with significant memory loss [132, 133]. Moreover, it has been reported that this transgenic mouse has behavioural and motor deficiencies [134]. Furthermore, recent studies have shown that 5xFAD mice have early inner retina impairment, which precedes neuronal loss in other parts of the brain [135]. This may be a valuable model for studying the processes related to the formation of senile plaques, synaptic loss and cognitive decline. This model has the advantage of producing a large amount of Aβ deposition in a short time. However, this model does not produce the same NFTs that are characteristic of AD in humans.

Triple—Transgenic Model

In 2003, a triple-transgenic model was described for the first time in which both senile plaques and NFT called 3xTg-AD were present [136]. This mouse expresses extracellular Aβ deposits before the formation of NFT. This phenotype is in keeping with the natural history of AD in humans, where there is progressive loss of synaptic plasticity followed by extracellular deposits of Aβ and the deposition of NFTs associated with Aβ immunoreactivity [137, 138]. Therefore, it is considered that this particular type of transgenic mouse is useful for studying the impact of Aβ and tau protein accumulation on synaptic plasticity. Moreover, this model presents with behavioural and cognitive deficits that increase with ageing. These characteristics are similar to those in humans with AD [139]. Since the creation of the 3xTg-AD mouse, various research projects have been initiated which seek to elucidate our understanding of AD.

It has been demonstrated that the accumulation of Aβ, which triggers tau deposition, occurs before it undergoes hyperphosphorylation [140, 141]. In 2005, a study showing that chronic nicotine administration exacerbates tauopathy in this model was published [142, 143]. The relationship between Aβ, tau and synaptic dysfunction was also assessed [136]. Likewise, the ratio of Aβ deposition and cognitive deficits was also demonstrated [144]. The 3xTg-AD model has been correlated with glial activation and Aβ deposition [145] and has also been used to study the inflammation in specific areas of the CNS to evaluate potential inflammatory markers of AD [145].

Furthermore, recent studies have shown the accumulation of Tau proteins in the retina in this model, which promotes anterograde axonal transport impairment [146]. In a paper published in 2005, primary cultures of 3xTgAD were used to study calcium release induced by caffeine [147]. The triple-transgenic mouse has proven to be a valuable model for studying the development of AD, and its neurobiochemical, neuropathological and neuropharmacological characteristics. Studies with this model outnumber those made with other types of models. However, there will always be controversy about the extent to which animal models are representative of the disease in humans.

Although an age-dependent increase in RGC apoptosis has been documented histologically in the double AD (APP/PS1) mouse [148], this has not yet been confirmed in real time. Using the triple transgenic mouse model of AD (3xTgAD), it has been attempted to assess both apoptosis and necrosis simultaneously in vivo. Both RGC apoptosis and necrosis are present in the retina of AD mice, and quantitative analysis revealed that the majority of apoptotic RGCs are in their early phase of apoptosis rather than in the late phase or necrosis, compared with age matched controls. This would suggest that early phase apoptosis of RGCs may be characteristic in 3xTgAD mice, and they could be reversed or rescued in this early stage of degeneration.

Increased evidence shows that oxidative stress is heavily implicated in AD pathology, along with increased Aβ accumulation and deposition in the brain [149]. As Aβ accumulation in the retina has been demonstrated in this AD model [150, 151].

Thus, the novel approach of *in-vivo* retinal imaging not only provides a means to detect RGC death, which could reflect the changes in the brain but also enables differentiation of apoptosing and necrosing processes simultaneously in the same living eye over time.

TgF334-AD Rat Model

The TgF344-AD rat model was developed by Cohen et al. [152]. The TgF344-AD rat displays the five characteristic features of AD without the need for additional human transgenes—(1) Aβ plaques, (2) cognitive deficits, (3) neurofibrillary tangles (NFTs), (4) neuronal loss, and (5) chronic neuroinflammation [153]. Beta-amyloid accumulates in an age-dependent manner with up to 82 times more beta-amyloid deposition seen in the model rat brain than in wild-type rats. The TgF344-AD rat also shows the formation of NFTs, probably due to rats expressing the full complement of the 6 tau isoforms present in humans compared to mice, who only express three [153]. The production of amyloid plaques and NFT's makes the TgF334-AD rat model a highly relevant model of AD.

19.6 Animal Models of Parkinson's Disease

Although the use of L-DOPA has revolutionised the treatment of PD, this is only a symptomatic treatment, which cannot arrest or delay the degeneration of dopaminergic neurons. The most significant obstacle to developing new neuro-protective drugs is the lack of knowledge of the specific molecular events that lead to neurodegeneration in PD [154]. The development of animal models represents a valuable tool for testing therapeutic strategies. In PD, studies in a wide range of invertebrates have shown that AS usually is present in retinal cells [155]. Moreover, the genetic expression of AS mRNA and protein is distributed across the different retinal layers [156]. Compared to AD, there are fewer animal studies that focus on retinal changes in PD with more emphasis on understanding the molecular mechanisms involved in dopaminergic neuronal death in the brain. The rodent and non-human primates models of the PD retina can be broadly categorised into neuropharmacological agents targeting catecholaminergic neurons (neurotoxins) and those based on genetic manipulations relevant to PD or sometimes used in combination [157]. To date, the agents used to induce degeneration of cells producing dopamine include MPTP (1-Methyl-4-phenyl-1,2,3,6-tetrahydropyridine) [158], and pesticides such as rotenone [159].

Treating animals with neurotoxins such as rotenone, paraquat, 6 OHDA, MPTP and -synuclein, provides essential models for studying the causes and the molecular mechanisms involved in the death of dopaminergic neurons in PD. Although these toxins induce CNS neurodegeneration, each one produces different clinical and neuropathological effects. Each neurotoxic model of PD has its advantages and disadvantages, and currently, no one model can represent all aspects of PD. For this reason, the choice of toxins used to induce a PD model is related to the type of study to be undertaken [160]. A summary of models is presented in Table 19.2.

Paraquat (1,1′-Dimethyl-4,4′-bipyridinium dichloride)

When administered systemically in rodents, paraquat can induce reduced motor activity, a dose dependant loss of dopaminergic neurons in the SN, and a reduction of dopaminergic fibres in the striatum [161]. Rats treated with paraquat also express pathological levels of α-syn in the SN [162]. However, a limitation of this model is that paraquat also induces severe lung, liver, and kidney toxicity, causing a high mortality rate in treated animals [163].

Table 19.2 Comparing the common animal models of PD

Model	Administration route	Type of damage	Histological findings	Symptoms	Disadvantages	References
Paraquat	Systemic	Loss of striatal dopaminergic fibres	α-syn inclusions	Reduced motor activity	Active on other neurotensmitter	[90–92]
6-OHDA	Local, stereotaxic	Loss of striatal dopaminergic neurons	Absence of α-syn inclusions,	Rotational behaviours	Intracranial injections are fatal	[94–98]
MPTP	Systemic, subcutaneous, intravenous, intraperitoneal or intramuscular	Selective loss of Da neurons, reduced DA fibers	Absence of α-syn inclusions,	Reduced motor activity	Acute model, does not progress	[102, 108–110]
α-synuclein	Viral vectors, transgenic model	Selective degeneration of dopaminergic neurons	Overexpression of α-syn	Heavily educed motor activity	Scarce evidence of neuronal death	[111, 113–115]
Rotenone	Systemic, subcutaneous, intravenous, intraperitoneal or intramuscular	Loss of striatal dopaminergic neurons	α-syn inclusions, reduced tyrosine hydroxylase levels, nigrostriatal microglial activation	Reduced motor activity, altered posture, sleep and gastrointestinal alteration	Time consuming, high rate of mortality	[123, 143, 164–166]
LRRK-2	Transgenic	Minor loss of striatal dopaminergic neurons	Presence of Lewy bodies	Reduced motor activity	Absence of α-syn inclusions, poorly reproducible	[154, 155, 158]

19.6.1 6-OHDA (6-Hydroxyl Dopamine or 2,4,5-Trihydroxy Phenethylamine)

6-OHDA does not readily cross the Blood Brain Barrier (BBB) and, therefore, cannot reach toxic concentrations in the CNS following a systemic administration. However, systemic administration of 6-OHDA causes damage to the peripheral nervous system [164]. Due to its inability to cross the BBB, direct administration of 6-OHDA in different brain areas has been achieved using stereotactic methods to better model PD [160]. Used firstly on rats, the direct administration of 6-OHDA has subsequently been characterised in mice and monkeys [165–169]. The most common method to induce a lesion in the nigrostriatal pathway is the unilateral administration of 6-OHDA in the forebrain bundle (which includes the nigrostriatal tract), or in the striatum [170]; however, a bilateral lesion with 6-OHDA is fatal. After direct administration of 6-OHDA, apoptosis of dopaminergic neurons is reported to occur within 24 h [171]. The maximum reduction in the levels of striatal DA occurs between 3 and 4 days after lesion onset when the residual striatal DA neuron population is reduced to less than 20% of age matched controls [172]. Therefore, this is a rapid model but very invasive. The presence of Lewy Bodies (LB) has yet to be documented in this model.

19.6.2 MPTP (1-Methyl-4-Phenyl-1,2,3,6-Tetrahydropyridine)

Neuropathological data, derived mainly from experiments on non-human primates, has demonstrated that administration of MPTP causes damage to the nigrostriatal dopaminergic pathway similar to that found in PD [173]. The most reliable and reproducible disease model is induced through systemic administration of MPTP via intranasal [174], subcutaneous [175], intravenous [176], intra-peritoneal [177] or intramuscular [178] injections. As in human PD, a significant loss of dopaminergic neurons in the CNS and ventral tegmental area is reported in this model [179, 180]. However, MPTP induced models of PD do not present with LBs [181].

19.6.3 α-Synuclein

Chronologically, this is the most recent model of PD, which is based on the genetic link between Parkinson's disease and the neuropathological effect of α-synuclein (α-syn) [182]. There are two types of α-syn animal models, either transgenic or non- transgenic. Transgenic model organisms in Drosophila and mice have been developed that over-express both the human wild-type α-syn and the mutated (A3OP and A53T) forms [183]. In models of Drosophila, a significant loss of DA neurons is reported, while murine models do not demonstrate significant anomalies in dopaminergic neurons [184]. Non-transgenic models are based instead on the insertion of α-syn encoding genes into the SNPC using viral vectors [185, 186].

The mutation of α-syn in this way is reported to cause the selective degeneration of dopaminergic neurons in the rat SNPC, with the formation of cytoplasmic structures containing a-syn, which are very similar to LBs [187].

19.6.4 Rotenone ((2R, 6aS, 12aS)-1,2,6,6a,12,12a-hexahydro-2-isopropenyl-8, 9-dimethoxy chromeno [3,4-b] furo (2,3-h) chromen-6-one)

Among the various models of PD, the rotenone model has recently drawn particular attention because it reproduces most of the motor defect symptoms and the histopathological features of PD [188, 189].

This insecticide found in the roots of leguminous plants, interacts specifically with the mitochondrial respiratory chain complex [190]. Rotenone acts by blocking the mitochondrial electron transport from complex I to CoenzymeQ10, leading to energy starvation and cellular death.

Rotenone may have initially been used by Indians as a poison when hunting for fish [191]. Today, it is commonly used as a pesticide due to its high biodegradability, degrading within days. It is highly lipophilic, so it quickly passes through the cell membrane and the blood brain barrier and accumulates in subcellular organelles such as mitochondria [192]. Both pulsatile [193] and chronic [194] administration of rotenone *in-vivo* and *in-vitro* models induces degeneration of nigrostriatal neurons, with formation of cytoplasmic inclusions similar to Lewy bodies, oxidative damage and parkinsonian bradykinesia and rigidity.

The mechanism by which complex I dysfunction induces neurotoxicity is still not known. The most common pathway seems to involve increased levels of oxidative stress [195], resulting in reduced levels of glutathione and oxidative modification of DNA, lipids, proteins and antioxidants such as α-tocopherol [196, 197]. Inhibition of Complex I was also demonstrated to increase levels of H_2O_2 and inhibition of Reactive Oxygen Species (ROS) [198]. It is believed that increased levels of ROS are mediated by microglia, which are also activated by rotenone [199]. This massive oxidative stress alters mitochondrial function and activation of the apoptotic cascade [198]. The resulting decrease in intracellular levels of ATP causes the opening of Na^+K^+-ATP channels [200]. It has been shown that the hyperpolarisation induced by the application of rotenone on dopamine cells of the CNS is mediated by the opening of these channels. In addition, the dopaminergic cells that contain the SUR-1 subunit of the Na^+ K^+-ATP channels are more sensitive to metabolic changes induced by the toxin [201].

The selectivity of rotenone on the dopaminergic system has been explained based on the cytotoxic effect mediated by the same endogenous mechanism [202]. It has been shown that rotenone induced blockade of mitochondrial complex I occurs in all cells indiscriminately [203], but this inhibition does not induce cell death in non-dopaminergic cells. The association between ROS–dopamine in dopaminergic cells could be the basis of the initial apoptotic process [204].

Biehlmaier et al. have demonstrated that rotenone-treated rats show a depletion of DA in the striatum and substantia nigra (SN) in association with a significant reduction in retinal dopaminergic amacrine cells, similar to that found in PD patients [205].

In 2000, it was first reported that chronic systemic rotenone exposure in rats produced phenotypical features of PD [194]. Rotenone is reported to exert highly selective toxicity on DA neurons in vitro [206, 207] and in vivo [208, 209].

The mechanisms of action of rotenone are various [210]; rotenone is reported to inhibit mitochondrial complex 1, impeding the oxidation of NADH to NAD^+ causing a reduction in cellular respiration [210]. The consequence of complex 1 inhibition is a cascade of events which leads to elevated oxidative stress [211] and ultimately apoptosis [212].

In-vivo models have been obtained through different routes of rotenone administration.

Oral administration (via food), is reported to cause only mild neurotoxicity [213]. Stereotactic administration of rotenone in the medial forebrain bundle is reported to cause depletion of striatal DA neurons [214]. Systemic administration, including intravenous (i.v.), subcutaneous (s.c.), or intraperitoneal (I.P.), has been found to induce the formation of α-syn cytoplasmatic particles in the substantia nigra of treated rats in a similar manner to the typical LBs found in PD [194, 215]. Systemic administration of rotenone is also reported to promote the production of pro inflammatory factors and microglial activation triggering further oxidative insult to DA neurons [216, 217].

Rotenone administration also causes symptomatic changes in rodents including motor rigidity, behavioural alterations, catalepsy, sleep and gastrointestinal alterations. L-DOPA therapy can temporarily reverse the motor deficits reported in these models [218, 219]. Furthermore, systemic rotenone administration frequently causes neurotoxicity and mortality in a dose-dependent manner.

Systemic rotenone administration has been reported, through its ability to penetrate all cells, to act also on non-dopaminergic neurons such as Retinal Ganglion Cells (RGCs) [220]. Additional supporting evidence for using rotenone as a PD model can be found in epidemiological studies which demonstrated a correlation between PD and rotenone exposure in humans [221, 222].

19.6.5 LRRK2 Model (Table 19.3)

Leucine Rich Repeat Kinase (LRRK2) is a gene responsible for coding an enzyme called dardarin, which has kinase activities and is responsible for signal transmission, protein–protein interaction, and amino acid phosphorylation [223]. Mutation of the *lrrk2* gene has been implicated in the pathogenesis of familial PD [224]. *lrrk2* was associated with the locus Park8 (Parkinson family of type 8) for the first time in 2002 in a large Japanese family that presented Parkinsonian symptoms with autosomal dominant inheritance but without the appearance of Lewy bodies [225]. Since 2004, mutations in *lrrk2*-linked to PD have been found in

Table 19.3 Mutation involved in genetic PD

	Locus	Gene	Transmission	Number of family	References
PARK 1	4q21-23	α-synuclein	AD	18	Polimeropulos, 1997
PARK 2	6q25-27	Parkin	AR	Many	Kitada, 1998
PARK 3	2p13	–	AD	6	Gasser, 1998
PARK 4	4q21-23	α-synuclein	AD	Many	Singleton, 2003
PARK 5	4p14	Ubiquitin	AD	1	Leroy, 1998
PARK 6	1p35-36	Pink-1	AR	Sporadic cases	Valente, 2001
PARK 7	1p36	DJ-1	AR	2 (?)	Bonifati, 2003
PARK 8	12p11-q13	Dardarin (LRKK2)	AD	Many + sporadic cases	Funayama, 2002 Bonifati, 2005
PARK 9	1p36	–	AR	Kulford-Rakeb Syndrome	Hampshire, 2001

many families, which also included cases with the presence of LBs [224]. The relationship between PD and *lrrk2* was later confirmed by gene sequencing, which revealed numerous pathogenic amino acid substitutions [226]. The *lrrk2* mutation Gly2019Ser is the most frequent replacement in the Caucasian population, which is statistically present in 0.5–2% of sporadic cases and 5% of MP in familial Parkinsonism [227]. The probability that a heterozygote manifests symptoms below the age of 50 is less than 20%, but this increases with age to more than 80% after 75 years [228]. Biopsies of the substantia nigra of patients with PD caused by the expression of mutated LRRK2 show the presence of Lewy bodies [229, 230]. La Morgia and colleagues have also shown retinal modifications in patients affected by the mutation of *lrrk2* [231] and reported the same RNFL thinning that occurs in patients with sporadic PD [232]. Retinal modifications have also been shown in a LRRK2 transgenic drosophila melanogaster model [233]. Using this model, Hindle et al. demonstrated a loss of visual response and concomitant photoreceptor degeneration.

19.7 Conclusion

Accessibility and cost efficiency combined with the great accessibility of the eye make animal models a precious tool for studying the natural history of neuro-ophthalmological diseases. This suggests these models could provide a source of novel biomarkers for the early diagnosis and follow up of neurodegenerative diseases. Nevertheless, due to anatomical and physiological differences, the validity of animal models is closely related to the level of similarity with human pathology. Therefore, prudence should always be applied in choosing the appropriate model for each neuro-ophthalmolgocial condition.

References

1. Sormani MP, Bruzzi P. Can we measure long-term treatment effects in multiple sclerosis? Nat Rev Neurol. 2014.
2. Stimmer L, Fovet C-M, Serguera C. Experimental models of autoimmune demyelinating diseases in nonhuman primates. Vet Pathol. 2017;55:27–41. https://doi.org/10.1177/0300985817712794.
3. Gold R, Hartung HP, Toyka KV. Animal models for autoimmune demyelinating disorders of the nervous system. Mol Med Today. 2000;6(2):88–91.
4. Hoglund RA, Maghazachi AA. Multiple sclerosis and the role of immune cells. World J Exp Med. 2014;4(3):27–37.
5. Klaren RE, Motl RW, Woods JA, Miller SD. Effects of exercise in experimental autoimmune encephalomyelitis (an animal model of multiple sclerosis). J Neuroimmunol. 2014;274(1–2):14–9.
6. Robinson AP, Harp CT, Noronha A, Miller SD. The experimental autoimmune encephalomyelitis (EAE) model of MS: utility for understanding disease pathophysiology and treatment. Handb Clin Neurol. 2014;122:173–89.
7. Kuerten S, Lehmann PV. The immune pathogenesis of experimental autoimmune encephalomyelitis: lessons learned for multiple sclerosis? J interferon Cytokine Res. 2011;31(12):907–16.
8. Handel AE, Lincoln MR, Ramagopalan SV. Of mice and men: experimental autoimmune encephalitis and multiple sclerosis. Eur J Clin Investig. 2011;41(11):1254–8.
9. Vesterinen HM, Sena ES, ffrench-Constant C, Williams A, Chandran S, Macleod MR. Improving the translational hit of experimental treatments in multiple sclerosis. Multiple Sclerosis. 2010;16(9):1044–55.
10. Pryce G, O'Neill JK, Croxford JL, Amor S, Hankey DJ, East E, et al. Autoimmune tolerance eliminates relapses but fails to halt progression in a model of multiple sclerosis. J Neuroimmunol. 2005;165(1–2):41–52.
11. Gogoleva VS, Atretkhany K-S, Drutskaya MS, et al. Cytokines as mediators of neuroinflammation in experimental autoimmune encephalomyelitis. Biochem Mosc. 2018;83:1089–103. https://doi.org/10.1134/s0006297918090110.
12. Inoue M, Williams KL, Oliver T, et al. Interferon-β therapy against EAE is effective only when development of the disease depends on the NLRP3 inflammasome. Sci Signal. 2012. https://doi.org/10.1126/scisignal.2002767.
13. Lalive PH, Neuhaus O, Benkhoucha M, et al. Glatiramer acetate in the treatment of multiple sclerosis. CNS Drugs. 2011;25:401–14. https://doi.org/10.2165/11588120-000000000-00000.
14. Friese MA, Montalban X, Willcox N, Bell JI, Martin R, Fugger L. The value of animal models for drug development in multiple sclerosis. Brain. 2006;129(Pt 8):1940–52.
15. Wiendl H, Hohlfeld R. Therapeutic approaches in multiple sclerosis. BioDrugs. 2002;16:183–200. https://doi.org/10.2165/00063030-200216030-00003.
16. Noseworthy JH, Wolinsky JS, Lublin FD, et al. Linomide in relapsing and secondary progressive MS: Part I: Trial design and clinical results. Neurology. 2000;54:1726–33. https://doi.org/10.1212/wnl.54.9.1726.
17. Martinez NE, Karlsson F, Sato F, Kawai E, Omura S, Minagar A, et al. Protective and detrimental roles for regulatory T cells in a viral model for multiple sclerosis. Brain Pathol. 2014;24(5):436–51.
18. Zhang J, Lipton HL, Perelson AS, Dahari H. Modeling the acute and chronic phases of Theiler murine encephalomyelitis virus infection. J Virol. 2013;87(7):4052–9.
19. Mecha M, Carrillo-Salinas FJ, Mestre L, Feliu A, Guaza C. Viral models of multiple sclerosis: neurodegeneration and demyelination in mice infected with Theiler's virus. Prog Neurobiol. 2013;101–102:46–64.

20. Joly S, Mdzomba JB, Rodriguez L, et al. B cell-dependent EAE induces visual deficits in the mouse with similarities to human autoimmune demyelinating diseases. J Neuroinflammation. 2022. https://doi.org/10.1186/s12974-022-02416-y.
21. Horstmann L, Kuehn S, Pedreiturria X, et al. Microglia response in retina and optic nerve in chronic experimental autoimmune encephalomyelitis. J Neuroimmunol. 2016;298:32–41. https://doi.org/10.1016/j.jneuroim.2016.06.008.
22. Takizawa S, Kaneyama T, Tsugane S, Takeichi N, Yanagisawa S, Ichikawa M, et al. Role of the Programmed Death-1 (PD-1) pathway in regulation of Theiler's murine encephalomyelitis virus-induced demyelinating disease. J Neuroimmunol. 2014;274(1–2):78–85.
23. Jin Y-H, Kim CX, Huang J, Kim BS. Infection and activation of B cells by Theiler's murine encephalomyelitis virus (TMEV) leads to autoantibody production in an infectious model of multiple sclerosis. Cells. 2020;9:1787. https://doi.org/10.3390/cells9081787.
24. Tsunoda I, Fujinami RS. Two models for multiple sclerosis: experimental allergic encephalomyelitis and Theiler's murine encephalomyelitis virus. J Neuropathol Exp Neurol. 1996;55(6):673–86. Available at: https://doi.org/10.1097/00005072-199606000-00001
25. Tsunoda I, Fujinami RS. Inside-out versus outside-in models for virus induced demyelination: axonal damage triggering demyelination. Springer Semin Immunopathol. 2002;24:105–25. https://doi.org/10.1007/s00281-002-0105-z.
26. McCarthy DP, Richards MH, Miller SD. Mouse models of multiple sclerosis: experimental autoimmune encephalomyelitis and Theiler's virus-induced demyelinating disease. Methods Mol Biol. 2012;381–401. https://doi.org/10.1007/978-1-60761-720-4_19
27. DePaula-Silva AB, Hanak TJ, Libbey JE, Fujinami RS. Theiler's murine encephalomyelitis virus infection of SJL/J and C57BL/6J MICE: models for multiple sclerosis and epilepsy. J Neuroimmunol. 2017;308:30–42. https://doi.org/10.1016/j.jneuroim.2017.02.012.
28. Li L, Ulrich R, Baumgärtner W, Gerhauser I. Interferon-stimulated genes—essential antiviral effectors implicated in resistance to Theiler's virus-induced demyelinating disease. J Neuroinflammation. 2015. https://doi.org/10.1186/s12974-015-0462-x.
29. Murray PD, McGavern DB, Pease LR, Rodriguez M. Cellular sources and targets of IFN-γ-mediated protection against viral demyelination and neurological deficits. Eur J Immunol. 2002;32:606. https://doi.org/10.1002/1521-4141(200203)32:3%3c606::aid-immu606%3e3.0.co;2-d.
30. Bowen JL, Olson JK. IFNΓ influences type I interferon response and susceptibility to Theiler's virus-induced demyelinating disease. Viral Immunol. 2013;26:223–38. https://doi.org/10.1089/vim.2013.0004.
31. Dittmer U, Hasenkrug KJ. Functional impairment of CD8 T cells by regulatory T cells during persistent retroviral infection. Immunity. 2004;20:653. https://doi.org/10.1016/s1074-7613(04)00115-3.
32. Eggena MP, Barugahare B, Jones N, et al. Depletion of regulatory T cells in HIV infection is associated with immune activation. J Immunol. 2005;174:4407–14. https://doi.org/10.4049/jimmunol.174.7.4407.
33. Groux H, O'Garra A, Bigler M, et al. A CD4+T-cell subset inhibits antigen-specific T-cell responses and prevents colitis. Nature. 1997;389:737–42. https://doi.org/10.1038/39614.
34. He H, Messer RJ, Sakaguchi S, et al. Reduction of retrovirus-induced immunosuppression by in vivo modulation of T cells during acute infection. J Virol. 2004;78:11641–7. https://doi.org/10.1128/jvi.78.21.11641-11647.2004.
35. Richards MH, Getts MT, Podojil JR, et al. Virus expanded regulatory T cells control disease severity in the Theiler's virus mouse model of MS. J Autoimmunity. 2011;36:142–54. https://doi.org/10.1016/j.jaut.2010.12.005.
36. Tsunoda I, Kurtz CIB, Fujinami RS. Apoptosis in acute and chronic central nervous system disease induced by Theiler's murine encephalomyelitis virus. Virology. 1997;228:388–93. https://doi.org/10.1006/viro.1996.8382.
37. Oleszak EL, et al. Theiler's virus infection: a model for multiple sclerosis. Clin Microbiol Rev. 2004;17(1):174–207. https://doi.org/10.1128/CMR.17.1.174-207.2004

38. Schlitt BP, Felrice M, Jelachich ML, Lipton HL. Apoptotic cells, including macrophages, are prominent in Theiler's virus-induced inflammatory, demyelinating lesions. J Virol. 2003;77:4383–8. https://doi.org/10.1128/jvi.77.7.4383-4388.2003.
39. Tsunoda I, Fujinami RS. Neuropathogenesis of Theiler's murine encephalomyelitis virus infection, an animal model for multiple sclerosis. J Neuroimmune Pharmacol. 2009;5:355–69. https://doi.org/10.1007/s11481-009-9179-x.
40. Clatch RJ, Miller SD, Metzner R, et al. Monocytes/macrophages isolated from the mouse central nervous system contain infectious Theiler's murine encephalomyelitis virus (TMEV). Virology. 1990;176:244–54. https://doi.org/10.1016/0042-6822(90)90249-q.
41. Girard S, Gosselin A-S, Pelletier I, et al. Restriction of poliovirus RNA replication in persistently infected nerve cells. J Gen Virol. 2002;83:1087–93. https://doi.org/10.1099/0022-1317-83-5-1087.
42. Jelachich ML, Bandyopadhyay P, Blum K, Lipton HL. Theiler's virus growth in murine macrophage cell lines depends on the state of differentiation. Virology. 1995;209:437–44. https://doi.org/10.1006/viro.1995.1276.
43. Misra UK, Tan CT, Kalita J. Viral encephalitis and epilepsy. Epilepsia. 2008;49:13–8. https://doi.org/10.1111/j.1528-1167.2008.01751.x.
44. Rodriguez M, Leibowitz JL, Lampert PW. Persistent infection of oligodendrocytes in Theiler's virus-induced encephalomyelitis. Ann Neurol. 1983;13:426–33. https://doi.org/10.1002/ana.410130409.
45. Libbey JE, Fujinami RS. Viral mouse models used to study multiple sclerosis: past and present. Arch Virol. 2021;166:1015–33. https://doi.org/10.1007/s00705-021-04968-5.
46. Namekata K, Kimura A, Harada C, et al. Dock3 protects myelin in the cuprizone model for demyelination. Cell Death Dis. 2014. https://doi.org/10.1038/cddis.2014.357.
47. Praet J, Guglielmetti C, Berneman Z, Van der Linden A, Ponsaerts P. Cellular and molecular neuropathology of the cuprizone mouse model: clinical relevance for multiple sclerosis. Neurosci Biobehav Rev. 2014;47C:485–505.
48. Sachs HH, Bercury KK, Popescu DC, Narayanan SP, Macklin WB. A new model of cuprizone-mediated demyelination/remyelination. ASN Neuro. 2014;6(5).
49. van der Star BJ, Vogel DY, Kipp M, Puentes F, Baker D, Amor S. In vitro and in vivo models of multiple sclerosis. CNS Neurol Disord Drug Targets. 2012;11(5):570–88.
50. Nastasijevic B, Wright BR, Smestad J, Warrington AE, Rodriguez M, Maher LJ 3rd. Remyelination induced by a DNA aptamer in a mouse model of multiple sclerosis. PLoS ONE. 2012;7(6): e39595.
51. Waring MJ. Complex formation between ethidium bromide and nucleic acids. J Mol Biol. 1965;13:269–82. https://doi.org/10.1016/S00222836(65)80096-1.
52. Blakemore WF. Ethidium bromide induced demyelination in the spinal cord of the cat. Neuropathol Appl Neurobiol. 1982;8:365–75.
53. Sim FJ, Zhao C, Penderis J, Franklin RJM. The age-related decrease in CNS remyelination efficiency is attributable to an impairment of both oligodendrocyte progenitor recruitment and differentiation. J Neurosci. 2002;22:2451–9. https://doi.org/10.1097/00041327-200306000-00025.
54. McMurran CE, et al. Toxin-based models to investigate demyelination and remyelination. Methods Mol Biol (Clifton, N.J.). 2019;1936:377–396. https://doi.org/10.1007/978-1-4939-9072-6_21
55. Woodruff RH, Franklin RJM. Demyelination and remyelination of the caudal cerebellar peduncle of adult rats following stereotaxic injections of lysolecithin, ethidium bromide, and complement/anti-galactocerebroside: a comparative study. Glia. 1999;25:216–28. https://doi.org/10.1002/(SICI)1098-1136(19990201)25:3%3c216::AID-GLIA2%3e3.0.CO;2-L.
56. Zawadzka M, Rivers LE, Fancy SPJ, et al. CNS-resident glial progenitor/stem cells produce Schwann cells as well as oligodendrocytes during repair of CNS demyelination. Cell Stem Cell. 2010;6:578–90. https://doi.org/10.1016/j.stem.2010.04.002.

57. Monteiro De Castro G, Deja NA, Ma D, et al. Astrocyte activation via Stat3 signaling determines the balance of oligodendrocyte versus Schwann cell remyelination. Am J Pathol. 2015;185:2431–40. https://doi.org/10.1016/j.ajpath.2015.05.011.
58. Tsai R-K, Huang T-L, Lin K-H, Wang J-K. Treatment strategies for neuromyelitis optica. Tzu Chi Med J. 2018;30:204. https://doi.org/10.4103/tcmj.tcmj_102_18.
59. Jones MV, Collongues N, de Seze J, Kinoshita M, Nakatsuji Y, Levy M. Review of Animal Models of Neuromyelitis Optica. Multiple Sclerosis Relat Disord. 2012;1(4):174–9.
60. Frohman EM, Kerr D. Is neuromyelitis optica distinct from multiple sclerosis?: something for "lumpers" and "splitters." Arch Neurol. 2007;64(6):903–5.
61. Kinoshita M, Nakatsuji Y, Kimura T, Moriya M, Takata K, Okuno T, et al. Neuromyelitis optica: passive transfer to rats by human immunoglobulin. Biochem Biophys Res Commun. 2009;386(4):623–7.
62. Saadoun S, Waters P, Bell BA, Vincent A, Verkman AS, Papadopoulos MC. Intra-cerebral injection of neuromyelitis optica immunoglobulin G and human complement produces neuromyelitis optica lesions in mice. Brain. 2010;133(Pt 2):349–61.
63. Bettelli E, Baeten D, Jager A, Sobel RA, Kuchroo VK. Myelin oligodendrocyte glycoprotein-specific T and B cells cooperate to induce a Devic-like disease in mice. J Clin Investig. 2006;116(9):2393–402.
64. Zhang H, Verkman AS. Longitudinally extensive NMO spinal cord pathology produced by passive transfer of NMO-IGG in mice lacking complement inhibitor CD59. J Autoimmunity. 2014;53:67–77. Available at: https://doi.org/10.1016/j.jaut.2014.02.011
65. Duan T, Verkman AS. Experimental animal models of aquaporin-4-IgG-seropositive neuromyelitis optica spectrum disorders: progress and shortcomings. Brain Pathol (Zurich, Switzerland). 2020;30(1):13–25. https://doi.org/10.1111/bpa.12793.
66. Marignier R, et al. Neuromyelitis Optica Study Model based on chronic infusion of autoantibodies in rat cerebrospinal fluid. J Neuroinflammation. 2016;13(1). Available at: https://doi.org/10.1186/s12974-016-0577-8
67. Asavapanumas N, Ratelade J, Papadopoulos MC, et al. Experimental mouse model of optic neuritis with inflammatory demyelination produced by passive transfer of Neuromyelitis Optica-Immunoglobulin G. J Neuroinflammation. 2014. https://doi.org/10.1186/1742-2094-11-16.
68. Zeka B, Hastermann M, Kaufmann N, et al. Aquaporin 4-specific T cells and NMO-IGG cause primary retinal damage in experimental NMO/SD. Acta Neuropathol Commun. 2016. https://doi.org/10.1186/s40478-016-0355-y.
69. Arnold AC, Hepler RS. Natural history of nonarteritic anterior ischemic optic neuropathy. J Neuro-ophthalmol. 1994;14(2):66–9.
70. Arnold AC. Pathogenesis of nonarteritic anterior ischemic optic neuropathy. J Neuro-ophthalmol. 2003;23(2):157–63.
71. Albrecht MC. Comparative anatomy of the optic nerve head and inner retina in non-primate animal models used for glaucoma research. Open Ophthalmol J. 2008;2:94–101.
72. Bernstein SL, Guo Y, Kelman SE, Flower RW, Johnson MA. Functional and cellular responses in a novel rodent model of anterior ischemic optic neuropathy. Investig Ophthalmol Vis Sci. 2003;44(10):4153–62.
73. Williams RW, Strom RC, Rice DS, Goldowitz D. Genetic and environmental control of variation in retinal ganglion cell number in mice. J Neurosci. 1996;16(22):7193–205.
74. Perry VH, Henderson Z, Linden R. Postnatal changes in retinal ganglion cell and optic axon populations in the pigmented rat. J Comp Neurol. 1983;219(3):356–68.
75. Morrison JC, Cork LC, Dunkelberger GR, Brown A, Quigley HA. Aging changes of the rhesus monkey optic nerve. Investig Ophthalmol Vis Sci. 1990;31(8):1623–7.
76. Zhao BQ, Suzuki Y, Kondo K, Kawano K, Ikeda Y, Umemura K. A novel MCA occlusion model of photothrombotic ischemia with cyclic flow reductions: development of cerebral hemorrhage induced by heparin. Brain Res Protoc. 2002;9(2):85–92.
77. Mosinger JL, Olney JW. Photothrombosis-induced ischemic neuronal degeneration in the rat retina. Exp Neurol. 1989;105(1):110–3.

78. Bernstein SL, Johnson MA, Miller NR. Nonarteritic anterior ischemic optic neuropathy (NAION) and its experimental models. Prog Retinal Eye Res. 2011;30(3):167–87.
79. Goldenberg-Cohen N, Guo Y, Margolis F, Cohen Y, Miller NR, Bernstein SL. Oligodendrocyte dysfunction after induction of experimental anterior optic nerve ischemia. Investig Ophthalmol Vis Sci. 2005;46(8):2716–25.
80. Khalilpour S, Latifi S, Behnammanesh G, et al. Ischemic optic neuropathy as a model of Neurodegenerative Disorder: a review of pathogenic mechanism of axonal degeneration and the role of neuroprotection. J Neurol Sci. 2017;375:430–41. https://doi.org/10.1016/j.jns.2016.12.044.
81. Feng G, Mellor RH, Bernstein M, Keller-Peck C, Nguyen QT, Wallace M, et al. Imaging neuronal subsets in transgenic mice expressing multiple spectral variants of GFP. Neuron. 2000;28(1):41–51.
82. Chen CS, Johnson MA, Flower RA, Slater BJ, Miller NR, Bernstein SL. A primate model of nonarteritic anterior ischemic optic neuropathy. Investig Ophthalmol Vis Sci. 2008;49(7):2985–92.
83. Kokona D, Häner NU, Ebneter A, Zinkernagel MS. Imaging of macrophage dynamics with optical coherence tomography in anterior ischemic optic neuropathy. Exp Eye Res. 2017;154:159–67. https://doi.org/10.1016/j.exer.2016.11.020.
84. Ziccardi L, Sadun F, De Negri AM, Barboni P, Savini G, Borrelli E, et al. Retinal function and neural conduction along the visual pathways in affected and unaffected carriers with Leber's hereditary optic neuropathy. Investig Ophthalmol Vis Sci. 2013;54(10):6893–901.
85. Rasool N, Lessell S, Cestari DM. Leber hereditary optic neuropathy: Bringing the lab to the clinic. Semin Ophthalmol. 2016;31:107–16. https://doi.org/10.3109/08820538.2015.1115251.
86. La Morgia C, Carbonelli M, Barboni P, Sadun AA, Carelli V. Medical management of hereditary optic neuropathies. Front Neurol. 2014;5:141.
87. Zhang X, Jones D, Gonzalez-Lima F. Mouse model of optic neuropathy caused by mitochondrial complex I dysfunction. Neurosci Lett. 2002;326(2):97–100.
88. Qi X, Lewin AS, Hauswirth WW, Guy J. Suppression of complex I gene expression induces optic neuropathy. Ann Neurol. 2003;53(2):198–205.
89. Marella M, Seo BB, Thomas BB, Matsuno-Yagi A, Yagi T. Successful amelioration of mitochondrial optic neuropathy using the yeast NDI1 gene in a rat animal model. PLoS ONE. 2010;5(7): e11472.
90. Heitz FD, Erb M, Anklin C, et al. Idebenone protects against retinal damage and loss of vision in a mouse model of Leber's hereditary optic neuropathy. PLoS ONE. 2012. https://doi.org/10.1371/journal.pone.0045182.
91. Klopstock T, Yu-Wai-Man P, Dimitriadis K, et al. A randomized placebo-controlled trial of idebenone in Leber's hereditary optic neuropathy. Brain. 2011;134:2677–86. https://doi.org/10.1093/brain/awr170.
92. Ratican SE, Osborne A, Martin KR. Progress in gene therapy to prevent retinal ganglion cell loss in glaucoma and Leber's hereditary optic neuropathy. Neural Plast. 2018;2018:1–11. https://doi.org/10.1155/2018/7108948.
93. Lin CS, Sharpley MS, Fan W, Waymire KG, Sadun AA, Carelli V, et al. Mouse mtDNA mutant model of Leber hereditary optic neuropathy. Proc Natl Acad Sci USA. 2012;109(49):20065–70.
94. Yu H, et al. Mutant NADH dehydrogenase subunit 4 gene delivery to mitochondria by targeting sequence-modified adeno-associated virus induces visual loss and optic atrophy in mice. Mol Vision. 2012;18:1668–83.
95. Qi X, Sun L, Lewin AS, et al. The mutant human ND4 subunit of complex I induces optic neuropathy in the mouse. Investig Opthalmol Vis Sci. 2007;48:1. https://doi.org/10.1167/iovs.06-0789.
96. Yu H, Koilkonda RD, Chou T-H, et al. Consequences of zygote injection and germline transfer of mutant human mitochondrial DNA in mice. Proc Natl Acad Sci. 2015. https://doi.org/10.1073/pnas.1506129112.

97. Wan X, Pei H, Zhao M, et al. Efficacy and safety of RAAV2-ND4 treatment for Leber's hereditary optic neuropathy. Sci Rep. 2016. https://doi.org/10.1038/srep21587.
98. Newman NJ, Yu-Wai-Man P, Carelli V, et al. Efficacy and safety of intravitreal gene therapy for Leber hereditary optic neuropathy treated within 6 months of disease onset. Ophthalmology. 2021;128:649–60. https://doi.org/10.1016/j.ophtha.2020.12.012.
99. Yu-Wai-Man P, Newman NJ, Carelli V, et al. Bilateral visual improvement with unilateral gene therapy injection for Leber hereditary optic neuropathy. Sci Transl Med. 2020. https://doi.org/10.1126/scitranslmed.aaz7423.
100. Yu-Wai-Man P, Newman N, Subramanian P, et al. The phase 3 reflect trial: Efficacy and safety of bilateral gene therapy for Leber hereditary optic neuropathy (lhon). Acta Ophthalmol. 2022. https://doi.org/10.1111/j.1755-3768.2022.0226.
101. Musardo S, Saraceno C, Pelucchi S, Marcello E. Trafficking in neurons: searching for new targets for Alzheimer's disease future therapies. Eur J Pharmacol. 2013;719(1–3):84–106.
102. Nogueras-Ortiz CJ, De Jesus-Cortes HJ, Vaquer-Alicea J, Vega IE. Novel autoimmune response in a tauopathy mouse model. Front Neurosci. 2014;7:277.
103. Ni R, Gillberg PG, Bergfors A, Marutle A, Nordberg A. Amyloid tracers detect multiple binding sites in Alzheimer's disease brain tissue. Brain. 2013;136(Pt 7):2217–27.
104. Krantic S, Torriglia A. Retina: source of the earliest biomarkers for Alzheimer's disease? J Alzheimer's Dis: JAD. 2014.
105. Novak P, Kontsekova E, Zilka N, Novak M. Ten years of tau-targeted immunotherapy: the path walked and the roads ahead. Front Neurosci. 2018. https://doi.org/10.3389/fnins.2018.00798.
106. Paquet C, Boissonnot M, Roger F, et al. Abnormal retinal thickness in patients with mild cognitive impairment and Alzheimer's disease. Neurosci Lett. 2007;420:97–9. https://doi.org/10.1016/j.neulet.2007.02.090.
107. Thomson KL, Yeo JM, Waddell B, et al. A systematic review and meta-analysis of retinal nerve fiber layer change in dementia, using optical coherence tomography. Alzheimer's Dementia. 2015;1:136–43. https://doi.org/10.1016/j.dadm.2015.03.001.
108. Ning A, Cui J, To E, Ashe KH, Matsubara J. Amyloid-beta deposits lead to retinal degeneration in a mouse model of Alzheimer disease. Investig Ophthalmol Vis Sci. 2008;49(11):5136–43.
109. Perez SE, Lumayag S, Kovacs B, Mufson EJ, Xu S. Beta-amyloid deposition and functional impairment in the retina of the APPswe/PS1DeltaE9 transgenic mouse model of Alzheimer's disease. Investig Ophthalmol Vis Sci. 2009;50(2):793–800.
110. Liu B, Rasool S, Yang Z, Glabe CG, Schreiber SS, Ge J, et al. Amyloid-peptide vaccinations reduce {beta}-amyloid plaques but exacerbate vascular deposition and inflammation in the retina of Alzheimer's transgenic mice. Am J Pathol. 2009;175(5):2099–110.
111. Dutescu RM, Li QX, Crowston J, Masters CL, Baird PN, Culvenor JG. Amyloid precursor protein processing and retinal pathology in mouse models of Alzheimer's disease. Graefes Arch Clin Exp Ophthalmol. 2009;247(9):1213–21.
112. Koronyo-Hamaoui M, Koronyo Y, Ljubimov AV, Miller CA, Ko MK, Black KL, et al. Identification of amyloid plaques in retinas from Alzheimer's patients and noninvasive in vivo optical imaging of retinal plaques in a mouse model. Neuroimage. 2011;54(Suppl 1):S204–17.
113. Loffler KU, Edward DP, Tso MO. Immunoreactivity against tau, amyloid precursor protein, and beta-amyloid in the human retina. Investig Ophthalmol Vis Sci. 1995;36(1):24–31.
114. Drummond E, Wisniewski T. Alzheimer's disease: experimental models and reality. Acta Neuropathol. 2017;133(2):155–75. https://doi.org/10.1007/s00401-016-1662-x.
115. Do Carmo S, Claudio Cuello A. Modeling Alzheimer's disease in transgenic rats. Mol Neurodegeneration. 2013;8:37. https://doi.org/10.1186/1750-1326-8-37
116. Tsai Y, et al. Ocular changes in TgF344-AD rat model of Alzheimer's disease. Investig ophthalmol Vis Sci. 2014;55(1):523–34. https://doi.org/10.1167/iovs.13-12888

117. de Lemos ML, de la Torre AV, Petrov D, Brox S, Folch J, Pallas M, et al. Evaluation of hypoxia inducible factor expression in inflammatory and neurodegenerative brain models. Int J Biochem Cell Biol. 2013;45(7):1377–88.
118. Duff K, Eckman C, Zehr C, Yu X, Prada CM, Perez-tur J, et al. Increased amyloid-beta42(43) in brains of mice expressing mutant presenilin 1. Nature. 1996;383(6602):710–3.
119. Park JH, Widi GA, Gimbel DA, Harel NY, Lee DH, Strittmatter SM. Subcutaneous Nogo receptor removes brain amyloid-beta and improves spatial memory in Alzheimer's transgenic mice. J Neurosci. 2006;26(51):13279–86.
120. Simard AR, Soulet D, Gowing G, Julien JP, Rivest S. Bone marrow-derived microglia play a critical role in restricting senile plaque formation in Alzheimer's disease. Neuron. 2006;49(4):489–502.
121. Yao J, Taylor M, Davey F, Ren Y, Aiton J, Coote P, et al. Interaction of amyloid binding alcohol dehydrogenase/Abeta mediates up-regulation of peroxiredoxin II in the brains of Alzheimer's disease patients and a transgenic Alzheimer's disease mouse model. Mol Cell Neurosci. 2007;35(2):377–82.
122. Holcomb L, Gordon MN, McGowan E, Yu X, Benkovic S, Jantzen P, et al. Accelerated Alzheimer-type phenotype in transgenic mice carrying both mutant amyloid precursor protein and presenilin 1 transgenes. Nat Med. 1998;4(1):97–100.
123. Schuessel K, Schafer S, Bayer TA, Czech C, Pradier L, Muller-Spahn F, et al. Impaired Cu/Zn-SOD activity contributes to increased oxidative damage in APP transgenic mice. Neurobiol Dis. 2005;18(1):89–99.
124. Esposito L, Raber J, Kekonius L, Yan F, Yu GQ, Bien-Ly N, et al. Reduction in mitochondrial superoxide dismutase modulates Alzheimer's disease-like pathology and accelerates the onset of behavioral changes in human amyloid precursor protein transgenic mice. J Neurosci. 2006;26(19):5167–79.
125. Duyckaerts C, Potier MC, Delatour B. Alzheimer disease models and human neuropathology: similarities and differences. Acta Neuropathol. 2008;115(1):5–38.
126. Hutton M, Lewis J, Dickson D, Yen SH, McGowan E. Analysis of tauopathies with transgenic mice. Trends Mol Med. 2001;7(10):467–70.
127. Gotz J, Chen F, van Dorpe J, Nitsch RM. Formation of neurofibrillary tangles in P3011 tau transgenic mice induced by Abeta 42 fibrils. Science. 2001;293(5534):1491–5.
128. Higuchi M, Ishihara T, Zhang B, Hong M, Andreadis A, Trojanowski J, et al. Transgenic mouse model of tauopathies with glial pathology and nervous system degeneration. Neuron. 2002;35(3):433–46.
129. Lewis J, McGowan E, Rockwood J, Melrose H, Nacharaju P, Van Slegtenhorst M, et al. Neurofibrillary tangles, amyotrophy and progressive motor disturbance in mice expressing mutant (P301L) tau protein. Nat Genet. 2000;25(4):402–5.
130. Terwel D, Lasrado R, Snauwaert J, Vandeweert E, Van Haesendonck C, Borghgraef P, et al. Changed conformation of mutant Tau-P301L underlies the moribund tauopathy, absent in progressive, nonlethal axonopathy of Tau-4R/2N transgenic mice. J Biol Chem. 2005;280(5):3963–73.
131. Gotz J, Deters N, Doldissen A, Bokhari L, Ke Y, Wiesner A, et al. A decade of tau transgenic animal models and beyond. Brain Pathol. 2007;17(1):91–103.
132. Oakley H, Cole SL, Logan S, Maus E, Shao P, Craft J, et al. Intraneuronal beta-amyloid aggregates, neurodegeneration, and neuron loss in transgenic mice with five familial Alzheimer's disease mutations: potential factors in amyloid plaque formation. J Neurosci. 2006;26(40):10129–40.
133. Ohno M, Cole SL, Yasvoina M, Zhao J, Citron M, Berry R, et al. BACE1 gene deletion prevents neuron loss and memory deficits in 5XFAD APP/PS1 transgenic mice. Neurobiol Dis. 2007;26(1):134–45.
134. Jawhar S, Trawicka A, Jenneckens C, Bayer TA, Wirths O. Motor deficits, neuron loss, and reduced anxiety coinciding with axonal degeneration and intraneuronal Abeta aggregation in the 5XFAD mouse model of Alzheimer's disease. Neurobiol Aging. 2012;33(1):196 e29–40.

135. Criscuolo C, Cerri E, Fabiani C, et al. The Retina as a window to early dysfunctions of Alzheimer's disease following studies with a 5xfad mouse model. Neurobiol Aging. 2018;67:181–8. https://doi.org/10.1016/j.neurobiolaging.2018.03.017.
136. LaFerla FM, Oddo S. Alzheimer's disease: Abeta, tau and synaptic dysfunction. Trends Mol Med. 2005;11(4):170–6.
137. Oddo S, Caccamo A, Shepherd JD, Murphy MP, Golde TE, Kayed R, et al. Triple-transgenic model of Alzheimer's disease with plaques and tangles: intracellular Abeta and synaptic dysfunction. Neuron. 2003;39(3):409–21.
138. Oddo S, Caccamo A, Kitazawa M, Tseng BP, LaFerla FM. Amyloid deposition precedes tangle formation in a triple transgenic model of Alzheimer's disease. Neurobiol Aging. 2003;24(8):1063–70.
139. Gimenez-Llort L, Blazquez G, Canete T, Johansson B, Oddo S, Tobena A, et al. Modeling behavioral and neuronal symptoms of Alzheimer's disease in mice: a role for intraneuronal amyloid. Neurosci Biobehav Rev. 2007;31(1):125–47.
140. Rissman RA, Poon WW, Blurton-Jones M, Oddo S, Torp R, Vitek MP, et al. Caspase-cleavage of tau is an early event in Alzheimer disease tangle pathology. J Clin Investig. 2004;114(1):121–30.
141. Oddo S, Billings L, Kesslak JP, Cribbs DH, LaFerla FM. Abeta immunotherapy leads to clearance of early, but not late, hyperphosphorylated tau aggregates via the proteasome. Neuron. 2004;43(3):321–32.
142. Oddo S, Caccamo A, Green KN, Liang K, Tran L, Chen Y, et al. Chronic nicotine administration exacerbates tau pathology in a transgenic model of Alzheimer's disease. Proc Natl Acad Sci USA. 2005;102(8):3046–51.
143. Smith IF, Green KN, LaFerla FM. Calcium dysregulation in Alzheimer's disease: recent advances gained from genetically modified animals. Cell Calcium. 2005;38(3–4):427–37.
144. Billings LM, Oddo S, Green KN, McGaugh JL, LaFerla FM. Intraneuronal Abeta causes the onset of early Alzheimer's disease-related cognitive deficits in transgenic mice. Neuron. 2005;45(5):675–88.
145. Janelsins MC, Mastrangelo MA, Oddo S, LaFerla FM, Federoff HJ, Bowers WJ. Early correlation of microglial activation with enhanced tumor necrosis factor-alpha and monocyte chemoattractant protein-1 expression specifically within the entorhinal cortex of triple transgenic Alzheimer's disease mice. J Neuroinflammation. 2005;2:23.
146. Chiasseu M, Alarcon-Martinez L, Belforte N, et al. Tau accumulation in the retina promotes early neuronal dysfunction and precedes brain pathology in a mouse model of Alzheimer's disease. Mol Neurodegeneration. 2017. https://doi.org/10.1186/s13024-017-0199-3.
147. Smith IF, Hitt B, Green KN, Oddo S, LaFerla FM. Enhanced caffeine-induced Ca^{2+} release in the 3xTg-AD mouse model of Alzheimer's disease. J Neurochem. 2005;94(6):1711–8.
148. Shimazawa M, Inokuchi Y, Okuno T, Nakajima Y, Sakaguchi G, Kato A, et al. Reduced retinal function in amyloid precursor protein-over-expressing transgenic mice via attenuating glutamate-N-methyl-d-aspartate receptor signaling. J Neurochem. 2008;107(1):279–90.
149. Lee CW, Shih YH, Kuo YM. Cerebrovascular pathology and amyloid plaque formation in Alzheimer's disease. Curr Alzheimer Res. 2014;11(1):4–10.
150. Alexandrov PN, Pogue A, Bhattacharjee S, Lukiw WJ. Retinal amyloid peptides and complement factor H in transgenic models of Alzheimer's disease. NeuroReport. 2011;22(12):623–7.
151. Savini G, Barboni P, Carbonelli M, Hoffer KJ. Comparison of methods to measure corneal power for intraocular lens power calculation using a rotating Scheimpflug camera. J Cataract Refract Surg. 2013;39(4):598–604.
152. Cohen RM, et al. A transgenic Alzheimer rat with plaques, tau pathology, behavioral impairment, oligomeric aβ, and frank neuronal loss. J Neurosci. 2013;33(15):6245–56. https://doi.org/10.1523/JNEUROSCI.3672-12.2013.
153. Bac B, et al. The TGF344-AD RAT: behavioral and proteomic changes associated with aging and protein expression in a transgenic rat model of Alzheimer's disease. Neurobiol Aging. 2023;123:98–110. Available at: j.neurobiolaging.2022.12.015

154. Worth PF. How to treat Parkinson's disease in 2013. Clin Med. 2013;13(1):93–6.
155. Martínez-Navarrete GC, Martín-Nieto J, Esteve-Rudd J, et al. Alpha synuclein gene expression profile in the retina of vertebrates. In: Molecular vision. 2007. https://www.ncbi.nlm.nih.gov/pmc/articles/PMC3380420/. Accessed 10 Oct 2023.
156. Brancato R, Pece A, Carassa R. Central retinal artery occlusion after local anesthesia for blepharoplasty. Graefe's Arch Clin Exp Ophthalmol. 1991;229:593–4. https://doi.org/10.1007/bf00203328.
157. Gubellini P, Kachidian P. Animal models of Parkinson's disease: an updated overview. Revue Neurologique. 2015;171:750–61. https://doi.org/10.1016/j.neurol.2015.07.011.
158. Nicklas WJ, Vyas I, Heikkila RE. Inhibition of NADH-linked oxidation in brain mitochondria by 1-methyl-4-phenyl-pyridine, a metabolite of the neurotoxin, 1-methyl-4-phenyl-1,2,5,6-tetrahydropyridine. Life Sci. 1985;36(26):2503–8.
159. McNaught KS, Perl DP, Brownell AL, Olanow CW. Systemic exposure to proteasome inhibitors causes a progressive model of Parkinson's disease. Ann Neurol. 2004;56(1):149–62.
160. Bove J, Prou D, Perier C, Przedborski S. Toxin-induced models of Parkinson's disease. NeuroRx. 2005;2(3):484–94.
161. Blesa J, Phani S, Jackson-Lewis V, Przedborski S. Classic and new animal models of Parkinson's disease. J Biomed Biotechnol. 2012;2012: 845618.
162. Manning-Bog AB, McCormack AL, Li J, Uversky VN, Fink AL, Di Monte DA. The herbicide paraquat causes up-regulation and aggregation of alpha-synuclein in mice: paraquat and alpha-synuclein. J Biol Chem. 2002;277(3):1641–4.
163. Freire C, Koifman S. Pesticide exposure and Parkinson's disease: epidemiological evidence of association. Neurotoxicology. 2012;33(5):947–71.
164. Zheng LF, Wang ZY, Li XF, Song J, Hong F, Lian H, et al. Reduced expression of choline acetyltransferase in vagal motoneurons and gastric motor dysfunction in a 6-OHDA rat model of Parkinson's disease. Brain Res. 2011;1420:59–67.
165. Annett LE, Torres EM, Clarke DJ, Ishida Y, Barker RA, Ridley RM, et al. Survival of nigral grafts within the striatum of marmosets with 6-OHDA lesions depends critically on donor embryo age. Cell Transpl. 1997;6(6):557–69.
166. Crofts HS, Dalley JW, Collins P, Van Denderen JC, Everitt BJ, Robbins TW, et al. Differential effects of 6-OHDA lesions of the frontal cortex and caudate nucleus on the ability to acquire an attentional set. Cereb Cortex. 2001;11(11):1015–26.
167. He Y, Appel S, Le W. Minocycline inhibits microglial activation and protects nigral cells after 6-hydroxydopamine injection into mouse striatum. Brain Res. 2001;909(1–2):187–93.
168. Ma KH, Huang WS, Chen CH, Lin SZ, Wey SP, Ting G, et al. Dual SPECT of dopamine system using [99mTc]TRODAT-1 and [123I]IBZM in normal and 6-OHDA-lesioned formosan rock monkeys. Nucl Med Biol. 2002;29(5):561–7.
169. Lundblad M, Picconi B, Lindgren H, Cenci MA. A model of L-DOPA-induced dyskinesia in 6-hydroxydopamine lesioned mice: relation to motor and cellular parameters of nigrostriatal function. Neurobiol Dis. 2004;16(1):110–23.
170. Javoy F, Sotelo C, Herbet A, Agid Y. Specificity of dopaminergic neuronal degeneration induced by intracerebral injection of 6-hydroxydopamine in the nigrostriatal dopamine system. Brain Res. 1976;102(2):201–15.
171. Jeon BS, Jackson-Lewis V, Burke RE. 6-Hydroxydopamine lesion of the rat substantia nigra: time course and morphology of cell death. Neurodegeneration. 1995;4(2):131–7.
172. Faull RL, Laverty R. Changes in dopamine levels in the corpus striatum following lesions in the substantia nigra. Exp Neurol. 1969;23(3):332–40.
173. Allen JM, Cross AJ, Crow TJ, Javoy-Agid F, Agid Y, Bloom SR. Dissociation of neuropeptide Y and somatostatin in Parkinson's disease. Brain Res. 1985;337(1):197–200.
174. Lao CL, Kuo YH, Hsieh YT, Chen JC. Intranasal and subcutaneous administration of dopamine D3 receptor agonists functionally restores nigrostriatal dopamine in MPTP-treated mice. Neurotoxicity Res. 2013;24(4):523–31.

175. Kim JI, Yang EJ, Lee MS, Kim YS, Huh Y, Cho IH, et al. Bee venom reduces neuroinflammation in the MPTP-induced model of Parkinson's disease. Int J Neurosci. 2011;121(4):209–17.
176. Liu K, Shi N, Sun Y, Zhang T, Sun X. Therapeutic effects of rapamycin on MPTP-induced Parkinsonism in mice. Neurochem Res. 2013;38(1):201–7.
177. Yabuki Y, Ohizumi Y, Yokosuka A, Mimaki Y, Fukunaga K. Nobiletin treatment improves motor and cognitive deficits seen in MPTP-induced Parkinson model mice. Neuroscience. 2013;259C:126–41.
178. Masilamoni GJ, Bogenpohl JW, Alagille D, Delevich K, Tamagnan G, Votaw JR, et al. Metabotropic glutamate receptor 5 antagonist protects dopaminergic and noradrenergic neurons from degeneration in MPTP-treated monkeys. Brain. 2011;134(Pt 7):2057–73.
179. Seniuk NA, Tatton WG, Greenwood CE. Dose-dependent destruction of the coeruleus-cortical and nigral-striatal projections by MPTP. Brain Res. 1990;527(1):7–20.
180. Sirinathsinghji DJ, Kupsch A, Mayer E, Zivin M, Pufal D, Oertel WH. Cellular localization of tyrosine hydroxylase mRNA and cholecystokinin mRNA-containing cells in the ventral mesencephalon of the common marmoset: effects of 1-methyl-4-phenyl-1,2,3,6-tetrahydropyridine. Brain Res Mol Brain Res. 1992;12(1–3):267–74.
181. Ovadia A, Zhang Z, Gash DM. Increased susceptibility to MPTP toxicity in middle-aged rhesus monkeys. Neurobiol Aging. 1995;16(6):931–7.
182. Blandini F, Armentero MT. Animal models of Parkinson's disease. FEBS J. 2012;279(7):1156–66.
183. Xun Z, Sowell RA, Kaufman TC, Clemmer DE. Quantitative proteomics of a presymptomatic A53T alpha-synuclein Drosophila model of Parkinson disease. Mol Cell Proteomics: MCP. 2008;7(7):1191–203.
184. Corti O, Lesage S, Brice A. What genetics tells us about the causes and mechanisms of Parkinson's disease. Physiol Rev. 2011;91(4):1161–218.
185. Lindgren HS, Lelos MJ, Dunnett SB. Do alpha-synuclein vector injections provide a better model of Parkinson's disease than the classic 6-hydroxydopamine model? Exp Neurol. 2012;237(1):36–42.
186. Recchia A, Debetto P, Negro A, Guidolin D, Skaper SD, Giusti P. Alpha-synuclein and Parkinson's disease. FASEB J. 2004;18(6):617–26.
187. Recchia A, Rota D, Debetto P, Peroni D, Guidolin D, Negro A, et al. Generation of a alpha-synuclein-based rat model of Parkinson's disease. Neurobiol Dis. 2008;30(1):8–18.
188. Betarbet R, Sherer TB, Greenamyre JT. Animal models of Parkinson's disease. BioEssays. 2002;24(4):308–18.
189. Schober A. Classic toxin-induced animal models of Parkinson's disease: 6-OHDA and MPTP. Cell Tissue Res. 2004;318(1):215–24.
190. Schuler F, Casida JE. Functional coupling of PSST and ND1 subunits in NADH:ubiquinone oxidoreductase established by photoaffinity labeling. Biochimica Biophys Acta. 2001;1506(1):79–87.
191. Prance G. The poisons and narcotics of the Amazonian Indians. J Royal Coll Phys Lond. 1999;33(4):368–76.
192. Talpade DJ, Greene JG, Higgins DS Jr, Greenamyre JT. In vivo labeling of mitochondrial complex I (NADH:ubiquinone oxidoreductase) in rat brain using [(3)H]dihydrorotenone. J Neurochem. 2000;75(6):2611–21.
193. Alam M, Schmidt WJ. Rotenone destroys dopaminergic neurons and induces parkinsonian symptoms in rats. Behav Brain Res. 2002;136(1):317–24.
194. Betarbet R, Sherer TB, MacKenzie G, Garcia-Osuna M, Panov AV, Greenamyre JT. Chronic systemic pesticide exposure reproduces features of Parkinson's disease. Nat Neurosci. 2000;3(12):1301–6.
195. Sherer TB, Betarbet R, Testa CM, Seo BB, Richardson JR, Kim JH, et al. Mechanism of toxicity in rotenone models of Parkinson's disease. J Neurosci. 2003;23(34):10756–64.
196. Alam ZI, Jenner A, Daniel SE, Lees AJ, Cairns N, Marsden CD, et al. Oxidative DNA damage in the parkinsonian brain: an apparent selective increase in 8-hydroxyguanine levels in substantia nigra. J Neurochem. 1997;69(3):1196–203.

197. Floor E, Wetzel MG. Increased protein oxidation in human substantia nigra pars compacta in comparison with basal ganglia and prefrontal cortex measured with an improved dinitrophenylhydrazine assay. J Neurochem. 1998;70(1):268–75.
198. Tada-Oikawa S, Hiraku Y, Kawanishi M, Kawanishi S. Mechanism for generation of hydrogen peroxide and change of mitochondrial membrane potential during rotenone-induced apoptosis. Life Sci. 2003;73(25):3277–88.
199. Beal MF. Mitochondria, oxidative damage, and inflammation in Parkinson's disease. Ann N Y Acad Sci. 2003;991:120–31.
200. Aguilar-Bryan L, Clement JPt, Gonzalez G, Kunjilwar K, Babenko A, Bryan J. Toward understanding the assembly and structure of KATP channels. Physiol Rev. 1998;78(1):227–45.
201. Liss B, Bruns R, Roeper J. Alternative sulfonylurea receptor expression defines metabolic sensitivity of K-ATP channels in dopaminergic midbrain neurons. EMBO J. 1999;18(4):833–46.
202. Stokes AH, Hastings TG, Vrana KE. Cytotoxic and genotoxic potential of dopamine. J Neurosci Res. 1999;55(6):659–65.
203. Spector S, Sjoerdsma A, Udenfriend S. Blockade of endogenous norepinephrine synthesis by alpha-methyl-tyrosine, an inhibitor of tyrosine hydroxylase. J Pharmacol Exp Ther. 1965;147:86–95.
204. Sakka N, Sawada H, Izumi Y, Kume T, Katsuki H, Kaneko S, et al. Dopamine is involved in selectivity of dopaminergic neuronal death by rotenone. NeuroReport. 2003;14(18):2425–8.
205. Biehlmaier O, Alam M, Schmidt WJ. A rat model of Parkinsonism shows depletion of dopamine in the retina. Neurochem Int. 2007;50(1):189–95.
206. Marey-Semper I, Gelman M, Levi-Strauss M. A selective toxicity toward cultured mesencephalic dopaminergic neurons is induced by the synergistic effects of energetic metabolism impairment and NMDA receptor activation. J Neurosci. 1995;15(9):5912–8.
207. Huang J, Liu H, Gu W, Yan Z, Xu Z, Yang Y, et al. A delivery strategy for rotenone microspheres in an animal model of Parkinson's disease. Biomaterials. 2006;27(6):937–46.
208. Feng Y, Liang ZH, Wang T, Qiao X, Liu HJ, Sun SG. Alpha-Synuclein redistributed and aggregated in rotenone-induced Parkinson's disease rats. Neurosci Bull. 2006;22(5):288–93.
209. Xiong N, Huang J, Zhang Z, Zhang Z, Xiong J, Liu X, et al. Stereotaxical infusion of rotenone: a reliable rodent model for Parkinson's disease. PLoS ONE. 2009;4(11): e7878.
210. Xiong N, Long X, Xiong J, Jia M, Chen C, Huang J, et al. Mitochondrial complex I inhibitor rotenone-induced toxicity and its potential mechanisms in Parkinson's disease models. Crit Rev Toxicol. 2012;42(7):613–32.
211. Testa CM, Sherer TB, Greenamyre JT. Rotenone induces oxidative stress and dopaminergic neuron damage in organotypic substantia nigra cultures. Brain Res Mol Brain Res. 2005;134(1):109–18.
212. Isenberg JS, Klaunig JE. Role of the mitochondrial membrane permeability transition (MPT) in rotenone-induced apoptosis in liver cells. Toxicol Sci. 2000;53(2):340–51.
213. Marking LL. Oral toxicity of rotenone to mammals. Investig Fish Control. 1988.
214. Heikkila RE, Nicklas WJ, Vyas I, Duvoisin RC. Dopaminergic toxicity of rotenone and the 1-methyl-4-phenylpyridinium ion after their stereotaxic administration to rats: implication for the mechanism of 1-methyl-4-phenyl-1,2,3,6-tetrahydropyridine toxicity. Neurosci Lett. 1985;62(3):389–94.
215. Schmidt WJ, Alam M. Controversies on new animal models of Parkinson's disease pro and con: the rotenone model of Parkinson's disease (PD). J Neural Transm Suppl. 2006;70:273–6.
216. Hu LF, Lu M, Tiong CX, Dawe GS, Hu G, Bian JS. Neuroprotective effects of hydrogen sulfide on Parkinson's disease rat models. Aging Cell. 2010;9(2):135–46.
217. Pan-Montojo F, Anichtchik O, Dening Y, Knels L, Pursche S, Jung R, et al. Progression of Parkinson's disease pathology is reproduced by intragastric administration of rotenone in mice. PLoS ONE. 2010;5(1): e8762.
218. Alam M, Schmidt WJ. L-DOPA reverses the hypokinetic behaviour and rigidity in rotenone-treated rats. Behav Brain Res. 2004;153(2):439–46.

219. Alam M, Mayerhofer A, Schmidt WJ. The neurobehavioral changes induced by bilateral rotenone lesion in medial forebrain bundle of rats are reversed by L-DOPA. Behav Brain Res. 2004;151(1–2):117–24.
220. Kamalden TA, Ji D, Osborne NN. Rotenone-induced death of RGC-5 cells is caspase independent, involves the JNK and p38 pathways and is attenuated by specific green tea flavonoids. Neurochem Res. 2012;37(5):1091–101.
221. Hancock DB, Martin ER, Mayhew GM, Stajich JM, Jewett R, Stacy MA, et al. Pesticide exposure and risk of Parkinson's disease: a family-based case-control study. BMC Neurol. 2008;8:6.
222. Dhillon AS, Tarbutton GL, Levin JL, Plotkin GM, Lowry LK, Nalbone JT, et al. Pesticide/environmental exposures and Parkinson's disease in East Texas. J Agromed. 2008;13(1):37–48.
223. Chan SL, Angeles DC, Tan EK. Targeting leucine-rich repeat kinase 2 in Parkinson's disease. Expert Opin Ther Targets. 2013;17(12):1471–82.
224. Houlden H, Singleton AB. The genetics and neuropathology of Parkinson's disease. Acta Neuropathol. 2012;124(3):325–38.
225. Gasser T. Molecular genetic findings in LRRK2 American, Canadian and German families. J Neural Transm Suppl. 2006;70:231–4.
226. Lesage S, Brice A. Parkinson's disease: from monogenic forms to genetic susceptibility factors. Hum Mol Genet. 2009;18(R1):R48-59.
227. Peeraully T, Tan EK. Genetic variants in sporadic Parkinson's disease: East vs West. Parkinson Relat Disord. 2012;18(Suppl 1):S63–5.
228. Farrer MJ. Genetics of Parkinson disease: paradigm shifts and future prospects. Nat Rev Genet. 2006;7(4):306–18.
229. Mamais A, Raja M, Manzoni C, Dihanich S, Lees A, Moore D, et al. Divergent alpha-synuclein solubility and aggregation properties in G2019S LRRK2 Parkinson's disease brains with Lewy Body pathology compared to idiopathic cases. Neurobiol Dis. 2013;58:183–90.
230. Healy DG, Falchi M, O'Sullivan SS, Bonifati V, Durr A, Bressman S, et al. Phenotype, genotype, and worldwide genetic penetrance of LRRK2-associated Parkinson's disease: a case-control study. Lancet Neurol. 2008;7(7):583–90.
231. La Morgia C, Barboni P, Rizzo G, Carbonelli M, Savini G, Scaglione C, et al. Loss of temporal retinal nerve fibers in Parkinson disease: a mitochondrial pattern? Eur J Neurol. 2013;20(1):198–201.
232. Satue M, Garcia-Martin E, Fuertes I, Otin S, Alarcia R, Herrero R, et al. Use of Fourier-domain OCT to detect retinal nerve fiber layer degeneration in Parkinson's disease patients. Eye. 2013;27(4):507–14.
233. Hindle SJ, Elliott CJ. Spread of neuronal degeneration in a dopaminergic, Lrrk-G2019S model of Parkinson disease. Autophagy. 2013;9(6):936–8.
234. Mastroberardino PG, Hoffman EK, Horowitz MP, Betarbet R, Taylor G, Cheng D, et al. A novel transferrin/TfR2-mediated mitochondrial iron transport system is disrupted in Parkinson's disease. Neurobiol Dis. 2009;34(3):417–31.
235. Lapointe N, St-Hilaire M, Martinoli MG, Blanchet J, Gould P, Rouillard C, et al. Rotenone induces non-specific central nervous system and systemic toxicity. FASEB J. 2004;18(6):717–9.
236. Drolet RE, Cannon JR, Montero L, Greenamyre JT. Chronic rotenone exposure reproduces Parkinson's disease gastrointestinal neuropathology. Neurobiol Dis. 2009;36(1):96–102.

OCT and OCTA in Glaucoma

20

Jo-Hsuan Wu, Sasan Moghimi, Harsha Rao, Kaweh Mansouri, and Robert N. Weinreb

Abstract

Optical coherence tomography (OCT) detects structural abnormalities in glaucoma by evaluating retinal thickness changes in the optic nerve head and macula. The structural abnormalities detected on OCT often precede detectable functional loss, enabling early diagnosis of glaucoma. Longitudinal assessment of structural parameters using OCT also helps in detecting glaucoma progression. OCT angiography (OCTA) shows promise for diagnosing and monitoring glaucoma and may complement OCT for clinical evaluation.

Keywords

Glaucoma • Optical coherence tomography • Glaucoma diagnosis • Glaucoma progression • Optical coherence tomography angiography

J.-H. Wu · S. Moghimi · R. N. Weinreb (✉)
Hamilton Glaucoma Center, Shiley Eye Institute, Viterbi Family Department of Ophthalmology, University of California, San Diego, 9500 Gilman Drive, La Jolla, CA 92093-0946, USA
e-mail: rweinreb@ucsd.edu

J.-H. Wu
e-mail: Jow009@health.ucsd.edu

S. Moghimi
e-mail: samoghimi@health.ucsd.edu

H. Rao
Narayana Nethralaya, Bangalore, India

K. Mansouri
Glaucoma Center, Montchoisi Clinic, Swiss Vision Network, Lausanne, Switzerland

A. Grzybowski and P. Barboni (eds.), *OCT and Imaging in Central Nervous System Diseases*, https://doi.org/10.1007/978-3-031-72156-4_20

20.1 Optical Coherence Tomography (OCT)

Glaucoma is a chronic optic neuropathy characterised by progressive loss of retinal ganglion cells (RGCs) [1]. It is the leading cause of irreversible blindness in the world. A systematic review and meta-analysis conducted in 2014 estimated that the number of people aged between 40 and 80 years with glaucoma worldwide was 64.3 million, and that it would increase to 111.8 million in 2040 [2]. Another meta-analysis reported in 2016 that the number of people blind due to glaucoma worldwide was 2.1 million and those visually impaired due to glaucoma was 4.2 million [3]. The meta-analysis also reported that between 1990 and 2010, the number of people blind due to glaucoma increased by 0.8 million or 62% and those visually impaired increased by 2.3 million or 83%, respectively [3]. As the loss of RGCs in glaucoma is irreversible, early detection of the disease is of utmost importance because appropriate treatment can prevent or slow disease progression and therefore, preserve vision.

Glaucoma is characterised by typical optic nerve head (ONH) and retinal nerve fiber layer (RNFL) changes with or without the presence of correlating visual field (VF) loss. Detection of VF loss by means of standard automated perimetry (SAP) has been one of the mainstays in the diagnosis and monitoring of glaucoma. However, the subjective nature of perimetry creates large variability in results, which make it difficult to reliably assess and monitor the disease. Structural changes in the ONH and RNFL often are visible before the appearance of detectable loss by SAP [4, 5]. The ability to detect structural loss at the level of the ONH and peripapillary RNFL is, therefore, fundamental in the diagnosis and management of glaucoma. Clinical examination of the ONH and RNFL is routinely done on a slit-lamp biomicroscope using a high powered convex lens. Although detecting glaucoma by this method is fairly simple in moderate and severe stages of the disease, identification of subtle ONH and RNFL changes in early glaucoma requires training and experience. Another method to detect glaucoma is the evaluation of optic disc stereo-photographs. Both these methods, however, are subjective, and the agreement even among experts in detecting glaucomatous changes either clinically or on disc photographs is far from excellent [6, 7]. The other major drawback of these methods is that changes can only be qualitatively assessed but cannot be quantified. These limitations are overcome by optical coherence tomography (OCT) imaging, which provides objective assessment of structural changes in glaucoma with high reproducibility [8, 9].

OCT technology has evolved from time-domain (TD-) to spectral-domain technology (SD-OCT) which is faster and provides greater resolution (axial resolution of 5 μm). As a result of improved resolution, it is now possible to evaluate each layer of the retina separately using SD-OCT. This has led to a renewed interest in evaluating the macular changes in glaucoma [10]. Macula contains approximately 50% of all RGCs. RGC layer in the macula contains seven layers of RGC bodies in contrast to the peripheral retina where the RGC layer is only one cell thick [11]. Therefore, evaluation of macula, especially the inner retinal layers (ganglion cell layer and the inner plexiform layer), along with ONH and RNFL, has gained importance in glaucoma [12].

Current OCT devices evaluate the ONH, peripapillary RNFL as well as the macula using cube scans for assessing the amount of structural damage in glaucoma. Below is a description of the way ONH, RNFL and macular analysis is performed by different OCT devices.

20.2 ONH Analysis of OCT

Glaucoma is a disease that primarily affects the RGCs and their axons, which travel through the ONH into the optic nerve. Loss of RGCs and their axons, therefore show typical features on the ONH, such as increased cup-to-disc ratio, thinning of the neuroretinal rim (NRR) and NRR notching. Clinical characteristics such as NRR thinning and increased optic disc cupping differentiate glaucoma from other optic neuropathies [13].

ONH analysis with OCT is performed by automated software. Different manufacturers of OCT devices have their own proprietary softwares for ONH analysis, which vary slightly from each other. A brief description of the automated ONH analysis performed in commonly used OCT devices is important to understand the differences between the reported measurements.

The software of one OCT device identifies the termination of Bruch's membrane as the disc margin from the 3-dimensional data set. The software then generates a set of vectors from the disc margin to points on the vitreoretinal interface for each radial direction and calculates a trapezoidal, cross-sectional area associated with each vector. For each point on the disc margin, the vector that produces the minimum cross-sectional area is identified and each of these vectors is geometrically transformed into the plane of the optic disc to provide a 2-D representation of the 3-D data acquired by the imaging software. In this manner, the cup margin is defined by a set of optimal vectors and the neuro-retinal rim area is calculated as a piece-wise sum of the corresponding minimum trapezoidal, cross-sectional areas. One of the difficulties in clinical assessment of the ONH is when the viewing angle of the ophthalmologist is not the same as the ONH axis, for example in tilted discs, where the neuro-retinal rim appears foreshortened. The 2-D representation of the ONH provided is as though the viewing angle is parallel to the ONH axis which minimizes the problem of foreshortening (Fig. 20.1) [14].

The software of another OCT device detects the retinal pigment epithelium (RPE) tips automatically and then delineates the optic disc margin by joining the RPE tips. The optic cup is defined by fitting a plane 150 μm parallel to and above the plane that fit the coordinates of the RPE tips. ONH tissue above the cup line and within the perpendicular lines drawn from the RPE tips to the surface of the retina is considered as the neuroretinal rim (Fig. 20.2).

The software of yet another OCT device identifies the termination of the Bruch's membrane and delineates the Bruch's membrane opening (BMO) which acts as a surrogate for the disc margin. It subsequently calculates a parameter

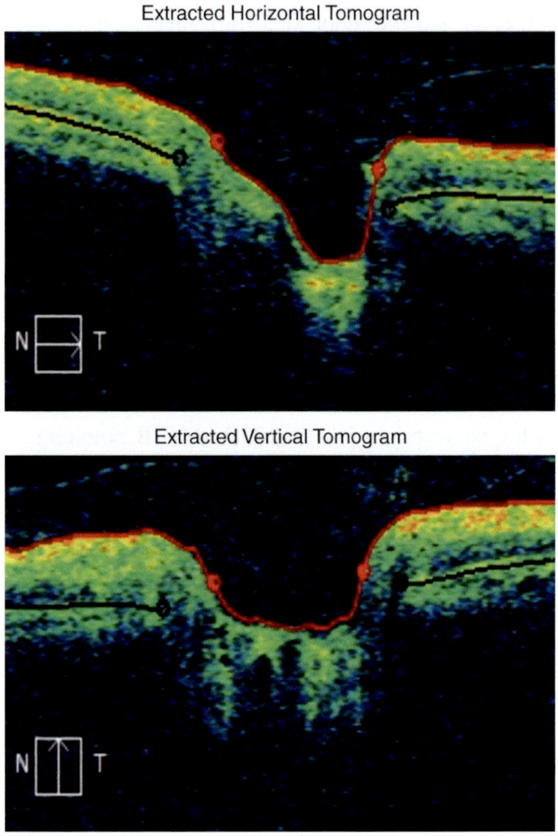

Fig. 20.1 Automated segmentation of the optic nerve head on an OCT device. Open black circles represent the termination of Bruch's membrane and the red circles represent the demarcation between neuroretinal rim and cup

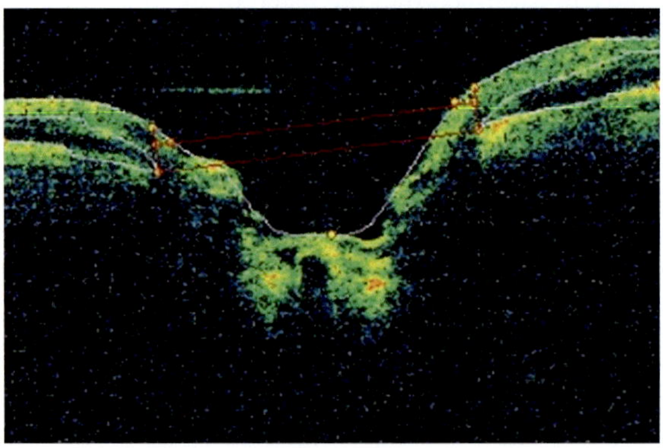

Fig. 20.2 Automated segmentation of the optic nerve head with another OCT software. The lower red straight line represents the line connecting the retinal pigment epithelium (RPE) tips and another red line is drawn 150 μm above and parallel to this plane. The optic nerve head tissue above the upper red line (between the 3 yellow colored circles) is defined as the neuroretinal rim tissue (source: Optovue.com)

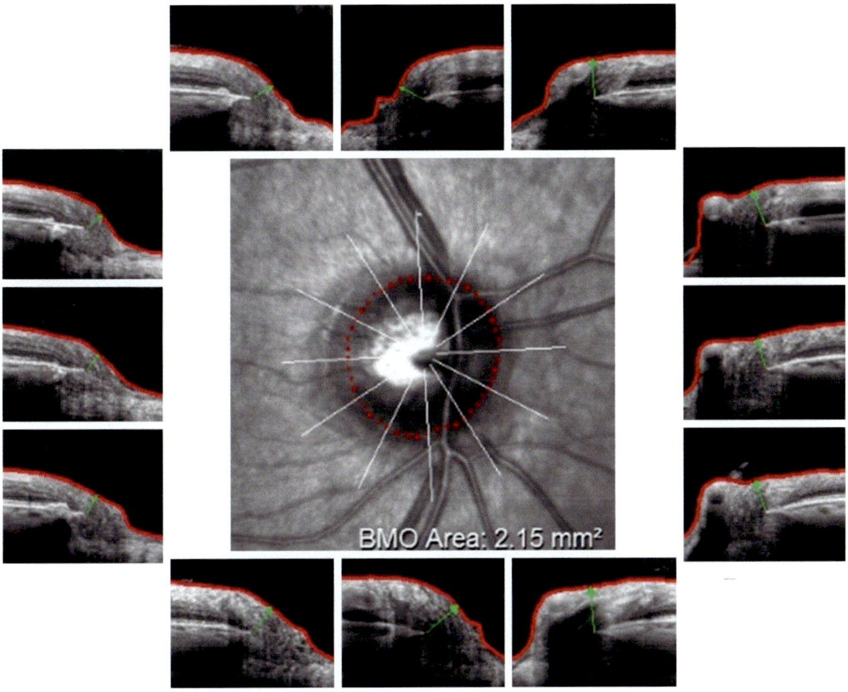

Fig. 20.3 The software of another OCT device identifies the termination of Bruch's membrane (Bruch's membrane opening, BMO) as the disc margin. The green lines represent the minimum rim width (MRW) which is the shortest distance between the BMO and the surface of the rim tissue at various locations

called minimum rim width (MRW) which is the minimum distance between the BMO line and the surface of the rim tissue (Fig. 20.3).

It is important to note that the ONH measurements of different imaging technologies are dependent on the segmentation performed by the propriety software and are not necessarily interchangeable with each other.

20.3 Peripapillary RNFL Analysis of OCT

RNFL contains the axons of the RGCs and the loss of the axons in glaucoma manifests as RNFL thinning and wedge shaped RNFL defects around the ONH (peripapillary region). Like for the ONH, different manufacturers of OCT devices have their own proprietary automated softwares for segmenting the peripapillary RNFL and measuring its thickness. Software of most OCT devices measure the RNFL thickness along a circle 3.46/3.45 mm in diameter positioned evenly around the center of the optic disc (Figs. 20.4 and 20.5). Software of another OCT device

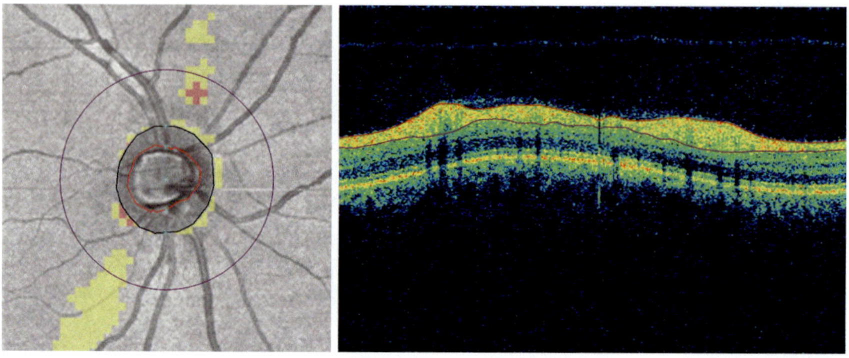

Fig. 20.4 Left image shows the circle scan along which peripapillary retinal nerve fiber layer (RNFL) thickness is measured on an OCT device. Right image shows the segmentation of RNFL; red line marks the internal limiting membrane and purple line marks the lower border of the RNFL

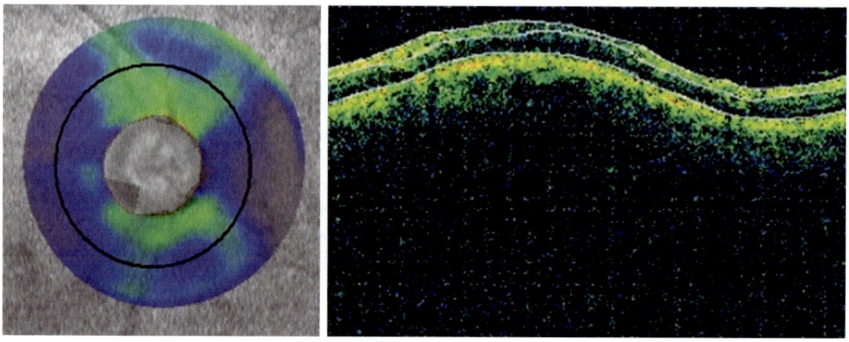

Fig. 20.5 Left image shows the circle scan along which retinal nerve fiber layer (RNFL) thickness is measured on a different OCT device. Right image shows the segmentation of RNFL displayed by the upper two white lines on the B scan image (source: Optovue.com)

uses Fovea-to-Disc alignment technology that automatically tracks and aligns circle scans of 3.45 mm diameter to overcome measurement errors due to changing head and /or eye position during scanning (Fig. 20.6). This alignment technology improves the reproducibility of RNFL measurements.

Studies have shown that the RNFL thickness values vary between different SD-OCT devices and cannot be used interchangeably [15, 16].

20.4 Macular Analysis of OCT

Macula contains the greatest density of RGCs and therefore, loss of RGCs result in thinning of the inner retinal layers at the macula. Thinning of inner retinal layers at the macula, however, cannot be assessed either clinically using slit-lamp

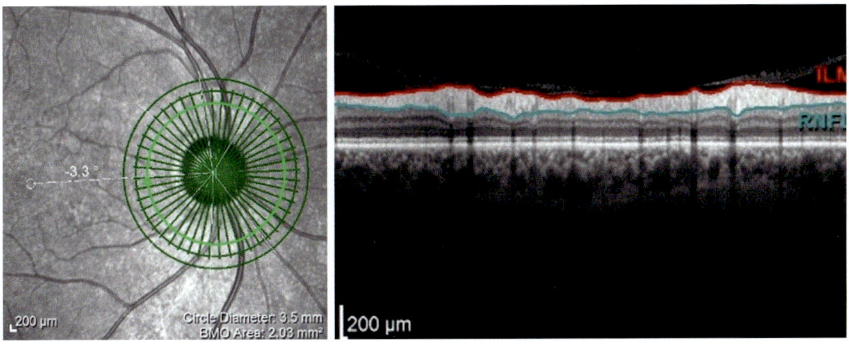

Fig. 20.6 Left image shows the circle scans (green) along which retinal nerve fiber layer (RNFL) thickness is measured on another OCT device. FoDi (fovea to disc) alignment technology (blue line) is used here to overcome the effect of eye rotation and head tilt on RNFL measurements and to match with alignment of the normative database. Right image shows the segmentation of RNFL; red line marks the internal limiting membrane and blue line marks the lower border of the RNFL

biomicroscope or on fundus photographs. This macular information provided by OCT therefore is unique.

Different manufacturers of OCT devices have different proprietary automated software for segmenting the inner retinal layers and measuring their thicknesses at the macula (which roughly is a region 8 degrees in radius from the center of the fovea). Software of one OCT device measures the GCL and IPL thickness together as ganglion cell-inner plexiform layer (GCIPL) thickness (Fig. 20.7) while that of another device measures the RNFL and GCIPL thickness together as ganglion cell complex (GCC, Fig. 20.8). Another OCT device measures the thicknesses of each retinal layer separately (Fig. 20.9).

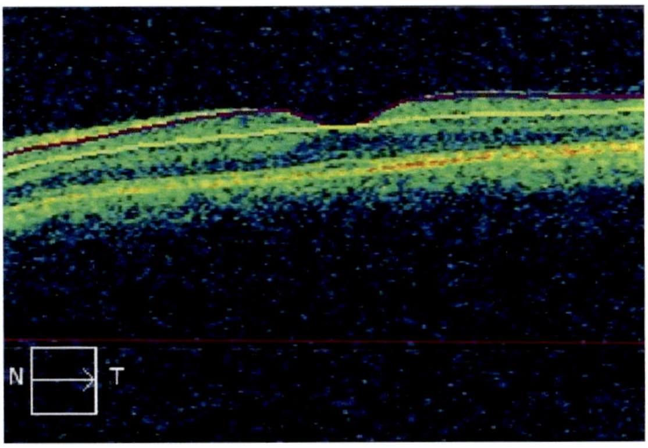

Fig. 20.7 Macular imaging of an OCT device which evaluates ganglion cell layer and inner plexiform layer together as ganglion cell-inner plexiform layer (GCIPL) thickness. Purple and yellow lines demonstrate the segmentation of GCIPL

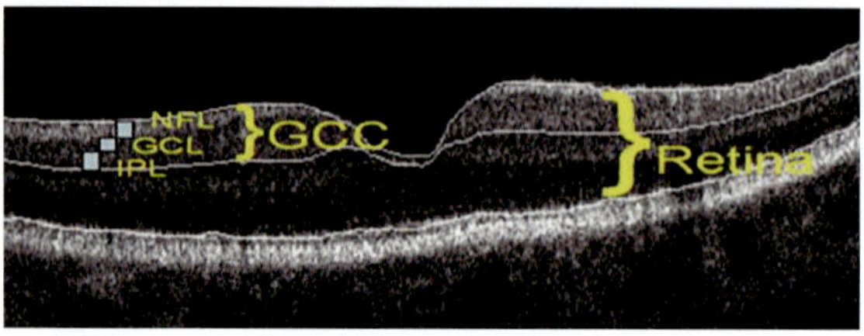

Fig. 20.8 Macular imaging of an OCT device which evaluates retinal nerve fiber layer, ganglion cell layer and inner plexiform layer together as ganglion cell complex (GCC) thickness. The two white lines on the top demonstrate the segmentation of GCC (source: Optovue.com)

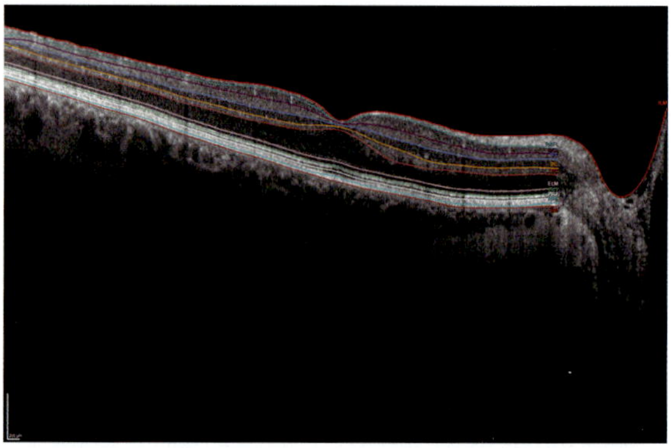

Fig. 20.9 Macular imaging from an OCT device which segments each layer of the retina and measures the thickness of each layer of retina separately (source: Heidelberg Engineering)

20.5 Interpreting the ONH, RNFL and Macular Measurements of OCT in Normal and Glaucoma Eyes

Once the ONH, RNFL and macular scans are acquired and segmentation performed, the software of the OCT calculates certain parameters. All these measurements are then compared with an age-matched reference database within the device to quantify glaucomatous damage and are interpreted either as "within normal limits (color-coded as green)" or "borderline (coded as yellow)" or "outside normal limits (coded as red)". The parameter is coded in green if the subject's measurement falls between the 5th and the 95th percentile values of the reference database ($p > 5\%$). The parameter is flagged in yellow if the measurement falls between the 5th and the 1st percentile values ($p < 5\%$ and $p > 1\%$) and "red" if the measurement falls below the lowest one percentile value ($p < 1\%$) of the reference database.

Figure 20.10 shows the ONH and RNFL report of a normal (Fig. 20.10a) and a glaucomatous (Fig. 20.10b) eye, and Fig. 20.11 shows the macular (GCIPL) analysis report of a normal (Fig. 20.11a) and a glaucoma (Fig. 20.11b) patient from a commercially available OCT device. Figure 20.12 shows the results of ONH, RNFL and macular imaging from another OCT device in a normal subject

(Fig. 20.12a) and a glaucoma patient (Fig. 20.12b). Figures 20.13, 20.14 and 20.15 show the ONH, RNFL and macular analysis report, respectively, of a normal (a) and a glaucomatous (b) patient from yet another OCT device.

Most of these reports show (i) a thickness map: in which RNFL/macular thickness measurements are represented in pseudocolors (hot colors such as red and orange represent thicker measurements, while cool colors such as green and blue represent thinner measurements), (ii) deviation and sector/clock-hour maps: in which the RNFL/macular thickness is compared with the reference database and coded either as green, yellow or red as described previously.

RNFL/macular thickness map is reported to be better than the deviation and the clock hour map to detect structural abnormalities in early glaucoma [17, 18]. Deviation and clock hour maps rely on the reference database to classify a measurement as normal, suspect or outside normal limits. The reference database has strict inclusion criteria and because of the wide range of "normal", significant reduction in the structural measurements is usually required before a measurement is labelled as "outside normal limits" of the reference database.

20.6 Role of OCT in Diagnosing Glaucoma

Multiple studies have evaluated the ability of OCT in diagnosing glaucoma. A Cochrane review of these studies found the ONH and RNFL measurements to have excellent abilities to diagnose glaucoma [19]. In clinical practice, OCT imaging has been found to be especially useful in eyes with suspicious optic discs and normal VF. Figure 20.16 shows an eye with a glaucomatous optic disc (showing neuroretinal rim thinning and the presence of a RNFL defect inferiorly) and normal VF. OCT confirms the presence of RNFL thinning and quantifies it, enabling monitoring over time for progression. A study by Kuang et al. found that OCT was able to detect RNFL thinning 8 years before the development of VF defects [20]. Figure 20.17 shows an eye with a suspicious optic disc and a probable nasal defect on VF. OCT confirms the presence of RNFL thinning inferiorly which aids in the diagnosis and monitoring of this patient.

Structural changes in glaucoma are detectable on the ONH, RNFL and macular scans of OCT. To clarify which of these parameters detects glaucoma early, some studies have compared the diagnostic performance of macular OCT measurements to that of ONH and RNFL measurements, and generally found RNFL, particularly peripapillary/circumpapillary RNFL thickness, to have the best diagnostic ability for glaucoma [21–23]. A systematic review including 150 studies also reported RNFL measurements to be better than the inner retinal measurements at macula for diagnosing glaucoma [24]. Whereas in a meta-analysis, RNFL and segmented macular thicknesses (GCIPL, GCC) were found to have similar diagnostic accuracy higher than that of total macular thickness [25]. However, it is still useful to evaluate glaucomatous damage both on the ONH/RNFL and macular OCT scans to better understand the severity and pattern of structural loss.

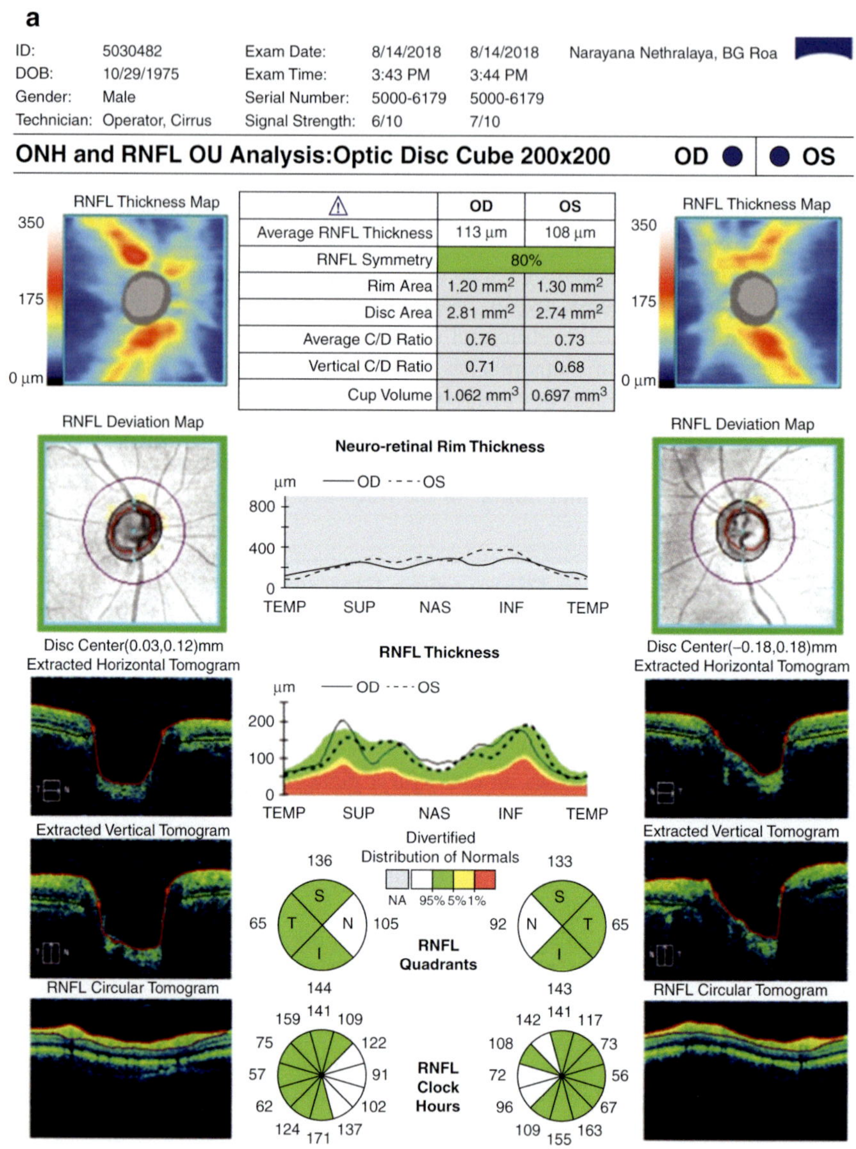

Fig. 20.10 Optic nerve head (ONH) and retinal nerve fiber layer (RNFL) reports of a normal subject (a) and a glaucoma patient (b). Compared to a normal eye, glaucomatous eye shows cool colors (blues, greens) on the "RNFL thickness map" representing thinning of RNFL (seen in the superior quadrant of the right eye and inferior quadrant of the left eye, b), red and yellow regions on the "deviation map" and "quadrant and clock hour maps" corresponding to the regions of RNFL thinning, RNFL and neuroretinal rim thickness falling in the red or yellow shaded region at corresponding locations around the disc on "TSNIT profile map" and reduction in the "summary parameters" in the tables which are color-coded in yellow or red

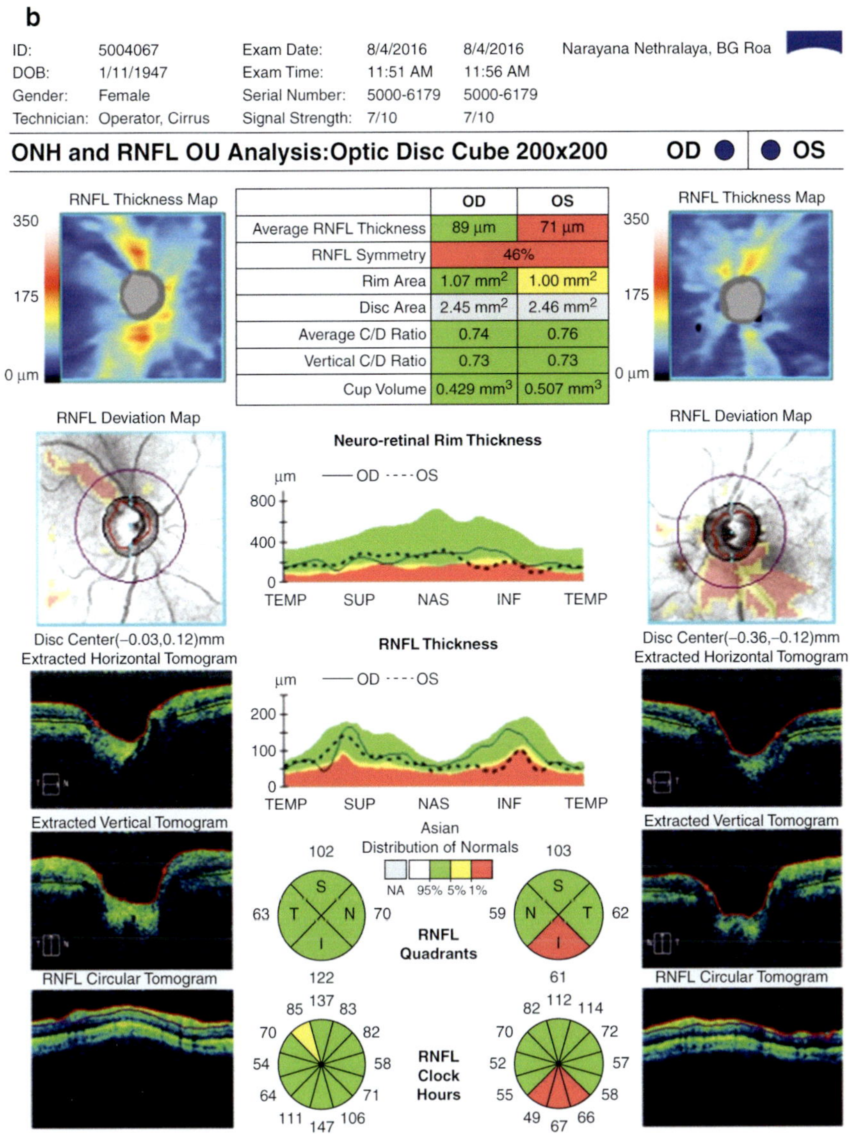

Fig. 20.10 (continued)

Using reference database-based criteria, El-Nimri et al. [26] investigated the glaucoma diagnostic performances of RNFL thickness and BMO-MRW in individuals of European descent (ED) and African descent (AD). With the significantly lower diagnostic performances found in AD individuals compared with ED individuals, the authors suggested that, with the current OCT reference database, both RNFL thickness and BMO-MRW criteria are not adequate for diagnosing

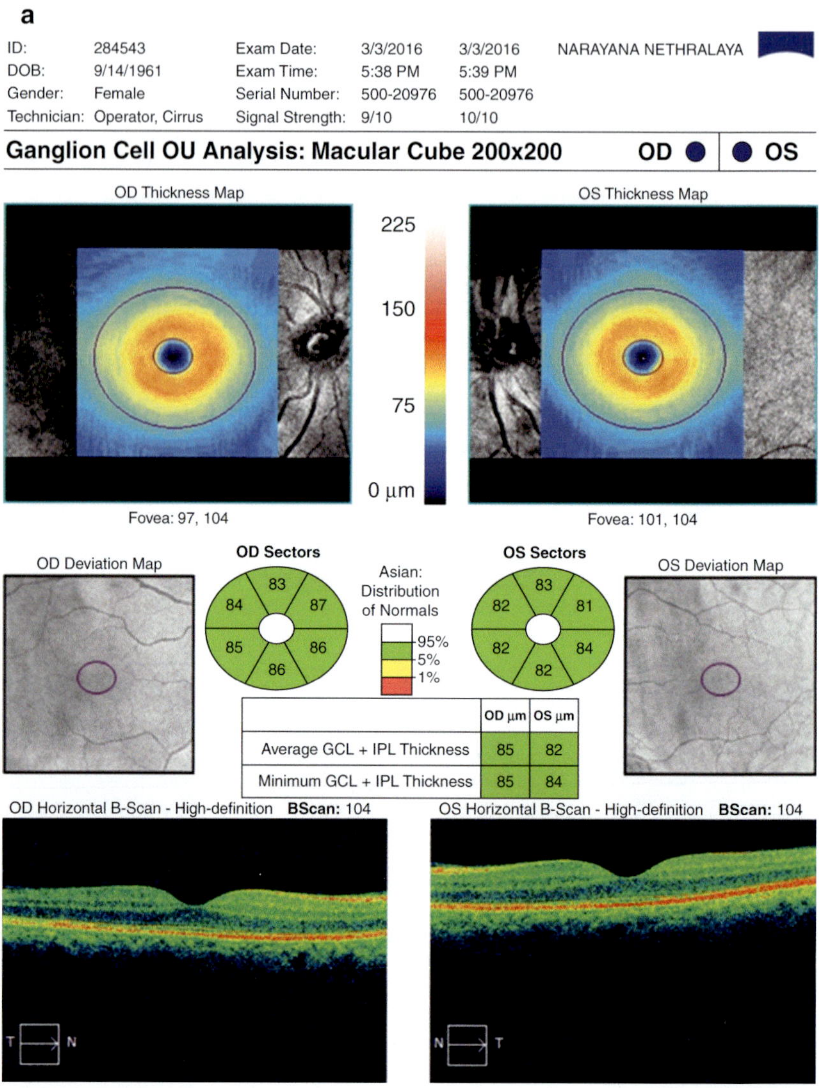

Fig. 20.11 Macular scan of a normal subject (a) and a glaucoma patient (b) showing the analysis of ganglion cell-inner plexiform layer (GCIPL) thickness. Interpretation of the macular report is similar to that described for the retinal nerve fiber layer (RNFL) report in Fig. 20.10. Figure (b) shows normal GCIPL thickness in right eye but superior GCIPL thinning in left eye, which is shown on GCIPL thickness, deviation and sector maps

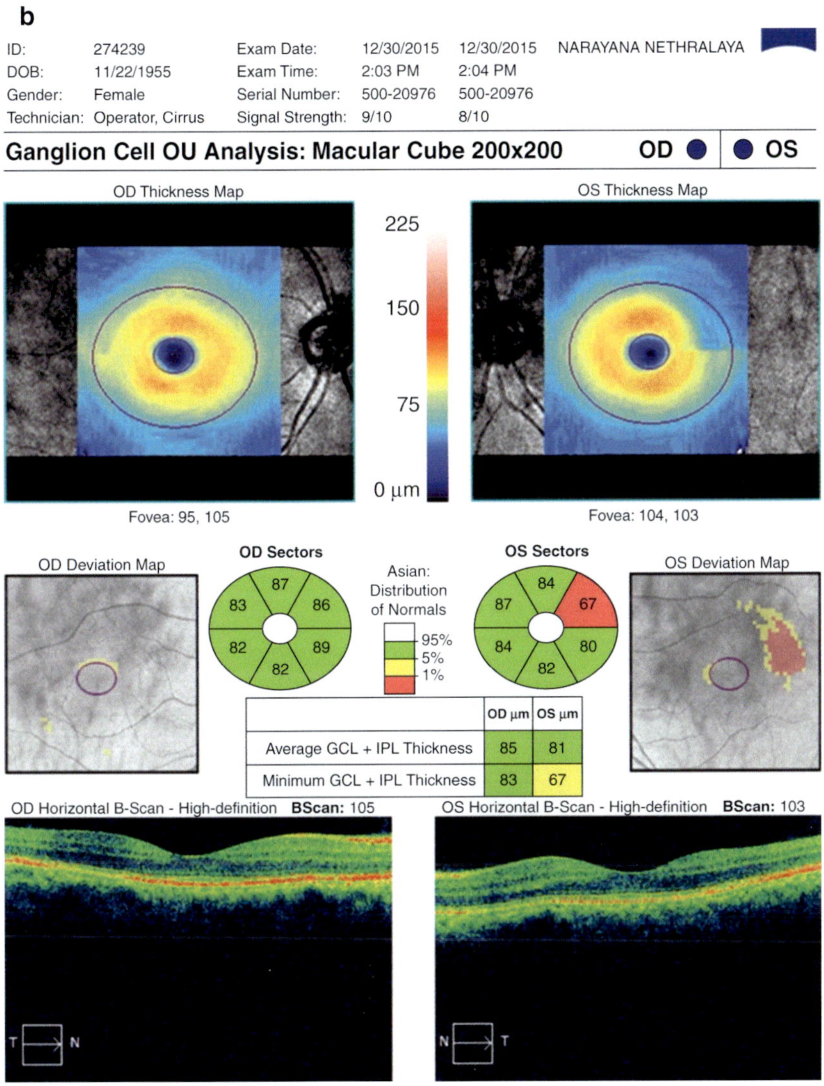

Fig. 20.11 (continued)

glaucoma in AD individuals [26]. More studies are needed to clarify the racial differences in the performance of OCT in detecting glaucoma.

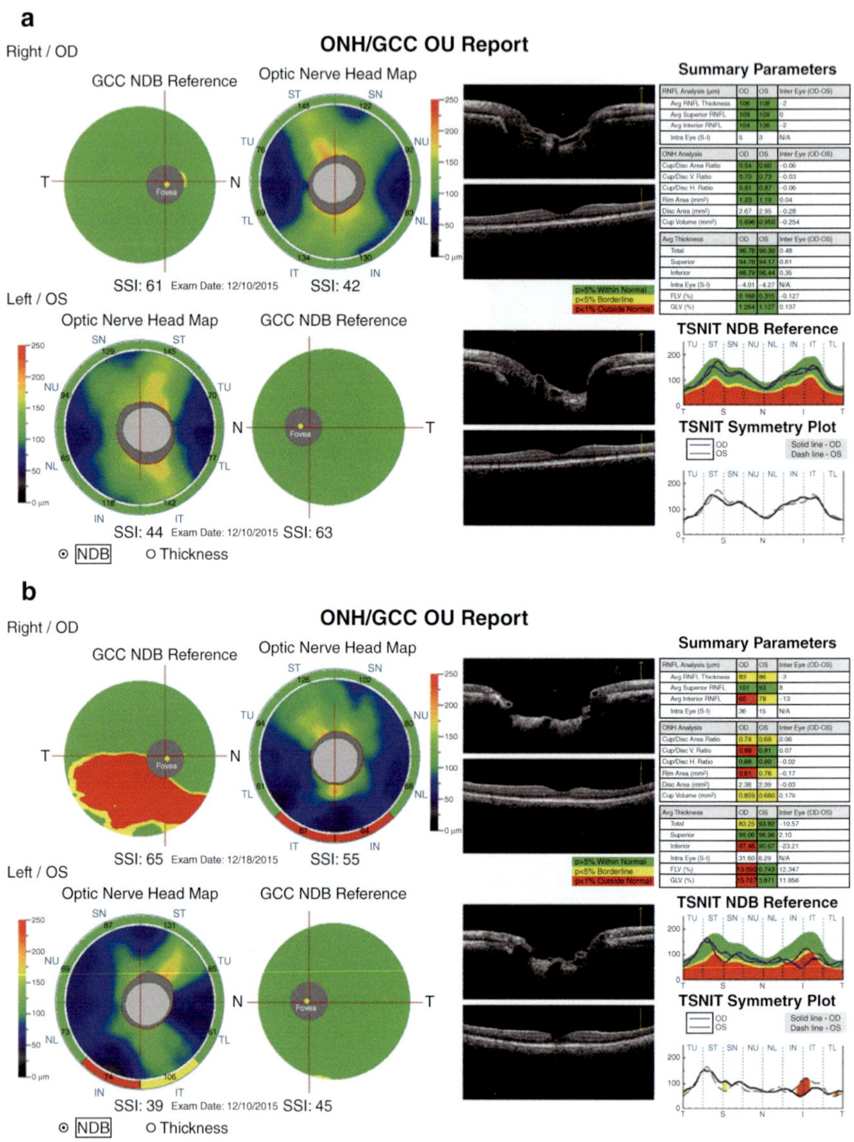

Fig. 20.12 Optic nerve head (ONH), retinal nerve fiber layer (RNFL) and ganglion cell complex (GCC) analysis report of a normal subject (a) and a glaucoma patient (b) from an OCT device. The interpretation of the report is similar to that described in Fig. 20.10. Figure (b) shows RNFL and GCC thinning in the inferior quadrant of right eye. Left eye in Figure (b) shows inferior quadrant RNFL thinning without any GCC abnormality

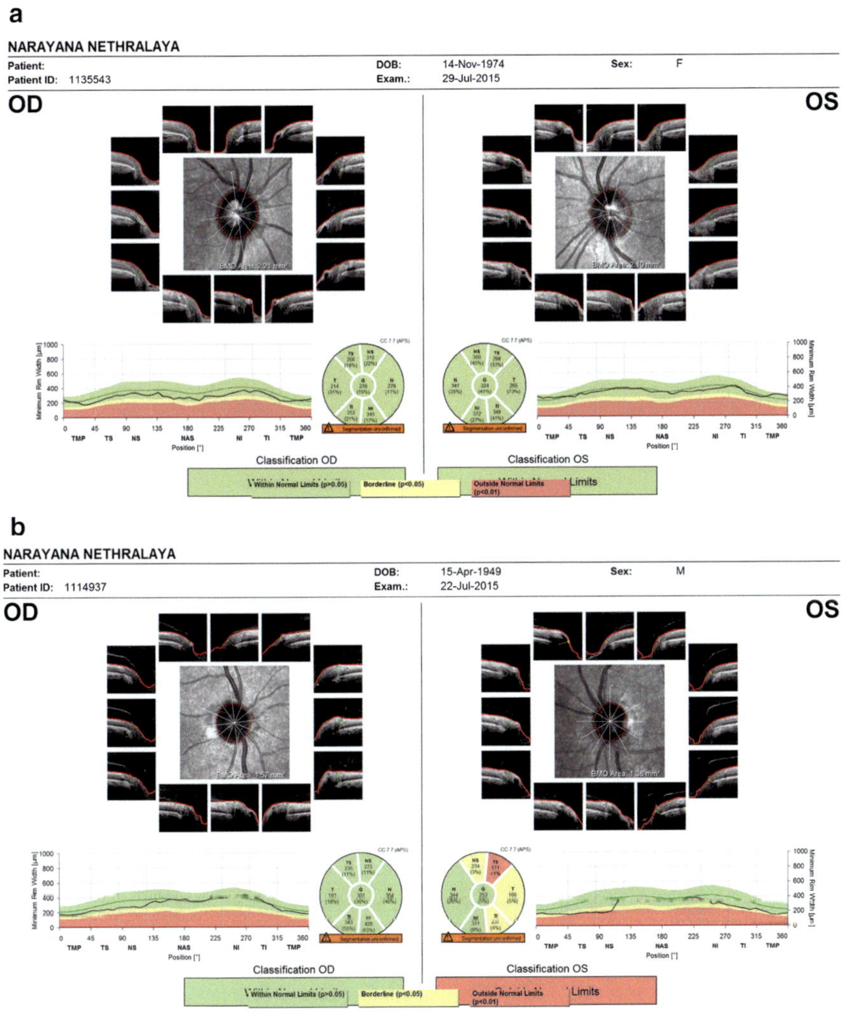

Fig. 20.13 Optic nerve head (ONH) report of a normal subject (a) and a glaucoma patient (b) from another OCT device showing the minimum rim width (MRW) at different sectors. Compared to the normal MRW measurements in Figures (a), Figure (b) shows MRW being thinner in the superior, temporal and inferior regions of left eye

20.7 OCT in Monitoring Glaucoma Progression

One of the most challenging aspects in the management of glaucoma is to diagnose progression early and accurately. Like for VF, software to detect progression on OCT also employ trend and event-based analyses. A trend-based analysis estimates the rate of change (slope) of the parameter over time. An event-based analysis

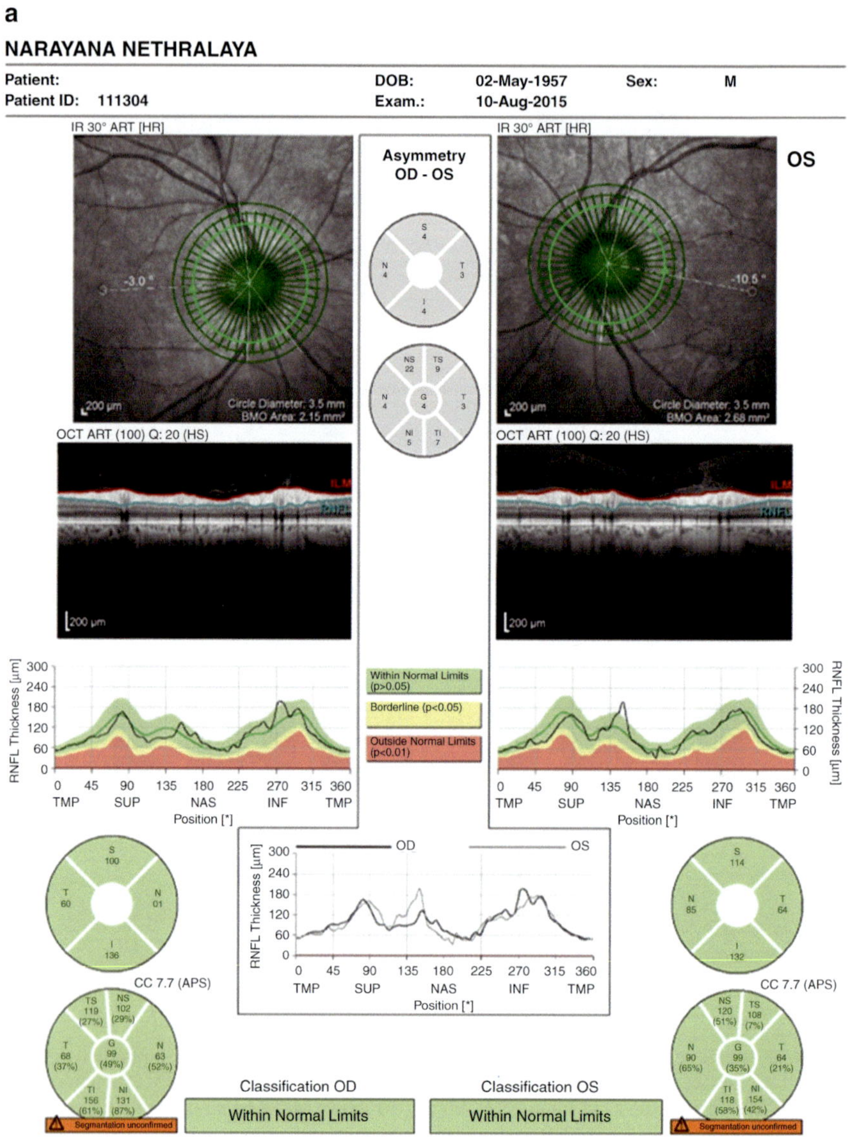

Fig. 20.14 Retinal nerve fiber layer (RNFL) report of a normal subject (a) and a glaucoma patient (b) from another OCT device. Compared to the RNFL report of the normal subject, glaucoma patient shows inferotemporal RNFL thinning in both eyes

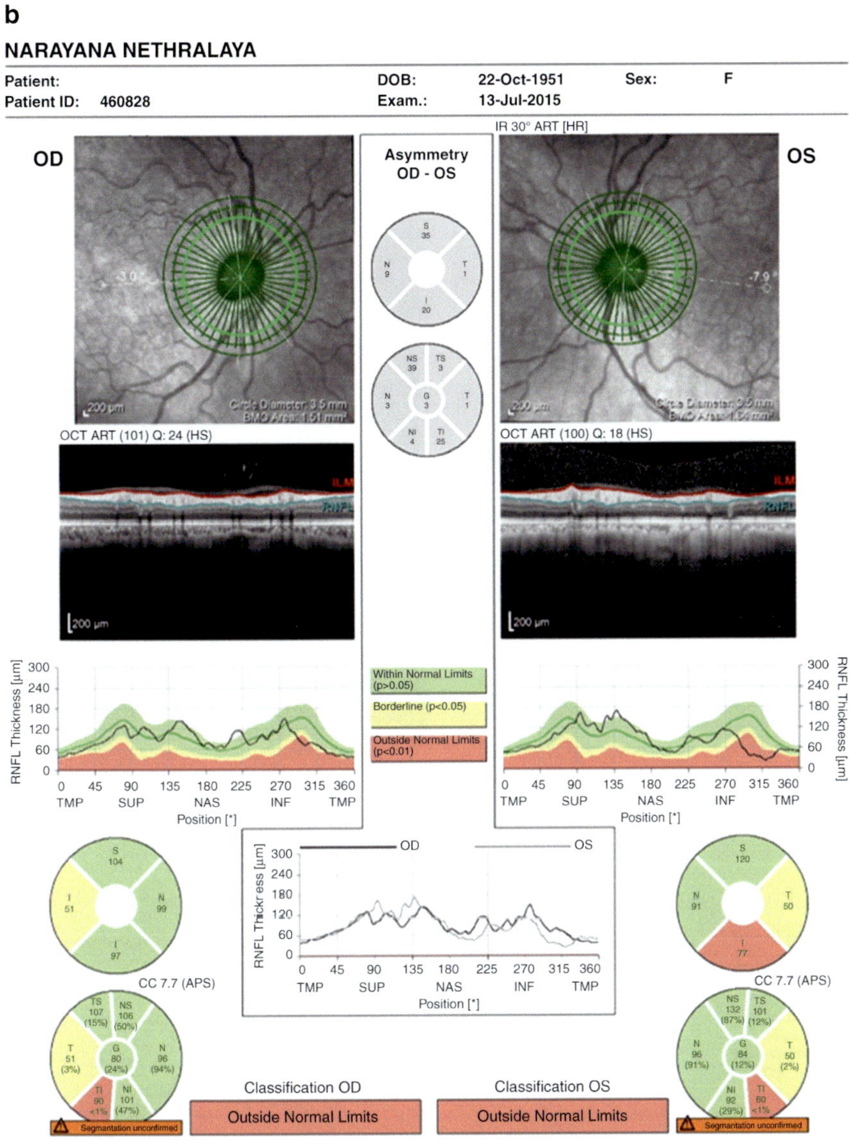

Fig. 20.14 (continued)

determines progression if the amount of change crosses a particular pre-set value (threshold).

Figure 20.18a shows the ONH/RNFL progression report of one OCT device which uses both the trend- and the event-based progression analyses. The report includes three analyses:

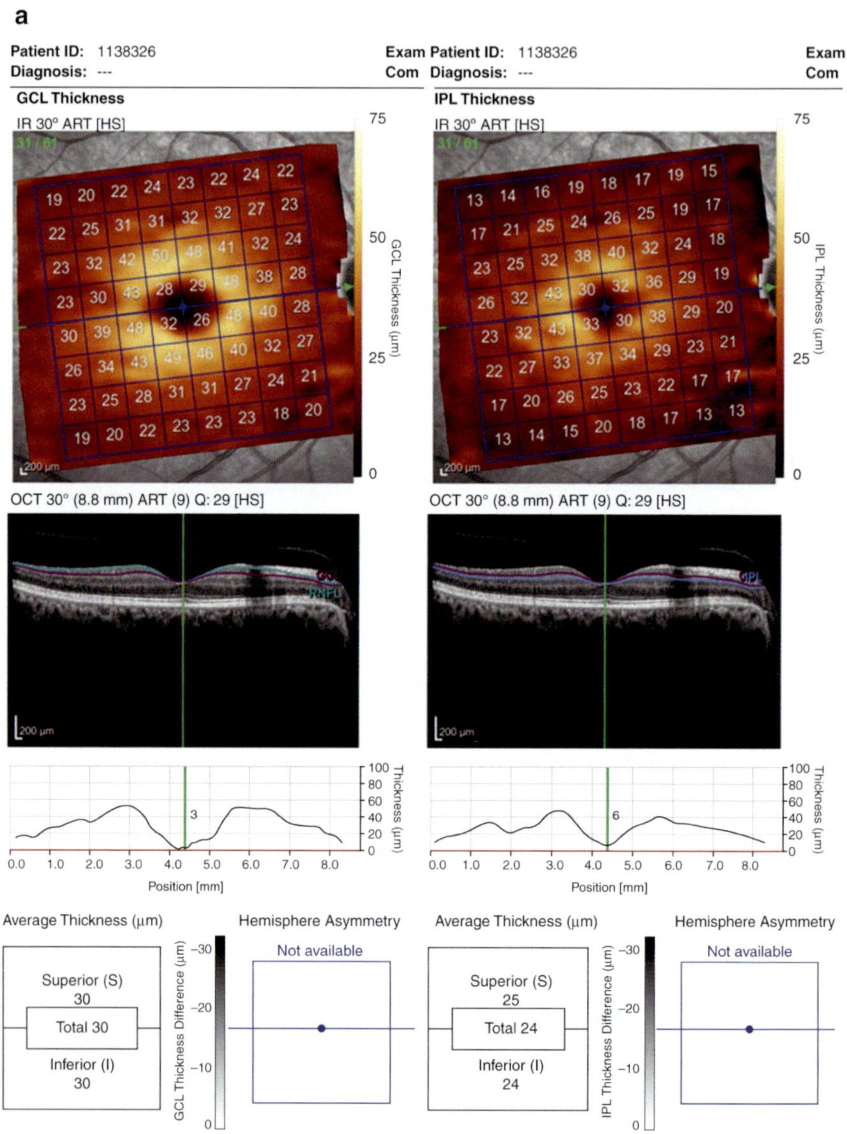

Fig. 20.15 Macular analysis report of a normal (a) and a glaucomatous eye (b) from another OCT device. Each layer of retina is analysed separately in this device, and ganglion cell layer (GCL) and inner plexiform layer (IPL) analysis is shown here. For each layer, the thickness is assessed at 64 cubes across the entire scan region and overlaid on the thickness map. The comparison between the superior and inferior hemispheres is also provided. Compared to the normal eye, the glaucomatous eye shows thinning of both the GCL and IPL in the inferior hemisphere

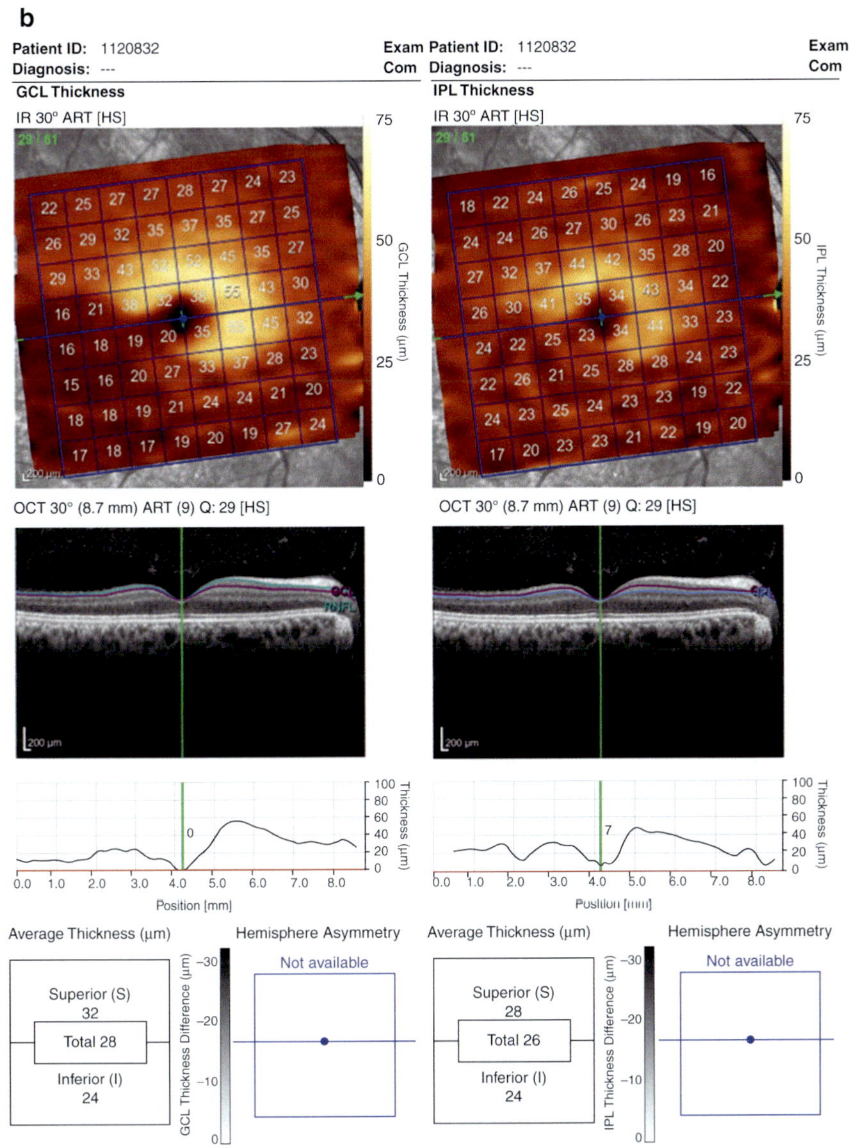

Fig. 20.15 (continued)

1. a chronological display of RNFL thickness maps and RNFL thickness change maps
2. average cup to disc ratio (CDR), superior, inferior and average RNFL thickness graphs representing rate of change, and
3. RNFL thickness profiles comparing the current exam to the baseline exams.

Two good quality baseline exams are required for these analyses, and two good quality follow-up exams are required to confirm likely change in the ONH and RNFL parameters. Statistically significant changes are summarized with color-codes for possible or likely RNFL thickness loss (or possible RNFL thickness increase).

RNFL thickness map and thickness change map are based on event-based analysis, which compares the follow-up exams with the baseline exams and marks out the RNFL regions which have changed by an amount greater than the test–retest variability. When a particular region exceeded the test–retest variability for the first time, it is flagged as a "possible loss" and coded in yellow. When the same region shows a change beyond the test–retest variability in a subsequent exam, it is flagged as a "likely loss" and coded in red. When a particular region shows an increase in RNFL thickness beyond the test–retest variability, it is flagged as a "possible increase" and coded in lavender. In the absence of concurrent retinal pathologies, "possible increase" generally occurs if the baseline exams include poor quality scans with an improvement in scan quality subsequently. RNFL thickness change map is preferred for the detection of focal changes.

RNFL thickness profile analysis is also an event-based analysis, which compares the RNFL profile of the current examination to that of the baseline exams. It detects the regions on the RNFL profile graph that have decreased beyond the expected test–retest variability. The regions showing the change are flagged as "possible loss", "likely loss" or "possible increase" as mentioned above. RNFL

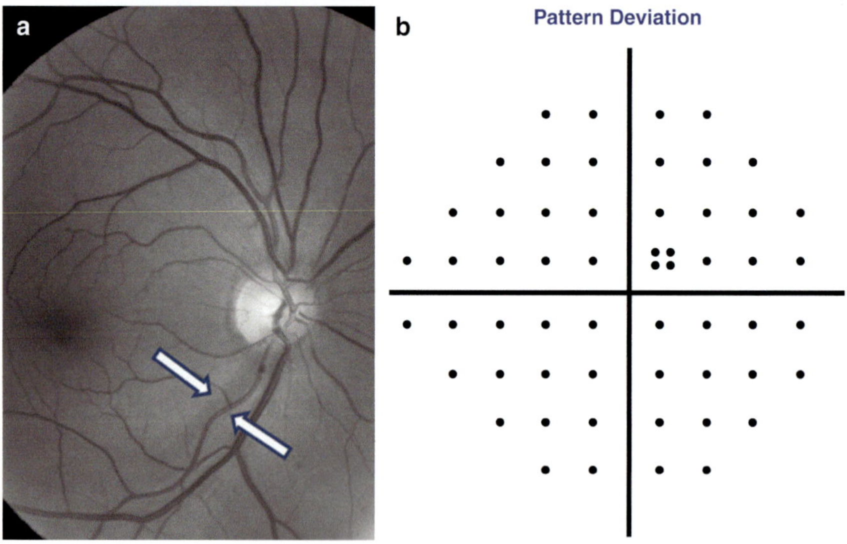

Fig. 20.16 An example of a right eye showing neuroretinal rim thinning and the presence of a retinal nerve fiber layer (RNFL) defect inferiorly on the optic disc photograph (a) but normal visual field (b). OCT confirms the presence of RNFL thinning on RNFL thickness map, deviation map and clock-hour map (c)

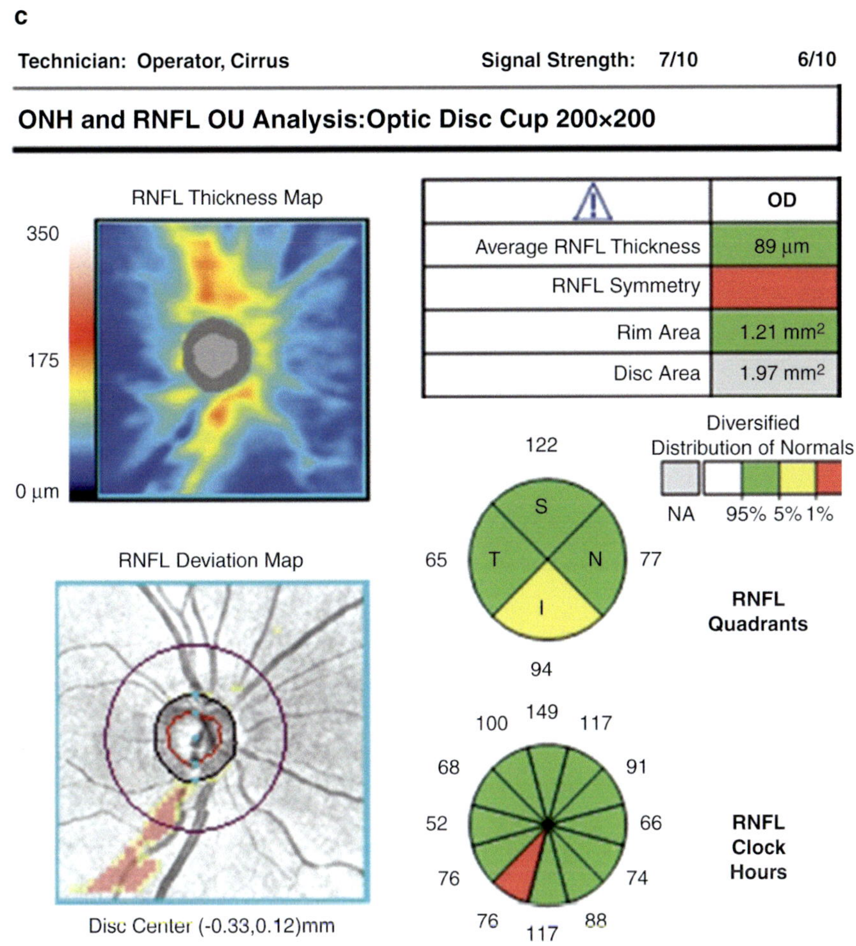

Fig. 20.16 (continued)

thickness profile analysis, like the RNFL thickness and change map, is preferred for detecting focal changes.

Average cup to disc ratio (CDR) and RNFL thickness graphs use trend-based analysis to evaluate the rate of change in average CDR, superior, inferior and average RNFL thickness measurements over time. Rate of change in these trend-based analyses is estimated using linear regression. The individual data points (from each examination) are highlighted (color-coded) to indicate when the amount of change in the parameter exceeds the test–retest variability. The result shows up as "possible loss" when the rate of loss is statistically significant for only a single visit and is indicated by a yellow symbol. The result shows up as "likely loss" when the rate of loss is statistically significant for two visits in a row and is indicated by a red symbol. Average thickness graphs are preferred for the detection

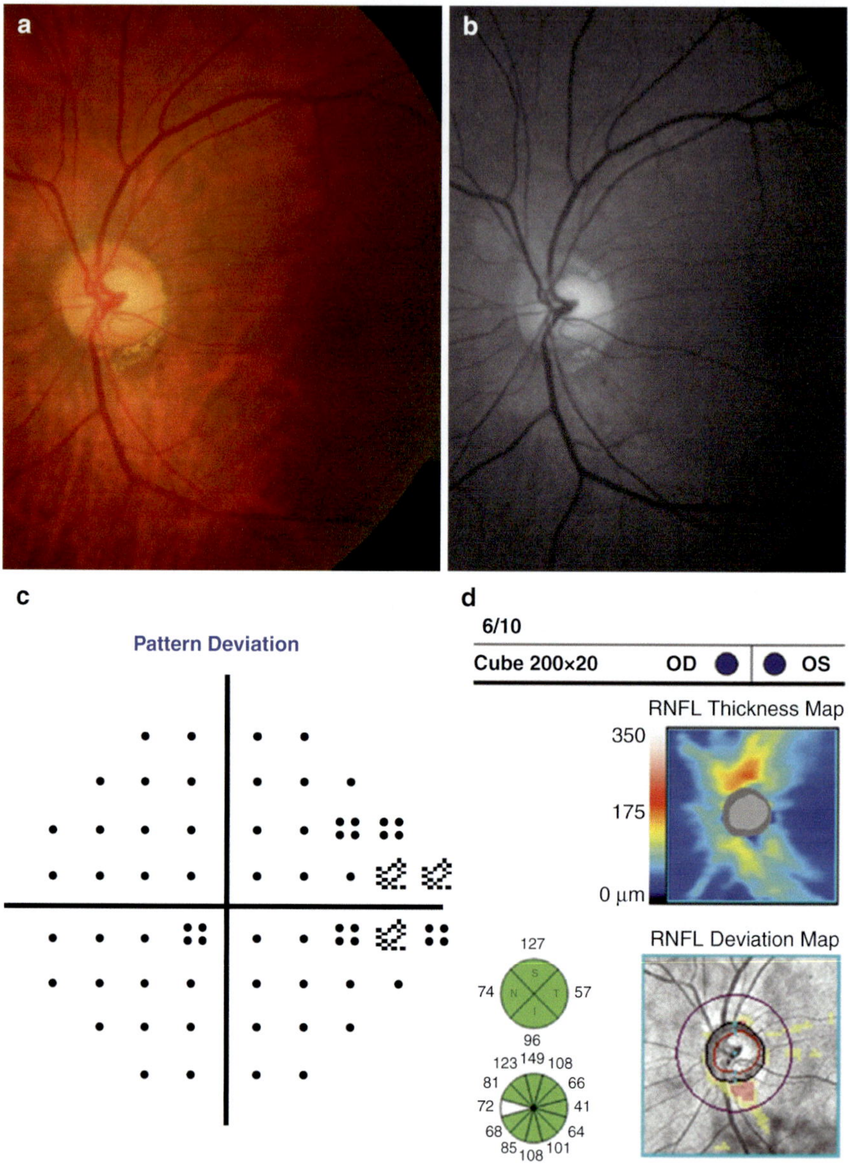

Fig. 20.17 An example of an eye showing suspicious optic disc (a), a possible inferotemporal retinal nerve fiber layer (RNFL) defect on red-free photograph (b) and a probable nasal defect on visual fields (c). OCT confirms the presence of inferotemporal RNFL thinning on the thickness map and deviation map (d). It can be noted that the clock-hour and quadrant maps do not show any RNFL abnormality; these maps are known to have a poorer diagnostic ability as compared to the thickness and deviation maps

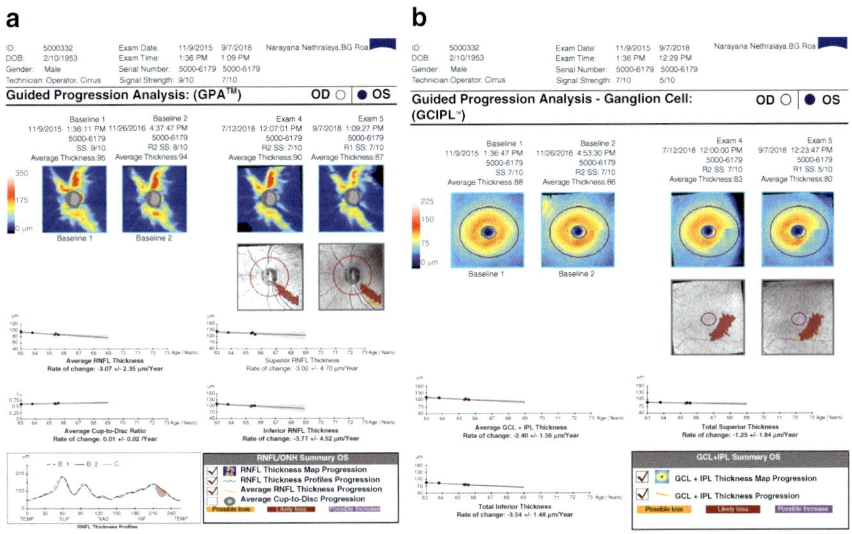

Fig. 20.18 Optic nerve head (ONH)/retinal nerve fiber layer (RNFL) progression analysis of an OCT device (a) showing disease progression on both event and trend-based methods. Two good quality baseline exams are required for all analyses and two good quality follow-up exams are required to confirm "likely change" in the ONH and RNFL parameters. The progression report includes "RNFL thickness change map", an event-based analysis, which marks out the RNFL regions which have changed by an amount greater than the test–retest variability, "RNFL thickness graphs", trend-based analyses, which evaluate the rate of change of superior, inferior and average RNFL thickness measurements over time and "RNFL thickness profile analysis", also an event-based analysis, which detects the regions on the RNFL profile graph that have decreased beyond the expected test–retest variability. Macular (GCIPL thickness) analysis (b) showing disease progression on both event and trend-based methods. The report of GCIPL progression analysis, similar to the ONH/RNFL report, includes "GCIPL thickness change map", an event-based analysis, and "GCIPL thickness graphs", a trend-based analysis

of diffuse changes, in contrast to the two maps mentioned previously for detecting focal changes. Figure 20.18b shows the macular progression analysis report, which is interpreted similarly as the RNFL progression report detailed above.

Figure 20.19 shows the progression analysis report from another OCT device which employs a trend-based method to evaluate the rates of change of RNFL and macular (GCC) thicknesses over time. The rate of change is high-lighted (as shown in the figure) according to the p value of the slope. In the example figure, both RNFL and GCC thicknesses are decreasing at a magnitude which is statistically significant.

Figure 20.20 shows the trend-based analysis of the global RNFL thickness (Fig. 20.20a) and the global MRW (Fig. 20.20b) of an OCT device. The analysis shows the magnitude of change in the parameters over time (the slope of change), as well as the *p* value associated with the slope.

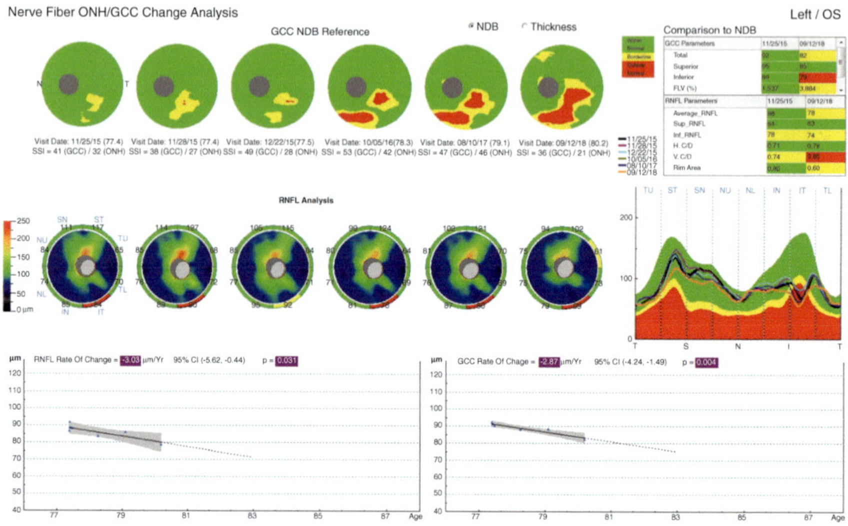

Fig. 20.19 Retinal nerve fiber layer (RNFL) and ganglion cell complex (GCC) thickness progression analysis of an OCT device showing significant deterioration of average RNFL and GCC thickness on the trend-based analysis

As demonstrated above, OCT analyses ONH, RNFL and macular parameters for progression; therefore, it is of interest to evaluate which of these parameters is useful in detecting progression early and at all stages of disease severity [27].

Kim et al. investigated the temporal relationship between GCIPL change and corresponding peripapillary RNFL thinning on the OCT deviation maps in early-stage POAG, and found the former is frequently detected before the latter [28]. They concluded that peripapillary RNFL analysis alone likely would overlook macular damage, and macular imaging should be included in longitudinal follow-up for glaucoma [28]. In the study by Hwang et al., progression was found to be more frequent in RNFL than GCIPL thickness [29]. Of the 106 eyes that showed either RNFL and/or GCIPL progression in a cohort of 527 glaucoma eyes, 51% showed RNFL progression earlier, 12% showed GCIPL progression earlier, and 37% showed simultaneous RNFL/GCIPL progression [29]. Another study by Hou et al. investigated the temporal relationship among progressive macular GCIPL thinning, progressive RNFL thinning, and VF progression in POAG eyes followed for ≥5 years [30]. GPA detected progressive thinning in GCIPL and RNFL in 25% and 29% of eyes at a specificity of 95.5% and 91.0%, respectively. In their study, progressive GCIPL thinning and progressive RNFL thinning are mutually predictive. Additionally, eyes with progressive GCIPL and RNFL thinning were at a higher risk of VF progression, although VF progression did not predict progressive RNFL or GCIPL thinning [30]. They concluded that integrating GCIPL and RNFL measurements is relevant to facilitate early detection of glaucoma deterioration [30]. Recently, Mohammadzadeh et al. studied a cohort of glaucoma suspect

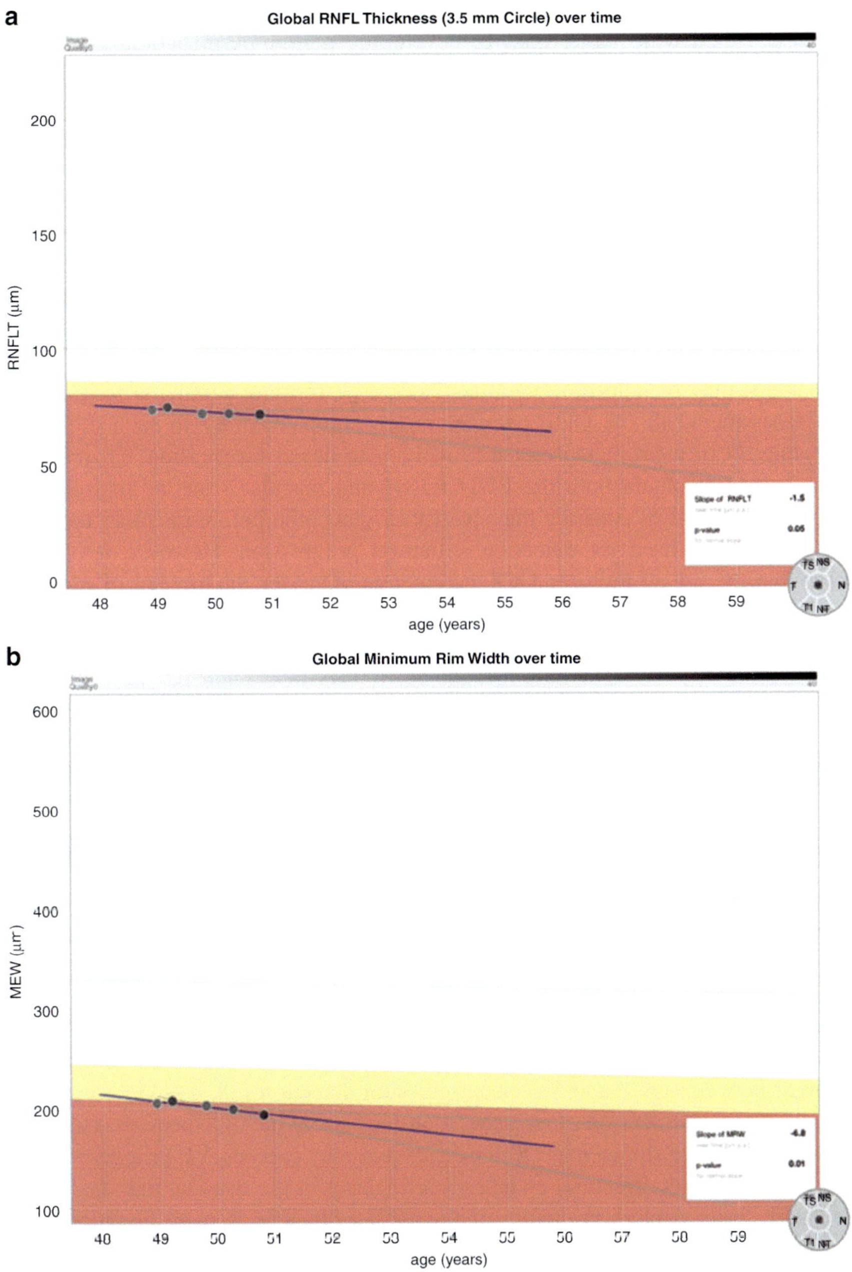

Fig. 20.20 Trend-based progression analysis of global retinal nerve fiber layer (RNFL) thickness and minimum rim width (MRW) of an OCT device (source: Dr. Sebastian Rausch, Heidelberg Engineering)

eyes and found faster rates of both GCIPL and circumpapillary RNFL thinning were associated with higher risks of developing perimetric glaucoma [31]. They suggested both parameters may be useful for monitoring VF deterioration in eyes with suspected glaucoma.

Interested to see whether OCT may readily detect progression as glaucoma worsens, Lavinsky et al. found that OCT macular and ONH parameters can detect progression even in advanced cases, where the RNFL thickness had reached a "floor" (explained below) [32]. The study by Rabiolo et al. further compared the rates of progression among macular OCT measurements [33]. They concluded that GCC thickness, in comparison to GCIPL, ganglion cell layer, outer retinal layer and full macular thicknesses, is most likely to detect structural worsening along the spectrum of glaucoma severity.

While it may be helpful to identify the best-performing parameter for progression assessment, all the OCT parameters are complementary to each other and analysing all of them increases the sensitivity to detect progression. Therefore, it is preferable to obtain both the RNFL/ONH and macular scans at all follow-up examinations, and to consider the severity of glaucoma before deciding the OCT parameter to be used for detecting structural progression. However, it is to be noted that the use of multiple OCT parameters increases the number of eyes that are falsely labelled as progressing [27].

The magnitude of decrease in OCT measurements that is clinically significant is also debatable. For example, a range from 1.88 to 6.5 μm has been reported for the test–retest variability (TRV) of OCT-measured RNFL thickness [9, 34–40]. Similarly, variable TRVs have been reported in different studies for macular OCT measurements. Such variability in the TRVs reported across studies might be associated with the differing OCT devices used and the discrepant study design, since the aging effect might be more pronounced when evaluating long-term TRV, as compared to short-term TRV. In general, a change of 3–4 μm for GCIPL, 4–5 μm for average RNFL, and 6–7 μm for inferior and superior sectoral RNFL thickness should be considered clinically significant, and this can be used as a thumb rule to aid decision making.

The relevance of structural progression detected by OCT is frequently questioned because it is believed that functional progression detected by VF is more important from the patients' perspective. Overall, a slight-to-fair agreement was reported between OCT and VF on progression detection [38, 41–43], suggesting only limited agreement on progressors identified using the two methods. However, some studies have shown that OCT progression may precede VF progression [44, 45], and that faster structural changes, particularly in the macula, may be associated with faster decline in quality of life (QoL) [46–48]. Recent literatures have shown structural change in the macula is associated with central VF (CVF) defect and visual acuity loss, both of which are pertinent to the vision-related QoL of glaucoma patients [48–51]. A higher risk of faster CVF worsening has been found for patients with thinner macular GCC measurement and more rapid GCC thinning [52, 53]. OCT therefore offers the possibility of detecting patients at high risk of VF progression, who should be followed more closely in order to provide augmenting treatment early.

The timing and number of OCT tests needed to detect progressive RNFL worsening has been investigated in several studies. In a computer simulation by Mahmoudinezhad et al., when OCT was performed 2 and 3 times per year, the time to detect progression in 80% of the glaucoma eyes with a circumpapillary RNFL thinning rate of -1 μm/year was 5.0 and 4.2 years, respectively [54]. The authors concluded that there was no difference between performing OCT two or three times annually for the time to progression detection. On the other hand, Bradley et al. suggested that increasing the number or frequency of OCT tests, as well as using a clustered measurement strategy, can help to more accurately capture RNFL worsening [55]. In their simulation, the accuracy of diagnosing moderate-to-rapid RNFL worsening (75–90th percentile) within a 2-year period was improved from less than 50% to 60% when the number of OCT scans increased from 3 to 7 with a clustered strategy. Furthermore, the accuracy of detecting an RNFL thinning rate of –3 μm/year or worse within 13 measurements can be improved from 58 to 75% with a clustered measurement strategy, rather than spaced measurement strategy [55].

Summary

It is important to note that the OCT progression analysis gives us statistically significant change, but not necessary clinically significant change. Furthermore, studies on clinical factors potentially affecting longitudinal OCT measurement change remain limited [9, 56]. Therefore, the results of OCT progression analysis should not be interpreted independently but in the context of the entire clinical picture. It is important to consider the results of the clinical evaluation (intraocular pressure, disease stage, occurrence of disc hemorrhage, increase in beta peripapillary atrophic region, etc.) and the VF along with the OCT findings while determining glaucoma progression.

20.8 Lamina Cribrosa Imaging

The lamina cribrosa (LC) is a multi-layered sieve-like structure in the sclera where retinal ganglion cell axons exit from the eye. The LC has been known to play a critical role in the pathogenesis of glaucoma [57]. Blockage of axonal transport within the LC has been proposed as a salient pathogenic mechanism for glaucoma. It is assumed that the LC provides mechanical support to the nerve fibers traversing the deeper ocular structures. Deformation of LC presumably from elevated IOP likely hinders axoplasmic flow and thus disrupts transport of trophic factors critical to retinal ganglion cells, thereby causing neuronal death that is characteristic of glaucoma. Furthermore, the LC represents a biomechanical discontinuity in the spherical casing of the eye, so that the globe is more vulnerable to stress loading that may play a role in glaucoma. Understanding such forces that affect the structure of the LC, through both focal and general morphologic changes, would clarify the mechanisms of glaucoma. A detailed study of the LC, however, requires accurate and clear visualization of this structure. Clinical examination of the LC structures cannot be performed routinely with current diagnostic methods.

Advances in OCT technology have enabled in vivo visualization of the LC now [58–60]. The enhanced depth imaging (EDI) technique for example, has provided better image contrast for the deep portion of the ONH [61, 62]. OCT light-attenuation software such as adaptive compensation has further improved LC visibility by effective blood-vessel shadow removal and better differentiation of tissue boundaries [63, 64]. Swept-source OCT (SS-OCT), which incorporates a longer-wavelength (1050 nm) light source than SD-OCT, reduces light dispersion from blood vessels, thereby allowing for high-resolution imaging of the LC [65].

LC findings on OCT are commonly categorized in terms of position (LC depth and LC insertion depth), curvature or shape, and microarchitectural change (LC defect) [66].

LC depth (LCD, Fig. 20.21) is defined as the maximum or mean vertical distance from the anterior LC surface to the reference plane of Bruch's membrane opening (BMO). Multiple studies have demonstrated that the LCD is greater in eyes with glaucoma compared to healthy eyes [67–69]. LCD was also noted to reduce when the IOP in glaucomatous eyes was lowered after the introduction of medical therapy [70], or after glaucoma filtration surgery [71, 72]. In prospective studies, greater LCD was also associated with greater visual field progression [73] and faster rates of retinal nerve fibre layer (RNFL) thinning [74]. However, one of the limitation of calculating LCD is that it requires the use of a reference plane and BMO, which is used as the reference plane commonly, includes choroidal thickness in its measurement. Choroidal thickness varies with age and other non-glaucomatous pathologies and therefore can affect the LCD measurement [75, 76].

Similar to LCD, lamina cribrosa insertion (LCI, Fig. 20.21), the region wherein the vascular perfusion from the capillaries of the short posterior ciliary artery drains to the LC [77], is reported to migrate posteriorly in glaucoma [78]. Determining LCI depth also requires the use of a reference plane.

To overcome the challenges of LCD and LCI depth determination, LC curvature, which does not require the use of a reference plane, has been proposed as an alternative structural parameter that is useful in glaucoma. LC curvature has been evaluated by measuring the difference between the mean LCD and the anterior LCI depth, in both the horizontal and vertical meridians [79]. The lamina cribrosa curvature index (LCCI), an indicator of the extent of LC curvature, is reported to have a significantly better diagnostic performance than LCD that is comparable to RNFL thickness. In another prospective study, a faster rate of RNFL loss was found associated with greater LCCI [80]. All the above LC parameters on OCT are based only on the anterior surface of LC and the posterior surface of LC is difficult to image on OCT [81].

Focal LC defect (FLD) is representative of focal LC-microstructural change. On OCT, it is seen as an anterior laminar surface irregularity manifesting as a laminar hole or disinsertion that violates the normal smooth curvilinear contours

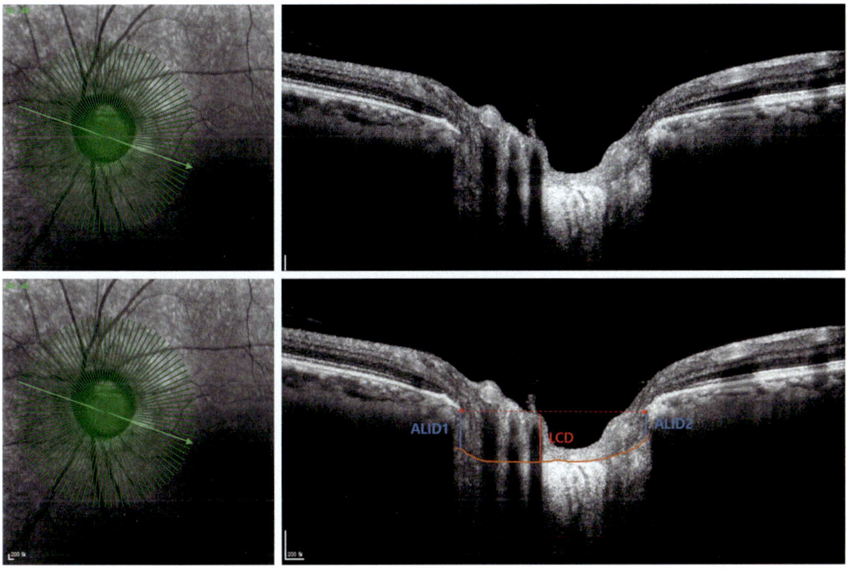

Fig. 20.21 The anterior laminar insertion depth (ALID) is defined as the perpendicular distance between the Bruch's membrane openings (BMO, red dots) and the anterior laminar insertion (ends of the orange line). The lamina cribrosa depth (LCD) is measured as the vertical distance between the BMO reference plane (red dotted line) and the maximally depressed point of the anterior laminar surface (orange line). (Image courtesy: Minh H. Suh, Department of Ophthalmology, Haeundae Paik Hospital, Inje University College of Medicine, Busan, South Korea)

of the LC (Fig. 20.22) [82]. FLD presents clinically as an acquired pit of optic nerve, rim thinning or notching, and has shown a spatial correlation with VF defect and localized RNFL defects [83, 84]. FLDs are also associated with presence of disc hemorrhages [85, 86]. Eyes with FLDs showed a faster rate of glaucoma progression [87–90].

20.9 Limitations of OCT

The quality of OCT scan is crucial to structural assessment in glaucoma. The segmentation algorithms of OCT software often fail in poor-quality scans, leading to erroneous measurements. It was reported that OCT segmentation error may cause underestimated (thinner) structural measurement, and a larger difference in measurement is associated with older age, thinner RNFL, and worse scan quality value [91]. As scan quality is known to significantly affect the ability of OCT to detect glaucomatous defects [92, 93], it is important to perform image quality review and manual refinement of segmentation, if needed, before interpreting OCT results. Using OCT in highly myopic eyes is also challenging as a result of the greater difficulty in obtaining a good-quality image and comparisons drawn using a

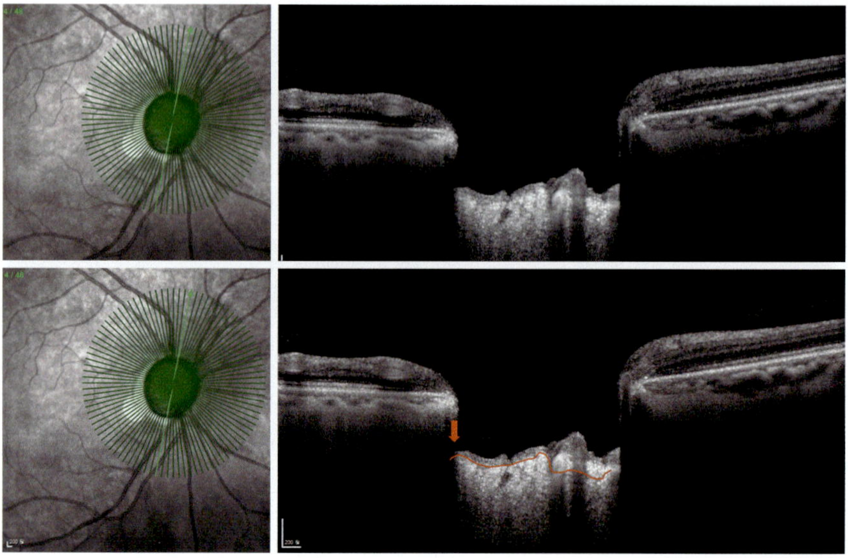

Fig. 20.22 Focal lamina cribrosa defect (FLD) observed in the inferotemporal region of the optic nerve head. (Image courtesy: Minh H. Suh, Department of Ophthalmology, Haeundae Paik Hospital, Inje University College of Medicine, Busan, South Korea)

dissimilar reference database. Additionally, certain clinical findings that are crucial in decision making, such as neuroretinal rim pallor and disc hemorrhages [94], are not picked up by the OCT.

OCT measurements are known to level off in more advanced stages of glaucoma. RNFL thickness, for example, levels off when the corresponding functional loss on automated perimetry reaches a severity of −10 to −15 dB [95, 96]. Further deterioration in the glaucoma severity causes little change in the RNFL thickness, resulting in a floor effect (Fig. 20.23). It has to be noted that the floor may be at different levels for different OCT parameters, and GCIPL and ONH measurements may still be able to detect progression in eyes where the RNFL thickness has reached a floor [32, 97]. Specifically, in the study by Bowd et al. on moderate-advanced glaucoma eyes, the average floors were 105 μm, 38 μm, and 38 μm for minimum rim width (MRW), GCIPL, and circumpapillary RNFL thickness, respectively [97]. Since more GCIPL tissue remained above the measurement floor compared to other measurements, they concluded GCIPL thickness might perform better in detecting structural progression in advanced cases [97]. Therefore, when assessing longitudinal structural thinning in eyes with more severe glaucoma by OCT, it is essential to consider the measurement floor of the parameters to prevent delayed detection of glaucoma progression.

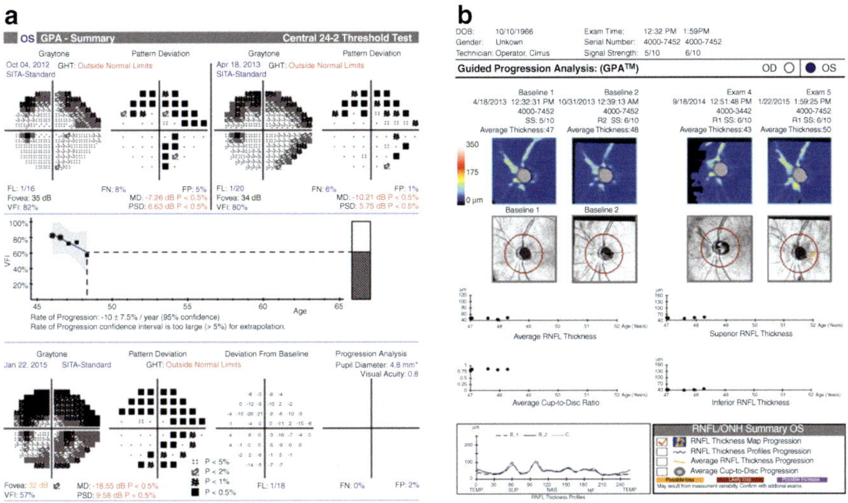

Fig. 20.23 An example of a left eye showing obvious progression on visual fields (a) but showing no progression on retinal nerve fiber layer (RNFL) analysis of OCT due to the 'floor effect'

20.10 OCT Angiography (OCTA)

OCT has also been used to non-invasively delineate the vasculature of the retina and ONH. Doppler OCT was one of the earliest techniques developed for vascular imaging. It assessed blood flow by comparing phase differences between adjacent A-scans [98]. Although Doppler OCT was appropriate for large vessels around the disc, it was not sensitive enough to measure accurately the low velocities in small vessels that make up the ONH and retinal microcirculation. The search for a simple, non-invasive, reproducible method of evaluating the ocular blood flow has led to the development of a technique called OCT angiography (OCTA).

OCTA is capable of imaging large vessels as well as microvasculature of the retina and ONH by performing multiple OCT scans of the same region. The variation in OCT signal at each location is then studied. Moving particles, such as red blood cells, result in a high variance of the OCT signal between repeated scans and this is used to identify blood vessels. Several algorithms have been developed to interpret the OCT signals and to delineate the blood vessels. Split spectrum amplitude decorrelation angiography (SSADA; Angiovue, RTVue-XR SD-OCT, Optovue Inc., Fremont, CA) is one such algorithm that uses the variation in the intensity of the OCT signal to identify blood vessels. The fluctuating value of OCT intensities is considered as the decorrelation (D). Thus, pixels in the B-scan frame where blood is flowing have fluctuating intensities and yield high D values (approaching 1). Pixels in the B-scan frames that contain static tissue yield small D values (approaching 0) [99]. The principles of SSADA have been explained in detail by Jia et al. [100]. The optical microangiography (OMAG), another algorithm that performs OCTA (Angioplex, Cirrus HD-OCT, Carl Zeiss Meditec Inc.,

Dublin, CA), uses the variation in intensity as well as the phase difference of the OCT signals for vessel delineation. As the time required to obtain the scan with OCTA is close to 3 s, involuntary saccades and changes in fixation during data acquisition can lead to motion artifacts that may confound the interpretation of the final OCT angiogram. Active eye tracking is therefore an essential feature of the OCTA devices.

Retina is segmented into different slabs, such as choriocapillaris, outer retina, deep retina and superficial retina, and vessels in each of these slabs is presented in 2-dimensional format. The macular OCTA scan is performed using a volumetric scan covering a 3 mm × 3 mm (Fig. 20.24) or a 6 mm × 6 mm areas (Fig. 20.25). The segmentation of retinal scan slabs differs slightly with different OCTA software versions [101]. In the Phase 7.0 software of Angiovue/RTVue-XR, the superficial retinal slab extends from the internal limiting membrane (ILM) to 10 μm below the inner plexiform layer (IPL). Deep retinal slab extends from 10 μm below IPL to 10 μm above the outer plexiform layer (OPL). Outer retinal slab extends from 10 μm above the OPL to 10 μm below the Bruch's membrane (BRM), and choroid capillary slab extends from 10 μm below the BRM to 30 μm below the BRM.

The optic disc OCTA scan is performed using volumetric scans covering an area of 4.5 mm × 4.5 mm. The optic disc region, similar to the macular region, is divided into several slabs for further analysis. Figure 20.26 shows the optic disc scan of one OCTA device. In the Phase 7.0 software of Angiovue/RTVue-XR, the most superficial "vitreous/retina" slab captures all the vasculatures above the OPL. The "radial peripapillary capillary (RPC)" slab extends from the ILM to the posterior boundary of the RNFL and is used for assessing the vascular supply of the RNFL layer of the peripapillary region. And the "choroidal slab" is used to assess the deep retinal and choroidal vasculature.

OCTA quantifies the ocular circulation using two parameters: flow index and vessel density. Flow index is defined as the average decorrelation values in the measured area, and vessel density (VD), which is the most widely used OCTA parameter, is defined as the percentage area occupied by vessels in the measured area [99]. The threshold decorrelation value used to separate blood vessel and static tissue is set at 0.125, which is two standard deviations above the mean decorrelation value in the foveal avascular zone (described below), a region devoid of vessels.

Quantification of VD can be performed in the vitreous/retina slab and the RPC slab of the optic disc scan, but not the choroidal slab. After acquiring the optic disc scan, the software automatically fits an ellipse to the optic disc margin. The region within this margin is referred to as the "inside disc' region. The circumpapillry/peripapillary region is defined as a 0.75 mm-wide elliptical annulus extending from the optic disc boundary. This region can be divided into 2 hemispheres of 180 degrees each (superior and inferior) and 4 sectors of 90 degrees each (nasal, inferior, superior, and temporal sectors). Additionally, it can be divided based on the Garway-Heath map and the temporal- superior-nasal-inferior-temporal (TSNIT) plot.

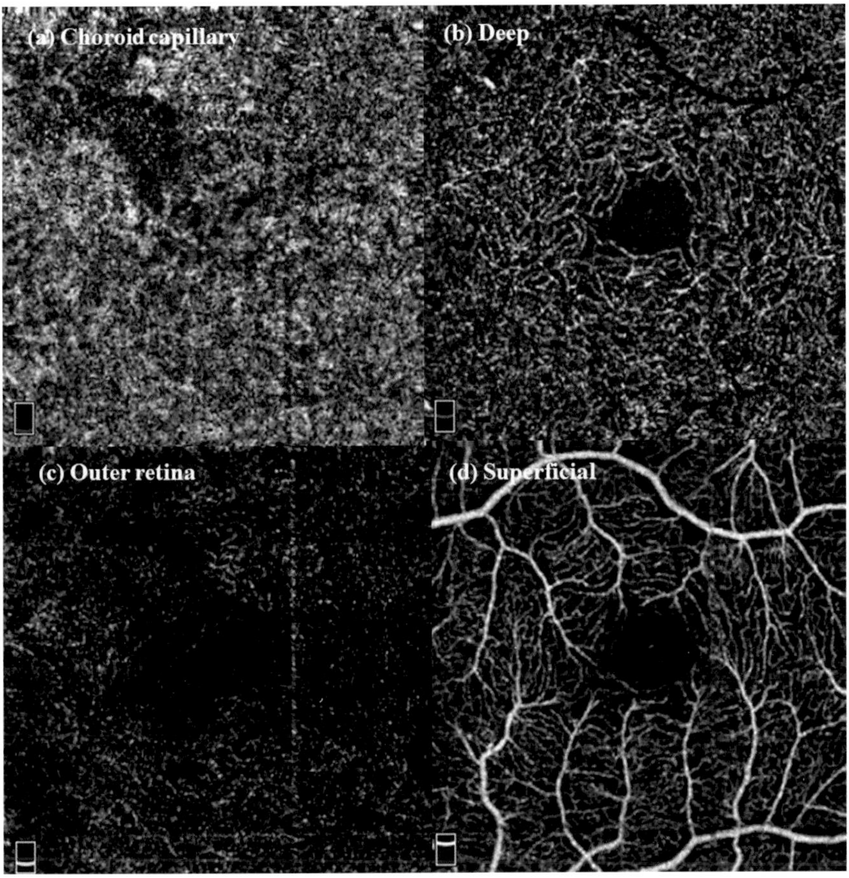

Fig. 20.24 Angiography slabs of the 3 mm × 3 mm macular scan obtained using spectral domain optical coherence tomography showing the choriocapillaris (a), deep retinal (b), outer retinal (c) and superficial retinal (d) slabs

Similarly, VD can also be determined for the superficial and deep vascular plexus of the macula scan. The macula is divided into the small central foveal area, the parafoveal region, and the perifoveal region (on 6 mm × 6 mm macular scan only) (Fig. 20.27). The parafoveal VD measurements are measured in both 3 mm × 3 mm and 6 mm × 6 mm macular scans, while the perifoveal VD measurements are only available from the 6 mm × 6 mm macular scan. Both parafoveal and perifoveal regions can be divided into superior/inferior hemispheres abd and nasal/inferior/superior/temporal sectors.

The current OCTA instruments do not contain a normative database for comparison of the patient's VD. Currently these comparisons are made in research studies using control eyes.

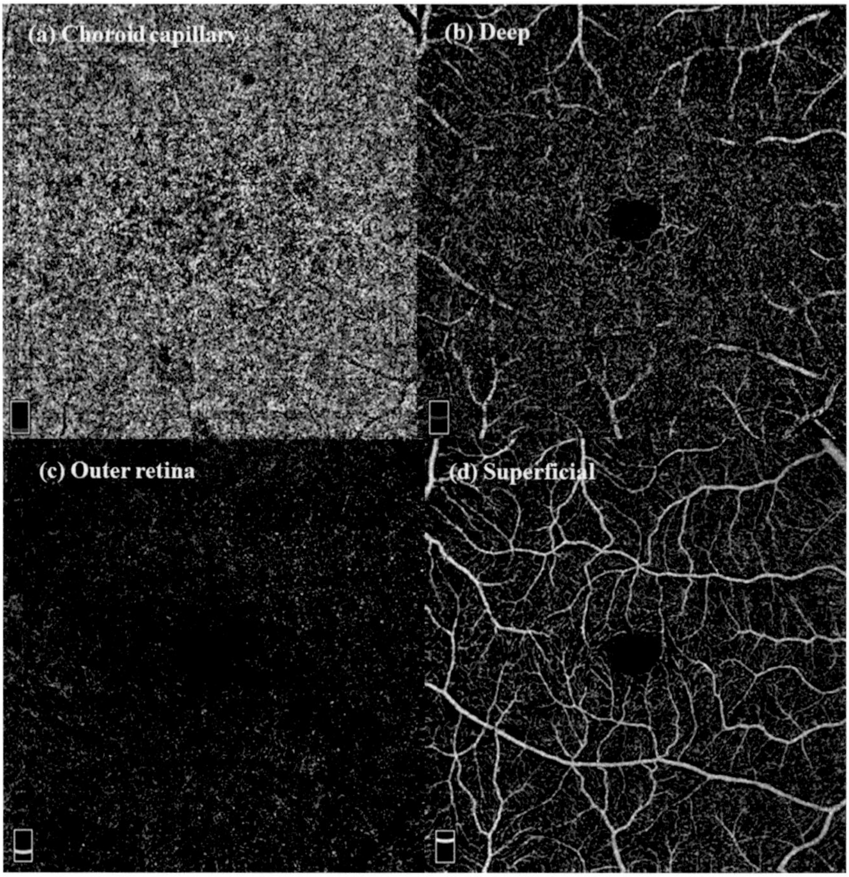

Fig. 20.25 Angiography slabs of the 6 mm × 6 mm macular scan obtained using spectral domain optical coherence tomography showing the choriocapillaris (a), deep retinal (b), outer retinal (c) and superficial retinal (d) slabs

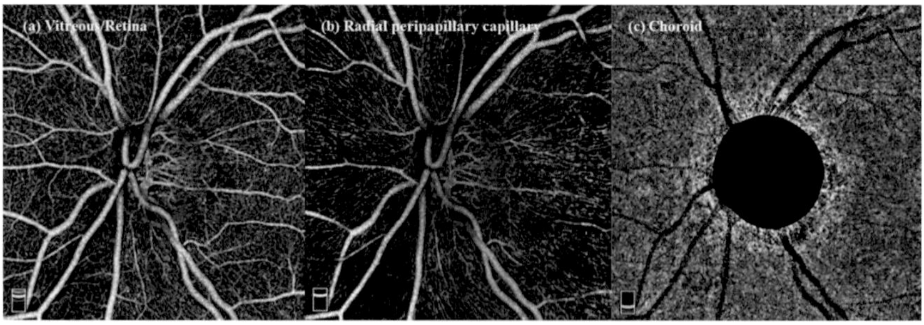

Fig. 20.26 Angiography slabs of the optic nerve head scan obtained using spectral domain optical coherence tomography showing the vitreous/retina (a), radial peripapillary capillary, RPC (b), and choroid (c) slabs

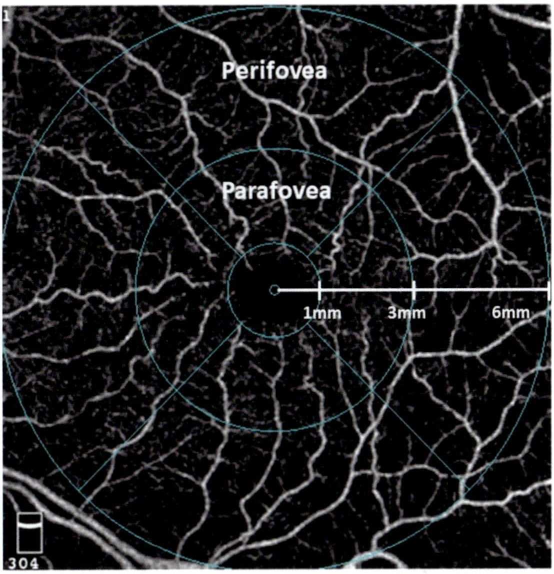

Fig. 20.27 Regions corresponding to the fovea, parafovea, and perifovea on the 6 mm × 6 mm macular OCTA scans. The parafovea is defined as the annular region with an inner diameter of 1 mm and an outer diameter of 3 mm centered on the fovea. The perifovea is defined as the annular region with an inner diameter of 3 mm and an outer diameter of 6 mm centered on the fovea

20.11 OCTA Report of a Normal Eye

Figure 20.28 shows the peripapillary OCTA report of a normal eye (showing normal optic disc and visual field). The OCTA report includes angiography image showing large vessels and a dense network of capillaries in the RPC segment (Fig. 20.28a); En face image (Fig. 20.28b); table showing the VD in the entire scan region and various sectors (Fig. 20.28c); B scan showing the segmentation lines (for the RPC segment) along with the blood vessels detected by the SSADA algorithm (Fig. 20.28d and e); heat map (Fig. 20.28f) showing dense network of vessels in the peripapillary region; represented by warm colors such as red and yellow.

Figure 20.29 shows a 3 mm × 3 mm macular OCTA report of a normal eye showing the superficial retinal vessels. The interpretation of this report is similar to that of the peripapillary OCTA report described earlier.

20.12 OCTA Report of a Glaucomatous Eye

Figure 20.30 shows a glaucomatous eye (mild severity of disease) with a superior neuroretinal rim notch and superotemporal RNFL defect (indicated by arrows on the disc photograph) with a correlating inferior hemifield defect on the visual fields. OCTA shows reduced VD in the superotemporal region on the angiography and the heat map, along with a decrease in the VD in the corresponding sector.

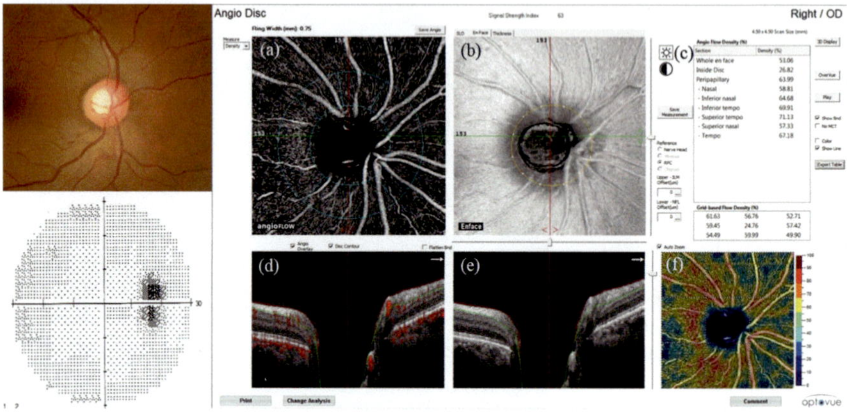

Fig. 20.28 Peripapillary OCTA report of an eye showing normal optic disc (upper left) and normal visual fields (lower left). The OCTA report shows dense radial peripapillary capillaries on the angiography image (a) and heat map (f) with vessel densities in different sectors quantified in the table (c)

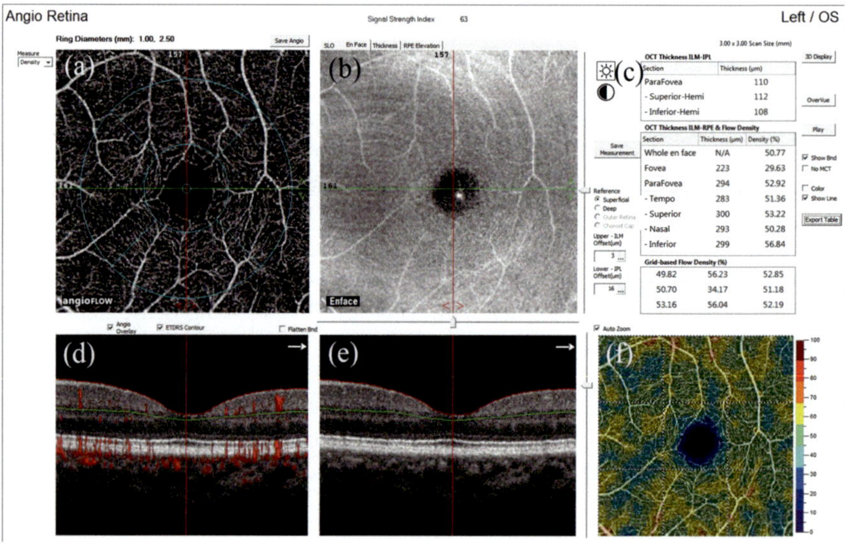

Fig. 20.29 Macular OCTA report (3 mm × 3 mm) showing the superficial retinal vessels of a normal eye. The OCTA report shows dense capillaries on the angiography image (a) and heat map (f) with vessel densities in different sectors quantified in the table (c)

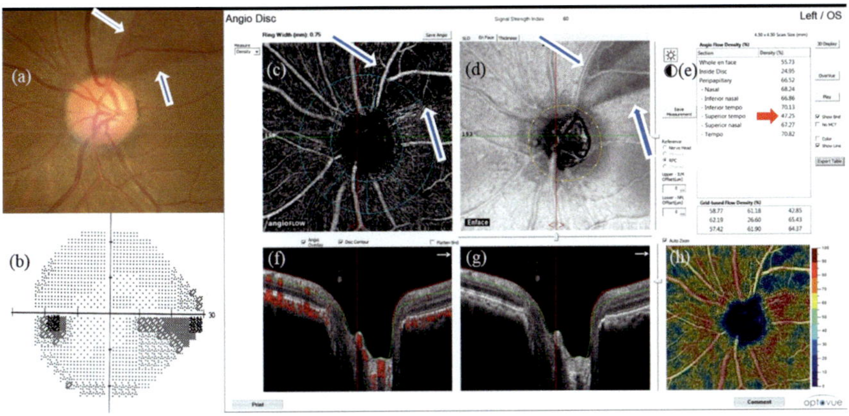

Fig. 20.30 Peripapillary OCTA report of a glaucomatous eyes with mild disease. Optic disc photograph (a) shows superior neuroretinal rim notch and superotemporal RNFL defect (indicated by arrows on the disc photograph) with a correlating inferior hemifield defect on the visual fields (b). OCTA report shows reduced vessel density in the superotemporal region as indicated by the arrows on the angiography (c) and heat map (h), along with a decrease in the vessel density in the corresponding region on the table (e, red arrow)

Figure 20.31 shows an eye with advanced glaucoma. OCTA shows gross loss of capillaries on the angiography and heat map, along with a decrease in the VD in all peripapillary sectors in the table.

Figure 20.32 shows a glaucomatous eye with superior hemifield defect and a corresponding inferior GCC thinning. Macular 3 mm × 3 mm OCTA scan shows reduced superficial retinal VD in the inferior macular region noted on the heat map. Figure 20.33 shows the heat map of macular OCTA scan of the same eye performed with 6 mm × 6 mm scan. Compared to the 3 mm × 3 mm scan, the vessel dropouts are more obvious on the 6 mm × 6 mm scan.

Figure 20.34 shows the 6 mm × 6 mm macular OCTA report of a mild POAG eye showing the superficial retinal vessels. The table include both parafoveal and perifoveal VD measurements, and more obvious vascular dropouts were observed in the perifoveal region.

20.13 OCTA Changes in Different Subtypes of Glaucoma

(i) POAG: All the initial studies with OCTA were performed in eyes with primary open angle glaucoma (POAG), and showed reduced flow index and VD inside the ONH and in the peripapillary region of eyes with POAG compared to controls [99, 102–104]. Multiple studies subsequently showed that the OCTA VD measured in the macular regions were also reduced in eyes with glaucoma compared to control eyes [105, 106]. Vascular theory of

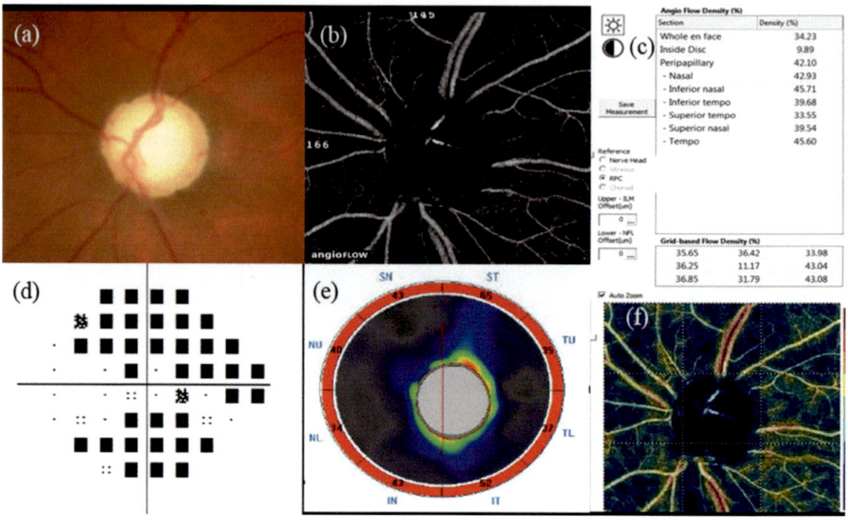

Fig. 20.31 Peripapillary OCTA report of a glaucomatous eyes with advanced disease. It shows advanced disc damage (a), bi-arcuate visual field loss (b) and diffuse RNFL thinning (e). OCTA report shows gross loss of capillaries on the angiography (b) and heat map (f), along with a decrease in the vessel densities in all peripapillary OCTA sectors in the table (c)

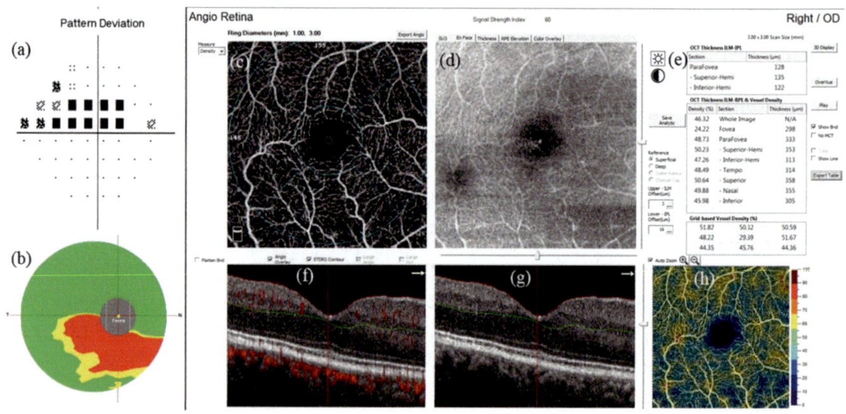

Fig. 20.32 Macular OCTA report (3 mm × 3 mm) of a glaucomatous eye which shows a superior hemifield defect (a) and a corresponding inferior ganglion cell complex thinning (b). OCTA shows reduced superficial macular vessel density in the inferior region better noted on the heat map (h) and quantified in the table (e)

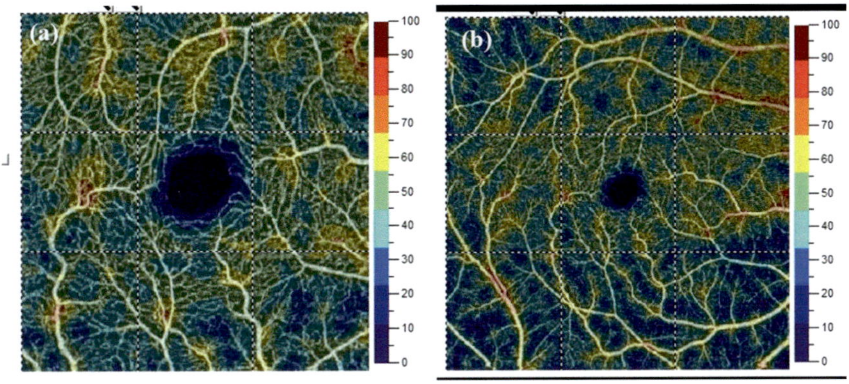

Fig. 20.33 Macular OCTA report of the eye shown in Fig. 20.30 imaged using a 3 mm × 3 mm (a) and a 6 mm × 6 mm scan (b). Compared to the 3 mm × 3 mm scan, the vessel dropouts are more obvious on the 6 mm × 6 mm scan

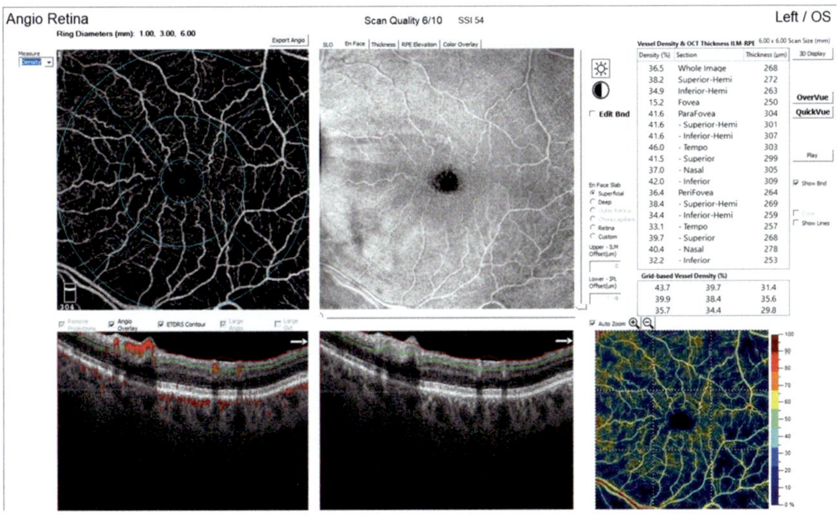

Fig. 20.34 Macular OCTA report (6 mm × 6 mm) of a mild POAG eyes. The table includes both parafoveal and perifoveal vessel density measurements. The vessel dropouts are more obvious in the perifoveal region, particularly the inferior and temporal perifoveal sectors, in comparison to the parafoveal region

glaucoma was considered to be more applicable in eyes developing glaucomatous damage at low/normal IOP. A few studies, therefore, have compared the OCTA measurements in POAG eyes showing damage at low/normal IOP and high IOP. However, no differences in OCTA measurements were seen between these two POAG groups [105, 107].

(ii) Angle closure glaucoma: OCTA measurements in primary angle closure glaucoma (PACG) were found to be similar to that in POAG when the severity of disease was matched [108, 109]. However, distinct patterns of VD loss between POAG and PACG have also been reported [110]. Hou et al. found a lower infero-temporal peripapillary VD in POAG eyes in comparison to PACG eyes, which showed a more even peripapillary VD reduction [110]. Like POAG (described below), OCT neuronal (NRR, RNFL and GCC) measurements seemed to have a better diagnostic ability compared to OCTA VD measurements (inside ONH, peripapillary and macular regions) in PACG [111]. A recent study by Rao et al. demonstrated a cross-sectional association between lower superficial VD and faster VF progression in PACG eyes, indicating OCTA may help detect past VF progression [112]. Other studies have shown early reductions in VD and long-term decrease in circumpapillary RNFL (cpRNFL) thickness after acute primary angle closure (APAC) attack after [113, 114]. A lower VD at 2 months after the attackwas the best predictor of conversion to an abnormal cpRNFL thickness, and glaucomatous progression should be suspected in eyes with lower VD after the remission of APAC episode [113, 114].

(iii) Pseudoexfoliation glaucoma (PXG): Prior studies have shown significant decreases of peripaillary VD and macular VD in PXG eyes in comparison to healthy eyes [115], and that OCTA can detect reduced capillary density before significant cpRNFL changes occurred to the fellow eyes of PXG patients [116]. However, it remains controversial whether OCTA changes differ between PXG eyes and POAG eyes [115]. Some studies revealed a greater reduction of superficial peripapillary VD and macular VD in PXG eyes [117–119], while others reported no significant difference [120, 121].

20.14 Relationship Among OCTA, OCT and VF Measurements

To determine whether OCTA changes observed in glaucoma may be clinically meaningful, many studies have assessed whether VD measurement correlates with OCT and VF measurements in glaucoma [122]. Generally, a moderate-to-strong correlation was found between ONH peripapillary VD and VF defects, and a moderate correlation between peripapillary VD and OCT thickness measurements [122]. The strength of correlation varies among different ONH sectors, with the infero-temporal peripapillary VD demonstrating the strongest association with the spatially corresponded regional RNFL and VF measurements [123]. The association of macular VD with OCT and VF measurements was found slightly weaker than that of ONH VD, although whether the difference is significant remains debatable [122, 124, 125]. Nonetheless, macular VD, particularly in the inferior area, may provide more help in assessing central VF than ONH VD due to its stronger association with central VF defects [52, 126–130].

Most studies to date used cross-sectional OCTA data to assess its relationship with OCT and VF, since longitudinal OCTA data is not yet widely available due to the recentness of this technique. Nevertheless, Mohammadzadeh et al. were able to examine the longitudinal functional association of serial macular VD and GCC measurements with serial 10-2 VF tests, and demonstrated comparable and significant functional associations for both measurements [131].

To help develop strategies that may detect glaucoma in the earliest stages, it is also important to determine the temporal relationship among VD reduction, RNFL thinning, and VF defects. A few cross-sectional studies have found reduced peripapillary VD and RNFL thickness in the hemiretina corresponding to the perimetrically intact hemifield in established perimetric glaucoma eyes, as compared to that in controls [132–134]. This suggested both OCT and OCTA changes might precede detectable VF defects. One of these studies also found the temporal sector of the perimetrically intact hemifield (corresponding to the region of papillomacular bundles) showed reduced VD despite a normal RNFL thickness [133]. This further suggested there may be regional variations in the alterations of RNFL thickness and VD, and OCTA changes may precede RNFL changes in some sectors.

Other retrospective cohort studies have shown cross-sectional VD measurements are predictive of subsequent nerve thinning detected by OCT. Moghimi et al. showed lower baseline macular and ONH VD were associated with faster RNFL thinning in mild-moderate glaucoma [125]. Similarly, Wu et al. showed baseline superficial parafoveal VD was associated with faster macular GCC thinning [135]. It is still unclear if OCTA-measured VD loss occurs before or after OCT-measured neuronal (NRR, RNFL and GCC) changes in glaucoma. More longitudinal studies examining the chronological sequence of OCTA changes in relation to OCT changes are needed to better clarify this.

As compared to deep VD loss, superficial VD loss is considered more likely associated with glaucomatous damage [136]. Many studies have found a stronger association of superficial VD than deep VD with OCT and VF defects [135, 137, 138], suggesting the OCTA evaluation of superficial capillary plexus may be more relevant to glaucoma assessment.

20.15 Comparing OCTA to OCT in Diagnosing Glaucoma

A number of studies have compared the diagnostic abilities (area under the receiver operating characteristic curves [AUC] and sensitivities at high specificities) of OCTA measurements (VD of the inside disc, ONH, and macular regions) with corresponding OCT measurements (ONH neuroretinal rim area, RNFL and macular thickness) in glaucoma [122].

Most studies found similar diagnostic abilities of peripapillary VD and RNFL thickness in POAG, with the AUC ranging mostly between 0.85 to 0.95 [103, 104, 108]. A few other studies have reported a better diagnostic ability of RNFL thickness compared to peripapillary VD [106, 139]. In spite of the similar AUCs, some studies suggested that the sensitivity to detect glaucoma in pre-perimetric or early stages of glaucoma was better with RNFL thickness compared to peripapillary VD [106, 140]. Meanwhile, the diagnostic abilities of VD measurements inside ONH were found to be significantly worse than that of the OCT measured NRR area [106].

The diagnostic abilities of macular VD and macular GCC thickness have also been compared, and an overall better performance was found for the latter (AUC: 0.85–0.95 vs macular VD: 0.70–0.85) [106, 122, 126]. Still, a few studies reported there was no significant difference in the discriminative power of macular OCT and OCTA measurements [141, 142]. Of note, macular VD assessed in these studies were mostly acquired from 3 mm × 3 mm scans. A better diagnostic performance of macular VD acquired from the 6 mm × 6 mm scans have been reported in subsequent studies [143], particularly when discriminating mild POAG eyes from healthy eyes [144].

When comparing the diagnostic abilities of macular versus ONH OCTA parameters, ONH peripapillary VD tended to achieve a higher AUC than macular VD in differentiating glaucomatous and normal eyes [106, 122, 145, 146], similar to that previously observed for OCT structural measurements.

Summary

The diagnostic performance of OCT thickness measurements was generally considered comparable to or better than that of OCTA VD measurements [106, 122, 142]. Nonetheless, some studies have observed variability in the preferential changes in VD/perfusion or thickness among glaucoma eyes [142, 147, 148], with about one third of eyes having a higher percentage of VD/perfusion change than the percentage of thickness change [142, 148]. Potential factors identified to affect such the phenomenon included OCT/OCTA signal strength, RNFL thickness, and female sex [148]. The presence of disc hemorrhage and optic disc phenotype were also found to affect the pattern of VD and thickness changes [149–151]. Considering these differences at individual level, obtaining both OCT and OCTA image may constitute a more comprehensive evaluation.

20.16 OCTA Versus OCT for Assessing VF Loss and Progression

With a robust diagnostic performance for glaucoma and a good correlation with VF defects [123, 152, 153], it is thus wondered if OCTA VD measurements may help to evaluate glaucomatous VF loss and progression, and how it compares to OCT.

One potential edge of OCTA over OCT in assessing VF loss is its greater dynamic range and less significant floor effect [96]. The measurement floor of perifoveal VD, ciucumpapillary capillary density, ciucumpapillary RNFL thickness, and GCC thickness has been estimated at VF mean deviation (MD) of approximately −26 dB, −19 dB, −18 dB, and −14 dB, respectively, implicating that when the VF MD is worse than −14 dB, OCTA may better detect progression than OCT [96]. Assessing glaucoma eyes along the whole spectrum of severity, a few studies have also found longitudinal retinal VD loss to have a stronger functional correlation than structural thinning as glaucoma worsens, and may be more suitable for VF progression detection in moderate-advanced glaucoma eyes [130, 154, 155].

As aforementioned, some studies have found a lower cross-sectional retinal VD may predict faster structural thinning [125, 135]. Similarly, some others have found lower cross-sectional VD measurements to be associated with faster VF loss and/or higher probability of VF progression [52, 138]. Notably, comparing macular GCC thickness to superficial macular VD for the association with past 10-2 VF loss, Wu et al. found a lower macular VD to be associated with both faster 10-2 VF worsening and higher risk of trend-based progression, while a thinner GCC was only associated with faster 10-2 VF worsening [52].

Interestingly, Nishida et al. examined whether faster macular VD loss during the initial follow-up period may be associated with faster VF loss during an extended follow-up period [156]. They reported that a rapid initial VD loss was associated with higher concurrent and subsequent rates of VF MD loss, and that OCTA may assist in clinical decision making for high-risk patients. Furthermore, the OCTA model in this study may better explain the variability of future VF loss as compared to OCT [156]. Similar observation was reported for rapid initial macular GCC thinning in the study by Mahmoudinedzah et al., which suggested macular OCT may also help identify patients at risk of subsequent central VF loss [53].

Since longitudinal OCTA data is very limited, information on the progression detection capability of OCTA remains scarce. Only one published study has assessed the progression detection capability of longitudinal OCTA measurements, although they included only advanced POAG eyes [38]. When comparing between VF progressors and non-progressors, the authors found the rates of ciucumpapillary RNFL and macular GCC thinning to be similar, while the rates of ciucumpapillary and macular VD loss to differ. Furthermore, VF showed stronger agreement with OCTA than with OCT on event-based analysis. The authors concluded that OCTA VD loss may better detect VF progression than OCT structural loss in advanced POAG [38].

To summarize, these results support the use of OCTA in assessing VF loss and/or progression, especially in moderate-advanced glaucoma. However, its performance on progression detection in relation to OCT remains to be confirmed when more longitudinal OCTA studies become available.

20.17 Combining OCT and OCTA for Glaucoma Evaluation

While OCT and OCTA individually have shown satisfactory performances in assessing glaucomatous change, some recent works have examined if including both OCT and OCTA measurements may further enhance clinical evaluation of glaucoma [157].

For the diagnosis of glaucoma, Bowd et al. used both standard OCT/OCTA measurements and gradient-boosting classifier (GBC), a machine learning (ML) classifier, to discriminate healthy eyes from mild-moderate glaucoma eyes [157]. It was reported the GBC combining both OCT and OCTA data (AUC = 0.93) showed the best diagnostic ability, which significantly outperformed GBCs based on only OCT data (AUC = 0.91) and only OCTA data (AUC = 0.90) [157]. Nonetheless, the study by Rabiolo et al. did not find the combined OCT-OCTA data to improve the diagnostic ability over OCT structural parameters alone when discriminating healthy, glaucoma suspect, and POAG eyes [158].

A few studies have suggested OCTA may complement OCT in assessing VF damage. Wong et al. tested the modeling of focal VF losses in early POAG eyes based on OCTA circumpapillary capillary density data, OCT circumpapillary RNFL data, and combined OCT-OCTA data [159]. They found the combined data to best model focal VF loss, and conclude that such combined approach may benefit VF evaluation in early glaucoma [159]. The study by Xu et al. also examined OCT, OCTA, and combined method in predicting paracentral VF total deviation, and found the combined method to best predict the severity of paracentral VF loss [160]. More recently, Kamalipour et al. used combined longitudinal OCT-OCTA data to detect VF progression via ML models, and again showed a higher classification accuracy of this approach than using either modality data alone [161].

20.18 OCTA of the Peripapillary Choroid

Peripapillary choroidal circulation is of particular interest in glaucoma as it may be a surrogate marker for the perfusion of the deep ONH structures. Choroidal microvasculature dropout (CMvD, Fig. 20.35), defined as the complete loss of choriocapillaris in localized regions of parapapillary atrophy (PPA), has been observed using OCTA [162, 163]. The prevalence of CMvD was higher in POAG than in in PACG and PXG [120, 164], suggesting its unique role in the pathophysiology of POAG.

CMvD has been shown to be a true perfusion defect using indocyanine green angiography [165]. In Micheletti et al., CMvD was detected in 58.2% of POAG eyes at baseline and in an additional of 18.6% eyes during follow-up. They also reported factors associated with CMvD enlargement in POAG, including greater IOP fluctuation, worse glaucoma severity, and greater number of glaucoma medications [166].

There appears to be a topographic association between the location of CMvD and structural defects (RNFL thinning and lamina cribrosa defects), as well as functional defects (VF loss), in POAG eyes [162, 167–170]. It has been argued that CMvD is likely to precede structural and functional damage [171]. A few studies have reported an association between the presence of CMvD at baseline and higher risk of subsequent faster or progressive structural thinning in POAG and normal tension glaucoma eyes [172–175]. Similar relationship was also found between baseline CMvD and subsequent VF progression [176]. Some other studies

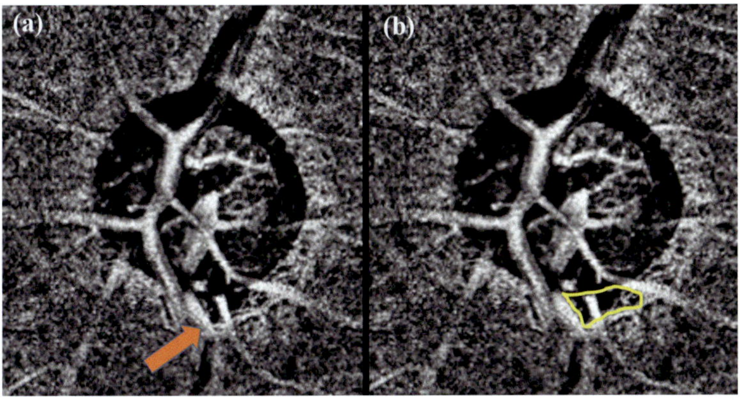

Fig. 20.35 Choroidal OCTA slab of a glaucomatous eye showing the presence of choroidal microvasculature dropout (CMvD) in the inferior region (a). Arrow points to the CMvD. Yellow line marks out the boundary of the CMvD (b)

have observed the enlargement or occurrence of CMvD during follow-up, and found these events to correlate with faster RNFL and VF worsening [177–179], providing longitudinal evidence for the clinical relevance of CMvD in glaucoma. Recently, a cross-sectional study found the presence of juxtapapillary CMvD to be associated with not only worse glaucoma severity but also 10-2 VF defect [180]. Furthermore, such CMvD was more prevalent and larger in POAG eyes with high myopia than in non-highly myopic POAG eyes.

The potentially differing roles of β- and γ-PPA and associated vasculature dropouts have also been investigated in a few recent works. Localized CMvD was found predictive of generalized loss of parapapillary choroidal VD within the β PPA in OAG eyes [181], which was reported to correlate with VF progression, but not structural progression [182]. Additionally, the presence of CMvD seemed associated with faster RNFL thinning only in POAG eyes with β-PPA, but not γ-PPA [183].

20.19 OCTA of the Foveal Avascular Zone (FAZ)

OCTA measurements of the FAZ, defined as the capillary-free region enclosed by the innermost macular arcade, have garnered attention in glaucoma evaluation due to its central location in the macula [50, 184]. It was hypothesized that impaired vascular perfusion to the central macula, which has the highest density of retinal ganglion cells, may be assessed by OCTA FAZ metrics. Figure 20.36 shows the regions corresponding to the commonly assessed FAZ metrics, including the FAZ area, FAZ perimeter/circumference, and foveal density 300 (FD300), on the macular scan of an OCTA device [50, 184].

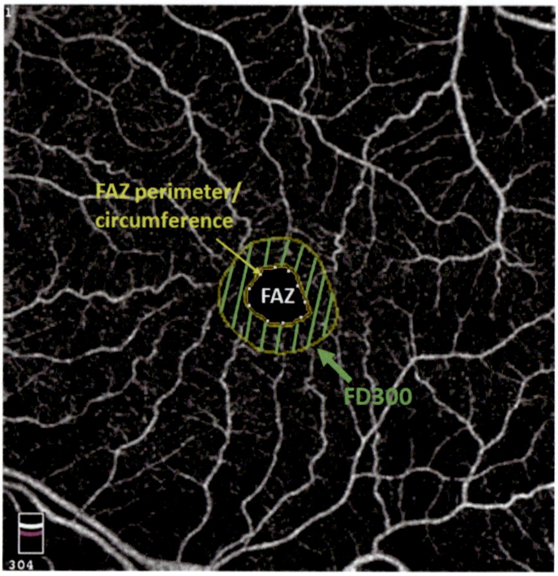

Fig. 20.36 Regions corresponding to the FAZ area, FAZ perimeter/circumference, and foveal density 300 (FD300), defined as the superficial vessel density of the 300 μm width ring surrounding the FAZ (c)

Changes to the FAZ metrics have been found to correlate with glaucomatous damage in multiple studies. Kown et al. showed the FAZ area and perimeter are associated with VD measurements in open-angle glaucoma (OAG) eyes [185], and larger FAZ area was spatially associated with worse central VF defects [186]. Igarashi et al. also found FAZ area to correlate negatively with retinal inner layer thickness, foveal sensitivity threshold, and 10-2 VF MD in OAG [187], although in another study, the FD300, but not FAZ area, was found associated with 10-2 VF MD and foveal threshold [184]. In a recent study, the FAZ area decreased after IOP-lowering surgery (e.g., trabeculectomy), and the change in FAZ area was significantly correlated with both pre-operative foveal sensitivity and change in IOP [188]. Longitudinal studies are needed to better determine the clinical implication of OCTA FAZ metrics in glaucoma.

20.20 OCTA Measurement Reproducibility and Its Determinants

The reproducibility of superficial OCTA VD has been evaluated. Generally, OCTA showed satisfactory short-term measurement reproducibility in both healthy and glaucoma eyes, although the variability of OCT measurement is still smaller [189–191]. OCTA also showed good long-term reproducibility, which was superior to that of VF test and slightly inferior to that of OCT [8, 9]. The test–retest variability (TRV) of global ONH or macular VD was reported to range between 3 and 5%, while the TRV of sectoral VD ranged between 4 and 7% [8, 9, 191].

Unlike the neuronal elements, vasculature is affected by multiple factors other than glaucoma, thus are the VD measurements. Various potential determinants of OCTA measurement variability have been identified, including subject-related (age, gender, systemic hypertension and diabetes), eye-related (refractive error, optic disc size, central corneal thickness [CCT]) and technology-related (signal strength index, [SSI] of the scans) factors, but with variable strengths [192]. Among them, age and SSI were usually considered the most relevant determinants. Generally, the variability of OCTA measurements increased with older age [8, 9]. While higher SSI is associated with higher VD measurement and lower OCTA variability [8, 9, 191, 192]. Other factors, such as VF MD, IOP and CCT, were found to affect OCTA TRV in some studies, but not others [8, 9]. These should be considered while analyzing OCTA VD.

20.21 Limitations and Recent Advances in OCTA

Artifacts are common with OCTA imaging, particularly motion artifacts, due to the prolonged time required to acquire the scans [193]. In spite of methods available to account for the artifacts (Fig. 20.37), multiple studies have reported high numbers of poor-quality images with OCTA due to the presence of artifacts [191, 194–197]. Media opacities, especially vitreous opacities, can significantly affect the quality of OCTA scans and the quantification of VD (Fig. 20.38). Analyzing 5263 OCTA images, Kamalipour et al. reported around 34% of them were of poor quality [197]. This indicates the necessity of scan quality review prior to interpreting VD for glaucoma evaluation, as well as the need for better measures to overcome the issue of poor quality.

Two technical improvements incorporated in OCTA software to enhance scan quality are (i) real time eye tracking technology, for controlling the motion artifacts more effectively [198] and, (ii) high-density (HD) scanning mode, for improving the resolution of the scans. Prior study comparing the reproducibility of HD and non-HD OCTA scans has reported that the number of poor-quality scans significantly decreased with the incorporation of these improvements [199]. A recent study also showed a higher risk of acquiring poor-quality scans without eye tracking [197].

OCTA technology evaluates the superficial retinal vessels well, but not the deeper retinal and choroidal vasculature. This is because the signals from the superficial retinal vessels project on to the deeper layers, causing artifacts known as the projection artifacts [100]. Detection of CMvD, for example, is often affected by the presence of projection artifacts. Therefore, methods to correct/remove projection artifacts have been incorporated to OCTA during recent software updates [101, 200]. Such projection-artifact removal algorithm has been found to better quantify not only the deeper retinal and choroidal vasculature, but also the superficial vasculature, thus improving the reliability of OCTA in glaucoma evaluation [201, 202].

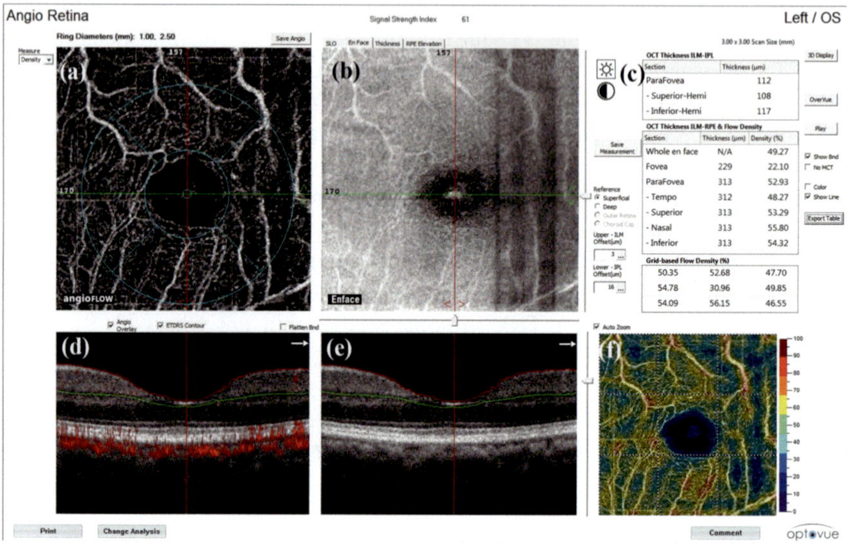

Fig. 20.37 Macular OCTA scan showing two types of artifacts; motion artifacts, recognized as vertical bands temporally on the en face map (b) and duplication of vessels, recognized inferiorly and nasally on the angiography map (a). These artifacts cause a decrease in vessel density in the temporal sector and increase in vessel density in the nasal and inferior sectors (noted on the heat map [f] and table [c])

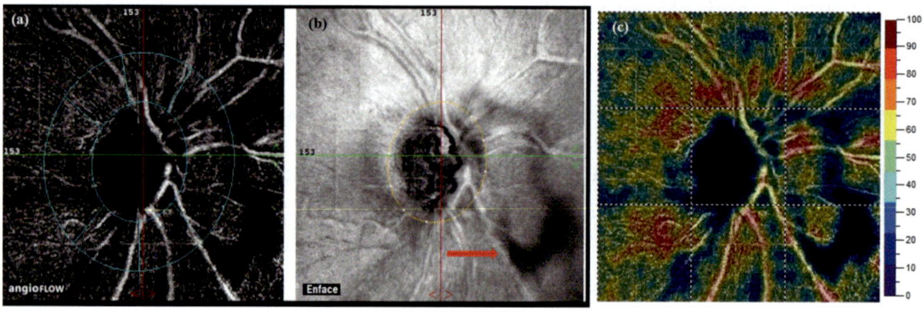

Fig. 20.38 Vitreous opacity (red arrow on en face map [b]) casting a shadow, as seen on the angiography map (a) and causing a falsely reduced vessel density on the heat map (c)

20.22 Conclusion

The introduction of OCT has caused a paradigm shift in glaucoma diagnosis and monitoring and has shown the benefits of incorporating structural assessment in addition to clinical examination and VF test in managing this disease. Additionally, as an emerging technique, the use of OCTA may complement OCT and provide further insights assisting with the clinical evaluation of glaucoma.

Acknowledgements This work is supported in part by NIH grant R01EY029058 and R01EY034148, UC Tobacco Related Disease Research Program (T31IP1511), and an unrestricted grant from Research to Prevent Blindness (New York, NY).

References

1. Weinreb RN, Aung T, Medeiros FA. The pathophysiology and treatment of glaucoma: a review. JAMA. 2014;311(18):1901–11.
2. Tham YC, Li X, Wong TY, et al. Global prevalence of glaucoma and projections of glaucoma burden through 2040: a systematic review and meta-analysis. Ophthalmology. 2014;121(11):2081–90.
3. Bourne RR, Taylor HR, Flaxman SR, et al. Number of people blind or visually impaired by glaucoma worldwide and in world regions 1990–2010: a meta-analysis. PLoS ONE. 2016;11(10): e0162229.
4. Quigley HA, Addicks EM. Quantitative studies of retinal nerve fiber layer defects. Arch Ophthalmol. 1982;100(5):807–14.
5. Harwerth RS, Carter-Dawson L, Smith EL 3rd, et al. Neural losses correlated with visual losses in clinical perimetry. Invest Ophthalmol Vis Sci. 2004;45(9):3152–60.
6. Abrams LS, Scott IU, Spaeth GL, et al. Agreement among optometrists, ophthalmologists, and residents in evaluating the optic disc for glaucoma. Ophthalmology. 1994;101(10):1662–7.
7. Jampel HD, Friedman D, Quigley H, et al. Agreement among glaucoma specialists in assessing progressive disc changes from photographs in open-angle glaucoma patients. Am J Ophthalmol. 2009;147(1):39–44e1.
8. Nishida T, Moghimi S, Hou H, et al. Long-term reproducibility of optical coherence tomography angiography in healthy and stable glaucomatous eyes. Br J Ophthalmol. 2021.
9. Wu J-H, Moghimi S, Nishida T, et al. Evaluation of the long-term variability of macular OCT/OCTA and visual field parameters. Br J Ophthal. 2022:bjo-2022–322470.
10. Zeimer R, Asrani S, Zou S, et al. Quantitative detection of glaucomatous damage at the posterior pole by retinal thickness mapping. A pilot study. Ophthalmology. 1998;105(2):224–31.
11. Curcio CA, Allen KA. Topography of ganglion cells in human retina. J Comp Neurol. 1990;300(1):5–25.
12. Mohammadzadeh V, Fatehi N, Yarmohammadi A, et al. Macular imaging with optical coherence tomography in glaucoma. Surv Ophthalmol. 2020;65(6):597–638.
13. Burgoyne C. The morphological difference between glaucoma and other optic neuropathies. J Neuroophthalmol. 2015;35(Suppl 1):S8-s21.
14. Mwanza JC, Oakley JD, Budenz DL, Anderson DR. Ability of cirrus HD-OCT optic nerve head parameters to discriminate normal from glaucomatous eyes. Ophthalmology 2011;118(2):241–8 e1.
15. Leite MT, Rao HL, Weinreb RN, et al. Agreement among spectral-domain optical coherence tomography instruments for assessing retinal nerve fiber layer thickness. Am J Ophthalmol. 2011;151(1):85–92 e1.
16. Pierro L, Gagliardi M, Iuliano L, et al. Retinal nerve fiber layer thickness reproducibility using seven different OCT instruments. Invest Ophthalmol Vis Sci. 2012;53(9):5912–20.
17. Hwang YH, Kim YY, Kim HK, Sohn YH. Ability of cirrus high-definition spectral-domain optical coherence tomography clock-hour, deviation, and thickness maps in detecting photographic retinal nerve fiber layer abnormalities. Ophthalmology. 2013;120(7):1380–7.
18. Hwang YH, Jeong YC, Kim HK, Sohn YH. Macular ganglion cell analysis for early detection of glaucoma. Ophthalmology. 2014;121(8):1508–15.
19. Michelessi M, Lucenteforte E, Oddone F, et al. Optic nerve head and fibre layer imaging for diagnosing glaucoma. Cochrane Database Syst Rev. 2015(11):CD008803.

20. Kuang TM, Zhang C, Zangwill LM, et al. Estimating lead time gained by optical coherence tomography in detecting glaucoma before development of visual field defects. Ophthalmology. 2015;122(10):2002–9.
21. Medeiros FA, Zangwill LM, Bowd C, et al. Evaluation of retinal nerve fiber layer, optic nerve head, and macular thickness measurements for glaucoma detection using optical coherence tomography. Am J Ophthalmol. 2005;139(1):44–55.
22. Leung CK, Chan WM, Yung WH, et al. Comparison of macular and peripapillary measurements for the detection of glaucoma: an optical coherence tomography study. Ophthalmology. 2005;112(3):391–400.
23. Nakatani Y, Higashide T, Ohkubo S, et al. Evaluation of macular thickness and peripapillary retinal nerve fiber layer thickness for detection of early glaucoma using spectral domain optical coherence tomography. J Glaucoma. 2011;20(4):252–9.
24. Oddone F, Lucenteforte E, Michelessi M, et al. Macular versus retinal nerve fiber layer parameters for diagnosing manifest glaucoma: a systematic review of diagnostic accuracy studies. Ophthalmology. 2016;123(5):939–49.
25. Kansal V, Armstrong JJ, Pintwala R, Hutnik C. Optical coherence tomography for glaucoma diagnosis: an evidence based meta-analysis. PLoS ONE. 2018;13(1): e0190621.
26. El-Nimri NW, Moghimi S, Nishida T, et al. Racial differences in detection of glaucoma using retinal nerve fiber layer thickness and bruch membrane opening minimum rim width. Am J Ophthalmol. 2023;246:223–35.
27. Tatham AJ, Medeiros FA. Detecting structural progression in glaucoma with optical coherence tomography. Ophthalmology. 2017;124(12s):S57-s65.
28. Kim YK, Ha A, Na KI, et al. Temporal relation between macular ganglion cell-inner plexiform layer loss and peripapillary retinal nerve fiber layer loss in glaucoma. Ophthalmology. 2017;124(7):1056–64.
29. Hwang YH, Kim Y, Chung JK, Lee KB. Glaucomatous progression in the retinal nerve fibre and retinal ganglion cell-inner plexiform layers determined using optical coherence tomography-guided progression analysis. Clin Exp Optom. 2018;101(5):666–73.
30. Hou HW, Lin C, Leung CK. Integrating macular ganglion cell inner plexiform layer and parapapillary retinal nerve fiber layer measurements to detect glaucoma progression. Ophthalmology. 2018;125(6):822–31.
31. Mohammadzadeh V, Moghimi S, Nishida T, et al. Association of rates of ganglion cell and inner plexiform thinning with development of glaucoma in eyes with suspected glaucoma. JAMA Ophthalmol. 2023.
32. Lavinsky F, Wu M, Schuman JS, et al. Can macula and optic nerve head parameters detect glaucoma progression in eyes with advanced circumpapillary retinal nerve fiber layer damage? Ophthalmology. 2018.
33. Rabiolo A, Mohammadzadeh V, Fatehi N, et al. Comparison of rates of progression of macular OCT measures in glaucoma. Transl Vis Sci Technol. 2020;9(7):50.
34. Vazirani J, Kaushik S, Pandav SS, Gupta P. Reproducibility of retinal nerve fiber layer measurements across the glaucoma spectrum using optical coherence tomography. Indian J Ophthalmol. 2015;63(4):300–5.
35. Reis ASC, Jammal AA, Zangalli C, et al. Repeatability of macular and optic nerve head OCT parameters in advanced glaucoma. Invest Ophthalmol Vis Sci. 2019;60(9):1423.
36. Wu H, de Boer JF, Chen TC. Reproducibility of retinal nerve fiber layer thickness measurements using spectral domain optical coherence tomography. J Glaucoma. 2011;20(8):470–6.
37. Tan BB, Natividad M, Chua KC, Yip LW. Comparison of retinal nerve fiber layer measurement between 2 spectral domain OCT instruments. J Glaucoma. 2012;21(4):266–73.
38. Lee A, Sung KR, Shin JW. Progression detection capabilities of circumpapillary and macular vessel density in advanced glaucomatous eyes. Sci Rep. 2022;12(1):12109.
39. Mwanza JC, Chang RT, Budenz DL, et al. Reproducibility of peripapillary retinal nerve fiber layer thickness and optic nerve head parameters measured with cirrus HD-OCT in glaucomatous eyes. Invest Ophthalmol Vis Sci. 2010;51(11):5724–30.

40. Kim KE, Yoo BW, Jeoung JW, Park KH. Long-term reproducibility of macular ganglion cell analysis in clinically stable glaucoma patients. Invest Ophthalmol Vis Sci. 2015;56(8):4857–64.
41. Leung CK, Chiu V, Weinreb RN, et al. Evaluation of retinal nerve fiber layer progression in glaucoma: a comparison between spectral-domain and time-domain optical coherence tomography. Ophthalmology. 2011;118(8):1558–62.
42. Nguyen AT, Greenfield DS, Bhakta AS, et al. Detecting glaucoma progression using guided progression analysis with OCT and visual field assessment in eyes classified by international classification of disease severity codes. Ophthalmol Glaucoma. 2019;2(1):36–46.
43. Zhang X, Dastiridou A, Francis BA, et al. Comparison of glaucoma progression detection by optical coherence tomography and visual field. Am J Ophthalmol. 2017;184:63–74.
44. Miki A, Medeiros FA, Weinreb RN, et al. Rates of retinal nerve fiber layer thinning in glaucoma suspect eyes. Ophthalmology. 2014;121(7):1350–8.
45. Yu M, Lin C, Weinreb RN, et al. Risk of visual field progression in glaucoma patients with progressive retinal nerve fiber layer thinning: a 5-year prospective study. Ophthalmology. 2016;123(6):1201–10.
46. Gracitelli CP, Abe RY, Tatham AJ, et al. Association between progressive retinal nerve fiber layer loss and longitudinal change in quality of life in glaucoma. JAMA Ophthalmol. 2015;133(4):384–90.
47. Nishida T, Moghimi S, Mohammadzadeh V, et al. Association between ganglion cell complex thinning and vision-related quality of life in glaucoma. JAMA Ophthalmol. 2022;140(8):800–6.
48. Nishida T, Moghimi S, Yamane MLM, et al. Vision-related quality of life among healthy, preperimetric glaucoma, and perimetric glaucoma patients. Am J Ophthalmol. 2023;248:127–36.
49. Yamazaki Y, Sugisaki K, Araie M, et al. Relationship between vision-related quality of life and central 10° of the binocular integrated visual field in advanced glaucoma. Sci Rep. 2019;9(1):14990.
50. Wu J-H, Moghimi S, Nishida T, et al. Association of macular OCT and OCTA parameters with visual acuity in glaucoma. British Journal of Ophthalmology 2022:bjophthalmol-2022-321460.
51. Latif K, Nishida T, Moghimi S, Weinreb RN. Quality of life in glaucoma. Graefe's Arch Clin Experiment Ophthalmol. 2023.
52. Wu J-H, Moghimi S, Nishida T, et al. Association of macular vessel density and ganglion cell complex thickness with central visual field progression in glaucoma. Br J Ophthal. 2022:bjophthalmol-2022-321870.
53. Mahmoudinezhad G, Moghimi S, Nishida T, et al. Association between rate of ganglion cell complex thinning and rate of central visual field loss. JAMA Ophthalmol. 2023;141(1):33–9.
54. Mahmoudinezhad G, Moghimi S, Proudfoot JA, et al. Effect of testing frequency on the time to detect glaucoma progression with optical coherence tomography (OCT) and OCT angiography. Am J Ophthalmol. 2023;245:184–92.
55. Bradley C, Hou K, Herbert P, et al. Evidence-based guidelines for the number of peripapillary OCT scans needed to detect glaucoma worsening. Ophthalmology. 2023;130(1):39–47.
56. Nishida T, Moghimi S, Chang AC, et al. Association of intraocular pressure with retinal nerve fiber layer thinning in patients with glaucoma. JAMA Ophthalmol. 2022;140(12):1209–16.
57. Quigley HA, Addicks EM. Regional differences in the structure of the lamina cribrosa and their relation to glaucomatous optic nerve damage. Arch Ophthalmol. 1981;99(1):137–43.
58. Kagemann L, Ishikawa H, Wollstein G, et al. Ultrahigh-resolution spectral domain optical coherence tomography imaging of the lamina cribrosa. Ophthalmic Surg Lasers Imaging. 2008;39(4 Suppl):S126–31.
59. Inoue R, Hangai M, Kotera Y, et al. Three-dimensional high-speed optical coherence tomography imaging of lamina cribrosa in glaucoma. Ophthalmology. 2009;116(2):214–22.

60. Lee EJ, Kim TW, Weinreb RN, et al. Three-dimensional evaluation of the lamina cribrosa using spectral-domain optical coherence tomography in glaucoma. Invest Ophthalmol Vis Sci. 2012;53(1):198–204.
61. Lee EJ, Kim TW, Weinreb RN, et al. Visualization of the lamina cribrosa using enhanced depth imaging spectral-domain optical coherence tomography. Am J Ophthalmol. 2011;152(1):87–95.e1.
62. Park SC, De Moraes CG, Teng CC, et al. Enhanced depth imaging optical coherence tomography of deep optic nerve complex structures in glaucoma. Ophthalmology. 2012;119(1):3–9.
63. Girard MJ, Strouthidis NG, Ethier CR, Mari JM. Shadow removal and contrast enhancement in optical coherence tomography images of the human optic nerve head. Invest Ophthalmol Vis Sci. 2011;52(10):7738–48.
64. Mari JM, Strouthidis NG, Park SC, Girard MJ. Enhancement of lamina cribrosa visibility in optical coherence tomography images using adaptive compensation. Invest Ophthalmol Vis Sci. 2013;54(3):2238–47.
65. Mansouri K, Nuyen B, Weinreb RN. Improved visualization of deep ocular structures in glaucoma using high penetration optical coherence tomography. Expert Rev Med Devices. 2013;10(5):621–8.
66. Kim YW, Jeoung JW, Kim YK, Park KH. Clinical implications of in vivo lamina cribrosa imaging in glaucoma. J Glaucoma. 2017;26(9):753–61.
67. Furlanetto RL, Park SC, Damle UJ, et al. Posterior displacement of the lamina cribrosa in glaucoma: in vivo interindividual and intereye comparisons. Invest Ophthalmol Vis Sci. 2013;54(7):4836–42.
68. Park SC, Brumm J, Furlanetto RL, et al. Lamina cribrosa depth in different stages of glaucoma. Invest Ophthalmol Vis Sci. 2015;56(3):2059–64.
69. Lee SH, Kim TW, Lee EJ, et al. Diagnostic power of lamina cribrosa depth and curvature in glaucoma. Invest Ophthalmol Vis Sci. 2017;58(2):755–62.
70. Lee EJ, Kim TW, Weinreb RN, Kim H. Reversal of lamina cribrosa displacement after intraocular pressure reduction in open-angle glaucoma. Ophthalmology. 2013;120(3):553–9.
71. Reis AS, O'Leary N, Stanfield MJ, et al. Laminar displacement and prelaminar tissue thickness change after glaucoma surgery imaged with optical coherence tomography. Invest Ophthalmol Vis Sci. 2012;53(9):5819–26.
72. Lee EJ, Kim TW, Weinreb RN. Reversal of lamina cribrosa displacement and thickness after trabeculectomy in glaucoma. Ophthalmology. 2012;119(7):1359–66.
73. Wu Z, Lin C, Crowther M, et al. Impact of rates of change of lamina cribrosa and optic nerve head surface depths on visual field progression in glaucoma. Invest Ophthalmol Vis Sci. 2017;58(3):1825–33.
74. Lee EJ, Kim TW, Kim M, Kim H. Influence of lamina cribrosa thickness and depth on the rate of progressive retinal nerve fiber layer thinning. Ophthalmology. 2015;122(4):721–9.
75. Rhodes LA, Huisingh C, Johnstone J, et al. Variation of laminar depth in normal eyes with age and race. Invest Ophthalmol Vis Sci. 2014;55(12):8123–33.
76. Johnstone J, Fazio M, Rojananuangnit K, et al. Variation of the axial location of Bruch's membrane opening with age, choroidal thickness, and race. Invest Ophthalmol Vis Sci. 2014;55(3):2004–9.
77. Hayreh SS. Blood flow in the optic nerve head and factors that may influence it. Prog Retin Eye Res. 2001;20(5):595–624.
78. Lee KM, Kim TW, Weinreb RN, et al. Anterior lamina cribrosa insertion in primary open-angle glaucoma patients and healthy subjects. PLoS ONE. 2014;9(12): e114935.
79. Kim YW, Jeoung JW, Kim DW, et al. Clinical assessment of lamina cribrosa curvature in eyes with primary open-angle glaucoma. PLoS ONE. 2016;11(3): e0150260.
80. Kim J-A, Kim T-W, Weinreb RN, et al. Lamina cribrosa morphology predicts progressive retinal nerve fiber layer loss in eyes with suspected glaucoma. Sci Rep. 2018;8(1):738.
81. Girard MJ, Tun TA, Husain R, et al. Lamina cribrosa visibility using optical coherence tomography: comparison of devices and effects of image enhancement techniques. Invest Ophthalmol Vis Sci. 2015;56(2):865–74.

82. Kiumehr S, Park SC, Syril D, et al. In vivo evaluation of focal lamina cribrosa defects in glaucoma. Arch Ophthalmol. 2012;130(5):552–9.
83. You JY, Park SC, Su D, et al. Focal lamina cribrosa defects associated with glaucomatous rim thinning and acquired pits. JAMA Ophthalmol. 2013;131(3):314–20.
84. Tatham AJ, Miki A, Weinreb RN, et al. Defects of the lamina cribrosa in eyes with localized retinal nerve fiber layer loss. Ophthalmology. 2014;121(1):110–8.
85. Sharpe GP, Danthurebandara VM, Vianna JR, et al. Optic disc hemorrhages and laminar disinsertions in glaucoma. Ophthalmology. 2016;123(9):1949–56.
86. Kim YK, Park KH. Lamina cribrosa defects in eyes with glaucomatous disc haemorrhage. Acta Ophthalmol. 2016;94(6):e468–73.
87. Faridi OS, Park SC, Kabadi R, et al. Effect of focal lamina cribrosa defect on glaucomatous visual field progression. Ophthalmology. 2014;121(8):1524–30.
88. Moghimi S, Zangwill LM, Manalastas PIC, et al. Association between lamina cribrosa defects and progressive retinal nerve fiber layer loss in glaucoma. JAMA Ophthalmol. 2019;137(4):425.
89. Park HL, Lee J, Jung Y, Park CK. Optic disc hemorrhage and lamina cribrosa defects in glaucoma progression. Sci Rep. 2017;7(1):3489.
90. Ghassibi MP, Chien JL, Patthanathamrongkasem T, et al. Glaucoma diagnostic capability of circumpapillary retinal nerve fiber layer thickness in circle scans with different diameters. J Glaucoma. 2017;26(4):335–42.
91. Mansberger SL, Menda SA, Fortune BA, et al. Automated segmentation errors when using optical coherence tomography to measure retinal nerve fiber layer thickness in glaucoma. Am J Ophthalmol. 2017;174:1–8.
92. Rao HL, Addepalli UK, Yadav RK, et al. Effect of scan quality on diagnostic accuracy of spectral-domain optical coherence tomography in glaucoma. Am J Ophthalmol 2014;157(3):719–27 e1.
93. Rao HL, Addepalli UK, Yadav RK, et al. Factors affecting the ability of the spectral domain optical coherence tomograph to detect photographic retinal nerve fiber layer defects. PLoS ONE. 2014;9(12): e116115.
94. David RCC, Moghimi S, Do JL, et al. Characteristics of central visual field progression in eyes with optic disc hemorrhage. Am J Ophthalmol. 2021;231:109–19.
95. Hood DC, Kardon RH. A framework for comparing structural and functional measures of glaucomatous damage. Prog Retin Eye Res. 2007;26(6):688–710.
96. Moghimi S, Bowd C, Zangwill LM, et al. Measurement floors and dynamic ranges of OCT and OCT angiography in glaucoma. Ophthalmology. 2019;126(7):980–8.
97. Bowd C, Zangwill LM, Weinreb RN, et al. Estimating optical coherence tomography structural measurement floors to improve detection of progression in advanced glaucoma. Am J Ophthalmol. 2017;175:37–44.
98. Wang Y, Bower BA, Izatt JA, et al. Retinal blood flow measurement by circumpapillary Fourier domain Doppler optical coherence tomography. J Biomed Opt. 2008;13(6): 064003.
99. Jia Y, Morrison JC, Tokayer J, et al. Quantitative OCT angiography of optic nerve head blood flow. Biomed Opt Exp. 2012;3(12):3127–37.
100. Jia Y, Tan O, Tokayer J, et al. Split-spectrum amplitude-decorrelation angiography with optical coherence tomography. Opt Express. 2012;20(4):4710–25.
101. Sampson DM, Ali N, Au Yong A, et al. RTVue XR angiovue optical coherence tomography angiography software upgrade impacts on retinal thickness and vessel density measurements. Transl Vis Sci Technol. 2020,9(3).10.
102. Jia Y, Wei E, Wang X, et al. Optical coherence tomography angiography of optic disc perfusion in glaucoma. Ophthalmology. 2014;121(7):1322–32.
103. Liu L, Jia Y, Takusagawa HL, et al. Optical coherence tomography angiography of the peripapillary retina in glaucoma. JAMA Ophthalmol. 2015;133(9):1045–52.
104. Yarmohammadi A, Zangwill LM, Diniz-Filho A, et al. Optical coherence tomography angiography vessel density in healthy, glaucoma suspect, and glaucoma eyes. Invest Ophthalmol Vis Sci 2016;57(9):OCT451–9.

105. Rao HL, Pradhan ZS, Weinreb RN, et al. Regional comparisons of optical coherence tomography angiography vessel density in primary open-angle glaucoma. Am J Ophthalmol. 2016;171:75–83.
106. Rao HL, Pradhan ZS, Weinreb RN, et al. A comparison of the diagnostic ability of vessel density and structural measurements of optical coherence tomography in primary open angle glaucoma. PLoS ONE. 2017;12(3): e0173930.
107. Scripsema NK, Garcia PM, Bavier RD, et al. Optical coherence tomography angiography analysis of perfused peripapillary capillaries in primary open-angle glaucoma and normal-tension glaucoma. Invest Ophthalmol Vis Sci. 2016;57(9):Oct611–Oct20.
108. Rao HL, Kadambi SV, Weinreb RN, et al. Diagnostic ability of peripapillary vessel density measurements of optical coherence tomography angiography in primary open-angle and angle-closure glaucoma. Br J Ophthalmol. 2017;101(8):1066–70.
109. Mohammadi M, Mohammadi SS, Tabatabaei SM, et al. Comparison of vascular density and structural patterns between primary open angle glaucoma and primary angle closure glaucoma. J Glaucoma 2022;31(8):645–650.
110. Hou T-Y, Kuang T-M, Ko Y-C, et al. Optic disc and macular vessel density measured by optical coherence tomography angiography in open-angle and angle-closure glaucoma. Sci Rep. 2020;10(1):5608.
111. Venugopal JP, Rao HL, Weinreb RN, et al. Repeatability of vessel density measurements of optical coherence tomography angiography in normal and glaucoma eyes. Br J Ophthalmol. 2017;102:352–7.
112. Rao HL, Srinivasan T, Pradhan ZS, et al. Optical coherence tomography angiography and visual field progression in primary angle closure glaucoma. J Glaucoma. 2021;30(3):e61–7.
113. Moghimi S, SafiZadeh M, Xu BY, et al. Vessel density and retinal nerve fibre layer thickness following acute primary angle closure. Br J Ophthalmol. 2020;104(8):1103–8.
114. Moghimi S, SafiZadeh M, Fard MA, et al. Changes in optic nerve head vessel density after acute primary angle closure episode. Invest Ophthalmol Vis Sci. 2019;60(2):552–8.
115. Chatziralli I, Milionis I, Christodoulou A, et al. The role of vessel density as measured by optical coherence tomography angiography in the evaluation of pseudoexfoliative glaucoma: a review of the literature. Ophthalmol Ther. 2022;11(2):533–45.
116. Safizadeh M, Shaabani A, Kamalipour A, et al. Optic nerve head vessel density in different stages of pseudoexfoliation disease. Br J Ophthalmol. 2022;106(2):223–8.
117. Suwan Y, Geyman LS, Fard MA, et al. Peripapillary perfused capillary density in exfoliation syndrome and exfoliation glaucoma versus POAG and healthy controls: an OCTA study. Asia Pac J Ophthalmol (Phila). 2018;7(2):84–9.
118. Park JH, Yoo C, Girard MJA, et al. Peripapillary vessel density in glaucomatous eyes: comparison between pseudoexfoliation glaucoma and primary open-angle glaucoma. J Glaucoma. 2018;27(11):1009–16.
119. Philip S, Najafi A, Tantraworasin A, et al. Macula vessel density and foveal avascular zone parameters in exfoliation glaucoma compared to primary open-angle glaucoma. Invest Ophthalmol Vis Sci. 2019;60(4):1244–53.
120. Pradhan ZS, Rao HL, Dixit S, et al. Choroidal microvascular dropout in pseudoexfoliation glaucoma. Invest Ophthalmol Vis Sci. 2019;60(6):2146–51.
121. Lommatzsch C, Rothaus K, Koch JM, et al. Vessel density in glaucoma of different entities as measured with optical coherence tomography angiography. Clin Ophthalmol. 2019;13:2527–34.
122. WuDunn D, Takusagawa HL, Sit AJ, et al. OCT angiography for the diagnosis of glaucoma: a report by the American Academy of Ophthalmology. Ophthalmology. 2021;128(8):1222–35.
123. Rao HL, Pradhan ZS, Weinreb RN, et al. Relationship of optic nerve structure and function to peripapillary vessel density measurements of optical coherence tomography angiography in glaucoma. J Glaucoma. 2017;26(6):548–54.
124. Manalastas PIC, Zangwill LM, Daga FB, et al. The association between macula and ONH optical coherence tomography angiography (OCT-A) vessel densities in glaucoma, glaucoma suspect, and healthy eyes. J Glaucoma. 2018;27(3):227–32.

125. Moghimi S, Zangwill LM, Penteado RC, et al. Macular and optic nerve head vessel density and progressive retinal nerve fiber layer loss in glaucoma. Ophthalmology. 2018;125(11):1720–8.
126. Penteado RC, Zangwill LM, Daga FB, et al. Optical coherence tomography angiography macular vascular density measurements and the central 10-2 visual field in glaucoma. J Glaucoma. 2018;27(6):481–9.
127. Xu H, Yu J, Kong X, et al. Macular microvasculature alterations in patients with primary open-angle glaucoma: a cross-sectional study. Medicine (Baltimore). 2016;95(33): e4341.
128. Tao A, Liang Y, Chen J, et al. Structure-function correlation of localized visual field defects and macular microvascular damage in primary open-angle glaucoma. Microvasc Res. 2020;130: 104005.
129. Ghahari E, Bowd C, Zangwill LM, et al. The association between regional macula vessel density and central visual field damage in advanced glaucoma eyes. J Glaucoma. 2022;31(9):734–43.
130. Shin JW, Lee J, Kwon J, et al. Relationship between macular vessel density and central visual field sensitivity at different glaucoma stages. Br J Ophthalmol. 2019;103(12):1827–33.
131. Mohammadzadeh V, Moghimi S, Nishida T, et al. Longitudinal structure-function relationship between macular vessel density and thickness and central visual field in early glaucoma. Ophthalmol Glaucoma. 2022;5(6):648–57.
132. Yarmohammadi A, Zangwill LM, Diniz-Filho A, et al. Peripapillary and macular vessel density in patients with glaucoma and single-hemifield visual field defect. Ophthalmology. 2017;124(5):709–19.
133. Pradhan ZS, Dixit S, Sreenivasaiah S, et al. A sectoral analysis of vessel density measurements in perimetrically intact regions of glaucomatous eyes: an optical coherence tomography angiography study. J Glaucoma. 2018;27(6):525–31.
134. Chen CL, Bojikian KD, Wen JC, et al. Peripapillary retinal nerve fiber layer vascular microcirculation in eyes with glaucoma and single-hemifield visual field loss. JAMA Ophthalmol. 2017;135(5):461–8.
135. Wu J-H, Moghimi S, Nishida T, et al. Correlation of ganglion cell complex thinning with baseline deep and superficial macular vessel density in glaucoma. Br J Ophthalmol. 2022:bjophthalmol-2021-320663.
136. Lee J, Park CK, Park H-YL. Determinants of vessel defects in superficial and deep vascular layers in normal-tension glaucoma using optical coherence tomography angiography. Sci Rep. 2021;11(1):9941.
137. El-Nimri NW, Manalastas PIC, Zangwill LM, et al. Superficial and deep macula vessel density in healthy, glaucoma suspect, and glaucoma eyes. J Glaucoma. 2021;30(6):e276–84.
138. Kamalipour A, Moghimi S, Hou H, et al. Multilayer macula vessel density and visual field progression in glaucoma. Am J Ophthalmol. 2022;237:193–203.
139. Chihara E, Dimitrova G, Amano H, Chihara T. Discriminatory power of superficial vessel density and prelaminar vascular flow index in eyes with glaucoma and ocular hypertension and normal eyes. Invest Ophthalmol Vis Sci. 2017;58(1):690–7.
140. Chen C-L, Zhang A, Bojikian KD, et al. Peripapillary retinal nerve fiber layer vascular microcirculation in glaucoma using optical coherence tomography–based microangiography. Invest Ophthalmol Vis Sci. 2016;57(9):OCT475–OCT85.
141. Chen HS, Liu CH, Wu WC, et al. Optical coherence tomography angiography of the superficial microvasculature in the macular and peripapillary areas in glaucomatous and healthy eyes. Invest Ophthalmol Vis Sci. 2017;58(9):3637–45.
142. Hou H, Moghimi S, Zangwill LM, et al. Macula vessel density and thickness in early primary open-angle glaucoma. Am J Ophthalmol. 2019;199:120–32.
143. Takusagawa HL, Liu L, Ma KN, et al. Projection-resolved optical coherence tomography angiography of macular retinal circulation in glaucoma. Ophthalmology. 2017;124(11):1589–99.

144. Penteado RC, Bowd C, Proudfoot JA, et al. Diagnostic ability of optical coherence tomography angiography macula vessel density for the diagnosis of glaucoma using difference scan sizes. J Glaucoma. 2020;29(4):245–51.
145. Triolo G, Rabiolo A, Shemonski ND, et al. Optical coherence tomography angiography macular and peripapillary vessel perfusion density in healthy subjects, glaucoma suspects, and glaucoma patients. Invest Ophthalmol Vis Sci. 2017;58(13):5713–22.
146. Chung JK, Hwang YH, Wi JM, et al. Glaucoma diagnostic ability of the optical coherence tomography angiography vessel density parameters. Curr Eye Res. 2017;42(11):1458–67.
147. Kamalipour A, Moghimi S, Jacoba CM, et al. Measurements of OCT angiography complement OCT for diagnosing early primary open-angle glaucoma. Ophthalmol Glaucoma. 2022;5(3):262–74.
148. Hirasawa K, Smith CA, West ME, et al. Discrepancy in loss of macular perfusion density and ganglion cell layer thickness in early glaucoma. Am J Ophthalmol. 2021;221:39–47.
149. Nishida T, Moghimi S, David RCC, et al. Rates of circumpapillary retinal nerve fiber layer thinning and capillary density loss in glaucomatous eyes with disc hemorrhage. Am J Ophthalmol. 2022;235:24–31.
150. Ekici E, Moghimi S, Bowd C, et al. Capillary density measured by optical coherence tomography angiography in glaucomatous optic disc phenotypes. Am J Ophthalmol. 2020;219:261–70.
151. David RCC, Moghimi S, Ekici E, et al. Rates of retinal nerve fiber layer thinning in distinct glaucomatous optic disc phenotypes in early glaucoma. Am J Ophthalmol. 2021;229:8–17.
152. Lin YH, Huang SM, Yeung L, et al. Correlation of visual field with peripapillary vessel density through optical coherence tomography angiography in normal-tension glaucoma. Transl Vis Sci Technol. 2020;9(13):26.
153. Yarmohammadi A, Zangwill LM, Diniz-Filho A, et al. Relationship between optical coherence tomography angiography vessel density and severity of visual field loss in glaucoma. Ophthalmology. 2016;123(12):2498–508.
154. Hou H, Moghimi S, Proudfoot JA, et al. Ganglion cell complex thickness and macular vessel density loss in primary open-angle glaucoma. Ophthalmology. 2020;127(8):1043–52.
155. Shin JW, Song MK, Kook MS. Association between progressive retinal capillary density loss and visual field progression in open-angle glaucoma patients according to disease stage. Am J Ophthalmol. 2021;226:137–47.
156. Nishida T, Moghimi S, Wu J-H, et al. Association of initial optical coherence tomography angiography vessel density loss with faster visual field loss in glaucoma. JAMA Ophthalmol. 2022;140(4):319–26.
157. Bowd C, Belghith A, Proudfoot JA, et al. Gradient-boosting classifiers combining vessel density and tissue thickness measurements for classifying early to moderate glaucoma. Am J Ophthalmol. 2020;217:131–9.
158. Rabiolo A, Fantaguzzi F, Sacconi R, et al. Combining structural and vascular parameters to discriminate among glaucoma patients, glaucoma suspects, and healthy subjects. Transl Vis Sci Technol. 2021;10(14):20.
159. Wong D, Chua J, Tan B, et al. Combining OCT and OCTA for focal structure-function modeling in early primary open-angle glaucoma. Invest Ophthalmol Vis Sci. 2021;62(15):8.
160. Xu C, Saini C, Wang M, et al. Combined model of OCT angiography and structural OCT parameters to predict paracentral visual field loss in primary open-angle glaucoma. Ophthalmol Glaucoma. 2022.
161. Kamalipour A, Moghimi S, Khosravi P, et al. Combining optical coherence tomography and optical coherence tomography angiography longitudinal data for the detection of visual field progression in Glaucoma. Am J Ophthalmol. 2023;246:141–54.
162. Suh MH, Zangwill LM, Manalastas PI, et al. Deep retinal layer microvasculature dropout detected by the optical coherence tomography angiography in glaucoma. Ophthalmology. 2016;123(12):2509–18.

163. Lee EJ, Kim TW, Lee SH, Kim JA. Underlying microstructure of parapapillary deep-layer capillary dropout identified by optical coherence tomography angiography. Invest Ophthalmol Vis Sci. 2017;58(3):1621–7.
164. Rao HL, Sreenivasaiah S, Riyazuddin M, et al. Choroidal microvascular dropout in primary angle closure glaucoma. Am J Ophthalmol. 2019;199:184–92.
165. Lee EJ, Lee KM, Lee SH, Kim TW. Parapapillary choroidal microvasculature dropout in glaucoma: a comparison between optical coherence tomography angiography and indocyanine green angiography. Ophthalmology. 2017;124(8):1209–17.
166. Micheletti E, Moghimi S, Nishida T, et al. Factors associated with choroidal microvascular dropout change. Br J Ophthalmol. 2022:bjophthalmol-2022-321157.
167. Lee EJ, Lee SH, Kim JA, Kim TW. Parapapillary deep-layer microvasculature dropout in glaucoma: topographic association with glaucomatous damage. Invest Ophthalmol Vis Sci. 2017;58(7):3004–10.
168. Shin JW, Kwon J, Lee J, Kook MS. Choroidal microvasculature dropout is not associated with myopia, but is associated with glaucoma. J Glaucoma. 2018;27(2):189–96.
169. Rao HL, Sreenivasaiah S, Riyazuddin M, et al. Choroidal microvascular dropout in primary angle closure glaucoma. Am J Ophthalmol. 2018.
170. Jo YH, Kwon J, Shon K, et al. Greater severity of glaucomatous damage in eyes with than without choroidal microvasculature dropout in open-angle glaucoma. Invest Ophthalmol Vis Sci. 2019;60(4):901–12.
171. Lee EJ, Kim TW, Kim JA, Kim JA. Central visual field damage and parapapillary choroidal microvasculature dropout in primary open-angle glaucoma. Ophthalmology. 2018;125(4):588–96.
172. Park HL, Kim JW, Park CK. Choroidal microvasculature dropout is associated with progressive retinal nerve fiber layer thinning in glaucoma with disc hemorrhage. Ophthalmology. 2018;125(7):1003–13.
173. Lee EJ, Kim J-A, Kim T-W. Influence of choroidal microvasculature dropout on the rate of glaucomatous progression: a prospective study. Ophthalmology Glaucoma. 2020;3(1):25–31.
174. Micheletti E, Moghimi S, El-Nimri N, et al. Relationship of macular ganglion cell complex thickness to choroidal microvasculature drop-out in primary open-angle glaucoma. Br J Ophthalmol. 2022:bjophthalmol-2021-320621.
175. Lin S, Cheng H, Zhang S, et al. Parapapillary choroidal microvasculature dropout is associated with the decrease in retinal nerve fiber layer thickness: a prospective study. Invest Ophthalmol Vis Sci. 2019;60(2):838–42.
176. Jo YH, Shin JW, Song MK, et al. Baseline choroidal microvasculature dropout as a predictor of subsequent visual field progression in open-angle glaucoma. J Glaucoma. 2021;30(8):672–81.
177. Lee JY, Shin JW, Song MK, et al. An increased choroidal microvasculature dropout size is associated with progressive visual field loss in open-angle glaucoma. Am J Ophthalmol. 2021;223:205–19.
178. Jo YH, Kwon J, Jeong D, et al. Rapid central visual field progression rate in eyes with open-angle glaucoma and choroidal microvasculature dropout. Sci Rep. 2019;9(1):8525.
179. Kim JA, Lee EJ, Kim TW. Evaluation of parapapillary choroidal microvasculature dropout and progressive retinal nerve fiber layer thinning in patients with glaucoma. JAMA Ophthalmol. 2019;137(7):810–6.
180. Micheletti E, El-Nimri N, Nishida T, et al. Central visual field damage in glaucoma eyes with choroidal microvasculature dropout with and without high axial myopia. Br J Ophthalmol. 2023:bjo-2022-322234.
181. Jo YH, Shin JW, Song MK, et al. Choroidal microvasculature dropout is associated with generalized choroidal vessel loss within the β-parapapillary atrophy in glaucoma. Am J Ophthalmol. 2020;215:37–48.
182. Park HY-L, Shin DY, Jeon SJ, Park CK. Association between parapapillary choroidal vessel density measured with optical coherence tomography angiography and future visual field progression in patients with glaucoma. JAMA Ophthalmol 2019;137(6):681–8.

183. Hwang HS, Lee EJ, Kim J-A, et al. Influence of choroidal microvasculature dropout on progressive retinal nerve fibre layer thinning in primary open-angle glaucoma: comparison of parapapillary β-zones and γ-zones. Br J Ophthalmol. 2023:bjo-2022-322505.
184. Nishida T, Oh WH, Moghimi S, et al. Central macular OCTA parameters in glaucoma. Br J Ophthalmol. 2023;107(2):207–14.
185. Kwon J, Choi J, Shin JW, et al. An optical coherence tomography angiography study of the relationship between foveal avascular zone size and retinal vessel density. Invest Ophthalmol Vis Sci. 2018;59(10):4143–53.
186. Kwon J, Choi J, Shin JW, et al. Alterations of the foveal avascular zone measured by optical coherence tomography angiography in glaucoma patients with central visual field defects. Invest Ophthalmol Vis Sci. 2017;58(3):1637–45.
187. Igarashi R, Ochiai S, Togano T, et al. Foveal avascular zone measurement via optical coherence tomography angiography and its relationship with the visual field in eyes with open-angle glaucoma. J Glaucoma. 2020;29(6):492–7.
188. Shoji T, Kanno J, Weinreb RN, et al. OCT angiography measured changes in the foveal avascular zone area after glaucoma surgery. Br J Ophthalmol. 2022;106(1):80–6.
189. Manalastas PIC, Zangwill LM, Saunders LJ, et al. Reproducibility of optical coherence tomography angiography macular and optic nerve head vascular density in glaucoma and healthy eyes. J Glaucoma. 2017;26(10):851–9.
190. Lim CW, Cheng J, Tay ELT, et al. Optical coherence tomography angiography of the macula and optic nerve head: microvascular density and test-retest repeatability in normal subjects. BMC Ophthalmol. 2018;18(1):315.
191. Venugopal JP, Rao HL, Weinreb RN, et al. Repeatability of vessel density measurements of optical coherence tomography angiography in normal and glaucoma eyes. Br J Ophthalmol. 2018;102(3):352–7.
192. Rao HL, Pradhan ZS, Weinreb RN, et al. Determinants of peripapillary and macular vessel densities measured by optical coherence tomography angiography in normal eyes. J Glaucoma. 2017;26(5):491–7.
193. Holmen IC, Konda SM, Pak JW, et al. Prevalence and severity of artifacts in optical coherence tomographic angiograms. JAMA Ophthalmol. 2020;138(2):119–26.
194. Suh MH, Zangwill LM, Manalastas PI, et al. Optical coherence tomography angiography vessel density in glaucomatous eyes with focal lamina cribrosa defects. Ophthalmology. 2016;123(11):2309–17.
195. Hollo G. Intrasession and between-visit variability of sector peripapillary angioflow vessel density values measured with the angiovue optical coherence tomograph in different retinal layers in ocular hypertension and glaucoma. PLoS ONE. 2016;11(8): e0161631.
196. Spaide RF, Fujimoto JG, Waheed NK. Image artifacts in optical coherence tomography angiography. Retina. 2015;35(11):2163–80.
197. Kamalipour A, Moghimi S, Hou H, et al. OCT angiography artifacts in glaucoma. Ophthalmology. 2021;128(10):1426–37.
198. Camino A, Zhang M, Gao SS, et al. Evaluation of artifact reduction in optical coherence tomography angiography with real-time tracking and motion correction technology. Biomed Opt Express. 2016;7(10):3905–15.
199. Venugopal JP, Rao HL, Weinreb RN, et al. Repeatability and comparability of peripapillary vessel density measurements of high-density and non-high-density optical coherence tomography angiography scans in normal and glaucoma eyes. Br J Ophthalmol. 2018.
200. Hormel TT, Huang D, Jia Y. Artifacts and artifact removal in optical coherence tomographic angiography. Quant Imaging Med Surg. 2021;11(3):1120–33.
201. Campbell JP, Zhang M, Hwang TS, et al. Detailed vascular anatomy of the human retina by projection-resolved optical coherence tomography angiography. Sci Rep. 2017;7:42201.
202. Liu L, Edmunds B, Takusagawa HL, et al. Projection-resolved optical coherence tomography angiography of the peripapillary retina in glaucoma. Am J Ophthalmol. 2019;207:99–109.

OCT in Amblyopia—2023 Version

21

Paolo Nucci, Andrea Lembo, Sofia Ginelli, and Francesco Pichi

Abstract

Purpose: To analyze the advantages of optical coherence tomography (OCT) or OCT angiography (OCTA) to detect retinal nerve fiber layer (RNFL) thickness abnormalities, changes in the macula and in the choroidal thickness in amblyopic patients. *Methods*: Studies were selected through an electronic search on PUBMED, EMBASE and GOOGLE SCHOLAR using the following terms: "Optical coherence tomography in amblyopia", "OCT and amblyopia", "Optical coherence tomography and anisometropic amblyopia", "Optical coherence tomography and strabismic amblyopia". *Results* Optical coherence tomography is a rapid, non-invasive imaging technique allowing objective quantification of retinal structures with high resolution; it can be successfully applied to young children, even those who are neurologically disabled or less cooperative. New generations devices, such as spectral domain OCT, have led to a dramatic increase in sensitivity that enables high-speed imaging. Furthermore, the OCT angiography advent has allowed us to study the retinal circulation in an accurate and non-invasive way. It can also be performed in children without technical and physical difficulties of fluorescein angiography. *Discussion*: OCT and OCT angiography could be useful technologies for evaluating progressive choroidal and RNFL thinning and changes in the macula in amblyopia. Evidence for direct retinal changes in eyes with amblyopia has been controversial, so that further studies with large sample are required.

P. Nucci (✉) · A. Lembo · S. Ginelli
Dipartimento di Scienze Biomediche, Chirurgiche e Odontoiatriche, University of Milan, Via San Vittore 12, 20123 Milan, Italy
e-mail: paolo.nucci@unimi.it

F. Pichi
Cleveland Clinic Abu Dhabi, Eye Institute, Abu Dhabi, United Arab Emirates

A. Grzybowski and P. Barboni (eds.), *OCT and Imaging in Central Nervous System Diseases*, https://doi.org/10.1007/978-3-031-72156-4_21

Keywords

Optical coherence tomography • Retinal nerve fiber thickness • Macular thickness • Amblyopia

Amblyopia is one of the most common causes of monocular visual loss in children and young adults in many countries and can be defined as a disorder characterized by a dysfunction of the processing of visual information [1]. It results from degradation of the retinal image during the period of visual development, which historically has been thought to be the first six years of life [2]. Therefore, amblyopia never occurs in isolation; the disease is not the cause, but the effect of another pathological process. Amblyopia can be seen as a result of either disuse, due to the absence of a clear image on the retina (anisometropia or deprivation), or misuse, due to abnormal binocular interaction (strabismus) [3]. In fact, primary types of amblyopia include anisometropia, strabismus, form deprivation and high bilateral refractive errors. In particular, the degradation of the image, and subsequent central suppression that leads to amblyopia results from one of the three causal processes.

In 2003, the American Association for Pediatric Ophthalmology and Strabismus (AAPOS) published a list of risk factors for amblyopia [4]; Arnold et al. [5] attempted to estimate cut-off found by the AAPOS in a meta-analysis. The following results were obtained: approximate prevalence of anisometropia of 1.2%, hyperopia of 6%, astigmatism of 15%, myopia of 0.6%, strabismus of 2.5%, and a visual acuity less than 20/40 of 6%. The mean combined prevalence found was $21\% \pm 2\%$ compared to a prevalence of amblyopia 20/40 and worse of 2.5%. The estimated prevalence of amblyopia in adults is 2–9% [6], and it still seems to be the leading cause of monocular vision loss in people aged between twenty and seventy years [7]. Considering these data, it is easy to think how important an early diagnosis of amblyopia is. The diagnosis of unilateral amblyopia is made when reduced visual acuity is recorded in the presence of an amblyogenic factor, and not explained by another ocular abnormality. Residual visual deficits after correction of any amblyogenic factor (for example by spectacles prescription) are assumed to be due to amblyopia [3]. A widely accepted definition of amblyopia based on visual acuity is two or more Snellen or logMAR lines difference between eyes in best-corrected visual acuity. A one-line difference is usually a normal result, based on test–retest variability [8]. One important feature of visual acuity testing to diagnose amblyopia is that there is a distribution or range of typical visual acuity in any population. This range changes with age because of neural maturational processes [3].

Although clinical ocular examination is most often normal in amblyopia, microscopic anatomical and structural abnormalities have been found, starting from Hubel and Wiesel's pioneering work [9] in the retina, lateral geniculate bodies, and visual cortex [10–12]. With the advent of OCT in ophthalmology, there have been numerous attempts to investigate the structural differences in macular and peripapillary retinal nerve fiber layer (RNFL) in amblyopic patients [13–15]. Despite the use of more and more advanced techniques, conflicting results have often been found.

Khan et al. [16] compared the anterior and posterior ocular architecture of amblyopic and normal fellow eyes in 14 patients with hyperopic anisometropic amblyopia. Subjects were children between 5 and 10 years of age, with hyperopia>1.5 D and unilateral amblyopia with an interocular difference in spherical equivalent of at least 1D. Patients were examined using two tools: corneal topography to measure anterior and posterior corneal curvature, corneal thickness and volume, anterior chamber volume and depth; and OCT for RNFL, central macular thickness and macular volume measurements. In these children, corneal topography and OCT revealed no differences ($P > 0.05$) in the anterior and posterior architecture between the amblyopic and the fellow eye.

Wu et al. [17] examined a larger sample, including 72 children (range 5–16 years) to compare the RNFL and macular thickness in amblyopic eyes with that in fellow eyes. All enrolled children had unilateral hyperopic anisometropic amblyopia and normal vision in the contralateral eye. After a full ophthalmological assessment, OCT scans were performed using a spectral domain OCT (3D-OCT 1000). The foveolar thickness, central macular thickness and four quadrants of the inner and outer macular thickness were measured for each subject. Peripapillary RNFL thickness was measured using the "fast RNFL thickness (3.4 mm diameter)" scan protocol, which consisted of six radial line scans. OCT measurements found thicker foveolas and peripapillary RNFL in eyes with hyperopic anisometropic amblyopia compared to the controlateral eyes, but no changes in 1-mm central macular thickness (Fig. 21.1). This difference between foveolar thickness and 1-mm central macular thickness needs further histopathologic investigation. No correlation was found between severity of anisometropia and differences of peripapillary RNFL thickness, or between central macular thickness and foveal thickness in the contralateral eyes, suggesting far more complex pathophysiologic mechanisms for anisometropic amblyopia than we currently know.

An interesting biological theory regarding differences in RNFL thickness in eyes with and without amblyopia proposes that in humans the total population of cells in the ganglion cell layer is at its highest approximately between 18 and 30 weeks of gestation and declines rapidly thereafter [18]. The number of axons in the human optic nerve decreases too during gestation [19]. Absence of normal visual stimulation may contribute to the reduced apoptosis of retinal ganglion cells in amblyopic eyes, eventually leading to thicker RNFL compared to non-amblyopic eye. Yen et al. [20] mentioned that the physiological postnatal ganglion cell reduction could be inhibited in amblyopia, while Kok et al. [21] concluded that a hypothetical arrest of the normal ganglion cell reduction is expected to lead to an abnormally thick retinal thickness, especially the pericentral retinal thickness. A second hypothesis seems to regard the macula, which becomes thicker rather than thinner in the perifoveal retina in six-month embryos, manifesting a slight protrusion. Wu et al. [17] found that the foveola was significantly thicker in amblyopic

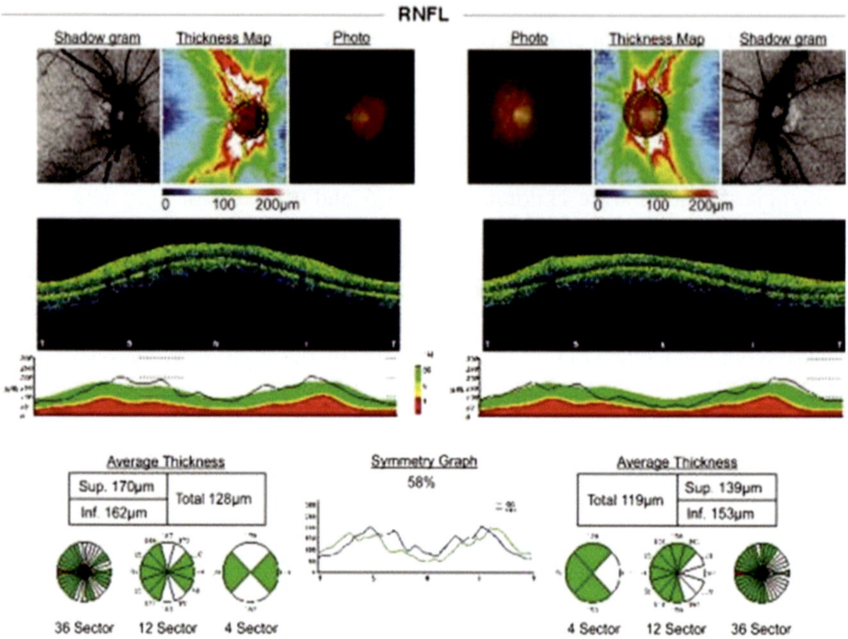

Fig. 21.1 OCT of retinal nerve fiber layer (RNFL) in a patient with hyperopic anisometropic amblyopia [17]

eyes than in the fellow eyes (181.4 ± 14.2 μm vs. 175.2 ± 13.3 μm, $P < 0.01$). In their studies, blurred vision could lead to insufficient stimulation in the amblyopic eye, affecting the normal maturation of the macula, including movement of Henle's fibers away from the fovea and a decrease in foveal cone diameter, which would result in increased foveolar thickness. In a more recent study Guagliano et al. [22] compared OCT parameters as peripapillary RNFL thickness, morphometric optic nerve head (ONH) parameters, central macular thickness, and ganglion cell complex (GCC) thickness between healthy and amblyopic eyes obtained from a population of 117 children (243 eyes) split into four group. Groupe A represented non-amblyopic subjects, group B fellow eyes of subjects affected by monolateral amblyopia, group C amblyopic eyes of subjects affected by monolateral amblyopia and group D with subjects affected by bilateral amblyopia. There was no statistically significant difference for RNFL thickness and GCC thickness values between amblyopic and healthy eyes, instead, analysis of ONH parameters showed statistically significant differences for rim area and disk area parameters, both smaller in monolateral amblyopic eyes compared to normal control eyes. In this study was found a significant difference in central macular thickness between group A and group C, whereas no differences were found in the macular thickness measured in the superior, inferior, nasal, and temporal sectors at 3- and 5-mm distances from the fovea. In conclusion, this study hypothesized that the amblyopic process has

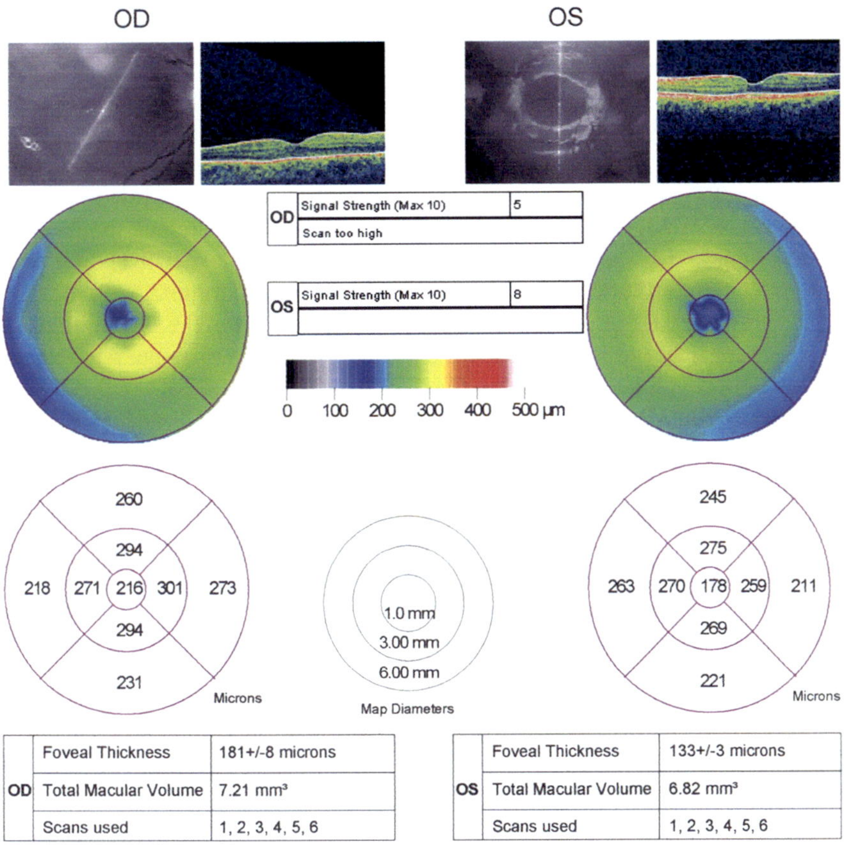

Fig. 21.2 OCT images from an amblyopic subject (OD: amblyopic eye; OS: fellow eye). Refractive error OD: − 6.00–1.25 × 165, OS: − 1.25 sph [22]

no significant effect on the RNFL and GCC development and this result disagrees with previously reported studies. Regarding myopic amblyopia, Pang et al. [23] conducted a study on 31 children with a mean age of 9.56 years and mean spherical equivalent in amblyopic eyes of -10.79 ± 3.40 diopters. Patients were scanned with OCT using the "Fast macular thickness protocol". The following ten parameters were measured for each subject: foveal minimum thickness, average foveal thickness, inner nasal, superior, temporal, and inferior macular thickness, outer nasal, superior, temporal, and inferior macular thickness. Pang et al. [23] found that amblyopic children with unilateral high myopia tend to have a thicker fovea and thinner inner and outer layers in the amblyopic eye compared to the normal fellow eye (Fig. 21.2).

Recently, Wan et al. [24] investigate changes in retinal and choroidal thickness in high myopic amblyopia (HMA). Using enhanced depth imaging (EDI) system of SD-OCT, retinal thickness (RT) and choroidal thickness (CT) were measured at different locations: subfoveal (SF), and at 0.5 mm/1.0 mm/1.5 mm/2.0 mm/2.5 mm/3.0 mm to the fovea in superior, nasal, inferior, and temporal sectors. These parameters were measured in five groups: high myopic amblyopia (HMA), low myopia (LM), moderate myopia (MM), high myopia (HM), and normal group (NG). In this study no statistical difference at SFRT was found between HMA and other groups. At 1.0 mm/1.5 mm/2.0 mm/2.5 mm/3.0 mm to fovea, HMA has thinner RT in all four sectors compared to NG, LW, and MM, except for two points. RT of HMA was thinner than HM at each measurement point in the four directions, and was more significant in the inferior, with statistical difference. Moreover, thinner CT was observed at 1.0 mm/1.5 mm/2.0 mm/2.5 mm/3.0 mm in the superior and inferior sectors of HMA compared with HM. In addition, the CT was thinner in the inferior sector compared to the superior one. At the same time, at the 0.5 mm area outside the fovea in the inferior sector, HMA had thinner RT compared to HM, while no significant difference in SFCT and SFRT were observed between the two groups. This was a novel finding that was not consistent with previous research and these data suggest that CT thinning is associated with RT thinning in HMA and amblyopia influences RT and CT. Thus, thinner choroid supplies less blood to the outer retina, resulting in thinning of the retina.

Another important parameter that can be detected at OCT and that can be investigated in amblyopic eyes is the thickness of the choroid. Nowadays, the EDI OCT makes it possible to have a clearer view of the choroid. Nishi et al. [25] showed a different choroidal profile in the amblyopic eyes and found the subfoveal choroid of eyes with hyperopic anisometropic amblyopia significantly thicker than that of the fellow eyes and the age-matched normal eyes (Fig. 21.3). Yu et al. [26] investigated the choroidal thickness (CT) in children with amblyopia through SD-OCT and found that in the subfoveal area, the choroid was thicker in amblyopic eyes than in fellow eyes and control eyes as well. In contrast, Niyaz et al. [27] found that the choroidal thickness was not significantly different between amblyopic and fellow eyes in strabismus 175 patients.

Moreover, Pang et al. [28] showed that the increased central macular thickness of eyes with myopic anisometropic amblyopia tended to decrease to the fellow eye level after amblyopia treatment (refractive correction and patching). These results indicate that anatomic changes may be present in the retinas of amblyopic children with unilateral high myopia and these changes could be partially reversible with proper treatment. Anisometropia as the most frequent cause of amblyopia has been evaluated in numerous studies. However, anisometropia associated with high myopia has often been excluded from these studies. The few studies investigating anisometropic amblyopia caused by unilateral high myopia have concluded that this type of amblyopia had poorer treatment outcomes [29]. Underlying structural abnormalities and macular hypoplasia have been proposed as causes for the poor treatment outcomes in myopic anisometropia [30, 31]. Knowledge of the macular structure and associated factors in amblyopia associated with unilateral high myopia will help the understanding of this disease and may assist clinicians in predicting treatment outcomes. Studies that have focused on comparison between strabismic and anisometropic amblyopia, have found differences between the two

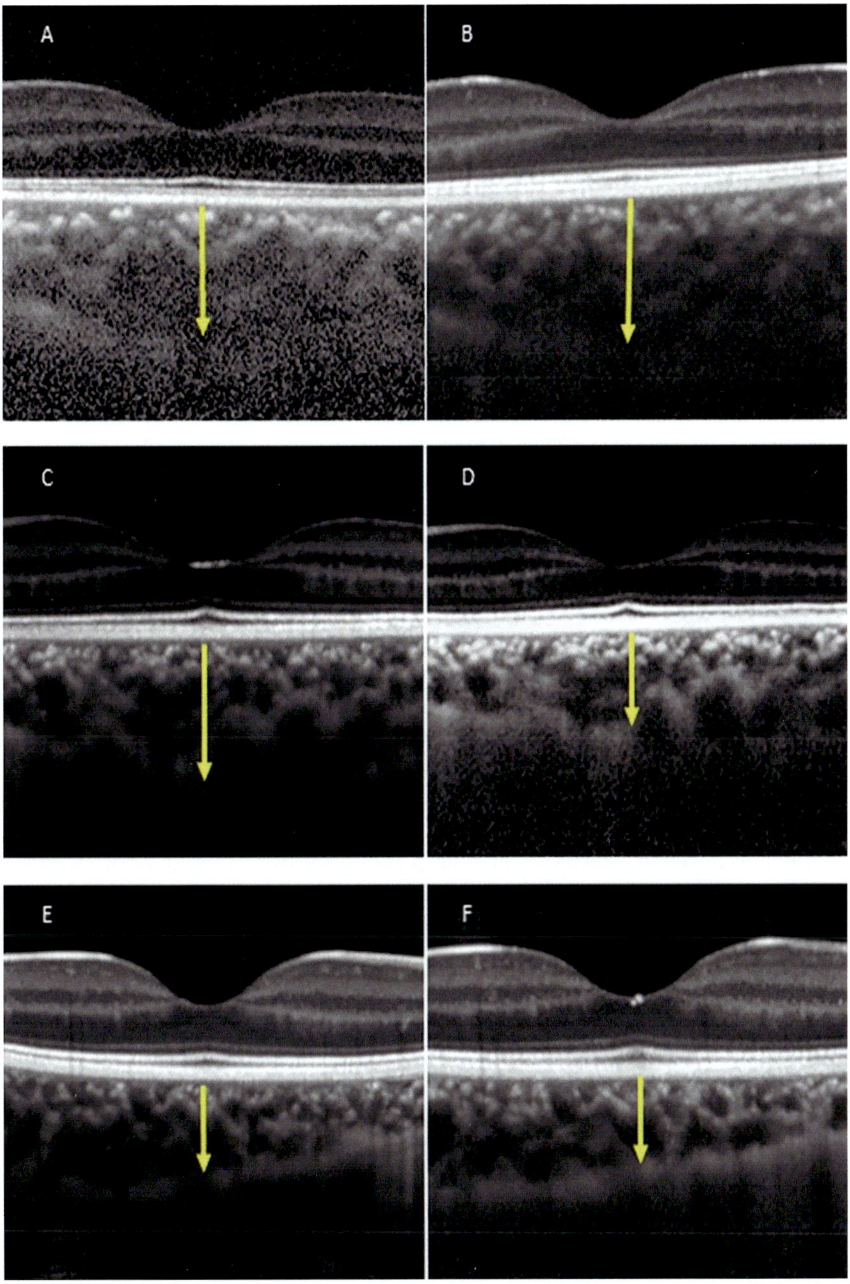

Fig. 21.3 Enhanced depth imaging spectral domain optical coherence tomographic (EDI-SD-OCT) images of an anisohypermetropic amblyopic eye and control eye [23]

defects. Dickmann et al. [32] conducted a study to determine whether RNFL thickness, macular thickness, and foveal volume in patients with unilateral amblyopia differed between the amblyopic and the fellow eye. Stratus OCT was performed on 80 eyes of 40 patients (mean age, 15.2 years; range, 5–56 years) with unilateral amblyopia divided into 20 strabismic and 20 anisometropic. OCT found that the difference in RNFL thickness between the amblyopic and fellow eyes was no statistically significant ($p > 0.05$) in both groups. Conversely, macular thickness and foveal volume in strabismic amblyopia were 5% lower in the fellow eye than in the amblyopic one. On the other hand, in the anisometropic group there was no significant difference between eyes in either macular thickness or foveal volume. Dickmann et al. [33] found similar results on 15 patients with strabismic anysometropia and 15 patients with anisometric amblyopia. In both groups, mean foveal volume and RNFL thickness did not differ significantly between eyes. Only macular thickness in the strabismic group differed significantly between the amblyopic and fellow eyes. This statistically significant difference, also established in other studies [15, 32], was not present in the refractive amblyopia group: amblyopia of different etiologies could therefore be associated with different changes of the retinal tissues. Thickening of the amblyopic fovea could be related to a developmental arrest, with incomplete formation of the foveal depression, even if it's difficult to determine whether this may be caused by a direct effect of abnormal sensory output or the consequence of primary alteration of visual cortex and the lateral geniculate nucleus (Fig. 21.2). There was also a significant correlation between RNFL thickness and macular sensitivity measured with microperimetry (strabismic group, $r = 0.84$, $P = 0.002$; anisometropic group, $r = 0.66$, $P = 0.02$). Although visual fields generally appear normal, amblyopia can be associated with small central and paracentral scotoma in an amblyopic eye but do not need further evaluations, especially if the patient is asymptomatic. If a deep focal deficit is found, causes of organic pathologies (for example optic neuropathy) should be investigated. Data from Dickmann et al. [33] study suggest that the anatomical differences of RNFL thickness between the amblyopic and the fellow eye could determine the difference in macular sensitivity between the two eyes. Additional studies with larger, more diverse cohorts are needed to reveal whether these findings can be confirmed. Szigeti et al. [34] used OCT imaging and image segmentation methodology on 38 patients (range 6–67 years) with different types of amblyopia (strabismus without anisometropia, anisometropia without strabismus, strabismus with anisometropia). They detected structural changes in the outer nuclear layer of the fovea, suggesting the possible involvement of photoreceptor**.** There is ***growing*** evidence showing that photoreceptors may be affected in amblyopia. For example, Enoch [35] using the Stiles-Crawford function suggested that photoreceptor orientation is abnormal in amblyopic eyes, while other Authors did not found indication of retinal dysfunction at the level of the cones in amblyopic eyes [27]. Nishi et al. [25] used SD OCT to analyze the thickness of the outer nuclear layer (ONL), photoreceptor inner segment (IS) layer and outer segment (OS) layer of 21 patients (mean 6.0 ± 2.3 years) with anisohypermetropic amblyopia and 25 age-mached controls (mean 5.6 ± 1.9 years). Additionally, they assessed the effects of optical treatments on the photoreceptor layer. Results showed that the length of the OS was significantly lower in the ambliopic eyes (42.4 ± 4.6 μm, $p = 0.03$) than in the fellow eyes (48.0 ± 6.6 μm). One year after the optical treatment, the best-corrected visual acuity (BCVA) improved, and the length of the OS was significantly increased ($p = 0.0001$). The change of BCVA was significantly correlated with the change of the length of the OS 1 year after the treatment ($r = 0.52$; $p = 0.0004$). Even if the number of patients is exiguous and children enrolled have only hyperopic anysometropic amblyopia, this study suggest that there are qualitative and quantitative differences in the microstructure of photoreceptors of amblyopic fovea from normal one. Furthermore, optical treatment in anisohypermetropic amblyopia can induce dynamic changes in photoreceptors (increase in the OS length in the amblyopic eyes after the optical treatment, with significant correlation between the increased OS length and better BCVA). Anyway, the relationship between these morpho-structural changes and the amplyopia is still far from being clearly understood. Further studies are warranted to investigate better these changes.

As we previously anticipated, various studies in the latest 5 years investigate the correlation between Choroidal Thickness (CT) changes and amblyopia (both anisometropic and strabismic amblyopia) in children through OCT. A Meta-Analysis by Liu et al. [36], which includes 11 clinical trials involving 449 patients, indicated that the amblyopic process may involve the choroid. The results showed that the CT was thicker in the amblyopic eyes than in both the fellow and control eyes from the fovea to the temporal and nasal cavities at different interval (range: 0.5 mm~3 mm) points. Sub-Foveal Choroideal Thickness (SFCT) did not differ between anisometropic and strabismic amblyopia. Congruously with previous study, foveola was thicker in the amblyopic eyes than that in the visually normal control eyes. In this regard, the authors provide a suggestive theory to explain the CT thicker in amblyopic eyes. A thicker retina may require additional blood for nourishment. Therefore, the CT may have to increase to supply additional blood to the retina. Increased choroidal blood flow can cause choroidal thickening.

Zha et al. [37] describe the distribution of choroidal structure in 31 patients with unilateral amblyopia (strabismic and anisometropic amblyopia) and compare the choroidal thickness (CT) of amblyopic eyes, measured by EDI–OCT, with fellow eyes and control eyes. In particular, CT was measured at 13 points: at subfoveal point (SFCT) and at 1/2/3 mm intervals to the superior (S1/S2/S3), inferior (I1/I2/I3), temporal (T1/T2/T3) and nasal (N1/N2/N3) to the fovea. This study depicted a more detailed distribution of amblyopic choroid demonstrating a significantly thicker choroid in amblyopic eyes than control eyes only at SFCT, N1 and S1. Using split-spectrum amplitude-decorrelation angiography OCT (SSADA-OCT), simply known as OCT-Angiography, Guo et al. [38] discovered that 86.4% of the amblyopic eyes displayed a blurry choroidocapillary network and that 68.2% of the amblyopic eyes had a dark atrophic patch. The authors said that it was possible that the choroidocapillary atrophy patch caused a wide range of compensatory dilatation of its surrounding capillaries, and because of this, blurry images occurred. Dilatation of the choroidal vessels may lead to increased CT. All the studies included in the Meta-Analysis by Liu used SD-OCT. This could be a potential bias if we consider that swept source OCT (SS-OCT) is recognized as the latest landmark in choroidal imaging. Up to date, Araki et al. [39] published the only study which investigate the macular retinal and choroidal thickness in amblyopic eyes using SS-OCT. The design of the study is similar to those included in the Meta-Analysis, but the results are quite surprising: although there were significant differences in CT with hyperopic anisometropic amblyopia group (CT significantly greater than that of amblyopic fellow and normal eyes), there was no significant difference in CT for the strabismic amblyopia group respect to amblyopic fellow and normal eyes. The discrepancy in CT between the two types of amblyopia may be due to both differences in ocular size and underlying mechanism.

Aslan Bayhan et al. [40] assess changes in CT during amblyopia treatment using (SD-OCT). 40 patients (aged 3–9 years) with hyperopic anisometropic amblyopia underwent treatment with refractive correction alone for 16 weeks and if needed, with refractive correction and patching treatment thereafter (6 months). CT was measured at the fovea, and at two different distances (1.5–3.00 mm) temporally and nasally to the fovea in the amblyopic eyes and fellow eyes during treatment and in the control subjects ($n = 22$). CT at all locations decreased significantly after treatment in the amblyopic eyes. These findings indicate that thicker CT in amblyopic eyes partially regresses after amblyopia treatment.

However, considering these results, further studies are necessary to clear the causal relationship and the mechanisms involved between amblyopia and changes in CT.

Recently, the OCT technology was implemented with the introduction of the Optical Coherence Tomographic Angiography (OCTA). This new technique provides a non-invasive visualization of the microvasculature of the retina, allowing the identification of the superficial retinal capillary plexus (SCP), the deep retinal capillary plexus (DCP), and the choroid. An increasing number of studies have been conducted with the use of OCTA in the field of retinal pathology. Some pioneering studies have extended OCTA application even to amblyopic eyes.

Lonngi et al. [41] examined 63 eyes of 59 children (age < 18 years), 13 (21%) were amblyopic (anisometropic and refractive amblyopia) and 50 (79%) were control eyes. The objective of the study was to evaluate SCP and DCP in terms of vessel density, as a percentage, at Macular as well as optic nerve localizations. No abnormality in papillary and peripapillary vessel density was found between the two groups: this result is consistent with the findings of the Pediatric Eye Disease Investigator Group which used OCT and reported no difference in global or quadrantic RNFL thickness compared with the fellow non amblyopic eyes [42]. However, OCTA revealed a significantly lower vessel density of the DCP, with a mean of a 5.7% reduction in the 6×6-mm macular scan in children with amblyopia. This reduction was a mean of 1.8% in the SCP.

The same group [43] also investigated choriocapillaris vessel density by OCTA in a total of 20 eyes of 16 patients with amblyopia and 25 eyes of 25 controls. Mean choriocapillaris vessel density was significantly higher (74.8 ± 5.8) in the amblyopic group than in the control group (71.1 ± 3.6), even after adjusting for

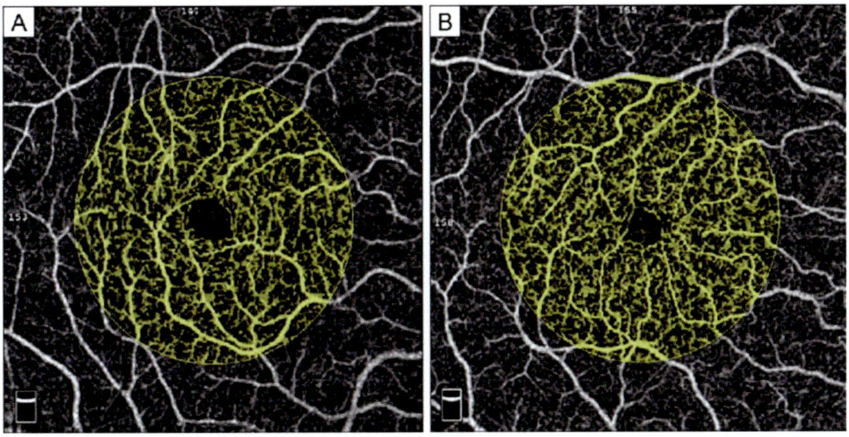

Fig. 21.4 Vessel density of SCP of an amblyopic eye (A) and a control eye (B). Vessel density of SCP is lower in the amblyopic eye [43]

age and refractive error (P = 0.012). Also, outer parafoveal macular thickness (the inner boundary of the inner nuclear layer to the retinal pigment epithelium outer boundary) was significantly greater in amblyopic eyes than in control eyes, congruously with previous studies [25].

Sobral et al. [44] evaluated the highest number of amblyopic children using OCT-A up to date (July 2018). They enrolled the largest cohort of amblyopic patients compared to the same number of control patients in order to overcome the limitations of sample size in the previous studies investigating the vascularization of amblyopic eyes in children using OCT-A [38, 42]. SCP and DCP were evaluated in terms of both vascular density (anatomical parameter) and flow area (functional parameter). They found a significant decreased macular vascular density of SCP ($53.07 \pm 2.55\%$ vs. $54.96 \pm 3.33\%$ [P = 0.0171]) and macular flow area of SCP (1.45 ± 0.11 mm^2 vs. 1.50 ± 0.09 [P = 0.0305]) in the amblyopic eyes compared with the fellow ones. Compared with randomly selected eyes of controls, amblyopic eyes showed a statistically significant decrease in the macular flow area of the SCP (P = 0.005) and of the DCP (P = 0.002), in the macula vascular density of the SCP (P = 0.022) and in the optic disk flow area (P = 0.004) (Fig. 21.4). Data on macular vascular density of the SCP and DCP are similar to the findings of Yilmaz, Lonngi and colleagues [41, 45]. Data on reduced macular and optic disk flow area in the amblyopic eyes represent original findings. However, the clinical significance and utility of these findings are thus far unknown.

It remains to be determined whether the documented microvascularization defect is the cause or a consequence of the amblyopia. The main limitations of these studies with OCT-A on amblyopia include lack of masking of observers and the absence of deprivational amblyopia cases in the amblyopia group. Future randomized, masked studies, with larger numbers of subjects will better confirm some

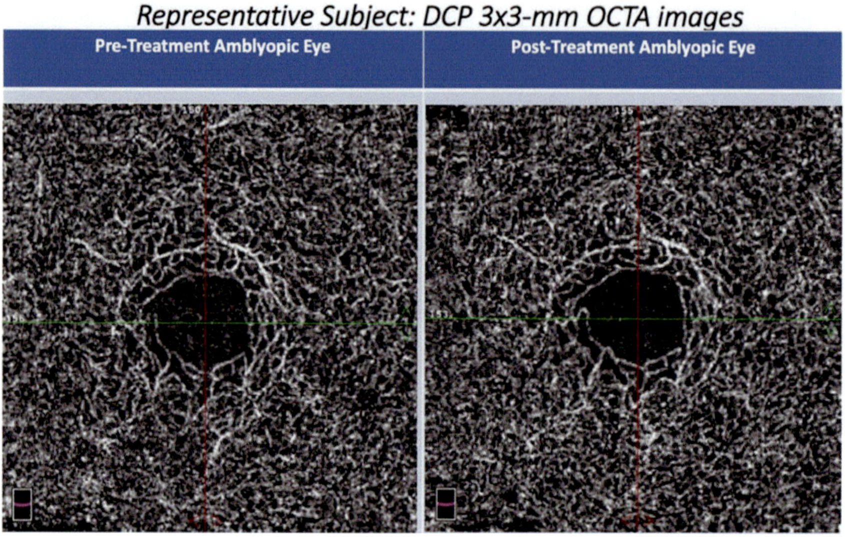

Fig. 21.5 3 × 3-mm OCTA image of pre and post treatment eye segmented at the deep capillary plexus (DCP) level from a subject whose vision improved with patching therapy

of these issues. It would be useful also to obtain follow-up studies after treatment to show if there is any change in these vascular parameters.

In a recent study Gunzenhauser et al. [46], using 3 × 3-mm OCTA scans, compare retinal vessel density (RVD) in pretreatment amblyopic eyes to those of amblyopic eyes following patching therapy. Deep capillary plexus (DCP) and superficial capillary plexus (SCP) in amblyopic eyes showed a significant post-treatment increase in RVD compared to pre-treatment in the whole image (Figs. 21.5 and 21.6).

Moreover, Araki et al. [47] investigate the area of foveal avascular zone (FAZ) and macular vessel density (VD) using OCTA in 15 patients with unilateral amblyopia, after correction of the images using individual axial length (AL). In this study FAZ area of SCP in amblyopic eyes was significantly smaller than that of fellow eyes ($P < 0.001$). Infact, the formation of FAZ is thought to be critical in the development of the foveal pit: if FAZ fails to form, the inner retinal layers may persist in the foveal center and foveal pit becomes shallow. In conclusion, there was no significant difference in macular VD between amblyopic eyes and fellow eyes.

As far as deprivation amblyopia in congenital cataract patients is concerned, the first study [48] investigating the structural difference of macular and peripapillary RNFL using OCT in this pathology has been conducted on a small sample. In Kim YW et al. work, 14 unilateral pseudophakic children with deprivational amblyopia and 14 age-matched normal children (mean age, 7.45 ± 2.57 years) were scanned with Cirrus HD-OCT. Macular, RNFL, and ganglion cell-inner plexiform layer thicknesses were measured and compared between the eyes after correction for axial length-related magnification errors. OCT demonstrated significant increase in

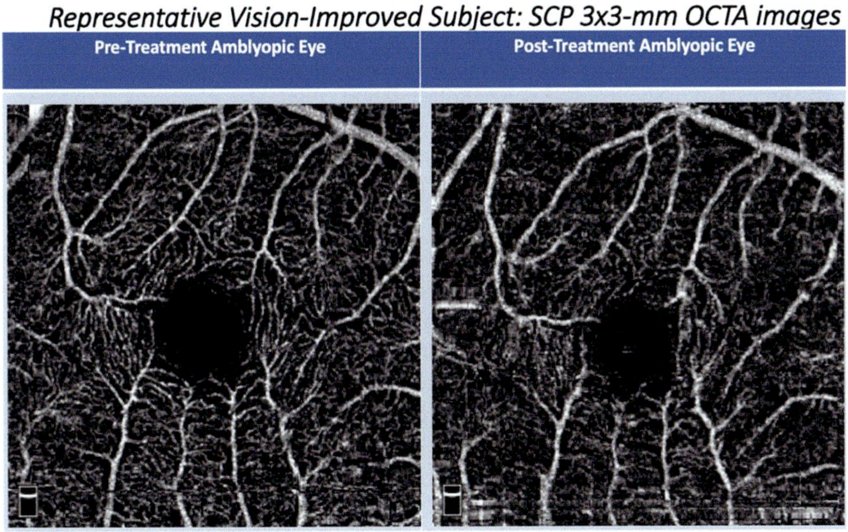

Fig. 21.6 3 × 3-mm OCTA images of the pre and post treatment eye segmented at the superficial capillary plexus (SCP) level from a subject whose vision improved with patching therapy

nasal RNFL thickness compared to fellow non-amblyopic eyes and age-matched normal eyes. The macular and macular ganglion cell-inner plexiform layer thickness did not show any significant difference. These results are quite contrasting if compared to data emerged from subsequent studies. Bansal et al. [49] compared the retinal nerve fiber layer thickness (RNFLT) and central macular thickness (CMT) in pediatric patients (age group 4–16 years) with unilateral congenital or developmental cataract (n = 15) and bilateral cataract (n = 15), and age-matched controls (n = 15). RNFLT and CMT were measured using SD-OCT in normal controls and 3 months postoperatively in children with unilateral and bilateral cataract. Children with unilateral cataract showed significant thinning of superior, nasal, and temporal RNFL compared to the fellow eyes as well as age-matched normal eyes on OCT. The CMT was inferior in deprivational amblyopic eyes than in age-matched normal eyes, but there was no significant difference compared to the fellow nonamblyopic eyes. In bilateral cataract, RNFLT was significantly thinner in superior and nasal quadrants as compared to age-matched normal eyes. Conversely, Al-Haddad et al. [50] found increased CMT in 14 eyes with deprivational amblyopia from pediatric cataract compared to 20 age-matched control eyes and this was correlated with the severity of amblyopia.

Several older studies reported a decrease in nasal visual fields in children treated for unilateral congenital cataract [51]. Kanamori et al. [52] demonstrated the relationship between visual field sensitivity at each tested location in standard automated perimetry and peripapillary RNFL thickness measured with Stratus OCT; the nasal sectoral RNFL corresponded well with nasal visual field area. Taken together, decreased nasal visual field in previous reports may have been due to increased nasal sectoral peripapillary RNFL thickness, as shown in Kim et al. study [35].

We can therefore conclude that OCT is certainly a rapid, non-invasive, office-based imaging technique allowing objective quantification of retinal structures with high resolution, including determination of peripapillary RNFL thickness, macular thickness, and choroidal thickness (CT) so that it can be successfully applied also in young children. The recent introduction of OCT-A represents a new fascinating method to evaluate the retinal microvasculature in a non-invasive way. Its application in amblyopia field is giving interesting new results regarding anatomical and functional changes of retinal vascular plexus which occurs in amblyopic eyes. These data have to be considered preliminary, but this new technology will improve, for sure, our knowledge on amblyopia mechanisms and related retinal changes. Nevertheless, evidence for direct retinal changes in eyes with amblyopia has been controversial: the results of these studies are equivocal with regard to whether macular, peripapillary RNFL and choroidal thicknesses differ in amblyopic eyes and between amblyopia subgroups (anisometropic, strabismic, deprivational). Moreover, the majority of the studies have been limited to strabismic or anisometropic amblyopia and analyzed the fellow non ambliopic eyes as control [48]. Further randomized, masked studies with larger sample are required, especially as regards myopic anisometropic and deprivational amblyopia.

References

1. McKee SP, Levi DM, Movshon JA. The pattern of visual deficits in amblyopia. J Vis. 2003;3(5):380–405.
2. Crawford ML, Harwerth RS, Smith EL, von Noorden GK. Keeping an eye on the brain: the role of visual experience in monkeys and children. J Gen Psychol. 1993;120(1):7–19.
3. Holmes JM, Clarke MP. Amblyopia. Lancet. 2006;367(9519):1343–51.
4. Donahue SP, Arnold RW, Ruben JB. Preschool vision screening: what should we be detecting and how should we report it? Uniform guideline for reporting results of preschool vision screening studies. J AAPOS. 2003;7(5):314–6.
5. Arnold RW. Amblyopia risk factor prevalence. J Pediatr Ophthalmol Strabismus. 2013;50(4):213–7.
6. Attebo K, Mitchell P, Cumming R, Smith W, Jolly N, Sparkes R. Prevalence and causes of amblyopia in an adult population. Ophthalmology. 1998;105(1):154–9.
7. National Eye Institute Office of Biometry and Epidemiology. Report on the national eye institute's visual acuity impairment survey Pilot Study. US Washington, DC: Department of Health and Human Services (1984).
8. Holmes JM, Beck RW, Repka MX, Leske DA, Kraker RT, Blair RC, et al. The amblyopia treatment study visual acuity testing protocol. Arch Ophthalmol. 2001;119(9):1345–53.

9. Wiesel TN, Hubel DH. Single-cell responses in striate cortex of kittens deprived of vision in one eye. J Neurophysiol. 1963;26:1003–17.
10. Williams C, Papakostopoulos D. Electro-oculographic abnormalities in amblyopia. Br J Ophthalmol. 1995;79(3):218–24.
11. Von Noorden GK, Crawford ML. The lateral geniculate nucleus in human strabismic amblyopia. Invest Ophthalmol Vis Sci. 1992;33(9):2729–32.
12. Horton JC, Hocking DR. Timing of the critical period for plasticity of ocular dominance columns in macaque striate cortex. J Neurosci. 1997;17(10):3684–709.
13. Dickmann A, Petroni S, Perrotta V, Parrilla R, Aliberti S, Salerni A, et al. Measurement of retinal nerve fiber layer thickness, macular thickness, and foveal volume in amblyopic eyes usingspectral-domain optical coherence tomography. J AAPOS. 2012;16(1):86–8.
14. Repka MX, Kraker RT, Tamkins SM, Suh DW, Sala NA, Beck RW. Retinal nerve fiber layer thickness in amblyopic eyes. Am J Ophthalmol. 2009;148(1):143–7.
15. Huynh SC, Samarawickrama C, Wang XY, Rochtchina E, Wong TY, Gole GA, et al. Macular and nerve fiber layer thickness in amblyopia: the Sydney Childhood Eye Study. Ophthalmology. 2009;116(9):1604–9.
16. Khan AO. A comparison between the amblyopic eye and normal fellow eye ocular architecture in children with hyperopic anisometropic amblyopia. J AAPOS. 2013;17(1):115–6.
17. Wu SQ, Zhu LW, Xu QB, Xu JL, Zhang Y. Macular and peripapillary retinal nerve fiber layer thickness in children with hyperopic anisometropic amblyopia. Int J Ophthalmol. 2013;6(1):85–9.
18. Provis JM, van Driel D, Billson FA, Russell P. Development of the human retina: patterns of cell distribution and redistribution in the ganglion cell layer. J Comp Neurol. 1985;233(4):429–51.
19. Provis JM, van Driel D, Billson FA, Russell P. Human fetal optic nerve: overproduction and elimination of retinal axons during development. J Comp Neurol. 1985;238(1):92–100.
20. Yen MY, Cheng CY, Wang AG. Retinal nerve fiber layer thickness in unilateral amblyopia. Invest Ophthalmol Vis Sci. 2004;45(7):2224–30.
21. Kok PH, de Kinkelder R, Braaksma-Besselink YC, Kalkman J, Prick LJ, Sminia ML, et al. Anomalous relation between axial length and retinal thickness in amblyopic children. J AAPOS. 2013;17(6):598–602.
22. Guagliano R, Barillà D, Bertone C, Montescani S, Vercellin ACV, Arpa C, Tinelli C, De Angelis G, Quaranta L. Evaluation of macular and optic nerve head parameters in amblyopic eyes: an optical coherence tomography study. Eur J Ophthalmol. 2022;32(4):1991–6.
23. Pang Y, Goodfellow GW, Allison C, Block S, Frantz KA. A prospective study of macular thickness in amblyopic children with unilateral high myopia. Invest Ophthalmol Vis Sci. 2011;52(5):2444–9.
24. Wan J, Zhang Z, Tian Y. Examination of macular retina and choroidal thickness in high myopic amblyopia using spectral-domain optical coherence tomography. Front Med (Lausanne). 2022;28(9): 808409.
25. Nishi T, Ueda T, Hasegawa T, Miyata K, Ogata N. Choroidal thickness in children with hyperopic anisometropic amblyopia. Br J Ophthalmol. 2014;98(2):228–32.
26. Xu J, Zheng J, Yu S, Sun Z, Zheng W, Qu P, Chen Y, Chen W, Yu X. Macular choroidal thickness in unilateral amblyopic children. Invest Ophthalmol Vis Sci. 2014;55(11):7361–8.
27. Niyaz L, Yücel OE, Arıtürk N, Terzi O. Choroidal thickness in strabismus and amblyopia cases. Strabismus. 2017;25(2):56–9.
28. Pang Y, Frantz KA, Block S, Goodfellow GW, Allison C. Effect of amblyopia treatment on macular thickness in eyes with myopic anisometropic amblyopia. Invest Ophthalmol Vis Sci. 2015;56(4):2677–83.
29. Kutschke PJ, Scott WE, Keech RV. Anisometropic amblyopia. Ophthalmology. 1991;98(2):258–63.
30. Nucci P, Drack AV. Refractive surgery for unilateral high myopia in children. J AAPOS. 2001;5(6):348–51.

31. Saw SM, Gazzard G, Shih-Yen EC, Chua WH. Myopia and associated pathological complications. Ophthalmic Physiol Opt. 2005;25(5):381–91.
32. Dickmann A, Petroni S, Salerni A, Dell'Omo R, Balestrazzi E. Unilateral amblyopia: an optical coherence tomography study. J AAPOS. 2009;13(2):148–50.
33. Dickmann A, Petroni S, Perrotta V, Salerni A, Parrilla R, Aliberti S, et al. A morpho-functional study of amblyopic eyes with the use of optical coherence tomography and microperimetry. J AAPOS. 2011;15(4):338–41.
34. Szigeti A, Tátrai E, Szamosi A, Vargha P, Nagy ZZ, Németh J, et al. A morphological study of retinal changes in unilateral amblyopia using optical coherence tomography imagesegmentation. PLoS ONE. 2014;9(2): e88363.
35. Enoch JM. Receptor amblyopia. Am J Ophthalmol. 1959;48(3):262–74.
36. Liu Y, Dong Y, Zhao K. A meta-analysis of choroidal thickness changes in unilateral amblyopia. J Ophthalmol. 2017;2017:2915261.
37. Zha Y, Zhuang J, Feng W, Zheng H, Cai J. Evaluation of choroidal thickness in amblyopia using optical coherence tomography. Eur J Ophthalmol. 2020;30(4):629–34.
38. Guo L, Tao J, Xia F, Yang Z, Ma X, Hua R. In vivo optical imaging of amblyopia: digital subtraction autofluorescense and split-spectrum amplitude-decorrelation angiography. Lasers Surg Med. 2016;48(7):660–7.
39. Araki S, Miki A, Goto K, Yamashita T, Takizawa G, Haruishi K, et al. Macular retinal and choroidal thickness in unilater amblyopia using swept source optical coherence tomography. BMC Ophthalmol. 2017;17(1):167.
40. Aslan Bayhan S, Bayhan HA. Effect of amblyopia treatment on choroidal thickness in children with hyperopic anisometropic amblyopia. Curr Eye Res. 2017;42(9):1254–9.
41. Lonngi M, Velez FG, Tsui I, Davila JP, Rahimi M, Chan C, et al. Spectral-domain optical coherence tomography angiography in children with amblyopia. JAMA Ophthalmol. 2017;135(10):1086–91.
42. Repka MX, Kraker RT, Tamkins SM, Suh DW, Sala NA, Beck RW, Pediatric Eye Disease Investigator Group. Retinal nerve fiber layer thickness in amblyopic eyes. Am J Ophthalmol. 2009;148(1):143–7.
43. Borrelli E, Lonngi M, Balasubramanian S, Tepelus TC, Baghdasaryan E, Pineles SL, et al. Increased choriocapillaris vessel density in amblyopic children: a case-control study. J AAPOS. 2018;pii: S1091-8531(18)30118-6.
44. Sobral I, Rodrigues TM, Soares M, Seara M, Monteiro M, Paiva C, et al. OCT angiography findings in children with amblyopia. J AAPOS. 2018;pii: S1091-8531(18)30121-6.
45. Yilmaz I, Ocak OB, Yilmaz BS, Inal A, Gokyigit B, Taskapili M. Comparison of quantitative measurement of foveal avascular zone and macular vessel density in eyes of children with amblyopia and healthy controls: an optical coherence tomography angiography study. J AAPOS. 2017;21:224–8.
46. Gunzenhauser RC, Tsui I, Velez FG, Fung SS, Demer JL, Suh SY, Sarraf D, Pineles SL. Comparison of pre-treatment vs. post-treatment retinal vessel density in children with amblyopia. J Binocul Vis Ocul Motil. 2020;70(3):79–85.
47. Araki S, Miki A, Goto K, Yamashita T, Yoneda T, Haruishi K, Ieki Y, Kiryu J, Maehara G, Yaoeda K. Foveal avascular zone and macular vessel density after correction for magnification error in unilateral amblyopia using optical coherence tomography angiography. BMC Ophthalmol. 2019;19(1):171.
48. Kim YW, Kim SJ, Yu YS. Spectral-domain optical coherence tomography analysis in deprivational amblyopia: a pilot study with unilateral pediatric cataract patients. Graefes Arch Clin Exp Ophthalmol. 2013;251(12):2811–9.
49. Bansal P, Ram J, Sukhija J, Singh R, Gupta A. Retinal nerve fiber layer and macular thickness measurements in children after cataract surgery compared with age-matched controls. Am J Ophthalmol. 2016;166:126–32.
50. Al-Haddad C, Mehanna CJ, Ismail K. High-definition optical coherence tomography of the macula in deprivational amblyopia. Ophthalmic Surg Lasers Imaging Retina. 2018;49(3):198–204.

51. Bowering ER, Maurer D, Lewis TL, Brent HP. Sensitivity in the nasal and temporal hemifields in children treated for cataract. Invest Ophthalmol Vis Sci. 1993;34(13):3501–9.
52. Kanamori A, Naka M, Nagai-Kusuhara A, Yamada Y, Nakamura M, Negi A. Regional relationship between retinal nerve fiber layer thickness and corresponding visual field sensitivity in glaucomatous eyes. Arch Ophthalmol. 2008;126(11):1500–6.

Pediatric Neuro-Ophthalmology and OCT

22

Maja Kostic, Gábor Mark Somfai, Edmund Arthur, and Delia Cabrera Debuc

Abstract

The abstract is published online only. If you did not include a short abstract for the online version when you submitted the manuscript, the first paragraph or the first 10 lines of the chapter will be displayed here. If possible, please provide us with an informative abstract. Embryology and neurodevelopment of the eyes are crucial for a better understanding of neuro-ophthalmic disorders. The field of pediatric neuro-ophthalmology has burgeoned over the past decade due to the more available diagnostic and therapeutic tools. This multidisciplinary field requires the collaborative work of a geneticist, pediatric ophthalmologist, pediatric ophthalmic-oncologists with coordination of a pediatric neuro-ophthalmologist. Embryology and early development of eyes as part of the brain can help us to understand developmental, degenerative and ocular pathology in ophthalmology better. Increasing evidence suggests that the changes of the retinal structure and microvasculature are correlated with neurodegenerative and cerebrovascular lesions, which in turn supports the view that the retina may serve as a window to the brain. Many problem-solving methods for diagnostics of disorders of the central nervous system in the childhood period need general anesthesia, which is a very stressful, time-consuming and high costly procedure. However, the introduction of low-cost diagnostic

M. Kostic · E. Arthur · D. Cabrera Debuc (✉)
Bascom Palmer Eye Institute, University of Miami Miller School of Medicine, Miami, FL, USA
e-mail: dcabrera2@med.miami.edu

M. Kostic
e-mail: mkostic@miami.edu

E. Arthur
e-mail: exa647@med.miami.edu

G. M. Somfai
Augenzentrum, Pallas Kliniken, Olten, Switzerland

A. Grzybowski and P. Barboni (eds.), *OCT and Imaging in Central Nervous System Diseases*, https://doi.org/10.1007/978-3-031-72156-4_22

ophthalmic instruments has facilitated the use of retinal imaging for the detection and management of neurodevelopmental disorders in the infanthood period. In this chapter, we will give an overview of embryology, ocular and neurological development, as well as an overview of the use of Optical Coherence Tomography in Neonatology and Pediatric Neuro- ophthalmology.

Keywords

Embryology • Neurodevelopment • Neuro-ophthalmic disorders • Optical coherence tomography • Neonatology and pediatric neuro-ophthalmology

22.1 Introduction

Eyes are one of the vital organs that provide more than 80% of all information we received and that help us to grow and develop.

Embryology and early development of eyes as part of the brain can help us to better understand developmental, degenerative and ocular pathology in ophthalmology. The changes of the retinal structure and microvasculature are seemingly correlated with neurodegenerative and cerebrovascular lesions, which in turn supports the view that the retina may serve as a window to the brain.

The changes of the retinal structure and microvasculature are seemingly correlated with neurodegenerative and cerebrovascular lesions, which in turn supports the view that the retina may serve as a window to the brain. It can be postulated that retinal microvascular structure could be mirroring that of the brain while the substructure of the retina may be like the structure of the brain.

Many diagnostic methods for diagnostics of the central nervous system in childhood period needs general anesthesia of kids, which are very stressful for kids, time-consuming and high costly depending. However, discovering low-cost diagnostic instruments whereas retinal imaging could provide a meaningful surrogate marker for disease detection and disease management that could be available not only for institutions and big clinic, and also for all doctors in primary care.

In this chapter, we will give an overview of embryology and ocular and neurological development, as well as overview of Optical Coherence Tomography (OCT) in neonatology and pediatric neuro-ophthalmology as an emerging technology in neurology applications and express our view about how retinal imaging could serve the above goals and open a window, which could serve as a direct view to the brain in the earlier ages.

22.2 Ocular and Neurological Development

The eye is a very complex organ from the embryogenic standpoint since its development involves diencephalic neuroectoderm, surface ectoderm and extraocular mesenchyme (Fig. 22.1) [1]. During the development, the retina, trabecular meshwork, the epithelium of the ciliary body and the iris, as well as the optic nerve shall form from the neuroectoderm. The lens, anterior surface of the cornea, eyelids, and skin shall emerge from surface ectoderm. Ectomesenchyme originates from the neural crest, and it is involved in the genesis of the sclera, part of the cornea, choroid, ciliary body, blood vessels and the muscles of the eye [22.2].

In the human embryo, the structures of the eye start appearing around the 22nd day of development, before the closing of neural folds into the neural tube (Fig. 22.2). Early in the 4th week of gestation, the optic recesses start appearing within the diencephalon [1, 2]. After closing of the rostral neuropore (anterior opening), around the 24th day of gestation, the primordial eye can be observed, in the form of an evagination being shaped as a vesicle, known as an optic vesicle [2]. The optic vesicle is connected to the diencephalon through a thin, hollow optic stem, the future optic nerve (Fig. 22.3). The distal anterior part of the optic vesicle grows externally, approaching the ectoderm, from which, during this phase of development, it is separated by a thin layer of ectomesenchyme. Upon approaching the ectoderm, the optic vesicle initially flattens and later, around the 32nd day of gestation, the distal anterior part of the optic vesicle creates an invagination,

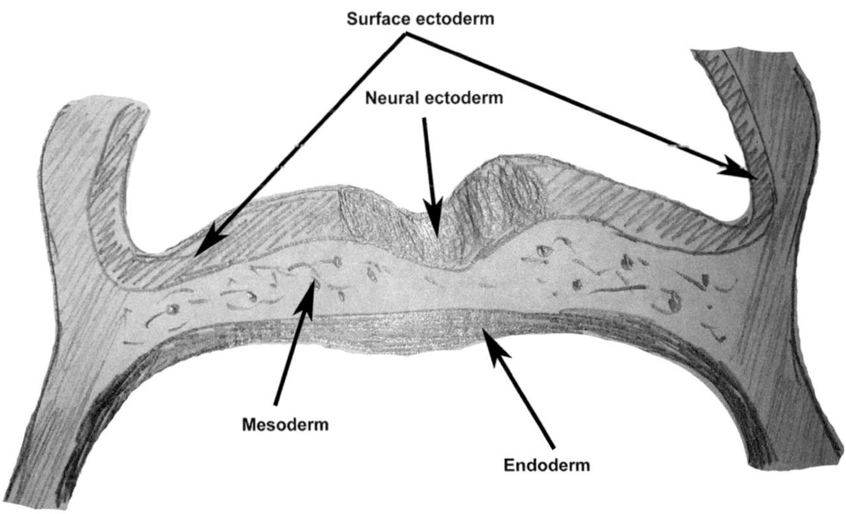

Fig. 22.1 Drawing of an about 16-day-old embryo. Note that ectoderm is differentiated into surface ectoderm on the lateral part (light gray part) and neural ectoderm in the middle (dark gray part) (*Image courtesy of* Maja Kostic, M.*D., Ph.D.; drawing inspired from images in "Pediatric Ophthalmology and Strabismus", K. Wright and P. Spiegel* [3], *second edition, ISBN 978-0-387-21753-6)*

and the vesicle transforms into the optic cup. During its development, the optic cup takes the shape of an asymmetric invagination. On the ventral, inferior side of the optic stalk, before the complete adhesion of its walls, the choroidal or retinal fissure is created [2, 3]. Through this fissure, the hyaloid artery reaches the optic cup (Fig. 22.4). Due to these changes, the optic vesicle transforms into a two-layer optic cup. The tissue invagination increases, and the cavity of the optic vesicle decrease during the development. The cavity of the vesicle finally changes into the fissure separating the outer pigmented layer of the retina from the inner neural layer. All layers of the optical part of retina shall develop from the posterior internal layers of the optic cup.

The blind part of the retina, covering internal surfaces of ciliary body and iris, shall form from the ridges of the optic cup [2, 3]. The external epithelial part of the ciliary body derives from the pigmented layer of the optic cup and the internal one, from the neural retina, as was mentioned previously. The ciliary body stroma originates from ectomesenchyme, as well as the muscle cells of the ciliary muscle. The iris stroma also originates from ectomesenchyme, whereas the muscle

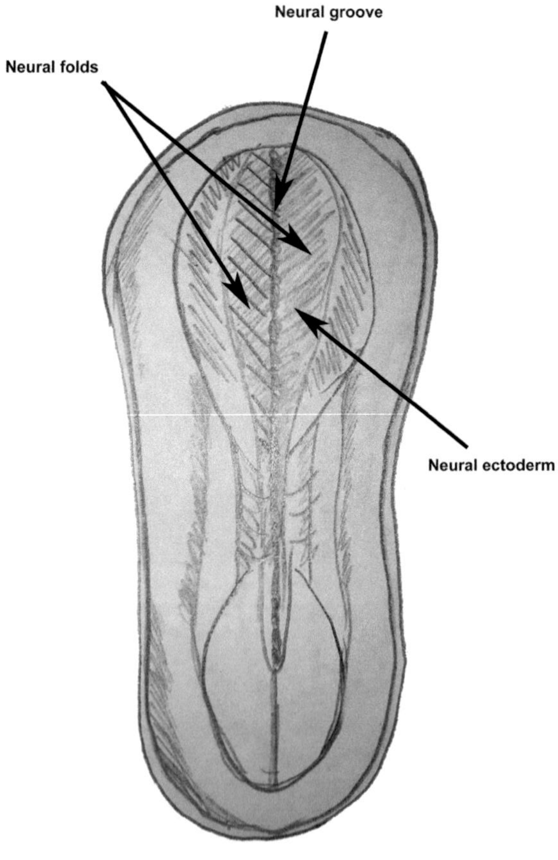

Fig. 22.2 Drawing of human embryo about 20 days' gestation. Neural groove originates from the neural plate, represent neural ectoderm (black line), and on each side of the groove are neural folds and represents surface ectoderm (*Image courtesy of Maja Kostic, M.D., Ph.D.; drawing inspired from images in "Pediatric Ophthalmology and Strabismus", K. Wright and P. Spiegel* [3], *second edition, ISBN 978-0-387-21753-6*)

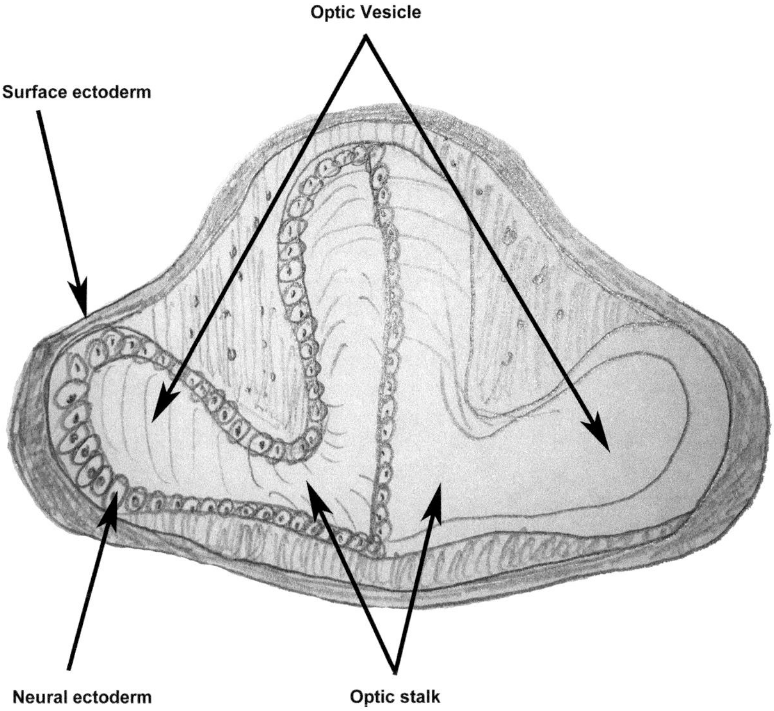

Fig. 22.3 Drawing of the optical vesicle of the about 25-day-old embryo. Optic vesicles and optic stalk are formed. Lens placode is formed from surface ectoderm (*Image courtesy of Maja Kostic, M.D., Ph.D.; drawing inspired from images in "Pediatric Ophthalmology and Strabismus", K. Wright and P. Spiegel* [3], *second edition, ISBN 978-0-387-21753-6*)

cells arise from the neuroectoderm of the optic cup. The external part of ectomesenchyme, surrounding the optic vesicle, shall transform into the external tunic of the bulb of the eye and its components, cornea, and sclera, while the internal part shall form the choroid.

Hyaloid blood vessels passing through the choroid fissure and vitreous chamber and reaching the lens shall form from the ectomesenchyme as well [3, 4].

Lens genesis starts around the 30th day in the form of superficial ectoderm thickening in the region of the optic cup. Thickened surface ectoderm shall transform into the lens placode during differentiation.

Invagination of the lens placode shall create the fovea of the lens, which will completely separate from surface ectoderm and shall become the lens vesicle during growth [4]. In this stage, the lens vesicle is confined within the optic cup, practically in mesenchyme. Differentiation of mesenchyme on its internal side shall create the gelatinous structure from which the primary vitreous shall emerge. Primary vitreous is located between the lens and the internal layer of the optic cup.

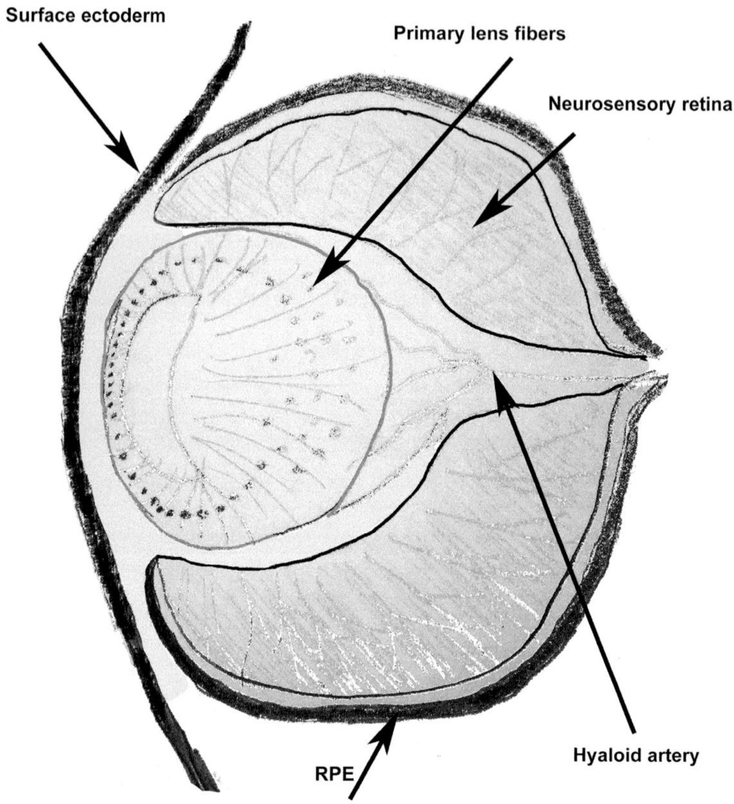

Fig. 22.4 Drawing of the embryonic eye in about 45 days. The hyaloid artery is seen in the posterior part of the eye between the lens and neurosensory retina. The posterior fibers (cells) of lens elongate from posterior towards anterior and make future lens (*Image courtesy of Maja Kostic, M.D., Ph.D.; drawing inspired from images in "Pediatric Ophthalmology and Strabismus", K. Wright and P. Spiegel* [3], *second edition, ISBN978-0-387-21753-6*)

Ectodermal cells covering the optic cup surface shall create its capsule. By the end of the 7th week of gestation, the lens turns into a solid structure, vascularized in the beginning by the branches of the hyaloid artery. Later, during fetal growth, it becomes avascular. Initially, the lens fills the optic cup almost completely, while later it takes only the smaller part of it with the vitreous body occupying most of it [5, 6].

The vitreous body originates from the cells of the internal layer of the optic cup and the base of the optic vesicle. The lens capsule is formed from the cells of the lens epithelium [6]. Differentiation of the retina starts at the end of 6th weeks when the two layers of the optic cup when the outer retinal pigment epithelium (RPE) and the inner neural retina began to form. Bruch's membrane which is a basal lamina of the RPE forms a functional unit with RPE and choriocapillaris

[7]. Ganglion cells, horizontal cells, and cone photoreceptors are born first, followed by amacrine and bipolar cells. Rod photoreceptors and Muller cells are last retinal cells to differentiate [8]. A foveal region started to develop at about 10–11 weeks' gestation when in the central region of retina only cone photoreceptors are detected. According to primate retinal studies, the fovea is the initiation point for most developmental events in the retina, including mitosis, apoptosis, opsin expression, and synaptogenesis [9] and development of retina radiates from this region across the retina. In week 34, cones and rods near the cone area of fovea have outer segments and forming elongated axons which terminate in the OPL [9].

Optic nerve develops from the edge of the optic fissure that is divided into two parts: the optic groove that originates from the optic stalk and the retinal fissure originates from the ventral optic vesicle. The optic disc will form at the transition between the optic groove and retinal fissure [10]. Type I astrocytes arise from neuroepithelial cells of the optic stalk and migrate onto the retinal surface where they associate with the surface vasculature to form blood/retinal barrier [10]. Retinal ganglion cells axons grow in close contact with Muller glial cells and with vitreal basal lamina [2, 11]. In the 29 gestational weeks, there is about 1.1 million retinal ganglion cell axons that entering the optic nerve.

All cranial nerves are formed by the seventh week of gestation. The cranial motor neurons are organized within individual or pairs rhombomeres (neuromeres of the rhombencephalon). The oculomotor (III) nucleus is located in the posterior midbrain, the trochlear (IV) nucleus in the anterior part of rhombomere 1, trigeminal (V) in rhombomeres 2 and 3, the abducens (VI) nucleus in rhombomere 4 and 5, the facial in 5 and 6 [12]. Normal development of efferent cranial nerves is critical for normal development of extraocular muscles [13]. Extraocular muscles develop from unsegmented prechordal and paraxial mesoderm form craniofacial muscles. Eye movement depends on the unique way of connectivity between cranial motor axons and the extraocular muscles [14]. The development of the eye bulb doesn't finish with birth. The axial length (AL) of the child's eye is around 17 mm and around 24 mm in adults. The growth of the eye is generally completed by age 5–8.

22.2.1 Embryonic Development of the Retinal Blood Vessels

The vascular system originates from mesoderm and appears in very early stages of development. At the basis of the vascular system development is the processes of vasculogenesis and angiogenesis [15], the apoptosis of blood vessels and their maturation [16]. In the early stages of retinal development, the necessary amount of oxygen is provided by the choroidal and hyaloid vascular systems, and later by the retinal ones.

22.2.1.1 Choroidal Vascular Plexus

Up to the 6th week of gestation, the retina is nourished exclusively through the choroid by diffusion [17]. In the 5 mm long human embryo, the primitive dorsal ophthalmic and primitive ventral ophthalmic arteries are separated from the internal carotid artery. The hyaloid artery originates from the primitive dorsal ophthalmic artery, passes through the embryonal fissure and reaches the indent in the region of the future optic nerve head.

The choroidal vascular plexus is observed in the human embryo of 4–5 mm in length. Its occurrence corresponds to the time of optic vesical genesis. It develops from the mesoderm and cranial part of the neural fold. Endothelial cells originate from mesoderm, while melanocytes, pericytes, and stromal cells originate from the neural fold [18]. The choroidal vascular plexus is composed of large primitive blood vessels that originate from the vascular system surrounding the neural tube and spreading up to the superficial layers of the optical cupulas. In the 13 mm long human embryo, choroidal capillaries surround the optical cupulas.

They are separated from the retina by the membrane of the retinal pigmented layer. The complex vascular plexus connecting with the posterior ciliary arteries, forming varicose veins and choriocapillary layer originates from the primitive vascular plexus during the 2nd and 3rd month of intrauterine growth [15]. The choroidal vascular plexus is of greatest importance for normal retinal function. It nourishes the retinal pigmented layer and photoreceptors [18].

22.2.1.2 Hyaloid Plexus

During the eye's development, the multiplication of retina cells causes an increase in its metabolic needs, which then leads to a demand that choroidal circulation cannot meet. As a result, a temporary hyaloid plexus which exists only during the first 4 months of intrauterine development, start developing [17]. The hyaloid plexus or the hyaloid artery starts developing at the beginning of the 4th gestation week off the dorsal ophthalmic artery. The development of the hyaloid artery is induced by retinal hypoxia.

As the hyaloid artery develops and reaches the cup of the future optic disc, it creates a vascular network which carries nutrients to the eye structures. When the embryo grows to 7 mm, the hyaloid artery has already made its way through the vitreous body and reaches the lens' back end. Once the embryo is 8–9 mm long, a dense capillary plexus can be observed, and it connects to the choroid plexus at the level of the front edge of the optic cup. This dense capillary plexus is called tunica vasculosa lentis, and through anastomosis, it is connected to the choroid plexus.

The hyaloid plexus has no veins, meaning the hyaloid system is solely made of arteries, whereas the vein part of the system is made of choroid veins. During its development, the hyaloid artery reaches the front side of the lens and builds the pupil membrane. In the 9th gestation week, or when the embryo is 60–80 mm long, the hyaloid plexus is fully developed and supplies the eye with needed nutrients. Parallel with the full development of the hyaloid network, the early start of the retinal plexus can be seen, as well as the beginning of the regression of the hyaloid vascular system [15].

The regression of the hyaloid vascular system starts around the 2nd month of intrauterine development, which is followed by the macrophage capillary occlusion. As the vascular structures start regrading, the primary vitreous body retracts. During the 5th month of intrauterine development, the back part of the eye is filled with the secondary vitreous body, while the primary vitreous body is S-shaped and positioned horizontally in the center [19].

22.2.2 The Retinal Vasculature

Further complexity of retinal growth and development is followed by the increased metabolic needs, which choroid and hyaloid vasculature cannot satisfy, so at the beginning of the 14th gestation week, a network of individual retinal blood vessels starts developing, which eventually creates the retinal vasculature [20]. The development of the retinal blood vessels begins with the occurrence of astrocytes, which play the active role in directing the blood vessels' endothelial cells during the 16th gestation week. It is the first time that the astrocytes can be seen in proximity of the hyaloid artery and around the optic nerve papilla. There, they are organized into a four-lobe formation, of which the two larger ones are temporal, and the two smaller ones are nasal. They all mark the pathways for the future main arteries and veins.

The early retina is made of only one undifferentiated layer. At the same time as the retina layers evolve and mature, the retinas' complex or network starts forming. The formation of the early vessel network of the central two-thirds of the retina is formed by vasculogenesis. The remainder of the vessels is formed by angiogenesis—by the creation of new blood vessels and sprouting of endothelial cells from the existing vessels, or by splitting of an existing blood vessel. Research indicates that both mentioned processes, vasculogenesis as well as angiogenesis, are essential for the development of the nerve/vessel network [21].

22.2.2.1 Vasculogenesis and Angiogenesis

Retinal blood vessels are created by the process of vascular and angiogenesis. This dual way of creation of the retinal vessel network, indicates its uniqueness, complexity, high differentness and dynamics of its development. The development of the retinal cells, primarily photoreceptors, and ganglion cells requires fast and extensive metabolic processes [16]. Retina's high demand for energy during its evolution/development/growth also requires an adequate blood vessel network, which can meet these needs [16].

The process of vasculogenesis in the embryo starts on the 17th day of its life. Chorion mesenchymal cells, yolk sac, mesenchymal stems, form blood islands. From the superficial mesenchymal cells of the angioblast blood islands, primitive angioblasts will develop [1]. Vasculogenesis is the process of "*de novo*" blood vessel formation. In the process of vasculogenesis, the differentiation of primitive angioblasts leads to the creation of a primitive blood vessel network responsible for the formation of large blood vessels, like the central retinal artery and its branches due to the positioning of the end part of the central retinal artery and the optic disc, nasal retinal blood vessels reach the ora serrata on the 36th week of gestation, whereas temporal retinal blood vessels reach it on the 40th week of gestation [16, 22].

Angiogenesis is the formation and growth of the new blood vessels from pre-existing vasculature. During this process, new blood vessels are formed by the sprouting of endothelial cells of the existing vessels, or by splitting angiogenesis, the process where a new blood vessel is created by splitting of an existing blood vessel (*intussusceptive growth*). This process represents proliferation and migration of vascular endothelial cells, as well as the processes that enable growth and blood vessel remodeling [15, 16]. As a physiological process, angiogenesis is typical in the areas with swift capillary growth [23]. The main inducer of the process of angiogenesis is hypoxia [24]. Angiogenesis is initiated by the VEGF via retinal Muller glia cells and astrocytes growth [24]. By this process of angiogenesis, perifoveal regions and blood vessels of deep retinal layers are formed.

As astrocytes lead the way for the direction and growth of endothelial cells into the retinal tissue, they play the crucial role in the development of retinal blood vessels. Along with the maturity of retinal cells, which occurs in the period of 14–15 gestation week, the development of the superficial, deep and radial peripapillary capillary plexus that originate from a central retinal artery [23]. Superficial blood plexus is made of arterioles, capillaries, and post-capillary venules. This plexus is located in the layer of nerve fibers and the ganglion cell layer. Deep blood plexus is located between the inner nuclear layer (INL) and the OPL. It is mostly made of capillary size blood vessels. Superficial and deep blood plexus stretch to the FAZ area where the retina is extremely thin and where all the needs are satisfied by the choroid plexus.

Radial peripapillary plexus forms a tiny ring-shaped area, which is surrounded by the optic disc. Same as the superficial blood plexus, it is also located in the layer of nerve fibers. Radial peripapillary plexus is developed into a capillary network on the 21st week of gestation. In the 26–27-week-old embryo, it is located in the superficial layers of the nerve fibers and from the optic disc, it stretches radially in all directions. It is created by the process of angiogenesis [23].

Retinal capillaries are made of endothelial cells, basement membranes and intramural pericytes. Endothelial capillary cells are connected by strong protein links, which represent a hemato-retinal barrier known as adherents' junctions. The hemato-retinal barrier is a highly selective functional barrier. The inner hemato-retinal barrier operates at the level of endothelial capillaries and represents a circulation barrier. Outer hemato-retinal barrier operates at the level of RPE and is a barrier to choroid circulation. Pigment epithelial cells are connected by occluding junctions, which are strong connections based on protein. High concentrations of VEGF lead to destabilization of intercellular connections, the breakdown of the hemato- retinal barrier, and cause a wide range of retinal diseases, which include retinopathy of prematurity (ROP) [24, 25]. Pericytes are contractile cells on the capillary Ocular and neurological development endothelium of retina, which play an essential role in the stabilization of the vascular retina.

22.3 OCT in Neonatology and Pediatric Neuro-Ophthalmology

Extremely preterm neonates who develop severe ROP are more likely than their equals unaffected by ROP to have evidence of brain damage, including severe disability, developmental delay, cerebral palsy, and lower scores on measures of verbal and performance IQ, general conceptual ability, and spatial ability [26–29]. OCT as a diagnostic tool for different neuro-ophthalmological diseases, it is in everyday practice in adults. However, neonates and small children were excluded, until a new handheld spectral-domain OCT (HH-SDOCT) was developed and optimized in neonatology and pediatric ophthalmology [30–33].

Nowadays, there are multiple applications in prematurity and neonatology in ROP, retinal dystrophies and dysplasia, optic nerve pathology, nystagmus, different injuries or trauma and in diagnosis and monitoring ocular tumors [34–36].

The natural development of the retina and foveal region is a complicated procedure, comprising centripetal migration of the cone photoreceptors into the central fovea and elongation of the outer retinal layers (ORLs), outer nuclear layer (ONL), and photoreceptor inner and outer segments (IS, OS), as well as centrifugal migration of the inner retinal layers (IRLs), RNFL, GCL, IPL, inner nuclear layer (INL), and OPL away from the central fovea with increasing age [34, 37–39].

22.3.1 Retinopathy of Prematurity

ROP is an abnormal development of retinal blood vessels in premature infants that can potentially lead to blindness [40–43]. Early diagnosis, an area where the application of OCT has been most investigated, is the key for detection, follow-up, and decision-making regarding the need for treatment.

There are many characteristic features of the infant's eye compared with the adult eye. All those characteristics are challenging factors for OCT application in neonatology. Premature babies and neonates have greater astigmatism and higher refractive errors, predominantly myopia, and between 40–52 weeks they shift to hyperopia [30, 44, 45]. The AL is shorter; investigations with ocular echography have estimated the ocular AL of the premature infant as 15 mm at 31 weeks' postmenstrual age (PMA) and reported the fastest growth to take place from 32 to 52 weeks PMA [46]. The cornea is steeper than the adult cornea, decreasing to adult values by 3 months [43, 47–51].

The typical features observed in the retina of babies with ROP are the persistence of the IRLs, reduction of foveal pit depth, reduction in the diameter of the foveal avascular zone (FAZ), with global decreases and segmental (temporal) increases in RNFL thickness measurements [52–55], increase in central macular thickness (CMT) measurements, thinning of the GCC, delay in photoreceptor development, and thinning of the photoreceptor layers [56–60]. Also, choroidal thickness is reduced in preterm children [61–63]. According to Maldonado et al. increased central foveal, IRL and foveal to parafoveal retinal thickness are associated with a higher risk of developing plus disease or ROP stage 3 [64]. Moreover, a new handheld SDOCT (HH-SDOCT) has played a very important role in detecting pre-retinal tissue, epiretinal membranes, cystoid macular edema (CME), retinal layer schisis, vascular abnormalities, and foveal architectural abnormalities not visible on conventional clinical examination. Interestingly, CME is reported in all stages in ROP with an incidence of more than 87.5% in stage three of ROP [65, 66]. The macular or foveal involvement in ROP, that can be detected by OCT has been very helpful as part of the decision-making process and in predicting visual and neurodevelopmental outcome in babies with ROP [67–69].

22.3.2 Infantile Nystagmus, Retinal Dystrophies and Dysplasia

Except induced by trauma or disease, nystagmus practically always is instigated by neurological complications in most people with nystagmus which usually are born with the condition or develop it early in life. Retinal dystrophies are chronic and progressive diseases characterized by defective color vision and night blindness due to neuronal death and consequent loss of functional connections. Retinal dysplasia is a congenital malformation of the retina, with the formation of folds or rosettes that appear clinically as retinal folds or larger areas of geographic dysplasia.

Congenital (infantile) nystagmus is characterized by involuntary rhythmic eye movements. The waveform, amplitude, and frequency of the oscillations, which are typically horizontal in direction but may be primarily vertical, torsional, or any combination of these three, can vary with changes in focal distance, the direction of gaze, and under monocular or binocular viewing conditions. Often, infantile nystagmus is associated with other ocular conditions (e.g., bilateral congenital cataracts) that impair visual acuity and sometimes can create life-threatening conditions [70]. OCT can be very helpful in identifying the etiology of infantile nystagmus syndrome (INS), a heterogeneous group of disorders, with multiple causes and different prognoses [71].

Lee et al. [71] recommended dividing INS into four diagnostic categories: typical foveal hypoplasia, atypical foveal hypoplasia, abnormal foveal morphology, and normal foveal morphology. The etiology of nystagmus can be anticipated, and diagnostic exams can be designated to confirm the diagnosis based on the presence or absence of foveal hypoplasia or the presence or absence of other abnormal macular morphology as visualized by OCT. If there is a typical foveal hypoplasia, it is most likely associated with albinism and PAX6 mutations. Retinal development is ongoing in early childhood, characterized by foveal hypoplasia and a reduction in ORL thickness measurements *as demonstrated by* longitudinal OCT imaging studies in albinism [72].

Also, achromatopsia (ACHM) is characterized by atypical foveal hypoplasia which is the foveal hypoplasia associated with photoreceptor disruption and/or the presence of a hyporeflective zone located between the external limiting membrane (ELM) and RPE at the fovea. OCT imaging has also demonstrated that there is evidence that retinal development is not arrested but is ongoing in ACHM, at a reduced rate and magnitude in comparison to controls [73]. This expresses as foveal hypoplasia, and reductions in total retinal thickness, ORL thickness and parafoveal IRL, IPL, and OPL thickness measurements [73]. Intriguingly, there is a primary decrease in CMT in early infancy in albinism because of ongoing regression of the IRLs from the fovea, which can indicate that there is a period of retinal developmental plasticity in childhood in both ACHM and albinism, that might help normalize retinal development and optimize vision. Abnormal morphology of fovea (category 3) is characteristic of retinal dystrophies, which are typically associated with abnormal lamination of the IRLs and ORLs, loss or disruption of photoreceptor integrity, and thinning of the ONL and RPE [67]. The fourth category in this group is idiopathic manifest latent nystagmus, characterized by normal foveal morphology.

22.3.3 Optic Nerve Pathology

OCT has also been used as a diagnostic and monitoring tool in wide pediatric optic nerve pathology like glaucoma, optic nerve atrophy or hypoplasia, and pseudotumor cerebri.

Hypoplasia of the optic nerve is the most usual hereditary disorder of the optic nerve which can be diagnosed by OCT with the following features: significantly smaller discs, horizontal cup diameter, thinning of the RNFL, GCL, IPL, ONL with increasing grade of glaucoma damage [74]. HH-SDOCT can be used as a marker of visual function to differentiate measurements between RNFL, GCL, and IPL in children with and without vision loss [74, 75].

Pseudotumor cerebri is idiopathic intracranial hypertension, which is a condition characterized by increased ICP without a detectable cause [76]. The main symptoms are headache, vision disturbances, pulsatile ringing in the ears, and shoulder pain [76, 77]. Complications may include vision loss [77]. OCT characteristics in pseudotumor cerebri are an increased central macular, temporal, and superior RNFL thickness. Moreover, optic atrophy and photoreceptor loss in OCT are findings associated with irreversible visual loss [78, 79]. Likewise, OCT can be used to diagnose and monitor pediatric pseudotumor cerebri and is potentially useful as a visual prognostic tool in this condition [78, 79].

22.3.4 Non-accidental Injury or Trauma

Abusive head trauma known as shaken baby syndrome (SBS) is characterized by many body injuries including broken bones, skull fractures, brain hemorrhage and retinal hemorrhages [80, 81]. SBS occurs when a baby is shaken repeatedly, often by a frustrated caretaker trying to quiet an inconsolable baby [82, 83]. The eyes of babies are more vulnerable to bleeding due to shaking because of a disproportionally large head and fragile blood vessels [83]. Symptoms may range from subtle to obvious that can lead to death [84]. However, very often there are no detectable signs of trauma with many complications in later life that include epileptic seizures, changes in visual acuity, or permanent visual loss, changes in cognitive functions as well as cerebral palsy [82, 83]. OCT has been reported to be helpful as a diagnostic tool in SBS with posterior vitreous separation and multilayered retinoschisis [84]. Also, it can be used to guide treatment in infants with shaken baby syndrome by providing additional morphologic information [85].

22.3.5 Pediatric Neuro-Oncology

In early childhood, the incidence of tumors is around 1 in 12,000 to 1 in 27,500 babies [86, 87]. Most ocular and orbital tumors of childhood are distinct from tumors that occur in adults. Many are congenital with early presentations. Most pediatric orbital tumors are benign like a dermoid cyst and capillary hemangiomas. A dermoid cyst is characterized by a sac that contains fluid and tissue that is not part of the eye or its surrounding area. The benign growth of tiny blood vessels, capillary hemangiomas along with a dermoid cyst are the most common benign lesions in the first months of life. The most common orbital malignancy is rhabdomyosarcoma, a cancerous tumor that develops in muscle or connective tissue. Also, a cancerous tumor that grows inside the retina of the eye known as retinoblastoma, is the most common intraocular malignant lesion.

Signs of orbital and ocular tumors differ depending on their location and whether they are benign or malignant. These symptoms may include bulging or crossed eye, redness or swelling near the eye, a bright red birthmark on or near the eye, and white pupillary reflex, mydriasis, or a red painful eye.

The role of OCT in neuro-oncology is a differentiation between types of tumors of the retina and RPE, to detect the degree of involvement of individual retinal layers and differentiate between abnormal and normal retina [88–90]. OCT images reveals the retinoblastoma lesions as isodense or hyperdense features, which are associated with patches of calcification, and usually have an abrupt transition toward uninvolved retina (Fig. 22.5) [89, 90].

In smaller tumors, depending on the lesion size, there is a different degree of retinal layer involvement from the inner nuclear and middle retinal layers. In larger tumors, there is involvement of the full thickness of the retina [36]. Also, small lesions- the pre-retinal seeds are located superficial to the retina, appear isodense

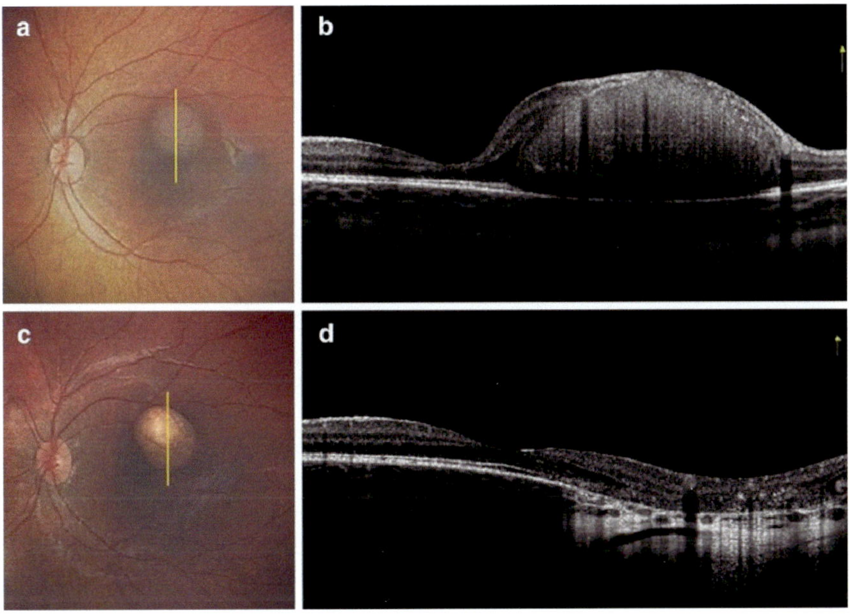

Fig. 22.5 Clinical case demonstrating the application of the Spectral domain hand-held optical coherence tomography (HH-OCT) system in a retinoblastoma patient (3-week-old girl), with a family history of maternal unilateral retinoblastoma [89]. (**a**) The left eye demonstrated a small dome-shaped, outer retinal tumor recurrence of (**b**) 2750 μm in basal dimension and 792 μm thickness in the para-foveolar region following 6 cycles of intravenous chemotherapy for bilateral retinoblastoma; and with adjacent shallow sub-retinal fluid. The mass was 615 μm from the foveola. (**c**) The tumor showed complete regression following 1 cycle of intra-arterial chemotherapy, (**d**) A concave scar of 120 μm in thickness and located 663 μm from foveolar documented by the HH-OCT. There was OCT light transmission through atrophic retinal pigment epithelial accentuating the underlying thin choroid. The foveola remained intact (*Image taken from Yarovaya et al. Int J Retin Vitr (2017) 3:43*)

and smooth, and are associated with shadowing of the underlying structures on OCT [36].

OCT has been demonstrated to be useful for monitoring tumor progression, identifying new lesions and recurrences, monitoring treatment response, and guiding further management of ocular and orbital tumor complications [36, 91, 92].

22.4 Controversies and Challenges in Neonatology and Pediatric Neuro-Ophthalmology

Although, the OCT can be very helpful for diagnosing retinal and optic nerve diseases in infants and young children, there are many neuro-ophthalmological conditions that are very difficult to diagnose in early childhood due to the limited ability of this age group to cooperate with standard adult diagnostic and monitoring tools. Some challenges for the use of OCT still exist in pediatric ophthalmology. For example, the OCT scan of the retina works by rotating the OCT beam in the iris plane, but because of the shorter AL in children's eyes, the scanning procedure should be corrected by shortening the OCT reference [30].

Maldonado et al. suggested that to correct for any refractive errors, the image should be further optimized by adjusting the focus of the handheld probe (range, 10–12 diopters) [30]. Also, to facilitate comparisons at specific locations across different age groups, the lateral scales for the OCT data need to be adjusted based on age-specific AL estimates [30]. Gerth and Chong, in their research, suggested that images obtained using the handheld probe may also contain movement artifacts caused by the examiner and/or the child [34, 93].

Moreover, the HH-SDOCT imaging is limited by its lack of automatic registration for serial measurements.

In addition, it is important to adjust OCT to the age of the child when assessing foveal morphology, because of age-related variations in measurements of each retinal layer due to ongoing foveal development [38].

Another very important technique to consider in testing the youngest kids is to prepare a friendly decorated environment for the performance of OCT testing and keep the area controlled from noise and light [94].

Besides the OCT challenges and controversies in children, the emerging applications of the OCT technology in neonatology and pediatric neuro-ophthalmology can be, potentially, an objective and noninvasive diagnostic and monitoring tool helpful in providing additional information that can assist in management decisions.

22.5 Final Remarks

Development of the human visual system is a complex process. Over the past decade, considerable progress has been made in our understanding of the developmental, degenerative and ocular pathology in the childhood period. OCT is a valuable diagnostic tool that can be very helpful in everyday practice to improve our understanding of all physiological and pathological changes in disorders commonly observed in pediatric neuro-ophthalmology and pediatric ophthalmic-oncology assessments. With that understanding, our knowledge of the eye defects that cause neuro-ophthalmic disease has significantly expanded. Continuous improvement of non-invasive, easy-applicable OCT technology can widely enable application in youngest ages. There is no doubt that the upcoming years offer great promise for the further characterization of neurodevelopmental disorders of the visual system.

References

1. Fuhrmann S. Eye morphogenesis and patterning of the optic vesicle. Curr Top Dev Biol. 2010;93:61–84. https://doi.org/10.1016/B978-0-12-385044-7.00003-5.
2. Fitzpatrick DR, van Heyningen V. Developmental eye disorders. Curr Opin Genet Dev. 2005;15:348–53. https://doi.org/10.1016/j.gde.2005.04.013.
3. Wright K, Spiegel P. Pediatric ophthalmology and strabismus. 2nd ed. New York: Springer; 2003.
4. Lovicu F, McAvoy J, de Iongh R. Understanding the role of growth factors in embryonic development: insights from the lens. Philos Trans R Soc Lond Ser B Biol Sci. 2011;366:1204–18. https://doi.org/10.1098/rstb.2010.0339.
5. Ponsioen TL, Hooymans JM, Los LI. Remodeling of the human vitreous and vitreoretinal interface—a dynamic process. Prog Retin Eye Res. 2010;29:580–95. https://doi.org/10.1016/j.preteyeres.2010.07.001.
6. Gunhaga L. The lens: a classical model of embryonic induction providing new insights into cell determination in early development. Philos Trans R Soc Lond Ser B Biol Sci. 2011;366:1193–203. https://doi.org/10.1098/rstb.2010.0175.
7. Booij JC, Baas DC, Beisekeeva J, Gorgel TG, Bergem AA. The dynamic nature of Bruch's membrane. Prog Retin Eye Res. 2010;29:1–18. https://doi.org/10.1016/j.preteyeres.2009.08.003.
8. Provis M, Penfold PL, Cornish EE, Sandercoe TM, Madigan MC. Anatomy and development of the macula: specialization and the vulnerability to macular degeneration. Clin Exp Optom. 2005;88:269–81.
9. Hendrickson A, Bumsted-O'Brien K, Natoli R, Ramamurthy V, Possin D, Provis J. Rod photoreceptor differentiation in fetal and infant human retina. Exp Eye Res. 2008;87:415–26. https://doi.org/10.1016/j.exer.2008.07.016.
10. Morcillo J, Martínez-Morales JR, Trousse F, Fermin Y, Sowden JC, Bovolenta P. Proper patterning of the optic fissure requires the sequential activity of BMP7 and SHH. Development. 2006;133:3179–90. https://doi.org/10.1242/dev.02493.
11. Mann F, Harris WA, Holt CE. New views on retinal axon development: a navigation guide. Int J Dev Biol. 2004;48:957–64. https://doi.org/10.1387/ijdb.041899fm.
12. Irving C, Malhas A, Guthrie S, Mason I. Establishing the trochlear motor axon trajectory: role of the isthmic organizer and Fgf8. Development. 2002;129:5389–98.
13. Nugent AA, Kolpak AL, Engle EC. Human disorders of axon guidance. Curr Opin Neurobiol. 2012;22:837–43. https://doi.org/10.1016/j.conb.2012.02.006.
14. Zacharias AL, Lewandoski M, Rudnicki MA, Gage PJ. Pitx2 is an upstream activator of extraocular myogenesis and survival. Dev Biol. 2011;349:395–405. https://doi.org/10.1016/j.ydbio.2010.10.028.
15. Saint-Geniez M, D'Amore PA. Development and pathology of the hyaloid, choroidal and retinal vasculature. Int J Dev Biol. 2004;48:1045–58. https://doi.org/10.1387/ijdb.041895ms.
16. Hughes S, Yang H, Ling C. Vascularisation of the human fetal retina: roles of vasculogenesis and angiogenesis. Invest Ophthalmol Vis Sci. 2000;41:1217–28.
17. Das A, McGuire PG. Retinal and choroidal angiogenesis: pathophysiology and strategies for inhibition. Prog Retin Eye Res. 2003;22:721–48.
18. Zhao S, Overbeek PA. Regulation of choroid development by retinal pigment epithelium. Mol Vis. 2001;7:277–82.
19. Anand-Apte B, Hollyfield JG. Developmental anatomy of the retinal and choroidal vasculature. Cleveland: Elsevier; 2010.
20. Jakobiec FA. Ocular anatomy, embryology, and teratology. Philadelphia: Harper and Row; 1982.
21. Provis JM, Hendrickson AE. The foveal avascular region of developing human retina. Arch Ophthalmol. 2008;126:507–11. https://doi.org/10.1001/archopht.126.4.507.

22. Fruttiger M. Development of the retinal vasculature. Angiogenesis. 2007;10:77–88. https://doi.org/10.1007/s10456-007-9065-1.
23. Penn J, editor. Retinal and choroidal angiogenesis. Dordrecht: Springer; 2008.
24. Chan-Ling T, McLeod DS, Hughes S, Baxter L, Chu Y, Hasegawa T, et al. Astrocyte/endothelial cell relationships during human retinal vascular development. Invest Ophthalmol Vis Sci. 2004;45:2020–32.
25. Jonssen AM, Gardner TW, Kirchof B, Ryan SJ. Retinal vascular disease. Cambridge: Cambridge University Press; 2006.
26. Hungerford J, Stewart A, Hope P. Ocular sequelae of preterm birth and their relation to ultrasound evidence of cerebral damage. Br J Ophthalmol. 1986;70:463–8.
27. Msall ME, Phelps DL, DiGaudio KM, Dobson V, Tung B, McClead RE, The Cryotherapy for Retinopathy of Prematurity Cooperative Group, et al. Severity of neonatal retinopathy of prematurity is predictive of neurodevelopmental functional outcome at age 5.5 years. Pediatrics. 2000;106:998–1005.
28. Cooke RW, Foulder-Hughes L, Newsham D, Clarke D. Ophthalmic impairment at 7 years of age in children born very preterm. Arch Dis Child Fetal Neonatal Ed. 2004;89:F249–53.
29. Stephenson T, Wright S, O'Connor A, Fielder A, Johnson A, Ratib S, et al. Children born weighing less than 1701 g: visual and cognitive outcomes at 11–14 years. Arch Dis Child Fetal Neonatal Ed. 2007;92:F265–70. https://doi.org/10.1136/adc.2006.104000.
30. Maldonado RS, Izatt JA, Sarin N, Wallace DK, Freedman S, Cotten CM, et al. Optimizing hand-held spectral domain optical coherence tomography imaging for neonates, infants, and children. Invest Ophthalmol Vis Sci. 2010;51:2678–85. https://doi.org/10.1167/iovs.09-4403.
31. Maldonado RS, O'Connell RV, Sarin N, Freedman SF, Wallace DK, Cotten CM, et al. Dynamics of human foveal development after premature birth. Ophthalmology. 2011;118:2315–25. https://doi.org/10.1016/j.ophtha.2011.05.028.
32. Lee H, Proudlock F, Gottlob I. Is handheld optical coherence tomography reliable in infants and young children with and without nystagmus? Invest Ophthalmol Vis Sci. 2013;54:8152–9. https://doi.org/10.1167/iovs.13-13230.
33. Avery RA, Cnaan A, Schuman JS, Chen CL, Glaug NC, Packer RJ, et al. Intra- and inter-visit reproducibility of ganglion cell-inner plexiform layer measurements using handheld optical coherence tomography in children with optic pathway gliomas. Am J Ophthalmol. 2014;158:916–23. https://doi.org/10.1016/j.ajo.2014.07.029.
34. Gerth C, Zawadzki RJ, Héon E, Werner JS. High-resolution retinal imaging in young children using a handheld scanner and Fourier-domain optical coherence tomography. J AAPOS. 2009;13:72–4. https://doi.org/10.1016/j.jaapos.2008.09.001.
35. Maldonado RS, Toth CA. Optical coherence tomography in retinopathy of prematurity: looking beyond the vessels. Clin Perinatol. 2013;40:271–96. https://doi.org/10.1016/j.clp.2013.02.007.
36. Rootman DB, Gonzalez E, Mallipatna A, Vandenhoven C, Hampton L, Dimaras H, et al. Hand-held high-resolution spectral domain optical coherence tomography in retinoblastoma: clinical and morphologic considerations. Br J Ophthalmol. 2013;97:59–65. https://doi.org/10.1136/bjophthalmol-2012-302133.
37. Vajzovic L, Hendrickson AE, O'Connell RV, Clark LA, Tran-Viet D, Possin D, et al. Maturation of the human fovea: correlation of spectral-domain optical coherence tomography findings with histology. Am J Ophthalmol. 2012;154:779-89.e2. https://doi.org/10.1016/j.ajo.2012.05.004.
38. Lee H, Purohit R, Patel A, Papageorgiou E, Sheth V, Maconachie G, et al. In vivo foveal development using optical coherence tomography. Invest Ophthalmol Vis Sci. 2015;56:4537–45. https://doi.org/10.1167/iovs.15-16542.
39. Hendrickson AE, Yuodelis C. The morphological development of the human fovea. Ophthalmology. 1984;91:603–12.
40. Oros A. Retinopathy of prematurity. Belgrade: Endowment Andrejevic; 2003.
41. Phelps DL. Retinopathy of prematurity: history, classification, and pathophysiology. NeoReviews. 2001;2:e153–66. https://doi.org/10.1542/neo.2-7-e153.

42. Terry TL. Extreme prematurity and fibroblastic overgrowth of persistent vascular sheath behind each crystalline lens. Preliminary report. Am J Ophthalmol. 1942;25:203–4.
43. Friling R, Weinberger D, Kremer I, Avisar R, Sirota L, Snir M. Keratometry measurements in preterm and full-term newborn infants. Br J Ophthalmol. 2004;88:8–10.
44. Cook A, White S, Batterbury M, Clark D. Ocular growth and refractive error development in premature infants with or without retinopathy of prematurity. Invest Ophthalmol Vis Sci. 2008;49:5199–207. https://doi.org/10.1167/iovs.06-0114.
45. Gordon RA, Donzis PB. Refractive development of the human eye. Arch Ophthalmol. 1985;103:785–9. https://doi.org/10.1001/archopht.1985.01050060045020.
46. Harvey PS, King RA, Summers CG. Spectrum of foveal development in albinism detected with optical coherence tomography. J AAPOS. 2006;10:237–42. https://doi.org/10.1016/j.jaapos.2006.01.008.
47. Wallman J, Winawer J. Homeostasis of eye growth and the question of myopia. Neuron. 2004;43(4):447–68. https://doi.org/10.1016/j.neuron.2004.08.008.
48. Isenberg S, Del Signore M, Chen A, Wei J, Christenson P. Corneal topography of neonates and infants. Arch Ophthalmol. 2004;122:1767–71. https://doi.org/10.1001/archopht.122.12.1767.
49. Inagaki Y. The rapid change of corneal curvature in the neonatal period and infancy. Arch Ophthalmol. 1986;104:1026–7.
50. Mohindra I, Held R, Gwiazda J, Brill S. Astigmatism in infants. Science. 1978;202:329–31.
51. Howland HC, Atkinson J, Braddock O, French J. Infant astigmatism measured by photorefraction. Science. 1978;202:331–3.
52. Wang J, Spencer R, Leffler JN, Birch EE. Characteristics of peripapillary retinal nerve fiber layer in preterm children. Am J Ophthalmol. 2012;153:850-855.e1. https://doi.org/10.1016/j.ajo.2011.10.028.
53. Pueyo V, González I, Altemir I, Pérez T, Gómez G, Prieto E, et al. Microstructural changes in the retina related to prematurity. Am J Ophthalmol. 2015;159:797–802. https://doi.org/10.1016/j.ajo.2014.12.015.
54. Åkerblom H, Holmström G, Eriksson U, Larsson E. Retinal nerve fibre layer thickness in school-aged prematurely-born children compared to children born at term. Br J Ophthalmol. 2012;96:956–60. https://doi.org/10.1136/bjophthalmol-2011-301010.
55. Park KA, Oh SY. Retinal nerve fiber layer thickness in prematurity is correlated with stage of retinopathy of prematurity. Eye. 2015;9:1594–602. https://doi.org/10.1038/eye.2015.166.
56. Ecsedy M, Szamosi A, Karkó C, Zubovics L, Varsányi B, Németh J, et al. A comparison of macular structure imaged by optical coherence tomography in preterm and full-term children. Invest Ophthalmol Vis Sci. 2007;48:5207–11.
57. Lago AD, Matieli L, Gomes M, Baba NT, Farah ME, Belfort Junior R, et al. Stratus optical coherence tomography findings in patients with retinopathy of prematurity. Arq Bras Oftalmol. 2007;70:19–21.
58. Hammer DX, Iftimia NV, Ferguson RD, Bigelow CE, Ustun TE, Barnaby AM, et al. Foveal fine structure in retinopathy of prematurity: an adaptive optics Fourier domain optical coherence tomography study. Invest Ophthalmol Vis Sci. 2008;49:2061–70. https://doi.org/10.1167/iovs.07-1228.
59. Akerblom H, Larsson E, Eriksson U, Holmström G. Central macular thickness is correlated with gestational age at birth in prematurely born children. Br J Ophthalmol. 2011;95:799–803. https://doi.org/10.1136/bjo.2010.184747.
60. Wu WC, Lin RI, Shih CP, Wang NK, Chen YP, Chao AN, et al. Visual acuity, optical components, and macular abnormalities in patients with a history of retinopathy of prematurity. Ophthalmology. 2012;119:1907–16. https://doi.org/10.1016/j.ophtha.2012.02.040.
61. Park KA, Oh SY. Analysis of spectral-domain optical coherence tomography in preterm children: retinal layer thickness and choroidal thickness profiles. Invest Ophthalmol Vis Sci. 2012;53:7201–7. https://doi.org/10.1167/iovs.12-10599.
62. Chrzanowska B, Szumiński M, Oziebło-Kupczyk M, Bakunowicz-Łazarczyk A. Macular morphology and peripapillary retinal nerve fiber layer thickness in children with regressed retinopathy of prematurity. Klin Ocz. 2013;115:280–4 (in Polish).

63. Moreno TA, O'Connell RV, Chiu SJ, Farsiu S, Cabrera MT, Maldonado RS, et al. Choroid development and feasibility of choroidal imaging in the preterm and term infants utilizing SD-OCT. Invest Ophthalmol Vis Sci. 2013;54:4140–7. https://doi.org/10.1167/iovs.12-11471.
64. Maldonado RS, O'Connell R, Ascher SB, Sarin N, Freedman SF, Wallace DK, et al. Spectral-domain optical coherence tomographic assessment of severity of cystoid macular edema in retinopathy of prematurity. Arch Ophthalmol. 2012;130:569–78. https://doi.org/10.1001/archopthalmol.2011.1846.
65. Scott AW, Farsiu S, Enyedi LB, Wallace DK, Toth CA. Imaging the infant retina with a hand-held spectral-domain optical coherence tomography device. Am J Ophthalmol. 2009;147:364–73.e2. https://doi.org/10.1016/j.ajo.2008.08.010.
66. Erol MK, Ozdemir O, Turgut Coban D, Bilgin AB, Dogan B, Sogutlu Sari E, et al. Macular findings obtained by spectral domain optical coherence tomography in retinopathy of prematurity. J Ophthalmol. 2014;2014:468653. https://doi.org/10.1155/2014/468653.
67. Lee AC, Maldonado RS, Sarin N, O'Connell RV, Wallace DK, Freedman SF, et al. Macular features from spectral-domain optical coherence tomography as an adjunct to indirect ophthalmoscopy in retinopathy of prematurity. Retina. 2011;31:1470–82. https://doi.org/10.1097/IAE.0b013e31821dfa6d.
68. Joshi MM, Trese MT, Capone A Jr. Optical coherence tomography finding in stage 4A retinopathy of prematurity: a theory for visual variability. Ophthalmology. 2006;113:657–60. https://doi.org/10.1016/j.ophtha.2006.01.007.
69. Patel CK. Optical coherence tomography in the management of acute retinopathy of prematurity. Am J Ophthalmol. 2006;141:582–4. https://doi.org/10.1016/j.ajo.2005.10.002.
70. Ehrt O. Infantile and acquired nystagmus in childhood. Eur J Pediatr Neurol. 2012;16:567–72. https://doi.org/10.1016/j.ejpn.2012.02.010.
71. Lee H, Sheth V, Bibi M, Maconachie G, Patel A, McLean RJ, et al. Potential of hand-held optical coherence tomography to determine cause of infantile nystagmus in children by using foveal morphology. Ophthalmology. 2013;120:2714–24. https://doi.org/10.1016/j.ophtha.2013.07.018.
72. Lee H, Purohit R, Sheth V, Papageorgiou E, Maconachie G, McLean RJ, et al. Retinal development in albinism: a prospective study using optical coherence tomography in infants and young children. Lancet. 2015;385(Suppl 1):S14. https://doi.org/10.1016/S0140-6736(15)60329-4.
73. Lee H, Purohit R, Sheth V, McLean RJ, Kohl S, Leroy BP, et al. Retinal development in infants and young children with achromatopsia. Ophthalmology. 2015;122:2145–7. https://doi.org/10.1016/j.ophtha.2015.03.033.
74. Pilat A, Sibley D, McLean RJ, Proudlock FA, Gottlob I. High-resolution imaging of the optic nerve and retina in optic nerve hypoplasia. Ophthalmology. 2015;122:1330–9. https://doi.org/10.1016/j.ophtha.2015.03.020.
75. Gu S, Glaug N, Cnaan A, Packer RJ, Avery RA. Ganglion cell layer-inner plexiform layer thickness and vision loss in young children with optic pathway gliomas. Invest Ophthalmol Vis Sci. 2014;55:1402–8. https://doi.org/10.1167/iovs.13-13119.
76. Wall M. Update on idiopathic intracranial hypertension. Neurol Clin. 2017;35:45–57. https://doi.org/10.1016/j.ncl.2016.08.004.
77. National Eye Institute. Idiopathic intracranial hypertension. 2018. https://nei.nih.gov/health/iih/intracranial. Accessed 12 Dec 2018.
78. Gospe SM, Bhatti MT, El-Dairi MA. Anatomic and visual function outcomes in paediatric idiopathic intracranial hypertension. Br J Ophthalmol. 2015;100:505–9. https://doi.org/10.1136/bjophthalmol-2015-307043.
79. El-Dairi MA, Holgado S, O'Donnell T, Buckley EG, Asrani S, Freedman SF. Optical coherence tomography as a tool for monitoring pediatric pseudotumor cerebri. J AAPOS. 2007;11:564–70.
80. Shaahinfar A, Whitelaw KD, Mansour KM. Update on abusive head trauma. Curr Opin Pediatr. 2015;27:308–14. https://doi.org/10.1097/MOP.0000000000000207.
81. Chiocca E. Advanced pediatric assessment. 2nd ed. New York: Springer; 2014. p. 484.

82. Barr RG. Preventing abusive head trauma resulting from a failure of normal interaction between infants and their caregivers. Proc Natl Acad Sci. 2012;109(Suppl 2):17294–301. https://doi.org/10.1073/pnas.1121267109.
83. Christian CW, Block R, Committee on Child Abuse and Neglect, American Academy of Pediatrics. Abusive head trauma in infants and children. Pediatrics. 2009;123:1409–11. https://doi.org/10.1542/peds.2009-0408.
84. Muni RH, Kohly RP, Sohn EH, Lee TC. Hand-held spectral domain optical coherence tomography finding in shaken-baby syndrome. Retina. 2010;30:S45-50. https://doi.org/10.1097/IAE.0b013e3181dc048c.
85. Scott AW, Farsiu S, Enyedi LB, Wallace DK, Toth CA. Imaging the infant retina with a hand-held spectral-domain optical coherence tomography device. Am J Ophthalmol. 2009;147:364–373.e2. https://doi.org/10.1016/j.ajo.2008.08.010.
86. Isaacs H Jr. Tumors of the fetus and newborn. Philadelphia: WB Saunders; 1997.
87. Moore SW, Satge D, Sasco AJ, Zimmermann A, Plaschkes J. The epidemiology of neonatal tumours. Report of an international working group. Pediatr Surg Int. 2003;19:509–19. https://doi.org/10.1007/s00383-003-1048-8.
88. Huot CS, Desai KB, Shah VA. Spectral domain optical coherence tomography of combined hamartoma of the retina and retinal pigment epithelium. Ophthalmic Surg Lasers Imaging. 2009;40:322–4.
89. Yarovaya V, Sioufi K, Shields CL. Parafoveolar retinoblastoma regression with foveal preservation following intraarterial chemotherapy documented on hand-held optical coherence tomography in a newborn. Int J Retin Vitr. 2017;3:43.
90. Goel N, Pangtey B, Bhushan G, Raina UK, Ghosh B. Spectral-domain optical coherence tomography of astrocytic hamartomas in tuberous sclerosis. Int Ophthalmol. 2012;32:491–3. https://doi.org/10.1007/s10792-012-9586-5.
91. Takahashi A, Otto S, Yoshimura N. High-penetration optical coherence tomography and enhanced depth imaging in presumed retinal pigment epithelial hamartoma. Retin Cases Brief Rep. 2013;7:179–82. https://doi.org/10.1097/ICB.0b013e31827aee75.
92. Yousef YA, Shroff M, Halliday W, Gallie BL, Héon E. Detection of optic nerve disease in retinoblastoma by use of spectral domain optical coherence tomography. J AAPOS. 2012;16:481–3. https://doi.org/10.1016/j.jaapos.2012.05.010.
93. Chong GT, Farsiu S, Freedman SF, Sarin N, Koreishi AF, Izatt JA, et al. Abnormal foveal morphology in ocular albinism imaged with spectral-domain optical coherence tomography. Arch Ophthalmol. 2009;127:37–44.
94. Lambert V, Coad J, Hicks P, Glacken M. Young children's perspectives of ideal physical design features for hospital-built environments. J Child Health Care. 2013;18:57–71. https://doi.org/10.1177/1367493512473852.

23 Machine Learning Approaches in OCT: Application to Neurodegenerative Disorders

Rui Bernardes, Lília Jorge, Ana Nunes, Pedro Guimarães, and Miguel Castelo-Branco

Abstract

The use of machine learning (ML) in medicine is gaining momentum. In this chapter, we address the use of optical coherence tomography (OCT) to image the ocular fundus of the human eye, and the ocular fundus of wild-type and animal models of neurodegenerative disorders. The use of image texture analysis to describe the central nervous system status from OCT data and ML towards the use of the retina as a window into the brain in neurodegenerative disorders are discussed.

Keywords

Machine learning • Optical coherence tomography • Retina • Alzheimer's disease • Parkinson's disease • Diagnosis • Texture analysis • Animal models of disease

R. Bernardes · L. Jorge · A. Nunes · P. Guimarães · M. Castelo-Branco (✉)
Coimbra Institute for Biomedical Imaging and Translational Research (CIBIT), Institute of Nuclear Sciences Applied to Health (ICNAS), University of Coimbra, Coimbra, Portugal
e-mail: mcbranco@fmed.uc.pt

R. Bernardes · P. Guimarães · M. Castelo-Branco
Clinical Academic Center of Coimbra (CACC), Faculty of Medicine (FMUC), University of Coimbra, Coimbra, Portugal

A. Grzybowski and P. Barboni (eds.), *OCT and Imaging in Central Nervous System Diseases*, https://doi.org/10.1007/978-3-031-72156-4_23

23.1 The Classical Approach: Univariate Comparisons of Thickness Measures and Potential Sources of Bias

Studying the visual system in neurodegenerative disorders both at the retinal and cortical level has been justified by the fact that visual impairments are among the initial manifestations of Alzheimer's disease (AD), especially in which concerns the loss of contrast sensitivity and motion perception [1–5]. Furthermore, the pathological mechanisms underlying the neurodegenerative process appear to be consistent across the retina and the brain [6].

If the tenet that the retina is a mirror for cortical neurodegeneration holds, then it might be feasible to use it to diagnose neurodegenerative disorders [7–10]. Indeed, published data suggest that the retinal structure itself might be altered in AD [11–14], Parkinson's disease (PD) [15–19], and multiple sclerosis (MS) [20–25] further supporting the use of the retina towards the establishment of image-based biomarkers for these disorders.

Optical coherence tomography (OCT) represents an inexpensive tool to assess neuronal changes at the retinal level. However, simple univariate approaches based on the traditionally performed thickness measurements remain problematic. There are three main reasons for this:

1. Results are not consistent across the literature. While several studies do not report retinal thickness differences between AD or PD patients and healthy subjects [16, 26, 27], others have found significant thinning for different retinal layers [11, 28–30];
2. Information about degeneration may be distributed across the tissue and not captured by simple thickness measurements;
3. There are still issues of reproducibility across sites.

We first review some of the reported findings in the literature. Peripapillary retinal nerve fiber layer (RNFL) thickness has been claimed to be reduced in patients with AD and mild cognitive impairment (MCI) [31]. Similar promising findings have been reported concerning the reduced combined thickness of the ganglion cell layer (GCL) and inner plexiform layer (IPL) in MCI patients [32]. If this holds, retinal changes occur before MCI conversion to AD. Importantly, this conversion rate has been estimated to be up to 87% in prediction models [33]. However, MCI is notably challenging to diagnose due to its rather mild symptoms of cognitive impairment, which can overlap with the structural and functional alterations occurring in normal aging [34, 35]. Retinal thickness-based findings thus encourage the use of OCT as a neuroimaging aid, in the study of the early stages of the neurodegeneration process, as a complement to the recommended approaches [36], contributing to earlier diagnoses.

Overall, OCT studies in AD do, in general, indicate a significant decline in peripapillary (not macular) RNFL in all quadrants [11, 37] and overall macular thickness [11], while [32] reports macular GCL-IPL reduction. On the other hand,

Ascaso et al. [12] and Iseri et al. [38] found a decline in peripapillary and macular RNFL thickness in an AD sample with mild-to-moderate dementia. However, explicitly segmented retinal layers have been little investigated so far.

Concerning the macular RNFL thickness, significant differences between patients and controls were found by Larrosa et al. in [39]. Haan et al. [40] did not find significant differences in any of the 7 segmented sublayers (RNFL, GCL, IPL, inner nuclear layer (INL), outer plexiform layer (OPL), outer nuclear layer (ONL), and retinal pigment epithelium (RPE)).

Some other studies using other imaging techniques have also provided evidence against RNFL thinning in AD [41–43]. For instance, resorting to scanning laser polarimetry, Kergoat et al. [42] assessed the RNFL thickness near the optic nerve head center in 30 individuals with mild-to-moderate AD and respective controls. They found no significant differences between both groups and suggested that this layer seems unlikely to be affected in the initial stages of the disease.

The significance of these findings would need to be reevaluated by studies assessing OCT measurements together with other biomarkers of neurodegeneration in AD. However, these types of studies are still scarce [11].

With the notable exceptions mentioned above, most of these studies have been conducted in patients in later stages of the disease: in mild-to-moderate or severe AD stages. A consensus remains, therefore, difficult to achieve. A sizable number of studies have reported a decrease in retinal layer thickness [12, 37, 38, 44–50], but others failed to report this difference [11, 16, 27–30, 38, 40–43].

Regarding the RNFL, inconsistencies may also derive from the fact that some studies have been conducted on the peripapillary RNFL, while others were performed in the macular region. Moreover, inconsistencies are also present concerning histological work [51–54].

Sources of potential bias in aging populations also must be considered. For example, in [49], Marziani et al. found that the thickness of the RNFL + GCL complex and the manually segmented RNFL were reduced in the AD sample. In contrast, the external layers did not show significant differences. Although the study population had mild-to-moderate dementia, with less than 3 years of diagnosis, the authors noted that their sample might include glaucoma patients. Such sources of bias are often not disclosed.

The fact that the primary visual cortex has been claimed to be spared in the early stages of the disease [55–62] does also not favor a direct imaging approach to the retina, at least in terms of the concept of a "window to the brain".

It is nevertheless still possible that a significant amount of information discriminating between multiple neurodegenerative states is conveyed by OCT imaging of the human retina, even when differences in average thickness are not yet present. In other words, approaches capturing multivariate information, which is just not possible with simple thickness-based univariate comparisons, may still detect early changes.

In [41], Jentsch et al. suggest that fluorescence lifetime imaging ophthalmoscopy (FLIO) may reveal retinal changes earlier than OCT, in a wide range of mild-to-moderate forms of AD, possibly because of earlier disease-specific changes in cellular metabolism. Even though OCT cannot directly capture these, potentially associated changes in the local biological environment may induce changes in the medium that are OCT-measurable.

Whether the detailed assessment of separate retinal layers will help identify earlier changes in OCT data remains a question. Most studies exploring AD macular integrity have focused on the RNFL, occasionally extending to the RNFL + GCL and GCL + IPL complexes. A notable exception is the work described by Haan et al. in [40], in which authors analyzed 7 sublayers.

Given all the discrepancies and sources of bias mentioned above, it remains a fundamental question whether data-driven machine learning approaches would allow identifying biomarkers of brain neurodegeneration.

23.2 Machine Learning

In a recent paper by Ahmed et al. [63] regarding the use of machine learning (ML) in neuroimaging modalities for dementia diagnosis, the current focus on using this type of applications in medicine in general and in clinical neurosciences in particular, is quite clear, with 16 of the referenced papers having been published from 2013 to 2018 [63]. Magnetic resonance imaging (MRI) is the preferred imaging modality by far, with 14 of the 16 studies using it. It has been argued by [64] that the popularity of the MRI modality, in particular where the ML-aided study of neurodegeneration (e.g., in AD and MCI) is concerned, is due to the AD neuroimaging initiative (ADNI) dataset [65].

Machine learning can broadly be defined by the famous quote attributed to Arthur Samuel, in 1959 [66], as the "Field of study that gives computers the ability to learn without being explicitly programmed," even though the exact quote is "Programming computers to learn from experience should eventually eliminate the need for much of this detailed programming effort." Actual and more accurate definitions do actually exist now, like IBM's definition [67]: "Machine learning is a branch of artificial intelligence (AI) and computer science which focuses on the use of data and algorithms to imitate the way that humans learn, gradually improving its accuracy."

Two major approaches can be thought of, the unsupervised and the supervised learning methods. For both types of algorithms, a set of examples that algorithms can learn from are required.

In unsupervised learning, the algorithm looks for structure in the data and aggregates similar cases in clusters. The measure of similarity plays a fundamental role, and distinct similarity metrics may lead to significantly different clustering results.

The supervised learning algorithm, on the other hand, requires a set of labeled examples. The algorithm looks, at the training phase, for the best way to split the set of cases according to the provided data for each one and the respective label. After that, new instances in which the labels are unknown will be labeled, for a classification problem, according to its data and the decision boundary established at the training phase. The above algorithm does not require an explicit definition of

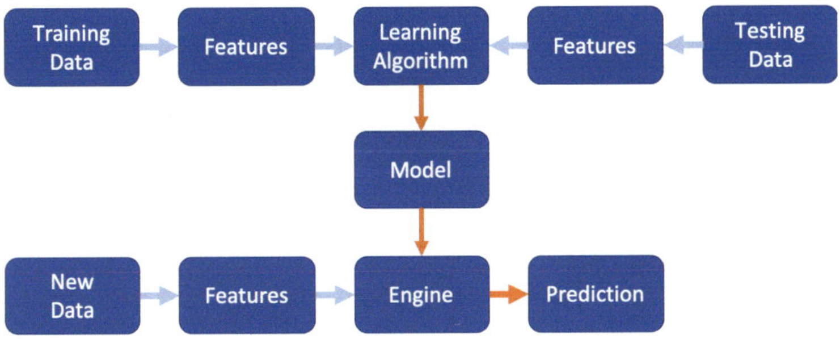

Fig. 23.1 Schematic of a machine learning model

how to proceed. It will come to the best decision based on the provided examples only (Fig. 23.1).

It is crucial to bear in mind that machine learning can only provide answers to a specific question and according to the metric used to measure the success in classifying the examples provided for the training (learning) phase.

In medical imaging applications of ML, most studies are classification-based ones, but a growing interest in pattern regression to estimate disease stages, namely by combining neuroimaging data with cognitive scores obtained from neuropsychological assessments, has been recognized [64].

A good insight on machine learning and its use in medical imaging can be found in the work of Erickson et al. [68]. In contrast, the potential challenges and pitfalls of such use—and recommendations on how to address them—have been recently discussed by Varoquaux and Cheplygina [69].

One widely used machine learning method in dementia diagnosis is the support vector machines (SVM) approach. Vapnik and Chervonenkis [70, 71] proposed this method which is based on the linear separation between two classes (binary classification). The SVM algorithm identifies the hyperplane that makes most of the cases of one class lay on one side of it and most of the cases of the other class on the other side while maximizing the distance between the hyperplane and the cases closer to it.

Individual cases are characterized by a set of values (features) that convey pertinent information on the case regarding the classification of interest. For example, the height and weight of a person would make sense for the classification of people in regular and overweight classes, while the iris color would not. Henceforth, it is required to compute/gather information relevant to the aimed classification.

Different machine learning approaches, like convolution neural networks (CNN) [72, 73], are possible and are based on a distinct rationale. The number of training cases is typically higher when compared to the SVM approach, where the rule of thumb to avoid overtraining is to have the number of training cases equal to ten times the number of classes times the number of features.

The application of machine learning is vast and can range from image segmentation and gene expression inference [74] to drug name recognition [75].

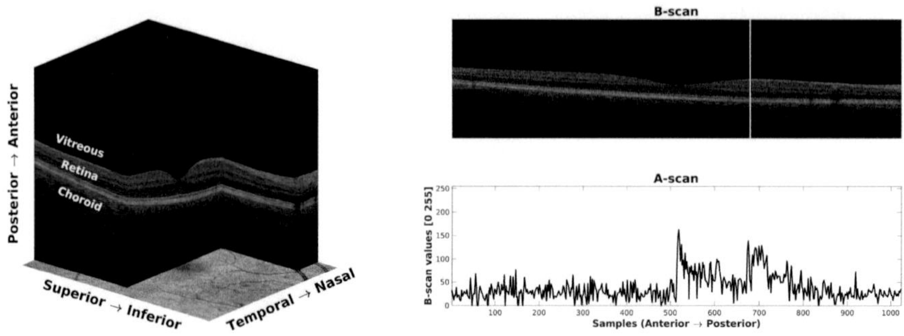

Fig. 23.2 Optical coherence tomography (OCT). Left: volumetric OCT data shown over an eye fundus reference computed from the inner limiting membrane (ILM) to the retinal pigment epithelium (RPE). Right: a B-scan (top) from the volume on the left and an A-scan profile (bottom) from the B-scan

Using the retina as a window to the brain means using it as a source of information that may convey the status of the brain concerning some aspect of interest, like the presence of signs of AD, PD disease, or any other neurodegenerative disorder of interest for a particular study. The rationale supporting this approach is that the retina is the visible part of the central nervous system (CNS) readily available for optical imaging. OCT is of particular interest for these studies because of its ability to detect changes in the refractive index, within the retina, with high sensitivity. The question remains if OCT data can be leveraged in a scalable way as a staple modality for imaging the CNS. In this regard, online public OCT databases [76, 77] are becoming increasingly available, mimicking the widespread availability of MRI neuroimaging datasets.

The traditional way to visualize OCT data from the ocular fundus is the direct visualization of B-scans, a form of presenting a set of A-scans taken side-by-side in the retina along a line, allowing for direct assessment of the structure of the retina (Fig. 23..2).

In addition to the structure, one can postulate that information not perceivable to the user, by direct observation of OCT data from the retina, may be present and may turn possible to identify differences between two different statuses based on the statistics of backscattered light. One possible way to compute information out of the appearance of an image is through the use of texture.

Texture analysis methods [78, 79] may provide additional insights into such changes. Image texture relates to the relative distribution of the image's intensity values [80], which can be quantified using several different metrics (often called "textural features"). In brief, texture analysis allows determining how values of pixel intensity aggregate in an image or regions of an image and compute metrics conveying information on the distinct ways pixels' intensity aggregate. Two types of texture exist: the texture pattern and the random pattern. The former is where it is possible to identify patterns like squares, diamond shapes, or akin visually. On the other hand, a random pattern is one where it is not possible to visually identify a pattern, the typical case of a fundus image for an individual layer computed from an OCT retinal scan.

Texture-based methods, which have been used in medical applications since the 1970s [81–83], have recently trespassed into the field of OCT imaging. In his doctoral thesis, Gao [84] explored some of these features in addition to thickness measurements and other metrics on optical properties and reported that his combination of different methods yields additional insights into the macular pathology of diabetic retinopathy (DR) patients. González et al. [85] used co-occurrence [78] texture analysis methods to detect cysts in OCT retinal images automatically, achieving a classification accuracy of 80%. In another classification study based on the SVM algorithm [86], the different explored texture-based methods confirmed that texture carries valuable information that can be used in addition to thickness measurements to detect changes caused by glaucoma. Subsequent studies by Varga et al. [21] and Morgan et al. [87] used texture analysis in OCT data to derive changes in the retinal tissue in MS and to detect retinal ganglion cell damage, respectively.

Besides the traditional OCT images (B-scans), fundus images can be computed for each retinal layer. Through image processing techniques, it is possible to determine the interfaces between consecutive retinal layers, like the RNFL-GCL and the GLC-IPL. Therefore, the region between these two interfaces is the GCL, meaning it is possible to isolate a layer of interest from the rest of the gathered data. Imaging the retina, e.g., the macular region, allows collecting information on the retinal tissue of interest across the imaged region by performing a series of B-scans side-by-side and isolating the same layer in each B-scan. Averaging the values of this layer along each A-scan allows computing a mean fundus (MVF) image [88] of a particular layer—the GCL in the current example. The same principle can be applied to any of the layers of interest (Fig. 23.3) and allows analyzing each of these images using well-known image analysis techniques, like texture analysis.

Other possibilities for texture analysis, besides the co-occurrence-based texture analysis, are the use of other statistical-based methods such as the run-length matrix [89] and local binary patterns [90]. This category of texture analysis methods is the most used in different fields of application, including medical image analysis. However, other classes of methods are available: image transforms, like the wavelet transform, as in [91]; or the well-known Fourier transform; model-based methods, which identify mathematical models that reflect the texture contents of an image; and structural methods, which look for the atomic elements that constitute image textures and their interrelationships. Beyond these four approaches (statistical, transform-based, model-based, and structural) to texture analysis, newer perspectives and methods for the characterization and quantification of image textures have recently been proposed [92, 93].

The use of specific texture metrics from MVF images of individual retinal layers is in line with [94], where particular layers of the retina and computed parameters were used, and utterly distinct from the approach of using CNNs, where the entire image is used and no explicit computation of parameters from the image are predefined. Recent research has been moving towards the latter approach, focusing

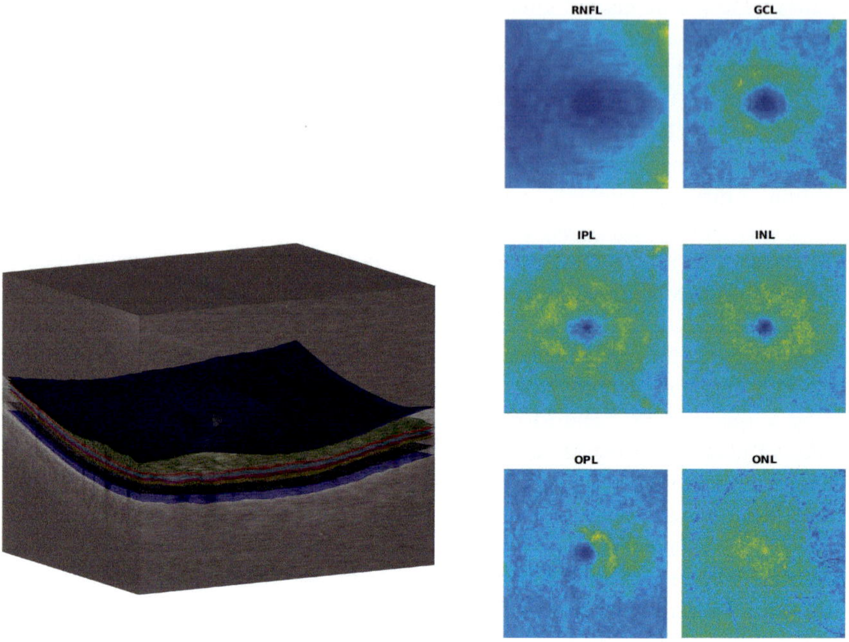

Fig. 23.3 An OCT volume (left) is shown with interfaces displayed in color, e.g., the interface vitreous-retina in blue. Pseudo-color fundus images (right) are shown for retinal layers composing the neuroretina. Pseudo-color is used for the ease of visualization only

on "learned texture," e.g., the textural elements within images learned by CNNs. A "texture hypothesis," which states that CNNs may be relying more on textural elements than object shapes, has actually been proposed by Geirhos et al. [95]. Notwithstanding it, a transition from pre-selected texture features towards deep-learned ones appears to be underway [92, 93, 96].

Exploratory studies performed on the retinas of mouse models of AD, using the techniques mentioned above, hint at the hypothesis that early changes associated with this disorder can be identified in specific layers of the retina[97, 98]. Naturally, studies performed on animal models of disease have the advantages of allowing OCT data to be collected in the early stages of the disease, on the one hand, and making it possible, on the other hand, for the neurodegenerative process to be tracked at regular intervals of the disease's course. The key to identifying biomarkers of neurodegeneration in OCT human data may thus be found by leveraging the information contained in the corresponding animal data and comparing datasets in both species.

OCT and machine learning techniques have been used to assess different health conditions through the retina at least since 2011 [99]. In this work, OCT was used to distinguish between the eyes of healthy controls (HC), eyes of patients diagnosed with diabetes and with no signs of DR (Early Treatment Diabetic

Retinopathy Study level 10 eyes), and eyes diagnosed with diabetic macular edema (DME) [99].

In this initial work bringing together OCT and ML, OCT data from the whole retina (from the inner limiting membrane (ILM) to the RPE) within the macular region, and SVM for the classification of cases into one of the three possible classes (HC, DR, and DME), it was possible to demonstrate that the retina may hold relevant information concerning the different statuses, even though that is not apparent from the traditional visual inspection, and that ML techniques may help gather information embedded in OCT data.

Following the same rationale and the same way of computing data to be used by the SVM classification algorithm, a subsequent work allowed to demonstrate, for the first time, the possibility of assessing healthy aging from OCT data, with the system being able to correctly classify HC into one of two possible age groups with an overall accuracy of 70% [100].

Recently, our research group focused on using these techniques and approaches to assess changes in the retina associated with neurodegenerative disorders. To get an insight into which layer(s) of the retina changes are predominant, the methodology developed by Guimarães et al. [88] was applied to compute a MVF image per retinal layer (Fig. 23.3).

In this exploratory work, using OCT data from healthy controls' retinas and OCT data from patients diagnosed with MS, texture analysis was applied to MVF images [88]. Data were gathered by a Cirrus SD-OCT 5000 (Carl Zeiss Meditec, Dublin, CA, USA) using the 512×128 macular cube protocol, and the layer segmentation was performed using the OCT Explorer software (Retinal Image Analysis Lab, Iowa Institute for Biomedical Imaging, Iowa City, IA, USA) [101–103].

For texture description, grey-level co-occurrence matrices (GLCM) [78] were computed, from which 20 texture features were calculated for each MVF image and block [78, 104, 105] (Fig. 23.4).

SVM with radial basis function (RBF) kernel [106, 107] was used after each variable had been z-score transformed at the preprocessing stage to eliminate differences in scale that may interfere with the system performance. A twofold cross-validation (50% of the cases for training and 50% for testing) was used to assess the system's performance in classifying unknown cases.

The accuracy of the discrimination was over 75% for the GCL and under 72% for any of the remaining layers when using only features of the layer under analysis. These results allowed us to put forward the possibility of identifying changes present in the retina of patients diagnosed with neurodegenerative disorders, on the one hand, and, on the other hand, that changes do not spread equally across the retina.

These approaches are significantly distinct from the ones that have been pursued so far, where the thickness of the retina or the thickness of specific layers of the retina are used to help diagnose neurodegenerative disorders. MS-related damage in the retina has been addressed by measuring the thickness of distinct layers [22, 23], with a particular focus on the thickness of the RNFL that has been

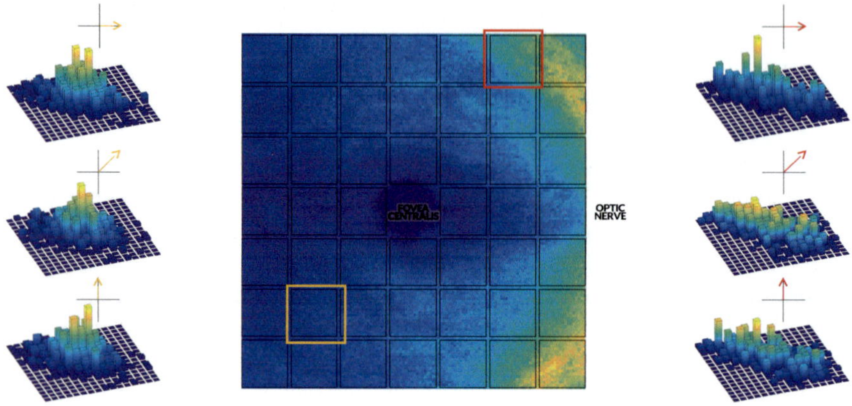

Fig. 23.4 The image in the center shows a pseudo-color fundus image from the retinal nerve fiber layer (RNFL). The grid delimits individual regions for texture analysis over the fundus image. Gray level co-occurrence matrices are plotted (left and right) for the two marked regions, respectively, the marker region in the 6th row and the marked region in row one. The arrows indicate the direction of texture analysis using the grey-level co-occurrence matrix (GLCM) [78]. As shown, pixels' intensities aggregate differently in different regions conveying different texture characteristics

correlated to measures of brain atrophy in MRI [24, 25]. In a recent study [108], Nunes et al. showed that texture-based metrics are not a surrogate for thickness measurements. In this study [108], it was shown that 16 out of the 20 texture features present statistically significant differences ($p \leq 0.05$) between the HC and MS groups in at least one of the retinal quadrants (Fig. 23.5). Fourteen of the 16 texture features present highly statistically significant differences ($p \leq 0.01$) and 5 of the 14 even higher ($p \leq 0.001$), while the correlation between texture metrics and RNFL thickness is moderate, ranging from 0.50 to 0.62, for two features in the MS group and seven features in the HC group.

Feeding machine learning techniques with data and class labels means that it is required to have a prior classification of known cases using currently accepted diagnosis methods. However, these can only provide a probable diagnosis at a particular disease stage, which for AD is thought to be 10–15 years after disease onset [109]. Hence, we may be teaching ML systems to detect what is currently known instead of teaching them to detect early signs of disease.

Pushing the limits, our research group put forward a study aiming to discriminate between HC, AD, and PD patients simultaneously (Fig. 23.6). The analysis of texture from the MVF images of the neuroretina, comprising layers from the RNFL to the ONL, allowed the classification system to identify eyes of healthy controls with a sensitivity (SEN) of 87.7% and specificity (SPE) of 83.9%, eyes of AD patients with 79.5% (SEN) and 92.5% (SPE), and eyes of PD patients with 75.9% (SEN) and 97.8% (SPE). Of utmost importance, though, is that 74.6% of the subjects have received the same classification in both eyes and that 92.8% of these people were classified in the correct group.

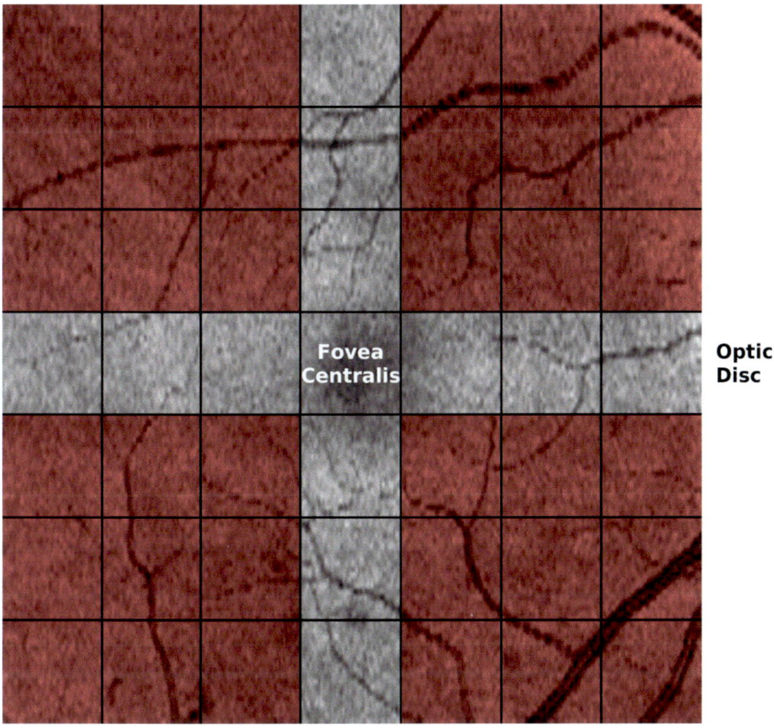

Fig. 23.5 Texture metrics are aggregated into retinal quadrants as shown by the reddish areas over the computed fundus image from the volumetric macular cube OCT scan of the right eye of a healthy control subject. Each of the 7×7 blocks shows the individual analyzed areas. Image axes are: x-axis (horizontal)—temporal (left) to nasal (right) and y-axis (vertical) superior (top) to inferior (bottom)

These findings suggest that information conveyed by texture analysis of OCT data from the human retina is specific to differentiate between neurodegenerative disorders instead of merely signaling a difference from the health status. These results hint at the potential of texture-based approaches for identifying localized changes in specific regions of the retina and for capturing microstructural alterations that cannot be quantified through thickness measurements alone. Texture analysis can thus help develop a more comprehensive neurodegeneration map of the retina, e.g., disease-specific texture profiles or "signatures" [110]. Such profiles could provide detailed information on the specific changes in the retinal tissue caused by a particular neurodegenerative disorder, provide further insight into the conflicting thickness-based research findings mentioned above, and, more importantly, assist in the differential diagnosis of neurodegenerative disorders.

Some authors have proposed integrating texture-based methods into the clinical decision workflow after adequate validation [111–113] to balance out the subjectivity variability involved when visually interpreting medical images. The use of

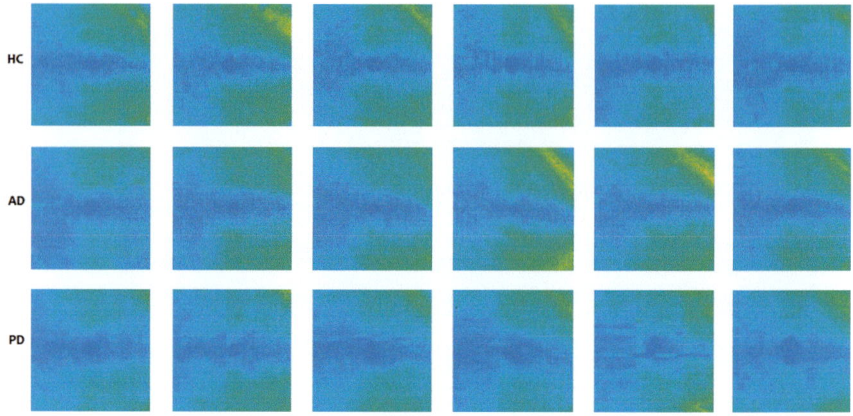

Fig. 23.6 Pseudo-color retinal nerve fiber layer (RNFL) fundus images of six eyes of healthy controls (HC) (top), six eyes of patients diagnosed with Alzheimer's disease (AD) (middle), and six eyes of patients diagnosed with Parkinson's disease (PD) (bottom) are shown. Through visual inspection, identifying characteristics distinguishing these groups would not be possible. All cases are age-matched

texture as a systematic and robust diagnostic aid may prove to be particularly relevant in longitudinal studies targeting disease progression, treatment response, and the normal aging process.

Our research group recently used the same retinal texture metrics (GLCM) to study sex-based retina interocular differences in healthy adults, e.g., to determine if women and men have the same retina texture characteristics in both eyes [114]. These features were tested for group mean differences between the right and left eye, demonstrating that texture differences exist only in the female group. This work illustrates how special care should be taken when designing research protocols that assess retina differences: the participant groups being compared should be sex-balanced, as was previously addressed by Shaqiri et al. in [115].

To address the possibility of identifying early signs of AD based on texture metrics from OCT data, our research group set a study using wild-type and mice models of AD and imaged those every 4 months starting at the age of 4 months. The system used in this study to image mice's retinas is the Micron IV OCT (Phoenix Research Labs, Pleasanton, CA, USA), which is tailored to image mouse and rat retinas and allows scanning the posterior pole of the eye gathering $512 \times 512 \times 1024$ voxels over 50° field of view. Because mice do not possess a macula, all scans were performed at the same retinal location, above the optic disc and horizontally centered in this region.

After the acquisition, images were processed as in [99]. Features computed from the histograms of OCT intensity distribution were fed into an SVM algorithm to find the possibility of classifying mice into the wild-type (WT) and AD-transgenic groups. This classifier achieved a median accuracy of 83% at the age of 4 months and 94% at the age of 8 months. We further tested texture information to find differences between groups, even using a gross split of the mouse retina into 3 layers. These findings paved the way for further ongoing studies.

Because of the suggested parallel between changes in the mice retina of the AD-transgenic model and those occurring in the human retina, we put forward another study where mice models of AD (born transgenic) and WT controls were continuously monitored until 16 months of age. Animals were frequently imaged by OCT to enlighten retinal changes induced by healthy aging (WT) and aging and familial AD-associated genes (transgenic mice). For the first time, mice's retinas have been carefully imaged from an early age (1-month-old), revealing surprising changes at the very beginning of these animals' lives. We have investigated quantifiable alterations, such as retinal thickness, and information embedded in the OCT data that could be used for early detection and diagnosis possible to be translated to humans, the ultimate goal.

WT and AD-transgenic mice showed a progressive decrease in total retinal thickness with age [116]. Nevertheless, significantly lower total retinal thickness values in AD-transgenic mice compared to age-matched WT animals were observed since the first month of age.

MVF images (see above) were computed from the RNFL-GCL complex, and INL, IPL, ONL, and OPL layers and texture parameters were determined for each layer to look for potential differences between WT and AD-transgenic mice retinas. The rationale is that minor changes at the molecular level can lead to changes in the tissue refractive index detectable by OCT and translatable into textural differences, as put forward above for the human retina, again resorting to GLCM metrics.

For every time point and layer, statistically significant differences were found between the two groups ($p < 0.001$) using the t-test when normality was not rejected (at a significance level of 10%) and the non-parametric alternative Mann–Whitney U-test otherwise. Achieved results indicate that changes are widespread across the retina (all layers present differences between groups) and persistent in time (differences in all layers at all time points). Therefore, the genes defining the mouse model of familial AD have an enormous phenotypic impact on the retina, which OCT could easily capture. Because the retina is part of the CNS, these results suggest that there may be a wide-reaching effect, including the brain, and that these can be non-invasively assessed by imaging the retina.

This study found statistically significant differences for both retinal thickness and texture at the first imaging time point (1-month-old mice). At this stage of development, the two groups already showed widespread differences across the retina. This is a limitation of the study as it was impossible to identify a point where WT and AD-transgenic mice started to diverge. One can speculate that early neurodevelopmental differences exist around or even before birth. For future studies, these results show that the assumption of parity between WT and AD-transgenic mice at early stages may not hold and that this should be considered when studying progression.

Age-related changes in the brain, such as neural tissue thinning, neural activity, and functional connectivity impairments, have been associated with AD [117–119]. Also, brain-predicted age has been reported as a significant predictor of dementia progression [120]. To shed light on the differences between the two animal groups mentioned above, WT and AD-transgenic mice, two CNNs were trained and tuned to predict mice age from retinal OCT data (B-scans) to understand if similar changes were present in the retina of both groups [121]. To eliminate training bias, one CNN was trained using only WTs' OCT B-scans, while the other relied on AD-transgenic mice data. Both CNNs could predict mice age for both WT and AD-transgenic mice. Moreover, achieved results indicate that the presence of the genes associated with the familial form of AD impact retinal aging. Both CNNs consistently and surprisingly predicted ages for WT mice older than 4 months above the ones predicted for AD-transgenic mice (Fig. 23.7).

These findings were somewhat unexpected as they appear to contradict what has been observed in the brain, which may partly be explained by a background of early neurodevelopmental changes. Overall, the underlying biological changes leading to age-dependent alterations are complex. Several age-dependent cellular and molecular changes have been previously reported in the retina, such as photoreceptor mislocalization [122], vascular and RPE changes [123], an increase in tissue autofluorescence at the photoreceptor-RPE interface [124], and scattering diversity [125]. Nevertheless, OCT does not directly capture these changes, and a straightforward comparison of results is not possible. Indeed, we can infer that

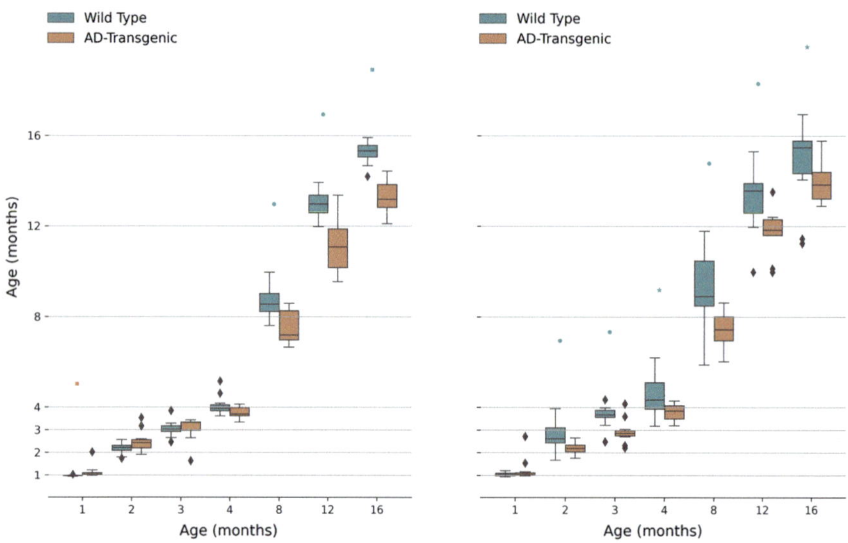

Fig. 23.7 Box plots of predicted ages, separated per class (wild-type vs. Alzheimer's disease(AD)-transgenic mice), for each acquisition time-point. From left to right, results for the wild-type and the Alzheimer's disease-transgenic trained models. * $p < 0.05$; ● $p < 0.01$; ■ $p < 0.001$. The color of the symbol indicates a higher median value

age-dependent neuronal adaptations that naturally correlate with age are captured by the method used. Thus, we can theorize that these healthy adaptations may be altered in AD-transgenic animals. Moreover, biological interpretations are further hindered by the complex interactions between inserted mutated genes and the mice's background. Additional functional and molecular tests are necessary to determine the factors responsible for these findings.

In conclusion, texture biomarkers from computed fundus images from OCT data are of paramount importance as they will likely turn possible to identify patients at risk of developing AD before they can be diagnosed using currently available methods and an imaging technique that is widely available, inexpensive, and non-invasive.

References

1. Gilmore GC, Groth KE, Thomas CW. Stimulus contrast and word reading speed in Alzheimer's disease. Exp Aging Res. 2005;31(1):15–33. https://doi.org/10.1080/03610730590882828.
2. Graewe B, Lemos R, Ferreira C, Santana I, Farivar R, Weerd PD, Castelo-Branco M. Impaired processing of 3D motion-defined faces in mild cognitive impairment and healthy aging: an fMRI study. Cereb Cortex. 2013;23(10):2489–99. https://doi.org/10.1093/cercor/bhs246.
3. Javaid FZ, Brenton J, Guo L, Cordeiro MF. Visual and ocular manifestations of Alzheimer's disease and their use as biomarkers for diagnosis and progression. Front Neurol. 2016;7:55. https://doi.org/10.3389/fneur.2016.00055.
4. Lemos R, Figueiredo P, Santana I, Simões MR, Castelo-Branco M. Temporal integration of 3D coherent motion cues defining visual objects of unknown orientation is impaired in amnestic mild cognitive impairment and Alzheimer's disease. J Alzheimer's Dis. 2012;28(4):885–96. https://doi.org/10.3233/jad-2011-110719.
5. Risacher SL, WuDunn D, Pepin SM, MaGee TR, McDonald BC, Flashman LA, Wishart HA, Pixley HS, Rabin LA, Paré N, Englert JJ, Schwartz E, Curtain JR, West JD, O'Neill DP, Santulli RB, Newman RW, Saykin AJ. Visual contrast sensitivity in Alzheimer's disease, mild cognitive impairment, and older adults with cognitive complaints. Neurobiol Aging. 2013;34(4):1133–44. https://doi.org/10.1016/j.neurobiolaging.2012.08.007.
6. Masland RH. The neuronal organization of the retina. Neuron. 2012;76(2):266–80. https://doi.org/10.1016/j.neuron.2012.10.002.
7. Cordeiro MF. Eyeing the brain. Acta Neuropathol. 2016;132(6):765–6. https://doi.org/10.1007/s00401-016-1628-z.
8. London A, Benhar I, Schwartz M. The retina as a window to the brain—from eye research to CNS disorders. Nat Rev Neurol. 2013;9(1):44–53. https://doi.org/10.1038/nrneurol.2012.227.
9. Svetozarskiy SN, Kopishinskaya SV. Retinal optical coherence tomography in neurodegenerative diseases (review). Sovremennye Tehnologii v Med. 2015;7(1):116–123. https://doi.org/10.17691/stm2015.7.1.14
10. Cheung CY, Ikram MK, Chen C, Wong TY. Imaging retina to study dementia and stroke. Prog Retin Eye Res. 2017;57:89–107. https://doi.org/10.1016/j.preteyeres.2017.01.001.
11. den Haan J, Verbraak FD, Visser PJ, Bouwman FH. Retinal thickness in Alzheimer's disease: a systematic review and meta-analysis. Alzheimer's Dementia Diagnosis Assess Dis Monit. 2017;6(1):162–70. https://doi.org/10.1016/j.dadm.2016.12.014.
12. Ascaso FJ, Cruz N, Modrego PJ, Lopez-Anton R, Santabárbara J, Pascual LF, Lobo A, Cristóbal JA. Retinal alterations in mild cognitive impairment and Alzheimer's disease:

an optical coherence tomography study. J Neurol. 2014;261(8):1522–30. https://doi.org/10.1007/s00415-014-7374-z.

13. Hart NJ, Koronyo Y, Black KL, Koronyo-Hamaoui M. Ocular indicators of Alzheimer's: exploring disease in the retina. Acta Neuropathol. 2016;132(6):767–87. https://doi.org/10.1007/s00401-016-1613-6.
14. Cheung CY, Ong YT, Ikram MK, Ong SY, Li X, Hilal S, Catindig JS, Venketasubramanian N, Yap P, Seow D, Chen CP, Wong TY. Microvascular network alterations in the retina of patients with Alzheimer's disease. Alzheimer's Dementia. 2014;10(2):135–42. https://doi.org/10.1016/j.jalz.2013.06.009.
15. Archibald NK, Clarke MP, Mosimann UP, Burn DJ. The retina in Parkinson's disease. Brain. 2009;132(5):1128–45. https://doi.org/10.1093/brain/awp068.
16. Archibald NK, Clarke MP, Mosimann UP, Burn DJ. Retinal thickness in Parkinson's disease. Parkinsonism Relat Disord. 2011;17(6):431–6. https://doi.org/10.1016/j.parkreldis.2011.03.004.
17. Tian T, Zhu X-H, Liu Y-H (n.d.). Potential role of retina as a biomarker for progression of Parkinson's disease. Int J Ophthalmol. 4(4):433–8. https://doi.org/10.3980/j.issn.2222-3959.2011.04.21.
18. Garcia-Martin E, Larrosa JM, Polo V, Satue M, Marques ML, Alarcia R, Seral M, Fuertes I, Otin S, Pablo LE. Distribution of retinal layer atrophy in patients with parkinson disease and association with disease severity and duration. Am J Ophthalmol. 2014;157(2):470-478.e2. https://doi.org/10.1016/j.ajo.2013.09.028.
19. Chorostecki J, Seraji-Bozorgzad N, Shah A, Bao F, Bao G, George E, Gorden V, Caon C, Frohman E, Bhatti MT, Khan O. Characterization of retinal architecture in Parkinson's disease. J Neurol Sci. 2015;355(1–2):44–8. https://doi.org/10.1016/j.jns.2015.05.007.
20. Calabresi PA, Balcer LJ, Frohman EM. Retinal pathology in multiple sclerosis: insight into the mechanisms of neuronal pathology. Brain. 2010;133(6):1575–7. https://doi.org/10.1093/brain/awq133.
21. Varga BE, Gao W, Laurik KL, Tátrai E, Simó M, Somfai GM, DeBuc DC. Investigating tissue optical properties and texture descriptors of the retina in patients with multiple sclerosis. PLoS ONE. 2015;10(11): e0143711. https://doi.org/10.1371/journal.pone.0143711.
22. Britze J, Pihl-Jensen G, Frederiksen JL. Retinal ganglion cell analysis in multiple sclerosis and optic neuritis: a systematic review and meta-analysis. J Neurol. 2017;264(9):1837–53. https://doi.org/10.1007/s00415-017-8531-y.
23. Saidha S, Syc SB, Ibrahim MA, Eckstein C, Warner CV, Farrell SK, Oakley JD, Durbin MK, Meyer SA, Balcer LJ, Frohman EM, Rosenzweig JM, Newsome SD, Ratchford JN, Nguyen QD, Calabresi PA. Primary retinal pathology in multiple sclerosis as detected by optical coherence tomography. Brain. 2011;134(2):518–33. https://doi.org/10.1093/brain/awq346.
24. Petzold A, de Boer JF, Schippling S, Vermersch P, Kardon R, Green A, Calabresi PA, Polman C. Optical coherence tomography in multiple sclerosis: a systematic review and meta-analysis. Lancet Neurol. 2010;9(9):921–32. https://doi.org/10.1016/s1474-4422(10)70168-x.
25. Henderson APD, Trip SA, Schlottmann PG, Altmann DR, Garway-Heath DF, Plant GT, Miller DH. An investigation of the retinal nerve fibre layer in progressive multiple sclerosis using optical coherence tomography. Brain. 2008;131(1):277–87. https://doi.org/10.1093/brain/awm285.
26. Lad EM, Mukherjee D, Stinnett SS, Cousins SW, Potter GG, Burke JR, Farsiu S, Whitson HE. Evaluation of inner retinal layers as biomarkers in mild cognitive impairment to moderate Alzheimer's disease. PLoS ONE. 2018;13(2):e0192646. https://doi.org/10.1371/journal.pone.0192646.
27. Aaker GD, Myung JS, Ehrlich JR, Mohammed M, Henchcliffe C, Kiss S. Detection of retinal changes in Parkinson's disease with spectral-domain optical coherence tomography. Clin Ophthalmol. 2010;4:1427–32. https://doi.org/10.2147/opth.s15136.
28. Garcia-Martin E, Bambo MP, Marques ML, Satue M, Otin S, Larrosa JM, Polo V, Pablo LE. Ganglion cell layer measurements correlate with disease severity in patients with Alzheimer's disease. Acta Ophthalmol. 2016;94(6):e454–9. https://doi.org/10.1111/aos.12977.

29. Hajee ME, March WF, Lazzaro DR, Wolintz AH, Shrier EM, Glazman S, Bodis-Wollner IG. Inner retinal layer thinning in parkinson disease. Arch Ophthalmol. 2009;127(6):737–41. https://doi.org/10.1001/archophthalmol.2009.106.
30. Altintaş Ö, Işeri P, Özkan B, Çağlar Y. Correlation between retinal morphological and functional findings and clinical severity in Parkinson's disease. Doc Ophthalmol. 2008;116(2):137–46. https://doi.org/10.1007/s10633-007-9091-8.
31. Thomson KL, Yeo JM, Waddell B, Cameron JR, Pal S. A systematic review and meta-analysis of retinal nerve fiber layer change in dementia, using optical coherence tomography. Alzheimer's Dementia Diagnosis Assess Dis Monit. 2015;1(2):136–43. https://doi.org/10.1016/j.dadm.2015.03.001.
32. Cheung CY, Ong YT, Hilal S, Ikram MK, Low S, Ong YL, Venketasubramanian N, Yap P, Seow D, Chen CLH, Wong TY. Retinal ganglion cell analysis using high-definition optical coherence tomography in patients with mild cognitive impairment and Alzheimer's disease. J Alzheimer's Dis. 2015;45(1):45–56. https://doi.org/10.3233/jad-141659.
33. Chen Y, Qian X, Zhang Y, Su W, Huang Y, Wang X, Chen X, Zhao E, Han L, Ma Y. Prediction models for conversion from mild cognitive impairment to Alzheimer's disease: a systematic review and meta-analysis. Front Aging Neurosci. 2022;14:840386. https://doi.org/10.3389/fnagi.2022.840386.
34. Lopez OL. Mild cognitive impairment. CONTINUUM Lifelong Learn Neurol. 2013;19(2, Dementia):411–24. https://doi.org/10.1212/01.con.0000429175.29601.97.
35. Eshkoor SA, Hamid TA, Mun CY, Ng CK. Mild cognitive impairment and its management in older people. Clin Interv Aging. 2015;10:687–93. https://doi.org/10.2147/cia.s73922.
36. Chen Y-X, Liang N, Li X-L, Yang S-H, Wang Y-P, Shi N-N. Diagnosis and treatment for mild cognitive impairment: a systematic review of clinical practice guidelines and consensus statements. Front Neurol. 2021;12:719849. https://doi.org/10.3389/fneur.2021.719849.
37. Coppola G, Renzo AD, Ziccardi L, Martelli F, Fadda A, Manni G, Barboni P, Pierelli F, Sadun AA, Parisi V. Optical coherence tomography in Alzheimer's disease: a meta-analysis. PLoS ONE. 2015;10(8):e0134750. https://doi.org/10.1371/journal.pone.0134750.
38. Iseri PK, Altina Ö, Tokay T, Yüksel N. Relationship between cognitive impairment and retinal morphological and visual functional abnormalities in Alzheimer disease. J Neuroophthalmol. 2006;26(1):18–24. https://doi.org/10.1097/01.wno.0000204645.56873.26.
39. Larrosa JM, Garcia-Martin E, Bambo MP, Pinilla J, Polo V, Otin S, Satue M, Herrero R, Pablo LE. Potential new diagnostic tool for Alzheimer's disease using a linear discriminant function for fourier domain optical coherence tomography. Investig Opthalmol Visual Sci. 2014;55(5):3043. https://doi.org/10.1167/iovs.13-13629.
40. den Haan J, Janssen SF, van de Kreeke JA, Scheltens P, Verbraak FD, Bouwman FH. Retinal thickness correlates with parietal cortical atrophy in early-onset Alzheimer's disease and controls. Alzheimer's Dementia Diagnosis Assess Dis Monit. 2017;10(1):49–55. https://doi.org/10.1016/j.dadm.2017.10.005.
41. Jentsch S, Schweitzer D, Schmidtke K, Peters S, Dawczynski J, Bär K, Hammer M. Retinal fluorescence lifetime imaging ophthalmoscopy measures depend on the severity of Alzheimer's disease. Acta Ophthalmol. 2015;93(4):e241–7. https://doi.org/10.1111/aos.12609.
42. Kergoat H, Kergoat M, Justino L, Chertkow H, Robillard A, Bergman H. An evaluation of the retinal nerve fiber layer thickness by scanning laser polarimetry in individuals with dementia of the Alzheimer type. Acta Ophthalmol Scand. 2001;79(2):187–91. https://doi.org/10.1034/j.1600-0420.2001.079002187.x.
43. Kurna SA, Akar G, Altun A, Agirman Y, Gozke E, Sengor T. Confocal scanning laser tomography of the optic nerve head on the patients with Alzheimer's disease compared to glaucoma and control. Int Ophthalmol. 2014;34(6):1203–11. https://doi.org/10.1007/s10792-014-0004-z.
44. Berisha F, Feke GT, Trempe CL, McMeel JW, Schepens CL. Retinal abnormalities in early Alzheimer's disease. Investig Opthalmol Vis Sci. 2007;48(5):2285. https://doi.org/10.1167/iovs.06-1029.

45. Gao L, Liu Y, Li X, Bai Q, Liu P. Abnormal retinal nerve fiber layer thickness and macula lutea in patients with mild cognitive impairment and Alzheimer's disease. Arch Gerontol Geriatr. 2015;60(1):162–7. https://doi.org/10.1016/j.archger.2014.10.011.
46. Kesler A, Vakhapova V, Korczyn AD, Naftaliev E, Neudorfer M. Retinal thickness in patients with mild cognitive impairment and Alzheimer's disease. Clin Neurol Neurosurg. 2011;113(7):523–6. https://doi.org/10.1016/j.clineuro.2011.02.014.
47. Kirbas S, Turkyilmaz K, Anlar O, Tufekci A, Durmus M. Retinal nerve fiber layer thickness in patients with Alzheimer disease. J Neuroophthalmol. 2013;33(1):58–61. https://doi.org/10.1097/wno.0b013e318267fd5f.
48. Liu J, Harris A, Kanwisher N. Perception of face parts and face configurations: an fMRI study. J Cogn Neurosci. 2010;22(1):203–11. https://doi.org/10.1162/jocn.2009.21203.
49. Marziani E, Pomati S, Ramolfo P, Cigada M, Giani A, Mariani C, Staurenghi G. Evaluation of retinal nerve fiber layer and ganglion cell layer thickness in Alzheimer's disease using spectral-domain optical coherence tomography. Investig Opthalmol Vis Sci. 2013;54(9):5953. https://doi.org/10.1167/iovs.13-12046.
50. Paquet C, Boissonnot M, Roger F, Dighiero P, Gil R, Hugon J. Abnormal retinal thickness in patients with mild cognitive impairment and Alzheimer's disease. Neurosci Lett. 2007;420(2):97–9. https://doi.org/10.1016/j.neulet.2007.02.090.
51. Blanks JC, Torigoe Y, Hinton DR, Blanks RHI. Retinal pathology in Alzheimer's disease. I. Ganglion cell loss in foveal/parafoveal retina. Neurobiol Aging. 1996;17(3):377–84. https://doi.org/10.1016/0197-4580(96)00010-3.
52. Blanks JC, Schmidt SY, Torigoe Y, Porrello KV, Hinton DR, Blanks RHI. Retinal pathology in Alzheimer's disease. II. Regional neuron loss and glial changes in GCL. Neurobiol Aging, 1996;17(3), 385–95. https://doi.org/10.1016/0197-4580(96)00009-7.
53. Curcio CA, Drucker DN. Retinal ganglion cells in Alzheimer's disease and aging. Ann Neurol. 1993;33(3):248–57. https://doi.org/10.1002/ana.410330305.
54. Davies DC, McCoubrie P, McDonald B, Jobst KA. Myelinated axon number in the optic nerve is unaffected by Alzheimer's disease. Br J Ophthalmol. 1995;79(6):596. https://doi.org/10.1136/bjo.79.6.596.
55. Benson D. The use of positron emission scanning techniques in the diagnosis of Alzheimer's disease. In: Corkin S, David K, Growdon J, Usdin E, Wurtman R, editors. Alzheimer's disease: a report of progress in research. New York: Raven Press; 1982. p. 79–82
56. Brun A, Gustafson L. Distribution of cerebral degeneration in Alzheimer's disease. Arch Psychiatr Nervenkr. 1976;223(1):15–33. https://doi.org/10.1007/bf00367450.
57. Buckner RL, Snyder AZ, Sanders AL, Raichle ME, Morris JC. Functional brain imaging of young, nondemented, and demented older adults. J Cogn Neurosci. 2000;12(Supplement 2):24–34. https://doi.org/10.1162/089892900564046.
58. Busatto GF, Diniz BS, Zanetti MV. Voxel-based morphometry in Alzheimer's disease. Expert Rev Neurother. 2008;8(11):1691–702. https://doi.org/10.1586/14737175.8.11.1691.
59. Lerch JP, Pruessner JC, Zijdenbos A, Hampel H, Teipel SJ, Evans AC. Focal decline of cortical thickness in Alzheimer's disease identified by computational neuroanatomy. Cereb Cortex. 2005;15(7):995–1001. https://doi.org/10.1093/cercor/bhh200.
60. Orwin A, Wright CE, Harding GF, Rowan DC, Rolfe EB. Serial visual evoked potential recordings in Alzheimer's disease. Br Med J (Clin Res Ed). 1986;293(6538):9. https://doi.org/10.1136/bmj.293.6538.9.
61. Prvulovic D, Hubl D, Sack AT, Melillo L, Maurer K, Frölich L, Lanfermann H, Zanella FE, Goebel R, Linden DEJ, Dierks T. Functional imaging of visuospatial processing in Alzheimer's disease. Neuroimage. 2002;17(3):1403–14. https://doi.org/10.1006/nimg.2002.1271.
62. Rizzo M, Anderson SW, Dawson J, Nawrot M. Vision and cognition in Alzheimer's disease. Neuropsychologia. 2000;38(8):1157–69. https://doi.org/10.1016/s0028-3932(00)00023-3.
63. Ahmed MR, Zhang Y, Feng Z, Lo B, Inan OT, Liao H. Neuroimaging and machine learning for dementia diagnosis: recent advancements and future prospects. IEEE Rev Biomed Eng. 2019;12:19–33. https://doi.org/10.1109/rbme.2018.2886237.

64. Arbabshirani MR, Plis S, Sui J, Calhoun VD. Single subject prediction of brain disorders in neuroimaging: promises and pitfalls. Neuroimage. 2017;145(Pt B):137–65. https://doi.org/10.1016/j.neuroimage.2016.02.079.
65. Jack CR, Bernstein MA, Fox NC, Thompson P, Alexander G, Harvey D, Borowski B, Britson PJ, Whitwell JL, Ward C, Dale AM, Felmlee JP, Gunter JL, Hill DLG, Killiany R, Schuff N, Fox-Bosetti S, Lin C, Studholme C, Study A. The Alzheimer's disease neuroimaging initiative (ADNI): MRI methods. J Magn Resonance Imaging. 2008;27(4):685–91.
66. Samuel AL. Some studies in machine learning using the game of checkers. IBM J Res Dev. 1959;3(3):210–29. https://doi.org/10.1147/rd.33.0210.
67. What is Machine Learning? IBM. www.ibm.com. Retrieved 2023-06-27.
68. Erickson BJ, Korfiatis P, Akkus Z, Kline TL. Machine learning for medical imaging. Radiographics. 2017;37(2):160130. https://doi.org/10.1148/rg.2017160130.
69. Varoquaux G, Cheplygina V. Machine learning for medical imaging: methodological failures and recommendations for the future. NPJ Digital Med. 2022;5(1):48. https://doi.org/10.1038/s41746-022-00592-y.
70. Vapnik VN. An overview of statistical learning theory. IEEE Trans Neural Netw. 2021;10(5):988–99. https://doi.org/10.1109/72.788640.
71. Vapnik N. Theory of pattern recognition. Moscow, Russia: Nauka; 1974 (in Russian). German translation: W. N. Wapnik and A. Ja. Chervonenkis Theorie der Zeichenerkennung. Berlin, Germany: Akademia-Verlag; 1979. p. 353.
72. Anwar SM, Majid M, Qayyum A, Awais M, Alnowami M, Khan MK. Medical image analysis using convolutional neural networks: a review. J Med Syst. 2018;42(11):226. https://doi.org/10.1007/s10916-018-1088-1.
73. Bakator M, Radosav D. Deep learning and medical diagnosis: a review of literature. Multimodal Technol Interact. 2018;2(3):47. https://doi.org/10.3390/mti2030047.
74. Cao C, Liu F, Tan H, Song D, Shu W, Li W, Zhou Y, Bo X, Xie Z. Deep learning and its applications in biomedicine. Genom Proteom Bioinform. 2018;16(1):17–32. https://doi.org/10.1016/j.gpb.2017.07.003.
75. Chalapathy R, Borzeshi EZ, Piccardi M. An investigation of recurrent neural architectures for drug name recognition. In: Proceedings of the seventh international workshop on health text mining and information analysis; 2016. 1–5. https://doi.org/10.18653/v1/w16-6101.
76. Kermany DS, Goldbaum M, Cai W, Valentim CCS, Liang H, Baxter SL, McKeown A, Yang G, Wu X, Yan F, Dong J, Prasadha MK, Pei J, Ting MYL, Zhu J, Li C, Hewett S, Dong J, Ziyar I, Zhang K. Identifying medical diagnoses and treatable diseases by image-based deep learning. Cell. 2018;172(5):1122-1131.e9. https://doi.org/10.1016/j.cell.2018.02.010.
77. Melinščak M, Radmilović M, Vatavuk Z, Lončarić S. Annotated retinal optical coherence tomography images (AROI) database for joint retinal layer and fluid segmentation. Automatika. 2021;62(3–4):375–85. https://doi.org/10.1080/00051144.2021.1973298.
78. Haralick RM, Shanmugam K, Dinstein I. Textural features for image classification. IEEE Trans Syst Man Cybern. 1973;SMC-3(6):610–21. https://doi.org/10.1109/tsmc.1973.4309314.
79. Kassner A, Thornhill RE. Texture analysis: a review of neurologic MR imaging applications. Am J Neuroradiol. 2010;31(5):809–16. https://doi.org/10.3174/ajnr.a2061.
80. Meyer-Bäse A. Pattern recognition for medical imaging. San Diego: Elsevier; 2004. ISBN: 978-0124932906.
81. Ledley RS. Texture problems in biomedical pattern recognition. In: Proceedings of the 1972 IEEE conference on decision and control and 11th symposium on adaptive processes; 1972. 590–5. https://doi.org/10.1109/cdc.1972.269080.
82. Hall EL, Kruger RP, Dwyer SJ, Hall DL, Mclaren RW, Lodwick GS. A survey of preprocessing and feature extraction techniques for radiographic images. IEEE Trans Comput. 1971;C-20(9):1032–44. https://doi.org/10.1109/t-c.1971.223399.
83. Harlow CA, Eisenbeis S A. The analysis of radiographic images. IEEE Trans Comput. 1973;C–22(7):678–89. https://doi.org/10.1109/tc.1973.5009135.

84. Gao W. Improving the quantitative assessment of intraretinal features by determining both structural and optical properties of the retinal tissue with optical coherence tomography. Doctoral thesis; 2012. https://scholarship.miami.edu/esploro/outputs/991031447274702976.
85. González A, Remeseiro B, Ortega M, Penedo MG, Charlón P. Automatic cyst detection in OCT retinal images combining region flooding and texture analysis. In: Proceedings of the 26th IEEE international symposium on computer-based medical systems; 2013. 397–400. https://doi.org/10.1109/cbms.2013.6627825.
86. Anantrasirichai N, Achim A, Morgan JE, Erchova I, Nicholson L. SVM-based texture classification in optical coherence tomography. In: 2013 IEEE 10th international symposium on biomedical imaging; 2013:1332–5. https://doi.org/10.1109/isbi.2013.6556778.
87. Morgan JE, Tribble J, Fergusson J, White N, Erchova I. The optical detection of retinal ganglion cell damage. Eye. 2017;31(2):199–205. https://doi.org/10.1038/eye.2016.290.
88. Guimarães P, Rodrigues P, Lobo C, Leal S, Figueira J, Serranho P, Bernardes R. Ocular fundus reference images from optical coherence tomography. Comput Med Imaging Graph. 2014;38(5):381–9. https://doi.org/10.1016/j.compmedimag.2014.02.003.
89. Galloway MM. Texture analysis using gray level run lengths. Comput Graphics Image Process. 1975;4(2):172–9. https://doi.org/10.1016/s0146-664x(75)80008-6.
90. Ojala T, Pietikäinen M, Harwood D. A comparative study of texture measures with classification based on featured distributions. Pattern Recogn. 1996;29(1):51–9. https://doi.org/10.1016/0031-3203(95)00067-4.
91. Zhang Y, Dong Z, Wu L, Wang S. A hybrid method for MRI brain image classification. Expert Syst Appl. 2011;38(8):10049–10053. https://doi.org/10.1016/j.eswa.2011.02.012.
92. Humeau-Heurtier A. Texture feature extraction methods: a survey. IEEE Access. 2019;7:8975–9000. https://doi.org/10.1109/access.2018.2890743.
93. Ghalati MK, Nunes A, Ferreira H, Serranho P, Bernardes R. Texture analysis and its applications in biomedical imaging: a survey. IEEE Rev Biomed Eng. 2021;15(99):222–46. https://doi.org/10.1109/rbme.2021.3115703.
94. Choi SH, Park SJ, Kim NR. Macular ganglion cell-inner plexiform layer thickness is associated with clinical progression in mild cognitive impairment and Alzheimers disease. PLoS ONE. 2016;11(9):e0162202. https://doi.org/10.1371/journal.pone.0162202.
95. Geirhos R, Rubisch P, Michaelis C, Bethge M, Wichmann FA, Brendel W. ImageNet-trained CNNs are biased towards texture; increasing shape bias improves accuracy and robustness; 2018. https://doi.org/10.48550/arxiv.1811.12231.
96. Liu L, Chen J, Fieguth P, Zhao G, Chellappa R, Pietikäinen M. From BoW to CNN: two decades of texture representation for texture classification. Int J Comput Vision. 2019;127(1):74–109. https://doi.org/10.1007/s11263-018-1125-z.
97. Bernardes R, Silva G, Chiquita S, Serranho P, Ambrósio AF. Retinal biomarkers of Alzheimer's disease: insights from transgenic mouse models. In: Karray F, Campilho A, Cheriet F, editors. Image analysis and recognition. ICIAR 2017. Lecture notes in computer science, vol. 10317. Cham: Springer; 2017. https://doi.org/10.1007/978-3-319-59876-5_60.
98. Nunes A, Ambrósio AF, Castelo-Branco M, Bernardes R. Texture biomarkers of Alzheimer's disease and disease progression in the mouse retina. In: 2018 IEEE 18th international conference on bioinformatics and bioengineering (BIBE); 2018. 41–6. https://doi.org/10.1109/bibe.2018.00016.
99. Bernardes R. Optical coherence tomography: health information embedded on OCT signal statistics. In: 2011 annual international conference of the IEEE engineering in medicine and biology society, 1; 2011. 6131–33. https://doi.org/10.1109/iembs.2011.6091514.
100. Bernardes R, Serranho P, Santos T, Gonçalves V, Vaz JC. Optical coherence tomography—automatic retina classification through support vector machines. Euro Ophthalmic Rev. 2012;06(04):200. https://doi.org/10.17925/eor.2012.06.04.200.
101. Garvin MK, Abràmoff MD, Wu X, Russell SR, Burns TL, Sonka M. Automated 3-D intraretinal layer segmentation of macular spectral-domain optical coherence tomography images. IEEE Trans Med Imaging. 2009;28(9):1436–47. https://doi.org/10.1109/tmi.2009.2016958.

102. Abràmoff MD, Garvin MK, Sonka M. Retinal imaging and image analysis. IEEE Rev Biomed Eng. 2010;3:169–208. https://doi.org/10.1109/rbme.2010.2084567.
103. Li K, Wu X, Chen DZ, Sonka M. Optimal surface segmentation in volumetric images—a graph-theoretic approach. IEEE Trans Pattern Anal Mach Intell. 2006;28(1):119–34. https://doi.org/10.1109/tpami.2006.19.
104. Soh L-K, Tsatsoulis C. Texture representation of SAR sea ice imagery using multi-displacement co-occurrence matrices. In: IGARSS'96. 1996 international geoscience and remote sensing symposium, 1; 1996. 112–4. https://doi.org/10.1109/igarss.1996.516261.
105. Clausi DA. An analysis of co-occurrence texture statistics as a function of grey level quantization. Can J Remote Sens. 2002;28(1):45–62. https://doi.org/10.5589/m02-004.
106. Duda RO, Hart PE, Stork DG. Pattern classification. 2nd ed. New York: Wiley; 2000. ISBN: 978-0-471-05669-0.
107. Chang C-C, Lin C-J. LIBSVM: a library for support vector machines. ACM Trans Intell Syst Technol (TIST). 2011;2(3):27. https://doi.org/10.1145/1961189.1961199.
108. Nunes A, Silva G, Alves C, Batista S, Sousa L, Castelo-Branco M, Bernardes R. Textural information from the retinal nerve fibre layer in multiple sclerosis. In: IEEE Portuguese meeting in bioengineering (ENBENG); 2019. 1–4. https://doi.org/10.1109/ENBENG.2019.8692454.
109. Krantic S, Torriglia A. Retina: source of the earliest biomarkers for Alzheimer's disease? J Alzheimer's Dis. 2014;40(2):237–43. https://doi.org/10.3233/jad-132105.
110. Tourassi GD. Journey toward computer-aided diagnosis: role of image texture analysis. Radiology. 1999;213(2):317–20. https://doi.org/10.1148/radiology.213.2.r99nv49317.
111. Scalco E, Rizzo G. Texture analysis of medical images for radiotherapy applications. Br J Radiol. 2017;90(1070):20160642. https://doi.org/10.1259/bjr.20160642.
112. Varghese BA, Cen SY, Hwang DH, Duddalwar VA. Texture analysis of imaging: what radiologists need to know. Am J Roentgenol. 2019;212(3):520–8. https://doi.org/10.2214/ajr.18.20624.
113. Eun NL, Kang D, Son EJ, Park JS, Youk JH, Kim J-A, Gweon HM. Texture analysis with 3.0-T MRI for association of response to neoadjuvant chemotherapy in breast cancer. Radiology. 2019;294(1):31–41. https://doi.org/10.1148/radiol.2019182718.
114. Bernardes R, Nunes A, Guimarães P, Serranho P, Castelo-Branco M. Central nervous system interocular sex differences spotted at the retina by texture analysis. Invest Ophthalmol Vis Sci. 2023;64(8):3721.
115. Shaqiri A, Roinishvili M, Grzeczkowski L, Chkonia E, Pilz K, Mohr C, Brand A, Kunchulia M, Herzog MH. Sex-related differences in vision are heterogeneous. Sci Rep. 2018;8(1):7521. https://doi.org/10.1038/s41598-018-25298-8.
116. Batista A, Guimarães P, Serranho P, Nunes A, Martins J, Moreira PI, Ambrósio AF, Morgado M, Castelo-Branco M, Bernardes R. Retinal imaging in animal models: Searching for biomarkers of neurodegeneration. Front Ophthalmol. 2023;3:1156605. https://doi.org/10.3389/fopht.2023.1156605.
117. Fox NC, Schott JM. Imaging cerebral atrophy: normal ageing to Alzheimer's disease. Lancet. 2004;363(9406):392–4. https://doi.org/10.1016/s0140-6736(04)15441-x.
118. Sperling R. Functional MRI studies of associative encoding in normal aging, mild cognitive impairment, and Alzheimer's disease. Ann NY Acad Sci. 2007;1097(1):146–55. https://doi.org/10.1196/annals.1379.009.
119. Toepper M. Dissociating normal aging from Alzheimer's disease: a view from cognitive neuroscience. J Alzheimer's Dis. 2017:1–22. https://doi.org/10.3233/jad-161099.
120. Gaser C, Franke K, Klöppel S, Koutsouleris N, Sauer H, Initiative ADN. BrainAGE in mild cognitive impaired patients: predicting the conversion to Alzheimer's disease. PLoS ONE. 2013;8(6):e67346. https://doi.org/10.1371/journal.pone.0067346.
121. Guimarães P, Serranho P, Martins J, Moreira PI, Ambrósio AF, Castelo-Branco M, Bernardes R. Retinal aging in 3× Tg-AD mice model of Alzheimer's disease. Front Aging Neurosci. 2022;14:832195. https://doi.org/10.3389/fnagi.2022.832195.

122. Sugita Y, Yamamoto H, Maeda Y, Furukawa T. Influence of aging on the retina and visual motion processing for optokinetic responses in mice. Front Neurosci. 2020;14:586013. https://doi.org/10.3389/fnins.2020.586013.
123. Hermenean A, Trotta MC, Gharbia S, Hermenean AG, Peteu VE, Balta C, Cotoraci C, Gesualdo C, Rossi S, Gherghiceanu M, D'Amico M. Changes in retinal structure and ultrastructure in the aged mice correlate with differences in the expression of selected retinal miRNAs. Front Pharmacol. 2021;11:593514. https://doi.org/10.3389/fphar.2020.593514.
124. Ferdous S, Liao KL, Gefke ID, Summers VR, Wu W, Donaldson KJ, Kim Y-K, Sellers JT, Dixon JA, Shelton DA, Markand S, Kim SM, Zhang N, Boatright JH, Nickerson JM. Age-related retinal changes in wild-type C57BL/6J mice between 2 and 32 months. Invest Ophthalmol Vis Sci. 2021;62(7):9. https://doi.org/10.1167/iovs.62.7.9.
125. Gardner MR, Baruah V, Vargas G, Motamedi M, Milner TE, Rylander HG. Scattering angle resolved optical coherence tomography detects early changes in 3xTg Alzheimer's disease mouse model. Transl Vis Sci Technol. 2020;9(5):18. https://doi.org/10.1167/tvst.9.5.18.

Optical Coherence Tomography Angiography in Neurology and Neuro-Ophthalmology

24

Julia Fallon, Alexander Pinhas, Valerie I. Elmalem,
Maria Castanos Toral, Davis B. Zhou, Jorge S. Andrade Romo,
Alexander Barash, and Richard B. Rosen

Abstract

Optical coherence tomography angiography (OCT-A) is a recent advancement in retinal imaging that uses high-speed OCT and advanced processing algorithms to generate en face angiographic images of the retinal and choroidal microcirculation, utilizing the non-invasive motion-contrast of intra-luminal erythrocyte flow. This chapter offers a review of the recent translational and clinical applications of OCT-A in the fields of neurology and neuro-ophthalmology, focusing on non-glaucomatous optic neuropathies and other central neurological disorders. In Alzheimer's dementia and Parkinson's disease, retinal microvascular loss detected by OCT-A may be a sensitive indicator of progressive vascular impairment that precedes neuronal death. OCT-A findings in multiple sclerosis suggest vascular involvement in the inflammatory disease process, leading to ischemia of neural tissues. Migraine with aura patients show a decreased retinal perfusion bilaterally with OCT-A, implying a systemic vascular involvement that may explain their increased risk for cardiovascular disease. OCT-A studies on non-arteritic anterior ischemic optic neuropathy suggest that peripapillary microvascular attenuation is secondary to an initial transient ischemic insult in the short posterior ciliary arteries, causing optic nerve edema that propogates anteriorly, in turn compressing the retinal microvasculature. OCT-A has allowed insight into the suspected vasculopathy associated with Leber's hereditary optic neuropathy, which may be due to mitochondrial dysfunction

J. Fallon · A. Pinhas · V. I. Elmalem · M. C. Toral · D. B. Zhou · J. S. A. Romo · A. Barash · R. B. Rosen (✉)
Department of Ophthalmology, New York Eye and Ear Infirmary of Mount Sinai, New York, NY, USA
e-mail: rrosen@nyee.edu

A. Pinhas
Department of Ophthalmology, State University of New York Downstate Medical Center, Brooklyn, NY, USA

A. Grzybowski and P. Barboni (eds.), *OCT and Imaging in Central Nervous System Diseases*, https://doi.org/10.1007/978-3-031-72156-4_24

influencing endothelial cell and vascular smooth muscle viability. Superficial optic nerve head drusen may cause focal areas of poor superficial retinal perfusion as detected by OCT-A, which may in turn lead to nerve fiber ischemia and rarefaction. OCT-A shows promise in becoming an important tool for researchers and clinicians in their multimodal approach in detecting pathological changes, monitoring disease progression and evaluating response to treatment in these disorders.

Keywords

Optical coherence tomography angiography • Neurology • Neuro-ophthalmology • Alzheimer's dementia • Parkinson's disease • Multiple sclerosis • Migraine • Amblyopia • Non-arteritic anterior ischemic optic neuropathy • Leber's hereditary optic neuropathy • Optic nerve head drusen • Dysthyroid optic neuropathy

24.1 Introduction

Alterations to blood circulation in the central nervous system and optic nerve in neurological and neuro-ophthalmological disease have been well documented by CT, MRI and Doppler in vivo, and histology ex vivo. It is unclear, however, whether the vascular alterations are secondary to neuronal loss from decreased metabolic demand and neurovascular coupling, or a pathogenic step preceding neurodegeneration. Studies using new tools and biomarkers involving the vasculature can help elucidate the relationship between the neuronal and vascular tissues in these diseases, as well as help diagnose disease earlier and monitor treatment efficacy.

Given the similarities between brain and retinal tissues, retinal imaging offers a readily accessible, non-invasive window into the vascular changes that accompany the pathophysiologic developments of neurological and neuro-ophthalmological diseases. Classical retinal vascular features including vascular attenuation, tortuousity and foveal avascular zone (FAZ) alterations, as well as structural optical coherence tomography (OCT) changes in retinal and choroidal layer thickness have received increasing attention in the setting of neurological and neuro-ophthalmological diseases.

OCT angiography (OCT-A) is a recent advancement in retinal imaging that uses high-speed OCT and advanced processing algorithms to generate *en face* angiographic images of the retinal and choroidal microcirculation utilizing the non-invasive motion-contrast of intra-luminal erythrocyte flow [1]. OCT-A images have enabled the in vivo study of retinal arterioles, venules and capillary beds at resolution rivaling the histologist's microscope (Fig. 24.1). This technology opens up a new world of possibilities for in situ analysis of the retinal microvasculature and correlation to ocular and systemic disease.

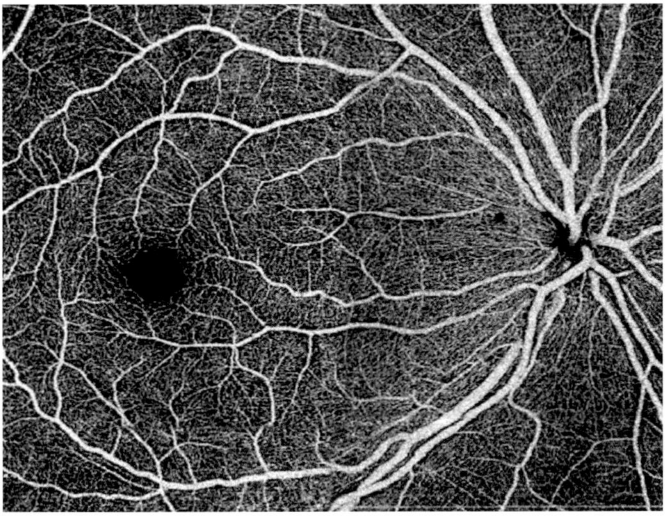

Fig. 24.1 OCT-A montage of the superficial capillary circulation of the macular and peripapillary retina in a healthy individual. Reproduced with permission from Elsevier, Spaide et al. [1]

This chapter offers a review of the recent translational and clinical applications of OCT-A in the fields of neurology and neuro-ophthalmology, focusing on non-glaucomatous optic neuropathies and other human neurological disorders.

24.2 Neurology

24.2.1 Alzheimer's Dementia

Alzheimer's dementia (AD) is a chronic progressive neurodegenerative disease resulting in cognitive impairment. It is the most common cause of dementia (60–70%), with a prevalence of 5.4 million among US residents, affecting 1 in every 5 individuals at age 85 worldwide. AD is characterized by deep brain atrophy due to accumulation of misfolded protein, namely extracellular amyloid-beta plaques and intracellular tau neurofibrillary tangles.

The presence of a vasculopathy in AD has been supported by a growing body of evidence. A number of cardiovascular risk factors have been associated with AD, including increasing age, diabetes, hypertension, stroke, atherosclerosis, smoking, physical inactivity and obesity, in addition to genetic predisposition, depression and cognitive inactivity. AD has been associated with cerebral hypoperfusion, decreased cerebral vascular density and increased tortuosity. The term cerebral amyloid angiopathy has been used to describe the presence of amyloid-beta deposits in vessel walls of AD cerebral tissue.

Visual problems in AD, including color vision deficits, depth misperception, visual field defects, and reduced contrast sensitivity have traditionally been attributed to cortical lesions. The retina, however, may be more directly involved in the pathogenic process. Studies have shown presence of amyloid-beta plaques and tau proteins, decreased angiogenesis, activated microglia and proinflammatory molecules and decreased neuronal activity in the retinas of AD patients. Morphological changes to the retina in AD patients have been well documented, including the presence of optic disc pallor and neuroretinal rim thinning, arteriolar narrowing, venular widening, as well as OCT evidence of choroidal, retinal nerve fiber layer (RNFL) and ganglion cell-inner plexiform layer (GC-IPL) thinning.

OCT-A evaluation of AD patients demonstrated significantly lower macular microvascular densities and choroidal thicknesses, and larger FAZ sizes, compared to controls [2]. Mini Mental State Examination (MMSE) scores correlated significantly with these changes. Preclinical AD is a period prior to symptom onset but with measureable amyloid burden. O'Bryhim et al. imaged 30 asymptomatic participants ranging in age from 62 to 92 years using OCT-A, along with PET scans and/or cerebrospinal fluid (CSF) testing to determine presence of amyloid (Fig. 24.2) [3]. Fourteen of 30 asymptomatic participants had biomarkers positive for AD. OCT-A revealed increases in FAZ size and decreases in inner foveal thickness in these preclinical AD patients (Figs. 24.2 and 24.3). However, no significant differences in vascular density were detected between the two groups. More recent studies have found statistically significant lower choriocapillaris vessel density in AD patients compared to patients with other major forms of dementia [4].

Pathological changes at the tissue level prior to symptom onset is a consistent finding in many AD studies. Microvascular compromise due to age and/or cardiovascular disease has been proposed as the cause of impaired autophagy and accumulation of amyloid deposits. Lumen stenosis, vessel dropout, and blood–brain barrier compromise are the result of accumulation of deposits in internal vessel walls. Binding and confining of trophic factors such as VEGF within the deposits may lead to decreased angiogenesis.

Mild cognitive impairment (MCI) is a clinical entity that describes patients prior to AD onset that have mild cognitive function decline but are still able to perform their activities of daily living. Using OCT-A, a statistically significant trend of decreasing capillary densities from healthy controls to MCI patients to AD patients was found [5]. Interestingly, MCI macular capillary density decreases were positively related to lower MMSE scores, but were not reflected in structural GC-IPL changes. In contrast, AD capillary density decreases were related to GC-IPL thinning. Prior longitudinal studies have demonstrated that decreased cerebral perfusion in MCI can predict progression to AD. Retinal microvascular loss in MCI as revealed by OCT-A may be a sensitive indicator of progressive vascular impairment that precedes neuronal death, and may be a useful tool in predicting the risk of potential conversion from MCI to AD.

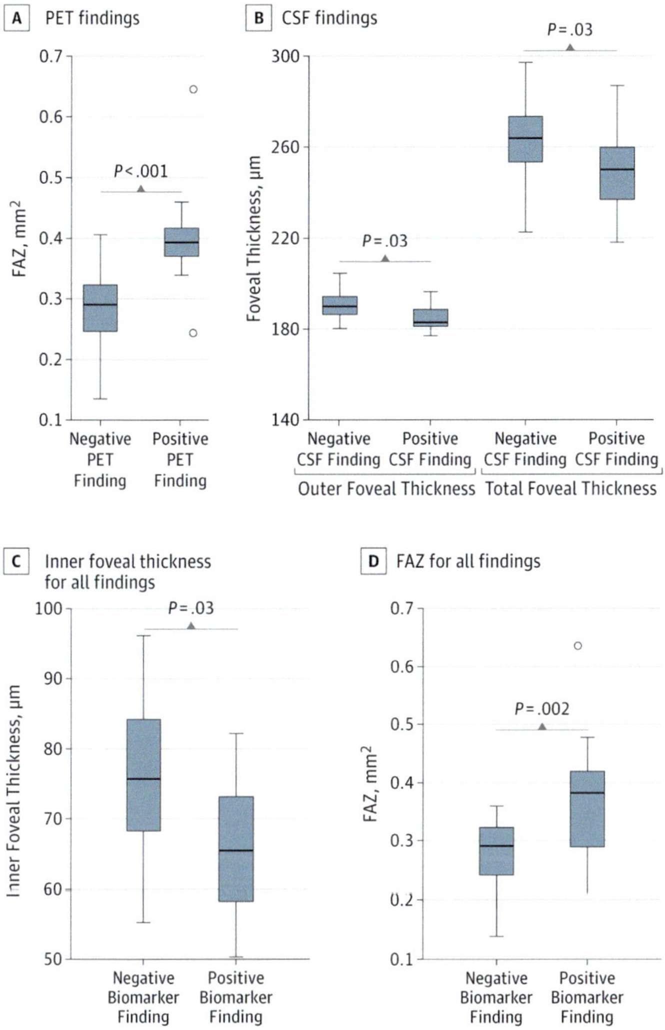

Fig. 24.2 Data are shown as box and whisker plots, where whiskers represent 1.5 times the interquartile range. (**A**) Positron emission tomography (PET) imaging results are shown for fluorine 18–labeled florbetapir compound testing. Open circles indicate outliers. (**B**) CSF analysis results are shown for β-amyloid 42 and τ protein biomarkers. (**C**) and (**D**) Participants with negative findings for all biomarkers (PET and/or CSF) were compared with those with positive findings for at least 1 test. Reproduced with permission from American Medical Association, O'Bryhim et al. [3]

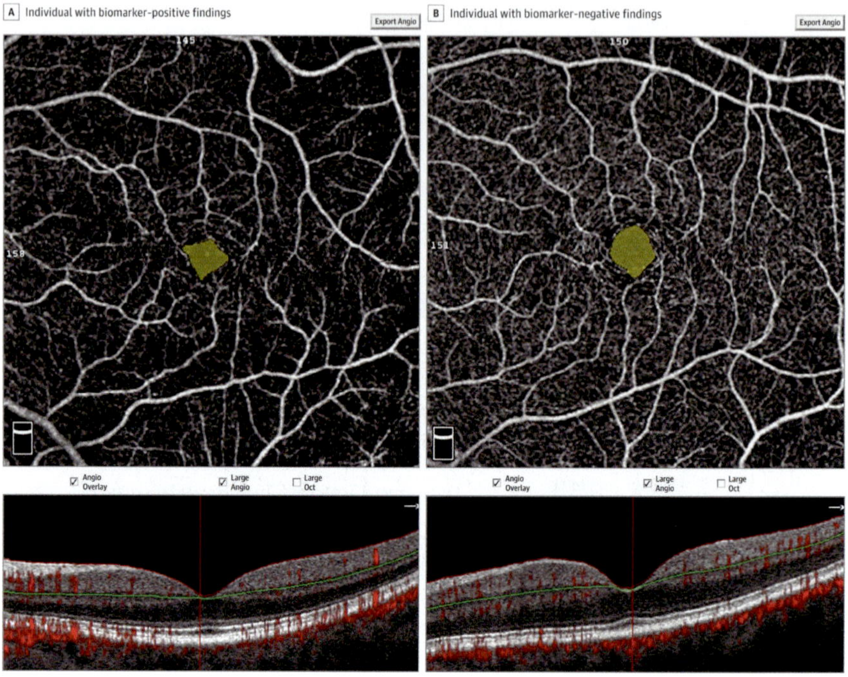

Fig. 24.3 Top images depict macular OCT-As with FAZ areas of (**A**) 0.212 mm^2 in an individual with biomarker-positive findings in preclinical AD, and (**B**) 0.311 mm^2 in an individual with biomarker negative findings. Bottom images depict their respective OCT scans. Reproduced with permission from American Medical Association, O'Bryhim et al. [3]

24.2.2 Parkinson's Disease

Parkinson's disease (PD) is a chronic progressive neurodegenerative disease resulting in cognitive impairment. It is the second most common neurodegenerative condition in the aging human population, with a prevalence of 1 million persons in the United States. PD is characterized by the loss of dopaminergic neurons in the central nervous system, leading to brain atrophy and irreversible deterioration in cognitive function. Risk factors for PD include male gender, increased age, genetic predisposition, Hispanic and non-Hispanic white races, and history of head trauma.

Visual problems such as decreased visual acuity, visual hallucinations, and deficits in visuospatial orientation have been associated with PD. As in AD, these problems have traditionally been considered to be of central origin. Recent studies have shown that retinal dopamine, which serves a vital role in retinal visual processing, is deficient in PD patients. Furthermore, OCT studies have shown inner retinal thinning in PD patients.

PD appears to have an impact largely on foveal vascularity. A recent large cross-sectional study looking at OCTA in PD patients and control subjects found significant FAZ abnormalities in PD patients including a smaller overall FAZ in PD patients. In non-adjusted models, this FAZ area was then found to be negatively associated with cognition [6].

OCT-A images of early PD patients were recently shown to have a significantly lower macular superficial capillary plexus density compared to controls, showing a positive correlation with GC-IPL thinning (Figs. 24.4 and 24.5) [7]. A major limitation of the study was that all PD patients were already on levodopa therapy at the time of imaging. The local impact of levodopa on microvascular density measures is not well understood.

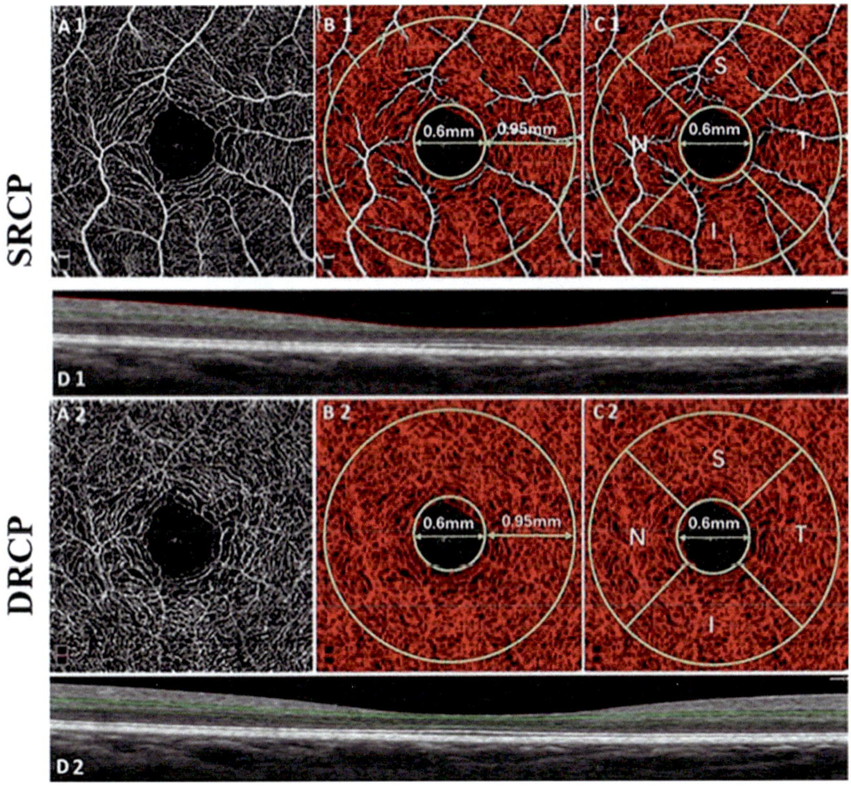

Fig. 24.4 Representative OCT-A images and diagrammatic sketch showing the microvascular density analysis of the superifical retinal capillary plexus (SRCP) and deep retinal capillary plexus (DRCP) in patients with PD. Original OCT-A images of both the SRCP (A1) and DRCP (A2). Binary images of the microvascular network after removing the large vessels with a width ≥ 25 μm and background noise in the SRCP (B1) and DRCP (B2). Microvascular density was performed on the total annulus zone with a diameter of 2.50 mm after excluding the FAZ (diameter 1/4 0.60 mm) in both the SRCP (B2) and DRCP (B2). Images of the capillaries are shown with microvascular density performed in the parafoveal four quadrant sectors, S, T, I, and N, of a circular zone with a diameter of 2.50 mm after excluding the FAZ in the SRCP (C1) and DRCP (C2). Reproduced with permission from IOVS, Kwapong et al. [7]

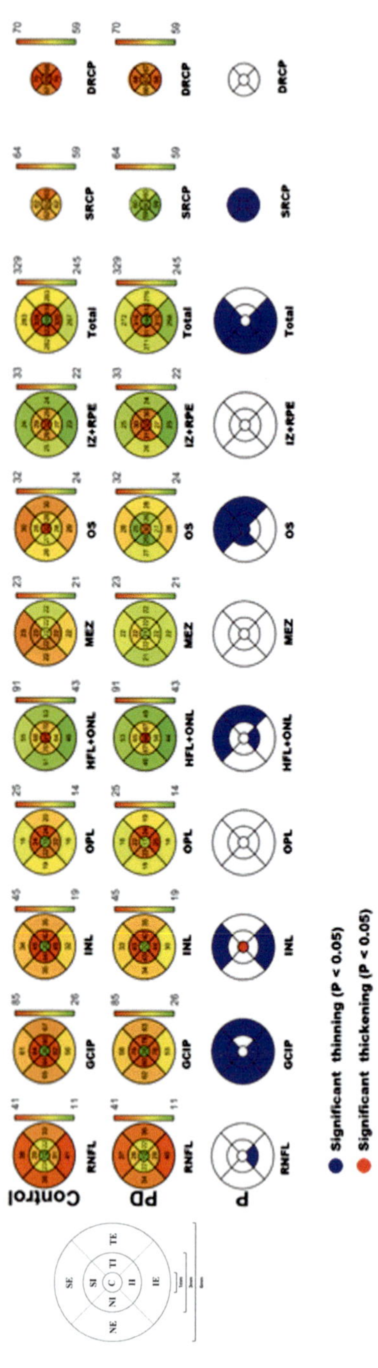

Fig. 24.5 Comparison of the microvascular density and retinal thickness between patients with PD and healthy controls. The first two rows represent the retinal thickness maps and microvascular density of healthy controls and PD patients, respectively. The retinal thickness and microvascular density are indicated by the colors shown in the color bar for each row. The third row shows the corresponding parameters between the healthy controls and the PD patients; blue represents significant thinning ($P < 0.05$), red represents significant thickening ($P < 0.05$). Reproduced with permission from IOVS, Kwapong et al. [7]

Microvascular compromise may contribute to the pathophysiology of PD. The mechanism may involve alpha-synuclein deposits in vessel walls, leading to lumen stenosis, vessel dropout, and blood–brain barrier compromise. It is yet unclear whether microvascular changes precede neuronal loss or are secondary to the neuronal loss.

24.2.3 Multiple Sclerosis

Multiple sclerosis (MS) is an inflammatory demyelinating disorder of the CNS associated with progressive neurodegeneration. An estimated 1 million individuals in the US and 2.5 million worldwide have MS. Optic neuritis is the initial manifestation of MS in approximately 25% of patients, and occurs in approximately 50% of patients at some point in the disease course. Other ocular findings include ocular motility dysfunction, peripheral vasculitis, retinitis and pars planitis.

Patients with MS have decreased cerebral perfusion, and increased ischemic risk. Comorbid vascular risk factors result in more rapid progression of neurodegeneration and disability in MS. In the retina, OCT has been used to show decreased total blood vessel diameter and number in MS, with associated ganglion cell loss. It is unclear whether the vasculopathy present in MS plays a causative role in progressive neurodegeneration, or whether it is secondary.

A number of recent OCT-A studies attempted to elucidate the relationship between retinal vasculopathy, neuronal death and disease burden in MS. Figure 24.6 shows representative examples of optic nerve head (ONH) and macular OCTA images in a healthy control, a patient with multiple sclerosis without optic neuropathy, and a patient with multiple sclerosis with a history of optic neuropathy. Compared to healthy controls, MS patients with a mean disease duration of 11 years, with or without history of optic neuritis, had significantly decreased parafoveal vessel densities as measured by OCT-A, along with RNFL and ganglion cell complex (GCC) thinning as measured by SD-OCT, compared to healthy controls [8]. The study found that OCT-A parafoveal vessel density was inversely correlated with the Expanded Disability State Scale (EDSS), while RNFL and GCC thicknesses were inversely correlated with the Multiple Sclerosis Severity Score. More recent studies have showed similar findings with MS patients regardless of prior history of ON [9, 10]. One study showed a significant difference in capillary flow density of both the superficial capillary plexus as well as choriocapillaris in MS patients compared to controls. This was found to be independent of a previous history of ON [9]. Similarly, MS patients were found to have decreased vascular density in the superficial parafovea, again independent of history of prior ON [10].

At 1-year follow up, a small but significant increase in parafoveal vessel density occurred in the MS patients on average, which the authors postulated may have been due to therapy [11]. Patients with decreased parafoveal vessel density also demonstrated higher accrual of disability, as measured by EDSS. Despite the observed vessel density variations at 1-year follow up, no significant structural

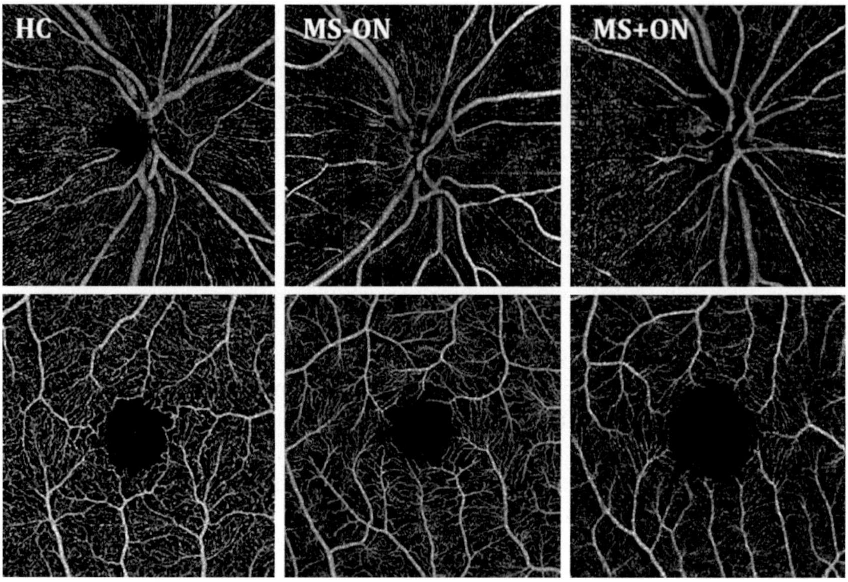

Fig. 24.6 Representative en face ONH and macular OCT-As of a 45 year old healthy control male (HC), a 34 year old male with multiple sclerosis without optic neuritis (MS−ON) and a 47 year old male with multiple sclerosis with history of optic neuritis (MS+ON)

changes were seen, as indicated by stable RNFL thickness measurements. Thus, the authors concluded that reduced retinal vessel density correlated well with progressive disability. Additionally, microcirculation may improve with treatment and over time, without structural changes to the inner retina, indicating that blood flow and neuronal death may reflect different aspects of MS pathology.

At a shorter mean disease duration of 2 years, MS or clinically isolated syndrome (CIS) patients with history of optic neuritis were shown to have reduced deep and superficial vessel densities, correlating with inner retinal layer thinning, while those without a history of optic neuritis did not show such changes [12]. Two studies, at a mean disease duration of 14 years [13] and 14.5 years [14], showed that MS patients with a history of optic neuritis had more significant reductions in their ONH flow index and inner retina layer thickness compared to MS patients without history of optic neuritis. These results indicate that in longstanding MS, both cellular layer and vasculature of the retina seem to show alterations regardless of optic neuritis history. Although, optic neuritis might cause a more rapid and more significant decrease in vessel density.

Higher choriocapillary vessel densities have been associated with ongoing inflammatory disease activity within 24 months of imaging [12]. It is postulated that this may be a consequence of inflammation-induced microvascular dilatation, and/or endothelial pro-angiogenetic factor upregulation occurring during MS activity. This evidence suggests a possible mechanism of the progressive neurodegeneration seen in MS, where inflammation-induced endothelial cell dysfunction causes vascular alteration and attenuation, leading to poor blood flow and ischemia of the neural tissue. Regardless of which occurs first in MS—vascular attenuation or neuronal death—combination indices of retinal angiographic and structural parameters have been shown to significantly improve the diagnostic accuracy of detecting prior history of optic neuritis in MS patients when compared to separate flow and structural indices [13].

24.2.4 Migraine

Migraine is a primary headache disorder characterized by recurrent, pulsating, moderate to severe headaches that typically include one half of the head. Migraines may be associated with nausea, vomiting, and sensitivity to light, sound or smell. Migraines affect about 15% of the world's population, and are approximately twice as prevalent in women as they are in men.

The pathophysiology of migraines is poorly understood, but may involve a vascular ischemic component. About one-third of migraine patients experience auras that immediately precede the migraines. Auras are focal neurological disturbances that are typically visual, and are thought to be secondary to cerebral transient focal ischemia. Migraine is furthermore associated with ischemic events such as stroke and myocardial infarction, as well as retinal vascular occlusion, ischemic optic neuropathy, normal tension glaucoma and paracentral acute middle maculopathy. Stroke and myocardial infarction associations are stronger for migraine with aura than without. Studies have also found a higher incidence of retinopathy in migraine patients compared to those without migraine.

OCT-A has the potential to reveal ocular perfusion changes in migraine patients, which may explain the predisposition of these patients to ischemic complications. Female migraine patients with aura, in a recent OCT-A study, had significantly lower superficial parafoveal and peripapillary vessel densities, and significantly enlarged FAZs, compared to female migraine patients without aura and female controls [15]. No significant differences were found between female migraine patients without aura and female controls, between male participants across the groups, or in structural OCT parameters including RNFL and GCC thicknesses across the groups. A major limitation of the study was that seven out of fifteen migraine with aura and six out of twelve migraine without aura patients were taking triptans, which is a class of migraine medications associated with vasoconstriction. The authors of the study concluded that the pathophysiology of the relationship between gender and ischemia in migraine may be related to the effect of estrogen and progesterone on endothelial cells. This may possibly mediate increased risk of ocular and systemic vascular complications in these patients.

Following 3 migraine patients at their baseline without migraine, and then during visual aura and post-aural migraine with 6×6 mm OCT-A macular scans, Barash et al. recently found that macular perfusion density was bilaterally and

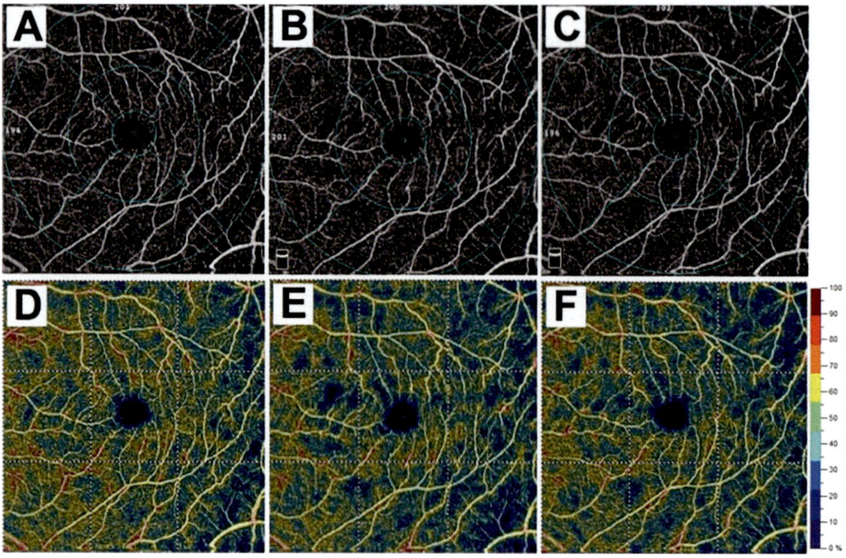

Fig. 24.7 OCT-A 6 × 6mm superficial macular scans of a 32-year-old male with ocular migraine during (**A**) baseline, (**B**) visual aura, and (**C**) post-aural migraine, with respective (**D**, **E**, **F**) perfusion density color maps

significantly decreased during post-aural migraine when compared to baseline and during visual aura (Fig. 24.7) [16]. A case report showed similar findings with decreased radial peripapillary capillary and foveal vessel density during the acute phase of visual aura associated with migraine [17]. Although the pathophysiology that may explain these changes remains unclear, these results imply systemic vascular involvement in migraine with aura patients and may explain their increased risk for cardiovascular disease. More studies using OCT-A are needed to confirm and expand on these results.

24.2.5 Amblyopia

Amblyopia represents an insult to the visual system during a critical period of neuronal plasticity and development, resulting in decreased visual acuity, color vision, contrast sensitivity and motion perception in one or both eyes. It affects approximately 3–5% of children, making it the most common cause of visual loss in children.

Although an ocular pathology such as strabismus, anisometropia, ptosis or cataract may cause the incongruence of visual information received by the eyes, amblyopia has classically been understood as a central nervous system disorder, involving neuronal structural and functional alterations in the lateral geniculate body as well as the visual cortex. More recent studies however implicate a larger role of the retina and choroid in the development of amblyopia.

Studies on amblyopic eyes have demonstrated an increased number of amacrine synapses and reduced number of bipolar synapses in the inner plexiform layer, as well as thinning of the RNFL, inner plexiform layer and outer nuclear layer, and a diminished Mueller fiber density. Amblyopic eyes have also been shown to have subfoveal choroidal thickening as compared to nonamblyopic eyes. Some studies have conversely reported an increased thickness of the outer nuclear layer in amblyopic eyes. Furthermore, amblyopic eyes have been shown to have abnormally orientated photoreceptors.

Recent studies using OCT-A have shown that superficial and deep capillary plexus densities of amblyopic eyes were lower than those in their nonamblyopic fellow eyes and age-matched control eyes (Figs. 24.8 and 24.9) [18–20]. Amblyopic eyes were found to have atrophic choroidal capillary perfusion with increased subfoveal choroidal thickness compared to their nonamblyopic fellow eyes [21]. The subfoveal choroidal thickening was found to be moderately and negatively correlated with visual acuity.

The decreased retinal and choroidal microvascular density in amblyopic eyes may be a secondary change due to neuronal atrophy and underuse. Choroidal capillary atrophy may induce malfunction of the outer retina, which may explain the observed increase in subfoveal choroidal thickness as a compensatory mechanism.

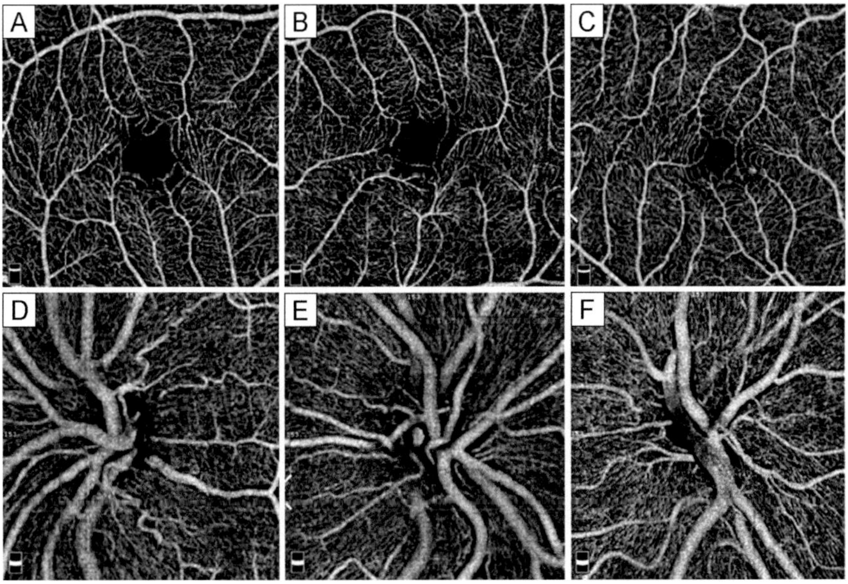

Fig. 24.8 Examples of central 3 × 3mm macular superficial capillary plexus scans (top row) and optic nerve scans (bottom row) from children studied: amblyopic eye (**A**, **D**), contralateral eye (**B**, **E**), control eye (**C**, **F**). Reproduced with permission from Elsevier, Sobral et al. [20]

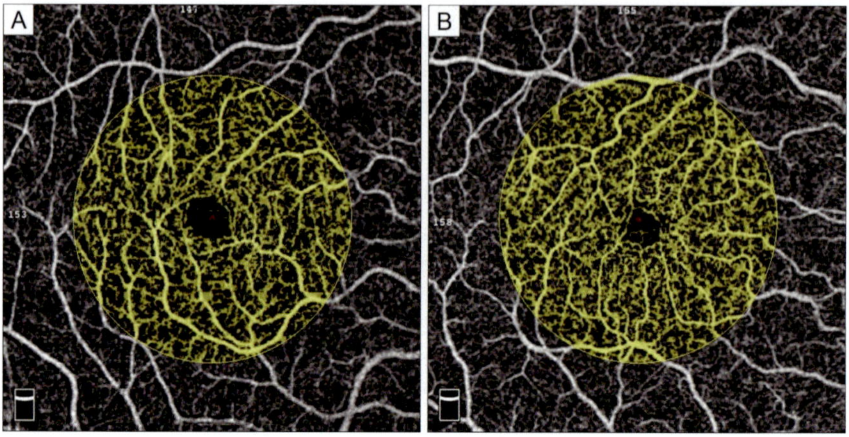

Fig. 24.9 2 mm diameter vessel density of superficial capillary plexus of an amblyopic eye (**A**) and a control eye (**B**). Vessel density is lower in the amblyopic eye, 6.059 mm^2 versus 6.617 mm^2. Reproduced with permission from Elsevier, Yilmaz et al. [18]

With growing evidence of retinal involvement in amblyogenesis, continued studies with OCT-A may shed light on the involvement of retinal and choroidal vessels. OCT-A may become a useful ancillary tool to help diagnose and monitor progression of amblyopia. Although a conflicting OCT-A study found no statistically significant differences in FAZ areas or retinal microvascular densities between amblyopic and nonamblyopic eyes [22]. The Hong Kong Children Eye Study (HKCES) recently found significant changes in FAZ circularity in children with amblyopia compared to controls which then corresponded with overall visual acuity [23].

24.3 Neuro-Ophthalmology

24.3.1 Non-arteritic Anterior Ischemic Optic Neuropathy

Non-arteritic anterior ischemic optic neuropathy (NAION) is the most common acute optic neuropathy over 50 years of age, affecting approximately 6 per 100,000 individuals per year. It is characterized by acute, painless unilateral vision loss or visual field loss in the presence optic disc edema. Optic disc pallor usually follows the resolution of edema. Patients typically have vascular risk factors such as hypertension, diabetes, hyperlipidemia, hypercoagulable disorders, anemia, sleep apnea and nocturnal hypotension. Other risk factors include optic disc drusen, and medications such as interferons and PDE-5 inhibitors.

The specific location of vasculopathy and pathophysiology of NAION is poorly understood. NAION usually occurs in a structurally crowded optic disc. It is believed to involve a transient hypoperfusion of the anterior optic disc microvasculature, which is chiefly contributed by the short posterior ciliary arteries. Histopathological studies have suggested that the probable location of the initial insult is the posterior laminar and retrolaminar optic nerve.

Doppler ultrasound, intravenous fluorescein angiography (FA) and indocyanine green angiography (ICGA) are limited in their ability to visualize the microcirculation in and surrounding the anterior optic nerve. Conventional OCT has shown choroidal thinning in NAION, indicating that the choroidal circulation may be involved in its pathogenesis. OCT-A, as a technology that is able to discern between different layers of microvasculature in and surrounding the anterior optic nerve, despite the possible presence of edema, may provide further insight on NAION.

Using OCT-A, non-acute NAION eyes were found to have significantly decreased perfusion through the optic disc, which was closely correlated with both central (best-corrected visual acuity) and peripheral (visual field) vision [24]. Additionally, in some NAION eyes, OCT-A revealed a significant decrease in perfusion through the optic disc without alteration of visual acuity or visual fields, suggesting that OCT-A changes in NAION may be at times subclinical and more sensitive in its diagnosis and monitoring. Not only can OCT-A yield information about perfusion in NAION, recent studies have also shown significant morphologic changes associated with peripapillary vasculature in NAION including vascular dropout in areas of edema as well as vascular tortuosity [25].

Acute and non-acute NAION (range 1 week—10 years, average 23 months since diagnosis) have been shown to have peripapillary perfusion deficits in both retinal and choroidal capillary beds, which correlate well with retinal structural (RNFL and GCC) and visual field defects [26, 27]. Retinal peripapillary perfusion deficits in acute and non-acute NAION have been shown to be significantly correlated to decreased visual acuity as well [28]. Furthermore, fellow eyes and healthy control eyes were shown to have no significant differences in retinal peripapillary or optic disc microvasculature.

Acute NAION imaged within 7 days of symptom onset was shown to have the presence of peripapillary retinal and choroidal perfusion deficits [29]. A prospective subset of these acute NAION patients was re-imaged after resolution of optic disc edema and shown to have a partial spontaneous recovery of the retinal and choroidal microcirculations. Atrophic NAION (at least 3 months after symptom onset) was shown to have significant retinal peripapillary capillary rarefaction that was strongly correlated with visual acuity, RNFL thickness and visual field parameters (Fig. 24.10) [30], and macular retinal capillary rarefaction that correlated with visual acuity [31]. Importantly, no differences in either peripapillary or macular choriocapillaris densities were detected at this time interval.

Gandhi et al. compared the peripapillary choroidal microvascular network and visual fields of unilateral acute NAION (with disc edema present at time of imaging) with their normal fellow eyes and non-ischemic papilledema eyes, in order to rule out the possible contribution of microvascular alterations by disc edema itself [32]. Compared to normal eyes, the authors found that both NAION and papilledema eyes showed diffuse loss of the microvasculature cuff surrounding the optic disc at the choroidal level. These changes were not related to visual field changes. The authors concluded that this pattern of microvascular loss was likely a result of disc edema itself, which could cause mechanical compression of blood vessels or affect scan acquisition. NAION eyes showed an additional area of sectoral loss of choroidal vasculature extending from the disc. These changes were not seen in papilledema eyes, and were strongly correlated with visual field defects (91.6% of the time). The authors concluded that this focal pattern of choroidal microvascular loss was more likely to represent true hypoperfusion.

The short posterior ciliary arteries supplying the posterior laminar and retrolaminar optic nerve are likely involved in the initial ischemic insult in NAION. Recent OCT-A studies show a decreased peripapillary choroidal perfusion in acute NAION, which may be the tributary circulation from the involved short posterior

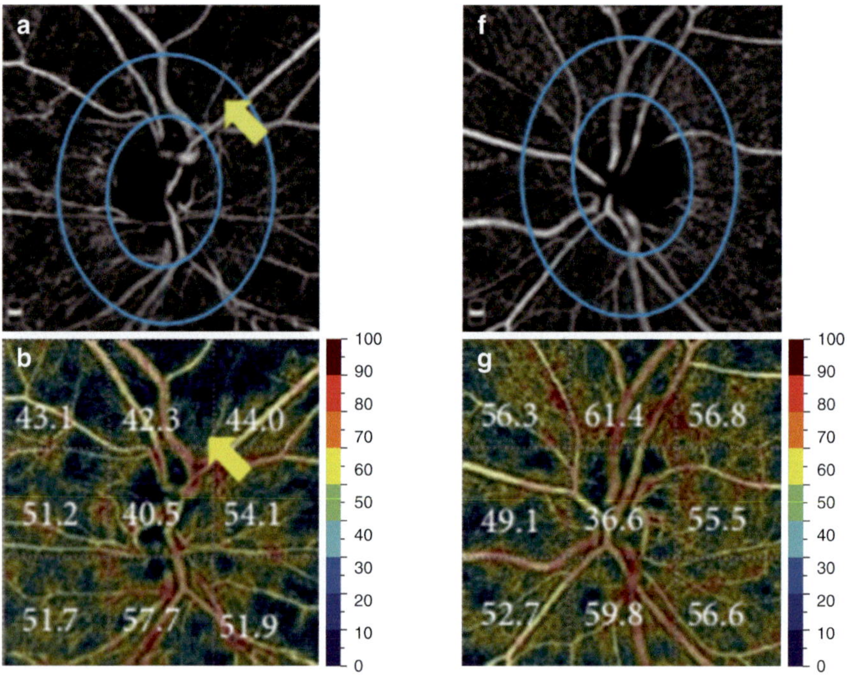

Fig. 24.10 Comparison of the peripapillary and parafoveal retinal angiograms: (**A**, **F**) en face OCT-A in the RPC layer, (**B**, **G**) vessel density (%) of RPCs with a color-coded map, (**C**, **H**) OCT-A in the parafoveal area, (**D**, **I**) vessel density (%) in the parafoveal area with a color-coded map, and (**E**, **J**) total deviation of the visual field in a representative NAION eye and the normal fellow eye. In the NAION eye (**A–E**), the microvascular network of the RPC layer was attenuated (arrow) compared with that of the normal fellow eye (**F–J**). The parafoveal microvascular networks in these examples showed no clear differences. The circles indicate the measured area for circumpapillary and parafoveal vessel density. Reproduced with permission from Hindawi, Liu et al. [30]

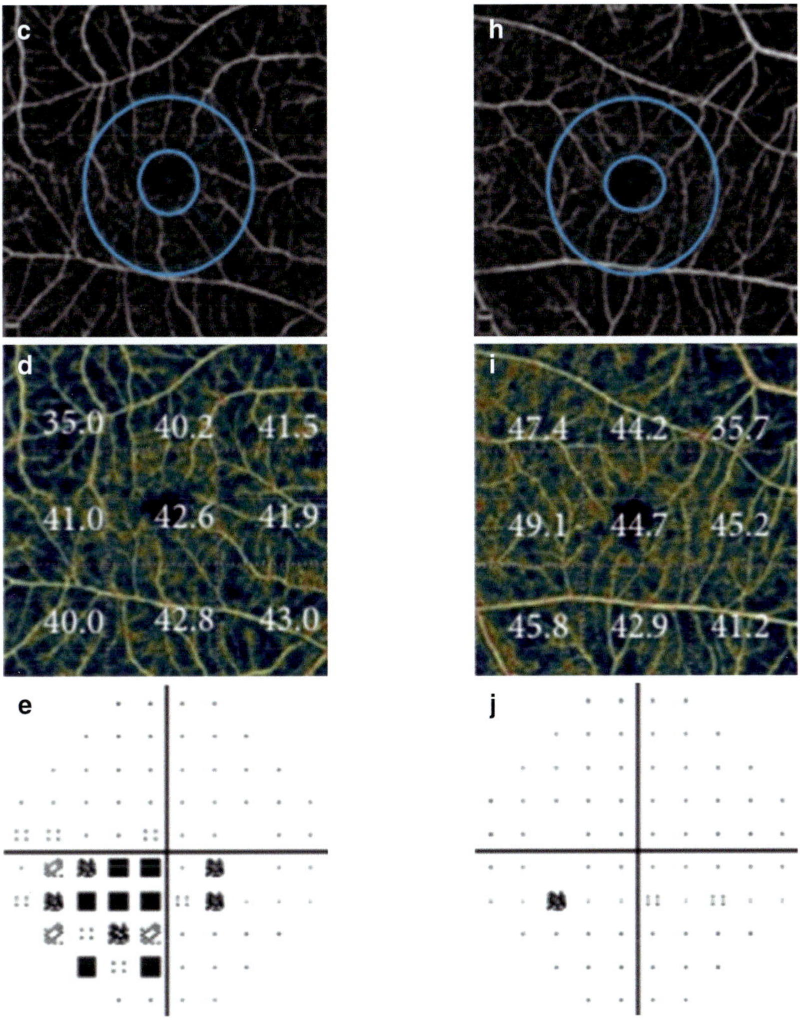

Fig. 24.10 (continued)

ciliary arteries. After the acute presentation resolves, the involved peripapillary choroidal perfusion seems to recover at least in part.

The OCT-A studies also showed rarefaction of the peripapillary retinal microcirculation. Since retinal capillaries depend on the central retinal artery and therefore should not be affected by abnormal posterior ciliary arteries, the mechanism by which they are altered must be different. Augstburger et al. propose that the resultant optic nerve edema due to swelling of ischemic axons from a transient ischemic insult in the short posterior ciliary arteries propagates anteriorly, compressing the retinal vessels and capillaries and aggravating tissue ischemia in a vicious cycle. This mechanism may explain findings that peripapillary capillary density in the temporal sector significantly decreased over 3 months following NAION, correlating with development of temporal nerve pallor and GC-IPL thinning [33].

Importantly, the OCT-A studies demonstrated that vessel density measurements correlate well with visual acuity and visual field parameters, suggesting that OCT-A could be of prognostic value in the assessment of ischemic severity in NAION patients. There are limits to OCT-A use in NAION, especially given the alteration of optic disc anatomy. A recent retrospective review found higher rates of segmentation error in discs affected by NAION versus healthy controls [34]. Thus, it is important to consider these changes when interpreting OCT-A images in NAION patients.

24.3.2 Leber's Hereditary Optic Neuropathy

Leber's Hereditary Optic Neuropathy (LHON) is the most common inherited mitochondrial disorder. Males are more likely to be affected than females, and age of onset is typically between 15–30 years. Mitochondrial DNA point mutations cause dysfunction in the mitochondrial respiratory chain, increasing reactive oxygen species (ROS) production. Given mitochondrial heteroplasmy, some individuals termed unaffected carriers remain asymptomatic throughout life. In individuals with a high enough mutation load, the increased ROS are thought to cause retinal ganglion cell and axonal injury and apoptosis, leading to a progressive optic neuropathy with initial optic disc swelling and subsequent RNFL thinning and optic nerve atrophy. Vision may worsen to less than 20/200, but rarely progresses to no light perception. There is no established medical therapy for LHON, and gene therapy studies are underway.

The optic disc microangiopathy in LHON is present with optic disc swelling and is characterized by an increase in tortuosity and size of the capillaries. The pathogenesis of the microangiopathy is unclear. It may be secondary to optic disc swelling and retinal ganglion cell damage, and may be involved in causing further RGC damage. OCT-A has been used to show that parafoveal vessel density is decreased in LHON patients compared to controls (Fig. 24.11) [35, 36]. Furthermore, microvascular density, as opposed to OCT-detectable structural changes, correlated well with visual acuity.

Several stages of LHON are recognized. The sub-acute stage involves a progressive evolution of optic disc and RNFL swelling for 3 months followed by thinning, resulting in a central scotoma that enlarges for a few months, becoming a stable defect within 6 months. The dynamic stage involves minor RNFL thinning after 6 months. Transition to the chronic stage occurs within 12 months of initial onset. OCT-A has recently been used to show that retinal peripapillary capillary density incrementally worsens over progressive stages of LHON [37]. Importantly, microvascular changes in the temporal sector were shown to precede RNFL changes, and mirrored GC-IPL changes.

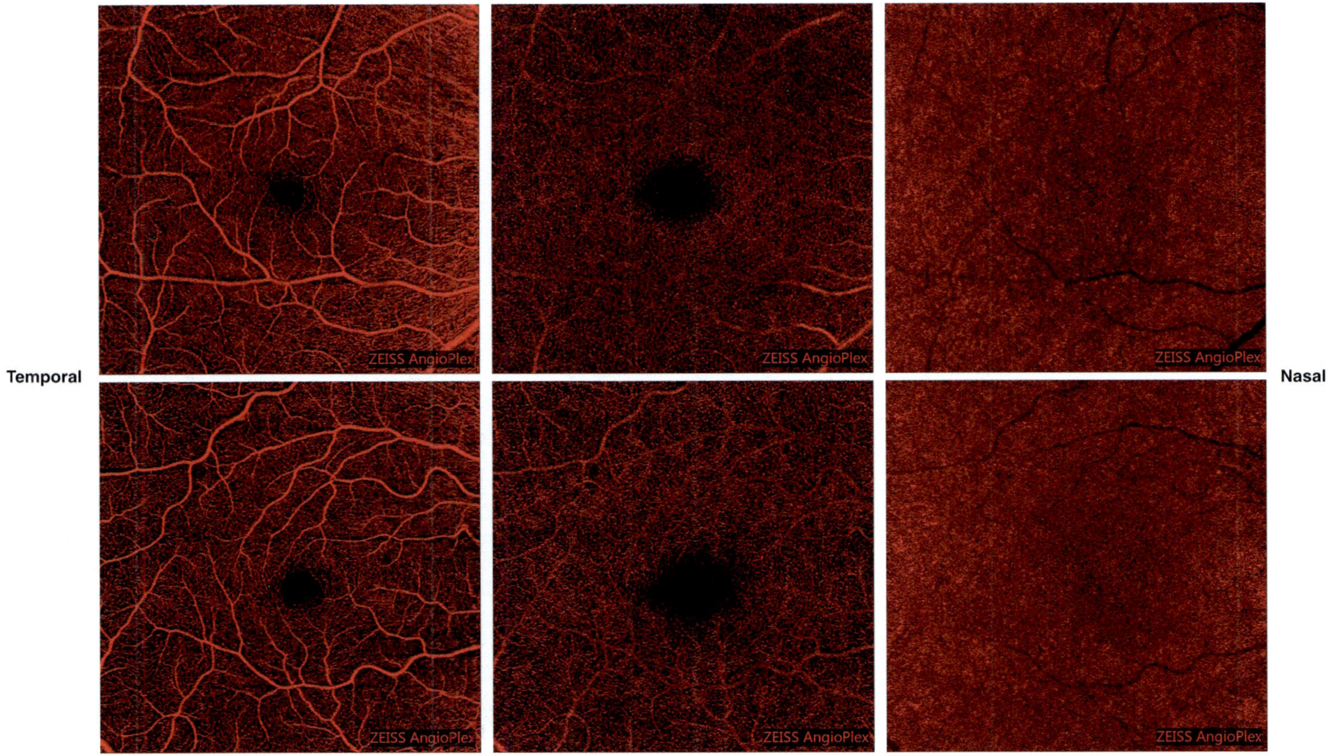

Fig. 24.11 Representation of LHON and healthy patients Representative OCTA 6 × 6 mm scans segmented at the level of the superficial capillary plexus (SCP; Left images), deep capillary plexus (DCP; Middle images). and choriocapillaris (CC, Right images) from a healthy subject (above) and an LHON patient (below). A reduced flow was demonstrated at the level of the SCP and DCP, especially in the nasal and inferior parafoveal sectors, in LHON patients. Reproduced with permission from Elsevier, Borrelli et al. [35]

Microvascular density appears to correlate with visual acuity better than structural changes, pointing to a microvascular dysfunction in LHON preceding neuronal dysfunction. This suggests that microvascular dysfunction may be an important contributor to retinal ganglion cell dysfunction and loss. One proposed mechanism includes mitochondrial dysfunction influencing endothelial cell and vascular smooth muscle viability, similar to its effect on retinal ganglion cells and their axons. OCT-A studies on LHON indicate that microvascular dysfunction may play a more important part than previously realized in the pathogenesis of LHON.

24.3.3 Optic Disc Swelling

Optic disc swelling is most commonly due to non-arteritic ischemic optic neuropathy (NAION), optic neuritis, or papilledema (swelling from elevated intracranial pressure). Clinically, optic disc swelling may appear similar across the three entities, while having different risk factor profiles, associated systemic diseases, prognosis and treatment. Bilateral NAION or optic neuritis may be mistaken for papilledema. Vice versa, papilledema may be mistaken for bilateral NAION or optic neuritis.

Using OCT-A, NAION and optic neuritis eyes have been shown to have a significantly lower retinal peripapillary vessel density compared to papilledema eyes and healthy control eyes (Fig. 24.12) [38]. No significant differences were found between NAION and optic neuritis eyes, or between papilledema and healthy control eyes. These results indicate that OCT-A can be employed, together with other imaging modalities and standard work up, in a clinical situation where it is otherwise difficult to differentiate NAION or optic neuritis from papilledema.

24.3.4 Optic Nerve Head Drusen

Optic nerve head drusen (ONHD) are calcium and phosphorus deposits within a filamentous protein matrix that accumulate in the optic nerve. ONHD occur in approximately 2% of the population, are usually asymptomatic, and are bilateral in 75% of cases. They can be buried or superficial. Superficial drusen can be directly visualized, while deeper drusen may need ultrasound for visualization, and can alter the contour of the optic nerve giving it an elevated, congested and swollen appearance. There are contradictory reports regarding which type of ONHD is more likely to cause visual field deficits with associated RNFL loss.

ONHD are associated with small and crowded optic discs. They are associated with optic nerve pallor and choroidal neovascularization, as well as vascular alterations and vascular occlusive disease such as NAION, central retinal artery occlusion and central retinal vein occlusion. ONHD can mimic several pathologies such as optic disc edema and glaucoma as signs and symptoms are similar.

The pathogenesis of ONHD is unclear. Some postulate that the deposits originate from extruded mitochondria, while others postulate that the primary pathology

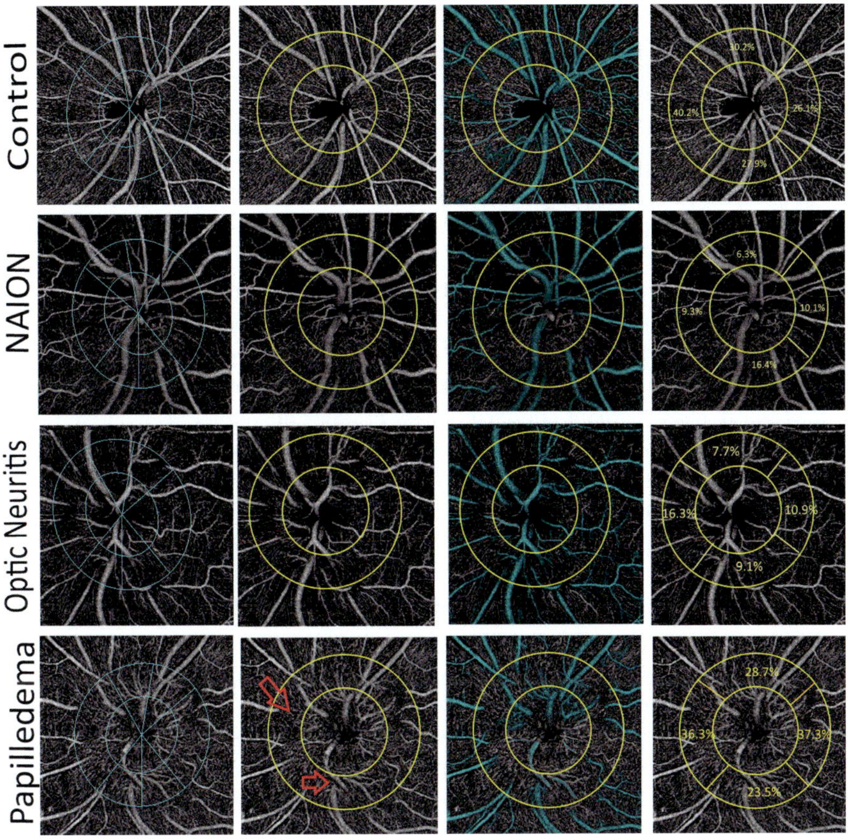

Fig. 24.12 OCT-A of peripapillary total vasculature and capillaries in eyes with optic disc swelling. (Left column) OCT-A sectors of peripapillary vasculature. (Second column) OCT-A images with 2 concentric circles with 3.45 and 1.95 mm diameter with customized software. (Third column) Major vessel (in cyan) removal using customized software. (Fourth column) Peripapillary capillary density (%) in each sector. Capillary density in NAION eyes is lower than papilledema and control eyes. OCT-A images of papilledema eyes show large vessel distortions and obscurations (arrows) compared to other disc swellings. Reproduced with permission from Elsevier, Fard et al. [38]

is an inherited dysplasia of the optic disc and its blood supply leading to abnormal transudation of plasma proteins and other extracellular materials.

The mechanisms by which ONHD cause visual damage are also poorly understood. It is unclear whether ONHD cause retinal nerve fiber injury directly through axonal compression or indirectly through vascular compression and resultant nerve fiber ischemia. Conventional microvasculature imaging modalities such as intravenous FA have not been successful in answering this question due to limitations in resolution of the retinal peripapillary capillary network. Doppler ultrasound has been used to show lower systolic and diastolic flow velocities in the central retinal artery and short posterior ciliary arteries, but not the ophthalmic artery, in eyes with ONHD, which correlated with visual field loss.

OCT-A has revealed that ONHD are associated with focal decreases in vessel density within their localization [39]. OCT-A was recently used to image a patient who developed decreased vision in the right eye and was then found to have a heavy burden of superficial ONHD [40]. In this patient, superficial microvascular attenuation was associated with most but not all drusen, while RNFL thinning corresponded to some but not all areas of microvascular attenuation. The authors concluded that superficial ONHD may cause focal areas of poor superficial retinal perfusion that may in turn lead to nerve fiber ischemia and rarefaction, causing visual acuity loss and visual field deficits. Further supporting the evidence of focality in disease burden of ONHD, a recent retrospective study looking at 44 eyes showed a statistically significant decrease in only temporal radial peripapillary vessel density, without similar findings in other quadrants [41]. These results indicate that OCT-A may be more sensitive than traditional peripapillary RNFL and visual field analysis for the earlier detection and monitoring of optic nerve and retinal injury from ONHD.

24.3.5 Thyroid Eye Disease and Dysthyroid Optic Neuropathy

Thyroid eye disease (TED) is an orbitopathy associated with thyroid dysfunction and a complex immunologic process. Treatment is aimed at ameliorating the resulting orbital congestion and inflammation. The most serious although infrequent (8–10%) vision-threatening complication of TED is dysthyroid optic neuropathy (DON). Clinical scoring systems such as the Clinical Activity Score have been used as assessment tools for guiding evaluation and treatment of TED, however no system prevails as the gold standard. Furthermore, none of the clinical scoring systems were designed to grade effectiveness of treatment of DON.

A number of studies using a variety of modalities have concluded that an important component of the pathophysiology of TED and DON is changes in blood flow in the orbit and optic nerve in the setting of compression and congestion/inflammation. Some have reported an increased blood flow through the ophthalmic artery and central retinal artery, while others have reported decreased chorioretinal perfusion, as well as congestion of the retinal veins and superior ophthalmic vein.

OCT-A may help shed light onto the perfusion status of the optic nerve head and retina in TED, and onto the early pathogenesis of DON. Earlier studies using OCT-A, eyes with active TED were found to have an increased retinal microvascular density compared to healthy controls [42]. The increase in density was moderately negatively correlated with visual acuity. Another study using OCT-A performed a prospective case series in a cohort of TED patients with and without DON who underwent bilateral orbital decompression [43]. The authors found that eyes with TED generally showed reduction in peripapillary microvascular density following decompression surgery, more so in eyes with DON (Fig. 24.13).

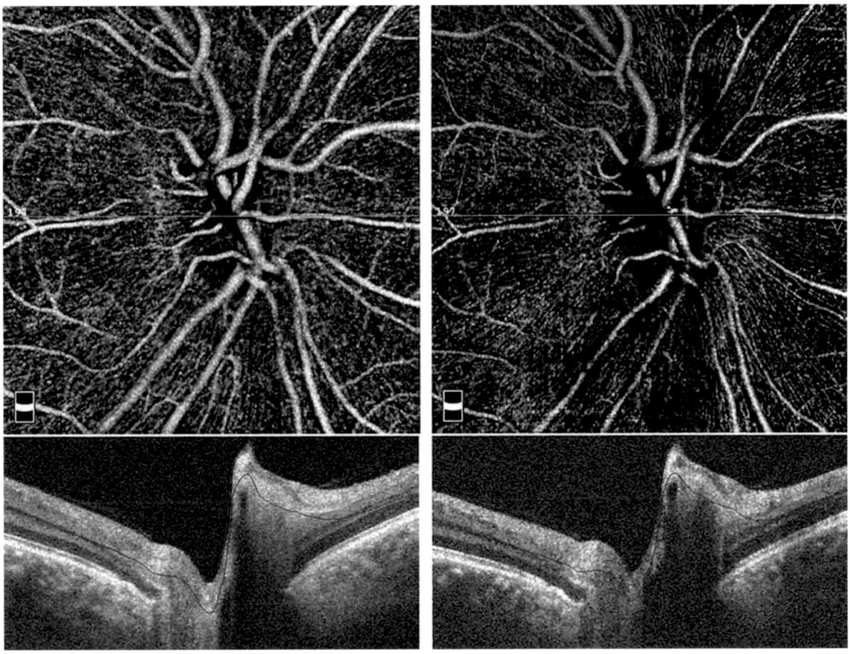

Fig. 24.13 Preoperative (left) and postoperative (right) OCT-A of the right eye in a patient with dysthyroid optic neuropathy. A significant reduction in blood vessel density was found after decompression (− 2.45 within the peripapillary ring and − 7.11 over the optic disk). Reproduced with permission from Taylor & Francis, Lewis et al. [43]

More recent studies have shown opposite trends. The peripapillary region has shown to have a decrease in vessel density in TED patients compared to controls, which further correlated with current activity of disease [44]. Similarly, a recent cohort study showed decreased both peripapillary and macular vessel density during active TED compared to controls as well as inactive TED patients [45]. Even with these seemingly conflicting reports to earlier data, it is evident that retinal blood flow is significantly impacted in TED patients and ongoing research may help us to determine what factors impact the increase or decrease in vessel density.

The choroid appears to be particularly sensitive to compression in TED. A case report in the literature describes a case with robust increase in choroidal perfusion using OCTA following treatment of TED with steroids and orbital decompression [46]. The authors hypothesize the susceptibility of the choroid may be secondary to absence of protection of the optic nerve sheath for the short posterior ciliary arteries as they travel to supply the choroid.

These studies demonstrate that OCT-A has potential to be a more sensitive and quantitative tool in grading clinical activity of TED, diagnosing DON earlier, and offering clinicians a tool to monitor response to treatment.

24.4 Summary

The early studies using OCT-A reviewed here demonstrate its potential for sorting out the interplay of vascular and neuronal changes in the pathophysiology of common neurological and neuro-ophthalmological disorders. OCT-A shows promise in becoming an important tool for researchers and clinicians in their multimodal approach in detecting pathological changes, monitoring disease progression and evaluating response to treatment in these disorders.

References

1. Spaide RF, Fujimoto JG, Waheed NK, Sadda SR, Staurenghi G. Optical coherence tomography angiography. Prog Retin Eye Res. 2018;64:1–55.
2. Bulut M, Kurtuluş F, Gözkaya O, Erol MK, Cengiz A, Akıdan M, et al. Evaluation of optical coherence tomography angiographic findings in Alzheimer's type dementia. Br J Ophthalmol. 2018;102(2):233–7.
3. O'Bryhim BE, Apte RS, Kung N, Coble D, Van Stavern GP. Association of preclinical Alzheimer disease with optical coherence tomographic angiography findings. JAMA Ophthalmol. 2018;136(11):1242–8.
4. Moussa M, Falfoul Y, Nasri A, El Matri K, Kacem I, Mrabet S, Chebil A, Gharbi A, Gouider R, El Matri L. Optical coherence tomography and angiography in Alzheimer's disease and other cognitive disorders. Eur J Ophthalmol. 2023;33(4):11206721221148952.
5. Jiang H, Wei Y, Shi Y, Wright CB, Sun X, Gregori G, et al. Altered macular microvasculature in mild cognitive impairment and Alzheimer disease. J Neuroophthalmol. 2018;38(3):292–8.
6. Murueta-Goyena A, Barrenechea M, Erramuzpe A, Teijeira-Portas S, Pengo M, Ayala U, Romero-Bascones D, Acera M, Del Pino R, Gómez-Esteban JC, Gabilondo I. Foveal remodeling of retinal microvasculature in Parkinson's disease. Front Neurosci. 2021;15: 708700.
7. Kwapong WR, Ye H, Peng C, Zhuang X, Wang J, Shen M, et al. Retinal microvascular impairment in the early stages of Parkinson's disease. Invest Ophthalmol Vis Sci. 2018;59(10):4115–22.
8. Lanzillo R, Cennamo G, Criscuolo C, Carotenuto A, Velotti N, Sparnelli F, et al. Optical coherence tomography angiography retinal vascular network assessment in multiple sclerosis. Mult Scler. 2018;24(13):1706–14.
9. Farci R, Carta A, Cocco E, Frau J, Fossarello M, Diaz G. Optical coherence tomography angiography in multiple sclerosis: a cross-sectional study. PLoS ONE. 2020;15(7): e0236090.
10. Cordon B, Vilades E, Orduna E, Satue M, Perez-Velilla J, Sebastian B, Polo V, Larrosa JM, Pablo LE, Garcia-Martin E. Angiography with optical coherence tomography as a biomarker in multiple sclerosis. PLoS ONE. 2020;15(12): e0243236.
11. Lanzillo R, Cennamo G, Moccia M, Criscuolo C, Carotenuto A, Frattaruolo N, et al. Retinal vascular density in multiple sclerosis: a 1-year follow-up. Eur J Neurol. 2018;26(1):198–201.
12. Feucht N, Maier M, Lepennetier G, Pettenkofer M, Wetzlmair C, Daltrozzo T, et al. Optical coherence tomography angiography indicates associations of the retinal vascular network and disease activity in multiple sclerosis. Mult Scler. 2018;25(2):1352458517750009.
13. Spain RI, Liu L, Zhang X, Jia Y, Tan O, Bourdette D, et al. Optical coherence tomography angiography enhances the detection of optic nerve damage in multiple sclerosis. Br J Ophthalmol. 2018;102(4):520–4.
14. Wang X, Jia Y, Spain R, Potsaid B, Liu JJ, Baumann B, et al. Optical coherence tomography angiography of optic nerve head and parafovea in multiple sclerosis. Br J Ophthalmol. 2014;98(10):1368–73.

15. Chang MY, Phasukkijwatana N, Garrity S, Pineles SL, Rahimi M, Sarraf D, et al. Foveal and peripapillary vascular decrement in migraine with aura demonstrated by optical coherence tomography angiography. Invest Ophthalmol Vis Sci. 2017;58(12):5477–84.
16. Barash AT, Pinhas MJ, Rosen A, Richard B. Macular and peripapillary retinal perfusion changes during migraine with aura detected by optical coherence tomography angiography. Paper presentation at the American Society of Retina Specialists. Chicago, Illinois; July 2019.
17. Bingöl Kızıltunç P, Atilla H. Vascular changes with optical coherence tomography angiography during aura of migraine: a case report. Eur J Ophthalmol. 2021;31(2):NP54–7.
18. Yilmaz I, Ocak OB, Yilmaz BS, Inal A, Gokyigit B, Taskapili M. Comparison of quantitative measurement of foveal avascular zone and macular vessel density in eyes of children with amblyopia and healthy controls: an optical coherence tomography angiography study. J AAPOS. 2017;21(3):224–8.
19. Lonngi M, Velez FG, Tsui I, Davila JP, Rahimi M, Chan C, et al. Spectral-domain optical coherence tomographic angiography in children with amblyopia. JAMA Ophthalmol. 2017;135(10):1086–91.
20. Sobral I, Rodrigues TM, Soares M, Seara M, Monteiro M, Paiva C, et al. OCT angiography findings in children with amblyopia. J AAPOS. 2018;22(4):286–9.
21. Guo L, Tao J, Xia F, Yang Z, Ma X, Hua R. In vivo optical imaging of amblyopia: digital subtraction autofluorescence and split-spectrum amplitude-decorrelation angiography. Lasers Surg Med. 2016;48(7):660–7.
22. Demirayak B, Vural A, Onur IU, Kaya FS, Yigit FU. Analysis of macular vessel density and foveal avascular zone using spectral-domain optical coherence tomography angiography in children with amblyopia. J Pediatr Ophthalmol Strabismus. 2018;56(1):1–5.
23. Wong ES, Zhang XJ, Yuan N, Li J, Pang CP, Chen L, Tham CC, Cheung CY, Yam JC. Association of optical coherence tomography angiography metrics with detection of impaired macular microvasculature and decreased vision in amblyopic eyes: the Hong Kong children eye study. JAMA Ophthalmol. 2020;138(8):858–65.
24. Ling JW, Yin X, Lu QY, Chen YY, Lu PR. Optical coherence tomography angiography of optic disc perfusion in non-arteritic anterior ischemic optic neuropathy. Int J Ophthalmol. 2017;10(9):1402–6.
25. Al-Nashar HY, Hemeda S. Assessment of peripapillary vessel density in acute non-arteritic anterior ischemic optic neuropathy. Int Ophthalmol. 2020;40(5):1269–76.
26. Wright Mayes E, Cole ED, Dang S, Novais EA, Vuong L, Mendoza-Santiesteban C, et al. Optical coherence tomography angiography in nonarteritic anterior ischemic optic neuropathy. J Neuroophthalmol. 2017;37(4):358–64.
27. Sönmez HK, Arda H, Gülmez SD. Evaluation of optic disc perfusion with optical coherence tomography angiography in acute non-arteritic anterior ischemic optic neuropathy. Turk J Ophthalmol. 2022;52(1):30–6.
28. Song Y, Min JY, Mao L, Gong YY. Microvasculature dropout detected by the optical coherence tomography angiography in nonarteritic anterior ischemic optic neuropathy. Lasers Surg Med. 2018;50(3):194–201.
29. Sharma S, Ang M, Najjar RP, Sng C, Cheung CY, Rukmini AV, et al. Optical coherence tomography angiography in acute non-arteritic anterior ischaemic optic neuropathy. Br J Ophthalmol. 2017;101(8):1045–51.
30. Liu CH, Kao LY, Sun MH, Wu WC, Chen HS. Retinal vessel density in optical coherence tomography angiography in optic atrophy after nonarteritic anterior ischemic optic neuropathy. J Ophthalmol. 2017;2017:9632647.
31. Augstburger E, Zéboulon P, Keilani C, Baudouin C, Labbé A. Retinal and choroidal microvasculature in nonarteritic anterior ischemic optic neuropathy: an optical coherence tomography angiography study. Invest Ophthalmol Vis Sci. 2018;59(2):870–7.
32. Gandhi U, Chhablani J, Badakere A, Kekunnaya R, Rasheed MA, Goud A, et al. Optical coherence tomography angiography in acute unilateral nonarteritic anterior ischemic optic neuropathy: a comparison with the fellow eye and with eyes with papilledema. Indian J Ophthalmol. 2018;66(8):1144–8.

33. Rebolleda G, Díez-Álvarez L, García Marín Y, de Juan V, Muñoz-Negrete FJ. Reduction of peripapillary vessel density by optical coherence tomography angiography from the acute to the atrophic stage in non-arteritic anterior ischaemic optic neuropathy. Ophthalmologica. 2018;240(4):191–9.
34. Anvari P, Sardarinia M, Zand A, Aghdam KA, Falavarjani KG. Accuracy of peripapillary OCTA in patients with acute nonarteritic anterior ischemic optic neuropathy. Can J Ophthalmol. 2022;58(6):577–81.
35. Borrelli E, Balasubramanian S, Triolo G, Barboni P, Sadda SR, Sadun AA. Topographic macular microvascular changes and correlation with visual loss in chronic leber hereditary optic neuropathy. Am J Ophthalmol. 2018;192:217–28.
36. Asanad S, Meer E, Fantini M, Borrelli E, Sadun AA. Leber's hereditary optic neuropathy: shifting our attention to the macula. Am J Ophthalmol Case Rep. 2018;13:13–5.
37. Balducci N, Cascavilla ML, Ciardella A, La Morgia C, Triolo G, Parisi V, et al. Peripapillary vessel density changes in Leber's hereditary optic neuropathy: a new biomarker. Clin Exp Ophthalmol. 2018;46(9):1055–62.
38. Fard MA, Jalili J, Sahraiyan A, Khojasteh H, Hejazi M, Ritch R, et al. Optical coherence tomography angiography in optic disc swelling. Am J Ophthalmol. 2018;191:116–23.
39. Flores-Reyes E, Hoskens K, Mansouri K. Optic nerve head drusen: imaging using optical coherence tomography angiography. J Glaucoma. 2017;26(9):845–9.
40. Gaier ED, Rizzo JF, Miller JB, Cestari DM. Focal capillary dropout associated with optic disc drusen using optical coherence tomographic angiography. J Neuroophthalmol. 2017;37(4):405–10.
41. Turker IC, Uzun SU, Dogan CU, Dirim AB, Ozyurek EBA, Yesiltas SK, Guven D. Evaluation of peripapillary and macular vascular flow changes with OCT-A in patients with superficial optic disk drusen. Sisli Etfal Hastan Tip Bul. 2022;56(2):196–201.
42. Ye L, Zhou SS, Yang WL, Bao J, Jiang N, Min YL, et al. Retinal microvasculature alteration in active thyroid-associated ophthalmopathy. Endocr Pract. 2018;24(7):658–67.
43. Lewis KT, Bullock JR, Drumright RT, Olsen MJ, Penman AD. Changes in peripapillary blood vessel density in Graves' orbitopathy after orbital decompression surgery as measured by optical coherence tomography angiography. Orbit. 2018;38:1–8.
44. Sabermoghaddam A, Shoeibi N, Jafarzadeh H, Bakhtiari E, Salahi Z, Saeidi Rezvani T, Heidarzadeh HR, Abrishami M. Optic nerve head optical coherence tomography angiography findings in patients with thyroid eye disease: a case-control study. Thyroid Res. 2022;15(1):17.
45. Dave TV, Laghmisetty S, Krishnamurthy G, Bejjanki K, Ganguly A, Jonnadula GB, Dave VP, Reddy PR. Retinal vascularity, nerve fiber, and ganglion cell layer thickness in thyroid eye disease on optical coherence tomography angiography. Orbit. 2022;41(2):170–7.
46. Mimura M, Nishikawa Y, Inagaki K, Sato Y, Fujita Y, Kikkawa DO. Change of intraocular blood flow during treatment for thyroid eye disease. Taiwan J Ophthalmol. 2022;12(1):97–100.

Flavoprotein Fluorescence in the Detection of Eye Disorders

25

Sofia Ahsanuddin and Richard B. Rosen

Abstract

Mitochondrial dysfunction is integral to the pathophysiology of a number of ocular disease states, including diabetic retinopathy, age-related macular degeneration, and glaucoma. In recent years, a novel non-invasive imaging modality has been developed that may detect pre-structural metabolic dysfunction that occurs in the retina in each of these disease states. This technology specifically quantifies mitochondrial stress and has been used to study both the macula and the optic nerve head. Most exciting is its use in monitoring treatment response in diabetic macular edema, suggesting its potential role in early detection of therapeutic efficacy or failure. In this book chapter, we will provide a clinical overview of mitochondrial dysfunction and its relevance in the pathogenesis across a spectrum of retinal disease states. We will discuss the rationale of flavoprotein fluorescence (FPF) quantification as a proxy for measuring retinal oxidative stress and current studies that have investigated its utility.

Keywords

Flavoprotein fluorescence • Retinal metabolic analysis • Mitochondrial dysfunction • Diabetic retinopathy • Age-related macular degeneration • Glaucoma • Retinal dystrophies • Central serous chorioretinopathy

S. Ahsanuddin · R. B. Rosen (✉)
Department of Ophthalmology, New York Eye and Ear Infirmary of Mount Sinai, New York, NY, USA
e-mail: rrosen@nyee.edu

Department of Ophthalmology, Icahn School of Medicine at Mount Sinai, New York, NY, USA

A. Grzybowski and P. Barboni (eds.), *OCT and Imaging in Central Nervous System Diseases*, https://doi.org/10.1007/978-3-031-72156-4_25

25.1 Introduction

Mitochondria are responsible for energy production, maintenance of homeostasis, and cellular signaling [1–3]. Retinal cells are highly metabolically active and require significant oxygen consumption. Thus, they are particularly vulnerable to mitochondrial stress or dysfunction leading to the release of reactive oxygen species (ROS) which can lead to apoptosis [4, 5]. Inadvertent induction of apoptosis can result in inappropriate loss of retinal cells and subsequent retinal tissue dysfunction [6].

Mitochondrial dysfunction associated with oxidative stress has been implicated in the pathogenesis of a wide spectrum of retinal diseases ranging from age-related macular degeneration (AMD), diabetic retinopathy (DR), and retinal vein occlusion (RVO) [7–10]. Mitochondrial leakage of reactive oxygen species (ROS) can result in excessive oxidative stress that exceeds the antioxidant defenses of the cell. In the presence of increasing oxidative stress, flavoproteins linked to mitochondrial enzymes in the electron transport chain become oxidized and emit a green fluorescence within the range of 520–540 nm in response to blue light excitation (430–470 nm) [11–13]. Thus, assessing levels of mitochondrial flavoprotein fluorescence (FPF) can be used as a proxy for measuring mitochondrial oxidative stress and potential dysfunction of the retina in vivo [1, 14].

Functional imaging of mitochondria can be used to detect response to therapeutic intervention. To isolate the specific fluorescence signal of mitochondrial flavoproteins in the presence of other retinal fluorophores such as lipofuscin, a novel device known as the OcuMet Beacon has been recently developed. The device is equipped with a narrow notch filter centered at the emission peak of flavoproteins which is shorter and at the shoulder of the shorter end of the lipofuscin emission curve. The filter bandwidth is designed to optimize signal-to-noise ratio and maximally isolate the signal emitted by the flavoproteins. The device provides an unprecedented picture of metabolic disturbances that precede the structural changes that occur later in disease [11, 12, 15]. An overview of the imaging acquisition workflow and comparison of FPF across several retinal disease states is illustrated in Figs. 25.1 and 25.2.

Several studies to date have utilized two indices, FPF intensity and FPF heterogeneity, to assess the severity of mitochondrial dysfunction in retinal disease. FPF intensity is a measure of average pixel intensity over a 5.5 mm-diameter region centered on either the macula or the optic nerve head [1, 16]. FPF heterogeneity reports the variation of signal intensity of all the pixels in the region of interest (ROI) in the imaged eye. Both elevated levels of FPF intensity and heterogeneity have been correlated with disease progression and may be of value for evaluating clinical severity, response to treatment, and predicting prognosis [15, 17, 18]. Here, we provide an overview of the literature describing FPF in quantifying mitochondrial dysfunction in various retinal pathologies.

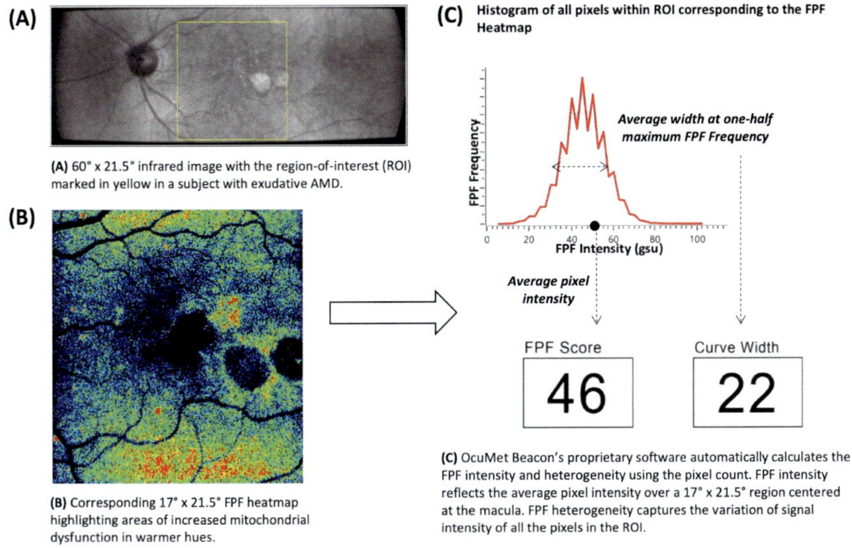

Fig. 25.1 Overview of the OcuMet Beacon® FPF imaging methodology. **(A)** 60° × 21.5° infrared image with the region-of-interest (ROI) marked in yellow in a subject with exudative AMD. **(B)** Corresponding 17° × 21.5° FPF heatmap highlighting showing areas of increased mitochondrial dysfunction in warmer hues. **(C)** OcuMet Beacon's proprietary software automatically calculates the FPF intensity and heterogeneity using the pixel count. FPF intensity reflects the average pixel intensity over a 17° × 21.5° region centered at the macula. FPF heterogeneity captures the variation of signal intensity of all the pixels in the ROI. *Reprinted with permission from Ahsanuddin et al. "Flavoprotein fluorescence elevation is a marker of mitochondrial oxidative stress in patients with retinal disease" (2023)*

25.2 In Vitro FPF Animal and Human Studies

Two in vitro studies involving animal and human models have assessed FPF in the retina. Elner et al. investigated FPF in cultured human retinal pigment epithelial (RPE) cells exposed to sublethal concentrations of hydrogen peroxide (H_2O_2) or C_2 ceramide with and without the presence of N-acetylcysteine or dihydroceramide C_2 [11, 12]. H_2O_2 and C_2 ceramide are known to induce apoptosis in RPE cells; N-acetylcysteine is an antioxidant and dihydroceramide C_2 is a competitive antagonist of ceramide. They observed that retinal fluorescence was significantly elevated in cells treated with H_2O_2 compared to control cells. Importantly, fluorescence was found to be significantly reduced in cells treated with both H_2O_2 and N-acetylcysteine compared to even control cells, suggesting that the presence of N-acetylcysteine can improve mitochondrial function. Similarly, increased fluorescence was observed in RPE cells treated with only C_2 ceramide in comparison to control cells and cells treated with both C_2 ceramide and dihydroceramide C_2. Field et al. built upon these findings and evaluated FPF in cultured human RPE cells [19]. They found that RPE cells treated with higher doses of

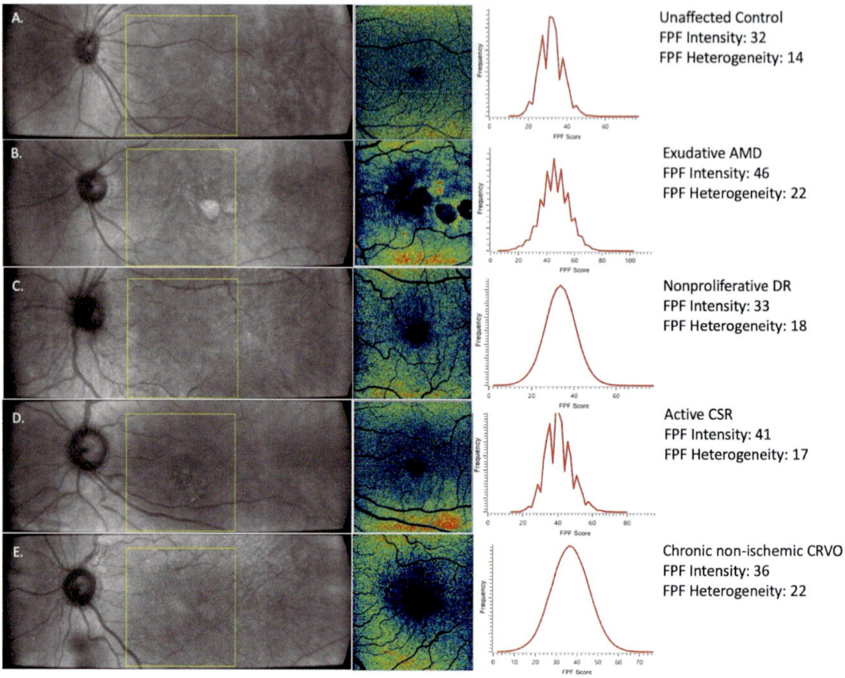

Fig. 25.2 Representative images of **(A)** healthy control, **(B)** exudative AMD, **(C)** nonproliferative DR, **(D)** active CSR, and **(E)** chronic non-ischemic CRVO. **(Left)** $60° \times 21.5°$ infrared images with the yellow box indicating the region of interest (ROI) at the macula for FPF measurements. **(Center)** $17° \times 21.5°$ FPF heat map. Warmer colors indicate higher FPF intensities. FPF heterogeneity is the average width of the histogram curve at one-half the maximum FPF frequency. **(Right)** Distribution of FPF intensities among all image pixels. *Reprinted with permission from Ahsanuddin et al. "Flavoprotein fluorescence elevation is a marker of mitochondrial oxidative stress in patients with retinal disease" (2023)*

H_2O_2 had significantly elevated levels of FPF in comparison to samples treated with lower doses of H_2O_2 and both N-acetylcysteine and H_2O_2. Increased FPF was correlated with both decreased mitochondrial membrane potential, increased apoptosis vis-à-vis significant elevations of oligonucleosomes, and expression of pro-inflammatory cytokines (such as interleukin-8 (IL-8) and monocyte chemotactic factor-1 (MCP1)) that have been previously associated with increased induction of oxidative stress. N-acetylcysteine has significant antioxidant properties and was found to inhibit FPF elevation and subsequent apoptosis in cultured RPE cells exposed to H_2O_2.

25.3 FPF in Glaucoma, Ocular Hypertension (OHT), and Pseudotumor Cerebri

In glaucoma, several complex cellular mechanisms contribute to the generation of excess reactive oxygen species (ROS) and mitochondrial dysfunction. The primary sites for glaucomatous damage occur within retinal ganglion cells (RGCs) and at the optic nerve head (ONH), both of which contain dense concentrations of mitochondria. Although the mechanisms are not completely elucidated, increased intraocular pressure (IOP) is hypothesized to result in increased mechanical stress, chronic hypoperfusion, and ischemia in the eye, thereby resulting in ROS production and RGC apoptosis [1]. Ju et al. demonstrated that elevated hydrostatic pressure can accelerate loss of ATP production and mitochondrial cristae in human RGC cultures [20]. In normal tension glaucoma, increased ROS production is thought to be caused by variants of nuclear genes encoding mitochondrial proteins that then contribute to impaired mitochondrial machinery. Due to these mechanisms, it has been suggested that restoration of antioxidant defense systems and inhibition of RGC apoptosis can prevent the progression of glaucoma. Similarly, in pseudotumor cerebri, RGC dysfunction is thought to result in vision loss [11, 12].

To investigate FPF in patients with mild visual dysfunction secondary to pseudotumor cerebri, Elner et al. published a case–control study comparing FPF between 6 age-matched control eyes and 6 eyes with pseudotumor cerebri [11, 12]. They found that the average FPF intensity and heterogeneity of patients with pseudotumor cerebri was 1.6 times more elevated compared to age-matched control subjects. They hypothesized that one potential mechanism for increased FPF in pseudotumor cerebri is RGC dysfunction.

In 2016, Geyman et al. analyzed FPF in 36 eyes from 18 healthy controls, 16 Ocular Hypertensive (OHT) eyes from 8 subjects, and 40 Primary Open Angle Glaucoma (POAG) eyes from 20 subjects [21]. Patients were diagnosed with POAG by glaucomatous ONH changes, circumpapillary retinal nerve fiber layer (cpRNFL) thickness below the bottom fifth percentile of the normative database, and visual field deficits on Humphrey visual field 24-2 tests (Fig. 25.3). They found that FPF at the macula and the macular FPF/RGC$^+$ layer thickness ratio [defined as including both the ganglion cell layer (GCL) and inner plexiform layer (IPL)] were significantly increased in OHT eyes despite the absence of glaucomatous damage or deterioration in visual acuity. In OHT eyes, increased FPF at the macula despite a lack of cpRNFL thinning or visual field changes suggests that FPF can potentially be used as a marker of substructural glaucomatous activity (Fig. 25.4). In POAG eyes, FPF was found to be moderately but insignificantly elevated compared to control eyes in the setting of greater cpRNFL and visual field defects. However, the ratio of FPF/RGC$^+$ thickness was found to be significantly elevated in POAG compared to control eyes. These findings suggest that mitochondrial dysfunction could potentially occur earlier on in the disease process.

Zhou et al. expanded on these findings by studying FPF in 50 eyes of 30 POAG patients and 36 eyes of 20 controls [22]. FPF was quantified by a software algorithm that identified the ONH margins on the infrared image (Fig. 25.5). FPF then

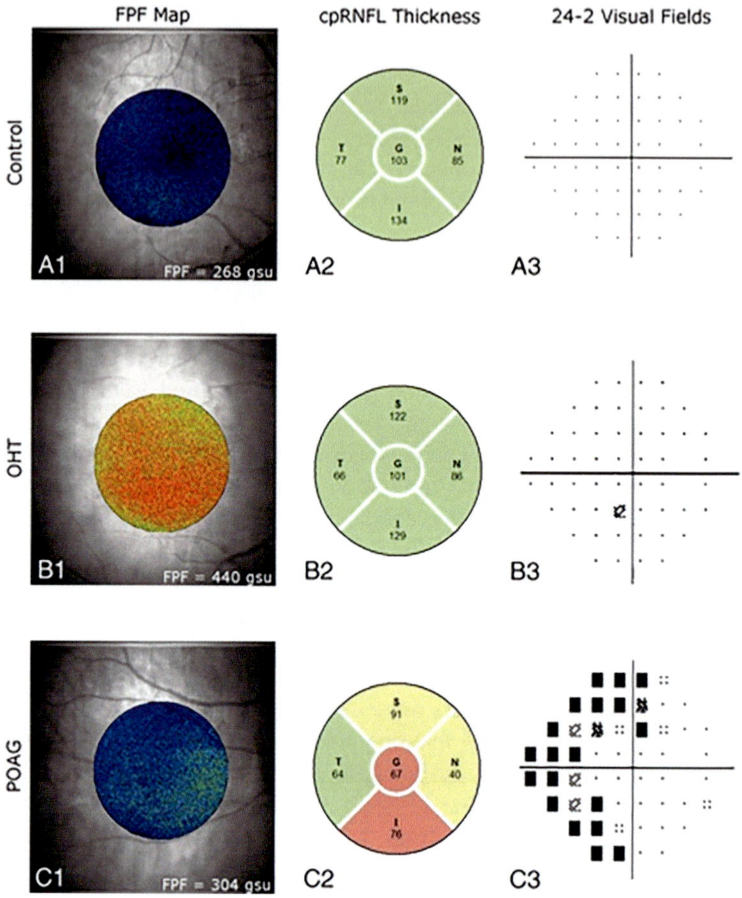

Fig. 25.3 FPF heatmaps and corresponding circumpapillary retinal nerve fiber layer (cpRNFL) thickness maps (column 2) and visual field pattern deviation plots in representative OHT and POAG eyes compared to healthy control eyes using an earlier generation of the OcuMet Beacon®. **(Left)** FPF heatmaps demonstrate mitochondrial dysfunction in OHT and POAG. **(B1)** Increased red–orange coloration in the OHT eye compared with the control eye **(A1)** suggests increased mitochondrial dysfunction at the macula despite a lack of cpRNFL thinning **(A2–B2)**) or visual field changes **(A3–B3)**. **(C1)** The POAG eye demonstrates lower levels of mitochondrial dysfunction compared to the OHT eye, but with greater cpRNFL loss **(C2)** and visual field defects **(C3)**, suggesting that mitochondrial dysfunction could potentially occur earlier on in the disease process. *Reprinted with permission from Dr. Lawrence Gayman, MD and Dr. Richard Rosen, MD's "Mitochondrial Dysfunction in Primary Open-angle Glaucoma Characterized by Flavoprotein Fluorescence at the Optic Disc Rim" in Investigative Ophthalmology and Visual Science (2021)*

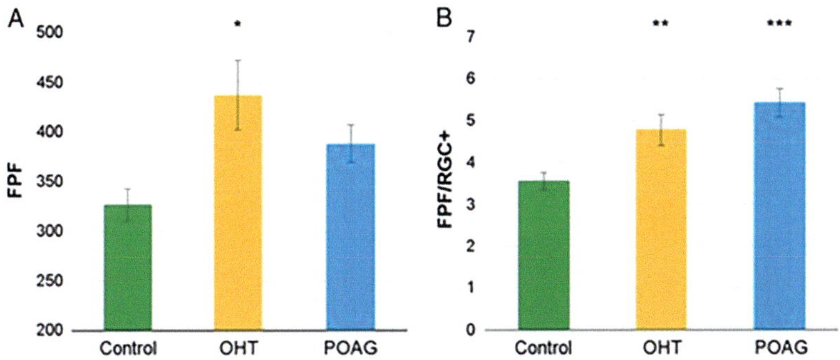

Fig. 25.4 FPF measurements in unaffected control, OHT, and POAG eyes. **(A)** FPF is significantly elevated in OHT eyes compared to control eyes. **(B)** FPF divided by retinal ganglion cell-plus layer (RGC+) thickness values are significantly elevated in POAG and OHT eyes compared to controls. Error bars correspond to the SEM. **p < 0.05, **p < 0.01, ***p < 0.001. Reprinted with permission from Dr. Lawrence Gayman, MD and Dr. Richard Rosen, MD's "Mitochondrial Dysfunction in Primary Open-angle Glaucoma Characterized by Flavoprotein Fluorescence at the Optic Disc Rim" in Investigative Ophthalmology and Visual Science (2021)*

was measured within an elliptical annulus around the ONH rim, with the inner and outer boundaries corresponding to 0.5–1.1 times the ONH rim size. After adjusting for age and intraocular pressure, they found that eyes with POAG displayed significantly increased FPF intensity in the temporal, superior, inferior, and nasal anatomic sectors compared to control subjects. In POAG eyes, FPF was significantly correlated with visual field mean deviation, visual field pattern standard deviation, and cpRNFL thickness.

25.4 FPF in Genetically Inherited Retinal Dystrophies

In degenerative retinal dystrophies, mitochondrial dysfunction is thought to be primarily caused by pathological alterations in mitochondrial DNA (mtDNA), downregulated mitochondrial function in mitochondrial dystrophies or increased production of reactive oxygen species in rod-cone retinal dystrophies. Elner et al. was the first to demonstrate that patients with retinitis pigmentosa possess significantly elevated FPF compared to age-matched controls [11, 12]. Most recently, Russell et al. studied FPF in 121 eyes from 61 patients with various retinal dystrophies [Rod-Cone dystrophies (Retinitis pigmentosa, Usher syndrome), 31 eyes with Stargardt disease, 4 eyes with Bardet-Biedl Syndrome, 6 eyes with mitochondrial encephalomyopathy, lactic acidosis, and stroke-like episodes (MELAS), and 2 eyes with Mitochondrial ATP synthase subunit 6 mutation (MT-ATP6)] compared to 121 eyes from 96 healthy control patients [23]. They demonstrated that patients with Bardet-Biedl Syndrome, rod-cone dystrophies, Stargardt's disease, and MT-ATP6 possess significantly increased FPF intensity compared to age-matched controls. Those patients with rod-cone dystrophies, Stargardt's disease, and BBS

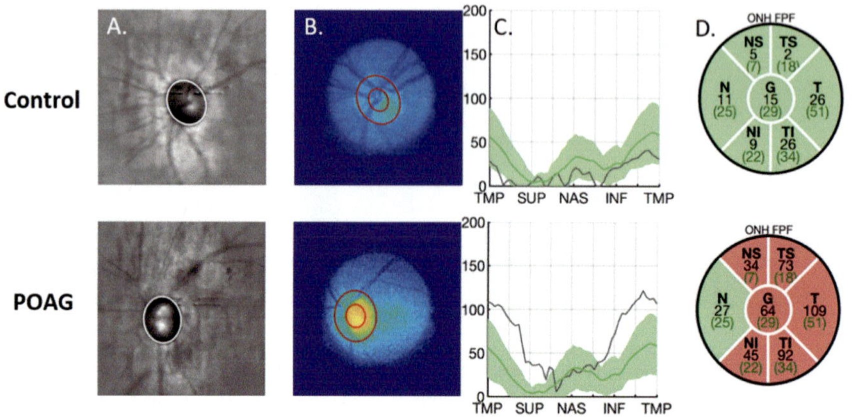

Fig. 25.5 FPF imaging at the optic nerve head (ONH) in primary open angle glaucoma (POAG). (A) A 23° × 23° infrared image of a representative control eye (upper row) versus a POAG eye (lower row). The white ellipse indicates the ONH and FPF capture field spanning 13° in diameter. (B) FPF measurement at the ONH was obtained by including the fluorescence signal between the inner and outer red ellipses generated at radiometric distances 0.5 and 1.1 times, respectively, of the white ONH ellipse perimeter. This annulus captures the highest concentration of FPF signal, which coincides with the distribution of mitochondria at the ONH. (C) FPF anatomic sector map with horizontal axis orientation following a circumferential format demonstrating FPF measurements in a representative control eye (upper) compared to a POAG eye (bottom). The green line and green area indicate the mean ± standard deviation (SD) of FPF in healthy controls. (D) Sectoral presentation of measurements with mean FPF profile in a POAG eye reflecting averaged measurements from each anatomic sector. Reference mean FPF values from healthy controls are indicated in the green text. The center region represents the global average of all FPF sectors. G = global; gsu = gray scale unit; I = inferior; INF = inferior; N = nasal; NAS = nasal; NI = nasal inferior; NS = nasal superior; S = superior; SUP = superior; T = temporal; TI = temporal inferior; TMP = temporal; TS = temporal superior. *Reprinted with permission from Dr. Davis Zhou, MD and Dr. Richard Rosen, MD's "Mitochondrial Dysfunction in Primary Open-angle Glaucoma Characterized by Flavoprotein Fluorescence at the Optic Disc Rim" in Investigative Ophthalmology and Visual Science (2021)*

also possessed significantly greater FPF heterogeneity compared to age-matched controls. Interestingly, no significant difference was noted between patients with MELAS and controls in terms of either FPF intensity or heterogeneity. Several potential explanations have been offered for this finding, including small sample size (6 eyes were included within the present study), the effect of pigment mottling on dilated fundus exam and color fundus photography, or some unknown aspect of the pathophysiology of MELAS. Patients with MELAS have tRNA mutations and thus may not have sufficiently impaired mitochondrial function to generate an FPF signal. Significant differences in FPF were also noted between patients with MELAS and Bardet Biedl Syndrome, rod-cone dystrophies and Bardet Biedl Syndrome, Stargardt's disease and Bardet Biedl Syndrome, and MT-ATP6. Of

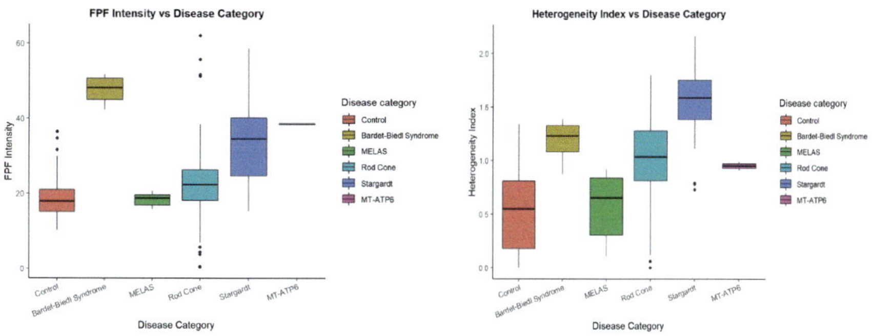

Fig. 25.6 Comparison of FPF intensity and heterogeneity of patients with various retinal dystrophies with age-matched healthy controls. Subjects with Bardet-Biedl Syndrome (BBS), rod cone dystrophies, Stargardt's disease, and MT-ATP6 possess significantly increased FPF intensity compared to age-matched controls. Those patients with Rod-cone dystrophies, Stargardt's disease, and BBS also possessed significantly greater FPF heterogeneity compared to age-matched controls. No significant difference in FPF was noted between patients with MELAS and controls. *Reprinted with permission from Dr. Rishi Singh, MD's "Functional imaging of mitochondria in genetically confirmed retinal dystrophies using flavoprotein fluorescence" and Taylor & Francis Online (2023)*

note, FPF signal was found to be correlated with the dystrophic lesions on fundus autofluorescence in representative patients with retinitis pigmentosa, Stargardt disease, and MT-ATP6 as well (Figs. 25.6 and 25.7).

25.5 FPF in Diabetes Mellitus with and Without Retinopathy

The pathophysiological mechanisms underlying mitochondrial dysfunction in diabetes mellitus are related to chronic hyperglycemia stimulating the production of advanced glycation end products (AGEs) and other toxic pro-inflammatory metabolites via the diacylglycerol protein kinase C (DAG-PKC) pathway and sorbitol via the polyol pathway [1]. Animal models of diabetic retinopathy have implicated increased production of mitochondrial superoxide in the apoptosis of retinal pericytes and endothelial cells [24, 25]. Compared to subjects with diabetes mellitus with no retinopathy, patients with diabetic retinopathy had significantly elevated FPF [11, 12]. Field et al. evaluated FPF in 42 eyes of 21 subjects with diabetes mellitus compared to control eyes and found that the diabetic subjects with retinopathy in at least one eye displayed significantly elevated FPF intensity and heterogeneity compared to diabetic subjects without retinopathy in either eye [26]. More recently, Andrade Romo et al. investigated the impact of anti-VEGF therapy on FPF in 8 diabetic retinopathy subjects and found that treatment significantly reduced FPF intensity in 5 out of 8 patients (Fig. 25.8, [15]). This reduction in FPF was found to be independent of structural changes at the macula, as evaluated by the central macular thickness (CMT) on optical coherence tomography

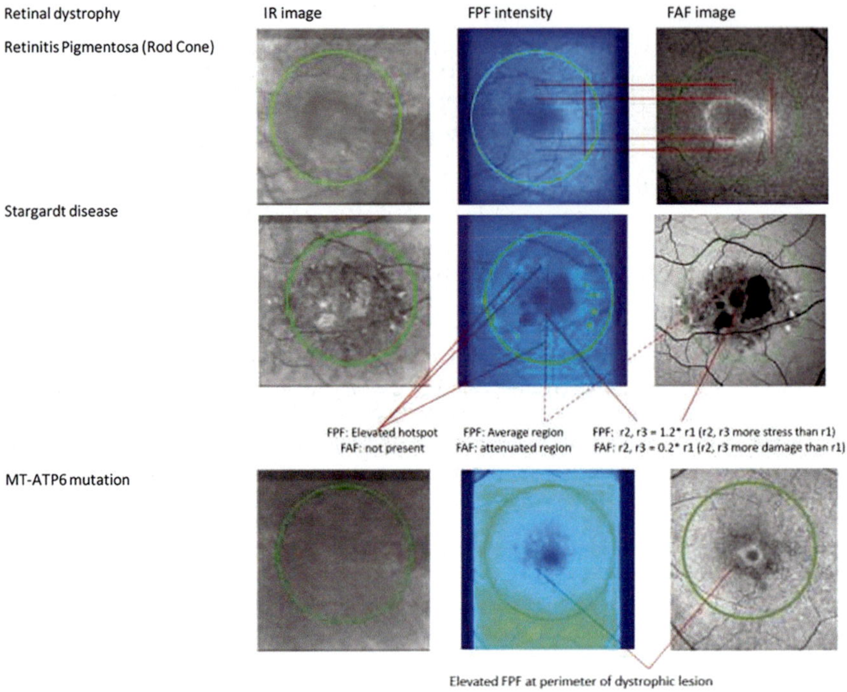

Fig. 25.7 Comparison of FPF signal strength with fundus autofluorescence (FAF) in three patients with retinal dystrophies. Areas with increased FPF signal were noted to correspond with lesions with decreased signal on FAF, further highlighting the difference between the autofluorescense of flavoprotein vs. lipofuscin. Elevated FPF at the perimeter of the dystrophic lesion was found in a representative patient with MT-ATP6. *Reprinted with permission from Dr. Rishi Singh, MD's "Functional imaging of mitochondria in genetically confirmed retinal dystrophies using flavoprotein fluorescence" and Taylor and Francis Online (2023)*

(OCT). In contrast, reduction in FPF in response to anti-VEGF therapy correlated with improvement in best corrected visual acuity (BCVA), more so than with improved CMT (Fig. 25.9). Chen et al. conducted the largest cohort study to date involving 117 diabetic eyes and 151 age-matched control eyes which found that FPF intensity and heterogeneity were significantly elevated in diabetic eyes compared to age-matched eyes [1]. Age and female gender were found to be predictive of elevated FPF intensity values and elevated FPF heterogeneity scores were found to be correlated with poorer visual acuity.

25.6 FPF in Age-Related Macular Degeneration

In age-related macular degeneration, advanced age is thought to predispose individuals to increased levels of oxidative stress and mitochondrial dysfunction particularly in the retinal pigment epithelium (RPE). Mitochondrial DNA

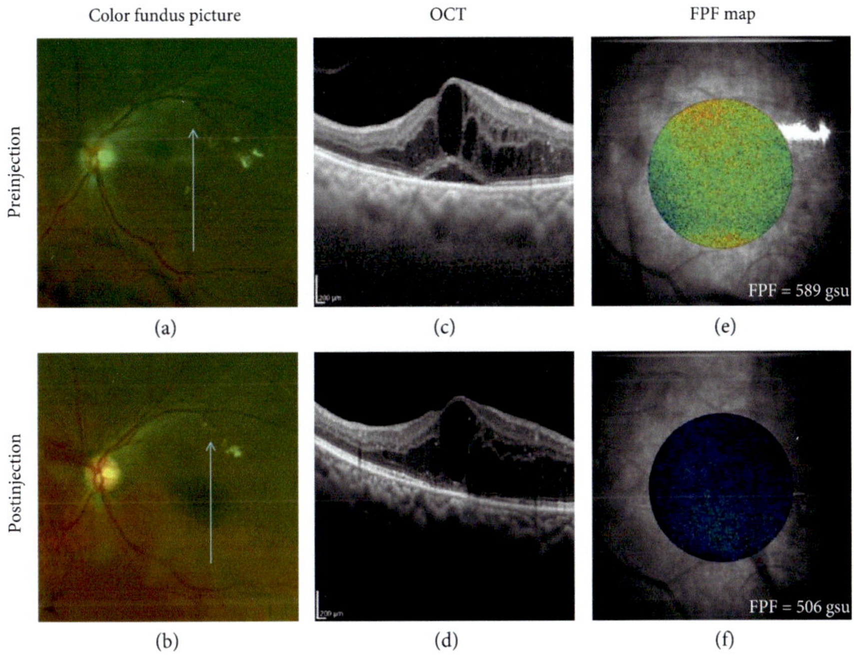

Fig. 25.8 Color fundus photos (**A** and **B**), OCT B-scan (**C** and **D**), and FPF maps (**E** and **F**) indicating structural and functional changes at the macula pre- and post-therapy with anti-VEGF administration in a 65-year-old male patient with proliferative diabetic retinopathy (PDR) and cystic macular edema (CME). Central macular thickness prior to injection was 574 μm (**C**) and 541 μm post-injection (**D**). The FPF maps indicate a transition from increased green-yellow coloration prior to injection (**E**) to dark blue coloration (**F**), indicating a reduction in FPF at the macula post-injection. *Reprinted with permission from Dr. Jorge Andrade Romo, MD and Dr. Richard Rosen, MD's "Flavoprotein Fluorescence Correlation with Visual Acuity Response in Patients Receiving Anti VEGF Injection for Diabetic Macular Edema (2018)*

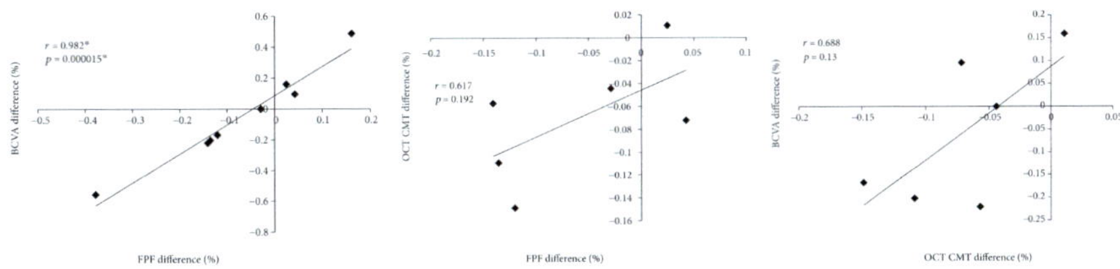

Fig. 25.9 Pearson correlation coefficients demonstrating a strong correlation (r = 0.98, p = 0.000015) between FPF difference and improvement in BCVA prior to and after anti-VEGF administration. The correlation between reduction in CMT and FPF (r = 0.617, p = 0.192) was not found to be statistically significant. *Reprinted with permission from Dr. Jorge Andrade Romo, MD and Dr. Richard Rosen, MD's "Flavoprotein Fluorescence Correlation with Visual Acuity Response in Patients Receiving Anti-VEGF Injection for Diabetic Macular Edema" (2018)*

(mtDNA) damage and decreased repair of retinal tissue predisposes individuals to significant reductions in RPE mitochondrial density and matrix density [1]. In patients with geographic atrophy (GA), oxidation of protein and DNA and lipid peroxidation have been observed in histochemical studies [27]. Inflammasome activation in the RPE has also been implicated in AMD [28]. Elner et al. was the first to observe elevations in FPF in a patient with exudative AMD [11, 12]. In 2012, Field et al. assessed FPF in 3 eyes with non-exudative age-related macular degeneration (AMD) with GA and 3 eyes without GA compared to 6 healthy age-matched controls. They found that all non-exudative AMD eyes with and without GA had significantly elevated FPF compared to control eyes [29]. Eyes with GA were found to possess higher FPF heterogeneity than eyes without GA, suggesting that there is increased variability in detectable levels of mitochondrial dysfunction in those patients with advanced disease. A more recent study enrolled 456 eyes (228 AMD eyes, 228 age-matched control eyes) to study FPF [30]. 31 eyes with early AMD, 107 eyes with intermediate AMD, 19 eyes with GA, and 21 eyes with neovascular AMD were included in this study. The authors found that intermediate, GA, and exudative AMD diagnoses correlated with significantly increased FPF intensity. All AMD stages significantly correlated with increased FPF heterogeneity. FPF intensity and heterogeneity were also found to be significant negative predictors of visual acuity (Fig. 25.10).

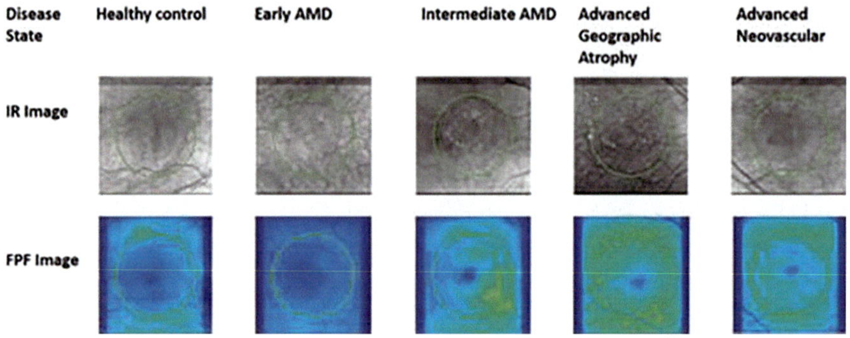

Fig. 25.10 Representative infrared (IR) and FPF images from each AMD stage compared to a healthy age-matched control. As the disease process progresses, FPF increases, as indicated by increased yellow-green coloration in the FPF image. In the GA case, the region of atrophy corresponds to a lack of FPF signal in the same anatomic location. Increased FPF signal is observed to correspond with areas of increased choroidal neovascularization in the exudative AMD case. *Reprinted with permission from Dr. Rishi Singh, MD's "Functional Imaging of Mitochondria in Age-Related Macular Degeneration Using Flavoprotein Fluorescence" (2023)*

25.7 FPF in Central Serous Chorioretinopathy (CSCR)

The pathogenesis of central serous chorioretinopathy (CSCR) is thought to involve dysfunction of the RPE and choriocapillaris and subsequent breakdown of the outer blood-retina barrier (oBRB). On optical coherence tomography (OCT), patients will classically present with neurosensory and retinal epithelial detachments and occasionally, cystic changes within the retina. Elner et al. imaged a 49-year-old patient with bilateral CSR without subretinal or sub-RPE fluid and found significant elevations in both FPF intensity and heterogeneity in both eyes [11, 12]. Field et al. extended the clinical investigation of FPF to 3 eyes with CSCR and found that eyes with CSCR had significantly elevated FPF intensity and heterogeneity compared to contralateral unaffected eyes and age-matched control eyes [31]. More recently, Ahsanuddin et al. found that a cohort of 10 CSR patients also exhibited FPF intensity values that were 1.7 times as high as the age-matched control group [17]. In contrast to standard fundus autofluorescence, which typically detects RPE abnormalities several weeks after disease onset, elevations in FPF could be detected as early as one week of disease onset in Field et al.'s study. Field et al. used these findings to support the notion that the FPF signal is not due to lipofuscin, but due to dysfunctional mitochondrial activity in early CSCR (but before photoreceptor apoptosis occurs). These findings suggest that FPF could be used as an early signal of CSCR-induced retinal metabolic stress or impending recurrence.

25.8 Summary and Future Directions

In summary, this book chapter highlights the potential utility of flavoprotein fluorescence as a rapid, noninvasive, and quantitative indicator of in vivo mitochondrial dysfunction in the human retina. FPF has been found to be a robust and sensitive metric for evaluating the severity of retinal disease states known to be mediated by oxidative stress, even prior to structural changes detected on OCT. FPF has the clinically useful diagnostic capability to differentiate healthy eyes from diseased eyes and for monitoring the effect of anti-VEGF therapy in diabetic macular edema. Future potential investigations will evaluate FPF's utility for monitoring new therapeutic approaches for geographic atrophy or glaucoma where structural deterioration follows insidious metabolic dysfunction.

References

1. Chen AX, Conti TF, Hom GL, Greenlee TE, Raimondi R, Briskin IN, et al. Functional imaging of mitochondria in retinal diseases using flavoprotein fluorescence. Eye. 2021;35:74–92. https://doi.org/10.1038/s41433-020-1110-y.
2. Kisilevsky E, Freund P, Margolin E. Mitochondrial disorders and the eye. Survey Ophthalmol. 2020;65:294–311. https://doi.org/10.1016/j.survophthal.2019.11.001.

3. Nascimento-dos-Santos G, de-Souza-Ferreira E, Lani R, Faria CC, Araújo VG, Teixeira-Pinheiro LC, et al. Neuroprotection from optic nerve injury and modulation of oxidative metabolism by transplantation of active mitochondria to the retina. BBA Mol Basis Dis. 2020;1866:165686. https://doi.org/10.1016/j.bbadis.2020.165686
4. Chan DC. Mitochondria: dynamic organelles in disease, aging, and development. Cell. 2006;125:1241–52. https://doi.org/10.1016/j.cell.2006.06.010.
5. Ferrington DA, Kenney MC, Atilano SR, Hurley JB, Brown EE, Ash JD. Mitochondria: the retina's achilles' heel in AMD. Adv Exp Med Biol. 2021;1256:237–64. https://doi.org/10.1007/978-3-030-66014-7_10.
6. Wang L-L, Yu Q-L, Han L, Ma X-L, Song R-D, Zhao S-N, et al. Study on the effect of reactive oxygen species-mediated oxidative stress on the activation of mitochondrial apoptosis and the tenderness of yak meat. Food Chem. 2018;244:394–402. https://doi.org/10.1016/j.foodchem.2017.10.034.
7. Avrutsky MI, Ortiz CC, Johnson KV, Potenski AM, Chen CW, Lawson JM, et al. Endothelial activation of caspase-9 promotes neurovascular injury in retinal vein occlusion. Nat Commun. 2020;11:3173. https://doi.org/10.1038/s41467-020-16902-5.
8. Feher J, Kovacs I, Artico M, Cavallotti C, Papale A, Balacco GC. Mitochondrial alterations of retinal pigment epithelium in age-related macular degeneration. Neurobiol Aging. 2006;27:983–93. https://doi.org/10.1016/j.neurobiolaging.2005.05.012.
9. Masuda T, Shimazawa M, Hara H. Retinal diseases associated with oxidative stress and the effects of a free radical scavenger (edaravone). Oxid Med Cell Longev. 2017;2017:9208489. https://doi.org/10.1155/2017/9208489.
10. Zhong Q, Kowluru RA. Epigenetic changes in mitochondrial superoxide dismutase in the retina and the development of diabetic retinopathy. Diabetes. 2011;60:1304–13. https://doi.org/10.2337/db10-0133.
11. Elner VM, Park S, Cornblath W, Hackel R, Petty HR. Flavoprotein autofluorescence detection of early ocular dysfunction. Arch Ophthalmol. 2008a;126(2):259–60. https://doi.org/10.1001/archophthalmol.2007.44.
12. Elner SG, Elner VM, Field MG, Park S, Heckenlively JR, Petty HR. Retinal flavoprotein autofluorescence as a measure of retinal health. Trans Am Ophthalmological Soc. 2008b;106:215–22.
13. Moon J, Yun J, Yoon YD, Park SI, Seo YJ, Park WS, et al. Blue light effect on retinal pigment epithelial cells by display devices. Integr Biol Quantitative Biosci Nano to Macro. 2017;9:436–43. https://doi.org/10.1039/C7IB00032D
14. Hsueh J, Raimondi R, Hom G, Conti T, Singh RP. Flavoprotein fluorescence is a marker of AMD progression. Invest Ophthalmol Visual Sci. 2019;60:9.
15. Andrade Romo JS, Lynch G, Liu K, Kim D, Jansen M, Field MG, et al. Flavoprotein fluorescence correlation with visual acuity response in patients receiving anti-VEGF injection for diabetic macular edema. Oxid Med Cell Longevity. 2018;2018:3567306. https://doi.org/10.1155/2018/3567306.
16. Zhou DB, Castanos MV, Geyman L, et al. Mitochondrial dysfunction in primary open-angle glaucoma characterized by flavoprotein fluorescence at the optic nerve head. Ophthalmol Glaucoma. 2022;5(4):413–20. https://doi.org/10.1016/j.ogla.2021.12.006.
17. Ahsanuddin S, Rios HA, Otero-Marquez O, Macanian J, Zhou D, Rich C, Rosen RB. Flavoprotein fluorescence elevation is a marker of mitochondrial oxidative stress in patients with retinal disease. Front Ophthalmol. 2023. https://doi.org/10.3389/fopht.2023.1110501.
18. Sun MT, Beykin G, Lee WS, Sun Y, Chang R, Nunez M, et al. Structural and metabolic imaging after short-term use of the balance goggles system in glaucoma patients: a pilot study. J Glaucoma. 2022;31:634–8. https://doi.org/10.1097/IJG.0000000000002066.
19. Field MG, Yang D, Bian ZM, Petty HR, Elner VM. Retinal flavoprotein fluorescence correlates with mitochondrial stress, apoptosis, and chemokine expression. Exp Eye Res. 2011;93(4):548–55. https://doi.org/10.1016/j.exer.2011.06.023.

20. Ju W-K, Liu Q, Kim K-Y, Crowston JG, Lindsey JD, Agarwal N, et al. Elevated hydrostatic pressure triggers mitochondrial fission and decreases cellular ATP in differentiated RGC-5 cells. Investig Ophthalmol Vis Sci. 2007;48:2145–51.
21. Geyman LS, Suwan Y, Garg R, Field MG, Krawitz BD, Mo S, Pinhas A, Ritch R, Rosen RB. Noninvasive detection of mitochondrial dysfunction in ocular hypertension and primary open-angle glaucoma. J Glaucoma. 2018;27(7):592–599. https://doi.org/10.1097/IJG.0000000000000980. PMID: 29750714.
22. Zhou DB, Castanos Toral MV, Geyman LS, Rich C, Tantraworasin A, Ritch R, Rosen RB. Mitochondrial dysfunction in primary open-angle glaucoma characterized by flavoprotein fluorescence at the optic disc rim. Investig Ophthalmol Vis Sci. 2021;62:1769.
23. Russell MW, Muste JC, Seth K, et al. Functional imaging of mitochondria in genetically confirmed retinal dystrophies using flavoprotein fluorescence. Ophthalmic Genet. 2022;43(6):834–40. https://doi.org/10.1080/13816810.2022.2144903.
24. Du Y, Miller CM, Kern TS. Hyperglycemia increases mitochondrial superoxide in retina and retinal cells. Free Rad Biol Med. 2003;35:1491–9.
25. Kowluru RA, Abbas SN. Diabetes-induced mitochondrial dysfunction in the retina. Invest Ophthalmol Vis Sci. 2003;44:5327–34.
26. Field MG, Elner VM, Puro DG, et al. Rapid, noninvasive detection of diabetes-induced retinal metabolic stress. Arch Ophthalmol. 2008;126(7):934–8. https://doi.org/10.1001/archopht.126.7.934.
27. Shen JK, Dong A, Hackett SF, Bell WR, Green WR, Campochiaro PA. Oxidative damage in age-related macular degeneration. Histol Histopathol. 2007;22:1301–8.
28. Piippo N, Korhonen E, Hytti M, Kinnunen K, Kaarniranta K, Kauppinen A. Oxidative stress is the principal contributor to inflammasome activation in retinal pigment epithelium cells with defunct proteasomes and autophagy. Cell Physiol Biochem. 2018;49:359–67.
29. Field MG, Comer GM, Kawaji T, Petty HR, Elner VM. Noninvasive imaging of mitochondrial dysfunction in dry age-related macular degeneration. Ophthalmic Surg Lasers Imaging. 2012;43(5):358–65. https://doi.org/10.3928/15428877-20120712-02.
30. Muste JC, Russell MW, Chen AX, et al. Functional imaging of mitochondria in age-related macular degeneration using flavoprotein fluorescence. Ophthalmic Surg Lasers Imaging Retina. 2023;54(1):24–31. https://doi.org/10.3928/23258160-20221214-03.
31. Field MG, Elner VM, Park S, et al. Detection of retinal metabolic stress resulting from central serous retinopathy. Retina. 2009;29(8):1162–6. https://doi.org/10.1097/IAE.0b013e3181a3b923.

Empowering Optical Coherence Tomography with AI: A New Era for Neuro-Ophthalmic and Neurological Disorders

26

Charis Y. N. Chiang, Dan Milea, and Michaël J. A. Girard

Abstract

Many neuro-ophthalmic and neurological disorders can lead to irreversible neurodegeneration, thereby impacting the visual pathways at various levels, from the retina to the visual cortex. Optical coherence tomography (OCT), particularly 3-D structural eye scans of the retina and optic nerve head, have recently described various abnormalities associated to neurodegeneration. However, interpreting these scans require significant expertise, time and resources. Alternatively, recent advances in artificial intelligence methods applied to OCT

C. Y. N. Chiang · M. J. A. Girard (✉)
Ophthalmic Engineering & Innovation Laboratory, Emory Eye Center, Emory School of Medicine, Emory Clinic Building B, 1365B Clifton Road, NE, GA Atlanta 30322, USA
e-mail: mgirard@ophthalmic.engineering
URL: https://www.ophthalmic.engineering

C. Y. N. Chiang
Department of Biomedical Engineering, National University of Singapore, Singapore, Singapore

D. Milea
Visual Neuroscience Group, Singapore Eye Research Institute, Singapore National Eye Centre, Singapore, Singapore

D. Milea · M. J. A. Girard
Duke-NUS Graduate Medical School, Singapore, Singapore

C. Y. N. Chiang · M. J. A. Girard
Singapore Eye Research Institute, Singapore National Eye Centre, Singapore, Singapore

M. J. A. Girard
Department of Biomedical Engineering, Georgia Institute of Technology/Emory University, Atlanta, GA, USA

Emory Empathetic AI for Health Institute, Emory University, Atlanta, GA, USA

D. Milea
Rothschild Foundation Hospital, Paris, France

A. Grzybowski and P. Barboni (eds.), *OCT and Imaging in Central Nervous System Diseases*, https://doi.org/10.1007/978-3-031-72156-4_26

scans present immense potential for detecting a wide range of neurological diseases that directly or indirectly affect the visual pathways. In this chapter, we will discuss a range of AI-based methods for diagnosis, prognosis, and screening, specifically focusing on the use of OCT images in various neurological disorders. These disorders encompass a wide range, including, but not limited to, multiple sclerosis, Alzheimer's disease, glaucoma, and papilledema.

Keywords

Artificial intelligence • Optical coherence tomography • Optic nerve head • Retina • Neurological and neuro-ophthalmic disorders • Multiple sclerosis • Glaucoma • Papilledema • Alzheimer's disease

Abbreviations

AD	Alzheimer's Disease
CNS	Central Nervous System
ICP	Intracranial Pressure
IIH	Intracranial Hypertension
MCI	Mild Cognitive Impairment
MS	Multiple Sclerosis
ODD	Optic Disc Drusen
ON	Optic Neuritis
PD	Parkinson's Disease
CSF	Cerebral Spinal Fluid
MRI	Magnetic Resonance Imaging
OCT	Optical Coherence Tomography
PET	Photon Emission Tomography
ONH	Optic nerve head
RNFL	Retinal Nerve Fiber Layer
GCL	Ganglion Cell Layer
GC-IPL	Ganglion Cell-Inner Plexiform Layer
IPL	Inner Plexiform Layer
INL	Inner Nuclear Layer
OPL	Outer Plexiform Layer
ONL	Outer Nuclear Layer
AI	Artificial Intelligence
AUC	Area Under the Curve
DL	Deep Learning
GAN	Generative Adversarial Network
ML	Machine Learning
MLP	Multi-Layer Perceptron
NN	Neural Network
SVM	Support Vector Machine

26.1 Background

The eye has been described as an extension to the brain, and it provides an accessible window to examine, diagnose and prognose neurological disorders that could prove indispensable [1, 2]. The central nervous system (CNS) and the eye, specifically the retina and optic nerve, share a common developmental origin from the neuroectoderm [3]. Thus, the eye is an anatomical and developmental extension of the CNS. Consequentially, these structures exhibit numerous similarities in terms of anatomy, physiology and biomechanisms [1, 2]. Thus, it is unsurprising that ocular symptoms and manifestations are frequently observed in a wide range of neurological disorders, including neurodegenerative disorders [4–6]. There is growing evidence to show that ocular biomarkers, in addition to neural markers, can be used for the detection of neurodegeneration [7, 8]. This could be ground-breaking for mass screening, prognosis and management of neurological conditions because of the increasing prevalence of neurological disorders and limitations of current neuroimaging tools.

In a recent study [9] that assessed the global burden of diseases, it was found that neurological disorders ranked as the leading cause of disability worldwide and the second most prevalent cause of death globally. As life-expectancy continues to rise, there will be a corresponding increase in the prevalence of age-related neurodegenerative and neuro-ophthalmic disorders [4]. In most brain-related disorders, the key pathophysiological change associated with disability is neurodegeneration; some of the most prevalent neurological disorders are Alzheimer's Disease (AD) and other dementias, Parkinson's Disease (PD), Multiple Sclerosis (MS), stroke and even glaucoma [9–12]. Many of these neurodegenerative conditions are considered non-reversible due to the limited capability of the CNS for self-repair and the absence of effective medical treatments [1]. Therefore, the current approach to managing these neurodegenerative conditions emphasizes early detection and treatment to prevent further debilitation and slow down or arrest worsening of the condition [10]. Another subset of neurological conditions are neuro-ophthalmic disorders, which encompass vision disorders related to the nervous system, these disorders include papilledema, optic neuritis (ON) and ischemic optic neuropathy [13]. Early diagnosis is also key in increasing the likelihood of successful treatment and potentially reversing the vision deterioration associated with these conditions [14, 15].

However, the existing screening and diagnostic methods for many neurological disorders are currently inadequate, particularly in the early stages where successful treatment is more feasible [4]. This is due to the limitations of the current procedures which often involve clinical assessments, biomarker tests such as cerebral spinal fluid (CSF) or blood sampling and neuroimaging such as magnetic resonance imaging (MRI), computed tomography and/or photon emission tomography (PET); these tests are limited by high cost, subjectivity in analysis, invasiveness, and/or limited accessibility [4, 16, 17].

Conversely, ocular imaging offers advantages such as affordability, time-efficiency and greater accessibility, making it a more suitable option for testing a larger population. Fundus photography is a standard clinical procedure for capturing 2D images of the optic-disc and macular surface [18]. A study conducted by Milea et al. demonstrated the potential of AI in detecting optic-disc abnormalities, such as papilledema, from fundus photographs [18]. While the simplicity and widespread availability of fundus photography make it a useful tool, especially for mass screening purposes, 3D imaging could offer additional information, particularly for studying subtle structural changes.

One particularly promising tool to image 3D ocular structures is optical coherence tomography (OCT). OCT is a non-invasive technology that can capture clearly differentiated signals corresponding to different tissues, and thus, produce three-dimensional cross-section images of various sections of the human eye, including the macula and the optic nerve head (ONH) [19]. OCTs can be taken in mere seconds and up to spatial resolutions of 3 microns, sometimes less, enabling the analysis of tissues from a general structural or geometrical level down to at an almost cellular level [20]. These tissue layers (as shown in Fig. 26.1) include the retinal nerve fiber layer (RNFL), ganglion cell layer (GCL), inner plexiform layer (IPL), inner nuclear layer (INL), outer plexiform layer (OPL), outer nuclear layer (ONL), photoreceptor layer, retinal pigment epithelium, choroid, sclera and in ONH scans, the lamina cribosa [21, 22].

In the last decade, OCT has become invaluable to the research and diagnosis of many eye disorders [23]. However, the challenge of using OCT lies in its analysis. Typically, major tissue layers and regions in OCT scans are segmented to measure parameters such as tissue layer thicknesses or tissue volumes. However, manual segmentation is time-consuming and subject to bias, while automated segmentation algorithms incorporated into commercial OCT devices used clinically are also prone to segmentation errors [22, 24]. Additionally, the performance of automatic segmentation models can vary across retinal regions and diseases [24] and lowered performances could be observed in scans where the same disease group was not incorporated into the training data as the algorithm may not have learnt to segment abnormal patterns associated with those diseases. This has led to the exploration of using Artificial Intelligence (AI) to automate OCT analysis of both healthy and diseased eyes in recent years [22, 25]. AI-based segmentation should eliminate the need for a trained professional such as neuro-ophthalmologists and neurologists to manually review each scan, thus removing the bottleneck in using OCT for mass-screening of neuro-ophthalmic disorders.

AI is the attempt at simulating human intelligence to solve problems autonomously, without human assistance. Machine learning (ML) algorithms have emerged as a powerful class of AI methods enabling highly accurate diagnosis and management of various diseases when provided with OCT data and relevant features [23]. Deep learning (DL) models are a subclass of ML that excel in analysing and extracting valuable insights from both 2D and 3D images. They leverage the hierarchical nature of image features, enabling precise localization and comprehensive understanding of the spatial information encoded within the images [26]. DL models particularly benefit from large datasets, as this enhances the accuracy and generalisability of the models [27]. As such, the ease and safety in obtaining

a
b
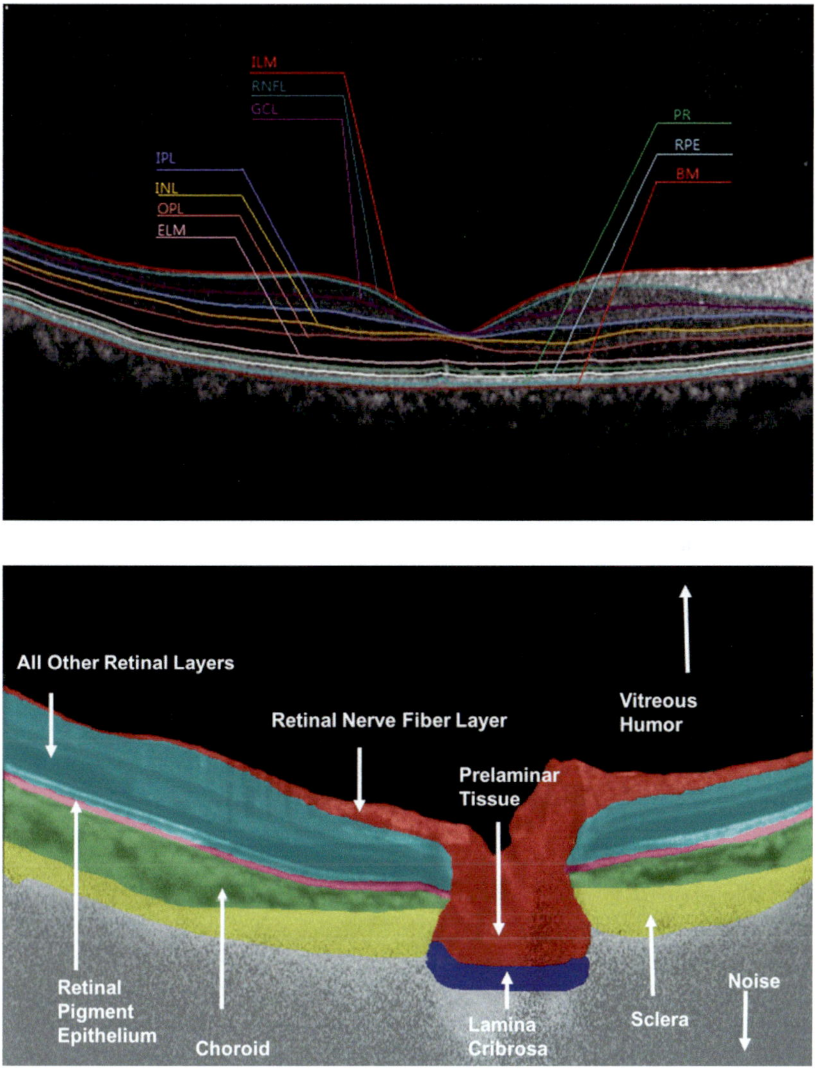

Fig. 26.1 Segmentation of tissue layers in optical coherence tomography for analysis of **a** macula scans, and **b** optic nerve head scans. The following tissue layers could be visible in OCT scans: (1) inner limiting membrane (ILM); (2) retinal nerve fiber layer (RNFL); (3) ganglion cell layer (GCL); (4) inner plexiform layer (IPL); (5) inner nuclear layer (INL); (6) outer plexiform layer (OPL); (7) outer nuclear layer (ONL); (8) photoreceptor (PR) layer; (9) retinal pigment epithelium (RPE); (10) Bruch's membrane (BM); (11) choroid; (12) sclera; (13) and in only ONH scans, the lamina cribosa. Panel **a** retrieved from Han et al. https://doi.org/10.1371/journal.pone.0197058 PLOS ONE [103]. Panel **b** retrieved from Devalla et al. https://doi.org/10.48550/arXiv.1803.00232 arXiv. [104]. Both panels were reproduced under the Creative Commons Attribution 4.0 International License (http://creativecommons.org/licenses/by/4.0/)

scans with OCT make it a prime tool for AI application in many ophthalmological studies [23]. Please refer to Appendix A for more detailed information about various ML and DL models used in OCT studies, as well as the performance metrics commonly used to evaluate these models.

Most studies investigating the application of AI to OCT scans for the diagnosis and prognosis of neurological disorders typically follow a two-stage process: feature extraction followed by classification. In the initial stage, these studies explore the extraction of key features from OCT scans, either statistical or AI methods [23]. Subsequently, in the second stage, the extracted features are used to classify the scans, serving diagnostic and prognostic purposes and facilitating an understanding of the disease pathology for effective disease management and treatment [23]. Similar methods are starting to be applied to the study of neurological disorders through OCT imaging of the eye, and it has emerged as a promising mass-screening tool [28, 29].

In this chapter, we will discuss how ML and DL approaches applied to OCT scans have shown immense potential in facilitating the automated detection, diagnosis, and prognosis of a variety of neurological and neuro-ophthalmic disorders. These disorders include multiple sclerosis, Alzheimer's disease, Parkinson's disease, bipolar disease, glaucoma, and papilledema. We will also explore the limitations of current works and potential future trends in this field.

26.2 Current Applications

Many studies using OCT and AI-based solutions have attempted to identify and classify neurological disorders (Table 26.1).

26.2.1 Multiple Sclerosis

Multiple sclerosis is a neurodegenerative disease characterized by demyelination and axonal degeneration in the CNS, resulting in progressive neurologic deficits [30, 31]. It is the number one cause of neurological disability amongst the global young and middle-aged adult population with rising prevalence over the past decade [32–34]. In 2020, an estimated 2.8 million people worldwide were suffering from MS [32]. MS presents with a wide range of symptoms, including motor and sensory dysfunction, as well as depression, anxiety, fatigue, chronic pain, and cognitive impairment [33, 34]. Inflammation associated with MS can also lead to optic neuritis, characterized by inflammation-induced damage to the optic nerve [35]. The diagnosis of MS is based on the McDonald criteria which involves clinical evaluation, neuroimaging (including MRI) and laboratory tests such as blood tests for serum markers and lumbar puncture for CSF analysis [30, 33, 36]. However, the McDonald criteria may not be applicable in the early stages of MS, it involves costly and invasive testing, and it requires the exclusion of MS mimics [37].

Table 26.1 Table of studies using AI and OCT for neurological disorders

Author	Year	Disorder	Task	AI models employed	Number of subjects	Results
Kenney et al.	2022	Multiple sclerosis (MS), with and without optic neuritis (ON)	Predict history of ON	Support vector machine and logistic regression	NC: 552 MS without ON: 874 MS with ON: 488	Sen: 81% Spe: 80% AUC = 0.89
Cavaliere et al.	2019	MS	Predict diagnosis	Support vector machine	NC: 48 MS: 48	Acc: 0.91 Sen: 0.89 Spe: 0.92 AUC: 0.97
Garcia-Martin et al.	2013	MS with ON	Predict diagnosis	Multi-layer perceptron neural networks	NC: 106 MS with ON: 115	Diagnostic precision: 88.5% Sen: 89.3% Spe: 87.6%
Lopez-Dorado et al.	2021	MS	Predict diagnosis	Convolutional neural networks, and data augmentation	NC: 48 MS: 48	Sen: 1.0 Spe: 1.0
Kavaklioglu et al.	2022	MS and other central nervous system demyelinating disorders	Predict diagnosis	Random forest; Multiclass distinction	NC: 69 MS: 57 MOGAD[a]: 27 MonoADS: 92 NMOSD: 11	Acc: 75% for DD Acc: 80% for MS Acc: 64% for multiclass distinction
Montolío et al.	2021	MS	Predict prognosis	Various machine learning models	NC: 104 MS: 108	Acc: 87.7% Sen: 87.0% Spe: 88.5% Precision 88.7% AUC: 0.8775

(continued)

Table 26.1 (continued)

Author	Year	Disorder	Task	AI models employed	Number of subjects	Results
Wang et al.	2022	Alzheimer's disease (AD)	Predict diagnosis	Various ML models	NC: 299 AD: 159	Acc, AUC, F1 score, recall: ~0.69 to 0.74
Chua et al.	2022	AD, Mild cognitive impairment (MCI)	Predict diagnosis	Multi-regression	NC: 55 eyes AD: 62 eyes MCI: 108 eyes	AUC: 0.80
Wisely et al.	2020	AD	Predict diagnosis	Convolutional neural networks	NC: 123 AD: 36	AUC: 0.836
Chrysou et al.	2020	Parkinson's disease (PD)	Predict diagnosis	Random forest	NC: 110 PD: 121	AUC: 0.82
Nunes et al.	2019	PD and AD	Predict diagnosis	Support vector machine	NC: 27 PD: 28 AD: 20	Acc: 0.82
Sánchez-Morla et al.	2021	Bipolar disorder (BD)	Predict diagnosis	Gaussian Naive Bayes, k-nearest neighbours and support vector machine	NC: 42 BD: 17	AUC: 0.97 Acc: 0.97
Devalla et al.	2020	Glaucoma	Segment ONH tissues	3D-U-NET	NC: 57 Glaucoma: 11	DC > 0.92
Russakoff et al.	2020	Referable glaucoma	Predict diagnosis	Convolutional neural networks	NC: 183 Referable glaucoma : 287	AUC: 0.88 for referable glaucoma
Panda et al.	2022	Glaucoma	Segment ONH tissues, Predict diagnosis	U-NET (segmentation), autoencoder (classification)	NC: 1548 Glaucoma: 2233	DC: 0.86 Acc: 0.92 Sen: 0.90

(continued)

Table 26.1 (continued)

Author	Year	Disorder	Task	AI models employed	Number of subjects	Results
Panda et al.	2022	Glaucoma	Segment retinal blood vessels, Predict diagnosis	DeepLabV3 model with a ResNet backbone (segmentation), 3D and 2D convolutional neural networks (classification)	NC: 2469 Glaucoma: 1639	DC: 0.81 $AUC_{3D\ CNN}$: 0.89 $AUC2_{D\ CNN}$: 0.90
Thompson et al.	2020	Primary open angle glaucoma (POAG)	Predict diagnosis	Convolutional neural networks	NC: 276 POAG: 359	Sen: 0.81 Spe: 0.95 AUC: 0.96
Asaoka et al.	2018	Early POAG	Predict diagnosis	Convolutional neural networks	NC: 166 POAG: 208	Sen: 0.90 Spe: 0.866 AUC: 0.937
Maetschke et al.	2019	POAG	Predict diagnosis	Convolutional neural networks	NC: 137 POAG: 432	AUC: 0.94
Zheng et al.	2020	Glaucoma	Predict diagnosis	Convolutional neural networks	NC: 446 Glaucoma: 203	Sen: 0.981 Spe: 0.981 AUC: 0.99
Thiery et al.	2022	Glaucoma	Predict diagnosis	PointNet, convolutional neural network	NC: 2296 Glaucoma: 477	$AUC_{PointNet}$: 0.95 AUC_{CNN}: 0.87
Braeu et al.	2023	Glaucoma	Predict diagnosis	PointNet, dynamic graph convolutional neural networks (DGCNN)	NC: 914 Glaucoma: 811	$AUC_{PointNet}$: 0.95 AUC_{DGCNN}: 0.97

(continued)

Table 26.1 (continued)

Author	Year	Disorder	Task	AI models employed	Number of subjects	Results
Braeu et al.	2023	Glaucoma	Identify the 3D structural changes in the ONH with increasing glaucoma severity	PointNet	NC: 213 Mild glaucoma: 204 Moderate glaucoma: 118 Advanced glaucoma: 118	Not applicable
Braeu et al.	2023	Glaucoma	Predict optic nerve head robustness	Random forest, autoencoder, dynamic graph convolutional neural networks	Glaucoma: 316	AUC_{RF}: 0.69 $AUC_{Autoencoder}$: 0/70 AUC_{DGCNN}: 0.76
Razaghi et al.	2022	Ischemic optic neuropathy (ION), Optic neuritis (ON)	Predict diagnosis	U-NET	NC: 210 eyes ION: 88 eyes ON: 79 eyes	DC: 0.87
Skau et al.	2013	Idiopathic intracranial hypertension (IIH)	Predict intracranial pressure	Linear regression	NC: 20 $IIH_{newly\ diagnosed}$: 20 $IIH_{long\text{-}term}$: 21	AUC: 0.869

(continued)

Table 26.1 (continued)

Author	Year	Disorder	Task	AI models employed	Number of subjects	Results
Girard et al.	2022	Papilledema, optic disc drusen (ODD)	Segment ONH tissues, predict diagnosis	U-NET++ (segmentation), random forest (classification)	NC: 100 Papilledema: 51 ODD: 105	DC: 0.93 AUC_{ODD}: 0.99 ± 0.001 $AUC_{Papilledema}$: 0.99 ± 0.005 AUC_{NC}: 0.98 ± 0.01
Jui-Kai et al.	2022	Papilledema caused by IIH	Characterise the changes in the swelling patterns of papilledema (longtitudinal study)	Variational autoencoder	125 subjects over multiple visits	Not applicable

NC: Normal Controls

Acc: Accuracy, Sen: Sensitivity, Spe: Specificity, DC: Dice Coefficient

[a]MOGAD: myelin oligodendrocyte glycoprotein associated disease; MonoADS: monophasic acquired demyelinating syndrome; NMOSD: neuromyelitis optica spectrum disease

Detection of Optic Neuritis History in MS Patients. Typically, OCT is primarily employed in MS patients with known acute optic neuritis to access optic nerve damage and monitor structural changes over time [38]. Kenney et al. investigated the potential of using OCT to identify a history of ON in MS patients using logistic regression and SVM models [39]. Their dataset included 488 MS patients with unilateral ON, 874 MS patients without ON and 552 healthy controls. Their findings indicated that intereye difference in macular GC-IPL thickness yielded the most accurate classification of unilateral ON history amongst all the other OCT measures they tested. When all the OCT measures were used in a ML model, logistic regression yielded a superior area under the curve (AUC) result of 0.91 as compared to using support vector machine (SVM) with linear kernel which achieved an AUC of 0.89; the SVM with a non-linear kernel performed relatively poorly. The stronger performance of the simpler models were likely attributable to the small sample sizes and limited number of feature variables used in their study, and larger studies would be necessary to validate the results. Nevertheless, the study demonstrated the potential utility of extracted OCT features, particularly intereye GC-IPL thickness differences, with simple AI models as a valuable test to confirm ON history in MS patients.

Automated MS Diagnosis with OCT parameters. Beyond using OCT solely for testing and monitoring ON in MS, which is directly linked to the eye, its potential utility for diagnosis of MS has also been explored. A common approach is to input extracted OCT measures into a ML classification model; Cavaliere et al. developed a SVM with a Gaussian quadratic kernel to classify 48 MS patients without ON and 48 normal controls [16]. The classification was based on three variables: total RNFL plus ganglion cell-inner plexiform layer (GC-IPL) thickness, macula inner nasal thickness and macula outer nasal thickness. These three variables were found to have the best discriminative capabilities out of all the retinal and choroidal thickness of the various macular and peripapillary areas, achieving a high AUC of 0.97. Interestingly, when testing a subsample of only females, the AUC of 0.97 was higher than the AUC of 0.92 obtained from testing a subsample of only males. This disparity in results by sex could be explained by additional observations made in the study: MS correlated with decreased macular inner nasal and macular outer nasal thickness in both sexes. However, while ageing correlated with macular inner nasal and macular outer nasal thickness loss in males, it correlated with increased macular inner nasal and macular outer nasal thickness in healthy females.

Automated MS Diagnosis with geometric OCT information. While Cavaliere et al. achieved good results, their method did not fully exploit the geometric information provided by 3D OCT scans. Recently, both Garcia-Martin et al. and Lopez et al. used DL models to better utilise the measurements taken by 3D OCT scans. Garcia-martin et used a circular peripapillary RNFL scan protocol which generated RNFL thickness measurements from 768 points (1 point per A-scan), these 768 points were then input to a multi-layer perceptron (MLP) neural network (NN) [40]. They trained one MLP NN to classify 115 MS patients and 106 normal control subjects achieving a sensitivity of 89.3% and specificity of 87.6%. Another

MLP NN was trained to classify MS patients without antecedent ON and MS patients with antecedent ON, achieving a sensitivity of 84.5% and a specificity of 83.2%. Since other studies found that mean peripapillary RNFL thickness is not as effective in discrimination of MS as other OCT variables, such as mean GC-IPL thickness [16, 39], Garcia-Martin et al.'s technique could have potentially yielded improved results if they had used a GC-IPL protocol.

In fact, Lopez-Dorado et al. did compare the discriminative capabilities of thickness maps of different tissue layers and found that the GCL-IPL layer was more discriminative than the RNFL and choroid layer [36]. They achieved 100% accuracy In classifying 48 normal control subjects from 48 MS patients (without history of ON) using a CNN with GC-IPL thickness maps as input. Although the DL models used by Garcia-Martin et al. and Lopez-Dorado et al. require higher computational capacity, their ability to exploit the geometric information from OCT scans is a great value-add and could potentially make OCT a valuable confirmatory test for patients with suspected MS even in the absence of visual manifestations of the disease. However, the excellent classification scores achieved by Lopez-Dorado et al. could be a result of their data augmentation method. Due to having a small dataset of 48 MS patient eyes and 48 control subject eyes, Lopez-Dorado et al. used data augmentation to generate 100 MS OCT scans and 100 control subject OCT scans; the synthetic data was generated using a separate generative adversarial network for the MS group and control group. The generative adversarial network framework is as follows: one, a generator model maps random noise to a synthetic image; two, both the synthetic images and real data are classified as either real or fake using a discriminator. Over time, the goal is for the synthetic images to become increasingly similar to the real data, to the point where the discriminator is unable to discriminate synthetic and real images, resulting in a discriminator loss of 0.5. However, given that the training dataset for the generative adversarial network was very small and the synthetic data constituted more than two-thirds of the data used to train the CNN, there is a possibility of significant overfitting which could explain the 100% classification rate. This could limit the clinical applicability of their findings. Therefore, although the utilization of extracted thickness maps and CNN as a diagnostic test for MS is very promising, it is essential to validate its effectiveness on a larger dataset.

Exclusion of MS Mimics. Another consideration to note about the aforementioned studies is that they focus on differentiating between MS and healthy controls, neglecting one criteria of the McDonald criteria for MS diagnosis: the exclusion of other MS mimics [37]. This exclusion is challenging because multiple clinical syndromes mimic MS. This could contribute to the problem of frequent MS misdiagnosis, which can hinder the patient from receiving proper treatment [36]. Though the true incidence and prevalence of MS misdiagnosis is unknown, studies by some MS centres have reported misdiagnosis rates as high as 30% or even up to 50% [41, 42]. As such, studies such as Kavaklioglu et al.'s are useful, where they attempted to differentiate MS from three other CNS demyelinating disorders using ML and OCT parameters, such as average RNFL thickness, average macular sector thickness, macular cube volume and average GC-IPL thickness [30]. Their study was performed using a population of children below 18 years of age, with 57 children having been diagnosed with MS, 130 being diagnosed with three other CNS demyelinating disorders and 69 being healthy controls. Their binary classification (MS vs other demyelinating disorders) resulted in an AUC of 0.73 using a random forest classifier which was a significantly poorer performance compared to their random forest classifier for MS vs healthy controls which achieved an AUC of 0.87. These results indicated that though OCT and AI may have utility in detecting MS, it is limited in its diagnostic capability. A further study incorporating geometric information such as thickness maps could reveal distinct retinal profiles in MS patients and subjects with MS mimics, although such investigations have not been explored extensively. Furthermore, a large cohort study involving a broader range of disease populations that mimic MS would be necessary to evaluate OCT and AI in MS diagnosis.

Automated MS Prognosis. The battery of tests required for the diagnosis of MS, including MRI and CSF testing, is typically repeated for monitoring and prognosis of the disease in order to determine an appropriate treatment plan. Montolio et al. presented a potential method for prognosis using an ML-based technique and extracted OCT parameters, such as peripapillary RNFL thickness and other macular area thicknesses [31]. They conducted a longitudinal cohort study spanning ten years, with annual follow-ups and classified 104 MS patients as either worsening or non-worsening based on their expanded disability status scale score. Ultimately their long short-term memory NN to classify MS patients resulted in an AUC of 0.82. While the binary classification used for prognosis is very simplistic, this study provided a proof-of-concept that OCT and AI could also be utilized for predicting the disability course of MS. If OCT and AI could replace one or more of the costly and invasive tests required for prognosis, it would greatly improve the accessibility of consultation and treatment for MS patients.

Conclusion on MS. In all, OCT has the potential to serve as a non-invasive test for a diagnostic biomarker for MS or for prediction of the MS course. By replacing costly or invasive testing, OCT can aid in preventing enabling early diagnosis with greater clinical certainty. This in turn would allow treatment to begin sooner, leading to a better quality of life for patients and mitigating the deterioration of their health [36]. However, further extensive testing is necessary to determine the clinical suitability of OCT and the use of automated decision-making using AI. In particular, more studies should focus on differentiating MS from other MS mimics, and even from other disorders that may exhibit similar effects on OCT features. These investigations are crucial to establish the reliability and specificity of OCT as a diagnostic tool in various clinical scenarios.

26.2.2 Alzheimer's Disease

Alzheimer's Disease is the world's leading neurodegenerative disorder, and the most common subtype of dementia [17]. AD causes cognitive decline and symptoms include loss of memory, language difficulties, mood swings, disorientation and impaired daily functioning [4]. While a definitive diagnosis of AD can only be confirmed through post mortem brain examination [43], various diagnostic criterion, including biological and symptomatic definitions, have been used to guide the clinical diagnosis of AD. The current clinical diagnosis involves a combination of cognitive testing, evaluation of symptoms, medical and family history, biomarker tests for brain amyloid using PET and CSF, and biomarker tests for neuronal injury using structural MRI [4, 44]. While AD is incurable, early treatment can slow disease progression [4, 17, 45]. However, the current testing methods for AD using PET, CSF and MRI are limited by their cost, invasiveness, subjectivity and low sensitivity and specificity [4, 45]. A more accessible means of testing which allows for earlier diagnosis could prove vital.

Automated AD Diagnosis with OCT parameters. Many studies have shown that AD is associated with several ocular changes as seen in ocular images (as depicted in Fig. 26.2). This includes significantly thinner peripapillary RNFL and GCC thicknesses and reduced macular volume as measured in OCT scans [4, 46]. These findings suggest that OCT parameters could be exploited for AD diagnosis using various machine learning techniques. Wang et al. conducted a study using extracted OCT parameters that were statistically significantly correlated with cognitive function, brain atrophy, CSF biomarkers and APOE genotypes [17]. The parameters included peripapillary RNFL thicknesses (average, superior and inferior), macular retinal thickness, total macular volume, macular RNFL, GCL and IPL which were all found to be significantly thinner in AD patients as compared to controls (seen in Fig. 26.3). These parameters were input into seven different ML models classifying 159 AD patients and 299 healthy controls. The best diagnostic performance was achieved using the extreme gradient boosting algorithm (AUC of 0.69), which outperformed other ML models including logistic regression (AUC of 0.52). Chua et al. explored the utility of OCT and a logistic regression model in the multi-class classification of three groups: 55 eyes from cognitively normal older adults, 108 eyes from subjects with mild cognitive impairment (MCI) and 62 eyes from subjects with symptomatic AD; MCI is the stage between normal cognitive decline due to ageing and significant decline in cognition due to dementia [47]. The study found that both circumpapillary thickness and macular layer thicknesses had greater diagnostic capabilities than retinal vessel density. Furthermore, their best performing model used a combination of macular layer thicknesses, compensated circumpapillary RNFL thickness and other extracted optic disc parameters, achieving an AUC of 0.80. This indicates that OCT parameters can be useful, not only for AD detection, but also for distinguishing normal cognitive decline from MCI and AD.

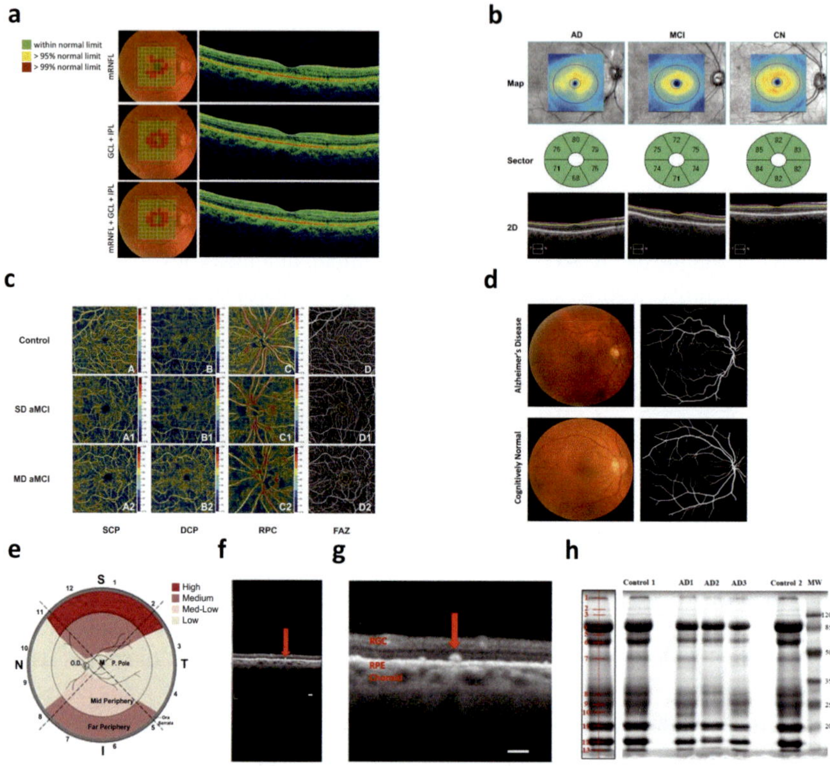

Fig. 26.2 Ocular imaging has revealed several biomarkers of Alzheimer's disease (AD): **a** macular retinal nerve fibre layer (mRNFL), ganglion cell layer (GCL) and inner plexiform layer (IPL) thinning in OCT images; **b** thinning of the GCL and IPL layers as shown in thickness maps extracted from OCT scans; **c** reduction of retinal vessel density in patients with amnestic mild cognitive impairment (aMCI) in OCT angiography images, aMCI can lead to AD; **d** retinal vessel morphology changes seen in segmented vessels from fundus photographs; **e** hotspot regions for retinal Aβ deposits in AD patients (S, superior; T, temporal; I, inferior; N, nasal); **f** amyloid plaques accumulation in optical coherence tomography (OCT) cross section; **g** curcumin-positive deposits above the retinal pigment epithelium (RPE) in high-magnification OCT images; and **h** changes in the tear proteome in gel images of tear proteins. Panel **e** modified from Cunha et al. https://doi.org/10.1186/s40942-016-0049-4 *Int J Retin Vitr* [105]. Panel **b** retrieved from Jiang et al. https://doi.org/10.1371/journal.pone.0192154 PLoS One [106]. Panel **c** retrieved from Criscuolo et al. https://doi.org/10.1371/journal.pone.0233975 PLoS One [107]. Panel **d** modified from Yousefzadeh et al. https://doi.org/10.48550/arXiv.2302.03008 arXiv [108] Panels **e**–**g** modified from Koronyo et al. https://doi.org/10.1172/jci.insight.93621 JCI Insight [109]. Panel **h** modified from Kallo et al. https://doi.org/10.1371/journal.pone.0158000 PLoS One [110]. All panels were reproduced under the Creative Commons Attribution 4.0 International License (http://creativecommons.org/licenses/by/4.0/)

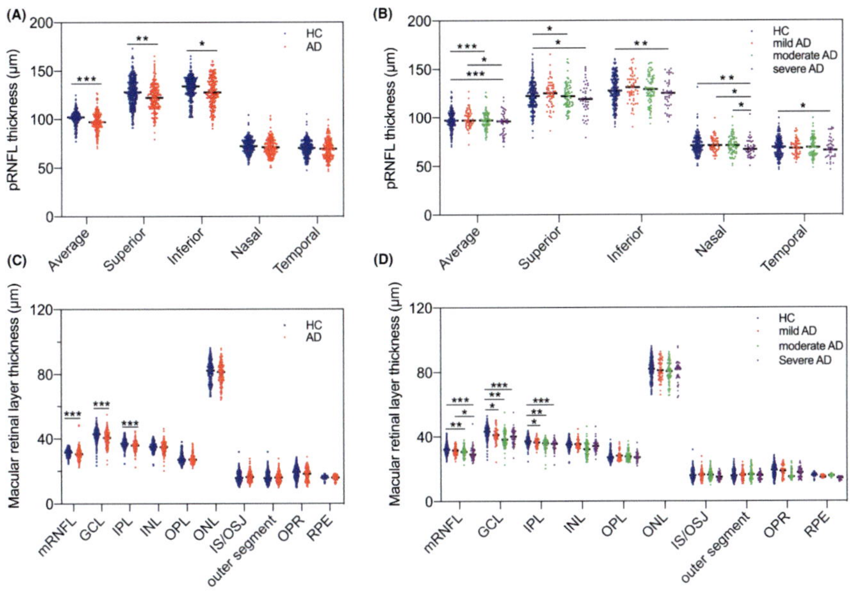

Fig. 26.3 There was a significant decrease in the average, superior, and inferior quadrant peripapillary retinal nerve fiber layer, macular retinal nerve fiber layer, ganglion cell layer (GCL), and inner plexiform layer (IPL) thicknesses in patients with Alzheimer's disease compared to healthy controls. Figure retrieved from Wang et al. https://doi.org/10.1111/cns.13963 CNS Neuroscience & Therapeutics [17]. Reproduced under the Creative Commons Attribution 4.0 International License (http://creativecommons.org/licenses/by/4.0/)

Automated AD Diagnosis with geometric OCT information. Chua et al.'s findings suggests that AD has a greater effect on tissue geometry than vessel density. However, both Chua et al. and Wang et al.'s ML methods are merely based on the on the average thicknesses without identifying the specific geometric changes in retinal tissue caused by or correlated with AD. DL-based methods, on the other hand, allow for the exploitation of the 3D image information obtained from OCT scan, as demonstrated in Wisely et al.'s study [45]. Wisely et al. performed the study using a cohort of 123 normal controls and 36 subjects. In their study, Wisely et al. tested various combinations of inputs including OCT angiography, ultra-widefield fundus, fundus autofluorescence, GC-IPL thickness maps generated by the OCT software, and a quantitative dataset consisting of OCT/OCTA numerical data and patient data. Each imaging modality was passed through a CNN-based feature-map extractor, and then each of the feature maps as well as the quantitative dataset were individually passed through modality-specific fully-connected layers outputting a pre-classification score. The final prediction result was based on an average of the pre-classification scores from the specific combination of modalities used input as input. The results of the study showed that among the models using a singular modality as input, the model using GC-IPL thickness maps had the highest predictive capability, followed by the model using only the quantitative dataset as input, with AUCs of 0.809 and 0.754 respectively. They also found that the best-performing model was achieved using a combination GC-IPL thickness maps and the quantitative dataset (0.841 AUC). Surprisingly, this model outperformed the one which used all the data as input (0.830 AUC). These results suggest that OCTA and fundus imaging modalities have limited utility in predicting AD diagnosis. These results and Chua et al.'s findings both support the notion that the classification decision is based on the geometric changes of the tissue. As such, it could be useful to perform OCT scanning and use a DL-based model during the clinical evaluation for AD diagnosis, eliminating the need for additional ocular imaging like fundus or OCTA.

However, Wisely et al. only extracted the GC-IPL thickness maps. AD has been associated with changes in the thickness of other tissue layers such as the macular RNFL or peripapillary RNFL [45]. As such, the study could have been enhanced by including the thickness maps of these other tissue layers in a similar multimodal DL model to allow the model to learn the structural changes associated with AD in these tissue layers as well. The additional analysis of the RNFL tissue layer could potentially result in a model with even higher predictive capability.

26.2.3 Parkinson's Disease

PD is a motor disorder with an average onset age of 60 [48, 49]. Similar to AD, early diagnosis of PD is crucial for initiating treatment to slow down disease progression. However, the diagnostic process is challenging due to the high-cost invasiveness of current testing methods. PD is characterised by the degeneration of dopaminergic neurons, which leads to reduced motor function [48]. It is possible that this dopamine degeneration could also affects retinal cell function and structure since dopamine plays a role in controlling visual functions [48]. Chrysou et al. discovered that retinal thinning occurs in patients with PD and can discriminate them from healthy individuals [50]. Their random forest classifier using ten tissue layer thicknesses as extracted from segmented OCT scans of 110 controls and 121 PD eyes achieved an AUC of 0.82. However, further research is needed to fully understand the pathophysiology.

Texture analysis could potentially uncover the specific local and global structural changes of the retina with neurodegenerative disorders such as PD. Nunes et al. investigated the use of retinal textual biomarkers, specifically the fray level co-occurrence matrix and wavelet-based texture features, for the classification of 28 patients with PD, 20 with AD and 27 healthy controls [51]. Nunes et al.'s non-linear SVM classification model used thickness and texture measures from five layers (GCL, IPL, INL, OPL and ONL layers) which resulted in a median accuracy of 0.82 using ten-fold cross validation. They observed that the textual biomarkers provided distinct information compared to the thickness measures, with global texture metrics, in particular, playing a significant role in the classification decision. These findings indicate that texture analysis of OCT data could be valuable input for AI-based classification models of neurodegenerative disorders, as it captures structural information that thickness measures alone cannot convey. Nunes et al.'s study is noteworthy as they conducted a multi-class classification involving two distinct neurodegenerative disease populations that exhibit retinal thinning. Their findings demonstrated that the AI model could effectively differentiate between these diseases using both thickness and textual measures, thereby serving as a disease-specific biomarker.

26.2.4 Bipolar Disorder

Bipolar Disorder is a chronic neurodegenerative disorder which manifests with a high variability in symptoms and neurobiology [52]. Few biomarkers for early diagnosis have been identified, leading to delays in treatment [52]. Sanchez-Moria et al. employed ML models to explore the classification of bipolar disorder from healthy eyes using thickness measurements from nine tissue layers in nine regions each [52]. They identified four thickness measurements to be the most discriminative: IPL and GCL thickness in the inner nasal region and INL thickness in the outer nasal and inner inferior regions. They conducted tests with several classifiers using different combinations of the four thickness measurements. Their SVM model using only GCL thickness in the inner nasal region as input achieved the highest AUC of 0.97. However, it is important to note that the sample size of only 17 patients with bipolar disorder was particularly small which likely contributed to an inflated AUC in the classification model. There was also quite a significant class imbalance issue with 42 normal controls which could have biased the model.

The study revealed that patients with bipolar disorder exhibited thinning in various retinal tissue layers, particularly the GCL and IPL layers. The authors also postulated that the reduction in retinal thickness could be attributed to neurological loss associated with inflammatory and oxidative activity during BP relapses. However, the extent of thickness reductions in patients with bipolar disorder was not found to be as significant as that in AD and MS patients. Furthermore, this finding might have been confounded by the fact that the patients with bipolar disorder in the study smoked heavily which could have been a contributing factor the observed retinal thinning. Nonetheless, this study indicates that bipolar disorder could indeed cause geometrical changes in the structure of the retina. Further studies should continue to explore the potential of using AI and OCT as a biomarker for the early diagnosis of bipolar disorder.

26.2.5 Glaucoma and Other Optic Neuropathies

Optic neuropathies encompass a group of neurological diseases characterised by degeneration of optic nerve tissue, potentially leading to partial or complete vision loss [12, 53]. Among these, glaucoma stands out as the leading cause of irreversible blindness in the world [53]. As of 2014, an estimated 3.54% of the global population over 40 years old were affected by this disease [54]. While early and appropriate treatment can manage the condition and prevent further vision loss, any vision already lost cannot be restored [55]. However, the current clinical procedures for glaucoma diagnosis involve a series of time-consuming tests that exhibit inter-observer and intra-observer variability [56]. This slow detection process hinders the timely initiation of treatment.

Automated Segmentation of OCT for Glaucoma Diagnosis. Extensive research into computer-aided diagnosis of glaucoma using OCT scans has been conducted in recent years [57]. AI models, like U-NETS, are commonly used for segmenting tissue layers in the ONH and macula, as demonstrated in the works of Devalla et al. and Russakoff et al. [58, 59]. Segmentation aids diagnosis models to detect subtle structural changes in the major neural and connective tissues caused by glaucoma, leading to improved diagnosis [58, 59]. For instance, Panda et al. processed segmented OCT scans using an autoencoder network to uncover ONH morphology changes and thus, identify novel glaucoma biomarkers [60]. Aside from neural and connective tissue layers, segmenting other structures could provide additional biomarkers for glaucoma diagnosis. Panda et al. trained a deep learning algorithm to segment the retinal blood vessels of the central retinal vessel trunk and its branches in OCT b-scans and used CNNs to diagnose glaucoma using the segmented structures achieving a high AUCs of 0.90 [61].

Segmentation-Free Glaucoma Diagnosis. While automatic segmentation algorithms have been tested with high performance, these algorithms are still be susceptible to errors and artifacts, which can introduce bias and errors into the classification models. It has been reported that such errors and artifacts can be present in up to 46.3% of spectral domain OCT scans of the RNFL [62]. Thus, other studies have also explored AI-based diagnosis solutions that do not rely on segmentation [55, 57, 63, 64]. In particular, Thompson et al. demonstrated the potential of AI and OCT scans to distinguish early-stage glaucoma from individuals without glaucoma using a segmentation-free approach. Detecting glaucoma at its early stages is crucial because vision loss caused by glaucoma is irreversible, and early detection and treatment can help preserve more vision [55]. In their study, Thompson et al. trained a residual deep CNN with raw OCT data in a two-step process: first, using transfer learning with a model pretrained on the ImageNet data set and training only the final two layers, and then finetuning all the model layers [57]. Transfer learning and finetuning allowed them to leverage the information learnt by the pretrained model on a large dataset, reducing computational resources and potentially requiring less training data. Their model, trained on raw OCT scans from 359 patients with glaucoma and 276 normal controls, achieved high AUCs of 0.92 in predicting preperimetric glaucoma, 0.92 in predicting mild perimetric glaucoma, and 0.99 in predicting both moderate and severe perimetric glaucoma. Moreover, their model exhibited significantly greater predictive capabilities than their tests using global or sectoral RNFL thickness parameters. These findings suggest that employing deep learning models with imaging modalities that capture more geometric information is more advantageous than relying solely on extracted numerical data, particularly in the early stages of glaucoma where structural changes are more subtle.

Geometric Deep Learning for Glaucoma Diagnosis. Deep learning applied to OCT research often focuses on utilizing 3D OCT scan volumes with CNN models. However, this approach has two limitations. One, it is computationally expensive, necessitating downsampling and resulting in the loss of important details. Two, it introduces a large number of redundant background pixels to the network, which could confuse the model. To address these challenges, Thiery et al. and Braeu et al. explored the use of point clouds, which are sets of points in a 3D coordinate space that efficiently capture only spatial information about the surfaces of tissues from OCT scans [65, 66]. They employed geometric deep learning methods, such as dynamic graph CNN and PointNet, designed to process 3D point clouds. In a study involving 477 glaucoma patients and 2296 controls, Thiery et al. compared the performance of CNN and PointNet, finding that PointNet outperformed CNN with AUCs of 0.95 and 0.87, respectively. Similarly, Braeu et al. classified 811 glaucoma subjects and 914 controls using PointNet and dynamic graph CNN, with the latter performing slightly better (AUCs of 0.95 and 0.97, respectively). This was also a superior performance compared to diagnosing glaucoma using RNFL thickness measurements alone (AUC of 0.92) [65]. In addition to the superior performance, an additional advantage of these geometric DL models is that it is designed to identify the points that were critical to the model's decision making. By projecting these points onto the ONH geometry, a 3D point cloud density map is generated, highlighting denser regions corresponding to significant 3D ONH structures for glaucoma diagnosis (Fig. 26.4). This makes it more interpretable and transparent. Braeu et al. conducted additional studies using similar techniques. One study included scans from glaucoma patients with varying severities to identify regions exhibiting distinct 3D structural changes with increasing severity [67]. In a separate study, Braeu et al. used the dynamic graph CNN to predict the robustness of an ONH solely from a single OCT scan of the ONH [65]. The model was trained and tested on scans from 316 patients and achieved an AUC of 0.76 in testing. With, further development to improve accuracy, this method holds great potential for assessing the biomechanical properties of ONH and macular tissues without the need to perform uncomfortable and potentially harmful biomechanical tests on subjects.

ONH Biomechanics and Beyond, Improved Glaucoma Understanding. Glaucoma comprises a complex group of subtypes which are not yet fully understood [68]. OCT and AI offer promising avenues, beyond tissue structure and thickness, to delve into diverse aspects of glaucoma, advancing diagnosis and prognosis. One area of interest which has been explored in recent years is the biomechanics of the ONH. In particular, several groups, including Chuangsuwanich et al., Midgett et al. and Kim et al., have explored the difference in 2D- and 3D-strain patterns in the ONH between different biomechanical states by taking OCT scans of glaucomatous eyes at baseline and at elevated or lowered intraocular pressures [69–71]. Furthermore, AI algorithms can analyse dynamic changes by capturing

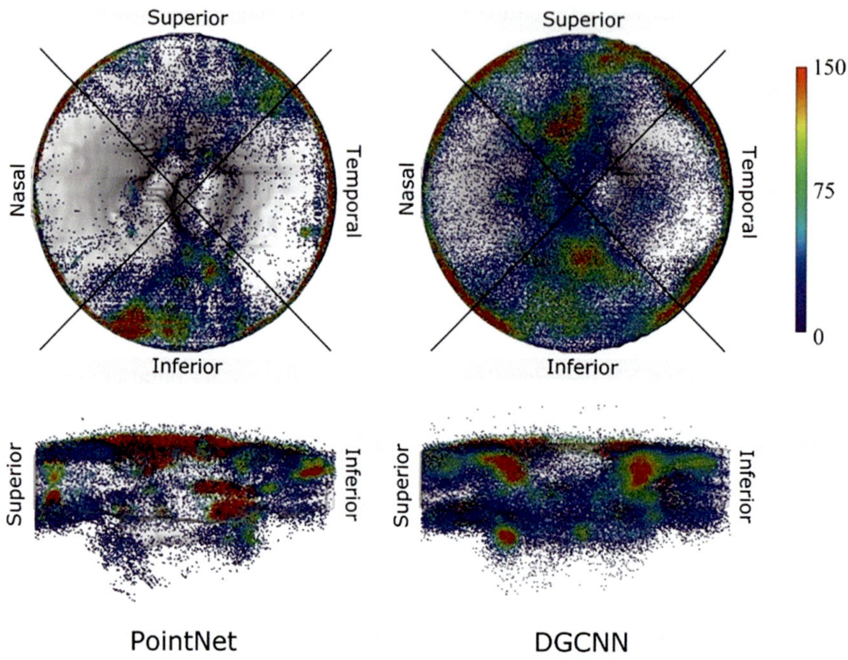

Fig. 26.4 Geometric deep learning models such as PointNet and dynamic graph convolutional neural network can be trained to diagnose glaucoma and identify the critical structural features used for diagnosis from point clouds representing optic nerve head tissues. The critical point density mapped onto the ONH geometry is shown, with denser regions corresponding to the structures that were more critical for glaucoma diagnosis. Figure retrieved from Braeu et al. https://doi.org/10.1016/j.ajo.2023.01.008 American Journal of Ophthalmology [65]

scans at different points, such as during eye movement [72]. Additionally, integrating OCT with other measurements, such as ocular blood flow [73], collagen fiber organisation [74, 75], ocular pulse amplitude [76], or intracranial pressures [77], and applying AI techniques could provide a holistic perspective of glaucoma. This synergistic approach has the potential to unveil novel biomarkers and patterns, deepening our understanding of glaucoma and paving the way for improved diagnostics and treatments.

Ischemic Optic Neuropathy and Optic Neuritis. Another type of optic neuropathy is ischemic optic neuropathy, Which occurs due to reduced blood flow to the optic nerve, leading to damage to the nerve fibres and potential vision loss [78]. In a study by Razaghi et al., a method was proposed to utilise a U-NET segmentation model for extracting more accurate RNFL thickness from OCT images to classify diagnose ischemic optic neuropathy and demyelinating optic neuritis (inflammation and damage to the myelin sheath surrounding the optic nerve) [79]. In this study, scans from 88 eyes with ischemic optic neuropathy, 79 eyes with optic neuritis and 210 normal control eyes were used. The developed automatic segmentation model demonstrated a good correlation with manual segmentation performed by experts on scans from both disease populations, resulting in more accurate thickness measurements compared to those obtained from the OCT machine. However, since retinal thinning occurs in both optic neuropathies as well as a host of other neurodegenerative disorders, this study could be further developed by using AI classifiers to aid in diagnosis of the disorders using RNFL thickness maps instead of using average measured RNFL thicknesses. Such an approach could aid in distinguishing between different disorders and determining the specific pattern of structural changes associated with each optic neuropathy.

26.2.6 Papilledema

Papilledema is a neuro-ophthalmic condition exclusively used to describe the swelling of the optic disc swelling which occurs as a result of increased intracranial pressure (ICP) [80]. Papilledema is indicative of a range of underlying conditions, including brain tumours, CNS inflammation, cerebral venous thrombosis and idiopathic intracranial hypertension (IIH) [14]. Depending on the severity of increased ICP and swelling, papilledema can lead to vision loss, which can be managed if detected and treated early [14]. Papilledema is typically diagnosed through a clinical examination which involves visual field testing, visual acuity testing, fundoscopy. Further investigations, such as brain imaging (MRI and magnetic resonance venography) and measurement of CSF opening pressure during lumbar puncture, are often conducted as part of the diagnostic work-up [14, 80].

IIH is the most common cause of papilledema, especially in patients presenting with papilledema under the age of fifty [14]. In most cases of IIH, ICP is elevated thus causing papilledema [81]. Skua et al. explored the potential of OCT markers, specifically, peripapillary RNFL thickness and total retinal thickness, in predicting ICP using multiple linear regression models [81]. Their study cohort included 20 normal controls, 20 patients newly diagnosed with IIH and 21 patients with long-term IIH. Their findings showed that a linear regression model adjusted for age and BMI achieved an AUC of 0.87 when using the OCT measures to predict ICP on a continuous scale. They also found that increased peripapillary RNFL and total retinal thicknesses were positively correlated with increased ICP levels. However, it is important to note that this study had a small sample size, with only 41 subjects diagnosed with IIH. Therefore, while the study suggests that OCT holds promise as a non-invasive tool for detecting elevated ICP levels and potentially replacing invasive procedures like lumbar puncture, in the clinical testing for papilledema, further evaluation is necessary to validate its effectiveness and reliability.

Another complication in the diagnosis of papilledema and its underlying causes is the difficulty in distinguishing early-stage papilledema from other causes of optic disc swelling, including pseudo-papilledema [80]. Jui-Kai et al. analysed papilledema patterns caused by IIH over time [82]. They scanned 1509 ONH OCT volumes from 125 subjects over multiple visits, extracting total retinal thickness maps. The thickness maps were input into a DL variational autoencoder which output a 2D latent space map to visualize and quantify swelling changes. These two latent variables encoded volumetric measures and spatial patterns of axon bundle swelling, aiding in differentiating papilledema from other causes of optic disc swelling. Separately, Girard et al. utilised an AI-based solution to distinguish papilledema (bilateral ONH swelling associated with confirmed raised ICP) and optic disc drusen (hyporeflective structures on ONH OCT scan) [80]. Optic disc drusen is a pseudo-papilledema which is particularly difficult to differentiate from papilledema. Girard et al. captured OCT scans from 51 subjects with papilledema, 105 subjects with optic disc drusen and 100 healthy subjects. Their three-stage process was as follows: one, automatic segmentation of all seven tissue layers and the drusen region in the ONH using a modified U-NET model; two, calculation of a drusen volume score and prelaminar swelling score based on the segmented regions; and three, random forest classifier to classify subjects as optic disc drusen, papilledema and healthy based on the two scores calculated. The U-NET was able to segment the scans with a high DC of 0.93 (as shown in Fig. 26.5). The random forest classifier was able to distinguish papilledema, optic disc drusen and healthy subjects with high AUCs between 0.98 and 0.99. A caveat to the high AUCs obtained is that relatively homogenous populations were used in the study; most of the scans of optic disc drusen (90 of the 105 scans) and papilledema (50 of the 51 scans) were taken from subjects imaged in Denmark, while all the healthy scans were taken from a population imaged in Singapore. Therefore, there may be other factors that biased the algorithm, particularly ethnicity which can significantly affect ONH morphology.

26.2.7 Limitations of Current Methods

There are a few limitations of the current AI-based solutions. Firstly, many of the studies have only established a correlation or association between the neurological conditions and ocular biomarkers [45]. Therefore, further research is needed to determine the causative pathways and the pathophysiological links between the eye and the brain in the context of neurological disorders. This lack of understanding contributes to low clinician confidence in AI models and hampers their clinical adoption rates.

Secondly, the black-box nature of AI models limits their transparency. This may make clinicians hesitant to rely on AI models for clinical decision-making and advice, particularly when the AI-based decisions disrupt the routines of clinicians at high-stake points [83]. However, this could be improved with interpretable AI techniques such as PointNet as discussed earlier [65].

Thirdly, many of the studies suffer from small sample sizes, particularly when it comes to the target diseases. This can be attributed to the limited availability of OCT instruments in neurology clinics, leading to a scarcity of data. However, this poses significant problems as a small study cohort fails to capture the true variability of real-world scenarios. Moreover, the AI models may become overly

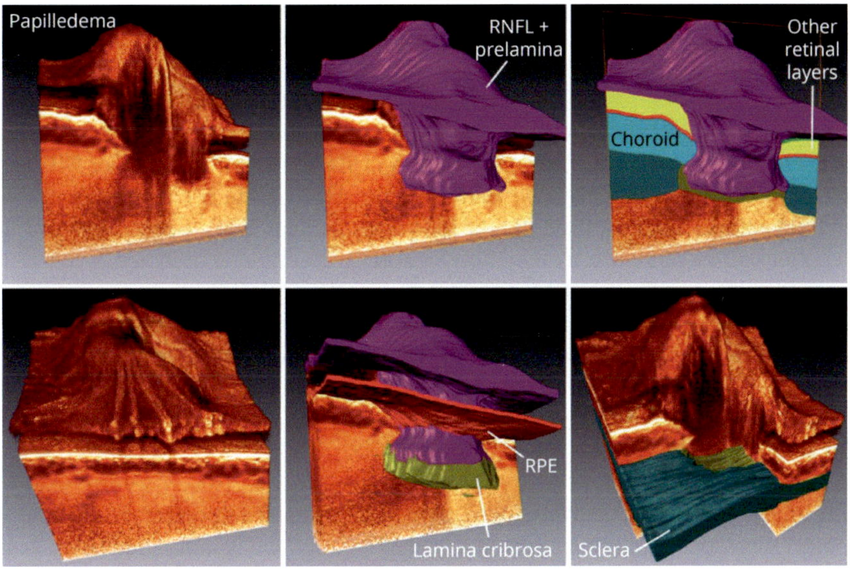

Fig. 26.5 A 3D rendering of an optical coherence tomography (OCT) scan of a subject with papilledema and a corresponding surface-mesh of the segmentation of several optic nerve head tissue layers. Figure retrieved from Girard et al. https://doi.org/10.1212/WNL.0000000000201350 Neurology [80]

specialized and prone to overfitting by learning patterns that are unique to the limited study population. Consequently, inflated performance metrics can arise, hindering the generalizability of the models to new populations. Additionally, studies with imbalanced classes, where the number of control subjects far outweighs the number of patients with the target disease, may introduce bias to the model or impede its ability to accurately predict the minority class. These challenges emphasize the pressing need for larger international consortia to address these issues effectively.

The robustness of many of the AI models reviewed are further limited by several factors. Firstly, strict exclusion criteria were often applied, including the exclusion of other common neurodegenerative and ocular disorders. Since many neurological disorders have similar effects on OCT parameters such as peripapillary RNFL thinning and GC-IPL thinning, the OCT plus AI models developed may not be disease specific tests. Secondly, the exclusion of low-quality OCT data [23, 45, 47, 52]. Thirdly, the studies are mostly retrospective and conducted on convenience samples rather than prospective studies, which limits their applicability to real world subjects. Fourthly, population demographics, including age, sex, and ethnicity, can influence the anatomical features of the optic nerve head and macula [84–87]. These demographic factors can have implications for the applicability of AI models in diagnosing diseases in populations with different characteristics from the ones on which the models were trained. All of these factors limit the generalisability of the models to new datasets and thus, limit the clinical applicability of the models for automated diagnosis [23, 52].

Finally, a general limitation of AI research is the difficulty in assessing the performance of AI networks. One of the challenges is that the area under the curve (AUC) values, which are commonly used to evaluate the performance of ML and DL models are not directly comparable across different studies if the algorithms and populations studied are different [68]. This comparability issue arises due to variations in factors such as the study cohort, preparation and choice of dataset, preprocessing techniques, feature selection, model architecture, hyperparameter tuning, and evaluation metrics used. These differences can lead to variations in AUC values even when evaluating similar tasks or algorithms.

26.2.8 Future Trends

The study of AI-based models for screening, diagnosis, and prognosis of neurological disorders with OCT scans is expected to continue gaining popularity. It is likely that other neurological disorders such as stroke, autism and Huntington's Disease will be explored in this context [88–91]. Ocular biomarkers have already shown promising associations to these diseases, providing a strong foundation for further research in these areas using AI methods [88, 89, 91]. Additionally, future studies could extend beyond the classification of diseased and non-diseased eyes to include prognosis and the development of personalised treatment plans. For example, Thompson et al.'s model successfully stratified the stage of glaucoma, which could be valuable in guiding the treatment decisions for managing the conditions [57].

A second possible direction this field might take is in the use of DL models and 2D or 3D imaging modalities in more studies. OCT scans offer a wealth of information beyond average thicknesses of tissue layers and regions. The raw scans can be input to DL models, and pre-processing could also be performed to produce texture markers, segmentation masks and thickness maps [22, 36, 45, 51]. These approaches enable DL models to detect specific structural and geometric changes in the ONH and macular tissues that may be associated with neurodegeneration.

Thirdly, there is likely to be an increasing focus on the explainability of AI-based models. This trend has already been observed in the study of glaucoma where efforts have been made to provide explanations for the decisions made by AI models, especially DL models [92–94]. This emphasis on explainability is expected to extend to the exploration of other neurological disorders, aiming to enhance the clinical relevance of these studies. Explainability is crucial as it enables clinicians to understand how AI models reach their decisions and helps build trust in these models [83]. Several approaches can be employed to achieve explainability in AI models. For instance, in the case of CNNs, activation maps and saliency maps can be used to visualize the features that the network focuses on when making a decision [92–94]. Wisely et al., Maetschke et al., and Thompson et al. all used class activation maps superimposed over the inputted imaging modalities in an attempt to identify regions of interest that might be more significant for the classification decision [45, 57, 63]. However, the limited resolution of the maps, resulting from down sampling in the final convolutional layers of the CNN models, poses a challenge to their accuracy. Therefore, it would be beneficial to explore more task- and model-specific visualization methods to achieve more accurate identification of key features in OCTs for DL-based decisions. One such example is the PointNet and dynamic graph CNN approach employed by Braeu et al. and Thiery et al. which captures critical structural features used by the models to diagnose glaucoma (Fig. 26.4) [65, 66, 95].

We could also expect an increase in the use of multi-classification models to detect and differentiate between multiple neurological and ophthalmological disorder. Given the overlapping structural effects and symptoms of many conditions, it is crucial not only to accurately detect a specific disease but also to distinguish it from similar disorders. In current clinical practice, the diagnosis of a particular neurological disorder often involves ruling out other similar conditions [4, 14]. Multi-classification models can aid in this process by classifying an OCT scan into one of several disease categories, rather than limiting the classification to a binary distinction between a specific disease or full-health. For example, a recent study by Kavaklioglu et al. used OCT imaging and AI to develop a multi-classification model for differentiating between healthy controls, MS and other CNS demyelinating disorders, achieving an accuracy of 64% [30]. Such models have the potential to enhance diagnostic accuracy and assist in identifying specific diseases within a broader spectrum of related disorders.

As this field gains more recognition, it will probably become easier to curate larger datasets for the studies. AI models, particularly DL models, require large datasets to train robust models. Smaller training datasets make the models more prone to overfitting, which limits the model's applicability to new unseen data [52]. In the field of neurology, curating large datasets of OCT scans can be challenging since it is not common practice to include an OCT scan for neurology patients. However, as the study of AI models with OCT scans for neurology gains more recognition, it will likely become easier to curate larger datasets for these studies. This, in turn, will improve the generalizability of these models, making them more valuable in clinical practice.

Finally, the advancement of this field could also encourage researchers to investigate parameters beyond structural measurements, to enhance our understanding of neurological disorders. In addition to thickness measurements and tissue structures, studies may delve into biomechanical testing, blood vessel morphology, blood flow, oxygenation, cellular behaviour, and other assessable parameters using ocular imaging techniques like OCT. Such exploration is crucial for unravelling the pathophysiology of neurological disorders within the brain and eye.

In conclusion, the exploration of using OCT scans and AI models as a test in screening, diagnosis and prognosis of neurological disorders is a rapidly evolving field. The success of current works in identifying ocular biomarkers for various neurological disorders suggests that the eye, via OCT scans, could be an easy-to-access point for studying these disorders. This potential of AI to discover ocular biomarkers in neurological disorders is ground-breaking. However, further research is needed to validate the findings, and the development of generalisable and explainable AI models is necessary for clinical adoption. The automated AI models have the potential to enable neurological clinics expertise in retinal imaging to use OCT scans as a screening tool. This would reduce the need for invasive procedures and subjective clinical interpretation, providing a cost-effective, efficient, and accurate tool which can improve access to care and reduce healthcare costs [19]. It also unlocks the potential for early detection through mass screening and more frequent monitoring of neurological disorders, which can be beneficial for early detection and timely intervention in irreversible neurodegenerative conditions. With continued research and development, AI-based models have the potential to revolutionize the diagnosis and management of neurological disorders, ultimately leading to improved patient outcomes.

26.3 Financial Support

We acknowledge the support from the donors of the National Glaucoma Research, a program of the BrightFocus Foundation (G2021010S [MJAG]) and the Tackling & Reducing Glaucoma Blindness with Emerging Technologies (TARGET) project that is supported by the National Medical Research Council (NMRC), Singapore (MOH-OFLCG21jun-0003 [MJAG]).

Conflict of Interest MJAG is a co-founder of the start-up company Abyss Processing Pte Ltd.

Appendix: AI Models and Performance Metrics

Machine Learning Models

The application of Artificial Intelligence (AI) to medical imaging is revolutionising both clinical and research capabilities. In particular, machine learning (ML) is a subfield of AI that enables systems to "learn" from data without being explicitly "taught" or programmed [96]. This offers a wide range of capabilities including automated analysis of big data and classification or segmentation of medical images, which facilitate diagnosis and prognosis [27, 58, 96]. ML models are input with user-provided features and return a predicted output [26]. In the context of optical coherence tomography (OCT) studies, the user-provided features are extracted from the OCT scans and may include parameters such as the thickness of specific tissue layers, the volume of those tissue layers and total macular volume [17, 27, 30, 80]. The ML models analyse these input features to make predictions or decisions based on the input data [23]. The outputs can take the form of continuous variables, such as intracranial pressure, or categorical classifications, such as distinguishing between healthy and glaucoma cases.

Classification. Classification is a problem whereby the algorithm learns to categorise input data [97]. Most of the AI models discussed in this review use classification models to categorise subjects into diseased or non-diseased populations [39, 40, 80].

Random Forest. One of the most popular machine learning techniques for classification is the random forest, which falls under the umbrella of ensemble learning and comprises multiple decisions trees [97]. In a random forest model, each decision tree takes a set of input features and learns a sequence of decisions that recursively split the data based on different features [98]. This recursive process ultimately leads to leaf nodes representing classification or prediction outcomes [98]. The random forest classifier combines the outputs of these individual decision trees to produce a final classification. By aggregating the predictions from multiple trees, the random forest classifier offers an accurate and robust classification model that is less susceptible to noise, mitigates overfitting and can handle large-scale datasets [99].

Support Vector Machine. Support vector machine (SVM) is another popular ML technique for classification tasks. The objective of SVM is to find the optimal decision boundary that maximizes the distance between different classes of data to separate them [31]. The algorithm identifies support vectors, which are a subset of training data points critical for defining the decision boundary, giving it its name. One of the key advantages of SVMs is its ability to handle non-linear boundaries through the use of support vectors and kernel functions, enabling them to achieve high accuracy and robustness [100]. Both SVM and random forest methods are particularly effective in categorizing data points with multiple input features, such as thickness measurements of each of the different tissue layers in different regions in OCT scans.

Logistic Regression. Logistic regression is a method specifically designed for binary classification tasks. It uses a logistic function to transform the linear relationship between independent variables and the log-odds of the binary prediction outcome [101]. While the simplicity of the model can be advantageous in terms of explainability, its applicability to complex non-linear relationships in the data is also restricted.

Linear Regression. Regression models are another ML approach which aim to learn a relationship between an output (dependent) variable and one or more input (independent variables). Some of the studies discussed in this chapter make use of regression models to predict specific continuous outcomes, such as intracranial pressure or other biological parameters, to aid in diagnosis and prognosis of neurological disorders [81]. The simplest regression method is linear regression which predicts outputs based on a learned linear relationship between the independent input variables and dependent output variables [31].

Deep Learning Models

Deep learning (DL) models are a subset of ML models which are typically more complex than conventional ML models. These models use neural networks which consist of layers of neurons stacked onto each other thereby adding depth [26]. Each layer of neurons takes in an input, performs computations to manipulate the data, and passes the output on to the next successive layer. In DL, the system learns which features to use for a given task in an unsupervised or semi-supervised way [26, 27]. As such, 2D or even 3D volumetric OCT scans be input to DL models without requiring prior pre-processing. However, the complexity of deep learning models also necessitates larger training datasets to prevent overfitting [27]. Limited availability of large datasets remains a challenge in the application of deep learning to medical images.

Convolutional Neural Network. One of the most widely used DL algorithms in medical image is the convolutional neural network (CNN) [36, 45, 55, 59, 63]. As with most DL models, the main advantage of CNN over traditional ML models is its ability to learn features from the data instead of requiring hand-crafted features [26]. CNNs are particularly effective for processing 2D or 3D images because their architecture is designed to exploit the hierarchical structure of image features. Each successive convolutional layer in a CNN utilizes convolutional operations to extract local features from the output of the previous layer [26]. CNNs can be employed to classify whole OCT scans into different disease categories or non-diseased populations. Additionally, they can be utilized for feature extraction tasks such as measuring tissue thickness, extracting textual features, or detecting specific objects within the OCT scans using techniques such as such as image segmentation or objection detection [23, 25].

U-NET. The U-NET is a CNN-based model commonly used for semantic segmentation tasks in medical images [102]. Segmentation involves classifying each pixel in a 2-D image or each voxel in a 3-D image into a specified label class; this means assigning each pixel or voxel a label indicating the tissue layer it belongs to [22]. The U-NET architecture forms a characteristic "U"-shaped framework. It is composed of an encoder followed by decoder with skip connections that enable precise localisation of objects in images [102]. The encoder extracts high-level features from the input image through convolutional layers and downsampling operations while the decoder, gradually recovers the spatial resolution of the feature maps through upsampling using transposed convolution [102].

Performance Metrics

AI models are typically evaluated on a separate test dataset, mutually exclusive from the data used to train and validate the model. Accuracy is one of the most common metrics to assess the overall performance of these models. It represents the proportion of correct predictions over total predictions [22].

In binary classification tasks, metrics such as sensitivity, specificity and AUC are often used. Sensitivity is a measure of the true positive rate, indicating the ability of a model to correctly identify positive cases. Specificity, on the other hand, represents the true negative rate, measuring the model's ability to correctly identify negative cases [22, 79]. Maximizing sensitivity is important when the goal is to detect all cases of a specific neurological disorder, while maximizing specificity is crucial in minimizing false predictions of the disorder in non-diseased individuals. AUC refers to the area under the receiver operating characteristic (ROC) curve, which plots the true positive rate against the false positive rate. An AUC value of 1 signifies perfect classification [16, 31, 47].

Finally, Dice coefficient is a common performance metric for evaluating medical image segmentation. It measures the overlap between the predicted segmentation and the ground truth segmentation; with a maximum DC score of 1 indicating perfect similarity [22, 79].

Though these metrics are useful for gauging performance of various models on a test dataset, one should note that the metrics, in particular AUC, should not be used to directly compare different studies unless either the methods or the population is the same in each both studies being compared [68].

References

1. De Groef L, Cordeiro MF. Is the eye an extension of the brain in central nervous system disease? J Ocul Pharmacol Ther. 2018;34:129–33. https://doi.org/10.1089/jop.2016.0180.
2. London A, Benhar I, Schwartz M. The retina as a window to the brain—from eye research to CNS disorders. Nat Rev Neurol. 2013;9:44–53. https://doi.org/10.1038/nrneurol.2012.227.
3. Yılmaz U, Küçük E, Ülgen A, Özköse A, Demircan S, Ulusoy DM, Zararsız G. Retinal nerve fiber layer and macular thickness measurement in patients with schizophrenia. Eur J Ophthalmol. 2016;26:375–8. https://doi.org/10.5301/ejo.5000723.
4. Colligris P, Perez de Lara MJ, Colligris B, Pintor J. Ocular manifestations of Alzheimer's and other neurodegenerative diseases: the prospect of the eye as a tool for the early diagnosis of Alzheimer's disease. J Ophthalmol. 2018;2018: e8538573. https://doi.org/10.1155/2018/8538573.
5. Biousse V, Skibell BC, Watts RL, Loupe DN, Drews-Botsch C, Newman NJ. Ophthalmologic features of Parkinson's disease. Neurology. 2004;62:177–80. https://doi.org/10.1212/01.wnl.0000103444.45882.d8.
6. Barnes D, McDonald WI. The ocular manifestations of multiple sclerosis. 2. Abnormalities of eye movements. J Neurol Neurosurg Psychiatry. 1992;55:863–8.
7. Rebolleda G, Diez-Alvarez L, Casado A, Sánchez-Sánchez C, de Dompablo E, González-López JJ, Muñoz-Negrete FJ. OCT: new perspectives in neuro-ophthalmology. Saudi J Ophthalmol. 2015;29:9–25. https://doi.org/10.1016/j.sjopt.2014.09.016.

8. Satue M, Obis J, Rodrigo MJ, Otin S, Fuertes MI, Vilades E, Gracia H, Ara JR, Alarcia R, Polo V, Larrosa JM, Pablo LE, Garcia-Martin E. Optical coherence tomography as a biomarker for diagnosis, progression, and prognosis of neurodegenerative diseases. J Ophthalmol. 2016;2016:1–9. https://doi.org/10.1155/2016/8503859.
9. Carroll WM. The global burden of neurological disorders. Lancet Neurol. 2019;18:418–9. https://doi.org/10.1016/S1474-4422(19)30029-8.
10. Lamptey RNL, Chaulagain B, Trivedi R, Gothwal A, Layek B, Singh J. A review of the common neurodegenerative disorders: current therapeutic approaches and the potential role of nanotherapeutics. Int J Mol Sci. 2022;23:1851. https://doi.org/10.3390/ijms23031851.
11. Gupta N, Yücel YH. Glaucoma as a neurodegenerative disease. Curr Opin Ophthalmol. 2007;18:110. https://doi.org/10.1097/ICU.0b013e3280895aea.
12. Chan JW, Chan NCY, Sadun AA. Glaucoma as neurodegeneration in the brain. Eye Brain. 2021;13:21–8. https://doi.org/10.2147/EB.S293765.
13. Pujari A, Bhaskaran K, Sharma P, Singh P, Phuljhele S, Saxena R, Azad SV. Optical coherence tomography angiography in neuro-ophthalmology: current clinical role and future perspectives. Surv Ophthalmol. 2021;66:471–81. https://doi.org/10.1016/j.survophthal.2020.10.009.
14. Xie JS, Donaldson L, Margolin E. Papilledema: a review of etiology, pathophysiology, diagnosis, and management. Surv Ophthalmol. 2022;67:1135–59. https://doi.org/10.1016/j.survophthal.2021.11.007.
15. Boomer J, Siatkowski M. Optic neuritis in adults and children. Semin Ophthalmol. 2003;18:174–80. https://doi.org/10.1080/08820530390895172.
16. Cavaliere C, Vilades E, Alonso-Rodríguez MC, Rodrigo MJ, Pablo LE, Miguel JM, López-Guillén E, Morla EMS, Boquete L, Garcia-Martin E. Computer-aided diagnosis of multiple sclerosis using a support vector machine and optical coherence tomography features. Sensors. 2019;19:5323. https://doi.org/10.3390/s19235323.
17. Wang X, Jiao B, Liu H, Wang Y, Hao X, Zhu Y, Xu B, Xu H, Zhang S, Jia X, Xu Q, Liao X, Zhou Y, Jiang H, Wang J, Guo J, Yan X, Tang B, Zhao R, Shen L. Machine learning based on optical coherence tomography images as a diagnostic tool for Alzheimer's disease. CNS Neurosci Ther. 2022;28:2206–17. https://doi.org/10.1111/cns.13963.
18. Milea D, Najjar RP, Jiang Z, Ting D, Vasseneix C, Xu X, Aghsaei Fard M, Fonseca P, Vanikieti K, Lagrèze WA, La Morgia C, Cheung CY, Hamann S, Chiquet C, Sanda N, Yang H, Mejico LJ, Rougier M-B, Kho R, Tran THC, Singhal S, Gohier P, Clermont-Vignal C, Cheng C-Y, Jonas JB, Yu-Wai-Man P, Fraser CL, Chen JJ, Ambika S, Miller NR, Liu Y, Newman NJ, Wong TY, Biousse V. Artificial intelligence to detect papilledema from ocular fundus photographs. N Engl J Med. 2020;382:1687–95. https://doi.org/10.1056/NEJMoa1917130.
19. Hrynchak P, Simpson T. Optical coherence tomography: an introduction to the technique and its use. Optom Vis Sci. 2000;77:347–56.
20. Al-Mujaini A, Wali UK, Azeem S. Optical coherence tomography: clinical applications in medical practice. Oman Med J. 2013;28:86–91. https://doi.org/10.5001/omj.2013.24.
21. Ko TH, Fujimoto JG, Schuman JS, Paunescu LA, Kowalevicz AM, Hartl I, Drexler W, Wollstein G, Ishikawa H, Duker JS. Comparison of ultrahigh- and standard-resolution optical coherence tomography for imaging macular pathology. Ophthalmol. 2005;112:1922.e1-1922.e15. https://doi.org/10.1016/j.ophtha.2005.05.027.
22. Devalla SK, Chin KS, Mari J-M, Tun TA, Strouthidis NG, Aung T, Thiéry AH, Girard MJA. A deep learning approach to digitally stain optical coherence tomography images of the optic nerve head. Investig Ophthalmol Vis Sci. 2018;59:63–74. https://doi.org/10.1167/iovs.17-22617.
23. Kapoor R, Whigham BT, Al-Aswad LA. Artificial intelligence and optical coherence tomography imaging. Asia-Pac J Ophthalmol. 2019;8:187. https://doi.org/10.22608/APO.201904.
24. Tian J, Varga B, Tatrai E, Fanni P, Somfai GM, Smiddy WE, Debuc DC. Performance evaluation of automated segmentation software on optical coherence tomography volume data. J Biophotonics. 2016;9:478–89. https://doi.org/10.1002/jbio.201500239.

25. Marques R, De Jesus DA, Breda JB, Van Eijgen J, Stalmans I, van Walsum T, Klein S, Vaz PG, Brea LS. Automatic segmentation of the optic nerve head region in optical coherence tomography: a methodological review. 2021. arXiv:210902322 [physics].
26. LeCun Y, Bengio Y, Hinton G. Deep learning. Nature. 2015;521:436–44. https://doi.org/10.1038/nature14539.
27. Ongsulee P. Artificial intelligence, machine learning and deep learning. In: 2017 15th international conference on ICT and knowledge engineering (ICT&KE); 2017. p. 1–6.
28. Turkan Y, Tek FB. A survey on automated diagnosis of Alzheimer's disease using optical coherence tomography and angiography. 2022.
29. Aslam N, Khan IU, Bashamakh A, Alghool FA, Aboulnour M, Alsuwayan NM, Alturaif RK, Brahimi S, Aljameel SS, Al Ghamdi K. Multiple sclerosis diagnosis using machine learning and deep learning: challenges and opportunities. Sensors. 2022;22:7856. https://doi.org/10.3390/s22207856.
30. Ciftci Kavaklioglu B, Erdman L, Goldenberg A, Kavaklioglu C, Alexander C, Oppermann HM, Patel A, Hossain S, Berenbaum T, Yau O, Yea C, Ly M, Costello F, Mah JK, Reginald A, Banwell B, Longoni G, Ann Yeh E. Machine learning classification of multiple sclerosis in children using optical coherence tomography. Mult Scler. 2022;28:2253–62. https://doi.org/10.1177/13524585221112605.
31. Montolío A, Martín-Gallego A, Cegoñino J, Orduna E, Vilades E, Garcia-Martin E, del Palomar AP. Machine learning in diagnosis and disability prediction of multiple sclerosis using optical coherence tomography. Comput Biol Med. 2021;133: 104416. https://doi.org/10.1016/j.compbiomed.2021.104416.
32. Walton C, King R, Rechtman L, Kaye W, Leray E, Marrie RA, Robertson N, La Rocca N, Uitdehaag B, van der Mei I, Wallin M, Helme A, Angood Napier C, Rijke N, Baneke P. Rising prevalence of multiple sclerosis worldwide: insights from the Atlas of MS, third edition. Mult Scler. 2020;26:1816–21. https://doi.org/10.1177/1352458520970841.
33. Dobson R, Giovannoni G. Multiple sclerosis—a review. Eur J Neurol. 2019;26:27–40. https://doi.org/10.1111/ene.13819.
34. Feinstein A. The neuropsychiatry of multiple sclerosis. Can J Psychiatry. 2004;49:157–63. https://doi.org/10.1177/070674370404900302.
35. Shindler KS, Guan Y, Ventura E, Bennett J, Rostami A. Retinal ganglion cell loss induced by acute optic neuritis in a relapsing model of multiple sclerosis. Mult Scler. 2006;12:526–32. https://doi.org/10.1177/1352458506070629.
36. López-Dorado A, Ortiz M, Satue M, Rodrigo MJ, Barea R, Sánchez-Morla EM, Cavaliere C, Rodríguez-Ascariz JM, Orduna-Hospital E, Boquete L, Garcia-Martin E. Early diagnosis of multiple sclerosis using swept-source optical coherence tomography and convolutional neural networks trained with data augmentation. Sensors. 2022;22:167. https://doi.org/10.3390/s22010167.
37. Hartung H-P, Graf J, Aktas O, Mares J, Barnett MH. Diagnosis of multiple sclerosis: revisions of the McDonald criteria 2017—continuity and change. Curr Opin Neurol. 2019;32:327. https://doi.org/10.1097/WCO.0000000000000699.
38. Olbert E, Struhal W. Retinal imaging with optical coherence tomography in multiple sclerosis: novel aspects. Wien Med Wochenschr. 2022;172:329–36. https://doi.org/10.1007/s10354-022-00925-2.
39. Kenney RC, Liu M, Hasanaj L, Joseph B, Abu Al-Hassan A, Blk LJ, Behbehani R, Brandt A, Calabresi PA, Frohman E, Frohman TC, Havla J, Hemmer B. The role of optical coherence tomography criteria and machine learning in multiple sclerosis and optic neuritis diagnosis. Neurology. 2022;99:e1100–12.
40. Garcia-Martin E, Herrero R, Bambo MP, Ara JR, Martin J, Polo V, Larrosa JM, Garcia-Feijoo J, Pablo LE. Artificial neural network techniques to improve the ability of optical coherence tomography to detect optic neuritis. Semin Ophthalmol. 2015;30:11–9. https://doi.org/10.3109/08820538.2013.810277.

41. Yamout BI, Khoury SJ, Ayyoubi N, Doumiati H, Fakhreddine M, Ahmed SF, Tamim H, Al-Hashel JY, Behbehani R, Alroughani R. Alternative diagnoses in patients referred to specialized centers for suspected MS. Mult Scler Relat Disord. 2017;18:85–9. https://doi.org/10.1016/j.msard.2017.09.016.
42. Solomon AJ, Bourdette DN, Cross AH, Applebee A, Skidd PM, Howard DB, Spain RI, Cameron MH, Kim E, Mass MK, Yadav V, Whitham RH, Longbrake EE, Naismith RT, Wu GF, Parks BJ, Wingerchuk DM, Rabin BL, Toledano M, Tobin WO, Kantarci OH, Carter JL, Keegan BM, Weinshenker BG. The contemporary spectrum of multiple sclerosis misdiagnosis: a multicenter study. Neurology. 2016;87:1393–9. https://doi.org/10.1212/WNL.0000000000003152.
43. Ash EL. 27—dementia. In: Marshall RS, Mayer SA, editors. On call neurology. 3rd ed. Philadelphia: W.B. Saunders; 2007. p. 401–17.
44. Yaari R, Fleisher AS, Tariot PN. Updates to diagnostic guidelines for Alzheimer's disease. Prim Care Companion CNS Disord. 2011;13:PCC.11f01262. https://doi.org/10.4088/PCC.11f01262.
45. Wisely CE, Wang D, Henao R, Grewal DS, Thompson AC, Robbins CB, Yoon SP, Soundararajan S, Polascik BW, Burke JR, Liu A, Carin L, Fekrat S. Convolutional neural network to identify symptomatic Alzheimer's disease using multimodal retinal imaging. Br J Ophthalmol. 2022;106:388–95. https://doi.org/10.1136/bjophthalmol-2020-317659.
46. Cipollini V, Abdolrahimzadeh S, Troili F, De Carolis A, Calafiore S, Scuderi L, Giubilei F, Scuderi G. Neurocognitive assessment and retinal thickness alterations in Alzheimer disease: is there a correlation? J Neuro-Ophthalmol. 2020;40:370. https://doi.org/10.1097/WNO.0000000000000831.
47. Chua J, Li C, Ho LKH, Wong D, Tan B, Yao X, Gan A, Schwarzhans F, Garhöfer G, Sng CCA, Hilal S, Venketasubramanian N, Cheung CY, Fischer G, Vass C, Wong TY, Chen CL-H, Schmetterer L. A multi-regression framework to improve diagnostic ability of optical coherence tomography retinal biomarkers to discriminate mild cognitive impairment and Alzheimer's disease. Alz Res Therapy. 2022;14:1–11. https://doi.org/10.1186/s13195-022-00982-0.
48. Inzelberg R, Ramirez JA, Nisipeanu P, Ophir A. Retinal nerve fiber layer thinning in Parkinson disease. Vis Res. 2004;44:2793–7. https://doi.org/10.1016/j.visres.2004.06.009.
49. Stern MB. Parkinson's disease: early diagnosis and management. J Fam Pract. 1993;36:439–47.
50. Chrysou A, Heikka T, van der Zee S, Boertien J, Jansonius N, van Laar T. Identifying de novo Parkinson's disease with optical coherence tomography of the retina: movement-disorder-society (MDS) international virtual congress. Mov Disord. 2020;35:S238.
51. Nunes A, Silva G, Duque C, Januário C, Santana I, Ambrósio AF, Castelo-Branco M, Bernardes R. Retinal texture biomarkers may help to discriminate between Alzheimer's, Parkinson's, and healthy controls. PLoS One. 2019;14: e0218826. https://doi.org/10.1371/journal.pone.0218826.
52. Sánchez-Morla EM, Fuentes JL, Miguel-Jiménez JM, Boquete L, Ortiz M, Orduna E, Satue M, Garcia-Martin E. Automatic diagnosis of bipolar disorder using optical coherence tomography data and artificial intelligence. J Pers Med. 2021;11:803. https://doi.org/10.3390/jpm11080803.
53. Guidoboni G, Sacco R, Szopos M, Sala L, Verticchio Vercellin AC, Siesky B, Harris A. Neurodegenerative disorders of the eye and of the brain: a perspective on their fluid-dynamical connections and the potential of mechanism-driven modeling. Front Neurosci. 2020;14:566428.
54. Tham Y-C, Li X, Wong TY, Quigley HA, Aung T, Cheng C-Y. Global prevalence of glaucoma and projections of glaucoma burden through 2040. Ophthalmol. 2014;121:2081–90. https://doi.org/10.1016/j.ophtha.2014.05.013.

55. Asaoka R, Murata H, Hirasawa K, Fujino Y, Matsuura M, Miki A, Kanamoto T, Ikeda Y, Mori K, Iwase A, Shoji N, Inoue K, Yamagami J, Araie M. Using deep learning and transfer learning to accurately diagnose early-onset glaucoma from macular optical coherence tomography images. Am J Ophthalmol. 2019;198:136–45. https://doi.org/10.1016/j.ajo.2018.10.007.
56. Raghavendra U, Fujita H, Bhandary SV, Gudigar A, Tan JH, Acharya UR. Deep convolution neural network for accurate diagnosis of glaucoma using digital fundus images. Inf Sci. 2018;441:41–9. https://doi.org/10.1016/j.ins.2018.01.051.
57. Thompson AC, Jammal AA, Berchuck SI, Mariottoni EB, Medeiros FA. Assessment of a segmentation-free deep learning algorithm for diagnosing glaucoma from optical coherence tomography scans. JAMA Ophthalmol. 2020;138:333–9. https://doi.org/10.1001/jamaophthalmol.2019.5983.
58. Devalla SK, Pham TH, Panda SK, Zhang L, Subramanian G, Swaminathan A, Yun CZ, Rajan M, Mohan S, Krishnadas R, Senthil V, de Leon JMS, Tun TA, Cheng C-Y, Schmetterer L, Perera S, Aung T, Thiery AH, Girard MJA. Towards label-free 3D segmentation of optical coherence tomography images of the optic nerve head using deep learning. 2020. arXiv:200209635 [cs, eess].
59. Russakoff DB, Mannil SS, Oakley JD, Ran AR, Cheung CY, Dasari S, Riyazzuddin M, Nagaraj S, Rao HL, Chang D, Chang RT. A 3D deep learning system for detecting referable glaucoma using full OCT macular cube scans. Transl Vis Sci Technol. 2020;9:12. https://doi.org/10.1167/tvst.9.2.12.
60. Panda SK, Cheong H, Tun TA, Devella SK, Senthil V, Krishnadas R, Buist ML, Perera S, Cheng C-Y, Aung T, Thiéry AH, Girard MJA. Describing the structural phenotype of the glaucomatous optic nerve head using artificial intelligence. Am J Ophthalmol. 2022;236:172–82. https://doi.org/10.1016/j.ajo.2021.06.010.
61. Panda SK, Cheong H, Tun TA, Chuangsuwanich T, Kadziauskiene A, Senthil V, Krishnadas R, Buist ML, Perera S, Cheng C-Y, Aung T, Thiery AH, Girard MJA. The three-dimensional structural configuration of the central retinal vessel trunk and branches as a glaucoma biomarker. Am J Ophthalmol. 2022;240:205–16. https://doi.org/10.1016/j.ajo.2022.02.020.
62. Nagarkatti-Gude N, Gardiner SK, Fortune B, Demirel S, Mansberger SL. Optical coherence tomography segmentation errors of the retinal nerve fiber layer persist over time. J Glaucoma. 2019;28:368–74. https://doi.org/10.1097/IJG.0000000000001222.
63. Maetschke S, Antony B, Ishikawa H, Wollstein G, Schuman J, Garnavi R. A feature agnostic approach for glaucoma detection in OCT volumes. PLOS ONE. 2019;14: e0219126. https://doi.org/10.1371/journal.pone.0219126.
64. Zheng C, Xie X, Huang L, Chen B, Yang J, Lu J, Qiao T, Fan Z, Zhang M. Detecting glaucoma based on spectral domain optical coherence tomography imaging of peripapillary retinal nerve fiber layer: a comparison study between hand-crafted features and deep learning model. Graefes Arch Clin Exp Ophthalmol. 2020;258:577–85. https://doi.org/10.1007/s00417-019-04543-4.
65. Braeu FA, Thiéry AH, Tun TA, Kadziauskiene A, Barbastathis G, Aung T, Girard MJA. Geometric deep learning to identify the critical 3D structural features of the optic nerve head for glaucoma diagnosis. Am J Ophthalmol. 2023;250:38–48. https://doi.org/10.1016/j.ajo.2023.01.008.
66. Thiéry AH, Braeu F, Tun TA, Aung T, Girard MJA. Medical application of geometric deep learning for the diagnosis of glaucoma. Transl Vis Sci Technol. 2023;12:23. https://doi.org/10.1167/tvst.12.2.23.
67. Braeu FA, Chuangsuwanich T, Tun TA, Perera SA, Husain R, Kadziauskiene A, Schmetterer L, Thiéry AH, Barbastathis G, Aung T, Girard MJA. The 3D structural phenotype of the glaucomatous optic nerve head and its relationship with the severity of visual field damage. 2023.
68. Girard MJA, Schmetterer L. Chapter 3—artificial intelligence and deep learning in glaucoma: current state and future prospects. In: Bagetta G, Nucci C, editors. Progress in brain research. Elsevier; 2020. p. 37–64.

69. Chuangsuwanich T, Tun TA, Braeu FA, Wang X, Chin ZY, Panda SK, Buist M, Strouthidis N, Perera S, Nongpiur M, Aung T, Girard MJA. Differing associations between optic nerve head strains and visual field loss in patients with normal- and high-tension glaucoma. Ophthalmol. 2023;130:99–110. https://doi.org/10.1016/j.ophtha.2022.08.007.
70. Midgett DE, Quigley HA, Nguyen TD. In vivo characterization of the deformation of the human optic nerve head using optical coherence tomography and digital volume correlation. Acta Biomater. 2019;96:385–99. https://doi.org/10.1016/j.actbio.2019.06.050.
71. Kim J, Gardiner SK, Ramazzotti A, Karuppanan U, Bruno L, Girkin CA, Downs JC, Fazio MA. Strain by virtual extensometers and video-imaging optical coherence tomography as a repeatable metric for IOP-induced optic nerve head deformations. Exp Eye Res. 2021;211: 108724. https://doi.org/10.1016/j.exer.2021.108724.
72. McDonald MA, Stevenson CH, Kersten HM, Danesh-Meyer HV. Eye movement abnormalities in glaucoma patients: a review. Eye Brain. 2022;14:83–114. https://doi.org/10.2147/EB.S361946.
73. Flammer J, Orgül S, Costa VP, Orzalesi N, Krieglstein GK, Serra LM, Renard J-P, Stefánsson E. The impact of ocular blood flow in glaucoma. Prog Retin Eye Res. 2002;21:359–93. https://doi.org/10.1016/S1350-9462(02)00008-3.
74. Coudrillier B, Pijanka JK, Jefferys JL, Goel A, Quigley HA, Boote C, Nguyen TD. Glaucoma-related changes in the mechanical properties and collagen micro-architecture of the human sclera. PLOS One. 2015;10: e0131396. https://doi.org/10.1371/journal.pone.0131396.
75. Pijanka JK, Coudrillier B, Ziegler K, Sorensen T, Meek KM, Nguyen TD, Quigley HA, Boote C. Quantitative mapping of collagen fiber orientation in non-glaucoma and glaucoma posterior human sclerae. Investig Ophthalmol Vis Sci. 2012;53:5258–70. https://doi.org/10.1167/iovs.12-9705.
76. Stürmer JP, Kniestedt C. Role of ocular pulse amplitude in glaucoma. Klinische Monatsblatter fur Augenheilkunde. 2015;232(2):162–8. https://doi.org/10.1055/s-0034-1396232.
77. Baneke AJ, Aubry J, Viswanathan AC, Plant GT. The role of intracranial pressure in glaucoma and therapeutic implications. Eye. 2020;34:178–91. https://doi.org/10.1038/s41433-019-0681-y.
78. Hayreh SS. Ischemic optic neuropathies. In: Hayreh SS, editor. Ocular vascular occlusive disorders. Cham: Springer International Publishing; 2015. p. 429–75.
79. Razaghi G, Hedayati E, Hejazi M, Kafieh R, Samadi M, Ritch R, Subramanian PS, Aghsaei Fard M. Measurement of retinal nerve fiber layer thickness with a deep learning algorithm in ischemic optic neuropathy and optic neuritis. Sci Rep. 2022;12:17109. https://doi.org/10.1038/s41598-022-22135-x.
80. Girard MJA, Panda S, Tun TA, Wibroe EA, Najjar RP, Aung T, Thiéry AH, Hamann S, Fraser C, Milea D. Discriminating between papilledema and optic disc drusen using 3D structural analysis of the optic nerve head. Neurology. 2023;100:e192–202. https://doi.org/10.1212/WNL.0000000000201350.
81. Skau M, Yri H, Sander B, Gerds TA, Milea D, Jensen R. Diagnostic value of optical coherence tomography for intracranial pressure in idiopathic intracranial hypertension. Graefes Arch Clin Exp Ophthalmol. 2013;251:567–74. https://doi.org/10.1007/s00417-012-2039-z.
82. Jui-Kai W, Deng W, Islam MS, Thurtell MJ, Kardon RH, Garvin MK. Differentiation of papilledema from non-arteritic anterior ischemic optic neuropathy (NAION) using 2D image-based features and 3D deep-learning-based shape features in color fundus photographs. Investig Ophthalmol Vis Sci. 2021;62:2407.
83. Winter PD, Carusi A. (De)troubling transparency: artificial intelligence (AI) for clinical applications. Med Humlties. 2023;49:17–26. https://doi.org/10.1136/medhum-2021-012318.
84. Rhodes LA, Huisingh C, Johnstone J, Massimo F, Smith B, Clark M, Downs C, Owsley C, Girard MJA, Mari JM, Girkin CA. Variation of laminar depth in normal eyes with age and race. Investig Ophthalmol Vis Sci (IOVS). 2014;55:8123–33. https://doi.org/10.1167/iovs.14-15251.

85. Kashani AH, Zimmer-Galler IE, Shah SM, Dustin L, Do DV, Eliott D, Haller JA, Nguyen QD. Retinal thickness analysis by race, gender, and age using stratus OCT. Am J Ophthalmol. 2010;149:496-502.e1. https://doi.org/10.1016/j.ajo.2009.09.025.
86. Rhodes LA, Huisingh C, Johnstone J, Fazio MA, Smith B, Wang L, Clark M, Downs JC, Owsley C, Girard MJA, Mari JM, Girkin CA. Peripapillary choroidal thickness variation with age and race in normal eyes. Investig Ophthalmol Vis Sci. 2015;56:1872–9. https://doi.org/10.1167/iovs.14-16179.
87. Knight OJ, Girkin CA, Budenz DL, Durbin MK, Feuer WJ, Cirrus OCT, Normative Database Study Group. Effect of race, age, and axial length on optic nerve head parameters and retinal nerve fiber layer thickness measured by cirrus HD-OCT. Arch Ophthalmol. 2012;130:312–8. https://doi.org/10.1001/archopthalmol.2011.1576.
88. Liu B, Hu Y, Ma G, Xiao Y, Zhang B, Liang Y, Zhong P, Zeng X, Lin Z, Kong H, Wu G, Du Z, Fang Y, Huang M, Wang L, Yang X, Yu H. Reduced retinal microvascular perfusion in patients with stroke detected by optical coherence tomography angiography. Front Aging Neurosci. 2021;13:628336.
89. Cameron JR, Tatham AJ. A window to beyond the orbit: the value of optical coherence tomography in non-ocular disease. Acta Ophthalmol. 2016;94:533–9. https://doi.org/10.1111/aos.12978.
90. Dusek P, Kopal A, Brichova M, Roth J, Ulmanova O, Klempir J, Preiningerova JL. Is retina affected in Huntington's disease? Is optical coherence tomography a good biomarker? PLOS One. 2023;18: e0282175. https://doi.org/10.1371/journal.pone.0282175.
91. Mazur-Michałek I, Kowalska K, Zielonka D, Leśniczak-Staszak M, Pietras P, Szaflarski W, Isalan M, Mielcarek M. Structural abnormalities of the optic nerve and retina in Huntington's disease pre-clinical and clinical settings. Int J Mol Sci. 2022;23:5450. https://doi.org/10.3390/ijms23105450.
92. Ko Y-C, Wey S-Y, Chen W-T, Chang Y-F, Chen M-J, Chiou S-H, Liu CJ-L, Lee C-Y. Deep learning assisted detection of glaucomatous optic neuropathy and potential designs for a generalizable model. PLOS One. 2020;15: e0233079. https://doi.org/10.1371/journal.pone.0233079.
93. Thakur A, Goldbaum M, Yousefi S. Predicting glaucoma before onset using deep learning. Ophthalmol Glaucoma. 2020;3:262–8. https://doi.org/10.1016/j.ogla.2020.04.012.
94. Zhou B, Khosla A, Lapedriza A, Oliva A, Torralba A. Learning deep features for discriminative localization. 2015.
95. Braeu FA, Chuangsuwanich T, Tun TA, Perera S, Husain R, Thiery AH, Aung T, Barbastathis G, Girard MJA. AI-based clinical assessment of optic nerve head robustness superseding biomechanical testing. Br J Ophthalmol. 2023. https://doi.org/10.1136/bjo-2022-322374.
96. Currie G, Hawk KE, Rohren E, Vial A, Klein R. Machine learning and deep learning in medical imaging: intelligent imaging. J Med Imaging Radiat Sci. 2019;50:477–87. https://doi.org/10.1016/j.jmir.2019.09.005.
97. Mung PS, Phyu S. Effective analytics on healthcare big data using ensemble learning. In: 2020 IEEE conference on computer applications (ICCA); 2020. p. 1–4.
98. Song Y, Lu Y. Decision tree methods: applications for classification and prediction. Shanghai Arch Psychiatry. 2015;27:130–135. https://doi.org/10.11919/j.issn.1002-0829.215044.
99. Breiman L. Random forests. Mach Learn. 2001;45:5–32. https://doi.org/10.1023/A:1010933404324.
100. Cortes C, Vapnik V. Support-vector networks. Mach Learn. 1995;20:273–97. https://doi.org/10.1007/BF00994018.
101. LaValley MP. Logistic regression. Circulation. 2008;117:2395–9. https://doi.org/10.1161/CIRCULATIONAHA.106.682658.
102. Ronneberger O, Fischer P, Brox T. U-Net: convolutional networks for biomedical image segmentation. In: Navab N, Hornegger J, Wells WM, Frangi AF, editors. Medical image computing and computer-assisted intervention—MICCAI 2015. Cham: Springer International Publishing; 2015. p. 234–41.

103. Han KJ, Lee YH. Optical coherence tomography automated layer segmentation of macula after retinal detachment repair. PLOS One. 2018;13: e0197058. https://doi.org/10.1371/journal.pone.0197058.
104. Devalla SK, Renukanand PK, Sreedhar BK, Perera S, Mari J-M, Chin KS, Tun TA, Strouthidis NG, Aung T, Thiery AH, Girard MJA. DRUNET: a dilated-residual u-net deep learning network to digitally stain optic nerve head tissues in optical coherence tomography images. 2018. arXiv:180300232 [cs].
105. Cunha LP, Almeida ALM, Costa-Cunha LVF, Costa CF, Monteiro MLR. The role of optical coherence tomography in Alzheimer's disease. Int J Retin Vitr. 2016;2:24. https://doi.org/10.1186/s40942-016-0049-4.
106. Jiang H, Liu Y, Wei Y, Shi Y, Wright CB, Sun X, Rundek T, Baumel BS, Landman J, Wang J. Impaired retinal microcirculation in patients with Alzheimer's disease. PLOS One. 2018;13: e0192154. https://doi.org/10.1371/journal.pone.0192154.
107. Criscuolo C, Cennamo G, Montorio D, Carotenuto A, Strianese A, Salvatore E, Tranfa F, Cennamo G, Lanzillo R, Morra VB. Assessment of retinal vascular network in amnestic mild cognitive impairment by optical coherence tomography angiography. PLOS One. 2020;15: e0233975. https://doi.org/10.1371/journal.pone.0233975.
108. Yousefzadeh N, Tran C, Ramirez-Zamora A, Chen J, Fang R, Thai MT. LAVA: Granular neuron-level explainable AI for Alzheimer's disease assessment from fundus images. 2023.
109. Koronyo Y, Biggs D, Barron E, Boyer DS, Pearlman JA, Au WJ, Kile SJ, Blanco A, Fuchs D-T, Ashfaq A, Frautschy S, Cole GM, Miller CA, Hinton DR, Verdooner SR, Black KL, Koronyo-Hamaoui M. Retinal amyloid pathology and proof-of-concept imaging trial in Alzheimer's disease. JCI Insight. 2017;2:16. https://doi.org/10.1172/jci.insight.93621.
110. Kalló G, Emri M, Varga Z, Ujhelyi B, Tőzsér J, Csutak A, Csősz É. Changes in the chemical barrier composition of tears in Alzheimer's disease reveal potential tear diagnostic biomarkers. PLOS One. 2016;11: e0158000. https://doi.org/10.1371/journal.pone.0158000.

Index

A. Grzybowski and P. Barboni (eds.), *OCT and Imaging in Central Nervous System Diseases*, https://doi.org/10.1007/978-3-031-72156-4

L

M

N

O

MIX
Papier aus verantwortungsvollen Quellen
Paper from responsible sources
FSC® C105338

If you have any concerns about our products,
you can contact us on
ProductSafety@springernature.com

In case Publisher is established outside the EU,
the EU authorized representative is:
Springer Nature Customer Service Center GmbH
Europaplatz 3, 69115 Heidelberg, Germany

Printed by Libri Plureos GmbH
in Hamburg, Germany